FIVE STEPS FOR FAST TREATMENT

1 Maintain an open airway.

Assess the patient's breathing. If he develops a sudden airway obstruction (from laryngeal edema), give mouth-to-mouth resuscitation, or insert an oral airway and apply mechanical ventilation. Keep an emergency tray on hand in case the doctor has to perform a tracheotomy.

2 Administer epinephrine.

Recommended dosage: 0.2 to 1 ml epinephrine 1:1,000 I.M. or subcutaneously. If needed, repeat the dose four or five times at 3- to 5-minute intervals. Vigorously massage the injection site to increase absorption. Epinephrine may produce complete reversal of the patient's symptoms.

3 Administer an antihistamine.

Recommended dosage: 50 to 100 mg diphenhydramine (Benadryl) P.O., I.M., or I.V., depending on patient's condition, size, and age. Giving an antihistamine with epinephrine may be the last treatment step the patient needs.

4 Administer fluids.

If symptoms of shock continue, start an I.V. with lactated Ringer's solution, using a large-bore catheter. This will support the patient's jeopardized circulatory system. The large-bore catheter makes it easier to give medications I.V.

5 Check blood pressure regularly.

If the patient's blood pressure drops rapidly, administer a vasopresser (such as norepinephrine) I.V. to constrict the vessels. *Recommended dosage:* 4 ml of the commercially prepared solution added to 1 liter of 5% dextrose in water. *Caution:* Watch the injection site carefully for signs of drug infiltration (redness and swelling) to prevent tissue necrosis.

Note: If the reaction's severe, the doctor may also order aminophylline to combat bronchospasms. *Recommended dosage:* 5.6 mg/kg (usually 250 to 500 mg in 500 shouldn't exceed 50 mg/minute. After loading dose, begin contir

For persistent bronchospasm, the doctor may order hydrocort dium succinate, I.V., 100 mg, repeated every 6 hours.

Important: Keep emergency drugs/equipment handy in either a

NURSE'S REFERENCE LIBRARY™

Drugs

Nursing82 Books
Intermed Communications, Inc.
Springhouse, Pa. 19477

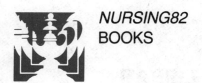

NURSE'S REFERENCE LIBRARY™ SERIES

PUBLISHER
Timothy B. King

EDITORIAL DIRECTOR
Maryanne Wagner

CLINICAL DIRECTOR
Minnie Bowen Rose, RN, BSN, MEd

Intermed Communications Book Division

CHAIRMAN
Eugene W. Jackson

PRESIDENT
Daniel L. Cheney

VICE-PRESIDENT
Timothy B. King

RESEARCH DIRECTOR
Elizabeth O'Brien

PRODUCTION AND PURCHASING DIRECTOR
Bacil Guiley

Library of Congress Cataloging in Publication Data

Main entry under title:

Drugs.

(Nurse's reference library)
"Nursing82 books."
Bibliography: p. 1361
Includes index.
1. Drugs. 2. Pharmacology. 3. Nursing. I. Series.
[DNLM: 1. Drugs—Nursing texts. QV 55 D7945]
RM300.D796 615'.1'024613 81-23206
ISBN 0-916730-38-7 AACR2

Staff for this volume

Drug Information Editor: Larry N. Gever, RPh, PharmD
Clinical Editor: Ann Moraca-Sawicki, RN, MSN
Special Projects Editor: Susan Rossi Williams
Senior Editor: Jerome Rubin
Assistant Editors: Nancy Holmes, Patricia E. McCulla, June T. Norris, Debra M. Rosenberg
Production Coordinator: Patricia Hamilton
Copy Chief: Jill Lasker
Copy Editors: Barbara Hodgson, Jo Lennon, David R. Moreau
Copyediting Assistants: Diane A. Dufresne, Sandra J. Purrenhage
Associate Designer: Kathaleen Motak Singel
Assistant Designers: Jacalyn Bove, Christopher Laird
Design Assistants: Jacquelyn Diotte, Darcy Feralio, Janet Schmoyer, Robert Walsh
Illustrators: Jean Gardner, Tom Herbert, Robert Jackson, Thomas Lewis, Kim Milnazik, John Murphy
Art Production Manager: Robert J. Perry, III
Art Assistants: Virginia Crawford, Diane Fox, Don Knauss, Peter Pizzo, Robert Renn, George Retseck, Sandra Simms, Craig T. Simon, Louise Stamper, Joan Walsh, Ron Yablon
Typography Manager: David C. Kosten
Typography Assistants: Janice Haber, Ethel Halle, Diane Paluba, Nancy Wirs
Production Manager: Wilbur D. Davidson
Quality Control Manager: Robert L. Dean
Editorial Assistants: Maree E. DeRosa, Bernadette Glenn, Sally Johnson
Researcher: Vonda Heller

Special thanks to Helen Hamilton, Jean Robinson, and Edward Quigley for their assistance, and to the following, no longer on the staff, who assisted in the preparation of this volume: Richard Eckersley; Linda S. Hewlings; Donna Monturo; Linda Roucken; Karen Dyer Vance, RN, BSN; Pat Weiser.

Contents

I General Information

II Antimicrobial and Antiparasitic Agents

III Cardiovascular System Drugs

IV Central Nervous System Drugs

V Autonomic Nervous System Drugs

VI Respiratory Tract Drugs

VII Gastrointestinal Tract Drugs

VIII Hormonal Agents

IX Agents for Fluid and Electrolyte Balance

X Hematologic Agents

XI Antineoplastic Agents

XII Eye, Ear, Nose, and Throat Drugs

XIII Dermatomucosal Agents

XIV Anesthetic Agents

XV Nutritional Agents

XVI Miscellaneous Drug Categories

XVII Appendices and Index

Nurse's Reference Library™

This volume is part of a new series conceived by the publishers of *Nursing82*® magazine and written by hundreds of nursing and medical specialists. This series, the NURSE'S REFERENCE LIBRARY, is the most comprehensive reference set ever created exclusively for the nursing profession. Each volume brings together the most up-to-date clinical information and related nursing practice. Each volume informs, explains, alerts, guides, educates. Taken together, the NURSE'S REFERENCE LIBRARY provides today's nurse with the knowledge and the skills that she needs to be effective in her daily practice and to advance in her career.

Other volumes in this reference series include the following: DISEASES, DIAGNOSTICS, ASSESSMENT, and PROCEDURES.

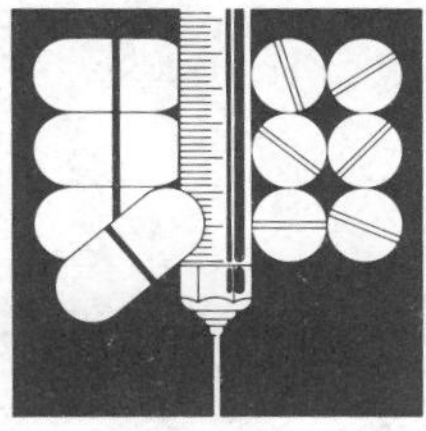

Advisory board

At the time of publication, the advisors, clinical consultants, and contributors held the following positions.

Lillian S. Brunner, RN, MSN, ScD, FAAN, Consultant in Nursing, Presbyterian–University of Pennsylvania Medical Center, Philadelphia.

Donald C. Cannon, MD, PhD, Professor, Pathology and Laboratory Medicine, the Medical School, University of Texas Health Science Center, Houston.

Luther Christman, RN, PhD, Dean, Rush College of Nursing; Vice-President, Nursing Affairs, Rush University, Chicago, Ill.

Kathleen A. Dracup, RN, MN, CCRN, Research Fellow, Medicine/Cardiology, University of California at Los Angeles.

Stanley J. Dudrick, MD, Professor and Chairman, Department of Surgery, University of Texas Medical School at Houston.

Halbert E. Fillinger, MD, Assistant Medical Examiner, Philadelphia County, Philadelphia, Pa.

M. Josephine Flaherty, RN, PhD, Principal Nursing Officer, Department of National Health and Welfare, Ottawa, Ont.

Joyce LeFever Kee, RN, MSN, Associate Professor, University of Delaware College of Nursing, Newark.

Dennis E. Leavelle, MD, Director, Mayo Medical Laboratories, Department of Laboratory Medicine, Mayo Clinic, Rochester, Minn.

Roger M. Morrell, MD, PhD, FACP, Professor, Neurology and Immunology/Microbiology, Wayne State University, School of Medicine, Detroit, Mich.; Chief, Neurology Service, Veterans Administration Medical Center, Allen Park, Mich.

Ara G. Paul, Dean, College of Pharmacy, University of Michigan, Ann Arbor.

Rose Pinneo, RN, MS, Associate Professor of Nursing and Clinician II, University of Rochester, N.Y.

Thomas E. Rubbert, JD, LLB, BSL, Attorney-at-Law, Los Angeles, Calif.

Maryanne Schreiber, RN, BA, Product Manager, Patient Monitoring, Hewlett Packard Co., Waltham Division, Waltham, Mass.

Frances J. Storlie, RN, PhD, Associate Professor of Nursing, University of Nevada, Reno.

Claire Watson, RN, Supervisor of I.V. Therapy, Hunt Memorial Hospital, Danvers, Mass.

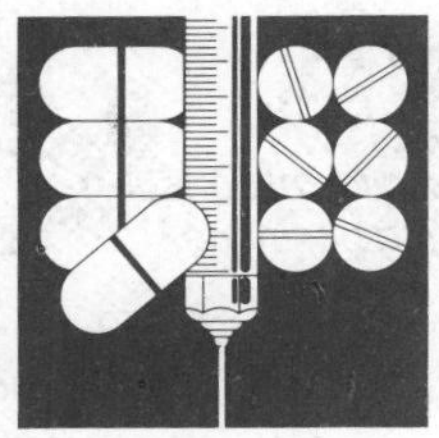

Clinical consultants

Beverly A. Baldwin, RN, MA, Assistant Professor, School of Nursing, University of Maryland, Baltimore.

Heather Boyd-Monk, RN, BSN, Educational Coordinator, Wills Eye Hospital, Philadelphia, Pa.

Nancy Burns, RN, PhD, Assistant Professor, University of Texas School of Nursing, Arlington.

Carla J. Burton, RN, BSN, Dermatology Nurse Clinician, Beth Israel Hospital, Boston, Mass.

Deborah Bussey, RN, BSN, Head Nurse, Thoracic Oncology Outpatient Clinic, M.D. Anderson Hospital and Tumor Institute, Houston, Tex.

Priscilla A. Butts, RN, MSN, Lecturer, University of Pennsylvania, Philadelphia.

Judy Donlen, RNC, MSN, Instructor, Perinatal Graduate Program, University of Pennsylvania School of Nursing, Philadelphia.

Jeanne Dupont, RN, Head Nurse, Emergency Department, Massachusetts Eye and Ear Infirmary, Boston.

Margarethe Hawkin, RN, MA, CNRN, Clinical Nurse Specialist in Neurology and Epilepsy, Seattle (Wash.) Veteran's Administration Medical Center.

Kathleen M. Hawkins, RN, Dermatology Nurse Specialist, University of Colorado, Health Sciences Center, Denver.

Carolyn Holt, RN, BSEd, Coordinator, Nursing Staff Development, Columbus-Cuneo-Cabrini Medical Center, Chicago, Ill.

Gail D'Onofrio Long, RN, MSN, Clinical Nurse Specialist in Medical Intensive Care and Coronary Care, University Hospital, Boston, Mass.

Elizabeth A. Phillips, RN, BA, BSN, Administrative Supervisor, Delaware Valley Medical Center, Bristol, Pa.

Turena Reeves, RN, Coordinator, Intravenous Therapy, Germantown Hospital and Medical Center, Philadelphia, Pa.

Despina Seremelis, RN, BSN, Staff Nurse, Oncology Unit, Temple University Hospital, Philadelphia, Pa.

Barbara Solomon, RN, MSN, Clinical Nurse Expert, Division of Arthritis and Metabolism, National Institute of Health, Bethesda, Md.

Robin Tourigan, RN, MSN, Nurse Clinician, Thomas Jefferson University Hospital, Philadelphia, Pa.

Paula Brammer Vetter, RN, BSN, Clinical Instructor in Coronary Intensive Care, Cleveland (Ohio) Clinic Hospital.

Carmen Brochu Wohrle, RN, MSN, Assistant Director of Nursing, Deaconess Hospital, Spokane, Wash.

Patricia H. Worthington, RN, BSN, Nutritional Support Nurse, Thomas Jefferson University Hospital, Philadelphia, Pa.

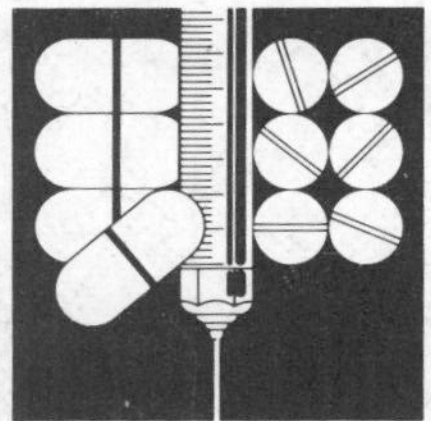

Contributors

Ron Ballentine, PharmD, Associate Professor and Chairman, Department of Clinical Pharmacy and Administration, University of Houston; Drug Information Specialist, M.D. Anderson Hospital and Tumor Institute, Houston, Tex.

Alan D. Barreuther, PharmD, Assistant Professor, Pharmacy Practice, College of Pharmacy; Instructor, Department of Pharmacology, College of Medicine, Arizona Health Sciences Center, Tucson.

Peter W. Chan, PharmD, Clinical Pharmacist, Aurora, Colo.

Bruce B. Clutcher, BS, Staff Pharmacist, University of Pennsylvania Hospital, Philadelphia.

Michael R. Cohen, BS, RPH, Director of Pharmacy, Quakertown (Pa.) Community Hospital; Assistant Clincial Professor of Pharmacy, Temple University School of Pharmacy, Philadelphia, Pa.

Lawrence J. Dwork, BS, Clinical Pharmacist, Grant Hospital, Columbus, Ohio.

DeAnn M. Englert, RN, MSN, Assistant Professor, Louisiana State University Medical Center School of Nursing, New Orleans.

Bruce M. Frey, PharmD, Clinical Pharmacist in Pediatrics, Thomas Jefferson University Hospital, Philadelphia, Pa.; Clinical Assistant Professor, Philadelphia (Pa.) College of Pharmacy and Science.

Matthew P. Fricker, BS, Clinical Pharmacist, Temple University Hospital, Philadelphia, Pa.

Steven J . Gilbert, BS, Staff Pharmacist, The Graduate Hospital, Philadelphia, Pa.

Dolores H. Heckenberger, RN, MS, Director of Professional Services, Community Health and Nursing Services of Greater Camden County, Collingswood, N.J.

James R. Hildebrand III, PharmD, Clinical Pharmacist Supervisor, Thomas Jefferson University Hospital, Philadelphia, Pa.

Jay H. Hoffman, BS, Clinical Pharmacist, Thomas Jefferson University Hospital, Philadelphia, Pa.

Alan W. Hopefl, PharmD, Assistant Professor of Clinical Pharmacy, St. Louis (Mo.) College of Pharmacy; Assistant Professor of Pharmacology in Medicine, St. Louis (Mo.) University School of Medicine.

Michael G. Krevitskie, BS, Staff Pharmacist, Lower Bucks Hospital, Bristol, Pa.

Joseph A. Linkewich, PharmD, Associate Professor of Clinical Pharmacy, Philadelphia (Pa.) College of Pharmacy and Science.

Steven Meisel, PharmD, Deputy Chief Pharmacist, Keams Canyon (Ariz.) Indian Hospital and Clinics, U.S. Public Health Service.

George Melnik, BS, Nutritional Support Service Pharmacist, Philadelphia (Pa.) Veterans Administration Medical Center.

Linda Nelson, PharmD, Instructor in Clinical Pharmacy, Philadelphia (Pa.) College of Pharmacy and Science.

David R. Pipher, PharmD, Clinical Pharmacist, Montefiore Hospital, Pittsburgh, Pa.

Susan Rogers, PharmD, Clinical Pharmacist, Radnor, Pa.

Joel Shuster, PharmD, Director of Pharmacy Services, The Fairmount Institute, Philadelphia, Pa.; Clinical Assistant Professor, Philadelphia (Pa.) College of Pharmacy and Science.

William Simonson, PharmD, Associate Professor of Pharmacy, Oregon State University School of Pharmacy, Corvallis.

Anthony P. Sorrentino, PharmD, Manager, Jefferson Apothecary, Philadelphia, Pa.

Joseph F. Steiner, PharmD, Assistant Professor of Clinical Pharmacy; Director of Clinical Pharmacy Program, University of Wyoming, Family Practice Residency Center, Casper.

Janet Louise Wagner, PharmD, Assistant Professor of Clinical Pharmacy, University of Cincinnati (Ohio) College of Pharmacy.

Frank F. Williams, PharmD, Drug Information Pharmacist, Temple University Hospital, Philadelphia, Pa.

Special thanks to those who contributed to past editions: Richard Bailey, BS; Marquette L. Cannon, PharmD; Judith Hopfer Deglin, PharmD; Betty H. Dennis, MS; Dina Dichek, BS; Teresa P. Dowling, PharmD; Dan R. Ford, PharmD; Lee Gardner, PharmD; Marie Gardner, PharmD; Philip P. Gerbino, PharmD; Patricia J. Hedrick, PharmD; Arthur I. Jacknowitz, PharmD; Sandra G. Jue, PharmD; Barbara H. Korberly, PharmD; Sheldon M. Leiman, BS; Lauren F. McKaig, BS; Kathryn Murphy, MSN; David W. Newton, PhD; George David Rudd, MS; Jamshid B. Tehrani, PhD; C. Wayne Weart, PharmD.

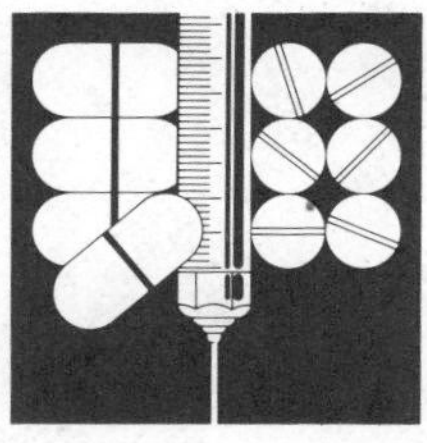

Foreword

As never before, you, the working nurse, have to accept greater personal responsibility for your clinical decisions. Peer review and assessment of the quality of nursing care are just two of the indicators of this trend. Likewise, the scientific knowledge you need to furnish effective nursing care is growing rapidly. And it's constantly being refined as we gain precise understanding of smaller and smaller details.

You can be keenly aware of this knowledge expansion in the daily administration of drugs. Besides the steady introduction of new drugs, there's a greater need for sophisticated understanding in the use of each drug. Each patient can be helped more than he would have been in the past as individual drug programs are tailored to his needs. So the effect of all this scientific productivity can be *better patient care,* if competently managed.

This book is a highly reliable tool to help you administer drugs with confidence. It contains what you need to know about more than 1,100 drugs. These drugs are grouped into 105 classes based on their pharmacologic actions, and into 16 major sections by clinical use or by the body system they influence.

In an easily read tabular format, each drug is identified by generic and trade name. Explicit dosage instructions, indications, side effects, and clinically significant interactions are listed. Nursing considerations include contraindications, special cautions, suggestions for administration and patient comfort, and proper drug storage and preparation.

Each chapter also covers major uses of drugs; mechanisms of action; and absorption, distribution, metabolism, and excretion of drugs. Numerous colorful charts, diagrams, and illustrations help you develop a better understanding of pharmacology and drug therapy.

In the general information section, you'll find comprehensive chapters on basic pharmacology; drug therapy in adults, children, and the elderly; calculations for nurses; principles of intravenous solution compatibility; and parenteral and enteral nutrition. An extensive, full-color identification section showing nearly 500 photos of drugs that can be abused adds to the usefulness of the volume.

Finally, there are several helpful appendices, and a single index for finding what you need quickly. In all, DRUGS is a valuable adjunct to your clinical practice. By answering your questions and easing your concerns about drug actions and effects on your patients, it lets you attend to other pressing areas of patient care.

LUTHER CHRISTMAN, PhD, RN
Vice-President, Nursing Affairs, and
Dean, College of Nursing, Rush University
Rush-Presbyterian-St. Luke's Medical Center
Chicago, Illinois

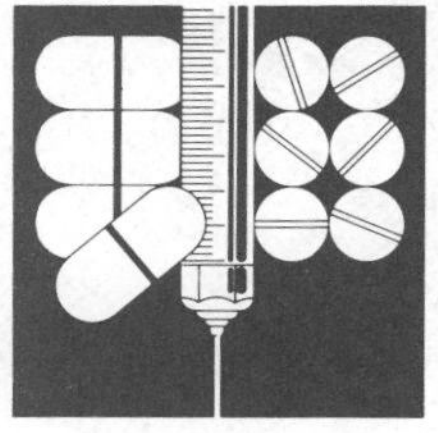

How to use this book

DRUGS represents a joint effort by clinical pharmacists and nurses to provide the nursing profession with comprehensive drug information. Although it emphasizes the clinical aspects of drug therapy, essential pharmacologic aspects of drugs are also presented in a clear, succinct, and graphic manner.

Introductory chapters

These seven chapters are included in the general information section:

- Chapter 1 summarizes *important general aspects of pharmacology* that will be referred to throughout the book.
- Chapter 2 discusses the *nursing implications of drug administration in adults.* This chapter describes the various routes of administration used in giving medications and offers expert advice for administering drugs.
- Chapters 3 and 4 discuss *the unique problems of administering drugs to pediatric and geriatric patients.* They help you avoid potential pitfalls and minimize problems in these areas.
- Chapter 5 presents a *summary of common dosage calculations* you can use when you administer drugs. This section includes sample problems complete with their solutions.
- Chapter 6 offers *information that will help you administer intravenous drugs effectively and safely, plus an updated I.V. compatibility chart.*
- Chapter 7 clarifies a subject of interest to more nurses every day—*parenteral and enteral nutrition.*

Drug identification section

Starting on page 76, you'll find a special full-color identification section on common drugs of abuse and misuse. Actual-sized photographs of common drugs, including controlled substances and others that you will want to identify, are arranged by color for fast identification. Specific details on how to use this section appear on page 78. In this section you'll also find helpful information on signs and effects of common drugs of abuse, managing overdose emergencies, schedules of controlled substances, over-the-counter drugs that can be misused, a list of "street" names, and additional resources.

Drug information

The remaining chapters (except Chapter 71, which explains the nursing implications of chemotherapy) are divided into sections. The first part of each chapter summarizes the known pharmacology of the drugs in that chapter. Specifically, this section includes:

- principal therapeutic uses
- mechanism of action, if known
- how drugs are absorbed, distributed, metabolized, and excreted
- how long they take to act, and how long their effects last
- principal combination products in which the drugs are found, if any.

The second part of each chapter consists of tabular information divided into five columns:

Column 1: *Name.* An alphabetic list of drugs by generic name, immediately followed by an alphabetic list of brand names. (Occasionally, a combination product appears in the tables under the name of its major ingredient.) Brands available in both the United States and Canada are designated with a diamond (♦); those available only in Canada with a double diamond (♦♦). A brand name with no symbol after it is available only in the United States. If a drug is a controlled substance, that too is clearly indicated (example: Controlled Substance Schedule II). The products listed, although generally available, may not be approved by the Food and Drug Administration. The mention of a brand name in no way implies endorsement or guarantees legality.

Column 2: *Indications and dosage.* Major indications and specific dosage instructions for adults and children, as applicable. Children's dosages are usually indicated in terms of mg/kg/day. Dosage instructions reflect current clinical trends in therapeutics and can't be considered absolute and universal recommendations. For individual application, dosage must be considered in context with the patient's condition.

Column 3: *Side effects.* Each drug's commonly observed side effects (and selected rare ones, if life-threatening). The most common and life-threatening side effects are italicized for easy reference. An exception to this rule is a side effect that, although normally considered quite hazardous, has been reported to be mild and reversible with the drug in question. For example, thrombocytopenia is considered a life-threatening side effect of mithramycin (a chemotherapeutic drug). However, the thrombocytopenia seen with methyldopa (Aldomet) is generally mild and reversible. Hence, thrombocytopenia listed as a side effect of mithramycin is italicized, whereas the same side effect under methyldopa is not. Side effects are grouped according to the body system in which they appear.

Column 4: *Interactions.* Each drug's confirmed, clinically significant interactions with other drugs, including additive effects, potentiated effects, and antagonistic effects. Also included are specific suggestions for dealing with dangerous drug interactions: reducing doses or monitoring certain laboratory tests, for example. Drug interactions are listed under the drug that is adversely affected. For example, magnesium trisilicate, an ingredient in antacids, interacts with tetracycline to cause decreased absorption of tetracycline. Therefore, this interaction is listed under tetracycline. To check on the possible effects of using two or more drugs simultaneously, refer to the interaction entry for each of the drugs.

Column 5: *Nursing considerations.* Contraindications and precautions, followed by monitoring techniques and suggestions for prevention and treatment of side effects. Also included in this column are investigational drug uses, when appropriate, and suggestions for promoting patient comfort, for patient teaching, and for preparing, administering, and storing each drug.

Appendices

Several appendices offer useful, supplementary information. Included are a section listing newly approved drugs; information to help identify, treat, and reverse toxic reactions, as well as relieve their symptoms; a list of substance abuse agencies and poison information services in the U.S. and Canada; a guide to drugs for cardiovascular emergencies; and an introduction to diagnostic imaging agents and a table summarizing the more common ones.

Another appendix lists selected drugs and describes their influence on laboratory test values. Also included in the appendix is "Selected References," which provides an annotated guide for further reading.

Index

A comprehensive index lists all drugs alphabetically by both generic and trade names. Monograph or tabular information appears in bold type; subentries are used, where appropriate, for easier reference, such as in cases of drugs with multiple uses. The index also includes combination products; teaching aids, nursing tips, and other learning aids; basic drug concepts; charts, photographs, and color plates. The index is printed on tinted paper so you can locate it easily.

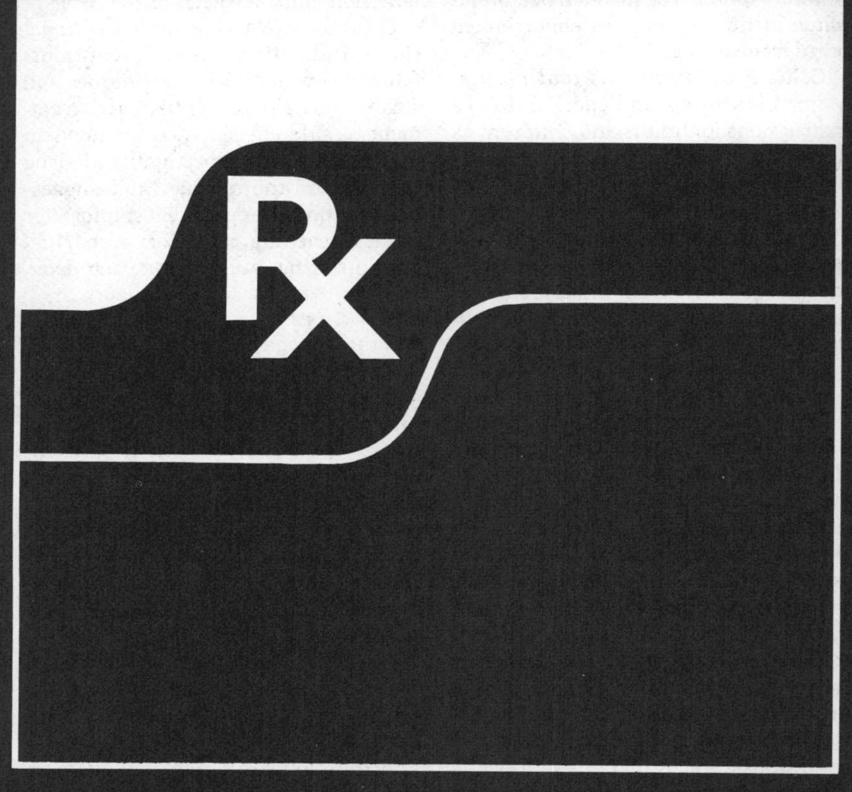

I General Information

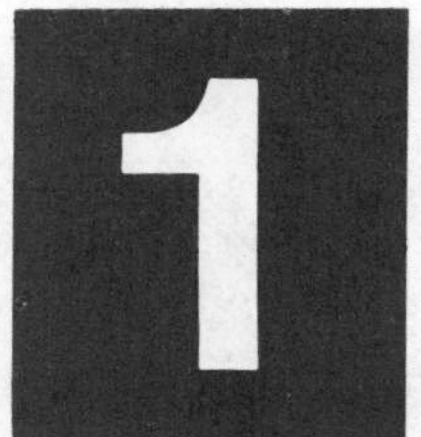

Pharmacology for nurses

Drug actions, reactions, and interactions explained

Administration of any drug provokes a series of physiochemical events within the body. The first event—the *drug action*—occurs when a drug reaches its site of action and combines with cellular drug receptors. The physiologic response to this action is the *drug effect.*

Depending on the number of different cellular drug receptors affected by a given drug, a drug effect can be local or systemic, or both. For example, the anti–peptic-ulcer drug cimetidine (Tagamet) acts solely by blocking histamine receptor cells in the parietal cells of the stomach. This is known as a local drug effect because the drug action is sharply limited to one area and doesn't spread to other parts of the body. However, diphenhydramine (Benadryl) produces a systemic effect in that it blocks histamine receptors in widespread areas of the body.

Furthermore, certain drugs may produce either type of effect depending on the route of administration. For example, epinephrine dilates the bronchioles when inhaled as an aerosol. However, I.V. administration of epinephrine produces a systemic effect on all adrenergic receptors.

Mechanisms of drug action

Understanding the principles of pharmacokinetics (the movement of a drug through the body as it is absorbed, distributed, metabolized, and excreted) helps you know the proper drug and dosage form required to produce the desired drug effect. The following summaries explain how each of these pharmacokinetic processes works.

1. *Absorption*
A drug must be absorbed into the bloodstream before it can act within the body. Several factors determine the speed and degree of absorption: various patient characteristics, the drug's physiochemical effects, dosage form, route of administration, and interactions with other substances in the gastrointestinal (GI) tract.

Drugs already in solution—such as syrups, elixirs, and injectables—are usually absorbed more rapidly than other dosage forms. This explains why some drugs, such as digoxin, produce higher blood levels when administered as solutions than they do as tablets.

If the drug's in tablet or capsule form, it must first disintegrate. Smaller particles of the disintegrated drug can dissolve in gastric juices and be absorbed into the bloodstream. When it is absorbed and circulating in the bloodstream, the drug is *bioavailable,* or ready to produce its effect.

Drugs administered intramuscularly are absorbed through the muscle before entering the bloodstream. This relatively fast process can be prolonged by administering the drug in an oil solution, or as a suspension, that is, by decreasing the solubility of the drug. For example, an intramuscular injection of penicillin G potassium is absorbed almost immediately; an intramuscular injection of penicillin G procaine takes several hours to be absorbed because its oily base makes the drug relatively lipid-insoluble.

Drugs administered intravenously are placed directly into the circulation and thus are immediately bioavailable.

For a drug to be absorbed when given other than intravenously, it must first pass through membranes by such methods as *active (carrier) transport* and *passive diffusion.*

- *Active transport* plays a minor role in drug absorption. The drug combines with a "carrier" on one side of the membrane and is taken through to the other side, where it dissociates from the carrier and is deposited in the bloodstream.
- *Passive diffusion* is the more common method of drug absorption. The rate of transfer during passive diffusion depends on the *concentration gradient* and the *lipid solubility* of the drug. If a drug's concentration in the GI tract is greater than its concentration in the bloodstream, the concentration gradient necessary for passive diffusion is set up. The drug will continue to pass through the GI membrane into the bloodstream until drug concentrations are equal in both areas. The higher concentration of drug in the GI tract maintains the concentration gradient until the drug is completely absorbed.

Lipid solubility also affects passive diffusion. The higher the lipid solubility of the drug, the greater and more rapid the absorption. The lipid solubility of a drug is due to several factors, including the degree of ionization of the drug in solution. Nonionized (uncharged) drugs have a higher degree of lipid solubility and are therefore more readily absorbed than ionized (charged) drugs, which are lipid-insoluble. Since most drugs are either weak acids or weak bases, their degree of ionization depends on their location in the GI tract.

Weak acids, such as aspirin, have a higher ratio of nonionized to ionized molecules in the acidic environment of the stomach, and thus are more readily absorbed from this area (see p. 6).

Weak bases, such as quinidine, however, have a higher proportion of nonionized molecules in the alkaline medium of the small intestine. Some nonionized molecules of the drug are present in both the stomach and the intestine, so absorption occurs to some extent in both locations. Only the ratio of nonionized to ionized molecules changes. Also, since the small intestine has a larger surface area than the stomach, a good blood supply, and a pH of 6.0 to 8.0, more absorption occurs there.

Gastric emptying time also affects absorption of medications from the GI tract. For instance, food or antacids in the stomach may prolong gastric emptying time and delay a drug's reaching the small intestine. However, if GI motility is increased, as in diarrhea, drugs may travel through the GI tract so rapidly that they're not completely absorbed. This condition would particularly undermine absorption of sustained-release preparations that are intended to be absorbed over 8 to 12 hours.

2. *Distribution*

As soon as a drug starts to be absorbed, it moves from the bloodstream into body fluids and tissues; this is distribution. Initially, tissues with a high blood flow—highly perfused organs such as the heart, liver, kidneys, and brain—receive most of the drug. Since absorption may take place over several hours, the processes of absorption, distribution, metabolism, and excretion can be occurring simultaneously.

A drug's ability to cross a lipid membrane influences its distribution to various sites in the body (for example, the central nervous system, the placenta, and breast milk). Since some drugs cannot pass through certain cell membranes, their distribution is limited. Other drugs, such as ethyl alcohol, can pass through virtually all cell membranes. Remember these points:

- *Plasma-protein binding* can greatly

influence the distribution and therefore the effectiveness and duration of drug action.

Many drugs are insoluble in plasma; these are transported as weak complexes bound to plasma proteins, especially albumin. (Drug binding can occur at sites of absorption, at extravascular sites, or, most commonly, in the blood.) Some drugs are highly bound to plasma proteins, many are moderately bound, and others may not be bound at all. All drugs bound to plasma proteins have a ratio of free, or unbound, drug to bound drug. For example, warfarin is 97% bound to plasma proteins. Only 3% is unbound, or free drug. Only free drug is pharmacologically active, or able to produce an effect at the drug receptor site; only free drug can be metabolized or excreted.

Bound drug acts as a reservoir; as free drug is eliminated, bound drug is released from the plasma proteins. Thus, drug binding is reversible. The binding process regulates the amount of free drug in circulation and prevents the drug from reaching its site of action fully concentrated.

• The *volume of distribution*—the total area to which a drug is distributed—depends on the individual

HOW IONIZATION AFFECTS ABSORPTION

Why are some drugs more lipid-soluble (and thus more readily absorbed) in the stomach, while others are more lipid-soluble in the intestine? A major reason is the ratio of nonionized to ionized molecules in a drug. This important ratio depends on whether the drug is a weak acid or a weak base, and what the pH of its environment is.

Ionized drug molecules are electrically charged. Since the lipid membrane itself is highly charged, it repels the ionized drug.

WEAK ACIDS
(such as aspirin, sulfonamides, and most barbiturates) are more readily absorbed from the acidic environment of the stomach, where a higher percentage of their molecules remains nonionized.

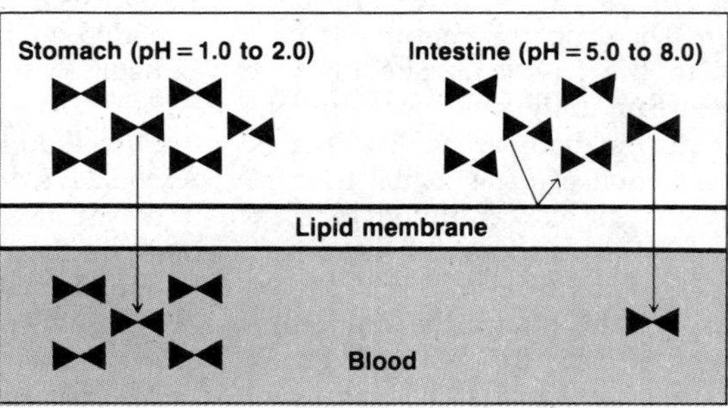

WEAK BASES
(such as amphetamine, quinidine, and ephedrine) are more readily absorbed from the alkaline environment of the intestine, where a higher percentage of their molecules remains nonionized.

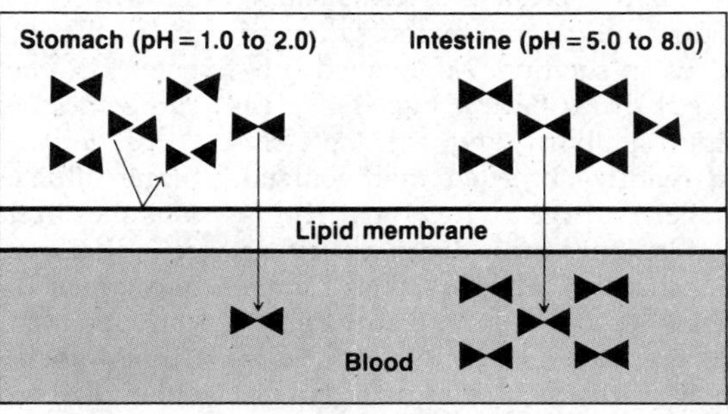

KEY: ▶◀ = nonionized (more lipid-soluble) ▶◀ = ionized (less lipid-soluble)

characteristics of the patient and the drug. For example, in an edematous patient, a given dose must be distributed to a larger volume than in a nonedematous patient; therefore, the drug amount may have to be increased. (Remember that the dosage should be decreased when edema is corrected.)

Conversely, in an extremely dehydrated patient, the drug is distributed to a much smaller volume, so the dose must be decreased.

Particularly obese patients may present another problem: Some drugs, such as digoxin, gentamicin, and tobramycin, are not well distributed to fatty tissue. For this type of drug, therefore, dosage based on actual body weight may lead to overdose and serious toxicity. In some cases, dosage must be based on lean body weight (which may be estimated from actuarial tables that give average weight range for height).

3. *Combination with receptors*
Through absorption and distribution, the drug reaches its site of action and combines with receptors in the cells. Certain drugs have an affinity for certain cells and not for others, so their biologic effect is produced selectively and specifically. When a drug combines with a receptor at a specific site, a series of biochemical and physiologic changes begin in response to the drug. Most receptors are proteins, such as enzymes of the body's metabolic or regulatory pathways or intracellular proteins of infecting bacteria. The receptor for penicillin, for example, is the enzyme transpeptidase. Penicillin renders this enzyme incapable of making the cell walls of the bacteria strong and rigid. Hence, the cell walls break down and the bacteria die.

Proteins also act as receptors for the body's regulatory chemicals, such as hormones and neurotransmitters. Drugs can mimic these chemicals or block their effects at the receptor sites.

A drug's ability to combine with a receptor is called *affinity; efficacy* refers to the drug's ability to activate the receptor. Drugs that have both characteristics are *agonists*. The degree of response to an agonist depends on the drug's affinity for the receptor site and its concentration there.

Drugs called *antagonists* may also combine with a receptor; these produce no pharmacologic response but inhibit actions of agonists for this receptor. An antagonist can be either competitive or noncompetitive. It's competitive if a sufficiently high dose of an agonist can overcome its effects. For example, enough histamine (agonist) can overcome antihistamine (antagonist). The process in this case is reversible.

An antagonist is noncompetitive if an agonist can't overcome it, regardless of dose. For example, organophosphates noncompetitively block cholinergic receptors. The process in this case is irreversible, since the antagonist inactivates the receptor.

Whether a drug is an agonist or antagonist, its affinity for the receptor depends on its specific molecular structure. Relatively small changes in the drug molecule may result in major differences in the pharmacologic effect. This relationship of molecular configuration to pharmacologic effect is called the *structure-activity relationship*. Modification of the drug's molecular structure may still permit the drug to interact with the receptor but may produce changes in the drug's pharmacokinetic or therapeutic effects.

Investigations of the structure-activity relationships of drugs and of endogenous substances such as hormones have led to the discovery of safer drugs and of new or more effective drugs. Good examples of products developed from this type of research are the nonsteroidal anti-inflammatory drugs. The drug ibuprofen's chemical structure can be manipulated to obtain a compound with similar therapeutic indications. Naproxen, one such compound, has some different pharmacokinetic characteristics than ibuprofen. For example, naproxen's longer duration of action may suit some patients' needs better than ibuprofen's short duration of action. Both drugs, however, produce the same therapeutic effect.

4. *Metabolism*
Some drugs are excreted virtually unchanged. Most drugs, however, are metabolized (biotransformed) by the liver before they're excreted by the kidneys. Hepatic metabolism usually produces a metabolite of the drug that is less lipid-soluble and more water-soluble, and thus able to be readily excreted by the kidneys.

A metabolite may be pharmacologically active or inactive. An *active* metabolite may produce effects similar to those of the drug itself or other, possibly toxic, effects.

In some cases, the drug being administered is pharmacologically *inactive* and must be metabolized to the active compound to be effective. Examples of this are cyclophosphamide, a cytotoxic drug, and chloral hydrate, a hypnotic. These inactive drugs must then undergo a second biotransformation before they can be excreted.

The liver is the main site of drug metabolism, but other tissues (for example, the lungs, kidneys, blood, and intestine) may also metabolize drugs. Orally administered drugs transverse the liver before reaching the systemic circulation. If they're significantly metabolized in this process, only a fractional amount of unmetabolized drug remains to cause the desired effect. This *first-pass effect* (biotransformation before the drug reaches general circulation) explains why oral doses of many drugs are much higher than parenteral doses. The oral dosage range of propranolol, for example, is 10 to 80 mg; the I.V. dose is 1 to 3 mg.

The rate at which a drug is metabolized varies with the patient. In some patients, drugs are metabolized so quickly that blood and tissue levels prove therapeutically inadequate. In others, metabolism is so slow that ordinary doses can produce toxic results.

Some drugs can alter the metabolism of other drugs. For example, a drug such as phenobarbital can stimulate hepatic-metabolizing enzymes to speed metabolism and change the effect of the other drugs metabolized by the liver.

Hepatic diseases may affect one or more of the liver's functions, resulting in increased, decreased, or unchanged drug metabolism. Patients with hepatic diseases, therefore, must be closely monitored for drug effect and toxicity.

5. *Excretion*
Some slight elimination takes place through perspiration, saliva, tears, feces, and breast milk. Certain volatile anesthetics, such as halothane, are eliminated primarily by exhalation. But most drugs are excreted by the kidneys either as the unchanged drug or as a metabolite. Renal excretion of drugs follows the usual pattern of excretion: passive glomerular filtration, active tubular secretion, and tubular reabsorption.

Some drugs (digoxin, gentamicin) are eliminated practically unchanged by the kidneys. For safe use of such drugs, renal function must be adequate or the drug will accumulate and produce toxic effects. In a patient with renal impairment, the route of drug excretion should be reviewed and dosage modifications made as necessary. Also, if a patient's renal function changes, all current medications in his regimen must be reevaluated.

Some drugs can alter the effect and excretion of other drugs. For example, probenecid can block renal excretion of penicillin, causing it to accumulate and enhancing its effects. Antacids speed excretion and thus diminish the effects of salicylates (aspirin).

A drug's excretion is also affected by its blood concentration, half-life, and accumulation in the body. Here's what you should know about these factors:

• *Blood concentration.* The ongoing processes of absorption, distribution, metabolism, and excretion are continuously affecting blood concentration of

THE IMPORTANCE OF HALF-LIFE

What it is:

The time required for the blood level of a drug to fall to half its peak amount. This diagram shows the time required (2½ hours) for the blood level of gentamicin to fall to 3 mcg/ml, one half its peak level of 6 mcg/ml. Intravenous injections, of course, produce peak blood levels immediately.

How it's determined:

Blood samples are taken from the patient at specific time intervals to determine the amount of drug in the blood. Standard data on drug half-life have helped establish the drug dosages required to achieve and maintain desired blood levels.

Thus, standard dosage intervals, such as every 4 hours, every 6 hours, and so on, give an indication of half-life. For some drugs, it's 30 minutes or less; for others, 8 hours or more.

What to watch for:

Body changes that may increase standard half-life, such as decreased ability to metabolize or excrete drugs. Patients with hepatic or renal disease, for example, may retain the drug in the blood or tissues for a longer time than normal. The half-life of the drug is extended in these cases; the dosage and/or frequency can be adjusted to prevent accumulation and toxicity.

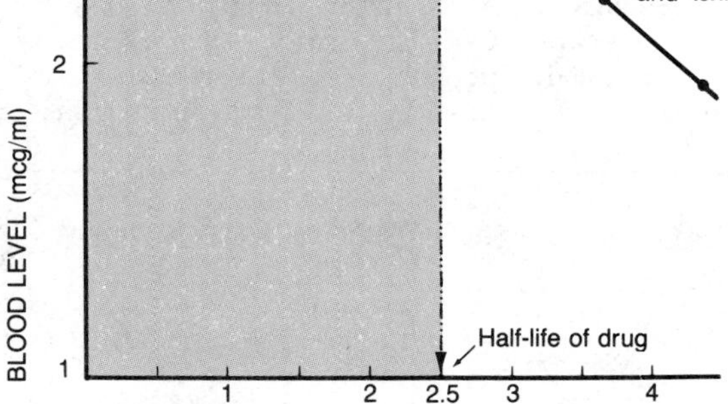

HALF-LIFE OF A GENTAMICIN INJECTION (I.V., 1 mg/kg)

a drug. Absorption of an oral drug is greater than its excretion until the peak blood level is reached. After this, more drug is excreted than absorbed, and the blood concentration of the drug falls. A drug administered by I.V. bolus is immediately bioavailable, rapidly distributed, and excreted.

• *Half-life.* This is the time required for the blood concentration of a drug to decrease by 50%. Half-life is an important drug characteristic used to establish optimum dosage regimens, such as loading dose, maintenance dose, and duration between doses. For example, a drug with a short half-life, such as penicillin G, must be given several times daily to maintain therapeutic effects; a drug like digoxin with a long half-life can be given once daily.

The figure above shows the half-life of an I.V. injection of gentamicin. Since for every half-life the concentration of the drug is halved, after five half-lives the drug will have been 95% eliminated.

• *Accumulation.* Many drugs reach a therapeutic blood level after the same dose is repeated several times. When an immediate response is required, a large or loading dose is given, followed by smaller maintenance doses. As shown in the figure below, the drug will accumulate if each successive dose is given before the previous dose has been completely excreted. This process continues until the dose given is equal to the amount of the drug being excreted. At this time *a steady state* exists, and the blood level will remain in this range as long as consecutive doses are given and no other pharmacokinetic processes (such as renal function, metabolism, or bioavailability) change.

The process of accumulation explains why the full effects of a drug may not be demonstrated for a few days to several weeks after therapy has started. This also explains how toxicity occurs. When a drug is excreted more slowly than it is absorbed, the amount of drug within the blood and organs increases. Unless dosage is adjusted, accumulative toxicity results.

Other modifying factors

• *The patient's age* is another important factor influencing a drug's action and effect. Elderly patients may have decreased muscle mass and diminished hepatic and renal functions. Consequently, lower doses and longer dosage intervals may be necessary to avoid toxicity in the elderly. (For more information on this subject, see Chapter 4, NURSING IMPLICATIONS OF DRUG THERAPY IN THE ELDERLY.)

Neonates have underdeveloped metabolic enzyme systems and reduced renal function, both slowing the excretion of some drugs. They need highly individualized dosing and careful monitoring. (See Chapter 3, NURSING IMPLICATIONS OF DRUG ADMINISTRATION AND THERAPY IN CHILDREN.)

• *An underlying disease* can also markedly affect drug action. For example, acidosis may cause insulin resistance, and hyperthyroidism may speed the metabolism of some drugs. Genetic diseases—such as glucose-6-phosphate dehydrogenase (G-6-PD) deficiency and hepatic porphyria—may

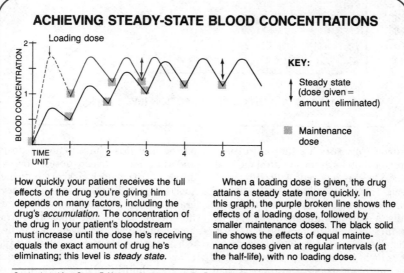

ACHIEVING STEADY-STATE BLOOD CONCENTRATIONS

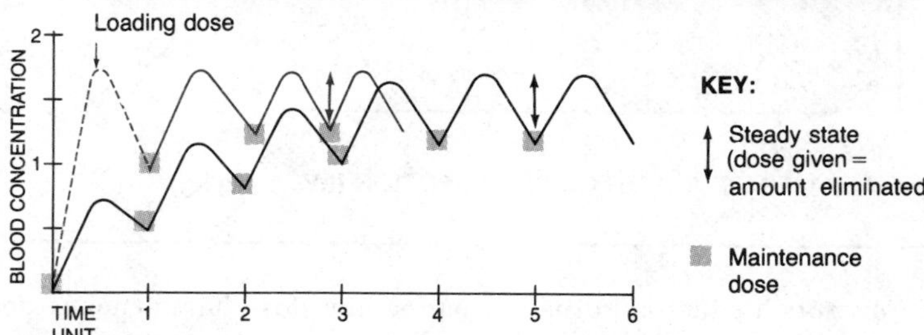

How quickly your patient receives the full effects of the drug you're giving him depends on many factors, including the drug's *accumulation.* The concentration of the drug in your patient's bloodstream must increase until the dose he's receiving equals the exact amount of drug he's eliminating; this level is *steady state.*

When a loading dose is given, the drug attains a steady state more quickly. In this graph, the purple broken line shows the effects of a loading dose, followed by smaller maintenance doses. The black solid line shows the effects of equal maintenance doses given at regular intervals (at the half-life), with no loading dose.

Graph adapted from Steven E. Mayer, et al., "Introduction: The Dynamics of Drug Absorption, Distribution, and Elimination," in *Goodman and Gilman's The Pharmacological Basis of Therapeutics,* 6th ed., edited by Alfred Goodman Gilman, et al.

turn drugs into toxins, with serious consequences. A patient with G-6-PD deficiency may develop hemolytic anemia when given sulfonamides or a number of other drugs. A genetically susceptible patient can develop an acute attack of porphyria if given a barbiturate or a sulfonamide. When treated with isoniazid, a patient with a highly active hepatic enzyme system (a rapid acetylator, for example) can develop hepatitis from the rapid intrahepatic buildup of a toxic metabolite.

• *Patient noncompliance* to the drug regimen can also affect the patient's response to the drug.

Things to consider about administration

• *Dosage forms do matter.* Some tablets and capsules are too large for very ill patients to swallow readily. You may request an oral solution or elixir of the same drug, but remember that the liquid is more easily and completely absorbed and produces higher blood levels than the tablet. When a potentially toxic drug, such as digoxin, is given in solution, the increased amount absorbed can cause toxicity. Also, enteric-coated tablets and sustained-release preparations may affect the degree of absorption of a drug and necessitate a dosage change to produce the desired effect.

• *Routes of administration are not therapeutically interchangeable.* For example, phenytoin (Dilantin) is readily absorbed orally, but slowly and erratically absorbed intramuscularly. Conversely, carbenicillin must be given parenterally because oral administration yields inadequate blood levels to treat systemic infections. Carbenicillin is given orally only to treat urinary tract infections because it concentrates in the urine.

• *The timing of drug administration can be important.* Sometimes, giving an oral drug during or shortly after mealtime decreases the amount of drug absorbed. This is not clinically significant with most drugs and may, in fact, be desirable with irritating drugs such as aspirin or indomethacin (Indocin). Certain penicillins and tetracyclines should not be given with meals because some foods can inactivate them. If in doubt about the effects of foods on a certain drug, check with a pharmacist.

• *Consider the patient's age, height, and weight.* The doctor will need this information when calculating the dose for many drugs. It should be accurately recorded on the patient's chart. The chart should also include current laboratory data, especially kidney and liver function studies, and whether the patient is edematous or dehydrated so that the doctor can adapt dosage.

• *Watch for metabolic changes.* Watch for any physiologic changes that might alter drug effect. Examples: depressed respiratory function or the development of acidosis or alkalosis.

• *Consider the possibility of pregnancy.* Many drugs may produce effects that are harmful to a developing fetus. Before giving a drug to a woman in her childbearing years, ask her whether she may be pregnant. (For more information on administering drugs to pregnant patients, see p. 15.)

• *Know the patient's history.* Whenever possible, obtain a comprehensive family history from the patient or his family. Consider past or present diseases that contraindicate a drug currently being used. Ask about past reactions to drugs, possible genetic traits that might alter drug response, and the concurrent use of other drugs. Multiple drug therapy can dramatically change the effects of many drugs or cause drug interactions.

Drug interactions

A drug interaction takes place when one drug administered in combination with or shortly after another drug alters the effect of one or both drugs. Usually, the effect of one drug is either increased or decreased. (In rare instances, an effect that cannot be attributed to either drug alone results.)

Drug interactions may result from al-

WITH FOOD OR NOT WITH FOOD?

Foods in the stomach may speed up, retard, or sometimes even prevent drug absorption. And some foods may affect one drug one way and another a different way.

Drugs given orally go through several processes before entering systemic circulation. Tablets, for example, must disintegrate and dissolve before they can be absorbed through the intestinal mucosa. But tablet breakdown is affected by the stomach's pH, so when food changes the pH, the rate and degree of breakdown—and of drug absorption—may also change.

Food stimulates various body secretions, including gastric acid and bile. For this reason, acid-labile drugs should be taken on an empty stomach, when gastric-acid secretions are minimal. Fat-soluble drugs, however, should be administered with meals because bile helps dissolve them.

Food delays stomach emptying, so a drug given with meals may remain in the stomach longer and delay therapeutic effect. So if a rapid effect is important, you'll do better to administer the drug when the patient's stomach is empty.

But sometimes a food buffer may be useful. It can, for example, reduce the gastrointestinal distress, nausea, and mucosal damage caused by ulcerogenic drugs such as aspirin and indomethacin (Indocin).

Before you administer medications, check possible drug and food interactions (see *Nursing Considerations* columns and inside back cover). You may help patients reduce unpleasant drug side effects, such as nausea, vomiting, dyspepsia, and diarrhea. You may even improve patient compliance and reduce the length (and cost) of a patient's hospital stay.

terations of the pharmocokinetics of absorption, distribution, metabolism, or excretion of one drug by another or from a combination of the drugs' actions or effects. For instance, one drug may inhibit or stimulate the metabolism or excretion of the other; or it may displace another from plasma-protein binding sites, freeing it for further action. Remember these points:

• *Combination therapy is based on drug interaction.* One drug, for example, may be given to potentiate, or increase, the effects of another. Probenecid, which blocks the excretion of penicillin, is sometimes given with penicillin to maintain adequate blood levels of penicillin for a longer period. Often, two drugs with similar actions are given together precisely because of the *additive effect* that results. For instance, aspirin and codeine, both analgesics, are given in combination because together they provide greater pain relief than either does alone.

• *Drug interactions are sometimes used to prevent or minimize certain side effects.* Hydrochlorothiazide and spironolactone, both diuretics, are administered in combination because the former is potassium-depleting and the latter, potassium-sparing.

• *Harmful drug interactions decrease efficacy or increase toxicity.* A hypertensive patient well controlled with guanethidine may see his blood pressure rise to its former high level if he takes the antidepressant amitriptyline (Elavil) at the same time. Drug combinations that produce antagonism between two drugs should be avoided if possible. Another kind of inhibiting effect occurs when tetracycline is administered with drugs or foods that contain calcium or magnesium (for example, antacids, milk). The calcium and magnesium ions combine with tetracycline in the GI tract and cause inadequate absorption of the tetracycline.

• *Several other factors may contribute to an adverse drug interaction:*

—use of more than one medication to treat a condition

—ingestion of alcohol along with medication

—self-medication with over-the-counter drugs or another person's prescription

—treatment by more than one doctor for different ailments.

Many adverse drug interactions can be prevented by appropriate modifications in dose, time, or route of administration. Patients receiving drugs that may interact must be monitored closely and taught to look for signs that may indicate adverse interaction.

Side effects

Any drug effect other than what is therapeutically intended is called a side effect. It may be expected and benign, or unexpected and potentially harmful. For example, during hay fever season, a patient may have to contend with the drowsiness caused by an antihistamine, such as chlorpheniramine, to obtain relief from hay fever symptoms. However, the woman who develops thrombophlebitis while taking oral contraceptives faces possible serious complications and hospitalization.

Thus, a side effect may be tolerated for the drug's therapeutic effect, or it may be so unacceptable or hazardous that the drug must be discontinued. Many dose-related side effects lessen or disappear when dosage is reduced (guanethidine-induced orthostatic hypotension is an example). Other side effects subside after continued drug use: Drowsiness associated with methyldopa (Aldomet) and orthostatic hypotension associated with prazosin (Minipress) usually subside after several days as the patient builds up a tolerance to these effects.

Although most side effects are therapeutically undesirable, occasionally one can be put to clinical use. For example, the drowsiness associated with diphenhydramine (Benadryl) makes this drug clinically useful as a mild hypnotic.

To deal with side effects correctly, you need to be alert to even minor changes in the patient's clinical status. Such minor changes may be an early warning of pending toxicity. Watch particularly for signs of hypersensitivity and for idiosyncratic reactions.

Hypersensitivity, a term sometimes used interchangeably with drug allergy, is the result of an antigen-antibody immune reaction that occurs when a drug is given to a susceptible patient. To be susceptible, the patient must have had prior exposure to the drug (or one of its derivatives).

Hypersensitivity can produce a relatively mild reaction such as urticaria, a more severe reaction such as serum sickness with symptoms of fever and lymphadenopathy, or a life-threatening anaphylactic reaction characterized by hypotension, bronchospasm, and laryngeal edema. One of the most common hypersensitivities is penicillin allergy, with patient response ranging from rash to anaphylaxis.

Idiosyncratic reactions occur rarely. These are highly unpredictable, individual, and unusual. Probably the best known is aplastic anemia, caused by the antibiotic chloramphenicol (Chloromycetin). This reaction develops in only 1 in 40,000 patients, but it's usually fatal. A more common idiosyncratic reaction is extreme sensitivity to very low doses of a drug, or insensitivity to higher-than-normal doses.

Recognizing drug allergies or serious idiosyncratic reactions can be lifesaving. Ask the patient about drugs he is taking or has taken in the past and what, if any, unusual effects he's experienced from taking them. If a patient claims to be allergic to a drug, ask him to tell you exactly what happened when he took it. He may be calling a harmless side effect, such as upset stomach, an allergic reaction, or he may have a true tendency to anaphylaxis. In either case, you and the doctor need to know this. Of course, you must record and report any clinical changes throughout the patient's hospital stay. If you suspect a hazardous side effect, withhold the drug until you can check with the pharmacist and the doctor.

Listen to the patient's complaints about how a drug makes him feel, and consider each complaint objectively. You may be able to reduce undesirable side effects in several ways. Obviously, reducing dosage helps in many cases, but so may simply rescheduling the same dose. For example, although pseudoephedrine (Sudafed) may stimulate a patient, this may not be a problem if it's given early in the day. Similarly, the drowsiness that occurs with antihistamines or tranquilizers can be acceptable—even desirable—to the patient if the dose is given at bedtime.

Most important, the patient needs to be told what side effects to expect so he won't become worried or stop taking the drug on his own. Of course, you should remind him to report any unusual or unexpected side effects.

Toxic reactions

Toxic reactions to drugs can be either *acute,* resulting from an excessive dose accidentally or deliberately taken, or *chronic,* from the accumulative effect of the drug buildup in the body. These toxic effects may be extensions of the desired pharmacologic effect. For example, barbiturates produce hypnotic and sedative effects by acting as nonspecific central nervous system (CNS) depressants. Toxic reactions to barbiturates are exhibited by an excessive degree of CNS depression, resulting in depressed respirations, decreased deep tendon reflexes, and possibly coma.

Drug toxicities may also result when drug blood levels rise because of impaired metabolism or excretion. For example, blood levels of theophylline rise when hepatic dysfunction impairs metabolism of the drug. Similarly, digoxin toxicity can follow impaired renal function because digoxin is excreted from the body almost exclusively by the kidneys (by glomerular filtration).

Of course, toxic blood levels also result from excessive dosage. Tinnitus (ringing in ears) caused by aspirin, for example, may be a sign that a safe dose has been exceeded. Most drug toxicity is predictable and dose-related; fortunately, most drug toxicity is also readily reversible with dosage adjustment.

Patients should be carefully monitored for physiologic changes that may alter drug effect. Watch especially for impaired hepatic or renal function. Tell the patient the signs of toxicity, and what to do if a toxic reaction occurs. Emphasize the importance of taking a drug exactly as prescribed: Warn the patient that serious problems may arise if he changes the dose or schedule. For detailed management of drug toxicity, see APPENDIX, *Drug Toxicities*.

Drugs and pregnancy

Ever since the thalidomide tragedy of the late 1950s—when thousands of infants were born malformed after their mothers used this mild sedative-hypnotic during pregnancy—use of drugs during pregnancy has been a source of controversy.

To identify drugs that may cause teratogenesis (the production of physical defects in offspring in utero), preclinical drug studies always include tests on pregnant laboratory animals. These tests point out gross teratogenicity but do not clearly establish safety. Different species react to drugs in different ways, and animal studies do not rule out possible teratogenic effects in humans. For example, the preliminary animal studies on thalidomide gave no warning of teratogenic effects, and it was subsequently released for general use in Europe.

To prevent such tragedies, almost all drugs carry a warning on the package insert. Such warnings state that safety in human pregnancy has not been established, and use of the drug in pregnancy requires that the expected therapeutic benefit be weighed against the possible hazard to mother and fetus. With the exception of vitamins and minerals, no drug is approved warning-free for use in pregnancy. Even Bendectin (a combination of the antihistamine doxylamine and the vitamin pyridoxine, for which nausea and vomiting of pregnancy are official indications) carries a warning for cautious use during pregnancy.

At one time, the placenta was thought to protect the fetus from drug effects, but today the idea of a placental barrier is considered a myth. Almost all drugs cross the placental membrane to some extent. Orally administered drugs that can cross the GI membrane can probably cross the placental membrane. Drugs with exceptionally large molecular structure, such as heparin, will not cross the placenta to a great extent; but use of these medications in pregnancy still requires caution. Just because drugs cross the placenta, however, does not necessarily mean the fetus will be harmed.

Actually, only one factor seems clearly related to exaggerated risk in drug therapy during pregnancy: the stage of fetal development. During two stages of pregnancy—the first and third trimesters—the fetus is especially vulnerable to damage from the mother's use of drugs. During these times, *all* drugs should be given with extreme caution. The most sensitive period for drug-induced fetal malformation is the first trimester, when fetal organs are differentiating (organogenesis). During this time, *all* drugs should be withheld unless doing so would jeopardize the mother's health. Theoretically, during this sensitive time, even aspirin could harm the fetus. So strongly advise your patients to avoid *all* self-prescribed drugs during the first trimester.

The other time of high fetal sensitivity to drugs is the last trimester. At birth, the newborn must rely on his own metabolism to excrete any drug remaining in his body. Since his detoxifying systems are not fully developed, any residual drug may take a long time to be metabolized—and thus may induce prolonged toxic reactions. Consequently, drugs should be used with caution during the last 3 months of pregnancy and only when absolutely necessary at term.

Nevertheless, in many circumstances, pregnant women must continue to take certain drugs. For example, a woman with epilepsy who is well controlled with an anticonvulsant should continue to take it even during pregnancy. Or a pregnant woman with a bacterial infection must receive antibiotics. In such cases, the potential risk to the fetus is outweighed by the mother's need for the drug.

NURSING TIPS

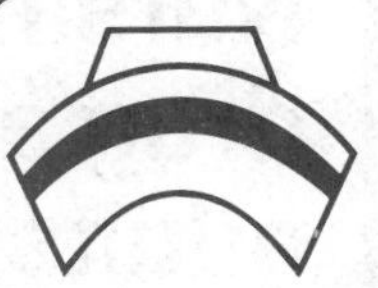

DRUGS AND YOUR PREGNANT PATIENT

To avoid adverse drug effects in your pregnant patient, follow these guidelines:
- Before administering any drug to a woman of childbearing age, ask the date of her last menstrual period and whether she could possibly be pregnant.
- Avoid administering all drugs except those essential to maintain the pregnancy or the mother's health. Be particularly cautious during the first and third trimesters when the fetus is most vulnerable.
- To minimize any harmful effect on the fetus, administer *the safest possible drug in the lowest possible dose.*
- Apply topical drugs cautiously. Many topically applied drugs can be absorbed in amounts large enough to harm the fetus.

As a precaution, remind your pregnant patient to check with her doctor before taking any drug. *Remember:* Alcohol and caffeine are drugs, too. Caution your pregnant patient to use them judiciously.

Drugs and lactation

Most drugs a nursing mother takes appear in breast milk. Drug levels in breast milk tend to be high when blood levels are high—generally, shortly after taking each dose. Therefore, advise the mother to breast-feed *before* taking medication, not *after*.

Breast-feeding should be temporarily interrupted and replaced with bottle-feeding when the mother must take:
- tetracyclines
- chloramphenicol
- sulfonamides (during first 2 weeks postpartum)
- oral anticoagulants
- iodine-containing drugs
- antineoplastics
- propylthiouracil

JOSEPH F. STEINER, PharmD

2 Nursing implications of drug administration in adults

To properly administer prescribed medications and monitor their effects, you must have a thorough knowledge of drug therapy and administration techniques. You should also understand the drug distribution system used in your institution. This chapter describes various drug distribution systems and provides important guidelines for safe drug administration.

Drug distribution systems

The drug distribution methods used in most hospitals today are almost always derived from one of these four basic systems:

- floor stock system
- individual prescription order system
- combination floor stock and individual prescription order system
- unit dose system.

Floor stock system

In the floor stock system, nearly all necessary medications are kept in stock at the nursing station. This makes each nursing unit almost a miniature pharmacy. Only special drugs like chemotherapeutic agents, certain antibiotics, and diagnostic agents are ordered from the pharmacy as needed.

Individual prescription order system

In this system, all medications are dispensed by the pharmacist for individual patients based on individual prescription orders. Normally a 5-day supply of medications is dispensed at one time.

Combination floor stock and individual prescription order system

This combination system is probably the most common one used in hospitals today. Most medications are *dispensed* as in the individual prescription order system, but the most frequently used medications are kept in floor stock.

Unit dose system

Many hospitals in the United States and Canada have initiated a unit dose system of drug distribution in the past 10 years. This system has been shown to be safer and more cost-effective and time-saving than traditional systems. The following characteristics are common to unit dose systems:

- The pharmacist receives a copy of all doctors' orders.
- The pharmacist maintains a patient medication profile for each patient. Before dispensing medications, he enters new orders on the profile, checking that each medication is appropriate.
- The pharmacist dispenses medications in properly labeled unit dose packages that contain the ordered amount of drug in a dosage form ready for administration to a particular patient by the prescribed route at a prescribed time.
- Medications are dispensed into patient-separated drug storage bins, usually in a drug cart.
- No more than a 24-hour supply of each medication is dispensed at one time.
- Floor stock of drugs is minimized.

COMPARING DRUG DISTRIBUTION SYSTEMS

SYSTEM	ADVANTAGES	DISADVANTAGES
Floor stock system	• Less delay because almost all drugs are readily available when ordered. Fewer orders need to be sent to the pharmacy.	• More work for the nurse, who must select the proper drug from a large floor stock • Chance of "pouring" errors because drugs aren't stored in separate containers for individual patients • Chance of medication errors because the pharmacist and nurse don't double-check each other whenever a drug is reordered and dispensed. Also, drugs may be used inadvertently after their expiration dates. • Increased costs of larger drug inventory throughout the hospital
Individual prescription order system	• Better pharmacy control of drug distribution than in the floor stock system • Less chance of medication errors because medication containers are identified by patient name. And both the nurse and the pharmacist double-check each other whenever a drug is reordered and dispensed.	• Potential delays in initiating therapy while waiting for ordered drugs • Waste of prescription medications due to changes or discontinuations after a drug is dispensed • Possibility of hoarding discontinued drugs on the nursing unit and using them for other patients • Potential for administering deteriorated doses • Chance of "pouring" errors because doses aren't stored individually • More nursing time spent in inventorying, ordering, and reordering prescribed drugs • Increased cost of inventory throughout the hospital
Combination floor stock and individual prescription order system	• Less delay in obtaining the most commonly ordered drugs because they're in stock on the unit	Same as those for the floor stock and individual prescription order systems
Unit dose system	• Less chance of medication and record-keeping errors because of numerous checks built into the system • Lower overall costs of drug distribution and inventory within the hospital • Lower costs for the patient: Unopened, discontinued doses may be returned to the pharmacy stocks and credited to the patient's bill. • More effective utilization of nurses and pharmacists	• Danger of errors caused by overconfidence if the nurse neglects to double-check the pharmacy • More expensive packaging • Increased pharmacy staff

Emergency medications, mouthwash, antiseptics, and frequently ordered p.r.n. medications are usually stocked.
• Nurses maintain a medication administration record. Before administering medication, the nurse compares what is written on the medication administration record with what the pharmacist has dispensed. Any discrepancies (extra doses, missing doses, wrong drugs or doses, and so on) must be resolved with the pharmacist. In this way, dispensing, administration, and record-keeping errors by pharmacists and nurses are minimized.

General guidelines for administering drugs to adults

• No medication, not even a placebo, should ever be administered to a patient without a doctor's order. Verbal orders should be taken only in emergencies, and then with extreme care to ensure accuracy. Such orders must follow established hospital policy.
• Avoid using the patient's own medications. Use them only if the doctor writes an appropriate order on the chart and the pharmacy cannot obtain the drugs. All such drugs must first be identified by a pharmacist. If they can't be identified, don't use them.
• Know why every drug you administer has been prescribed, its usual dosage range, its expected action, and its possible side effects.
• When storing drugs, keep preparations designed only for external use separate from those for internal use. Insist that the pharmacist affix "external use only" labels on containers of topical medications. Make sure the pharmacist uses appropriate auxiliary labels on eye and ear medications.
• Keep narcotics and other controlled substances under double lock.
• Remember that names of different drugs may have similar spellings. Check each very carefully. Never identify an item merely by its container, appearance, or customary shelf location. Check labels for expiration date. If the bottle has no label, return it to the pharmacy.
• Don't give medication that is discolored or in which a precipitate has formed unless the manufacturer's instructions indicate that doing so is not harmful. If in doubt, ask the pharmacist or check the manufacturer's directions.
• Always tightly cap any bottle of medication you open. Never leave a single capsule of a desiccant in a bottle—discard it to avoid giving it to a patient inadvertently.
• Never leave medications at a patient's bedside, except—on doctor's orders—antacids, various lotions and ointments, and nitroglycerin. Exceptions to this rule are medications that patients are permitted to administer to themselves (self-medication programs). Then make sure the patient understands the proper use of the medication, and monitor carefully.

Preparing and administering medications

• Always wash your hands thoroughly before preparing or administering medications.
• Only the nurse who prepares a medication should administer it.
• When preparing medication, guard against interruptions. If you have any doubt about a dose calculation, physical appearance, or name of a drug, ask the pharmacist, check a proper drug reference, or double-check calculations with another nurse.
• Don't hold tablets or capsules in your hands.
• Administer medication as close as possible (within hospital requirements) to the time officially prescribed. Be especially punctual when administering antibiotics, chemotherapeutic agents, and certain other drugs, such as those for myasthenia gravis, since a particular level of such drugs must be maintained in the blood.

Should any medication not be given as scheduled, record the reason in the nurse's notes, and report it to the pharmacist and the patient's doctor.
• Before administering a drug, read

the label three times (when taking the drug container from the shelf or cart bin, when preparing the dose, and when returning the drug to storage).

• Check the patient's wristband for proper identification; then address him by name. Or ask the patient his name.

• Always recheck when a patient expresses doubt or concern about the medication you're going to give him. There's *no* margin for error in administering drugs. Always go out of your way, therefore, to make certain that you're giving the *right dose* of the *right medication* to the *right patient* at the *right time* by the *right route*.

• Should a patient refuse to take his medication, try to find out why. In many situations, after you explain what the medication is and how it will help him, the patient will take the dose.

If he still refuses, report the matter to the head nurse and the doctor, and make a note in the patient's record. Discard the medication (except in a unit dose system; in this case, return the medication in its wrapper or container, along with proper documentation, to the pharmacy).

• When administering drugs p.r.n., always determine that enough time has passed since the last dose.

• Provide privacy as needed when administering medications such as suppositories and retention enemas.

Special considerations with a unit dose system

• If you're using a unit dose system, administer one patient's medications at a time. Never go into a room with more than one patient's medications.

• Compare the label on the dose against the medication administration record.

• If you need more than one or two dosage units (tablets, capsules, or ampuls) to prepare a single dose, question the order. Unless you're absolutely familiar with this need, check with a pharmacist before administering the dose. Something could be wrong. If large numbers of tablets or capsules are necessary, the pharmacist might be

LEGAL ADVICE

CAN YOU DISPENSE MEDICATIONS IN EMERGENCIES?

A patient is admitted to CCU at 2 a.m. Her doctor orders a heart stimulant to be given every 4 hours. You check and find the drug isn't available anywhere.

The doctor insists that you give the specific drug he ordered for the patient. Should you go to the pharmacy and get it? Nurses on evening and night shifts, especially supervisors, are likely to find themselves in this dilemma—do you practice pharmacy without a license or stick to the letter of the law?

Most state pharmacy acts specify that only pharmacists can dispense medications. Nurses are licensed and authorized to administer medications (defined as giving a single dose of a medication to a patient under order of a licensed medical doctor or other licensed practitioner).

According to some pharmacy acts, a nurse *may* remove one dose of a drug from the pharmacy for a patient. But even this may be dangerous. Instead:

• An *interdisciplinary hospital committee* should develop a written policy for the nurse to follow.

• The *pharmacist* should provide an emergency pharmaceutical kit containing drugs for the hospital when he's not there.

• The *nurse* should record when the drug was removed, the dose, the patient it's for, and her signature.

• If a drug that's ordered isn't available, the pharmacist designated for emergencies should be notified to provide the necessary emergency service of dispensing the medication.

Don't let yourself be put at legal risk. Take the necessary action to make sure you're authorized to act in your patient's best interest. And act in your own best interest by following a policy developed by the hospital interdisciplinary committee.

Adapted from Mary Dolores Hemelt and Mary Ellen Mackert, *Dynamics of Law in Nursing and Health Care*. Used with permission from Reston Publishing Co., a Prentice-Hall Co., 1978.

able to prepare a more convenient dosage form for the patient; for example, with the doctor's approval, the pharmacist may dispense the oral solution form of furosemide (Lasix).

• Don't remove drugs from unit dose packages until you are at the patient's bedside and he is ready to take the medication. This assures the drug's identification up to the time it is taken and its returnability if it's refused.

• After observing the patient take the drug, return to the medication administration record and record the dose given. Always chart *after* giving medication to each patient.

After administering medications

• Keep accurate records of all medication doses administered. Also, note the patient's reactions to medications, and when giving narcotics, routinely record the patient's pulse rate and respirations as well.

• Discard needles and syringes into proper containers.

• Include fluids taken with medication on the intake and output record.

Oral medications

• Unless authorized, don't leave oral medications at the patient's bedside for him to take later. Also, don't leave any medication for a patient who is not in his room; give him the dose when he returns.

• If a liquid or solid medication is prepackaged in a unit dose container, it should be opened and handed to the patient rather than first poured into a standard medication cup.

• Have the patient sit upright or at least in semi-Fowler's position before you administer any oral medication.

• If more than one medication has been prescribed, remain with the patient until all doses are swallowed.

• Unless contraindicated, give oral doses with cold water or juice, which may mask a medication's unpleasant taste.

• If a patient is vomiting, withhold oral medication and notify the doctor and pharmacist. Suggest substituting a parenteral or suppository form.

Tablets and capsules

• When preparing solid medication, transfer the correct number of tablets or capsules into the container's cap and then into a medication cup, unless you have a unit dose system.

• Do not break tablets unless they are scored.

• Should a patient have difficulty swallowing tablets or capsules, have him place the dose on the back of his tongue. Instruct the patient to tilt his head forward, not back. This action stimulates the back of the tongue and activates the swallowing mechanism.

• If your patient cannot swallow a tablet whole, you may be able to crush it for him and administer the drug in jelly or some other food. But first ask the pharmacist if a liquid form of the drug can be substituted.

• Remember that some tablets are enteric-coated to delay absorption or prevent the drug from irritating the stomach. Some capsules are designed to release medication over several hours. *Never crush or dissolve enteric-coated tablets or contents of sustained-release capsules.* Ask the pharmacist if you're in doubt as to whether or not you have an enteric-coated or sustained-release preparation. Some sugar-coated tablets appear to be enteric-coated.

• Instruct the patient not to chew enteric-coated tablets or sustained-release medications.

• Don't give enteric-coated tablets with milk or antacids, which may raise the pH level in the stomach and cause these tablets to dissolve prematurely.

• Should a patient vomit shortly after taking tablets or capsules, check the vomitus for undissolved particles; then notify the doctor. Don't give the patient another dose of the medication unless it's ordered.

Liquid medications

• When pouring liquid medication,

hold the bottle with the label against your palm so that if liquid runs down the bottle, it will not obscure the label. Then, wipe the bottle clean.

- If the liquid is a suspension, remember to shake it well before pouring.
- Hold a graduated medication cup at eye level to ensure accuracy of measure.
- If a medication is to be measured in drops, use a medicine dropper held at a 90° angle.
- Tell the patient to remove dentures before taking medications that may stain his teeth, such as liquid iron or iodides. Or these may be well diluted and taken through a straw.
- Give cough medicines last and undiluted. Do not dilute antacids or any other medication that's labeled not to be diluted.

Sublingual and buccal medications

- Sublingual and buccal routes of administration are used when a rapid action is desired, or when a drug is specifically designed to be easily absorbed into blood vessels under the tongue (sublingual route) or between the cheek and gums (buccal route). Examples are nitroglycerin, isosorbide dinitrate, and some male hormones. The tablets are completely soluble. These drugs cannot be given orally to obtain the same rapid effect.

  Drugs absorbed by these routes do not pass through the liver immediately after absorption as do orally administered drugs; therefore, metabolism is delayed.
- For sublingual administration, tell the patient to hold the tablet under his tongue until it's completely absorbed. Tell him not to move the tablet with his tongue to other parts of his mouth.
- For buccal administration, tell the patient to place the tablet between his cheek and gums, close his mouth, and hold the tablet there until it's absorbed.
- In both cases, remember to tell the patient not to drink water or swallow excessively until the tablet is completely absorbed.

Nasogastric tube medications

- Notify the pharmacist that the patient will be receiving medication by tube. The doctor's orders may not specify this.
- Drug action is the same as if given orally. However, all drugs must be in liquid form or crushed and well dissolved (when appropriate) just before administration.
- Supplies needed for nasogastric tube administration are:
  - —50-ml bulb syringe, syringe with plunger with adaptable tip (Toomey syringe) or funnel
  - —container with water
  - —medication
  - —stethoscope.
- Check on the possibility of administering the medication along with a tube feeding. If you can, give the medication first.
- Medication should be at room temperature.
- Avoid giving oily medications by this route: they'll cling to the side of the nasogastric tube.
- Dilute viscous medications, if possible, before introducing them through the tube.
- Measure the medication into a graduated medication cup unless it is in a unit dose container.
- Bring equipment and medication into the patient's room. Explain the procedure to the patient.
- Help the patient sit up or raise the bed to at least a 45° angle.
- Check for placement of nasogastric tube in the stomach with the following techniques:
  - —Attempt to aspirate the stomach contents with the syringe. Fluid should flow freely. Withdraw the tube slightly if you experience any difficulty. If you still cannot aspirate, the tube may be in the respiratory tract. If you have successfully aspirated stomach contents, flush the tube with 30 ml of normal saline solution to clear the tube.
  - —Place the stethoscope over the patient's stomach. Using the syringe,

inject air (about 15 ml). You should hear a "swoosh" sound as air enters the stomach.

- Close the tube with a hemostat or a clamp. Pour liquids into the syringe or funnel. Open the tube, and allow medication to flow by gravity. Don't force it down. To control flow rate, raise or lower syringe (funnel) height.
- Before air gets into the tubing, instill 30 to 50 ml of water to flush all medication through the tube. Keep in mind any fluid restrictions. Remember, the tubing will retain much of the medication unless flushed with water.
- Remove the syringe or funnel, and clamp the tube. Be sure the patient remains upright for at least 30 minutes.

Rectal medications

The rectal route is often used if the patient is unconscious or otherwise unable to swallow. Also, drugs administered rectally avoid destruction by digestive enzymes in the stomach and small intestine.

Suppositories

- Absorption of drug from rectal suppositories is unpredictable and often

NURSE'S GUIDE TO ENEMAS

Use this chart as a guide when you give your patient an enema. Before you decide which guidelines are appropriate, consider the type of medication the doctor has prescribed, as well as your patient's age, size, and condition. For instance, if your patient's a small 9-year-old child, use the smallest tube listed for his age-group. Physical size is more important than age.

Always use smaller tubing and less solution when you give a retention enema. This combination will create less pressure in the patient's rectum and make retention easier. *Note:* Never give a retention enema to an infant or young child. Neither will be able to retain it.

RETENTION ENEMAS

AGE-GROUP	RECTAL TUBE SIZE	AMOUNT OF TUBE TO INSERT	AMOUNT OF FLUID TO INTRODUCE
Adults	14 to 20 French	3″ to 4″ (7.5 to 10 cm)	150 to 200 ml
Children over age 6	12 to 14 French	2″ to 3″ (5 to 7.5 cm)	75 to 150 ml

NONRETENTION ENEMAS

AGE-GROUP	RECTAL TUBE SIZE	AMOUNT OF TUBE TO INSERT	AMOUNT OF FLUID TO INTRODUCE
Adults	22 to 30 French	3″ to 4″ (7.5 to 10 cm)	750 to 1,000 ml
Children over age 6	14 to 18 French	2″ to 3″ (5 to 7.5 cm)	500 to 1,000 ml
Children over age 2	12 to 14 French	1½″ to 2″ (3.75 to 5 cm)	500 ml or less
Infants	12 French	1″ to 1½″ (2.5 to 3.75 cm)	250 ml or less

poor. Except to relieve constipation, this route has been used less frequently in recent years. Supplies needed for rectal administration are:
—finger cot or disposable rubber glove
—suppository in wrapper or medication cup
—water-soluble lubricant.

• Explain the procedure to the patient and provide privacy; then have the patient turn on his left side, bend knees, and expose buttocks.

• Put on a glove or finger cot. Lubricate the suppository, if necessary. (Many suppositories are already moist enough to be inserted easily.) If a suppository seems too moist or melted to insert, hold it under cold running water or refrigerate it for a short time.

• With your ungloved hand, separate the patient's buttocks to expose the anus. Ask the patient to take a deep breath as you insert the suppository (tapered end first) into the rectum, past the anal sphincter.

• Hold the patient's buttocks together for a few moments until his urge to expel the suppository passes. Remove excess lubricant with a tissue. Urge the patient to retain the suppository for at least 20 minutes. However, if it is a glycerin suppository, tell him to defecate as soon as he feels the urge.

• Remove the glove or finger cot, and wash your hands.

Ointments, creams, foams, and lotions

• For external applications, wear gloves, and use a gauze pad to spread medication over the anal area.

• For internal applications, wear gloves, and attach the applicator supplied with the medication. Lubricate the tip before inserting it slowly into the rectum past the anal sphincter. Squeeze the tube to instill the medication.

• Follow the doctor's orders and instructions on the drug label to determine how much to administer.

• Remove the applicator, and place a folded 4″ x 4″ gauze pad between the patient's buttocks to absorb excess medication. Clean the applicator with water, and recap the tube.

Retention enemas

• Retention enemas of oil, magnesium sulfate, or glycerin and water are used for constipation, flatulence, and impaction. Sodium polystyrene sulfonate (Kayexalate) enemas treat hyperkalemia; neomycin enemas reduce intestinal bacteria that produce nitrogenous substances harmful to patients in hepatic coma.

• Take time to prepare the patient for the procedure. Make sure the patient understands the purpose of a retention enema and the importance of retaining it. Ask him to empty his bladder and rectum, if possible and appropriate, before you begin.

• For best results, warm solutions to at least body temperature. Wear gloves. Have a bedpan available.

• Position the patient on his left side, with knees flexed. Place bedsaver pads under his buttocks.

• Use a bulb syringe or bag connected to a rectal tube or Foley catheter with inflatable balloon. Flush air from the tube with solution, and clamp. Lubricate the end of the tube or catheter and insert it 4″ to 5″ (10 to 12.5 cm) past the anal sphincter. Inflate the balloon with sufficient fluid to hold it in the rectum and prevent leakage. Unclamp the tube, and slowly administer solution from a syringe or bag held about 5″ (12.5 cm) above the anus. Let solution flow by the force of gravity.

• After administering, clamp tubing and withdraw gently but quickly; or if using catheter with balloon, keep it in place for time specified for retention.

• The patient should retain the solution for at least 30 minutes—much longer if possible. Sodium polystyrene sulfonate enemas should be held for a minimum of at least 30 to 60 minutes and up to 6 to 10 hours, if possible.

• Usual maximum volume is 150 to 250 ml. However, volumes as large as 1 liter (dilute lactulose solutions) may be required. In this case, administer

PATIENT PREPARATION

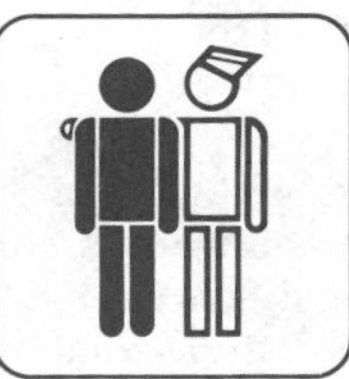

GIVING A MEDICATED RETENTION ENEMA

Always take enough time to thoroughly prepare your patient before giving him a medicated retention enema. You'll need his cooperation. Make sure he understands the purpose of the enema and the importance of retaining the medication until it's absorbed. Schedule the procedure before meals—a full stomach triggers peristalsis, making retention more difficult.

Finally, to reduce the risk of stimulating peristalsis during the procedure, ask him to empty his bladder and rectum before you begin.

Before giving the enema, check your patient's condition. Notify the doctor if:

• your patient's constipated. Feces in his rectum will interfere with drug absorption. The doctor may want you to administer a cleansing nonretention enema first.

• your patient has diarrhea. In this case, the drug may be expelled before it can be absorbed. The doctor may want you to check for fecal impaction before he treats the diarrhea. Then, he may want to choose another route of administration.

• your patient has an inflamed rectum. An enema may exacerbate the condition, so the doctor may choose another route.

250 ml of fluid at a time, every 30 minutes for 2 hours. Each time, ask the patient to retain the administered volume for 30 minutes.

• Retention enemas of small volume are more conveniently administered with prelubricated plastic squeeze bottles. Ask the pharmacist to supply the enema solution in these bottles, or prepackaged enemas.

Intradermal injections

• Intradermal injections are made into the dermis to produce a local effect or to give skin tests for allergy or anergy testing. See illustration on p. 26 for injection sites.

• A tuberculin syringe with a 26G to 27G needle is generally used.

Administration

• The ventral forearm is perhaps the most commonly used site for intradermal injection because of its easy access and lack of hair. Cleanse the area with an alcohol swab; apply pressure and use a circular, not a swiping motion. Hold the syringe at a 15° angle (almost flat against skin) with the bevel up. Insert the tip of needle just under the outer layer of skin and inject. If done properly, a small bleb will form. Withdraw the needle, but do not massage.

Subcutaneous injections

• Usually, subcutaneous injections are somewhat more slowly absorbed than intramuscular injections due to minimal blood flow in subcutaneous fat. Subcutaneous injections are made beneath the layers of the skin.

• The maximum volume injected is 2 ml. Needle length depends partly on the size of the patient. A child may require a ½" needle, an obese adult a ⅞" or 1" needle; however, a ⅝" needle can be used in most other patients.

• Any body surface area where there is loose connective tissue located away from large blood vessels and bones near the surface may be used as a site for injection. The outer aspects of the arms and the anterior lateral surfaces of the thighs, across the buttocks, and the lower abdomen above the iliac crest are common sites (see p. 27).

Administration

• Carefully draw up the prescribed dose of medication into the syringe. Some authorities advocate drawing 0.1 to 0.2 cc of air into the syringe to help clear all medication from the needle and prevent tracking when withdrawing the needle.

• Cleanse the injection site with an alcohol sponge or other antiseptic.

• Position the needle bevel up. To pre-

THE FOUR MAJOR INJECTION ROUTES

INJECTION ROUTE	SITE	COMMON NEEDLE SIZES	COMMON DOSAGE	DOSAGE RANGE
Intradermal	Skin	26G × ⅜″ (0.95 cm)	0.1 ml	0.01 to 0.1 ml
Subcutaneous	Subcutaneous fat beneath layers of skin	25G to 27G × ½″ to 1″ (1.27 to 2.54 cm)	0.5 ml	0.5 to 2 ml
Intramuscular	Mid-deltoid	23G to 25 G × ⅝″ to 1″ (1.59 to 2.54 cm)	0.5 ml	0.5 to 2 ml
	Gluteus medius (dorsogluteal)	20G to 23G × 1½″ to 3″ (3.81 to 7.62 cm)	2 to 4 ml	1 to 5 ml
	Gluteus medius and minimus (ventrogluteal)	20G to 23G × 1½″ to 3″ (3.81 to 7.62 cm)	1 to 4 ml	1 to 5 ml
	Vastus lateralis (preferred site for infants and children)	*Infants and children:* 22G to 25G × ⅝″ to 1″ (1.59 to 2.54 cm) *Adults:* 20G to 23G × 1½″ (3.81 cm)	1 to 4 ml	1 to 5 ml
	Rectus femoris (alternate site for infants)	22G to 25G × ½″ to 1″ (1.27 to 2.54 cm)	1 to 2 ml	1 to 3 ml
Intravenous	Basilic and cephalic veins	25G × ⅝″ (1.59 cm) for slow injections; 19G to 23G × 1″ to 1½″ (2.54 to 3.81 cm)	1 to 10 ml	0.5 to 50 ml

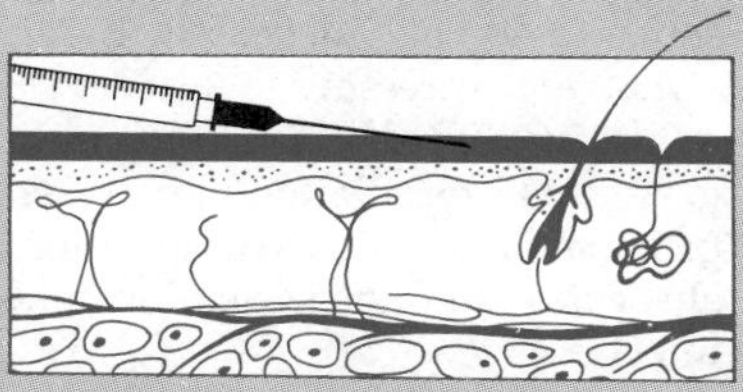

Intradermal

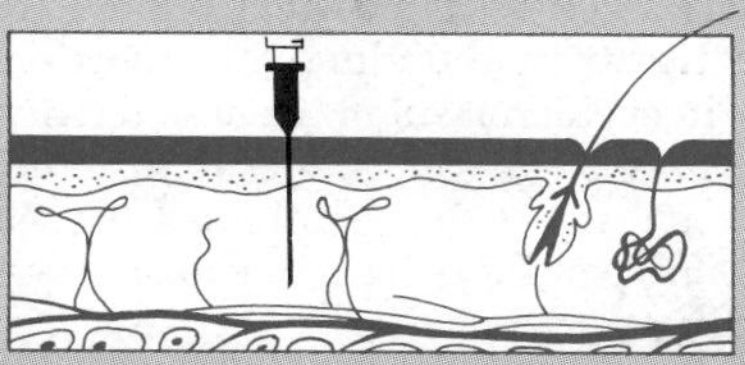

Subcutaneous

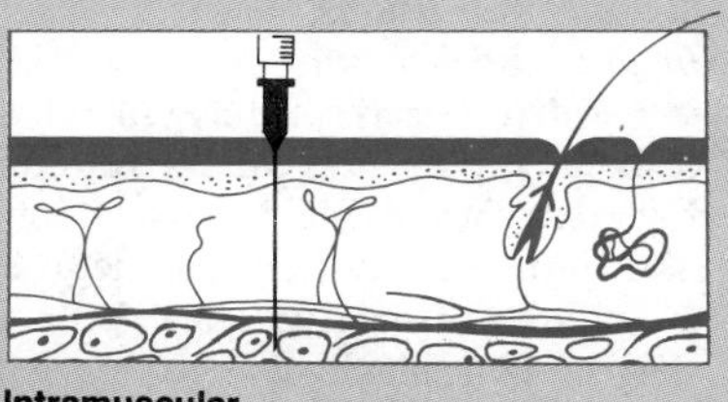

Intramuscular

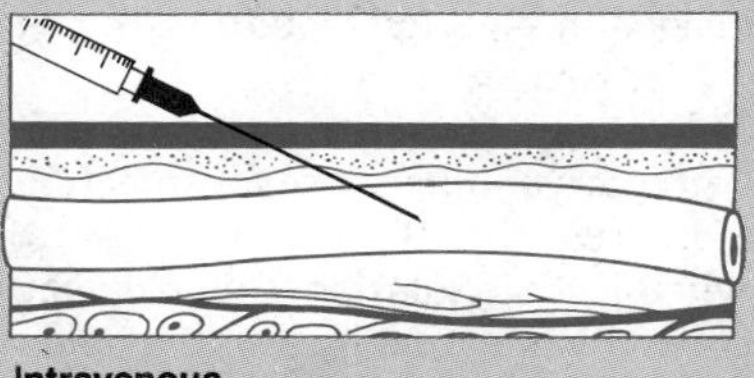

Intravenous

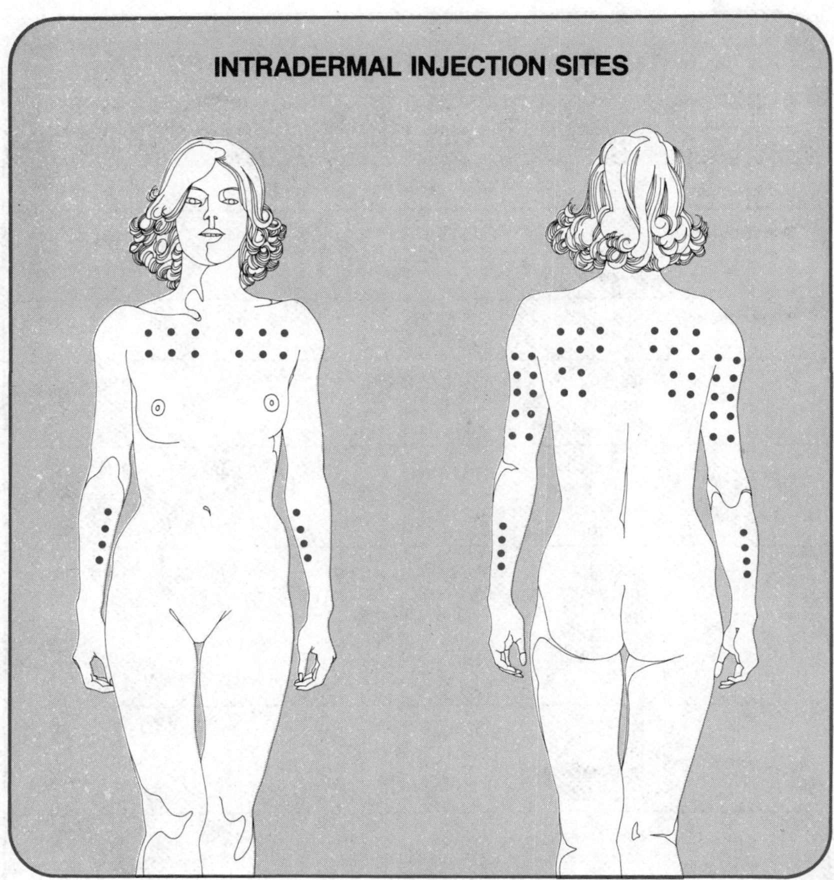

vent the needle from entering muscle, insert it at a 45° to 60° angle, and hold the tissue surrounding the injection site in cushion fashion. Release the tissue as soon as the needle is inserted or you'll inject the compressed tissue, causing painful pressure against nerve endings.

• To avoid injecting the drug into a blood vessel, pull back slightly on the plunger and look for blood *before you inject the drug.*

If blood appears, withdraw the needle and prepare another dose for injection at a different site. If no blood appears, slowly inject the solution. Complete the injection by injecting the small amount of air remaining in the syringe.

• Place an alcohol swab over the site and withdraw the needle quickly at the same angle you injected it. Using the swab, apply pressure to the site. Unless administering heparin, gently massage to stimulate circulation in the area and promote the solution's distribution and absorption into the system. Record the injection site.

Special precautions for insulin and heparin

• For drugs used routinely like insulin or heparin, have a plan for rotation of injection sites. Arms, thighs, abdomen, and buttocks together provide at least 56 different injection sites. Take care that the same site is not used more than once every 2 months; otherwise, changes in fatty tissue, such as lipodystrophy

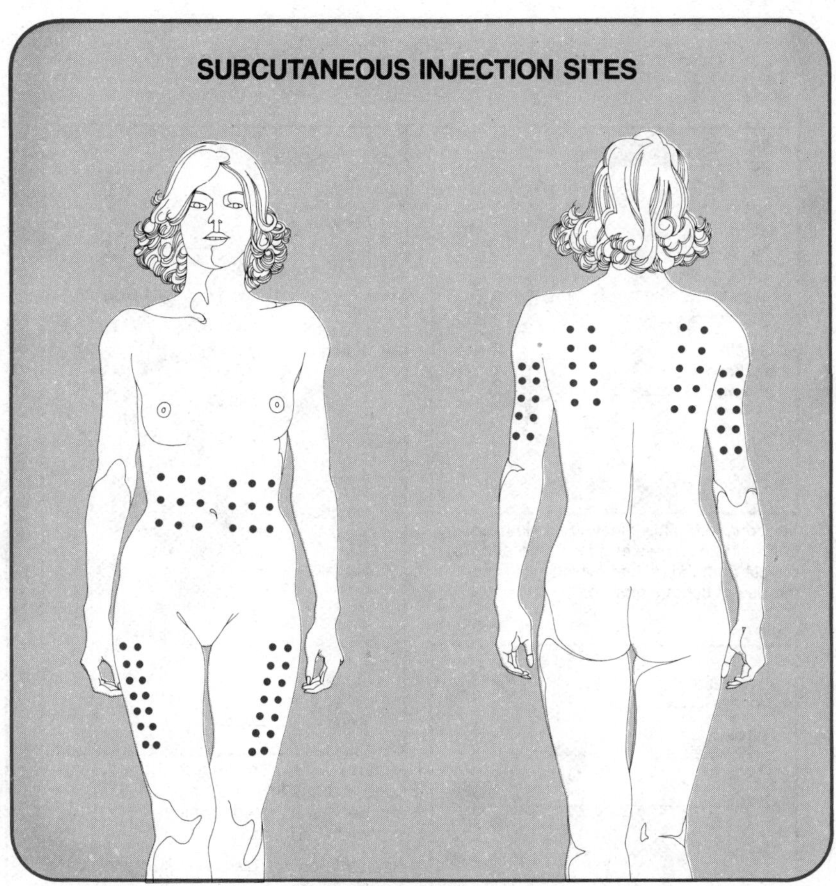
SUBCUTANEOUS INJECTION SITES

(dimpling) and hypertrophy (thickening), can make absorption of insulin more difficult.

• For heparin, make sure 0.1 to 0.2 cc of air is in the syringe to prevent heparin leaking and hemorrhage into intradermal tissues. Reduce possibility of a hematoma by injecting heparin into subcutaneous fat pad of the abdomen. The preferred site in this area is between the iliac crests. Do not check for blood backflow. Doing so may precipitate a hematoma. To avoid rupturing capillaries and causing a hematoma, do not massage the injection site. There is probably less chance of inducing hematoma if highly concentrated solutions of heparin are injected subcutaneously (20,000 units/ml), thus requiring smaller volumes (for example, 5,000 units/0.25 ml).

Intramuscular injections

• Absorption of an intramuscular (I.M.) dose is similar to that of drugs administered subcutaneously, but usually more rapid because muscle is more highly vascularized. However, some I.M. medications are in sustained-release form and are not supposed to be completely absorbed for several hours (penicillin G procaine) or several weeks (penicillin G benzathine, fluphenazine decanoate [Prolixin]). These medications have a prolonged effect.

Some drugs are not absorbed well by this route since microcrystals form at the injection site. Phenytoin is an ex-

INTRAMUSCULAR INJECTION SITES

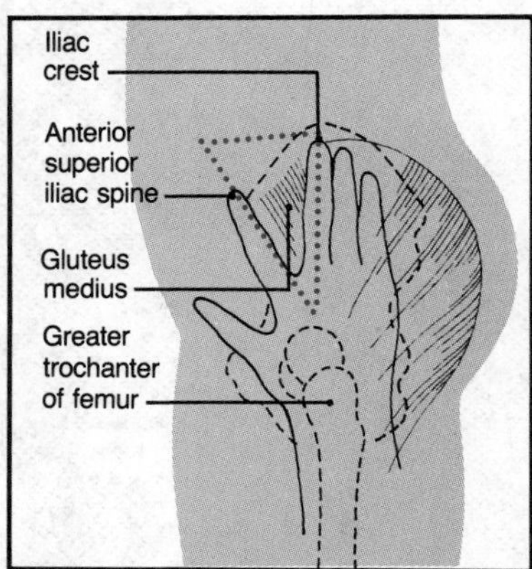

Ventrogluteal. This injection site is relatively free of large nerves and fat tissue and it's remote from the rectum (which minimizes the risk of contamination).

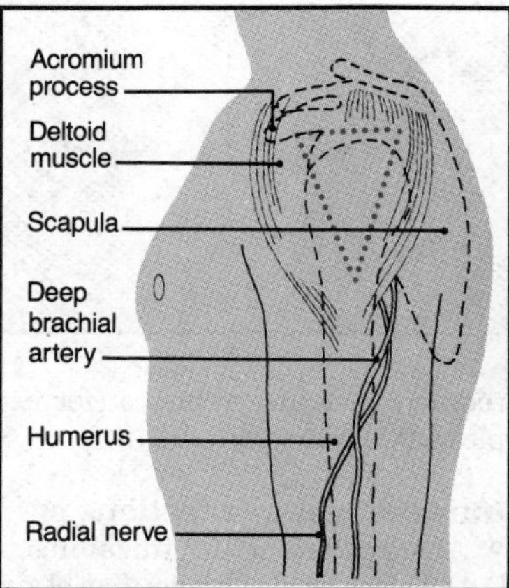

Deltoid. Because this muscle is small, this site is used only when small doses are administered. It's also dangerously close to the radial nerve. Seat the patient upright or have him lie flat, with his arms apart.

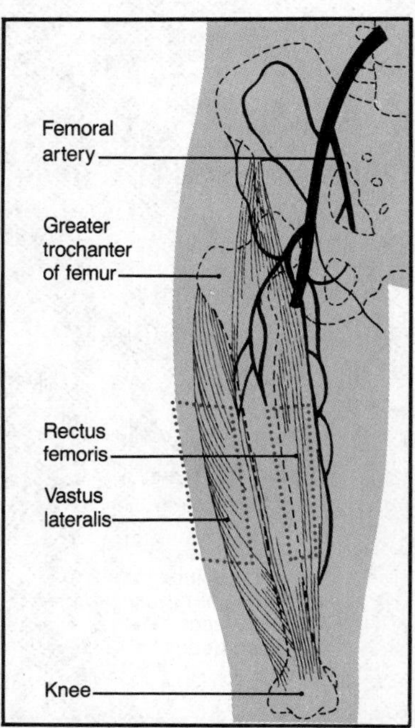

Vastus lateralis. This muscle is well developed and has few major blood vessels and nerves. It's used for all patients, especially children.

Rectus femoris. This site is frequently used for self-injection because of its accessibility. Position the patient in bed either sitting up or lying flat.

→

Dorsogluteal. These muscles aren't well developed in children under age 3, so they're most commonly used for adult patients. Position the patient flat on his stomach with his toes pointed inward, and his arms apart and flexed toward his head.

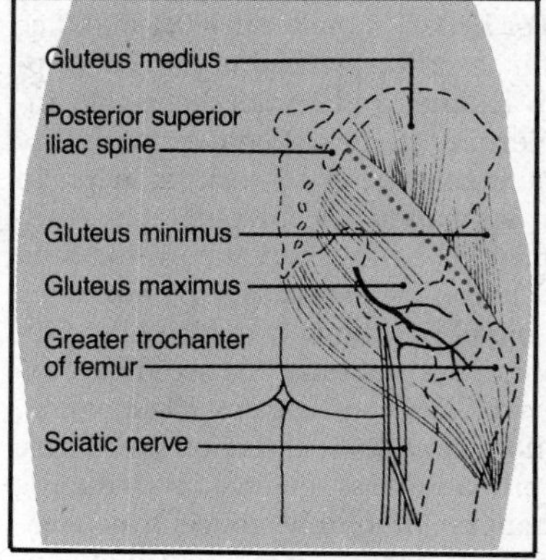

REDUCING THE PAIN OF I.M. INJECTIONS

You can reduce the pain of I.M. injections by following these tips:

- *Encourage your patient to relax the muscle you'll be injecting.* Injections into tense muscles cause more pain and bleeding than injections into relaxed muscles. (Give injections into the gluteal muscles while the patient lies face down with his toes pointed in, or on his side with the knee and hip of the upper leg flexed and anterior to the lower leg).
- *Avoid extra-sensitive areas.* When you choose the injection site, roll the muscle mass under your fingers and look for twitching. This indicates an extra-sensitive "trigger" area. Injections in this area may cause referred pain or a sharp pain as if the nerve were hit.
- *Wait until the skin antiseptic is dry.* If the antiseptic is still wet, it clings to the needle, creating pain when it reaches the sensory nerves of the subcutaneous tissues.
- *Always use a new needle.* The point and bevel of the needle can be dulled when they pass through the rubber stoppers in vials. Unless you change the needle, the dulled or rough edge that results causes more friction and pain during injection. Changing the needle also removes another source of pain—irritating medication that adheres to the outside of the needle when you draw the medication out of the vial.
- *Draw about 0.2 cc of air into the syringe.* This clears the needle bore of medication, which could leak out through the needle before or during insertion. When the needle is inverted for the injection, the air bubble rises to the plunger end of the syringe. Injecting this harmless air bubble reduces "tracking"—the leakage of medication from the needle injection path.
- *Dart the needle in rapidly and withdraw it rapidly to minimize puncture pain.*
- *Aspirate to be sure the needle isn't in a blood vessel.* Then, inject the medication slowly to allow it to spread into the tissue under less pressure.
- *Unless contraindicated, massage the relaxed muscle to distribute the medication better and increase its absorption.* This will reduce the pain caused by tissue stretching from a large-volume injection. (Physical exercise of the injected muscle serves the same purpose.)

ample of such a drug not recommended for administration by this route.

- Any body surface area with a significant amount of muscular tissue located away from large blood vessels and nerves may serve as an I.M. injection site. Sites include the mid-deltoid area, the gluteus medius, the ventrogluteal area, and the vastus lateralis.
- When giving large doses or irritating drugs, use the buttock muscles.
- The amount of an I.M. injection is normally up to 3 ml, but up may be to 5 ml of certain drugs (iron dextran [Imferon], paraldehyde). Syringe size depends on volume of solution; needle length and gauge depend on patient's size and may range from ½" to 1½" (2" for iron dextran) and from 21G to 23G. Needles of 18G to 20G may be required when administering thick suspensions such as penicillin G benzathine.

Administration

- Draw up 0.1 to 0.2 cc of air into a prepared syringe.
- When injecting in the gluteal region, avoid the sciatic nerve and the superior gluteal artery by proper site selection technique. For injections into muscles of buttocks, have the patient lie on his stomach with his toes pointing inward; this helps relax the muscles and provides maximum exposure. Ask the patient to relax beforehand by taking several slow, deep breaths.
- Cleanse a 2" (5 cm) diameter around area with an alcohol pad. Let alcohol evaporate before injecting.
- With one hand, stretch skin around the site until taut. Insert the needle at a 90° angle with a quick thrust to minimize pain.
- Aspirate gently before injecting to confirm correct needle placement. If blood appears, withdraw the needle and prepare another dose. If no blood

appears, inject the drug at a slow, even rate.

• After injecting the medication, inject the air to help clear the needle shaft and to prevent tracking of medication as the needle is withdrawn. Then, withdraw the needle quickly. Use an alcohol swab to apply pressure to the site, and then massage.

• For drugs like iron dextran and certain others that stain or irritate, use the Z-track technique for injection. Always use the patient's gluteus medius.

—Draw up 0.1 to 0.2 cc of air into the syringe after preparation.

—Then change the needle to one that is 2″ in length.

—Displace the skin laterally away from the intended injection site.

—Cleanse the site, introduce the needle at a 90° angle, aspirate to check for entry into a blood vessel, and inject the medication.

—After injection is completed (including air bubble), wait 10 seconds before withdrawing the needle.

—Withdraw the needle. Allow the retracted skin to resume its normal position. This prevents medication from tracking up needle line from one tissue layer to another. Do not massage. Alternate buttocks for subsequent injections.

Intravenous infusions

• Many hospitals keep lists of drugs that may or may not be administered I.V. by nurses. If you work in such a hospital, become familiar with this list, and check with the pharmacist about any drugs you aren't familiar with.

• When not already prepackaged from the manufacturer, unit doses are best prepared, diluted, and labeled under sterile conditions by the pharmacist.

• If unit dose–packaged syringes aren't available, dilute the medication according to directions, using only the exact diluent recommended by the manufacturer. If you're working with sterile water for injection, remember that ampuls are meant for single use only. Diluent in vials previously used for reconstitution of other drugs may be contaminated, so always use a fresh vial.

Many drugs prove irritating to the vein wall, but proper dilution can at least minimize such irritations.

Precautions

• Before administering any medication intravenously, consider possible incompatibility with fluids and other drugs given at the same time. (See Chapter 6, UNDERSTANDING INTRAVENOUS SOLUTION COMPATIBILITY.)

• Always clean the injection port with an alcohol swab or sponge before injecting medication, whether it's through a Y port of I.V. tubing, into an intermittent infusion device or a volume-control burette, or directly into an I.V. solution bottle or bag.

• When giving I.V. injections of any type, inspect the injection site for signs of extravasation and phlebitis.

• Change I.V. tubing and dressings according to hospital requirements, and apply antimicrobial ointment to the injection site. Record on the I.V. dressing and on the patient's chart the catheter (needle) type and gauge, date and time the catheter or needle was inserted, and your initials.

• Adverse reactions to drugs administered I.V. can occur almost immediately. In such cases, discontinue administration immediately and notify the doctor. Wherever I.V. therapy is used, emergency equipment and drugs should be readily available.

• Substances injected intravenously are absorbed into the system immediately. Take special care to prevent (or recognize) toxic reactions or shock caused by allergic reactions or by introducing too much solution too quickly.

The patient's condition and age, type of fluid or drug being administered, size of the administration set, and viscosity of the liquid are the principal factors determining the flow rate.

For greater accuracy, the flow rate should be measured in microdrops (requiring a special solution set) or regulated with an infusion control device. Of course, the infusion should be administered in strict accordance with the doctor's instructions.

• Should the flow of solution stop, first check for signs of infiltration. Then try to determine if the tubing is defective. Also, hold the bottle below the level of the injection site to backwash anything obstructing the flow.

If hospital procedure permits, irrigate the catheter with 1 ml of sterile saline solution. Keep in mind that if a filter is being used, it may be clogged and need to be changed.

• Administer supplemental drugs one at a time to prevent incompatibilities. Always flush the injection site on the tubing or intermittent infusion device with several milliliters of sterile saline solution between injections.

If an intermittent infusion device is used for administration of a drug other than heparin, a small amount of dilute heparin solution is placed into the lock after drug injection and saline flushing to maintain patency.

Always remember to flush this out of the lock before injecting another drug, as the two solutions may be incompatible.

Administration methods

Medication can be introduced intravenously by several methods. When a solution is being infused, medications can be added directly to the solution and infused continuously, or they can be infused intermittently using the bolus, volume-control burette, or the piggyback method.

• *Continuous infusions.* When medications are administered by continuous infusion to maintain therapeutic drug levels (aminophylline, heparin, thrombolytics, and others), an infusion control device is highly recommended, since you can control the rate of infusion best with this. A microdrip set may also be used, but it doesn't provide optimal accuracy for critical-care drugs.

If infusion pumps or rate controllers are used in your hospital, make certain you fully understand their operation before using them. Check the patient frequently during their use.

• *Bolus.* Before administering, assess the patient's condition. How are his vital signs? Is his urinary output sufficient?

Medication is injected into a Y port along the primary line tubing, into an intermittent infusion device (heparin lock) or directly into the vein.

Before injecting drugs by I.V. bolus, first pull back plunger of syringe to make sure blood flows freely.

Administer slowly. A good rule of thumb: Take not less than 1 minute (but make sure you know the administration rate before injecting). If a drug needs to be administered over a period longer than 5 minutes, consider using a volume-control burette set or piggyback bottle or bag.

• *Volume-control burette.* To administer small amounts (150 ml or less) of I.V. solution or diluted medication intermittently, you may use a volume-control set. This is usually piggybacked into a primary I.V. line (although it may actually be the primary line). The burette is labeled with the drug's name and dosage.

Change the set daily, and record date and time of change. To avoid incompatibilities, administer only one medication through any one burette.

• *Piggyback.* With this technique, you use minibags or minibottles containing a single dose prepared and labeled by the pharmacy. The usual volume is between 100 and 250 ml.

After checking the preparation, attach the bottle or bag to a secondary I.V. set, clear the line of air, cleanse the port, and piggyback the line into the primary I.V. set. Administer the dose over the time required. Set the secondary line to shut off automatically when the dose is completed and the primary line takes over. (Most doses run for 30 minutes to 1 hour.)

Dermatomucosal medications

Dermatomucosal medications are generally given for their local, not systemic, effects. With the notable exception of nitroglycerin ointment, their absorption through the skin is minimal.

Eye drops

- Explain the medication procedure to the patient. Then tell him to lie (or lean) back, with head tilted backward and to one side, so the unaffected eye is slightly higher. This helps prevent cross contamination in case of leakage and increases systemic absorption of drug by the lacrimal duct.
- Use a sterile, moistened gauze pad to wipe away any exudate. Using a clean pad for each eye, wipe from inner to outer canthus.
- Draw into the eyedropper no more than the amount actually needed. Hold the dropper perpendicular to the eye to ensure uniformity of drop size. Most ophthalmic preparations, however, do not require an eyedropper—you simply squeeze the bottle and a single drop is released.
- Ask the patient to look up and focus on an object. Hold the lower lid down with your forefinger, exposing the conjunctival sac, and instill the prescribed number of drops into the conjunctival sac. Be careful not to touch the eye with the dropper. Never drop the medication directly onto the cornea.
- Release the patient's eyelid, and let him blink to distribute the medication over the eye and inner lids. If more than one drop must be administered, have the patient blink before you instill the second drop.
- Expect some leakage of medication from the eye, and blot away excess with a tissue. Don't administer additional drops to replace any leakage.

Eye ointment

- Cleanse the patient's eyelids and lashes with a sterile gauze pad soaked with saline solution. As with eye drops, hold the lower lid down, and ask the patient to look up.
- Spread the ointment from inner to outer canthus along the conjunctival sac. Don't touch the tube to the eyelid. Body warmth will melt the ointment and help it spread.
- Have the patient close his eyes for 1 to 2 minutes to spread the medication; wipe away excess. Inform the patient that his vision will be blurred temporarily.

Ear drops

- Always use drops that are warmer than room temperature since cold drops are uncomfortable and may cause vertigo. Warm the solution by rolling the container between your hands.
- Explain the medication procedure to the patient, and position him on his side, with affected ear up.
- Straighten the auditory canal by gently pulling the auricle *up* and *back*. Be gentle if the ear is inflamed. (If the patient is a child, pull the auricle *down* and *back*.)
- Without touching the dropper to the ear, instill the prescribed number of drops along the canal. Do not drop them directly onto the tympanic membrane.
- Tell the patient to remain in this position for about 10 minutes to keep medication in the canal. Unless contraindicated, consider placing a medication-soaked cotton plug in the ear canal.

Nose drops

- Explain the medication procedure to the patient and warn him he may taste drops after instillation.
- Ask the patient to lie flat on his back, with a pillow placed under his shoulders. His head should be tilted slightly back.
- Push the tip of his nose slightly upward. Do not insert the dropper more than ½″ to ⅔″ (1.3 to 1.6 cm) into the nostril. Instill drops into each nostril.
- Tell the patient to breathe through his mouth temporarily and remain in this position for 2 to 3 minutes.

Nose sprays

- Have the patient sit upright, with his

PATIENT TEACHING

TEACHING YOUR PATIENT ABOUT NOSE DROPS

If the doctor has prescribed nose drops for your patient to use at home, show him how to instill them properly.

Tell your patient to position the dropper as shown in this illustration so the medication will flow down the back of his nose, not his throat. Be sure your patient:

- squeezes the dropper bulb to instill the correct number of drops into the nostril.
- repeats the process in the other nostril, if ordered.
- breathes through his mouth so the medication is not sniffed into his sinuses or aspirated into his lungs.

Be sure he knows the name of the medication and the prescribed dosage. In addition:

- Urge your patient to follow the doctor's orders exactly. Explain the dangers of overusing the medication.
- Because nose drops are easily contaminated, advise your patient not to buy more nose drops than he'll use in a short time. Instruct him to discard the medication if it contains sediment or looks discolored.
- Warn your patient not to share his medication with family members. Doing so may spread infection.
- Tell him to call the doctor if he notices any side effects.

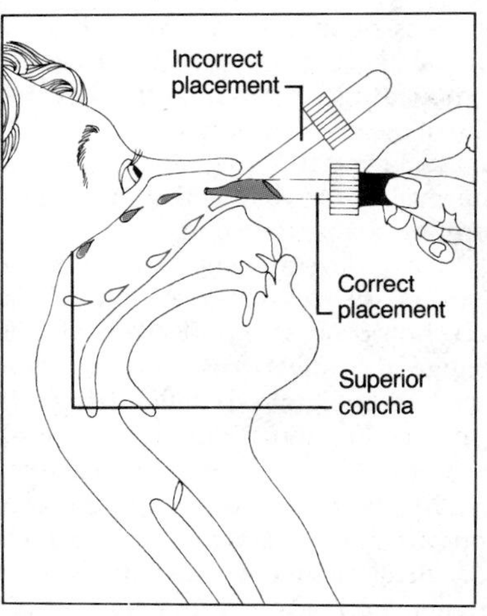

head tilted back.

- Spray medication horizontally into the nasal passages. After spraying once, ask the patient to tilt his head back further.
- Spray again, so medication reaches the interior passageway and other portions of the nasal passages. Tell the patient to hold his opposite nostril closed while breathing through the nostril that is being sprayed.

Vaginal suppositories and tablets

- To administer a vaginal suppository, first have the patient assume the lithotomy position. Remove the product from the wrapper, and lubricate the tip of the suppository with a small amount of water-soluble lubricant or water; then with a gloved hand or an applicator insert the suppository into the vagina. Have the patient keep her hips elevated for about 5 minutes.

Vaginal cream, ointment, or jelly

- Remove the cap from the tube of cream, ointment, or jelly, and fit the applicator on the tube. Fill the applicator and remove it from the tube.
- With patient in lithotomy position, gently insert applicator deep into vagina, and push plunger until all contents have been inserted.
- Remove applicator, wash with warm water, and return applicator and tube to box.

MICHAEL R. COHEN, BS

3 Nursing implications of drug administration and therapy in children

Administering medications to children can be more complex than it seems. Complicating the issue is the fact that 75% of the prescription drugs currently marketed in the United States lack full approval by the Food and Drug Administration for pediatric use.

During development, a child's absorption, distribution, metabolism, and excretion processes undergo profound changes that affect drug dosage. If these variables are ignored, underestimation or overestimation of dosage may result in therapeutic failure or subsequent toxicity, even death. Dosage calculations are only the starting point of therapy; drug regimens must be tailored to each patient's requirements to ensure optimal drug effect and minimal toxicity.

Absorption

Drug absorption in children depends on the form of the drug; its physical properties; other drugs or substances, such as food, taken simultaneously; physiologic changes; and concurrent disease.

- The pH of neonatal gastric fluid is neutral or slightly acidic and becomes more acidic as the infant matures. This affects drug absorption. For example, nafcillin and penicillin G, erratically absorbed or malabsorbed in an adult due to degradation by gastric acid, are better absorbed in an infant due to low gastric acidity.
- Various infant formulas or milk products may increase gastric pH and impede absorption of acidic drugs. So, if possible, give a child oral medications when his stomach is empty.
- Gastric emptying time and transit time through the small intestine—longer in children than in adults—can affect absorption. Also, intestinal hypermotility (as in diarrhea) can diminish the drug's absorption.
- A child's comparatively thin epidermis allows increased absorption of topical drugs.

Distribution

As with absorption, changes in body weight and physiology during childhood can significantly influence a drug's distribution and effects. In a premature infant, body fluid makes up about 85% of total body weight; in a full-term infant, 55% to 70%; and in an adult, 50% to 55%. Extracellular fluid (mostly blood) comprises 40% of a neonate's body weight, compared with 20% in an adult. Intracellular fluid remains fairly constant throughout life and has little effect on drug dosage.

Since most drugs travel through extracellular fluid to reach their receptors, however, extracellular fluid volume influences a water-soluble drug's concentration and effect. Children have a larger proportion of fluid to solid body weight, so their distribution area is proportionately greater.

Because the proportion of fat to lean body mass increases with age, the distribution of fat-soluble drugs is more limited in children than adults. As a result, a drug's lipid- or water-solubility affects the dosage for a child.

Binding to plasma proteins
As the result of a decrease in either albumin concentration or intermolecular attraction between drug and plasma protein, many drugs are less bound to plasma proteins in infants than in adults.

Furthermore, preparations that bind plasma proteins may displace endogenous compounds, such as bilirubin or free fatty acids. Conversely, an endogenous compound may displace a weakly bound drug. For example, displacement of bound bilirubin can cause a rise in unbound bilirubin, which can lead to increased risk of kernicterus at normal bilirubin levels.

Since only unbound, or free, drug has a pharmacologic effect, any alteration in ratio of protein-bound to unbound active drug can greatly influence effect.

Several diseases, such as malnutrition and nephrotic syndrome, can also decrease plasma protein and increase the concentration of unbound drug, intensifying the drug's effect or producing toxicity.

Metabolism

A newborn infant's ability to metabolize a drug depends on the integrity of his hepatic enzyme system, his intrauterine exposure to the drug, and the nature of the drug itself.

Certain metabolic mechanisms are underdeveloped in neonates. Glucuronidation, the mechanism that neutralizes drugs, for example, is insufficiently developed to permit full pediatric doses until the infant is 1 month old. Because of this, the use of chloramphenicol in a newborn infant may cause gray baby syndrome, illustrating the newborn's inability to metabolize the drug. Use of chloramphenicol in neonates, therefore, requires decreased dosage (25 mg/kg/day) and monitoring of blood levels.

Conversely, intrauterine exposure to drugs may induce precocious development of hepatic enzyme mechanisms, increasing the infant's capacity to metabolize potentially harmful substances.

Older children can metabolize some drugs (theophylline, for example) more rapidly than adults. This ability may be due to their increased hepatic metabolic activity. Larger doses than those recommended for adults may be required.

Also, preparations given concurrently to a child may alter hepatic metabolism and induce release of hepatic enzymes. Phenobarbital, for example, can induce hepatic enzyme production and accelerate metabolism of drugs given concurrently.

Excretion

Renal excretion of a drug is the net effect of glomerular filtration, active tubular secretion, and passive tubular reabsorption. Because so many drugs are excreted in the urine, the degree of renal development or presence of renal disease can profoundly affect a child's dosage requirements.

If a child is unable to excrete a drug renally, drug accumulation and possible toxicity may result unless dosage is reduced.

Physiologically, an infant's kidneys differ from an adult's in that they have:

- high resistance to blood flow and subsequent decreased renal fraction of cardiac output
- incomplete glomerular and tubular development and short, incomplete loops of Henle. (A child's glomerular filtration reaches adult values by age 2½ to 5 months; his tubular secretion may reach adult values by age 7 to 12 months.)
- low glomerular filtration rate. (Penicillins are eliminated by this route.)
- decreased ability to concentrate urine or reabsorb various filtered compounds
- reduced ability by the proximal tubules to secrete organic acids.

Both children and adults have diurnal variations in urine pH that correlate with sleep-wake patterns.

Calculating pediatric dosages

When calculating pediatric dosages, don't use formulas that modify adult dosages: a child is not a scaled-down version of an adult. Pediatric dosages should be calculated on the basis of either body weight (mg/kg) or body surface area (mg/m^2).

- Reevaluate dosages at regular intervals to ensure necessary adjustments as the child develops.
- Although useful for adults and older children, don't use dosages based on body surface area in premature or full-term infants. Use the body weight method instead.
- Don't exceed the maximum adult dose when calculating amounts per kilogram of body weight (except with certain drugs, such as theophylline, if indicated).
- A list of appropriate emergency drug dosages should be placed in all pediatric areas and on emergency equipment. For a summary of estimated emergency drug dosages, see pages 47 through 51.

Monitoring pediatric dosages

- Be alert to factors affecting the patient's blood levels of the drug.
- Monitor blood drug levels and vital signs.
- Study electrocardiogram and other diagnostic test results.
- To monitor drug response, know administration times and when to draw blood to measure drug levels. (Discuss findings with the doctor and pharmacist.)
- Obtain an accurate maternal drug history—prescription and nonprescription drugs, vitamins, and herbs or other health foods taken during pregnancy. In utero exposure may harm the neonate and hinder subsequent drug therapy.
- Drugs passed through breast milk can also have adverse effects on the nursing infant. Before a drug is prescribed for a breast-feeding mother, the

FLUID AND NUTRITION BALANCE: MEETING INFANTS' AND CHILDREN'S NEEDS

Maintaining proper fluid and electrolyte levels in infants is critical. Why? Because an infant's body is 70% to 75% water, whereas an adult's is only 50% to 60%. Therefore, gastrointestinal upset in an infant may lead to severe dehydration and dangerous disturbance of acid-base and electrolyte balance. Also, administering I.V. fluids too fast can lead to dangerous fluid overload. To help guard against severe dehydration or fluid overload, watch closely for these signs of fluid imbalance when the infant you're caring for is vomiting or has diarrhea.

Fluid overload

- Rapid pulse rate
- Hypertension
- Increased urinary output
- Decreased urine specific gravity
- Edema
- Fine rales

Dehydration

- Rapid pulse rate
- Hypotension
- Decreased urinary output
- Increased urine specific gravity
- Dry mucous membranes
- Depressed fontanelles
- Poor skin turgor
- Lethargy
- Refusal to eat
- Distended abdomen
- Weakness
- Absence of tearing and salivation

Remember, each patient's therapy must be adjusted to his individual needs and tolerance levels. When replacing fluid and electrolytes, the type and amounts you'll use may vary from one age-group to another. Nutritional requirements also change with changing growth patterns.

The tables at right contain some basic guidelines you can follow.

FLUID RECOMMENDATIONS

In Newborn Infants

1st day	60 to 80 ml/kg
2nd day	70 to 90 ml/kg
3rd day	80 to 100 ml/kg
4th day	100 to 120 ml/kg
5th day and thereafter	120 to 140 ml/kg

Note: Patent ductus arteriosus or other congenital cardiac conditions may require that fluids be given with greater caution. Also, increased losses may raise fluid requirements.

In Infants and Children

1 to 10 kg	100 ml/kg/day
10 to 20 kg	1,000 ml plus 50 ml/each kg over 10
20 to 30 kg	1,500 ml plus 20 ml/each kg over 20

Note: Increased losses raise fluid requirements. Also, fluid restriction or concurrent disease may limit fluid intake.

NUTRITIONAL REQUIREMENTS

Protein 1 to 3 g/kg/day

Carbohydrates Enough to supply necessary calories and, in combination with fat, to supply 20 to 50 nonprotein calories for every gram of protein.

Fats 1 to 4 g/kg/day to provide necessary calories in combination with carbohydrates. If patient's fat intake is restricted, supply 2% to 4% of the calories as linoleic acid to prevent essential fatty acid deficiency.

Electrolytes

Sodium	3 to 4 mEq/kg/day
Potassium	2 to 3 mEq/kg/day
Chloride	2 to 4 mEq/kg/day
Acetate	1 to 1.5 mEq/kg/day

Vitamins

Folic acid	50 to 75 mcg/kg/day
Vitamin B_{12}	5 to 10 mcg/kg/day
Vitamin K	150 to 200 mcg/kg/day
MVI	0.5 ml/kg/day

Minerals

Phosphate	1 to 3 millimoles/kg/day
Calcium	300 to 800 mg/kg/day as the gluconate salt
Magnesium	0.25 to 0.5 mEq/kg/day
Trace elements	
Zinc	300 mcg/kg/day in infants less than 3 kg; 100 mcg/kg/day over 3 kg
Chromium	0.14 mcg/kg/day
Manganese	2 mcg/kg/day
Copper	20 mcg/kg/day

DAILY CALORIC REQUIREMENTS

0 to 1 year	90 to 120 kcal/kg
1 to 7 years	70 to 100 kcal/kg
7 to 12 years	60 to 75 kcal/kg
12 to 18 years	30 to 60 kcal/kg

Caloric requirements may increase:

- 12% for each degree of fever over 37° C. (98.6° F.)
- 20% to 30% with major surgery
- 40% to 50% with severe sepsis
- 50% to 100% with long-term failure to thrive.

NOMOGRAM FOR ESTIMATING SURFACE AREA IN CHILDREN

If your patient is of average size, find his weight and corresponding surface area on the first, boxed scale. Otherwise, use the nomogram to the right. Lay a straight edge on the correct height and weight points for your patient, then see the intersecting point on the surface area scale.

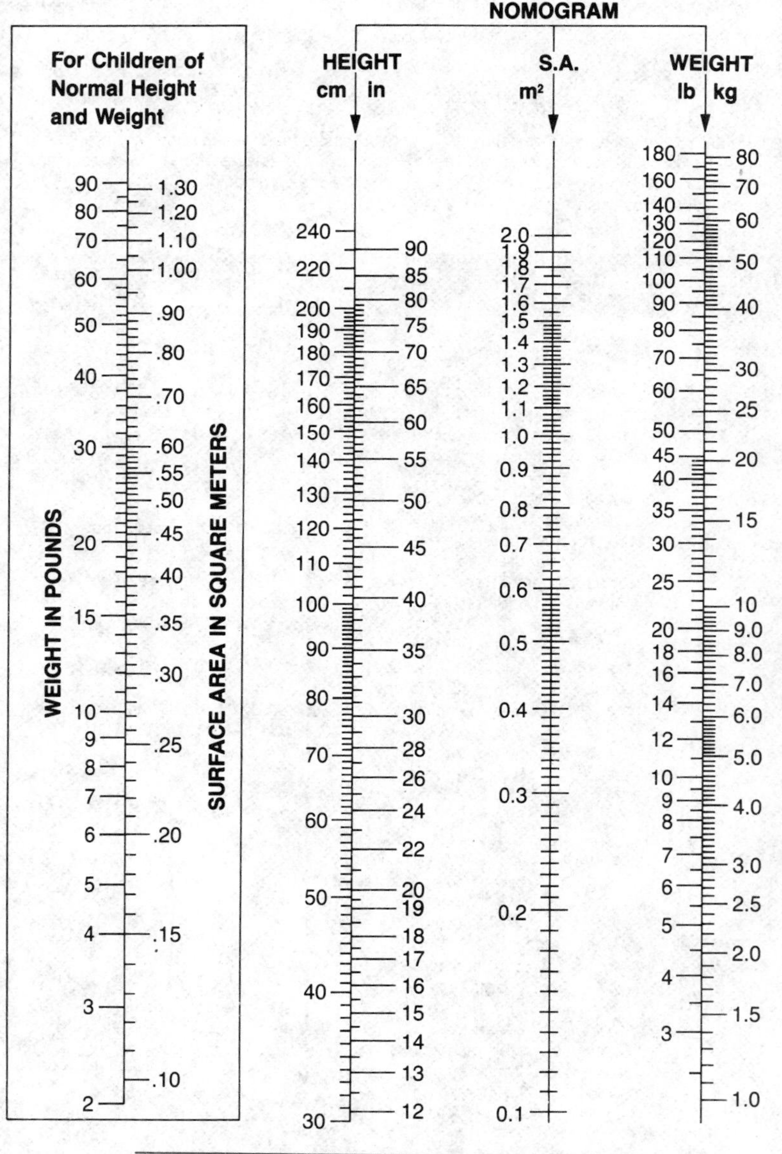

Reprinted with permission from Victor Vaughan, ed., *Nelson Textbook of Pediatrics* (11th ed.; Philadelphia: W.B. Saunders Co., 1979).

potential effects on the infant should be investigated. For example, sulfa drugs given to a breast-feeding mother for a urinary tract infection appear in breast milk and may cause kernicterus at lower-than-normal levels of unconjugated bilirubin. Also, high concentrations of isoniazid appear in breast milk. Since this drug is metabolized by the liver, an infant's immature hepatic enzyme mechanisms cannot metabolize the drug, and the infant may suffer central nervous system (CNS) toxicity.

Oral medications

- *When giving oral medication to an infant,* administer it in liquid form if possible. For accuracy, measure and give the preparation by syringe; never use a vial or cup.
- Lift the patient's head to prevent aspiration of the medication, and press down on his chin to prevent choking.
- You may also place the drug in a nipple and allow the infant to suck the contents.
- *If the patient is a toddler,* explain how you're going to give him the medication. If possible, have the parents enlist the child's cooperation.
- Don't mix medication with food or call it "candy" even if it has a pleasant taste.
- Let the child drink liquid medication from a calibrated medication cup rather than from a spoon: it's easier and more accurate. If the preparation is available only in tablet form, crush it and mix it with a compatible syrup. (Check with the pharmacist to make sure tablet can be crushed without losing its effectiveness.)
- *If the patient's an older child* who can swallow a tablet or capsule by himself, have him place the medication on the back of his tongue and swallow it with water or fruit juice. Remember, milk or milk products may interfere with drug absorption.
- Unless indicated to do otherwise, see that the patient receives all oral preparations on an empty stomach to maximize absorption.

Rectal medications

- Lubricate the tip of the suppository with a little water-soluble lubricating jelly.
- Insert the suppository; to prevent expulsion, hold the patient's buttocks closed for a few minutes.

Intravenous infusions

When administering I.V. infusions, be sure to record the volume, flow rate, and type of solution used. Check the I.V. setup hourly. Change the solution and I.V. administration set at least daily, and record the procedure. If a solution containing a new medication is started, be sure to change the I.V. tubing.

Setting up equipment

- If medication is to be added to the I.V. bottle, do this first. Before adding medication, check on its compatibility with the I.V. solution. In many cases, the pharmacist adds the medication.
- When setting up the I.V. administration tubing and volume-control burette, first attach the tubing to the I.V. solution.
- Next, open the clamp and let the fluid fill the burette and tubing, making sure that all the air is displaced.
- Close the clamp, and tape all connections to ensure that the tubing doesn't become disconnected and air doesn't enter the system (as little as 10 cc of air can cause a fatal embolus).

Protecting the insertion site

In infants, a peripheral vein or a scalp vein in the temporal region is used for I.V. infusions. The scalp vein is safest in that the needle is not likely to be dislodged; however, the head must be shaved around the site. Additional disfigurement may also result from the needle and infiltrated fluids. For these reasons, the scalp veins are not being used as frequently today as they have been in the past.

The extremities are the most accessible insertion sites; however, since patients may tend to move about, take

PROTECTING A SCALP INSERTION SITE

To protect a scalp I.V. insertion site, cut the top off a paper medication cup and tape the cup over the site.

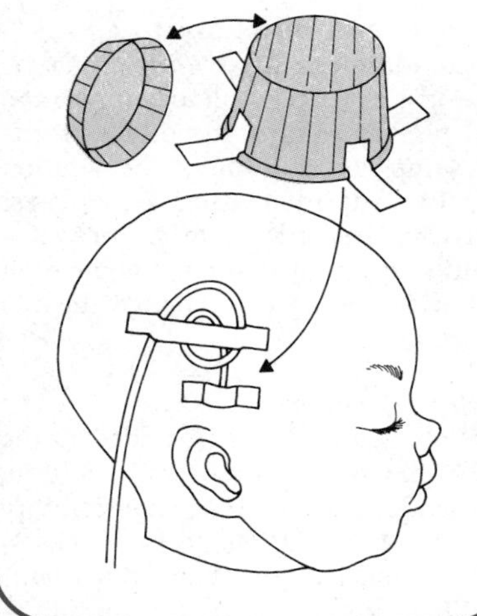

these precautions:

- Protect the insertion site to prevent catheter or needle dislodgment.
- Use a padded arm board to minimize dislodgment.
- Place the clamp out of the child's reach; if extension tubing is used to allow the child greater mobility, securely tape the connection.
- Restrain the child only when necessary.
- To allay anxiety, give a simple explanation to the child who must be restrained while asleep.

Maintaining flow rate and fluid balance

While administering a continuous I.V. infusion to a child, monitor flow rate and check the patient's condition and insertion site at least hourly—more frequently when giving medication intermittently.

- Adjust the flow rate only while the patient is composed; crying and emotional upset can constrict blood vessels. Flow rate may be retarded if a pump isn't used. Flow should be adequate because some drugs (calcium, for example) can be very irritating at low flow rates.
- Use an infusion pump for accurate administration. Remember, though, these pumps aren't foolproof; they continue to pump even if the needle becomes dislodged.
- Be sure to examine the insertion site for signs of infiltration or infection.
- Record intake and output carefully.
- Check the patient for fluid overload and dehydration each time you inspect the I.V. site. If flow rate is slower than was ordered, assess the patient's fluid balance and consult the doctor before increasing the rate.
- If an increase is necessary, correct the flow rate *slowly,* especially if glucose concentration of the solution is greater than 5%; infuse the additional volume as ordered.

Special considerations

To administer I.V. infusions correctly, you should know about solution compatibilities, dilution requirements, maximum administration times, and maximum infusion rates. Check these points before you begin:

- *What solution is the drug compatible with?*

If a medication is routine and compatible with the main I.V. vehicle, it may be diluted in enough fluid to run over 30 to 60 minutes regardless of the resulting concentration. (Administering a drug over 30 to 60 minutes can offset most concentration problems.)

Occasionally, a medication must be administered using a solution that is unfavorable to the child's condition or course of treatment. In such a case, use the minimum amount of solution and infuse it over 30 to 60 minutes regardless of the resulting concentration.

If a second drug is to be run through the same I.V. tubing, first flush the tubing with a small amount of solution that is compatible with the second drug.

• *What dilutions must be made?* Some drugs are hyperosmolar; in infants, these drugs must be diluted to prevent radical changes in fluid that might induce CNS hemorrhage. Sodium bicarbonate, for example, must be diluted to half strength to lower osmolality and lessen the risk of CNS bleeding.

In general, however, use the minimum amount of compatible fluid over the shortest recommended period of time. Remember also to check the total daily fluid intake and the amount allotted to medication.

• *What's the maximum administration time and infusion rate per minute?* Whether you're infusing a *stat* or regularly scheduled medication, you should know both the maximum total administration time and the maximum infusion rate per minute. Phenytoin, for example, should be infused at no more than 50 mg/minute.

If the medication has no maximum infusion rate or special concentration requirements, the drug may possibly be given I.V. push. If it has a maximum rate, follow the recommendation.

Discontinuing the I.V. infusion

When the prescribed volume of I.V. medication has been infused:

• Stop the flow by carefully closing the clamp or shutting off the pump.

• Hold the needle firmly with one hand, and gently remove the restraining tape.

• Then, while pressing a sterile sponge to the insertion site, slowly remove the needle, making sure that the hub is flush with the skin (to avoid tearing the vein's posterior wall).

• When the needle or catheter is removed, exert direct pressure on the site until bleeding stops.

SPECIAL CONSIDERATIONS

WHEN A CHILD NEEDS I.V. THERAPY

A child receiving I.V. therapy needs special care. Why? Because his anatomy and physiology differ significantly from an adult's. And because the procedure will probably be new and frightening for him.

A child's size increases the risk of both fluid and medication overdoses and decreases his ability to overcome them if they occur. His metabolism rate, which determines his body's water requirements, is about three times faster than an adult's. Thus, a child needs more water per kilogram of body weight than an adult and can easily become dehydrated.

The doctor will consider these factors when determining the correct drug dosage to be administered intravenously. You can help by:

• taking baseline readings
• keeping accurate intake and output records
• watching for complications.

Changes occur rapidly in children, so make sure your records are up to date.

You'll administer pediatric I.V. medication by the direct bolus method or with a volume-control set. A volume-control set is an I.V. line featuring a fluid chamber that allows you to accurately deliver medications that you've diluted in precise amounts of fluid. To ensure the correct flow rate, use an infusion pump.

You can help your young patient cope with his fears by:

• explaining the procedure in words he can understand
• answering his questions honestly
• giving him all the attention and support you can.

Intramuscular injections

Intramuscular injections are preferred when the drug cannot be given by other parenteral routes and rapid absorption is necessary. Before administering the drug, determine if it can be given I.M. Low platelets may preclude the use of the I.M. route. In the patient with volume depletion, fluid perfusion to muscle may be scanty; this will decrease the quantity of drug that is absorbed by the I.M. route. In such an instance,

I.V. infusion may be preferable.

In children under 2 years, the vastus lateralis muscle is the preferred injection site; in older children, either the ventrogluteal area or the gluteus medius muscle can be used. When giving I.M. injections, keep the following considerations in mind:

- If two drugs are to be given simultaneously, check their compatibility; determine the volume of the injectable dose and whether divided doses are necessary.
- To determine correct needle size, consider the patient's age, muscle mass, and nutritional status, and the drug's viscosity; record and rotate injection sites.
- Explain to the patient that the injection will hurt, but that the medication will help him. Restrain him during the injection and comfort him afterward.
- Cleanse the injection site with an alcohol swab, using a circular motion and moving from the center outward. If the drug is a suspension, shake it well just before administering.

Subcutaneous injections

The subcutaneous route is used to administer drugs such as heparin and insulin. The procedure is the same as for I.M. injection except that drug is injected into subcutaneous tissue. Make sure that the bevel of the needle faces up and that the angle of injection is at least 45°. See Chapter 2, NURSING IMPLICATIONS OF DRUG ADMINISTRATION IN ADULTS, for details of correct needle sizes for various age-groups.

Dermatomucosal medications

Dermatomucosal medications furnish local rather than systemic effects. Because drug absorption through skin or mucous membranes is limited, dermatomucosal medications are primarily confined to these applications:

- vasoconstriction, tissue contraction, and decreased secretion
- bacteriostatic action against surface microorganisms
- soothing and softening effects
- cleansing or removal of dirt and debris.

Ear drops

- Use drops warmed to room temperature; cold drops can cause considerable pain and possibly vertigo.
- To administer drops, turn the patient on his side, with the affected ear up. If he is younger than 3 years, pull the pinna down and back; if he is older than 3 years, pull the pinna up and back.
- Make sure the patient remains in the lateral position for at least 5 minutes.

Eye drops and ointment

- Use the same procedure as for an adult patient. You may, however, need help to restrain an uncooperative child.
- Make sure the applicator tip doesn't touch the conjunctiva.

Nose drops

- Hyperextend the patient's head to see the nostrils more easily.
- To minimize risk of bacterial contamination of the nose drops, make sure the dropper doesn't touch the nasal mucosa.
- Since nasal congestion can make feeding more difficult, administer decongestant drops 15 to 30 minutes before mealtime.

Inhalants

- Avoid using inhalants in very young children: obtaining their cooperation is difficult.
- Before attempting to administer medication through a metered-dose nebulizer to an older child, explain the inhaler to him. First have him hold the nebulizer upside down and close his lips around the mouthpiece. Have him exhale; pinch his nostrils shut; and when he starts to inhale, release one dose of medication into his mouth. Tell the patient to continue inhaling until his lungs feel full.
- Most inhaled agents are not useful if taken orally; therefore, if you doubt

NURSING TIPS

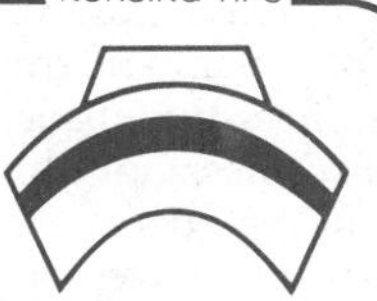

GIVING NOSE DROPS TO AN INFANT

Before you begin, check the medication order against the Kardex. Then, wash your hands and gather the following equipment: the bottle of medication, a medication dropper, and tissues. Choose a dropper with a protective rubber tip.

Important: Warm the medication by running warm water over the bottle for several minutes. Or warm it by carrying the bottle in your pocket for 30 minutes before you administer the medication.

Now, carefully position the infant so his head is tilted back on your arm, as shown.

Draw the medication into the dropper. Then, open the infant's nostrils by gently pushing up the tip of his nose. Instill the ordered number of drops in the nostril. Avoid touching the nostril with the dropper.

Repeat the process in the other nostril, if ordered.

After instilling the drops, keep the infant's head tilted back for 3 to 5 minutes, but stay alert for any sign of aspiration. If the infant begins to cough, sit him upright and pat his back until he has cleared his lungs.

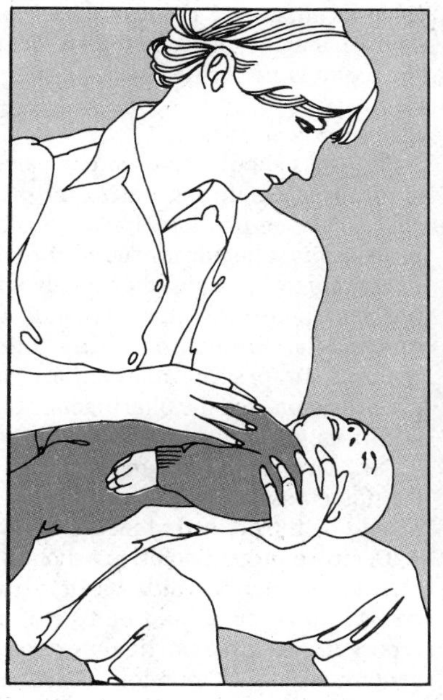

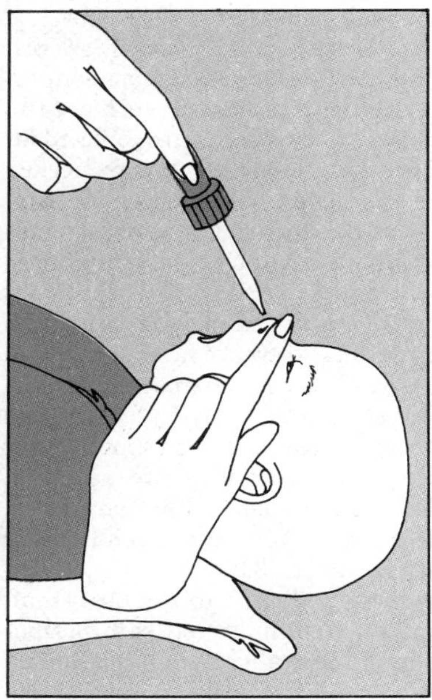

the patient's ability to use the inhalant correctly, don't use it.

- When using cromolyn sodium (for bronchial asthma), the capsule must first be pierced by the inhaler before it can be used.
- Always clean the inhaler after use to minimize bacterial contamination.

Parenteral nutrition

Intravenous nutrition—administered by either the central or peripheral route—is given to patients who can't or won't take adequate food orally and patients with hypermetabolic conditions who need I.V. supplementation. The latter group includes premature infants, and children who have burns or other major trauma, intractable diarrhea, malabsorption syndromes, gastrointestinal abnormalities, emotional disorders such as anorexia nervosa, and congenital abnormalities.

Components

Parenteral nutrition should not only reverse catabolism but also promote normal growth and development. Overall, the child has greater need than the adult for protein, carbohydrate, fat, electrolytes, trace elements, vitamins, and fluid. Accurate calculations of components and correct formulation of parenteral nutrition for children help prevent solution incompatibilities, which impair efficient delivery of nutrients to the patient.

Protein is supplied primarily as crystalline amino acids. Adequate nonprotein calories must also be furnished so that amino acids aren't metabolized for energy but rather synthesize needed protein. Nonprotein calories are supplied as dextrose solutions or fat emulsions, both of which have limitations.

Dextrose, started at 5% or 10%, is gradually increased in accordance with the patient's tolerance level. Peripheral veins can accept dextrose concentrations as high as 12.5%; phlebitis can develop at higher concentrations. These higher concentrations are administered through central venous lines. Central veins can accept solutions as concentrated as 35%.

Fats—supplied as 10% or 20% emulsions—are administered both peripherally and centrally. Their use is limited by the child's ability to metabolize them. An infant or child with a diseased liver cannot efficiently metabolize fats, for example.

Some fats, however, must be supplied both to prevent essential fatty acid deficiency and to permit normal growth and development. A minimum of calories (2% to 4%) must be supplied as linoleic acid—an essential fatty acid found in lipids. In the infant, fats are essential for normal neurologic development. Nevertheless, fat solutions may decrease oxygen perfusion and may adversely affect patients with pulmonary disease. This risk can be minimized by supplying only the minimum fat needed for essential fatty acid requirements and not the usual intake of 40% to 50% of the patient's total calories.

Fatty acids can also displace bilirubin bound to serum albumin, causing a rise in free, unconjugated bilirubin and an increased risk of kernicterus. However, fat solutions may interfere with some bilirubin assays and cause falsely elevated levels. To avoid this complication, a blood sample should be drawn 4 hours after infusion of the lipid emulsion; or if the emulsion is introduced over 24 hours, the blood sample should be centrifuged before the assay is performed.

Special precautions

- I.V. lines should be used exclusively for nutrient solutions unless all other routes for medication are exhausted. If drugs must be administered through the parenteral line simultaneously with nutrient solutions, first consult the pharmacist for compatibility information. To prevent interactions and precipitation, ask the pharmacist about additives you might mix with the solution. Only heparin can be added to the fat emulsion, and no other drug should be introduced at the same time.
- Dextrose-protein solutions should be filtered. Although fluids used in parenteral nutrition should be free of microorganisms and particulate matter, contamination is possible. Dextrose-protein solutions are efficient media for bacterial and fungal growth. Therefore, use a 0.22 aerophobic micron filter to prevent inadvertent administration of all microorganisms (except viruses) and particulate matter. Since air can't pass through the filter after it is primed, the filter prevents an air embolus from forming if the line has to be changed or the pump breaks down. Because fats cannot be filtered, the lipid emulsion

HOW A CATHETER IS INSERTED FOR PARENTERAL NUTRITION IN CHILDREN

To promote proper bone and tissue growth, parenteral nutrition solutions for children must contain higher concentrations of calcium, phosphorus, and magnesium than those for adults. Children also require higher proportions of vitamins.

Infants and small children are given central TPN solutions through a silicone rubber catheter inserted surgically under a general or local anesthetic. Here's the procedure:

- First, the doctor inserts the catheter by cutdown through the internal or external jugular vein into the superior vena cava, as shown in the illustration.
- Then, he tunnels the opposite end of the catheter subcutaneously along the scalp to exit behind the ear. *Note:* Leaving a generous length of catheter outside the scalp allows the child to move without putting too much tension on the catheter.
- Finally, to secure the catheter in the vein, the doctor attaches a silicone rubber sleeve with Dacron wings, stitches it internally, and closes the cutdown site with subcuticular sutures.

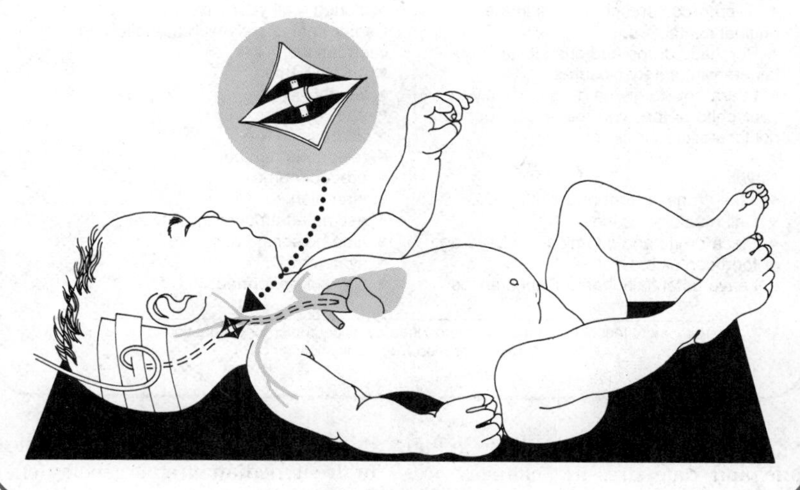

should be piggybacked into the line below the filter.

- Administer solutions at the prescribed rate; should the rate of administration fall behind, don't try to catch up. Before trying to adjust the rate, consult the doctor. With his permission, increase the rate up to 5% per hour if necessary.

Increasing the rate or making up for behind-schedule feedings can result in dextrose overload and subsequent osmotic diuresis, leading to rapid dehydration. Monitor intake and output closely, and be alert for disturbances in fluid balance.

Routine care

- Considering the patient's size, initially monitor electrolyte, BUN, and blood glucose levels daily, and cholesterol level weekly. To prevent osmotic diuresis, check for glycosuria every 6 hours. After these levels are stabilized, laboratory monitoring can be done less often.
- Since infection is a serious complication of parenteral nutrition, monitor vital signs closely.
- Scrutinize the catheter site for infection, inflammation, and infiltration.
- Change the tubing down to the catheter hub every 24 hours.

PARENT-TEACHING AID

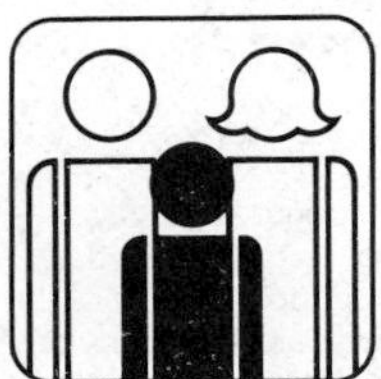

PREVENTING ACCIDENTAL POISONING: WHAT YOU SHOULD KNOW

Dear Parents:

Accidental poisoning has become a major cause of death in children. To help protect your child, follow these guidelines:

Always

- Place drugs and chemicals in locked cabinets.
- Keep drugs and chemicals in their original containers.
- Purchase drugs and chemicals in containers with safety closures.
- Learn how to give a drug correctly to your child before you leave the hospital, doctor's office, or clinic.

Never

- Take drugs in front of a child.
- Call medicine "candy."
- Place drugs and chemicals in beverage or food containers.
- Leave potentially harmful substances within a child's reach, even for a short time.
- Carry more than a 1-day supply of drugs in your purse or coat pocket.
- Leave safety caps off containers.

If you suspect your child has been poisoned, call your local Poison Control Center immediately with the following information:

- child's name
- weight
- age
- address
- telephone number
- product name
- ingredients
- estimated amount swallowed
- time poisoning occurred
- symptoms
- first aid performed.

- Initial the dressing, and include the time and date dressing changes are made.

Poisoning

Accidental poisoning occurs frequently among children. Many times it can be prevented by teaching adults to administer drugs correctly and store them safely. Use the parent-teaching aid on poison precautions, above. It tells parents how to minimize the risk of accidental poisoning and what to do if it does occur.

Emergency drug administration

To treat pediatric emergencies effectively, quick dosage calculation and administration are essential. *Common Drug Dosages for Pediatric Emergencies,* the chart beginning opposite, is a summary of critical dosage information by both weight (mg of drug/body weight) and volume (ml of drug/body weight). When referring to this chart, remember that individual circumstances may require different dosages.

BRUCE M. FREY, PharmD

COMMON DRUG DOSAGES FOR PEDIATRIC EMERGENCIES

This summary is intended only as a guide. Each emergency requires medical staff discretion.

DRUG OR MIXTURE	HOW SUPPLIED	ROUTE	DOSE BY WEIGHT	DOSE BY VOLUME
albumin, salt poor	25%, 12.5 g/50 ml, 50-ml vial	I.V.	0.5 to 1 g/kg	2 to 4 ml/kg
aminophylline	250 mg/10 ml, 10-ml ampul	I.V.	2 to 4 mg/kg over 15 to 20 min, then 0.9 mg/kg/hr up to 1.25 mg/kg/hr continuous I.V. infusion	0.08 to 0.16 ml/kg over 15 to 20 min
atropine	1 mg/ml, 1-ml ampul	I.V., S.C.	0.01 mg/kg Maximum single dose = 0.4 mg; may be repeated twice in 1 hr	0.01 ml/kg Maximum single dose = 0.4 ml; may be repeated twice in 1 hr
calcium gluconate	10%, 100 mg/ml, 10-ml ampul (4.6 mEq/10 ml)	I.V.	60 mg/kg up to 1 g/dose; may be repeated until a maximum of 200 mg/kg has been given *Caution: Do not administer if patient has received digoxin.*	0.6 ml/kg up to 10 ml/dose; may be repeated until a maximum of 2 ml/kg has been given
dexamethasone	10 mg/1 ml, 10-ml vial	I.V.	0.6 mg/kg I.V. initially, then 0.3 mg/kg/day given in divided doses (every 6 hr)	0.06 ml/kg I.V. initially, then 0.03 ml/kg/day given in divided doses (every 6 hr)
dextrose	50%, 500 mg/ml, 50-ml vial	I.V.	500 mg/kg up to 25 g/dose	1 ml/kg up to 50 ml/dose
dextrose/ insulin	dextrose 50%, 500 mg/ml, 50-ml vial insulin, regular 100 units/ml, 10-ml vial	I.V.	Add 8 units of insulin, regular to 50-ml vial of 50% dextrose; 0.5 to 1 ml/kg/dose of the dextrose/insulin mixture	
diazepam	5 mg/ml, 2-ml ampul	I.V.	*Acute anticonvulsant dose:* Slow I.V. 0.25 mg/kg at rate not to exceed 2 mg/min; may repeat every 15 min for 2 doses. Maximum dose for infants = 5 mg; maximum dose for older children = 15 mg	.05 ml/kg slow I.V Maximum dose for infants = 1 ml; maximum dose for older children = 3 ml
diazoxide	300 mg/20 ml, 20-ml ampul	I.V.	3 to 5 mg/kg/dose rapid I.V. push; dose may be repeated in 1 hr; usually recommended not to repeat in less than 1 hr; repeat doses every 4 to 24 hr	0.2 to 0.3 ml/kg/dose rapid I.V. push; dose may be repeated in 1 hr; usually recommended not to repeat in less than 1 hr; repeat doses every 4 to 24 hr

(continued on following page)

COMMON DRUG DOSAGES FOR PEDIATRIC EMERGENCIES *(continued)*

DRUG OR MIXTURE	HOW SUPPLIED	ROUTE	DOSE BY WEIGHT	DOSE BY VOLUME	
digoxin	Pediatric injection: 0.1 mg/1 ml, 1-ml ampul (100 mcg/ml) *Caution: Never use adult-strength digoxin.*		*Total digitalizing dose* (TDD):	*TDD*	*Initial dose* (0.3TDD)
		I.V.	**Premature infants** = 25 to 40 mcg/kg	0.25 to 0.4 ml/kg	0.08 to 0.13 ml/kg
		I.V.	**Infants 0 to 2 weeks** = 35 to 50 mcg/kg	0.35 to 0.5 ml/kg	0.11 to 0.17 ml/kg
		I.V.	**Infants 2 weeks to 2 years** = 40 to 65 mcg/kg	0.4 to 0.65 ml/kg	0.13 to 0.22 ml/kg
		I.V.	**Children 2 to 10 years** = 35 to 50 mcg/kg	0.35 to 0.5 ml/kg	0.12 to 0.17 ml/kg
			TDD may be divided equally in thirds and given at 8-hr intervals or less; total daily maintenance P.O. = ⅓ TDD based on original I.V. dosage.		
diphenhydramine	50 mg/ml, 1-ml syringe	I.V.	2 mg/kg slow I.V.	0.04 ml/kg slow I.V.	
dopamine	200 mg/5 ml, 5-ml ampul	I.V.	*Dilution:* add one ampul to 500 ml dextrose 5% in water (D_5W) to give final concentration of 400 mcg/ml *Dose:* start at 2 to 5 mcg/kg/min and increase by 5 to 10 mcg//kg/min increments after 15-min trial on each dose	See chart below	

Microdrops/min (200 mg/500 ml D_5W)

mcg/kg/min \ Patient wt (kg)	10	20	30	40
20	30	60	90	120
15	23	45	68	90
10	15	30	45	60
5	8	15	23	30
2	3	6	9	12

Dopamine dosage in microdrops/min (60 drops/ml minidripper); standard = 200 mg/500 ml D_5W (400 mcg/ml)

DRUG OR MIXTURE	HOW SUPPLIED	ROUTE	DOSE BY WEIGHT	DOSE BY VOLUME
epinephrine 1:1,000 *(anaphylaxis)*	1:1,000, 1-ml ampul (1,000 mcg/ml)	S.C.	**Newborns** = 10 mcg/kg every 15 to 20 min × 3 to 4 (500 mcg/dose, maximum)	0.01 ml/kg (of 1:1,000 epinephrine)
			Older children = 100 to 500 mcg every 15 to 20 min × 3 to 4	0.1 to 0.5 ml (of 1:1,000 epinephrine)
epinephrine 1:10,000 syringe *(cardiac)*	1:10,000, 10-ml syringe (100 mcg/ml)	I.V. or intracardiac	**Newborns** = 10 mcg/kg every 3 to 5 min	0.1 ml/kg (of 1:10,000 epinephrine)
			Older children = 100 to 500 mcg every 3 to 5 min	1 to 5 ml (of 1:10,000)

DRUG OR MIXTURE	HOW SUPPLIED	ROUTE	DOSE BY WEIGHT	DOSE BY VOLUME
epinephrine 1:1,000 *(infusion)*	1:1,000, 1-ml ampul (1,000 mcg/ml)	I.V.	*Dilution:* 3 ml epinephrine in 250 ml D_5W *Final concentration:* 12 mcg/ml *Dose:* 0.25 to 1 mcg/kg/min	*Microdrops/min (3 mg/250 ml D_5W)* mcg/kg/min **1**: 50 100 150 200 **0.75**: 38 75 113 150 **0.5**: 25 50 75 100 **0.25**: 13 25 38 50 **10 20 30 40** *Patient wt (kg)* Epinephrine dosage in microdrops/min (60 drops/ml minidripper); standard = 3 mg/250 ml D_5W (12 mcg/ml)
furosemide	10 mg/ml, 2-ml ampul	I.V.	0.5 to 1 mg/kg/dose	0.05 to 0.1 ml/kg/dose
insulin, regular	100 units/ml, 10-ml vial		1 unit for each 3 g (6 ml 50% dextrose) given	0.01 ml for each 3 g (6 ml 50% dextrose) given
isoproterenol	1:5,000, 0.2 mg/ml, 5-ml ampul (200 mcg/ml)	I.V.	*Dilution:* 10 ml isoproterenol in 250 ml D_5W *Final concentration:* 8 mcg/ml *Dose:* 0.25 to 1 mcg/kg/min	*Microdrops/min (2 mg/250 ml D_5W)* mcg/kg/min **1**: 75 150 225 300 **0.75**: 56 112 169 225 **0.5**: 38 76 113 150 **0.25**: 19 38 56 75 **10 20 30 40** *Patient wt (kg)* Isoproterenol dosage in microdrops/min (60 drops/ml minidripper); standard = 2 mg/250 ml D_5W (8 mcg/ml)
isoproterenol/ levarterenol (norepinephrine) *(alternative mixture)*		I.V.	*Dilution:* 1.25 ml/isoproterenol and 1 ml levarterenol to 250 ml D_5W *Final concentration:* isoproterenol = 1 mcg/ml; levarterenol = 4 mcg/ml *Dose:* titrate by blood pressure and heart rate (0.025 ml/kg/min; not to exceed 0.25 ml/kg/min)	
levarterenol (norepinephrine)	1 mg base/ml, 4-ml ampule	I.V.	*Dilution:* 1 ml (1 mg) in 250 ml D_5W *Final concentration:* 4 mcg/ml *Initial dose:* 0.1 mcg/kg/min; not to exceed 1 mcg/kg/min	0.025 ml/kg/min; not to exceed 0.25 ml/kg/min; with 60 drops/ml minidripper, instill 2 to 15 drops/kg/min (not to exceed 15 drops/kg/min)
lidocaine	1 g/25 ml, 25-ml vial	I.V.	0.5 to 1 mg/kg slow I.V. push; may be repeated every 5 to 10 min as needed; maximum total dose = 5 mg/kg	0.0125 to 0.025 ml/kg slow I.V. push; may be repeated every 5 to 10 min as needed

(continued on following page)

COMMON DRUG DOSAGES FOR PEDIATRIC EMERGENCIES *(continued)*

DRUG OR MIXTURE	HOW SUPPLIED	ROUTE	DOSE BY WEIGHT	DOSE BY VOLUME
lidocaine *(continued)*			*Infusion:* 20 to 50 mcg/kg/min; maximum total dose = 5 mg/kg *Dilution:* 1 g in 500 ml D_5W *Final concentration:* 2,000 mcg/ml	*Microdrops/min (1 g/500 ml D_5W)* — see chart below Lidocaine dosage in microdrops/min (60 drops/ml minidripper); standard = 1 g/500 ml D_5W (2,000 mcg/ml)

Microdrops/min (1 g/500 ml D_5W)

mcg/kg/min	10	20	30	40
50	15	30	45	60
40	12	24	36	48
30	9	18	27	36
20	6	12	18	24

Patient wt (kg)

DRUG OR MIXTURE	HOW SUPPLIED	ROUTE	DOSE BY WEIGHT	DOSE BY VOLUME
mannitol	25%, 250 mg/ml, 50-ml vial	I.V.	*Test dose:* 200 mg/kg I.V. single dose over 3 to 5 min *Edema:* (15% to 20% solution) 1 to 2 g/kg I.V. as slow I.V. infusion over 2 to 6 hr *Cerebral edema:* 1 to 2 g/kg I.V. over 30 to 60 min	*Test dose:* 0.8 ml/kg I.V. single dose over 3 to 5 min *Edema:* 15% solution—6.7 to 13.3 ml/kg I.V. as slow I.V. infusion over 2 to 6 hr; 20% solution—5 to 10 ml/kg I.V. as slow I.V. infusion over 2 to 6 hr *Cerebral edema:* 20% solution—5 to 10 ml/kg I.V. over 30 to 60 min
naloxone *(neonatal strength)*	0.02 mg/ml, 2-ml ampul (20 mcg/ml)	I.M. or I.V.	5 to 10 mcg/kg/dose; repeat every 2 to 3 min as needed × three doses	0.25 to 0.5 ml/kg/dose; repeat every 2 to 3 min as needed × three doses
naloxone *(adult strength)*	0.4 mg/ml, 1-ml ampul (400 mcg/ml)	I.M. or I.V.	5 to 10 mcg/kg/dose; repeat every 2 to 3 min as needed × three doses; maximum dose = 400 mcg	0.01 to 0.03 ml/kg/dose; repeat every 2 to 3 min as needed × three doses; maximum dose = 1 ml
nitroprusside *(for severe arterial hypertension only)*	50 mg/5 ml vial *Caution: Solution container should be protected from light with aluminum foil; solution should be discarded after 4 hr*	I.V.	*Dilution:* 50 mg nitroprusside to 500 ml D_5W *Final concentration:* 100 mcg/ml *Dose:* 0.5 to 2 mcg/kg/min	*Microdrops/min (50 mg/500 ml D_5W)* — see chart below Nitroprusside dosage in microdrops/min (60 drops/ml minidripper); standard = 50 mg/500 ml D_5W

Microdrops/min (50 mg/500 ml D_5W)

mcg/kg/min	10	20	30	40
2	12	24	36	48
1.5	9	18	27	36
1	6	12	18	24
0.5	3	6	9	12

Patient wt (kg)

DRUG OR MIXTURE	HOW SUPPLIED	ROUTE	DOSE BY WEIGHT	DOSE BY VOLUME
phenytoin *(anticonvulsant); therapeutic level = 10 to 20 mcg/ml*	100 mg/2 ml, 2-ml ampul 100 mg/capsule 50 mg/tablet 125 mg/5 ml suspension	I.V.	*Loading dose:* 8 mg/kg slow IV push at a rate not to exceed 25 mg/min. If seizures persist, another dose of 6 to 8 mg/kg may be administered; total loading dose not to exceed 16 mg/kg *Maintenance dose:* 5 to 8 mg/kg P.O. or I.V. given once daily or divided into two equal doses	*Loading dose:* 0.16 ml/kg at a rate not to exceed 0.5 ml/min. If seizures persist, another dose of 0.12 to 0.16 ml/kg may be administered; total loading dose not to exceed 0.32 ml/kg
phenytoin *(antiarrhythmic); therapeutic level = 5 to 18 mcg/ml*	100 mg/2 ml, 2-ml ampul	I.V.	1 to 5 mg/kg slow I.V. push; rate not to exceed 25 mg/min; repeat as needed; maximum total dose = 500 mg in 4 hr	0.02 to 0.1 ml/kg slow I.V. push; rate not to exceed 0.5 ml/min; repeat as needed; maximum total dose = 10 ml in 4 hr
propranolol *(use with extreme caution in congestive heart failure)*	1 mg/ml, 1-ml ampul	I.V.	0.025 to 0.1 mg/kg slow I.V. push over 10 min every 6 to 8 hr as needed; not to exceed 10 mg/dose (4 mg/dose if patient is anesthetized)	0.025 to 0.1 ml/kg slow I.V. push over 10 min, given every 6 to 8 hr as needed; not to exceed 10 ml/dose (4 ml/dose if patient is anesthetized)
sodium bicarbonate	44.6 mEq/50 ml, 50-ml syringe	I.V.	1 to 3 mEq/kg I.V. push every 10 min (dosage is empirical only if arterial blood gas data is not available) *Caution: Dilute solution to half strength for use in infants.*	1.1 to 3.4 ml/kg I.V. push every 10 min (dosage is empirical only if arterial blood gas data is not available)

COMMON PROCEDURES FOR PEDIATRIC EMERGENCIES

PROCEDURE	DOSE BY WEIGHT
Defibrillation	1 watt-second/lb (2.2 watt-second/kg)
Cardioversion	¼ to 1 watt-second/lb (0.55-2.2 watt-second/kg)

Courtesy of Thomas Jefferson University Hospital, Philadelphia, Pa. Compiled by Harris Koffer, BSc, Department of Pharmacy; Edmond J. Sacks, MD, Department of Pediatrics, and Director, Pediatric Cardiology and Pediatric ICU; Bruce M. Frey, PharmD, Department of Pharmacy.

4 Nursing implications of drug therapy in the elderly

Persons aged 65 or older make up one of the fastest-growing segments of the population. In the United States they comprised 11.3% of the population in 1980—up from 9.8% a decade before. Improved health care of the young and middle-aged has, of course, increased the number of elderly people.

If you're providing drug therapy for elderly patients, you'll want to understand patterns of drug use in the elderly; age-related pharmacokinetic and physiologic changes that may alter drug dosage; common adverse reactions; and how to improve patient compliance.

Medication consumption patterns

Medication consumption increases with age. In the United States, for example, a man between ages 25 and 44 takes 3.4 prescription medications annually, and a woman of the same age-group, 7.3. Men and women aged 65 and over take 11.2 and 14.3 prescription medications, respectively. In fact, the elderly population in the United States purchases about 25% of all prescription and nonprescription drugs sold.

The elderly consume more prescription and nonprescription drugs than the young because they have a greater variety of diseases requiring one or more medications. An elderly patient with congestive heart failure, for example, may take three prescription drugs: digoxin, to improve cardiac contractility; a diuretic, such as furosemide, to help eliminate excess body fluid; and potassium chloride, to replace potassium lost due to the diuretic's action.

Other diseases common to the elderly, such as arthritis and angina pectoris, also may require multiple medications. Besides major diseases, elderly persons may take medication for aches and pains, constipation and

MEDICATIONS TAKEN MOST FREQUENTLY BY THE ELDERLY

Cardiac drugs
digoxin (Lanoxin)
nitroglycerin
propranolol (Inderal)

Diuretics
furosemide (Lasix)
spironolactone

Sedatives/hypnotics
flurazepam (Dalmane)
chloral hydrate (Noctec)

Antidiabetics
insulin
tolbutamide (Orinase)

Psychotropics
chlorpromazine (Thorazine)
thioridazine (Mellaril)

Gastrointestinal drugs
cimetidine (Tagamet)
belladonna preparations

Laxatives and cathartics
magnesia magma (milk of magnesia)
bisacodyl (Dulcolax)

other gastrointestinal complaints, insomnia, and various skin disorders.

An older person's socioeconomic status, personal health, and health-care environment (extended-care facility or community living, for example) may affect his drug use. And his doctors and nurses have an influence as well, particularly in regard to p.r.n. medications.

Institutionalized elderly patients take more medications than outpatients. For example, elderly patients in nursing homes take between four and seven medications concurrently; elderly outpatients usually take between two and four different medications. For the medications taken most frequently by the elderly, see chart opposite.

Physiologic changes affecting drug action

As a person ages, gradual changes occur in his anatomy and physiology. Some of these age-related changes may alter the therapeutic and toxic effects of medications.

Body composition

Proportions of fat, lean tissue, and water in the body change with age. Total body mass and lean body mass tend to decrease; the proportion of body fat tends to increase. Although varying from person to person, these changes in body composition affect the relationship between a drug's concentration and solubility in the body.

For example, a *water-soluble* drug, such as gentamicin, is distributed mostly to the aqueous parts of the body and to lean tissue. The drug is *not* distributed to fat. Since there's less lean tissue for the drug to be distributed to in an elderly person, more of the drug remains in the bloodstream. This may result in an increased blood concentration unless the dosage is reduced.

The distribution of *fat-soluble* drugs, such as pentobarbital, may also be affected by age-related changes in body composition. As the proportion of body fat increases, fat-soluble drugs must be distributed to a greater volume of tissue. Accordingly, this increased volume may initially lower blood drug concentrations; however, after the body fat is saturated with drug, it may store the drug and slowly release it back into the general circulation, thus increasing the drug's duration of action. This phenomenon partially explains why pentobarbital and other fat-soluble sleep medications may produce residual drowsiness the morning after they're taken.

Gastrointestinal function

In the elderly, decreases in gastric acid secretion and gastrointestinal motility slow emptying of stomach contents and movement of intestinal contents through the entire tract. Furthermore, although inconclusive, research shows the elderly may have more difficulty absorbing medications. This is a particularly significant problem with drugs having a narrow therapeutic range, such as digoxin, in which any change in absorption can be crucial.

Hepatic function

Many drugs are either partially or entirely metabolized by the liver before they're excreted from the body. (See Chapter 1, PHARMACOLOGY FOR NURSES.) Although significantly reduced hepatic function normally isn't associated with the aging process, the liver's ability to metabolize certain drugs does decrease with age. This is probably due to diminished blood flow to the liver, which results from the age-related decrease in cardiac output. When an elderly patient takes certain sleep medications, such as secobarbital, his liver's reduced ability to metabolize the drug may produce a hangover effect due to central nervous system depression. Elimination of these medications is highly dependent on the liver. Decreased hepatic function may cause:

- more intense drug effects due to higher blood levels
- longer-lasting drug effects due to prolonged blood concentrations
- greater incidence of drug toxicity.

PATIENT-TEACHING AID

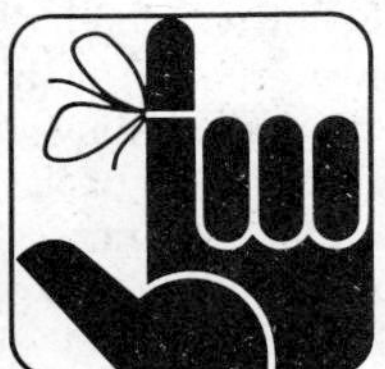

TAKING YOUR ORAL MEDICATIONS

Dear Patient:

For your drug therapy to be effective, you must take your medications exactly as your doctor directs, particularly when taking several medications at one time. Here are some helpful hints:

• **Sort your medications.** Label empty jars, extra prescription bottles (you can get these from your pharmacist), or envelopes with the times of day or the days of the week you must take medication. Use a separate container for each time. Each morning fill these containers with the appropriate dose of each medication.

Note: Some drugs may deteriorate when exposed to light. Before you remove drugs from their original containers, check with your pharmacist or doctor.

• **Make a medication calendar.** Use a calendar that has enough space to fill in the names of the drugs you need to take each day. Then put a check mark next to the name of the drug after you take each dose.

• **Make a chart.** List:
—name of drug
—what it's for
—what it looks like (shape, color)
—directions for taking the drug
—special cautions or side effects
—time of day to take drug.

Hang this chart near your medicine cabinet.

• **Set your alarm clock** or ask a relative or friend to remind you when to take your medications.

Renal function

Although an elderly person's renal function is usually sufficient to eliminate excess body fluid and waste, his ability to eliminate some medications may be reduced by 50% or more.

Many medications commonly used by the elderly, such as digoxin, are excreted primarily through the kidneys. If the kidneys' ability to excrete the drug is decreased, high blood concentrations may result. Digoxin toxicity, therefore, is relatively common.

Drug dosages can be modified to compensate for age-related decreases in renal function. Aided by laboratory tests, such as BUN and serum creatinine, clinical pharmacists and doctors can adjust medication dosages so the patient receives the expected therapeutic benefits without the risk of toxicity. You can help by carefully observing your patient for signs of toxicity or, when possible, by teaching him the signs to recognize. A patient taking digoxin, for example, may experience anorexia, nausea, and vomiting.

Adverse drug reactions

Although medications frequently cure or manage disease in the elderly, they may also cause adverse effects ranging from minor discomfort to total debilitation and even death.

The elderly reportedly have twice as many adverse drug reactions as younger people. This increased incidence of drug reactions, of course, is related to greater drug consumption, poor compliance, and physiologic changes.

Many times, signs and symptoms of adverse drug reactions—confusion, weakness, and lethargy—are mistakenly attributed to senility or disease. If the adverse reaction isn't identified, the patient may continue to receive the drug. And he may receive unnecessary additional medication to treat complications caused by the original drug.

Although any medication can cause adverse reactions, most serious adverse reactions in the elderly are caused by relatively few medications. When caring for the elderly, you should be particularly aware of toxicities resulting from diuretics, digoxin, corticosteroids, sleep medications, and nonprescription drugs.

Diuretic toxicity
The use of potassium-wasting diuretics, such as hydrochlorothiazide and furosemide, may result in fluid and electrolyte imbalance in the elderly patient. Because the average amount of total body water decreases with age, normal doses of these drugs may result in fluid loss and even dehydration in an elderly patient. These diuretics may deplete serum potassium, causing weakness in the patient; and they may raise blood uric acid and glucose levels, complicating preexisting gout and diabetes mellitus.

Digoxin toxicity
As the body's renal function and rate of excretion decline, digoxin concentrations in the blood may build to toxic levels, causing nausea, vomiting, diarrhea, and most serious, cardiac arrhythmias. You may be able to prevent severe toxicity in your patient by recognizing early signs such as appetite loss, confusion, or depression. If your patient cannot speak (aphasia) or has lost his hearing or sight, he may not be able to convey these symptoms to you. Therefore, observe him for changes in appetite, orientation, and mood.

Corticosteroid toxicity
Corticosteroids, such as prednisone, may also cause several adverse reactions in the elderly. Short-term effects include fluid retention and psychological manifestations ranging from mild euphoria to acute psychotic reactions. Long-term toxic effects, such as osteoporosis, can be especially severe in elderly patients who have been taking prednisone or related steroidal compounds for months or even years. To prevent serious toxicity, carefully monitor patients on long-term regimens. Observe them for subtle changes in appearance, mood, and mobility, as well as for signs of impaired healing and fluid and electrolyte disturbances.

Sleep medication toxicity
In some cases, sedatives or sleeping aids cause excessive sedation or residual drowsiness. For example, the hypnotic agent flurazepam causes residual drowsiness the morning after it's administered. Elderly patients may possibly fall or injure themselves—especially those who already have difficulty walking in the morning because of arthritic changes, hypotension, or reactions to other drugs. To help prevent serious injury to elderly patients taking sedatives or sleeping aids, institute precautionary measures, such as raising bed side rails whenever necessary. Obtain baseline data on their usual ability to walk after rising. After the medication has been started, observe and record any changes in their gait. Report these changes if they persist for any length of time so the dosage prescribed can be reevaluated.

Nonprescription drug toxicity
Although prescription drugs are more commonly recognized as the cause of adverse drug reactions, nonprescription drugs also can cause significant health problems for the elderly.

Aspirin and aspirin-containing an-

SENILITY OR SIDE EFFECTS?

Myth: *All elderly patients who exhibit symptoms associated with old age (such as drowsiness, forgetfulness, and confusion) are senile.*

Fact: *Many symptoms attributed to senility are actually side effects of drugs commonly prescribed for the elderly.*

Elderly patients themselves may assume that adverse drug reactions are due simply to aging. Thus, if the doctor doesn't warn them about side effects, they may ignore them or suffer through them needlessly. Here's what you can do to help distinguish drug effects from senility in your elderly patient:

- Check your patient's medication to be sure he's getting the lowest effective dose. You can help the doctor determine the lowest effective dose by monitoring your patient for therapeutic and adverse effects until steady-state blood concentrations have been attained, and by documenting your observations.
- Teach your patient to watch for possible side effects of his medications. Tell him to contact his doctor if they occur.
- Suggest that he have a thorough physical examination to rule out undiagnosed conditions, such as cardiac disease and nutritional deficiencies, that can contribute to senility.
- Review all his medications for possible drug interactions that may cause senility-like symptoms. Watch for these:

SYMPTOMS	POSSIBLE CAUSES
Confusion	Methyldopa, an antihypertensive agent; digoxin, a cardiac medication; and cimetidine, an anti-ulcer drug
Depression	Reserpine, an antihypertensive agent
Anorexia	Digoxin
Weakness	Certain diuretics, such as furosemide and hydrochlorothiazide, which can deplete body potassium
Lethargy and drowsiness	Various tranquilizers, analgesics, and sleep medications, including chlorpromazine, meperidine, and pentobarbital
Ataxia	Inappropriately high doses of flurazepam and other sedatives or hypnotics
Forgetfulness	Barbiturates
Constipation	Medications with anticholinergic properties, such as belladonna-containing drugs
Diarrhea	Various oral antacid preparations containing magnesium hydroxide
Gastrointestinal distress	Oral iron preparations or antiarthritic medications, such as aspirin, ibuprofen, or indomethacin

algesics are among the nonprescription drugs most commonly purchased by the elderly. The toxicity of these analgesics is minimal when used in moderation, but prolonged ingestion may cause gastrointestinal irritation and gradual blood loss resulting in severe anemia. Although anemia from chronic aspirin consumption can affect all age-groups, the elderly may be less able to compensate because of their already reduced iron stores.

Laxatives and cathartics are also commonly taken by the elderly, even though proper diet and exercise may preclude their use. Here are some of the problems they may cause:

- Diarrhea may occur if an elderly patient is extremely sensitive to a laxative such as bisacodyl.
- Chronic oral use of mineral oil as a lubricating laxative may result in lipid pneumonia due to aspiration of small residual oil droplets in the mouth.

Patient noncompliance

Noncompliance with prescribed drug therapy is a major problem in the elderly. It includes:

- failure to take prescribed doses
- consumption of inappropriate doses
- failure to follow the correct schedule
- premature discontinuance of medications
- consumption of medications prescribed for previous disorders
- indiscriminate use of medications ordered p.r.n. (To some, p.r.n. means taking several tablets at a time if considered necessary; to others, it may mean taking one tablet followed shortly by another and then another; to still others, it may mean continuing the drug long after it's actually required.)

Why do approximately one third of the elderly population fail to comply with their prescribed therapy? An age-related decline in sensory acuity is one reason for patient noncompliance. For example, an elderly patient with impaired vision may have difficulty reading prescription instructions. With hearing loss, the patient may not understand oral instructions. Also, physical disabilities, such as those produced by arthritis, may hinder him from opening "childproof" medication containers.

Since the patient may have received instructions for taking medications during a time of stress or anxiety, review the medication amount and the time and frequency of doses with him.

Also, explain how he should take each medication—whether with food or water, or by itself. *And make sure the patient understands your instructions.*

Proper nursing care can help manage, reduce, or overcome many drug therapy problems in the elderly patient. Don't wait for your patient to question you; instead, offer to review his medication regimen with him.

Ask the patient or his family about the medications he currently takes. When necessary, call the patient's pharmacy and his doctors to get a complete medication history.

Give the patient whatever help you can, and refer him to the pharmacist if he needs further information about his medications and their effects.

WILLIAM SIMONSON, PharmD

NURSING TIPS

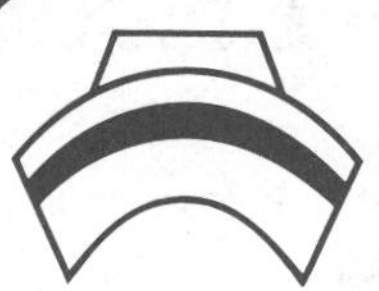

IMPROVING COMPLIANCE IN THE ELDERLY

An elderly patient may want to follow his doctor's orders but be hindered by age-related physical or financial problems. To help him overcome these problems and improve his compliance, ask these questions:

- *Can he open his medication bottles easily?* If he has arthritis or Parkinson's disease, he may need standard caps instead of childproof ones. Remind him to ask the pharmacist for standard caps whenever he needs his prescriptions refilled.
- *Is he on a fixed income?* If so, he may try to make his medications last longer. Stress the importance of following the doctor's orders exactly. If necessary, refer him to the social service representative for information on financial aid.
- *What are his eating habits?* Some of his medications may have to be taken with meals. If he habitually skips meals, he may miss those doses. Work together with your patient to plan a realistic schedule, then contact a social service program, such as Meals on Wheels, to help him begin eating properly.
- *Can he see well enough to read the medication labels?* If the medication's packaged in an amber container, tape the label on the outside so it won't be obscured by the tinted glass, or ask the pharmacist to package your patient's prescriptions in clear bottles (if not contraindicated). This way, your patient can identify his medication by its appearance. You can also print the dosage instructions and schedule on a separate sheet of paper (using large letters) and tape a sample tablet or capsule to the schedule. Then your patient, his family, or a visiting nurse can easily refer to them.

Calculations for nurses

Since you often have to interpret drug orders and solve problems of dosages and solutions quickly, you should know how to make certain mathematical calculations and conversions.

The unit dose system eliminates some of the mathematics involved in administering medications. In this system, the pharmacist dispenses the prescribed amount of medication—in individually labeled unit dose packages—ready for administration to a particular patient. (See Chapter 2, NURSING IMPLICATIONS OF DRUG ADMINISTRATION IN ADULTS, for more information on the unit dose system.) Even if this system is used in your hospital, you'll sometimes have to make calculations and conversions. Also, to double-check for accuracy, you'll have to know how to calculate a dispensed dose.

The three systems of measurement most often used are *metric, apothecary,* and *household.* Know how to make conversions from one system to another, since drugs or solutions on hand may not be in the same system as that written by the doctor. The metric and household systems include measures of weight, volume, and length; the apothecary system includes measures of weight and volume.

Metric system

The metric system—also called the decimal system—is most commonly used because of its accuracy. Any changes of units of measure can be made by multiplying or dividing by 10.

Apothecary system

The apothecary system, an old English method, is being replaced by the metric system. However, it is still used by some doctors and hospital staffs.

The terms *fluidram* and *fluidounce* are usually shortened to *dram* and *ounce,* with the understanding that drugs in liquid form are measured by volume and those in solid form by weight. When symbols are used, quantity is expressed in small Roman numerals placed after the symbol, for example, ii . If a fraction of a measure is ordered, a symbol is not used; instead, the amount is written out with the fraction first, for example, ⅕ ounce. An exception to this is one half, which has its own symbol ($\overline{ss}$). Thus an order for one half ounce can be written as ℥$\overline{ss}$ or ½ ounce.

Household system

Household measure, the least accurate system, is used only when it is impractical to calculate and measure doses by other systems. This may be the most convenient system for taking medications at home, for example. The household measure system is based on cooking utensils, such as the teaspoon and tablespoon. However, since a household teaspoon may hold from 3 to 8 ml, the American Standards Institute has established these standards:

60 drops (gtt)	=	1 teaspoonful
3 teaspoonfuls	=	1 tablespoonful
2 tablespoonfuls	=	1 fluidounce
8 fluidounces	=	1 glassful

FREQUENTLY USED EQUIVALENTS IN THE METRIC SYSTEM

Metric Weight

1 gram	=	0.001 kilogram (kg or Kg)
(g, gm, Gm)	=	0.01 hektogram (hg or Hg)
	=	0.1 dekagram (dag or Dg)
	=	10 decigrams (dg)
	=	100 centigrams (cg)
	=	1,000 milligrams (mg)

Metric Volume

1 liter (L or l)	=	0.001 kiloliter (kl or Kl)
	=	0.01 hektoliter (hl or Hl)
	=	0.1 dekaliter (dal or Dl)
	=	10 deciliters (dl)
	=	100 centiliters (cl)
	=	1,000 milliliters (ml)*

*1 ml = 1 cubic centimeter (cc); however, ml is the preferred measurement term today.

FREQUENTLY USED EQUIVALENTS IN THE APOTHECARY SYSTEM

Apothecary Weight

20 grains (gr)	=	1 scruple (℈)
3 scruples	=	1 dram (ʒ)
8 drams	=	1 ounce (℥)
12 ounces	=	1 pound (lb)

Apothecary Volume

60 minims* (♏)	=	1 fluidram (f ʒ)
8 fluidrams	=	1 fluidounce (f ℥)
16 fluidounces	=	1 pint (pt)
2 pints	=	1 quart (qt)
4 quarts	=	1 gallon (gal)

*A minim is *almost equal* to a drop. When a drug is prescribed in minims, it is best to measure it in minims. The minim is measured with a minim glass; the drop, with a medicine dropper.

APPROXIMATE METRIC AND APOTHECARY WEIGHT EQUIVALENTS

Metric		Apothecary
1 gram (g) (1,000 mg)	=	15 grains
0.6 g (600 mg)	=	10 grains
0.5 g (500 mg)	=	7½ grains
0.3 g (300 mg)	=	5 grains
0.2 g (200 mg)	=	3 grains
0.1 g (100 mg)	=	1½ grains
0.06 g (60 mg)	=	1 grain

Metric		Apothecary
0.05 g (50 mg)	=	¾ grain
0.03 g (30 mg)	=	½ grain
0.015 g (15 mg)	=	¼ grain
0.001 g (1 mg)	=	1/60 grain
0.6 mg	=	1/100 grain
0.5 mg	=	1/120 grain
0.4 mg	=	1/150 grain

APPROXIMATE HOUSEHOLD, APOTHECARY, AND METRIC VOLUME EQUIVALENTS

Household		Apothecary		Metric
1 teaspoonful (tsp)	=	1 fluidram (f ʒ)	=	4 or 5 ml*
1 tablespoonful (T or tbs)	=	½ fluidounce (f ℥)	=	15 ml
2 tablespoonfuls	=	1 fluidounce	=	30 ml
1 measuring cupful	=	8 fluidounces	=	240 ml
1 pint (pt)	=	16 fluidounces	=	473 ml
1 quart (qt)	=	32 fluidounces	=	946 ml
1 gallon (gal)	=	128 fluidounces	=	3,785 ml

*Although the fluidram is approximately 4 ml, in prescriptions it is considered equivalent to the teaspoon (which is 5 ml).

Converting measurements

Setting up a proportion may be the least complex method for converting measures either within the same system or from one system to another. A proportion is made up of two ratios, each indicating the relationship one quantity has to the other. It can be written as whole units or as a fraction:

A:B::C:D

2:3::4:6

$$\frac{A}{B}=\frac{C}{D}$$

$$\frac{2}{3}=\frac{4}{6}$$

The first and fourth terms (A and D) are called the extremes, and the second and third terms (B and C) are called the means. The product of the means equals the product of the extremes.

A:B::C:D	$\frac{A}{B} = \frac{C}{D}$
2:3::4:6	$\frac{2}{3} = \frac{4}{6}$
$2\times6=3\times4$	$2\times6=3\times4$
$12 = 12$	$12 = 12$

The proportion method can be helpful when one of your terms is unknown (x).

- Keep the unknown quantity on the left, the known on the right.
- Solve the proportion by equating the product of the means to the product of the extremes.
- For the value of x, simply divide the numerical value of the product containing the x into the product on the right of the equation.

Example: 2:x::4:6

or *Unknown* *Known*

$$\frac{2}{x} = \frac{4}{6}$$

$$4x = 2\times6$$

$$4x = 12$$

$$x = 3$$

- You can prove your answer when the problem is solved by substituting it in place of the x:

$$\frac{2}{3} = \frac{4}{6}$$

$$3\times4 = 2\times6$$

$$12 = 12$$

- When using proportion to solve medication problems, be sure the ratios are expressed in the same units of measure.

In the following practice problems, the proportions are set up as fractions.

<u>*Conversion within the same system*</u>

Example:

How many milligrams are in 4 grams?

Set up a proportion according to the information given.

$$\frac{g}{mg}=\frac{g}{mg}$$

NUMERICAL SYMBOLS COMMONLY USED WITH THE APOTHECARY SYSTEM

$\overline{\text{ss}}$	= ½	$\overline{\dot{\text{VI}}}$	= 6
$\overline{\dot{\text{I}}}$	= 1	$\overline{\ddot{\text{VII}}}$	= 7
$\overline{\ddot{\text{II}}}$	= 2	$\overline{\dddot{\text{VIII}}}$	= 8
$\overline{\dddot{\text{III}}}$	= 3	$\overline{\dot{\text{IX}}}$	= 9
$\overline{\dot{\text{IV}}}$	= 4	$\overline{\text{X}}$	= 10
$\overline{\text{V}}$	= 5	$\overline{\text{XV}}$	= 15

When apothecary symbols are used, the quantity is expressed in lower case Roman numerals, which are placed after the symbol: gr ii, ʒii, ℥iii. However, when fractions are indicated, or when pt, qt, and gal are written Arabic numerals are always used: gr ¼, qt 9. The only exception to this rule is the quantity ½, which is expressed as the symbol $\overline{\text{ss}}$ (Latin *semi* or *semisis*, meaning half).

METRIC WEIGHT AND VOLUME SCALE

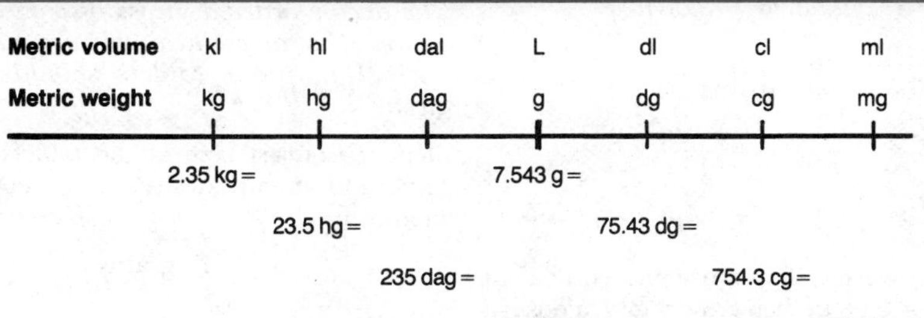

This graph shows the relationship between units of weight and units of volume in the metric system. And it provides an easy method of converting from one unit to another. When converting kilograms (kg) to grams (g), notice that the gram position is three steps to the right of the kilogram position, so move the decimal point three places to the right. When converting milligrams (mg) to grams, move the decimal point three places, but this time to the left. Use this same method to convert metric units of volume. See the table on frequently used metric equivalents (p. 59) for more information on the metric system.

Step 1: Check the reference tables on p. 59 to determine the relationship between grams and milligrams.

$$1 \text{ g} = 1{,}000 \text{ mg}$$

Step 2: *Unknown* *Known*

$$\frac{4 \text{ g}}{\text{x mg}} = \frac{1 \text{ g}}{1{,}000 \text{ mg}}$$

$$\text{x} = 4{,}000 \text{ mg}$$

Step 3: Prove your answer by substituting 4,000 for x.

$$\frac{4}{4{,}000} = \frac{1}{1{,}000}$$

$$4{,}000 = 4{,}000$$

Conversion from one system to another

Example:
How many grains are in 4 grams?
Set up a proportion.

$$\frac{\text{Metric}}{\text{Apothecary}} = \frac{\text{Metric}}{\text{Apothecary}}$$

Step 1: Check the reference tables to determine the relationship between grains and grams.

$$15 \text{ gr} = 1 \text{ g}$$

Step 2: *Unknown* *Known*

$$\frac{4 \text{ g}}{\text{x gr}} = \frac{1 \text{ g}}{15 \text{ gr}}$$

$$\text{x} = 60 \text{ gr}$$

Step 3: Prove your answer by substituting 60 for x.

$$\frac{4}{60} = \frac{1}{15}$$

$$60 = 60$$

Since reference tables aren't always available, you should memorize at least the following approximate equivalents:

$$1 \text{ g} = \text{gr } \overline{\text{xv}} \text{ (15 grains)}$$
$$1 \text{ gr (gr } \dot{\overline{\text{i}}}) = 0.06 \text{ g or 60 mg}$$

In the apothecary system, tablets and capsules are usually available in ½, 1, 1½, 5, or 7½ grains. Therefore the preferable equivalent is one that provides an answer in terms of an available form.

Example:
How many grains are in 0.3 grams?
If you use the equivalent 1 g = gr $\overline{\text{xv}}$,

then 0.3 g = gr $\dot{\overline{\text{ivss}}}$, a dosage form that's not available.

Unknown		*Known*
$\frac{g}{gr}$	=	$\frac{g}{gr}$
$\frac{0.3\ g}{x\ gr}$	=	$\frac{1\ g}{15\ gr}$
x	=	4.5 or gr $\dot{\overline{\text{ivss}}}$

However, if you use the equivalent gr $\dot{\bar{\text{i}}}$ = 0.06 g, then 0.3 g = gr $\bar{\text{v}}$, a dosage form that's available.

Unknown		*Known*
$\frac{g}{gr}$	=	$\frac{g}{gr}$
$\frac{0.3\ g}{x\ gr}$	=	$\frac{0.06\ g}{1\ gr}$
0.06x	=	0.3
x	=	5 grains or gr $\bar{\text{v}}$

Determining the number of tablets or capsules to give

You can determine the number of tablets required for a specific amount of medication in two steps:

Within the same system

Example:
How many ampicillin capsules containing 250 mg each do you need to give 1 g?

Step 1: Convert the amount desired and the size of the tablet on hand into a common unit.

1 g = 1,000 mg

Step 2: Set up a proportion.

$$\frac{mg}{caps} = \frac{mg}{caps}$$

Unknown		*Known*
$\frac{1,000\ mg}{x\ capsules}$	=	$\frac{250\ mg}{1\ capsule}$
250 x	=	1,000
x	=	4 capsules

From one system to another

Example:
The doctor ordered gr $\dot{\overline{\text{iss}}}$ of a medication. The tablets available are 0.2 g each. How many tablets should be given?

Step 1: Convert size of the tablet on hand and amount desired into a common unit.

1 g	=	15 grains
$\frac{g}{gr}$	=	$\frac{g}{gr}$
$\frac{0.2\ g}{x\ gr}$	=	$\frac{1\ g}{15\ gr}$
x	=	0.2 × 15
x	=	3 gr in each tablet

Step 2: Set up a proportion according to the information given.

$$\frac{gr}{tablets} = \frac{gr}{tablets}$$

Unknown		*Known*
$\frac{1.5\ gr}{x\ tablets}$	=	$\frac{3\ gr}{1\ tablet}$
3x	=	1.5
x	=	0.5 or ½ tablet

Determining the amount of drug to give in oral solution

Medications in dry form, such as crystals and powders, must first be weighed and then mixed into a solution. You're responsible for giving the volume of solution that contains (by weight) the amount of drug ordered for the patient. Oral solutions are prepared in many different concentrations. Therefore, read the label carefully to determine the amount of drug according to volume. This information will always be indicated on the drug label.

One-ounce containers, such as the medicine cup, are generally used for administering oral medications. Most of these are calibrated in the three commonly used systems of measurement—metric, apothecary, and household. For measuring smaller units, minim glasses, medicine droppers, or syringes without needles may be used.

Calculating oral solutions

The method for calculating oral solutions is the same as for any other medication problem.

Example 1.

The doctor ordered phenobarbital elixir gr $\overline{xv}$. On hand is a bottle labeled 1 g/dram. How much medication should be given?

Step 1: Convert amount desired and solution on hand into a common unit.

$$1 \text{ g} = \text{gr } \overline{xv}$$

Step 2: Set up a proportion.

$$\frac{\text{drug}}{\text{solution}} = \frac{\text{drug}}{\text{solution}}$$

Unknown *Known*

$$\frac{15 \text{ gr}}{x \text{ ʒ}} = \frac{15 \text{ gr}}{1 \text{ ʒ}}$$

$$15x = 15$$

$$x = 1 \text{ ʒ}$$

Example 2.

The doctor ordered gr $\bar{\text{v}}$ of Tylenol elixir. On hand is a bottle labeled 120 mg/5 ml. How much medication should be given?

Step 1: Convert amount desired and solution on hand into a common unit.

$$\text{gr } \dot{\bar{\text{i}}} = 60 \text{ mg}$$

$$\text{gr } \bar{\text{v}} = 300 \text{ mg}$$

Step 2: Set up a proportion according to the information given.

$$\frac{\text{drug}}{\text{solution}} = \frac{\text{drug}}{\text{solution}}$$

Unknown *Known*

$$\frac{300 \text{ mg}}{x \text{ ml}} = \frac{120 \text{ mg}}{5 \text{ ml}}$$

$$120x = 1{,}500$$

$$x = 12.5 \text{ ml}$$

Determining the amount of drug to give by parenteral administration

Ampuls and vials of medication (in solution, crystals, or powder) are used for intradermal, subcutaneous, intramuscular, and intravenous injections. Medications that deteriorate in solution are dispensed in dry form; then diluent is added immediately before the med-

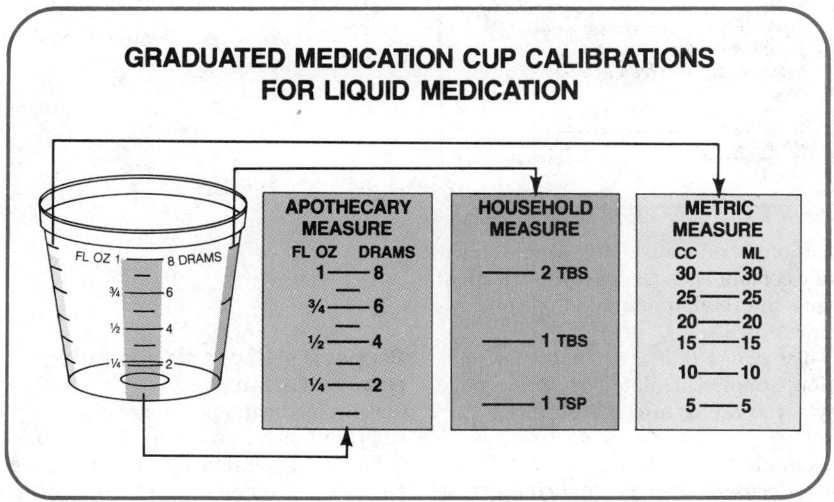

DRUG ERROR

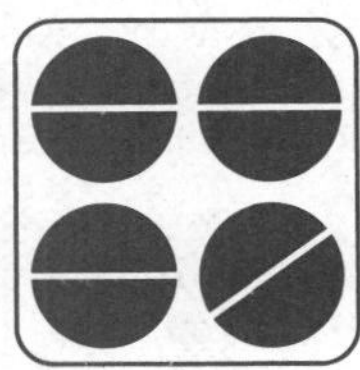

WATCH FOR MISPLACED DECIMAL POINTS

To eliminate confusion and ensure that your patient receives the best results from his drug therapy, watch for miscalculations and double-check illegible writing. These pitfalls are more common than you might think:

In a recent pediatric center study,* 1 out of every 12 doses computed by 95 registered nurses contained an error. Administering this inaccurate dose could have produced a serious drug error—a dose 10 times higher or lower than intended. Consider these cases:

- An infant became irritable and febrile after receiving 0.5 mg of atropine sulfate instead of the 0.05 mg that was ordered.
- Another infant developed digitalis intoxication when 0.09 mg of digoxin, instead of 0.009 mg, was administered.

Calculate doses carefully, write clearly, and follow these rules:

- *Always place a zero before a decimal point when referring to amounts less than 1; for example, 0.5 ml, not .5 ml.*
- *Don't use a zero when you have a round, whole number; for example, 2 mg, not 2.0 mg.*
- *Try to use fractions, not decimals, when expressing fractional doses; for example, 2½ ml, not 2.5 ml. Failure to see the decimal point can lead to a tenfold overdose.*

*Study results used with permission of Paul H. Peristein, MD, University of Cincinnati (Ohio) Medical Center.

ication is administered. Ampuls usually contain a single dose of medication; vials may contain either single or multiple doses.

For drugs that are already in solution, simply calculate dosage the same way you do for oral solutions.

Example 1.
The doctor ordered pentobarbital gr $\dot{\overline{\text{iss}}}$ I.M. On hand is a multiple-dose vial containing 40 mg/ml. How much medication should be given?

Step 1: Convert amount desired and solution on hand into a common unit.

$$\text{gr } \dot{\overline{\text{i}}} = 60 \text{ mg}$$

$$\text{gr } \dot{\overline{\text{iss}}} = 90 \text{ mg}$$

Step 2: Set up a proportion according to the information given.

$$\frac{\text{drug}}{\text{solution}} = \frac{\text{drug}}{\text{solution}}$$

$$\textit{Unknown} \quad \textit{Known}$$

$$\frac{90 \text{ mg}}{x \text{ ml}} = \frac{40 \text{ mg}}{1 \text{ ml}}$$

$$40x = 90$$

$$x = 2.25 \text{ ml}$$

Example 2.
The doctor ordered Thorazine 15 mg I.M. stat. On hand is a multiple-dose vial containing 25 mg/ml. How much medication should be given?

Step 1: No conversion necessary.

Step 2: Set up a proportion according to the information available.

$$\frac{\text{drug}}{\text{solution}} = \frac{\text{drug}}{\text{solution}}$$

$$\textit{Unknown} \quad \textit{Known}$$

$$\frac{15 \text{ mg}}{x \text{ ml}} = \frac{25 \text{ mg}}{1 \text{ ml}}$$

$$25x = 15$$

$$x = \frac{15}{25}$$

$$x = \frac{3}{5} \text{ ml or } 0.6 \text{ ml}$$

Preparing drugs that require reconstitution

Certain medications that are given parenterally, such as some antibiotics, are unstable in solution and therefore are packaged in crystal or powder form.

Before you administer these medications, you have to dissolve them in a correct diluent, such as sterile isotonic saline solution or bacteriostatic water. Use the same syringe to withdraw the diluent from one vial and add it to the vial or ampul containing the medication in dry form. If the entire amount of medication is to be administered, add enough diluent to dissolve the medication—at least 1 to 2 ml. This amount will vary with the type and amount of medication contained in the vial or ampul.

Directions for reconstituting are usually packaged with the medication; follow any specific directions included. Some medications are packaged by the manufacturer in "mix-o-vials," which contain the diluent in a sealed compartment within the neck of the vial. To make the solution, simply push the rubber stopper to remove the seal and then gently shake the vial.

With multiple-dose vials, if not otherwise specified, dissolve the medication in the amount of solution necessary to make 1 ml equal to the desired dose. Use this formula only when the amount of medication doesn't increase the amount of solution.

When the medication increases the amount of solution, follow the specific directions for the amount of diluent to be added. They will be packaged with the medication.

Example:
A vial contains 3 million units of aqueous penicillin G in dry powder. Your patient has an order for 300,000 units. How much sterile water would you add to the vial if specific directions haven't been included by the manufacturer?

Step 1: Set up a proportion with the information available.

$$\frac{\text{drug}}{\text{solution}} = \frac{\text{drug}}{\text{solution}}$$

$$\underset{\textit{Unknown}}{\frac{3{,}000{,}000 \text{ units}}{x \text{ ml}}} = \underset{\textit{Known}}{\frac{300{,}000 \text{ units}}{1 \text{ ml}}}$$

$$300{,}000x = 3{,}000{,}000$$

$$x = 10 \text{ ml added to the vial so that each ml contains } 300{,}000 \text{ units}$$

Whenever you reconstitute a medication in a multiple-dose vial, be sure to label it with the amount/ml as soon as it's prepared, and refrigerate the drug as required. Also, label the *date* and *time* that you reconstituted it. If it's not labeled, you have no way of knowing the concentration or expiration date of the solution.

Generally, directions for adding the correct amount of solution to make a specific concentration will be included with the medication. For a drug like penicillin for injection, several concentrations can be produced from the same vial of powder by adding different quantities of solution.

Example:
Penicillin G sodium for injection can be reconstituted as follows:

Amount of diluent to be added	*Concentration made*
23 ml	200,000 units/ml
18 ml	250,000 units/ml
8 ml	500,000 units/ml
3 ml	1,000,000 units/ml

Remember, label the vial *immediately* after reconstitution!

Administering insulin

Insulin is dispensed in different strengths indicating the number of units of insulin in 1 ml of solution. For example, U-40 has 40 units in every ml, and U-100 has 100 units in every ml.

The most accurate way to administer insulin is to use an insulin syringe calibrated in units per ml. Syringes are available in the scale U-100 as well as U-40. To draw up the correct dosage, use correlating insulin vials and syringes. When an insulin syringe isn't available, you may use a tuberculin syringe. Since you know the strength of insulin you are using (for example, U-40 contains 40 units/ml), use the formula for calculating any other parenteral medication.

Example:
You have an order to give 20 units of U-40 insulin, but you do not have an insulin syringe. How much medication must be given?

Set up a proportion using the information available.

$$\frac{\text{units}}{\text{ml}} = \frac{\text{units}}{\text{ml}}$$

Unknown *Known*

$$\frac{20\text{ units}}{x\text{ ml}} = \frac{40\text{ units}}{1\text{ ml}}$$

$$40x = 20$$

$$x = 0.5\text{ ml}$$

Administering I.V. fluids

When administering I.V. fluids, you must calculate and regulate the number of drops per minute to administer a prescribed amount of solution in a designated period of time. Maintaining proper flow rates for prescribed solutions is essential to prevent complications.

I.V. administration sets are constructed to deliver a specific number of drops per milliliter. This is called the drop factor, and can be found on the package containing the set.

Example:

10 drops/ml—Baxter (Travenol)
13 drops/ml—McGaw
15 drops/ml—Abbott
20 drops/ml—Cutter; IVAC
60 drops/ml—microdrip

Example:
The doctor ordered 1,000 ml of 5% dextrose in water to be infused in 8 hours. What is the rate of infusion?

Step 1: Convert hours into minutes, since you will need to figure drops/minute.

$$8 \times 60 = 480\text{ minutes}$$

Step 2: Set up a proportion using the available information.

$$\frac{\text{minute}}{\text{ml}} = \frac{\text{minute}}{\text{ml}}$$

Unknown *Known*

$$\frac{1\text{ minute}}{x\text{ ml}} = \frac{480\text{ minutes}}{1{,}000\text{ ml}}$$

$$480x = 1{,}000$$

$$x = 2.1\text{ ml/minute}$$

Next, calculate the number of drops/minute:

- Note the number of drops/ml the I.V. set you have delivers (10, 13, 15, 20, or 60).
- Convert the number of milliliters to drops by multiplying the two figures.

Examples:
Baxter set 10 drops/ml
2.1 ml/minute × 10 drops/ml = 21 drops/minute
Abbott set 15 drops/ml
2.1 ml/minute × 15 drops/ml = 32 drops/minute

Short formula for determining rate of infusion

$$\frac{\text{volume of solution}}{\text{time interval in minutes}} \times \text{drop factor} = \text{drops/minute}$$

$$\frac{1{,}000}{480}\ (= 2.1\text{ ml/minute}) \times 15\ (\text{Abbott}) = 32$$

Sometimes the doctor specifies the volume of I.V. solution to be infused each hour. In this case, use the hourly volume, not the container volume.

Example:
The orders read, "Give 500 ml 5% dextrose in water at 50 ml/hour." The drop factor of your I.V. microdrip set is 60 drops/ml.

$$\frac{\text{volume of solution}}{\text{time interval in minutes}} \times \text{drop factor} = \text{drops/minute}$$

$$\frac{50}{60} \times 60 = 50\text{ drops/minute}$$

DOLORES H. HECKENBERGER, RN, MS

FLOW RATE CONVERTERS

Here's what a standard I.V. flow rate converter might look like. Available from I.V. fluid manufacturers, these make flow rate determinations fast and easy.

Note that the drop factor for this set is listed at the bottom of the chart (15 drops = 1 ml).

STANDARD I.V. SET CONVERSION CHART

Drops per minute	Approximate volume infused in ml* per time interval				
	30 min	1 hr	2 hr	4 hr	8 hr
5	10	20	40	80	160
10	20	40	80	160	320
20	40	80	160	320	640
30	60	120	240	480	960
40	80	160	320	640	1,280
50	100	200	400	800	1,600
60	120	240	480	960	1,920
70	140	280	560	1,120	2,240
80	160	320	640	1,280	2,560
90	180	360	720	1,440	2,880
100	200	400	800	1,600	3,200
110	220	440	880	1,760	3,520
120	240	480	960	1,920	3,840
125	250	500	1,000	2,000	4,000

Approximately 15 drops = 1 ml

*Actual flow rate may vary as much as ± 10% with the following factors: viscosity of solution head pressure; rate of infusion; patient venous pressure; variation of drip orifice; patient position.

Note: Drip rates should be monitored periodically and control clamp adjustments made.

Adapted from American McGaw, Division of American Hospital Supply Corporation, Irvine, Calif.

6 Understanding intravenous solution compatibility

Administering medications by the parenteral route is common today. When medications are given parenterally on an intermittent basis, they're best administered using the piggyback method, a volume control burette, or an intermittent infusion device (heparin lock). Thus, you avoid multiple venipunctures and possible incompatibilities when adding medications to a large-volume parenteral solution. However, sometimes you *must* administer medications through a single I.V. line or give more than one medication at a time in a single solution. Whenever a drug is given I.V., you risk incompatibility—an undesired physical or chemical reaction between a drug and a solution or another drug.

Factors affecting compatibility

Many things influence the stability and compatibility of medications—some controllable and some not. Understanding these factors will help you administer I.V. medications more safely and accurately.

- *Concentration of drug:* For a chemical or physical reaction to occur, drugs must come into contact with one another. The higher the concentration of each drug mixed, the greater the chance for ion interaction, which produces incompatibility or instability. Proper dilution of drugs helps minimize this risk.
- *Length of time in solution:* Chemical reactions aren't necessarily instantaneous; reaction rates vary. For example, a reaction may occur in less than 1 second or after many days. However, the longer two drugs remain in contact with each other, the more likely a potential reaction will lead to an undesirable result. Minimize the time that drugs are in solution by mixing them just before administration.
- *Temperature:* A drug usually remains stable at a low temperature. Reaction rates double for each 10° C. (18° F.) rise in temperature. Many antibiotics in solution are four to eight times more stable under refrigeration (5° C. [41° F.]) than at room temperature (20° to 25° C. [68° to 77° F.]). Refrigerated antibiotics usually may be used for longer periods than those stored at room temperature. Check manufacturer's information or ask the pharmacist if the drug can be refrigerated.
- *pH:* A drug added to a solution may change the solution's pH or the drug's stability. For example, many antibiotics lose stability in alkaline (pH above 8.0) or acidic (pH below 4.0) solutions. Some solutions decompose if you add an alkaline drug like calcium, which causes the pH to exceed 7.0.

Physical incompatibility

A drug's physicochemical properties can cause solubility problems that visibly alter the solution: for example, precipitation, altered color, gas formation, turbidity, or cloudiness. Such changes are produced by physical or chemical reactions involving the drug's pH, the solvent, and the container holding the admixture.

USING A PIGGYBACK SET

When you can't mix a drug with the primary I.V. solution, one alternative is to use a piggyback set for intermittent solution delivery, as shown here.

The piggyback set includes a small I.V. bottle, short tubing, and usually a macro-drip system. This set connects into the primary line's upper Y-port, also called the piggyback port.

Use an extension hook to position the primary I.V. container at a lower level than the piggyback container. When the piggyback solution's incompatible with the primary solution, be sure to flush the primary I.V. line with saline solution before starting the piggyback solution and then again before restarting the primary solution.

Troubleshooting intermittent solution delivery

Problems can occur when you're administering a drug intermittently with the primary I.V. solution. To avoid them:

- Double-check the drip rate, and make sure the solution's running as calculated.
- Make sure the solution is clear. If a precipitate's forming in the bottle or tubing, you may have reconstituted the medication incorrectly, or a physical incompatibility reaction may be occurring. Discontinue the delivery and notify the pharmacist.
- Make sure that none of the junction sites are leaking. Check the piggyback port. Have you accidentally punctured the primary tubing with the secondary needle? Even if everything appears in working order, periodically double-check the entire set. If the patient moves, for example, he may dislodge a connection, disrupting his treatment.

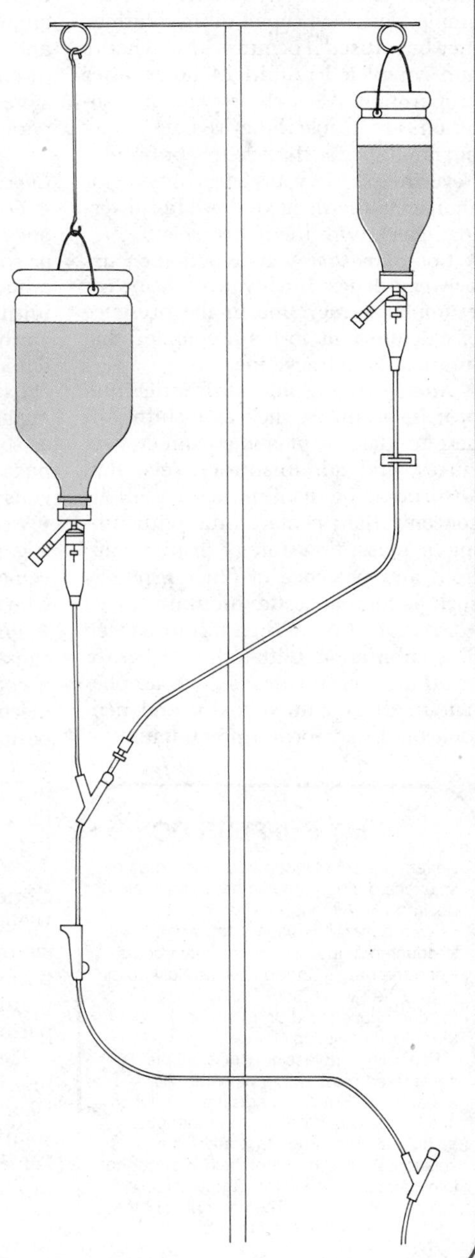

Physical incompatibility reactions

- *Color change:* Especially with cephalosporins and phenothiazines, color change or darkening may or may not indicate chemical breakdown. For example, darkened cephalothin solutions may be infused if begun within 6 hours and completed within 24 hours after preparation. Also, chlorpromazine solutions are usable if they're pale yellow but not if they're dark yellow or brown. Nevertheless, if you detect any color change in the drug you're administering, check with the pharmacist.
- *Complexation:* This reaction occurs between drugs, inactivating them. For example, tetracycline in the presence of calcium ions forms a complex that inhibits the tetracycline.
- *Adsorption:* Some antibiotics and protein products, such as insulin, adhere to glass or plastic containers, syringes, and administration sets. But, *ad*sorption of insulin varies with its concentration; contact time with tubing or glass; flow rate of insulin solution; and presence of other proteins, such as human serum albumin.
- *Precipitation:* When administered in combination with other drugs or solutions, certain drugs such as phenytoin, diazepam, digoxin, and pentobarbital may form a precipitate.

WHAT BUFFERS DO

Buffers are substances added to drugs or solutions during manufacture to maintain a desired pH. Although a drug may have its own buffer, it is usually too weak to counteract the pH change that occurs when the drug's added to a strongly acidic or alkaline I.V. solution. This change in pH can cause the drug to separate from the primary solution.

Penicillin G potassium, for example, is considered most stable between pH 6.0 and 7.0. But if you add it to a solution of 5% dextrose in water, along with other highly buffered drugs that make the solution alkaline (amphotericin B or cephalothin solution), penicillin G potassium rapidly deteriorates. The ideal pH of I.V. fluids is about 7.4, the pH of blood.

Chemical incompatibility

Chemical incompatibility causes a drug to degrade to a therapeutically inactive or toxic product. This irreversible breakdown isn't always visible: an example is the interaction of gentamicin and carbenicillin, and ampicillin sodium mixed in 5% dextrose in water stored for 4 hours or more at room temperature before administration.

Chemical incompatibility reactions

- *Oxidation:* A loss of electrons from one drug to another may turn the drug or solution pink, red, brown, or some other color, and make it therapeutically inactive. This reaction occurs especially with epinephrine, morphine, dopamine, and isoproterenol. The risk of oxidation can be minimized by adding an antioxidant (a preservative, such as sodium bisulfite) to the drug, or by packaging the drug in amber glass vials or ampuls.
- *Reduction:* A drug is reduced when it gains electrons from another drug. Penicillins, for example, are reduced when combined with other drugs.
- *Photolysis:* Exposure to light can cause hydrolysis (chemical splitting of a compound by water) or oxidation, discoloring the solution. Photolysis can be minimized in light-sensitive products such as nitroprusside by packaging them in amber glass and covering the container with aluminum foil during administration.

General guidelines

Whenever possible, administer medications separately. To minimize incompatibilities, use a heparin lock to infuse multiple doses of a drug that's incompatible with other parenteral drugs.

If several incompatible drugs must be infused through the same I.V. line, clear the tubing between doses with a solution compatible with each drug. For example, you may have an order to administer phenytoin I.V. to a patient receiving an infusion of 5% dextrose in one-half normal saline solution ($D_5\frac{1}{2}$ NS); the two are incompatible.

ABBREVIATIONS FOR I.V. SOLUTIONS

AA	Amino acids
D	Dextrose solution (percentage unspecified)
D5LR	Dextrose 5% in Ringer's injection, lactated
D5R	Dextrose 5% in Ringer's injection
D-S	Dextrose-saline combinations
D2.5½NS	Dextrose 2.5% in sodium chloride 0.45%
D2.5NS	Dextrose 2.5% in sodium chloride 0.9%
D5¼NS	Dextrose 5% in sodium chloride 0.225%
D5½NS	Dextrose 5% in sodium chloride 0.45%
D5NS	Dextrose 5% in sodium chloride 0.9%
D10NS	Dextrose 10% in sodium chloride 0.9%
D5W	Dextrose 5% in water
D10W	Dextrose 10% in water
DXN-NS	Dextran 6% in sodium chloride 0.9%
IS	Invert sugar
LR	Ringer's injection, lactated
NS	Sodium chloride 0.9%
PH	Protein hydrolysate
R	Ringer's injection
TPN	Total parenteral nutrition
W	Sterile water for injection

First stop the D_5½ NS, then clear the tubing with normal saline solution, administer the phenytoin, clear the tubing again with the normal saline solution, and finally restart the flow of D_5½ NS.

When medications must be administered concurrently or mixed in the same large-volume parenteral solution, refer to the *Intravenous Solution Compatibilities* chart on the next page, and the following guidelines:

- Chemical analogs or families of drugs react similarly. If one drug in a class is incompatible with the desired solution, others in this class may be incompatible too.
- When preparing a drug, follow manufacturer's instructions meticulously because the preservatives used in some diluents may be incompatible with the drug. For example, bacteriostatic normal saline solution contains benzyl alcohol, which is incompatible with a drug such as chloramphenicol sodium succinate.
- When reconstituting I.V. drugs and inspecting for a precipitate, don't shake the container; rotate or swirl it instead. This action prevents air bubble entrapment and foaming, which impair accurate drug dose measurement in syringes and trigger air exclusion alarms when solutions are administered by infusion pump. Also, air bubbles may be mistaken for particles in the solution.
- When reconstituting a drug, thoroughly mix it before administering or adding it to a solution.
- When mixing drugs in a large-volume parenteral solution, add one drug at a time; then mix and examine the solution before adding other drugs. Thorough mixing before adding other drugs prevents layering. Also, avoid adding more than two drugs whenever possible.
- Chemical reactions depend on concentration. Minimize these reactions by adding the most concentrated or most soluble drug to the large-volume parenteral solution first.
- Some precipitates are too fine or too clear to be detected, or are the same

INTRAVENOUS SOLUTION COMPATIBILITIES

Physical compatibility does not exclude the possibility of therapeutic incompatibility.

	albumin	amikacin	aminophylline	amino acid injection	amphotericin B	ampicillin	calcium gluconate	carbenicillin	cefamandole	cefazolin	cefoxitin	cephalothin	chloramphenicol	cimetidine	clindamycin	corticotropin (ACTH)	dexamethasone	dextrose 5% in water	dextrose 5% in lactated Ringer's	dextrose 5% in 0.45% NaCl	dextrose 5% in 0.9% NaCl	diazepam	diazoxide	diphenhydramine
albumin	X	○	○	○		○	○	○	○	○	○	○	○	○	○	○	○	C	C	C	C	●	NR	○
amikacin	○	X	8	○		●	24	8	NR	8	NR	●	24	24	24	○	●	24	24	24	24	●	NR	24
aminophylline	○	8	X	24		●	C	○	○	○	○	●	○	●	●	●	C	C	C	C	C	●	NR	C
amino acid injection	○	○	24	X		12	24	24	○	24	○	24	1	24	24	○	○	C	C	C	C	●	NR	○
amphotericin B						**T**	**O**		**B**	**E**		**P**	**R**	**E**	**P**	**A**	**R**	**E**	**D**		**B**	**Y**		**P**
ampicillin	○	●	●	●		X	●	●	○	○	○	○	1	C	●	○	○	2	4	4	4	●	NR	○
calcium gluconate	○	24	C	24		●	X	C	●	●	○	●	C	○	●	C	C	C	C	C	C	●	NR	C
carbenicillin	○	8	C	24		●	C	X	○	C	○	○	●	○	24	○	○	C	C	C	C	●	NR	○
cefamandole	○	NR	○	○		○	●	○	X	○	○	○	○	○	○	○	○	C	C	C	C	●	NR	○
cefazolin	○	8	○	24		○	●	C	○	X	○	○	24	24	○	○	C	C	C	C	C	●	NR	○
cefoxitin	○	NR	○	○		○	○	○	○	○	X	○	○	○	○	○	○	C	C	C	C	●	NR	○
cephalothin	○	●	●	24		○	●	○	○	○	○	X	C	24	24	○	○	C	C	C	C	●	NR	●
chloramphenicol	○	24	○	○	**T**	1	C	●	○	24	○	C	X	○	○	C	C	C	C	C	C	●	NR	C
cimetidine	○	24	●	24	**O**	C	●	○	○	24	○	24	○	X	24	24	○	C	C	C	C	●	NR	○
clindamycin	○	24	●	24		○	○	24	○	○	○	24	○	24	X	○	○	C	C	C	C	●	NR	○
corticotropin (ACTH)	○	○	●	○	**B**	●	C	○	○	○	○	○	C	○	○	X	○	C	C	C	C	●	NR	○
dexamethasone	○	●	●	○	**E**	○	C	○	○	C	○	○	C	○	○	○	X	C	C	C	C	●	NR	●
dextrose 5% in water	C	24	C	C		2	C	C	C	C	C	C	C	C	C	C	C	X	○	○	○	●	NR	C
dextrose 5% in lactated Ringer's	C	24	C	C	**P**	4	C	C	C	C	C	C	C	C	C	C	C	○	X	○	○	●	NR	C
dextrose 5% in 0.45% NaCl	C	24	C	C	**R**	4	C	C	C	C	C	C	C	C	C	C	C	○	○	X	○	●	NR	C
dextrose 5% in 0.9% NaCl	C	24	C	C	**E**	4	C	C	C	C	C	C	C	C	C	C	C	○	○	○	X	●	NR	C
diazepam	●	●	●	●	**P**	●	●	●	●	●	●	●	●	●	●	●	●	●	●	●	●	X	●	●
diazoxide	NR	NR	NR	NR	**A**	NR	NR	NR	NR	NR	NR	NR	NR	NR	NR	NR	NR	NR	NR	NR	NR	●	X	NR
diphenhydramine	○	24	C	○	**R**	○	C	○	○	○	○	●	C	○	○	○	●	C	C	C	C	●	NR	X
dopamine	○	○	●	24	**E**	●	24	24	○	○	○	6	24	○	○	○	○	C	C	C	C	●	NR	○
epinephrine	○	24	●	○	**D**	○	●	●	○	○	○	●	●	○	○	○	○	C	C	C	C	●	NR	○
erythromycin (I.V.) lactobionate	○	●	C	24		●	C	●	○	●	○	●	●	NR	○	C	○	C	C	C	C	●	NR	24
fat emulsion 10% & 20%	○	●	●	●	**B**	●	●	●	●	●	●	●	●	●	●	●	●	●	●	●	●	●	●	●
gentamicin	○	NR	NR	24	**Y**	●	NR	●	NR	NR	NR	●	●	24	24	NR	NR	C	C	C	C	●	NR	NR
heparin sodium	○	●	C	24		●	C	○	○	○	○	8	C	○	24	24	4	C	C	C	C	●	NR	○
hydrocortisone Na succinate	○	○	C	○	**P**	C	C	24	○	○	○	24	C	○	24	24	4	C	C	C	C	●	NR	●
insulin (regular)	○	○	●	24	**H**	○	○	○	○	○	○	8	○	24	○	○	○	○	○	○	○	●	NR	○
isoproterenol	○	○	●	24	**A**	○	C	○	○	○	○	C	○	○	○	○	○	C	C	C	C	●	NR	○
kanamycin	○	○	C	C	**R**	●	●	●	○	●	24	●	C	○	24	○	C	C	C	C	C	●	NR	○
lactated Ringer's	C	○	C	C	**M**	8	C	C	C	C	C	C	C	C	C	C	NR	○	○	○	○	●	NR	C
levarterenol (norepinephrine)	○	24	●	24	**A**	○	C	○	○	○	○	●	○	○	○	C	○	C	C	C	C	●	NR	○
lidocaine	○	○	C	24	**C**	●	C	C	C	○	○	●	C	○	○	○	C	C	C	C	C	●	NR	C
metaraminol	○	24	○	24	**Y**	●	○	○	○	○	○	C	C	○	○	○	●	C	C	C	C	●	NR	●
methicillin	○	●	C	24		●	C	○	○	○	○	●	1	○	○	C	C	6	6	6	6	●	NR	C
methylprednisolone	○	○	6	24	**O**	○	●	○	○	○	○	●	C	○	24	○	○	C	C	C	C	●	NR	●
miconazole	○	NR	NR	NR	**N**	NR	NR	NR	NR	NR	NR	NR	NR	NR	NR	NR	NR	C	NR	NR	NR	●	NR	NR
multiple vitamin infusion (MVI)	○	○	○	C	**L**	○	C	○	○	C	24	○	○	○	24	○	○	C	C	C	C	●	NR	○
nafcillin	○	○	12	○	**Y**	●	○	○	○	○	○	○	C	○	○	○	C	C	C	C	C	●	NR	C
nitroprusside	○	NR	NR	NR		NR	NR	NR	NR	NR	NR	NR	NR	NR	NR	NR	NR	C	NR	NR	NR	●	NR	NR
0.9% NSS	C	24	C	C		8	C	C	C	C	C	C	C	C	C	C	C	○	○	○	○	●	NR	C
oxacillin	○	8	●	24		●	○	○	○	C	○	●	●	○	○	○	○	C	C	C	C	●	NR	○
oxytocin	○	○	○	○		○	○	○	○	C	○	○	C	○	○	○	○	C	C	C	C	●	NR	○
penicillin G	○	8	●	24		●	C	○	○	C	○	●	C	24	24	C	C	C	C	C	C	●	NR	C
phenytoin	●	●	●	●		●	●	●	●	●	●	●	●	●	●	●	●	●	●	●	●	●	●	●
phytonadione	○	24	●	24		●	○	○	○	○	○	●	C	○	○	○	C	C	C	C	C	●	NR	C
polymyxin B	○	24	○	○		●	○	●	○	●	○	●	●	○	○	○	○	C	NR	NR	NR	●	NR	C
potassium chloride	○	4	C	24		C	C	24	○	C	○	C	C	24	24	C	4	C	C	C	C	●	NR	○
procainamide	○	NR	C	○		○	C	○	○	○	○	○	C	○	○	○	○	C	○	○	○	●	NR	C
sodium bicarbonate	○	24	C	○		○	●	24	○	○	24	C	C	C	24	●	○	C	C	C	C	●	NR	○
tetracycline	○	8	●	24		●	●	●	○	●	○	●	●	○	○	C	C	C	C	C	C	●	NR	C
thiamine	○	○	○	○		○	○	○	○	○	○	○	○	○	○	○	○	C	C	C	C	●	NR	○
ticarcillin	○	●	○	○		●	○	○	○	○	○	○	○	○	○	○	○	C	C	C	C	●	NR	○
tobramycin	○	○	○	○		○	●	●	NR	●	NR	●	○	○	●	○	○	C	C	C	C	●	NR	○
vancomycin	○	24	●	○		○	●	○	○	○	○	○	●	○	○	C	●	C	C	C	C	●	NR	C
vitamin B complex with C	○	24	●	○		●	C	●	○	C	24	C	●	24	24	C	4	C	C	C	C	●	NR	C

Key: **C** = Compatible ● = Incompatible **NR** = Not recommended by the manufacturer

dopamine	epinephrine	erythromycin lactobionate	fat emulsion 10% & 20%	gentamicin	heparin sodium	hydrocortisone Na succinate	insulin (regular)	isoproterenol	kanamycin	lactated Ringer's	levarterenol (norepinephrine)	lidocaine	metaraminol	methicillin	methylprednisolone	miconazole	multiple vitamin infusion (MVI)	nafcillin	nitroprusside	0.9% NSS	oxacillin	oxytocin	penicillin G	phenytoin	phytonadione	polymyxin B	potassium chloride	procainamide	sodium bicarbonate	tetracycline	thiamine	ticarcillin	tobramycin	vancomycin	vitamin B complex with C
○	○	○	○	○	○	○	○	○	○	C	○	○	○	○	○	○	○	○	○	C	○	○	○	●	○	○	○	○	○	○	○	○	○	○	○
●	24	●	●	○	●	○	○	○	○	○	24	○	24	●	○	NR	○	○	NR	24	8	○	8	●	24	24	4	NR	24	8	○	●	○	24	24
○	●	C	●	NR	C	C	●	●	C	C	●	C	○	C	6	NR	○	12	NR	C	●	○	●	●	●	○	C	C	C	●	○	○	○	●	●
24	○	24	●	24	24	○	24	24	C	C	24	24	24	24	24	NR	C	○	NR	C	24	○	24	●	24	○	24	○	○	24	○	○	○	○	○
H	A	R	M	A	C	Y		O	N	L	Y																								
●	○	●	●	●	●	C	○	○	●	8	○	●	●	●	○	NR	○	●	NR	8	●	○	●	●	●	●	C	○	○	●	○	●	○	○	●
24	●	C	●	NR	C	C	○	C	●	C	C	C	○	C	●	NR	C	○	NR	C	○	○	C	●	○	○	C	C	●	●	○	○	●	●	C
24	●	●	●	●	○	24	○	○	●	C	○	C	○	○	○	NR	○	○	NR	C	○	○	○	●	○	●	24	○	24	●	○	○	●	○	●
○	○	○	●	NR	○	○	○	○	○	C	○	C	○	○	○	NR	○	○	NR	C	○	○	○	●	○	○	○	○	○	○	○	○	NR	○	○
○	○	●	●	NR	○	○	○	○	●	C	○	○	○	○	○	NR	C	○	NR	C	C	C	C	●	○	●	C	○	○	●	○	○	●	○	C
○	○	○	●	NR	○	○	○	○	24	C	○	○	○	○	○	NR	24	○	NR	C	○	○	○	●	○	○	○	○	24	○	○	○	NR	○	24
6	●	●	●	●	8	24	8	C	●	C	●	●	C	●	●	NR	○	○	NR	C	●	○	●	●	●	●	C	○	C	●	○	○	●	○	C
24	○	●	●	●	C	C	○	○	C	C	●	C	C	1	C	NR	○	C	NR	C	●	C	C	●	C	●	C	C	C	●	○	○	○	●	●
○	○	NR	●	24	○	○	24	○	○	C	○	○	○	○	○	NR	○	○	NR	C	○	○	24	●	○	○	24	○	C	○	○	○	○	○	24
○	○	○	●	24	24	24	○	○	24	C	○	○	○	○	24	NR	24	○	NR	C	○	○	24	●	○	○	24	○	24	○	○	○	●	○	24
○	○	○	●	NR	24	24	○	○	○	C	C	○	○	C	○	NR	○	○	NR	C	○	○	C	●	○	○	C	○	●	C	○	○	○	C	C
○	○	○	●	NR	4	4	○	○	C	○	NR	C	●	C	○	NR	○	C	NR	C	○	○	C	●	C	○	4	○	○	C	○	○	○	●	4
C	C	C	●	C	C	C	○	C	C	○	C	C	C	6	C	C	C	C	NR	○	C	C	C	●	C	C	C	C	C	C	C	C	C	C	C
C	C	C	●	C	C	C	○	C	C	○	C	C	C	6	C	NR	C	C	NR	○	C	C	C	●	C	NR	C	○	C	C	C	C	C	C	C
C	C	C	●	C	C	C	○	C	C	○	C	C	C	6	C	NR	C	C	NR	○	C	C	C	●	C	NR	C	○	C	C	C	C	C	C	C
C	C	C	●	C	C	C	○	C	C	○	C	C	C	6	C	NR	C	C	NR	○	C	C	C	●	C	NR	C	○	C	C	C	C	C	C	C
●	●	●	●	●	●	●	●	●	●	●	●	●	●	●	●	●	●	●	●	●	●	●	●	●	●	●	●	●	●	●	●	●	●	●	●
NR	NR	NR	●	NR	NR	NR	NR	NR	NR	NR	NR	NR	NR	NR	NR	NR	NR	NR	NR	NR	NR	NR	NR	NR	NR	NR	NR	NR	NR	NR	NR	NR	NR	NR	NR
○	○	24	●	NR	○	●	○	○	○	C	○	C	●	C	●	NR	○	C	NR	C	○	○	C	●	C	C	○	C	○	C	○	○	○	C	C
X	○	○	●	6	24	○	○	○	24	C	○	24	○	○	18	NR	○	○	NR	C	24	○	6	●	○	○	24	○	●	24	○	○	○	○	○
○	X	○	●	NR	○	○	○	○	○	C	○	2	C	○	○	NR	○	○	NR	C	●	○	●	●	●	○	○	○	●	●	○	○	○	●	●
○	○	X	●	NR	●	C	○	○	○	C	○	C	●	C	○	NR	●	○	NR	C	○	○	C	●	○	C	C	○	24	●	●	○	○	○	●
●	●	●	X	●	●	●	●	●	●	●	●	●	●	●	●	●	●	●	●	●	●	●	●	●	●	●	●	●	●	●	●	●	●	●	●
6	NR	NR	●	X	●	NR	NR	NR	NR	C	NR	C	NR	NR	NR	NR	NR	●	NR	C	●	NR	NR	NR	NR	NR	NR	NR	NR	NR	NR	●	NR	NR	●
24	○	●	●	●	X	●	○	8	●	C	●	8	●	●	C	NR	○	C	NR	C	○	○	●	●	●	●	C	C	○	●	○	○	●	●	C
18	○	C	●	NR	●	X	8	○	●	C	C	C	●	●	4	NR	○	●	NR	C	○	○	C	●	○	○	C	C	C	●	○	○	○	●	C
○	○	○	●	NR	○	8	X	○	○	○	○	●	○	○	●	NR	○	○	NR	C	○	○	●	●	○	○	C	●	●	○	○	○	○	○	C
○	○	○	●	NR	8	○	○	X	○	C	○	●	○	○	○	NR	C	○	NR	C	○	○	○	●	○	○	C	○	●	C	○	○	○	○	C
24	○	○	●	NR	●	●	○	○	X	C	○	○	C	●	○	NR	●	NR	NR	C	NR	○	C	●	○	C	○	○	○	C	●	●	NR	NR	●
C	C	C	●	C	C	C	○	C	C	X	C	C	●	6	C	NR	C	C	NR	○	C	C	C	●	C	NR	C	○	C	C	C	C	C	C	C
○	○	○	●	NR	●	C	○	○	○	C	X	●	●	●	C	NR	C	C	NR	NR	●	●	●	●	○	○	C	○	●	●	○	○	C	○	C
24	2	C	●	C	8	C	●	●		C	●	X	C	○	○	NR	○	○	NR	C	○	○	C	●	○	○	C	○	●	C	○	○	○	○	C
○	C	●	●	NR	●	●	○	○	C	●	●	C	X	●	●	NR	●	●	NR	C	●	C	●	●	●	○	C	C	C	C	○	○	○	C	●
○	○	C	●	NR	●	●	○	○	●	6	●	○	●	X	○	NR	○	○	NR	6	○	○	●	●	●	C	C	NR	●	●	○	○	○	●	●
18	○	○	●	NR	C	4	●	○	○	C	C	○	●	○	X	NR	○	●	NR	C	○	○	●	●	○	○	C	○	C	●	○	C	○	○	●
NR	NR	NR	●	NR	NR	NR	NR	NR	NR	NR	NR	NR	NR	NR	NR	X	NR	NR	NR	C	NR	NR	NR	●	NR	NR	NR	NR	NR	NR	NR	NR	NR	NR	NR
○	○	●	●	NR	○	○	○	C	●	C	C	○	●	○	○	NR	X	○	NR	C	○	○	4	●	○	○	C	○	○	●	○	○	○	○	○
○	○	○	●	●	C	●	○	○	○	C	C	○	●	○	●	NR	○	X	NR	C	○	○	○	●	○	○	C	○	C	●	○	○	●	○	●
NR	NR	NR	●	NR	NR	NR	NR	NR	NR	NR	NR	NR	NR	NR	NR	NR	NR	NR	X	NR	NR	NR	NR	●	NR	NR	NR	NR	NR	NR	NR	NR	NR	NR	NR
C	C	C	●	C	C	C	C	C	C	○	NR	C	C	6	C	C	C	C	NR	X	C	C	C	●	C	C	C	○	C	C	C	C	C	C	C
24	●	○	●	●	○	○	○	○	NR	C	●	○	●	○	○	NR	○	○	NR	C	X	○	●	●	●	○	C	○	○	●	○	○	○	○	●
○	○	○	●	NR	○	○	○	○	○	C	●	○	C	○	○	NR	○	○	NR	C	○	X	C	●	C	○	○	○	○	C	○	○	○	○	○
6	●	C	●	NR	●	C	●	○	C	C	●	C	●	●	●	NR	4	○	NR	C	●	C	X	●	C	●	C	C	●	●	○	○	●	●	●
●	●	●	●	●	●	●	●	●	●	●	●	●	●	●	●	●	●	●	●	●	●	●	●	X	●	●	●	●	●	●	●	●	●	●	●
○	●	○	●	NR	●	○	○	○	NR	C	○	○	●	●	○	NR	○	○	NR	C	●	C	C	●	X	○	○	○	○	○	○	○	○	●	○
○	○	C	●	NR	●	C	○	○	C	○	○	○	○	C	○	NR	○	○	NR	C	○	○	●	●	○	X	○	○	○	●	○	○	○	○	C
24	○	C	●	NR	C	C	C	C	○	C	C	C	C	C	C	NR	C	C	NR	C	C	○	C	●	○	○	X	○	○	C	○	○	○	○	C
○	○	○	●	NR	C	C	●	○	○	○	○	○	C	NR	○	NR	○	○	NR	○	○	○	C	●	○	○	○	X	○	C	○	○	○	C	C
●	●	24	●	NR	○	C	●	●	○	C	●	●	C	●	C	NR	○	C	NR	C	○	○	●	●	○	○	○	○	X	●	○	○	○	●	●
24	●	●	●	NR	●	●	○	C	C	C	●	C	C	●	●	NR	●	●	NR	C	●	C	●	●	○	●	C	○	●	X	○	○	○	○	●
○	○	●	●	NR	○	○	○	○	●	C	○	○	○	○	○	NR	○	○	NR	C	○	○	○	●	○	○	○	○	○	○	X	○	○	○	C
○	○	○	●	●	○	○	○	○	●	C	○	○	○	○	C	NR	○	○	NR	C	○	○	○	●	○	○	○	○	○	○	○	X	●	○	○
○	○	○	●	NR	●	○	○	○	NR	C	○	○	○	○	○	NR	○	●	NR	C	○	○	●	●	○	○	○	○	○	○	○	●	X	○	○
○	●	○	●	NR	●	●	○	○	NR	C	○	○	C	●	○	NR	○	○	NR	C	○	○	●	●	●	○	C	C	●	○	○	○	○	X	●
○	●	●	●	●	C	C	C	C	●	C	C	C	●	●	●	NR	○	●	NR	C	●	○	●	●	○	C	C	C	●	●	C	○	○	●	X

○ = Data unavailable **2, 4, 8, 24** = Compatible only for the number of hours indicated **X** = Identical drug

COPING WITH INCOMPATIBILITIES WHEN USING I.V. BOLUS

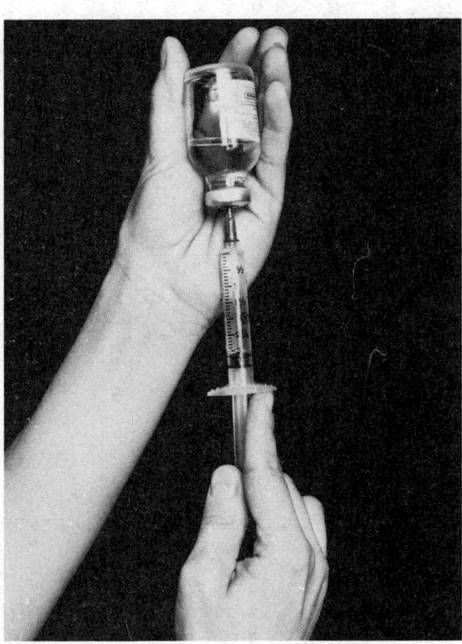

If the drug you're administering as an I.V. bolus injection is incompatible with the primary solution, you may follow these steps:

- Mix the drug with a diluent, and draw it up into a syringe. Then, draw saline solution into two other syringes.

  Important: This procedure does not apply when you're administering diazepam (Valium) or chlordiazepoxide (Librium); these drugs must not come in contact with saline solution under any circumstances.

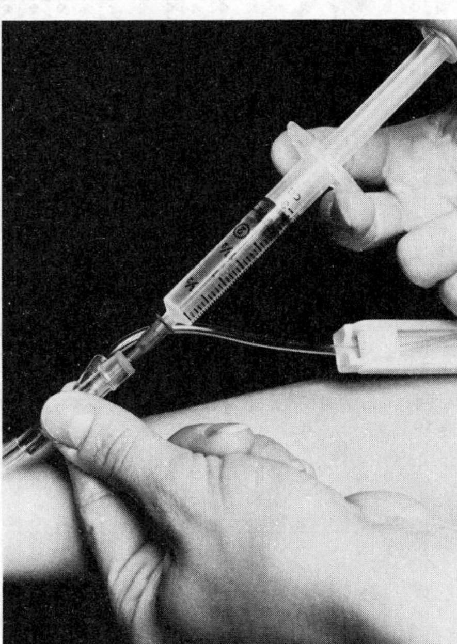

- Next, close the roller clamp on the primary I.V. tubing. Swab the injection port with alcohol. Insert the needle of one of the saline-filled syringes into the line's secondary injection port. After checking for blood backflow, make sure the I.V. needle's properly placed and there's no sign of infiltration. Then, flush the tubing with saline solution.
- Next, insert the needle of the syringe containing the medication into the injection port, and aspirate to check for blood backflow. Inject the medication at the prescribed rate. Don't open the roller clamp until you've flushed the tubing with the saline solution in the remaining syringe.

LAMINAR FLOW HOOD

To reduce the risk of airborne contamination, your hospital pharmacist will probably prepare admixtures under a laminar flow hood such as the one illustrated here. This hood keeps dust particles from entering the work area by providing a constant flow of microfiltered air. The laminar flow hood is one excellent reason why I.V.s should be made up in the pharmacy whenever possible.

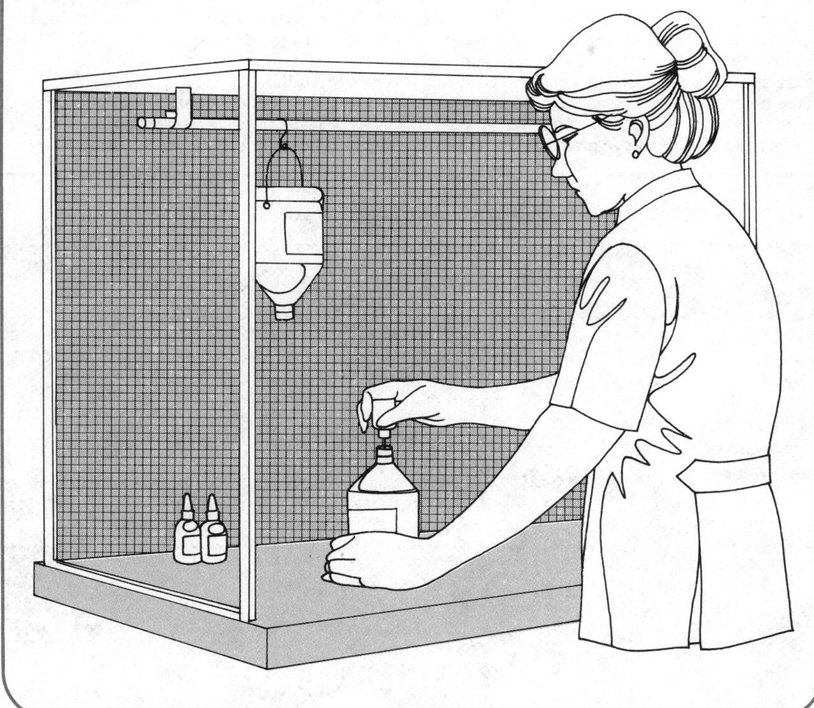

color as the solution. When you swirl or rotate the container, inspect for a precipitate in good light against both a dark and light background.

- Watch for color changes in the membrane of any I.V. filter device, indicating drug incompatibility not visible in the solution. This reaction becomes visible as the drug is trapped and accumulates in the filter chamber.
- If you detect a physical change, such as a precipitate or discoloration, don't administer the admixture. Notify the pharmacist.
- Avoid administering intermittent medications along with total parenteral nutrition solutions by a central venous catheter. Doing so risks contamination and incompatibilities. Use a secondary line for these drugs.
- Avoid administering medications through the same peripheral venous sites as amino acids and fat emulsions; instead, infuse them through a peripheral site not used for other drug therapy.
- Don't mix additives with blood or blood products.
- Avoid mixing drugs if no compatibility information is available. If you can't find such information, consult the pharmacist.

JAMES R. HILDEBRAND III, PharmD

Recognizing common drugs of abuse:

An identification guide and basic facts to help you

In your work, you may encounter addicts more often than you realize. That's because some are difficult—if not impossible—to identify. You should be cautious about basing an identification on only physical signs or abnormal behavior. For one thing, most symptoms suggesting drug abuse are common to various diseases. For another, the current popularity of mixed drug ingestion causes mixed symptoms. Taking stimulants and sedatives simultaneously, for instance, may cause antagonistic effects that defy interpretation. Also, differences in duration of effect may lead to withdrawal symptoms of one drug during the intoxicant phase of another.

Despite the difficulties of identifying drug abusers, you can spot certain signs of addiction and abuse. See the chart below for these and other related effects.

Types of addiction

As you can see in the chart, these drugs may cause physical or psychological dependence, or both. *Physical dependence* (or addiction) oc-

EFFECTS OF SOME COMMON DRUGS OF ABUSE

	CATEGORY/ DRUG	DEPENDENCE Physical	DEPENDENCE Psychological	POSSIBLE EFFECTS
Narcotics	**codeine**	Moderate	Moderate	Euphoria; respiratory depression; constricted pupils; nausea; risk of infection and hepatitis from I.V. (mainlined) drugs; wan, undernourished appearance; drowsiness and lethargy—user is on the "nod" (alternately dozing and waking) **Overdose:** Slow, shallow breathing; clammy skin; convulsions; coma; possibly death **Withdrawal:** Watery eyes, runny nose, yawning, anorexia, irritability, tremors, panic, chills and sweating, dilated pupils, piloerection (gooseflesh), cramps, nausea
	heroin	Strong	Strong	
	hydromorphone	Strong	Strong	
	meperidine	Strong	Strong	
	methadone	Strong	Strong	
	morphine	Strong	Strong	
Stimulants	**amphetamine**	Possible	Strong	Increased wakefulness, excitation, euphoria, talkativeness, irritability, dilated pupils, nervousness, increased pulse rate, elevated blood pressure **Overdose:** Agitation, fever, hallucinations, convulsions, possibly death **Withdrawal:** Apathy, long periods of sleep, irritability, depression, disorientation.
	cocaine	Possible	Strong	
	methylphenidate	Possible	Strong	
	phenmetrazine	Possible	Strong	
Depressants	**barbiturates**	Moderate to strong	Moderate to strong	Extreme drowsiness; slurred speech; disorientation; drunken behavior without alcohol use; slow, rapid, or shallow breathing; constricted pupils **Overdose:** Shallow breathing; cold, clammy skin; dilated pupils; weak, rapid pulse; coma; possibly death **Withdrawal:** Anxiety, insomnia, tremors, delirium, convulsions, possibly death
	chloral hydrate	Moderate	Moderate	
	glutethimide	Strong	Strong	
	methaqualone	Strong	Strong	
	other depressants	Moderate	Moderate	
	benzodiazepines	Little	Moderate	No significant effects
Hallucinogens	**lysergic acid diethylamide (LSD)**	None	Degree unknown	Illusions and hallucinations, poor perception of time and distance **Overdose:** Longer, more intense "trip" episodes, psychosis, possibly death **Withdrawal:** Withdrawal syndrome not reported
	mescaline and peyote	None	Degree unknown	
	phencyclidine (PCP)	Degree unknown	Strong	
	marijuana derivatives	Degree unknown	Moderate	Euphoria, increased appetite, disorientation **Overdose:** Fatigue, paranoia, possibly psychosis **Withdrawal:** Occasional insomnia, hyperactivity, and decreased appetite

curs when a person's body gets so accustomed to the drug that he cannot function normally without it. When the drug is withheld, physical and psychic withdrawal symptoms develop. A person may inadvertently become physically addicted, for example, when he takes certain drugs for a long-term illness.

Psychological dependence (or habituation) produces a desire to take drugs to feel good. The user has no physical compulsion to continue taking the drug. He may merely want to escape problems or situations he can't cope with, or he may seek pleasure and want to stimulate his senses.

Drug tolerance occurs when the user needs to take larger and larger doses to achieve the same effects. Accurate determination of tolerance levels is important in treatment programs.

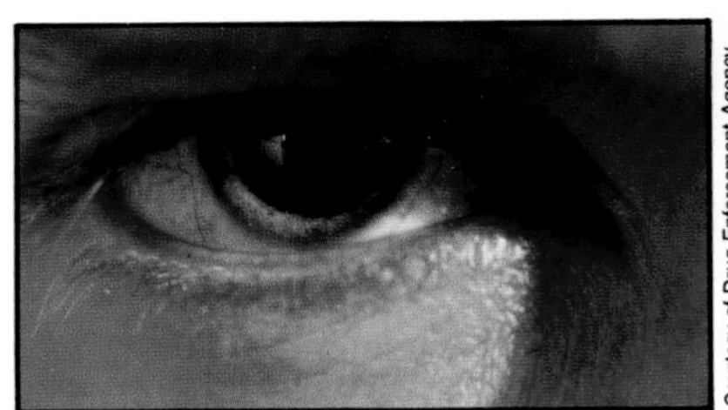
Courtesy of Drug Enforcement Agency

Someone using stimulants (amphetamines, for example) usually has dilated pupils.

Because you may see signs of drug abuse anywhere, you'll want to recognize drugs that can be abused, especially highly controlled substances. If you're working in a health-care

SPECIAL CONSIDERATIONS

Methadone is the drug of choice for withdrawal. As methadone maintenance becomes increasingly popular, more patients receiving methadone therapy are being admitted to general hospitals. This creates special medical and nursing problems. Some patients accurately report the dosage they're taking, but others don't know or exaggerate. A methadone-maintained patient may receive as much as 200 mg/day; the dosage must be verified by contacting the agency treating the patient for addiction. A patient on supervised daily doses of methadone has normal response to pain, so he requires the usual doses of analgesics for pain relief. But not all methadone treatment agencies give supervised daily doses; a patient taking methadone on a less controlled regimen may present all the classic problems of the street addict. So great is his tolerance that he may require massive doses of analgesics to relieve pain.

Abusers quickly develop tolerance, take massive doses, and after days without sleep or food, lapse into the abstinence syndrome. During withdrawal, the amphetamine user needs emotional support. Hospital emergency services would do well to study the crash-pad concept used effectively on college campuses. The crash pad is a haven where withdrawal is eased by generous amounts of kindness and understanding rather than drugs. Where staffing is inadequate for such a method, doctors may prescribe sedatives or tranquilizers to combat agitation and panic. They do so at some risk, because the patient may have already taken a sedative to ease the crash he anticipates when the stimulant wears off. So try to determine if your patient has taken a sedative to bring himself "down."

Patients develop great tolerance for barbiturates—they need to exceed their tolerance only slightly to precipitate a toxic reaction. The reaction poses great risk, because the main effect of barbiturates—CNS depression—is additive and synergistic to that of other sedatives and tranquilizers. Further, abrupt withdrawal from barbiturates poses a risk of major convulsive seizures; in fact, fatalities due to cardiovascular collapse have been reported. Thus, withdrawal must always be carried out under close supervision in a hospital.

In many cases, acute barbiturate intoxication is the result of a dose only slightly higher than the addictive level. After acute poisoning has been relieved, try to learn whether the barbiturates have been taken chronically. If so, gradual withdrawal is indicated. The withdrawal drug of choice is pentobarbital (Nembutal). However, the long-acting barbiturate phenobarbital can also be used.

When managing a patient on a bad "trip," exploit his hypersuggestible state for his own benefit by promising that he is safe from danger and that his reaction will soon pass. To reduce the intensity of the hallucinations, advise him to keep his eyes open. Rarely will you need to restrain him physically. Flashback phenomenon can occur weeks or months after ingestion of a hallucinogen (most commonly LSD, PCP). Once triggered, the flashback produces the same effects as drug ingestion. Medical treatment is symptomatic. If the doctor is reasonably sure the patient's intoxication is caused solely by hallucinogens, he may prescribe a phenothiazine. Doing so runs a risk: The patient may have taken an additional drug—an opiate, for instance—that would be potentiated by the phenothiazine.

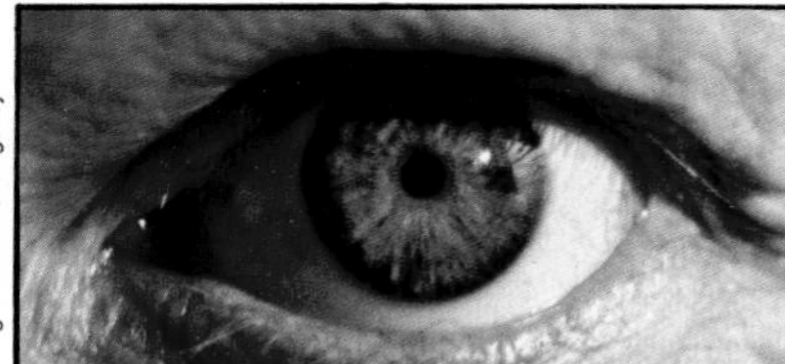
Drug Enforcement Agency

Someone using narcotics (heroin or morphine, for example) has constricted (pinpoint) pupils.

setting, you should be particularly aware of the abuse of prescription drugs, an increasingly serious problem. The health-care professional has to be more alert to the warning signs of abuse among patients and colleagues alike, as well as to drug thefts and substitutions.

To help you verify common drugs that can be abused or misused in tablet and capsule form, a full-color identification section follows. For more information about drug abuse, contact a drug abuse agency. You'll find a list of these agencies in the APPENDIX.

How to use this section

The color photos on the following pages will help you quickly identify almost 500 common drugs. Each drug is shown actual size. Because of printing limitations, colors may vary slightly from the actual tablets or capsules, although every effort has been made to reproduce the colors faithfully.

The section begins with white tablets and capsules, arranged by size, from smallest to largest. Then, beige, gray, yellow, brown, orange, red, pink, violet, blue, green, and multi-colored drugs follow.

The last page of photos contains some over-the-counter preparations that can be abused or misused.

Below each photo a caption gives as much of the following information as applicable: drug's trade name and dosage strength, generic name, controlled-substance schedule number, and manufacturer's name and code number. If the caption doesn't include a generic name, the drug is a combination product.

To identify an unfamiliar drug, turn to the page that contains drugs closest in color to the one you're trying to identify. When you think you've found the correct photo, compare *both* sides of the drug with the photo. In most cases, product markings are shown in the photos for easier identification. Remember, however, that handling may have removed some markings, especially on sugar-coated tablets. Markings and appearance may also have been changed by the manufacturer.

Tablet and capsule colors may vary from one batch of manufacturer's dye to another as well. Some products are sensitive to light and moisture, so their color and/or texture may change if stored for a long time. Color variation may also be affected by the light in which you view the tablets or capsules.

After identifying the drug, consult the index to find more information in this book. For additional details or confirming identification on the drug, please contact the manufacturer.

Except in emergencies, these photos should not be used as a substitute for a comprehensive chemical analysis, because visually similar products may differ markedly in contents.

Schedules of Controlled Substances, USA

Drugs regulated under the jurisdiction of the Controlled Substances Act of 1970 are divided into these five groups, or schedules.

Schedule I: No accepted medical use in the United States, with high potential for abuse. Examples: heroin, lysergic acid diethylamide (LSD), marijuana derivatives, mescaline, peyote, and psilocybin.

Schedule II: High potential for abuse, with severe psychic or physical dependence possible. Includes certain narcotic, stimulant, and depressant drugs. Examples: amobarbital, amphetamine, anileridine, cocaine, codeine, hydromorphone, meperidine, methadone, methamphetamine, methaqualone, methylphenidate, morphine, opium, oxycodone, oxymorphone, pentobarbital, phenmetrazine, and secobarbital.

Schedule III: Less abuse potential than drugs in Schedule II. Includes compounds containing certain narcotic and nonnarcotic drugs. Examples: barbituric acid derivatives (except those listed in another schedule), benzphetamine, chlorphentermine, clortermine, glutethimide, mazindol, methyprylon, Paregoric, and phendimetrazine.

Schedule IV: Less abuse potential than drugs in Schedule III. Examples: barbital, benzodiazepine derivatives, chloral hydrate, diethylpropion, ethchlorvynol, fenfluramine, ethinamate, meprobamate, methohexital, phenobarbital, paraldehyde, and phentermine.

Schedule V: Less abuse potential than drugs in Schedule IV. Consists of preparations containing limited quantities of certain narcotic drugs generally for antidiarrheal or antitussive purposes. Examples: diphenoxylate compound and expectorants with codeine.

Controlled Drugs, Canada

Schedule G: Drugs regulated under the jurisdiction of the Food and Drugs Act of 1952-1953 and regulations issued by the Health Protection Branch, Ottawa, Canada. All salts and derivatives of the following drugs are included: amphetamine, barbituric acid, benzphetamine, butorphanol, chlorphentermine, diethylpropion, methamphetamine, methaqualone, methylphenidate, pentazocine, phendimetrazine, phenmetrazine, phentermine, and thiobarbituric acid.

COMMON DRUGS THAT CAN BE ABUSED

Note: *The drugs pictured in this section, although usually prescribed for medicinal and therapeutic purposes, have the potential to be abused or misused under certain circumstances and by certain patients. They include both controlled and noncontrolled substances.*

CAPTION KEY:

Trade name (initial letter capitalized) or generic name (initial letter lower cased) and dosage strength
(generic name, when trade name has been listed)
Controlled-substance schedule number, if any
Manufacturer's name and code number, if any

morphine sulfate 10 mg Schedule II Lilly	**morphine sulfate 30 mg** Schedule II Lilly	**Ativan 0.5 mg** *(lorazepam)* Schedule IV Wyeth 81	**Lomotil** Schedule V Searle 61
codeine sulfate 15 mg Schedule II Lilly J09	**codeine sulfate 30 mg** Schedule II Lilly J10	**codeine sulfate 60 mg** Schedule II Lilly J11	**Cytomel 5 mcg** *(liothyronine sodium)* SKF D14
SK-Phenobarbital 15 mg *(phenobarbital)* Schedule IV SKF 136	**SK-Phenobarbital 30 mg** *(phenobarbital)* Schedule IV SKF 137	**Levo-Dromoran 2 mg** *(levorphanol tartrate)* Schedule II Roche 44	**Noludar 50 mg** *(methyprylon)* Schedule III Roche 16
Dolophine 5 mg *(methadone hydrochloride)* Schedule II Lilly J64	**Levothroid 0.05 mg** *(levothyroxine sodium)* Armour LL	**Demerol 50 mg** *(meperidine hydrochloride)* Schedule II Winthrop D35	**Synthroid 0.05 mg** *(levothyroxine sodium)* Flint
Desoxyn 5 mg *(methamphetamine hydrochloride)* Schedule II Abbott	**Haldol 0.5 mg** *(haloperidol)* McNeil	**Periactin 4 mg** *(cyproheptadine hydrochloride)* MSD 62	**Cylert 18.75 mg** *(pemoline)* Schedule IV Abbott TH
phenobarbital 16 mg Schedule IV Rugby	**phenobarbital 32 mg** Schedule IV Various manufacturers	**phenobarbital 65 mg** Schedule IV Various manufacturers	**Mebaral 32 mg** *(mephobarbital)* Schedule IV Breon M31

DRUGS THAT CAN BE ABUSED

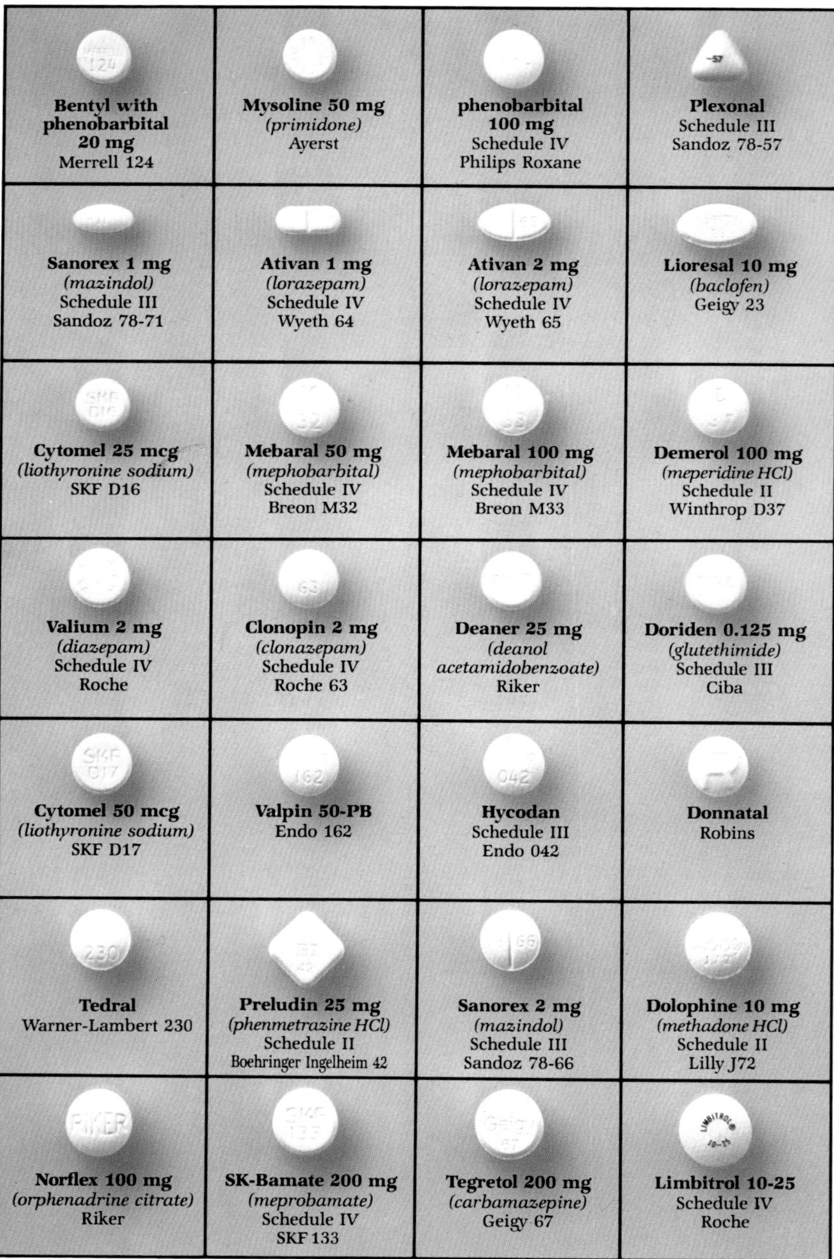
Bentyl with phenobarbital 20 mg Merrell 124
Mysoline 50 mg (primidone) Ayerst
phenobarbital 100 mg Schedule IV Philips Roxane
Plexonal Schedule III Sandoz 78-57
Sanorex 1 mg (mazindol) Schedule III Sandoz 78-71
Ativan 1 mg (lorazepam) Schedule IV Wyeth 64
Ativan 2 mg (lorazepam) Schedule IV Wyeth 65
Lioresal 10 mg (baclofen) Geigy 23
Cytomel 25 mcg (liothyronine sodium) SKF D16
Mebaral 50 mg (mephobarbital) Schedule IV Breon M32
Mebaral 100 mg (mephobarbital) Schedule IV Breon M33
Demerol 100 mg (meperidine HCl) Schedule II Winthrop D37
Valium 2 mg (diazepam) Schedule IV Roche
Clonopin 2 mg (clonazepam) Schedule IV Roche 63
Deaner 25 mg (deanol acetamidobenzoate) Riker
Doriden 0.125 mg (glutethimide) Schedule III Ciba
Cytomel 50 mcg (liothyronine sodium) SKF D17
Valpin 50-PB Endo 162
Hycodan Schedule III Endo 042
Donnatal Robins
Tedral Warner-Lambert 230
Preludin 25 mg (phenmetrazine HCl) Schedule II Boehringer Ingelheim 42
Sanorex 2 mg (mazindol) Schedule III Sandoz 78-66
Dolophine 10 mg (methadone HCl) Schedule II Lilly J72
Norflex 100 mg (orphenadrine citrate) Riker
SK-Bamate 200 mg (meprobamate) Schedule IV SKF 133
Tegretol 200 mg (carbamazepine) Geigy 67
Limbitrol 10-25 Schedule IV Roche

DRUGS THAT CAN BE ABUSED

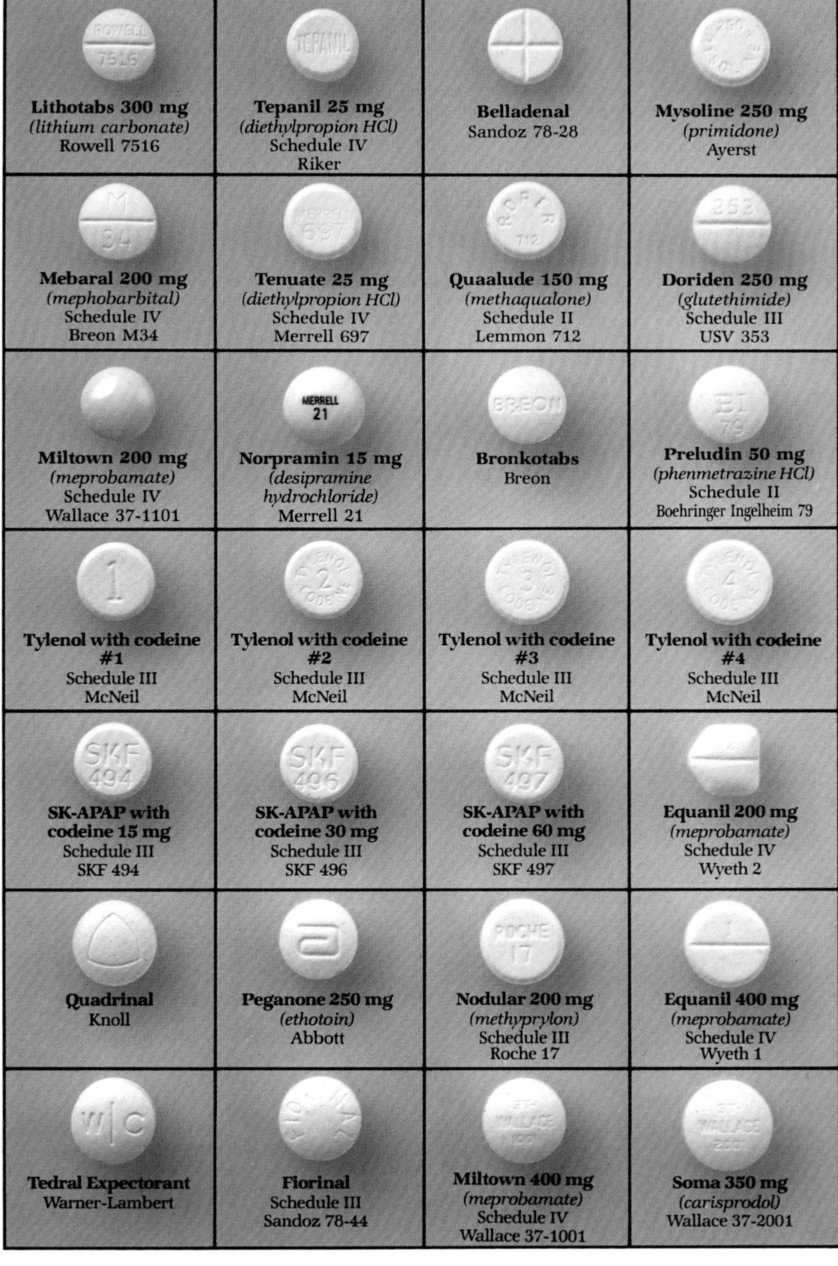
Lithotabs 300 mg
(lithium carbonate)
Rowell 7516
Tepanil 25 mg
(diethylpropion HCl)
Schedule IV
Riker
Belladenal
Sandoz 78-28
Mysoline 250 mg
(primidone)
Ayerst
Mebaral 200 mg
(mephobarbital)
Schedule IV
Breon M34
Tenuate 25 mg
(diethylpropion HCl)
Schedule IV
Merrell 697
Quaalude 150 mg
(methaqualone)
Schedule II
Lemmon 712
Doriden 250 mg
(glutethimide)
Schedule III
USV 353
Miltown 200 mg
(meprobamate)
Schedule IV
Wallace 37-1101
Norpramin 15 mg
(desipramine hydrochloride)
Merrell 21
Bronkotabs
Breon
Preludin 50 mg
(phenmetrazine HCl)
Schedule II
Boehringer Ingelheim 79
Tylenol with codeine #1
Schedule III
McNeil
Tylenol with codeine #2
Schedule III
McNeil
Tylenol with codeine #3
Schedule III
McNeil
Tylenol with codeine #4
Schedule III
McNeil
SK-APAP with codeine 15 mg
Schedule III
SKF 494
SK-APAP with codeine 30 mg
Schedule III
SKF 496
SK-APAP with codeine 60 mg
Schedule III
SKF 497
Equanil 200 mg
(meprobamate)
Schedule IV
Wyeth 2
Quadrinal
Knoll
Peganone 250 mg
(ethotoin)
Abbott
Nodular 200 mg
(methyprylon)
Schedule III
Roche 17
Equanil 400 mg
(meprobamate)
Schedule IV
Wyeth 1
Tedral Expectorant
Warner-Lambert
Fiorinal
Schedule III
Sandoz 78-44
Miltown 400 mg
(meprobamate)
Schedule IV
Wallace 37-1001
Soma 350 mg
(carisprodol)
Wallace 37-2001

DRUGS THAT CAN BE ABUSED

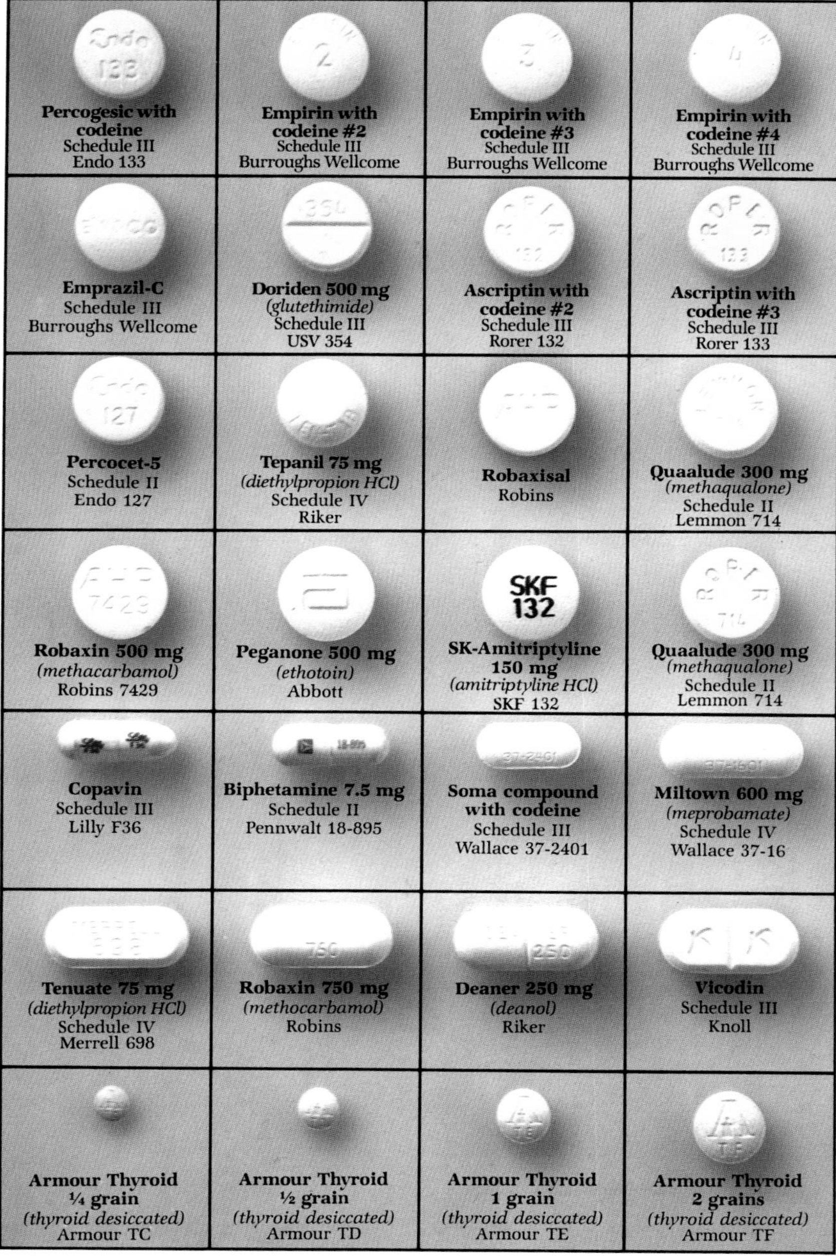

Percogesic with codeine Schedule III Endo 133	**Empirin with codeine #2** Schedule III Burroughs Wellcome	**Empirin with codeine #3** Schedule III Burroughs Wellcome	**Empirin with codeine #4** Schedule III Burroughs Wellcome
Emprazil-C Schedule III Burroughs Wellcome	**Doriden 500 mg** *(glutethimide)* Schedule III USV 354	**Ascriptin with codeine #2** Schedule III Rorer 132	**Ascriptin with codeine #3** Schedule III Rorer 133
Percocet-5 Schedule II Endo 127	**Tepanil 75 mg** *(diethylpropion HCl)* Schedule IV Riker	**Robaxisal** Robins	**Quaalude 300 mg** *(methaqualone)* Schedule II Lemmon 714
Robaxin 500 mg *(methacarbamol)* Robins 7429	**Peganone 500 mg** *(ethotoin)* Abbott	**SK-Amitriptyline 150 mg** *(amitriptyline HCl)* SKF 132	**Quaalude 300 mg** *(methaqualone)* Schedule II Lemmon 714
Copavin Schedule III Lilly F36	**Biphetamine 7.5 mg** Schedule II Pennwalt 18-895	**Soma compound with codeine** Schedule III Wallace 37-2401	**Miltown 600 mg** *(meprobamate)* Schedule IV Wallace 37-16
Tenuate 75 mg *(diethylpropion HCl)* Schedule IV Merrell 698	**Robaxin 750 mg** *(methocarbamol)* Robins	**Deaner 250 mg** *(deanol)* Riker	**Vicodin** Schedule III Knoll
Armour Thyroid ¼ grain *(thyroid desiccated)* Armour TC	**Armour Thyroid ½ grain** *(thyroid desiccated)* Armour TD	**Armour Thyroid 1 grain** *(thyroid desiccated)* Armour TE	**Armour Thyroid 2 grains** *(thyroid desiccated)* Armour TF

DRUGS THAT CAN BE ABUSED

Armour Thyroid 3 grains *(thyroid desiccated)* Armour TG

Armour Thyroid 5 grains *(thyroid desiccated)* Armour TI

Proloid ¼ grain *(thyroglobulin)* Warner-Lambert

Proloid ½ grain *(thyroglobulin)* Warner-Lambert

Proloid 1½ grains *(thyroglobulin)* Warner-Lambert 253

Proloid 1 grain *(thyroglobulin)* Warner-Lambert 252

Proloid 2 grains *(thyroglobulin)* Warner-Lambert 257

Proloid 3 grains *(thyroglobulin)* Warner-Lambert 254

Proloid 5 grains *(thyroglobulin)* Warner-Lambert 255

Mellaril 50 mg *(thioridazine hydrochloride)* Sandoz

Trilafon 2 mg *(perphenazine)* Schering 705

Trilafon 4 mg *(perphenazine)* Schering 940

Trilafon 8 mg *(perphenazine)* Schering 313

Trilafon 16 mg *(perphenazine)* Schering 077

Trilafon 8 mg Repetabs *(perphenazine)* Schering ADX

Eskalith 300 mg *(lithium carbonate)* SKF J09

SK-65 *(propoxyphene hydrochloride)* Schedule IV SKF 463

Tranxene 3.75 mg *(clorazepate dipotassium)* Schedule IV Abbott CI

Tranxene 15 mg *(clorazepate dipotassium)* Schedule IV Abbott CK

Euthroid-3 *(liotrix)* Warner-Lambert 263

Vesprin 25 mg *(triflupromazine)* Squibb 922

Zomax 100 mg *(zomepirac sodium)* McNeil

Dilantin Infatabs 50 mg *(phenytoin sodium)* Parke-Davis 007

Plegine 35 mg *(phendimetrazine tartrate)* Schedule III Ayerst

Pro-Banthine with phenobarbital Searle 631

Percodan Schedule II Endo 135

Dilaudid 4 mg *(hydromorphone HCl)* Schedule II Knoll

Voranil 50 mg *(clotermine hydrochloride)* Schedule III USV

DRUGS THAT CAN BE ABUSED

Desoxyn 15 mg *(methamphetamine hydrochloride)* Schedule II Abbott MF	**Levothroid 0.1 mg** *(levothyroxine sodium)* Armour LM	**Amytal 30 mg** *(amobarbital)* Schedule II Lilly T56	**Ritalin 5 mg** *(methylphenidate hydrochloride)* Schedule II Ciba 7
Haldol 1 mg *(haloperidol)* McNeil	**Valium 5 mg** *(diazepam)* Schedule IV Roche	**Synthroid 0.1 mg** *(levothyroxine sodium)* Flint	**Thyrolar 3 grains** *(liotrix)* Armour YH
Zactirin Compound-100 Wyeth 49	**Triavil 4-25** MSD 946	**Luminal 16 mg** *(phenobarbital)* Schedule IV Winthrop	**Prolixin 2.5 mg** *(fluphenaxine dihydrochloride)* Squibb 864
Etrafon 2-10 Schering 287	**Meprospan 200 mg** *(meprobamate)* Schedule IV Wallace 37-1401	**Nembutal 30 mg** *(pentobarbital sodium)* Schedule II Abbott	**Nembutal 100 mg** *(pentobarbital sodium)* Schedule II Abbott CH
Mellaril 150 mg *(thioridazine hydrochloride)* Sandoz	**Compazine 5 mg** *(prochlorperazine maleate)* SKF C66	**Compazine 10 mg** *(prochlorperazine maleate)* SKF C67	**Compazine 25 mg** *(prochlorperazine maleate)* SKF C69
Permitil Chronotab 1 mg *(fluphenazine hydrochloride)* Schering WKJ	**Elavil 25 mg** *(amitriptyline hydrochloride)* MSD 45	**Norpramin 25 mg** *(desipramine hydrochloride)* Merrell 11	**Ionamin 30 mg** *(phentermine)* Schedule IV Pennwalt 18-904
Aventyl 10 mg *(nortriptyline hydrochloride)* Lilly H17	**Aventyl 25 mg** *(nortriptyline hydrochloride)* Lilly H19	**Atarax 50 mg** *(hydroxyzine hydrochloride)* Roerig	**Janimine 25 mg** *(imipramine hydrochloride)* Abbott

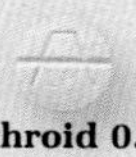

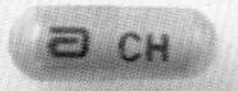

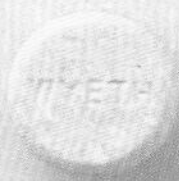

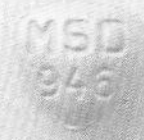

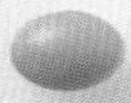

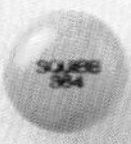

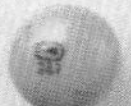

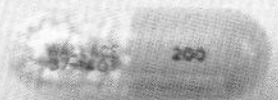

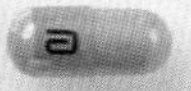

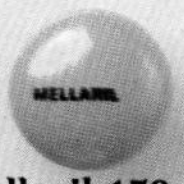

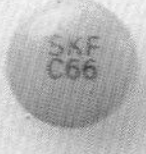

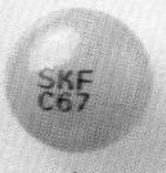

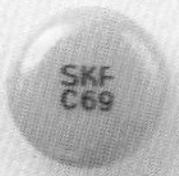

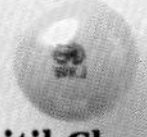

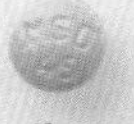

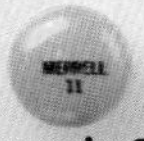

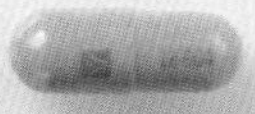

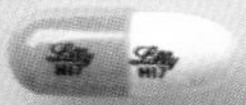

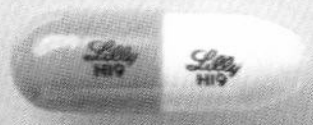

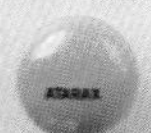

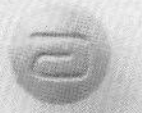

DRUGS THAT CAN BE ABUSED

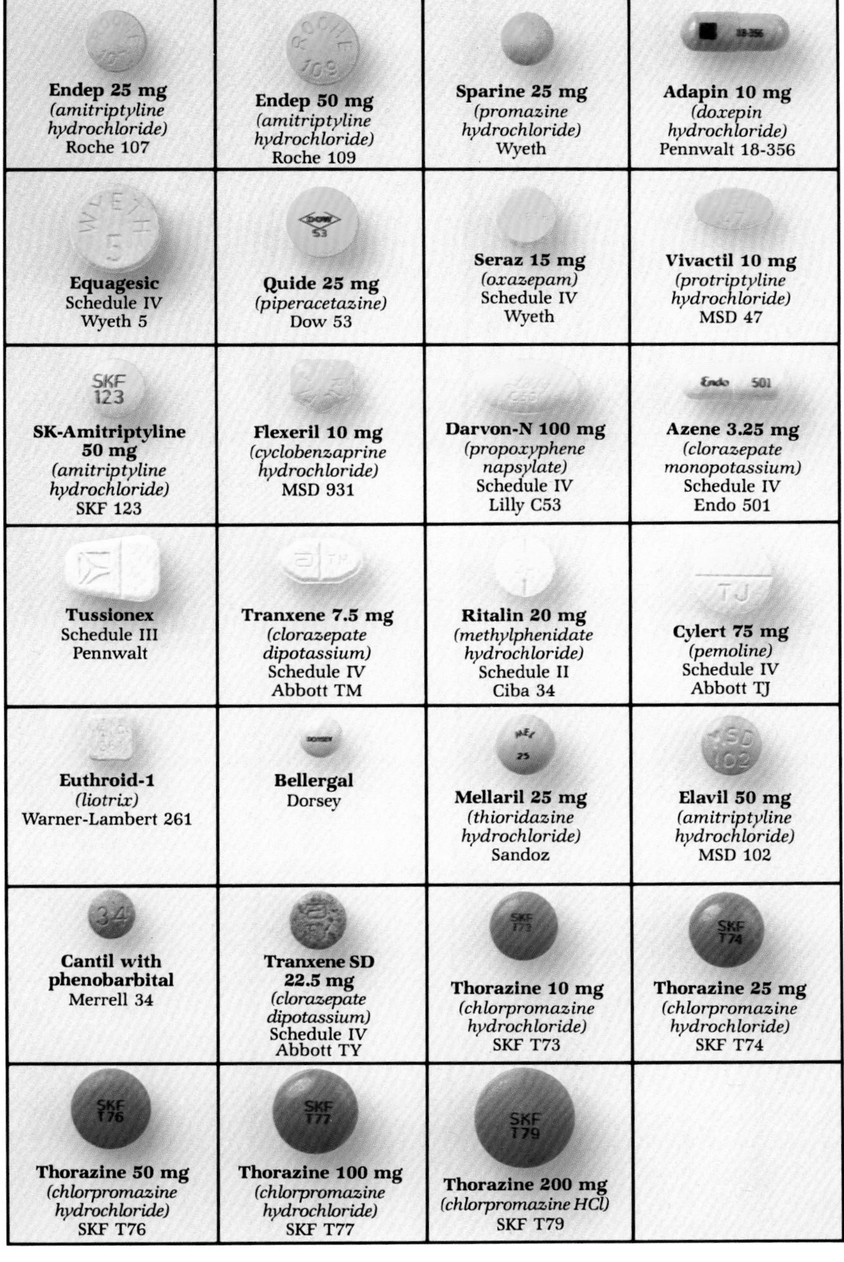

Endep 25 mg *(amitriptyline hydrochloride)* Roche 107	**Endep 50 mg** *(amitriptyline hydrochloride)* Roche 109	**Sparine 25 mg** *(promazine hydrochloride)* Wyeth	**Adapin 10 mg** *(doxepin hydrochloride)* Pennwalt 18-356
Equagesic Schedule IV Wyeth 5	**Quide 25 mg** *(piperacetazine)* Dow 53	**Seraz 15 mg** *(oxazepam)* Schedule IV Wyeth	**Vivactil 10 mg** *(protriptyline hydrochloride)* MSD 47
SK-Amitriptyline 50 mg *(amitriptyline hydrochloride)* SKF 123	**Flexeril 10 mg** *(cyclobenzaprine hydrochloride)* MSD 931	**Darvon-N 100 mg** *(propoxyphene napsylate)* Schedule IV Lilly C53	**Azene 3.25 mg** *(clorazepate monopotassium)* Schedule IV Endo 501
Tussionex Schedule III Pennwalt	**Tranxene 7.5 mg** *(clorazepate dipotassium)* Schedule IV Abbott TM	**Ritalin 20 mg** *(methylphenidate hydrochloride)* Schedule II Ciba 34	**Cylert 75 mg** *(pemoline)* Schedule IV Abbott TJ
Euthroid-1 *(liotrix)* Warner-Lambert 261	**Bellergal** Dorsey	**Mellaril 25 mg** *(thioridazine hydrochloride)* Sandoz	**Elavil 50 mg** *(amitriptyline hydrochloride)* MSD 102
Cantil with phenobarbital Merrell 34	**Tranxene SD 22.5 mg** *(clorazepate dipotassium)* Schedule IV Abbott TY	**Thorazine 10 mg** *(chlorpromazine hydrochloride)* SKF T73	**Thorazine 25 mg** *(chlorpromazine hydrochloride)* SKF T74
Thorazine 50 mg *(chlorpromazine hydrochloride)* SKF T76	**Thorazine 100 mg** *(chlorpromazine hydrochloride)* SKF T77	**Thorazine 200 mg** *(chlorpromazine HCl)* SKF T79	

DRUGS THAT CAN BE ABUSED

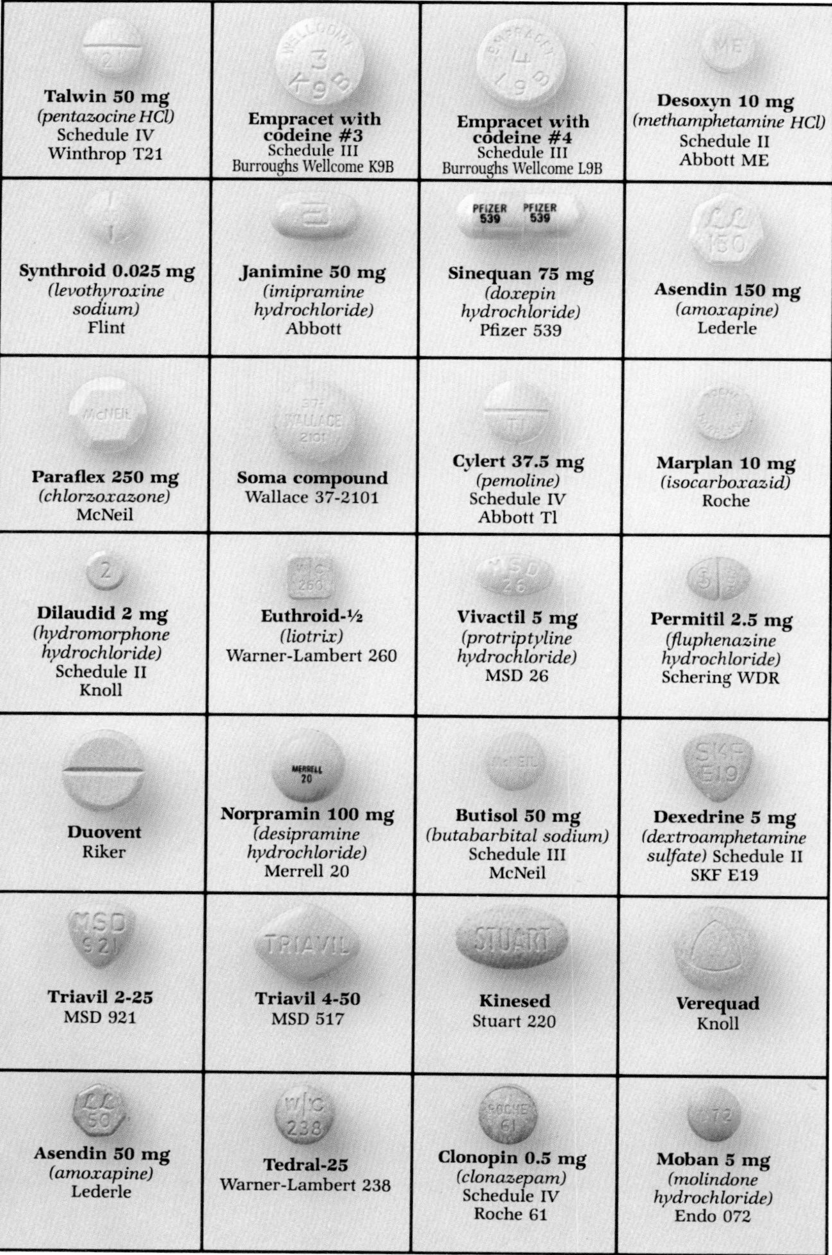

Talwin 50 mg (pentazocine HCl) Schedule IV Winthrop T21
Empracet with codeine #3 Schedule III Burroughs Wellcome K9B
Empracet with codeine #4 Schedule III Burroughs Wellcome L9B
Desoxyn 10 mg (methamphetamine HCl) Schedule II Abbott ME
Synthroid 0.025 mg (levothyroxine sodium) Flint
Janimine 50 mg (imipramine hydrochloride) Abbott
Sinequan 75 mg (doxepin hydrochloride) Pfizer 539
Asendin 150 mg (amoxapine) Lederle
Paraflex 250 mg (chlorzoxazone) McNeil
Soma compound Wallace 37-2101
Cylert 37.5 mg (pemoline) Schedule IV Abbott Tl
Marplan 10 mg (isocarboxazid) Roche
Dilaudid 2 mg (hydromorphone hydrochloride) Schedule II Knoll
Euthroid-½ (liotrix) Warner-Lambert 260
Vivactil 5 mg (protriptyline hydrochloride) MSD 26
Permitil 2.5 mg (fluphenazine hydrochloride) Schering WDR
Duovent Riker
Norpramin 100 mg (desipramine hydrochloride) Merrell 20
Butisol 50 mg (butabarbital sodium) Schedule III McNeil
Dexedrine 5 mg (dextroamphetamine sulfate) Schedule II SKF E19
Triavil 2-25 MSD 921
Triavil 4-50 MSD 517
Kinesed Stuart 220
Verequad Knoll
Asendin 50 mg (amoxapine) Lederle
Tedral-25 Warner-Lambert 238
Clonopin 0.5 mg (clonazepam) Schedule IV Roche 61
Moban 5 mg (molindone hydrochloride) Endo 072

DRUGS THAT CAN BE ABUSED

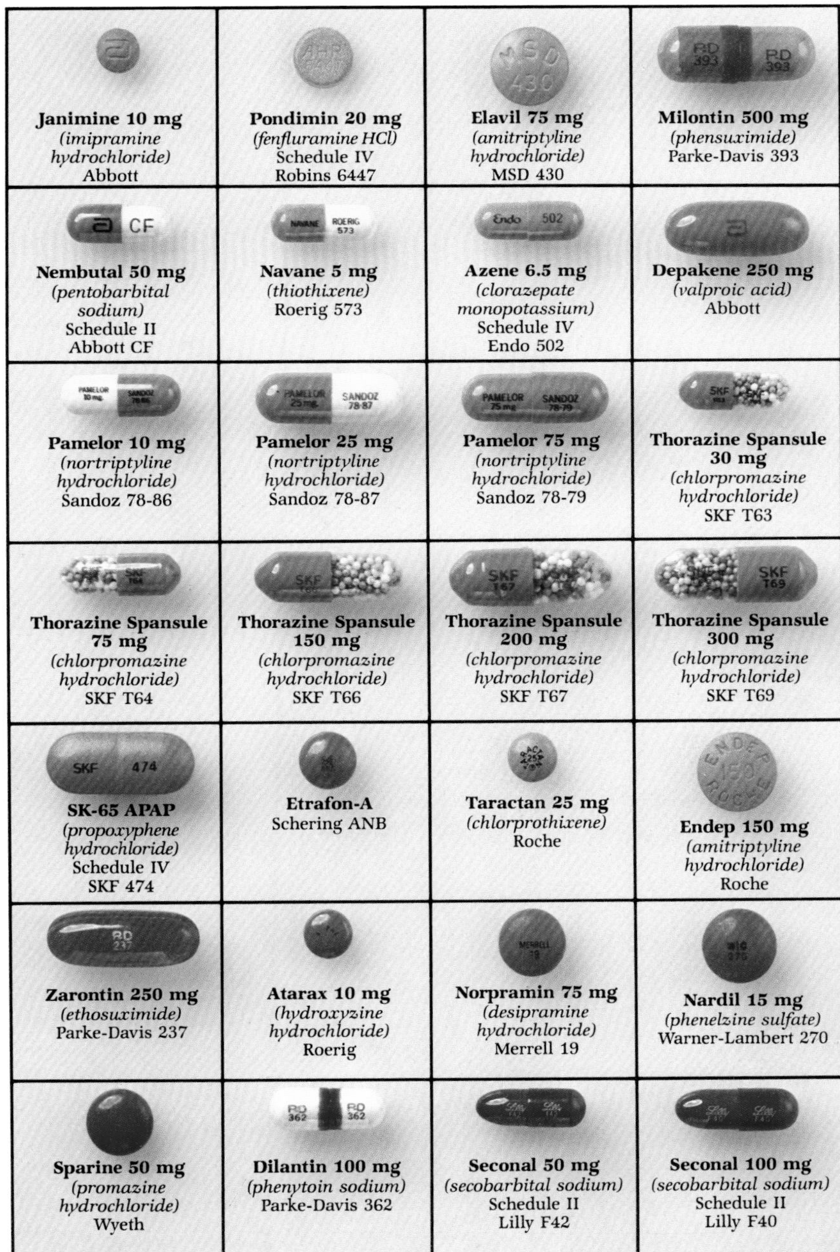

Janimine 10 mg *(imipramine hydrochloride)* Abbott	**Pondimin 20 mg** *(fenfluramine HCl)* Schedule IV Robins 6447	**Elavil 75 mg** *(amitriptyline hydrochloride)* MSD 430	**Milontin 500 mg** *(phensuximide)* Parke-Davis 393
Nembutal 50 mg *(pentobarbital sodium)* Schedule II Abbott CF	**Navane 5 mg** *(thiothixene)* Roerig 573	**Azene 6.5 mg** *(clorazepate monopotassium)* Schedule IV Endo 502	**Depakene 250 mg** *(valproic acid)* Abbott
Pamelor 10 mg *(nortriptyline hydrochloride)* Sandoz 78-86	**Pamelor 25 mg** *(nortriptyline hydrochloride)* Sandoz 78-87	**Pamelor 75 mg** *(nortriptyline hydrochloride)* Sandoz 78-79	**Thorazine Spansule 30 mg** *(chlorpromazine hydrochloride)* SKF T63
Thorazine Spansule 75 mg *(chlorpromazine hydrochloride)* SKF T64	**Thorazine Spansule 150 mg** *(chlorpromazine hydrochloride)* SKF T66	**Thorazine Spansule 200 mg** *(chlorpromazine hydrochloride)* SKF T67	**Thorazine Spansule 300 mg** *(chlorpromazine hydrochloride)* SKF T69
SK-65 APAP *(propoxyphene hydrochloride)* Schedule IV SKF 474	**Etrafon-A** Schering ANB	**Taractan 25 mg** *(chlorprothixene)* Roche	**Endep 150 mg** *(amitriptyline hydrochloride)* Roche
Zarontin 250 mg *(ethosuximide)* Parke-Davis 237	**Atarax 10 mg** *(hydroxyzine hydrochloride)* Roerig	**Norpramin 75 mg** *(desipramine hydrochloride)* Merrell 19	**Nardil 15 mg** *(phenelzine sulfate)* Warner-Lambert 270
Sparine 50 mg *(promazine hydrochloride)* Wyeth	**Dilantin 100 mg** *(phenytoin sodium)* Parke-Davis 362	**Seconal 50 mg** *(secobarbital sodium)* Schedule II Lilly F42	**Seconal 100 mg** *(secobarbital sodium)* Schedule II Lilly F40

DRUGS THAT CAN BE ABUSED

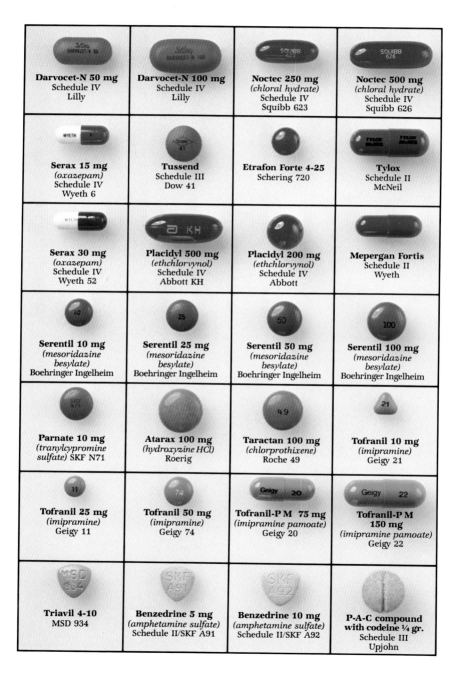

Darvocet-N 50 mg Schedule IV Lilly	**Darvocet-N 100 mg** Schedule IV Lilly	**Noctec 250 mg** *(chloral hydrate)* Schedule IV Squibb 623	**Noctec 500 mg** *(chloral hydrate)* Schedule IV Squibb 626
Serax 15 mg *(oxazepam)* Schedule IV Wyeth 6	**Tussend** Schedule III Dow 41	**Etrafon Forte 4-25** Schering 720	**Tylox** Schedule II McNeil
Serax 30 mg *(oxazepam)* Schedule IV Wyeth 52	**Placidyl 500 mg** *(ethchlorvynol)* Schedule IV Abbott KH	**Placidyl 200 mg** *(ethchlorvynol)* Schedule IV Abbott	**Mepergan Fortis** Schedule II Wyeth
Serentil 10 mg *(mesoridazine besylate)* Boehringer Ingelheim	**Serentil 25 mg** *(mesoridazine besylate)* Boehringer Ingelheim	**Serentil 50 mg** *(mesoridazine besylate)* Boehringer Ingelheim	**Serentil 100 mg** *(mesoridazine besylate)* Boehringer Ingelheim
Parnate 10 mg *(tranylcypromine sulfate)* SKF N71	**Atarax 100 mg** *(hydroxyzine HCl)* Roerig	**Taractan 100 mg** *(chlorprothixene)* Roche 49	**Tofranil 10 mg** *(imipramine)* Geigy 21
Tofranil 25 mg *(imipramine)* Geigy 11	**Tofranil 50 mg** *(imipramine)* Geigy 74	**Tofranil-P M 75 mg** *(imipramine pamoate)* Geigy 20	**Tofranil-P M 150 mg** *(imipramine pamoate)* Geigy 22
Triavil 4-10 MSD 934	**Benzedrine 5 mg** *(amphetamine sulfate)* Schedule II/SKF A91	**Benzedrine 10 mg** *(amphetamine sulfate)* Schedule II/SKF A92	**P-A-C compound with codeine ¼ gr.** Schedule III Upjohn

DRUGS THAT CAN BE ABUSED

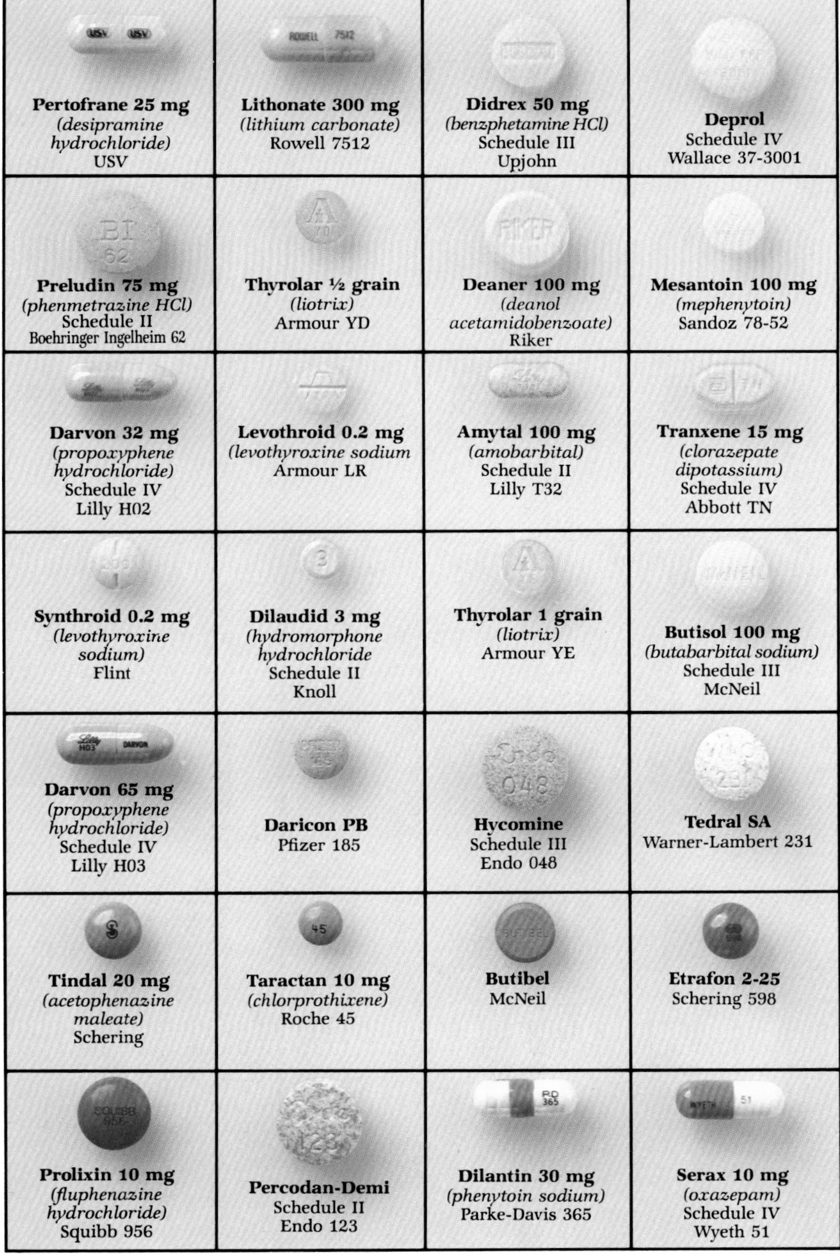

Pertofrane 25 mg
(desipramine hydrochloride)
USV
Lithonate 300 mg
(lithium carbonate)
Rowell 7512
Didrex 50 mg
(benzphetamine HCl)
Schedule III
Upjohn
Deprol
Schedule IV
Wallace 37-3001
Preludin 75 mg
(phenmetrazine HCl)
Schedule II
Boehringer Ingelheim 62
Thyrolar ½ grain
(liotrix)
Armour YD
Deaner 100 mg
(deanol acetamidobenzoate)
Riker
Mesantoin 100 mg
(mephenytoin)
Sandoz 78-52
Darvon 32 mg
(propoxyphene hydrochloride)
Schedule IV
Lilly H02
Levothroid 0.2 mg
(levothyroxine sodium
Armour LR
Amytal 100 mg
(amobarbital)
Schedule II
Lilly T32
Tranxene 15 mg
(clorazepate dipotassium)
Schedule IV
Abbott TN
Synthroid 0.2 mg
(levothyroxine sodium)
Flint
Dilaudid 3 mg
(hydromorphone hydrochloride
Schedule II
Knoll
Thyrolar 1 grain
(liotrix)
Armour YE
Butisol 100 mg
(butabarbital sodium)
Schedule III
McNeil
Darvon 65 mg
(propoxyphene hydrochloride)
Schedule IV
Lilly H03
Daricon PB
Pfizer 185
Hycomine
Schedule III
Endo 048
Tedral SA
Warner-Lambert 231
Tindal 20 mg
(acetophenazine maleate)
Schering
Taractan 10 mg
(chlorprothixene)
Roche 45
Butibel
McNeil
Etrafon 2-25
Schering 598
Prolixin 10 mg
(fluphenazine hydrochloride)
Squibb 956
Percodan-Demi
Schedule II
Endo 123
Dilantin 30 mg
(phenytoin sodium)
Parke-Davis 365
Serax 10 mg
(oxazepam)
Schedule IV
Wyeth 51

DRUGS THAT CAN BE ABUSED

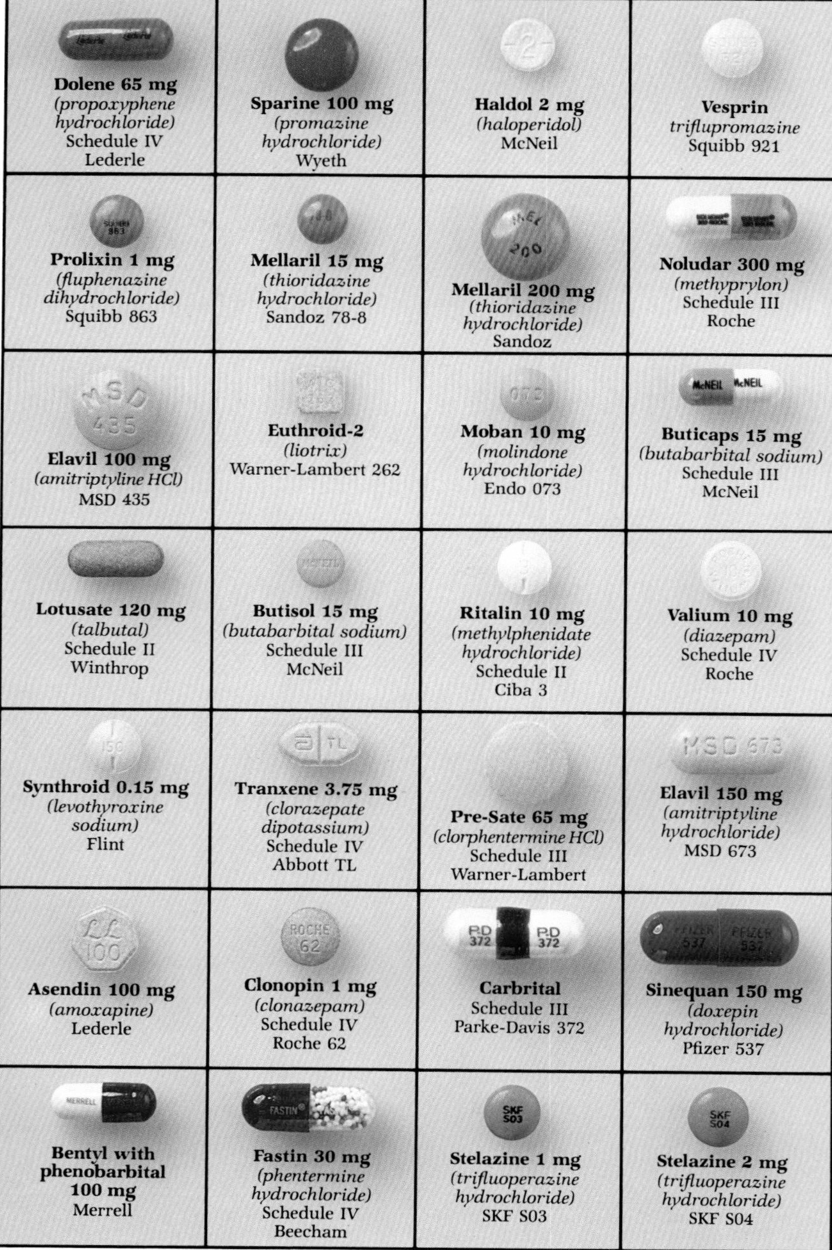

Dolene 65 mg *(propoxyphene hydrochloride)* Schedule IV Lederle	**Sparine 100 mg** *(promazine hydrochloride)* Wyeth	**Haldol 2 mg** *(haloperidol)* McNeil	**Vesprin** *triflupromazine* Squibb 921
Prolixin 1 mg *(fluphenazine dihydrochloride)* Squibb 863	**Mellaril 15 mg** *(thioridazine hydrochloride)* Sandoz 78-8	**Mellaril 200 mg** *(thioridazine hydrochloride)* Sandoz	**Noludar 300 mg** *(methyprylon)* Schedule III Roche
Elavil 100 mg *(amitriptyline HCl)* MSD 435	**Euthroid-2** *(liotrix)* Warner-Lambert 262	**Moban 10 mg** *(molindone hydrochloride)* Endo 073	**Buticaps 15 mg** *(butabarbital sodium)* Schedule III McNeil
Lotusate 120 mg *(talbutal)* Schedule II Winthrop	**Butisol 15 mg** *(butabarbital sodium)* Schedule III McNeil	**Ritalin 10 mg** *(methylphenidate hydrochloride)* Schedule II Ciba 3	**Valium 10 mg** *(diazepam)* Schedule IV Roche
Synthroid 0.15 mg *(levothyroxine sodium)* Flint	**Tranxene 3.75 mg** *(clorazepate dipotassium)* Schedule IV Abbott TL	**Pre-Sate 65 mg** *(clorphentermine HCl)* Schedule III Warner-Lambert	**Elavil 150 mg** *(amitriptyline hydrochloride)* MSD 673
Asendin 100 mg *(amoxapine)* Lederle	**Clonopin 1 mg** *(clonazepam)* Schedule IV Roche 62	**Carbrital** Schedule III Parke-Davis 372	**Sinequan 150 mg** *(doxepin hydrochloride)* Pfizer 537
Bentyl with phenobarbital 100 mg Merrell	**Fastin 30 mg** *(phentermine hydrochloride)* Schedule IV Beecham	**Stelazine 1 mg** *(trifluoperazine hydrochloride)* SKF S03	**Stelazine 2 mg** *(trifluoperazine hydrochloride)* SKF S04

DRUGS THAT CAN BE ABUSED

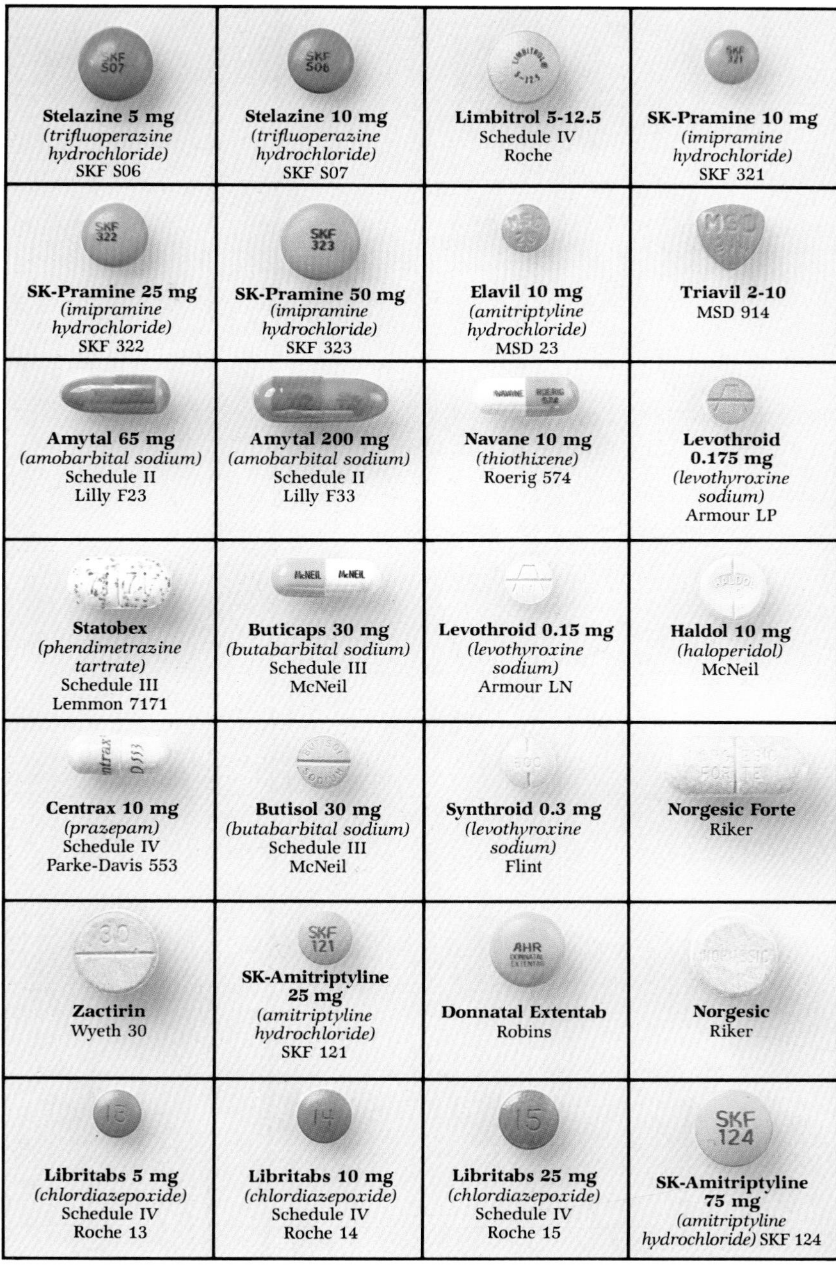

Stelazine 5 mg *(trifluoperazine hydrochloride)* SKF S06	**Stelazine 10 mg** *(trifluoperazine hydrochloride)* SKF S07	**Limbitrol 5-12.5** Schedule IV Roche	**SK-Pramine 10 mg** *(imipramine hydrochloride)* SKF 321
SK-Pramine 25 mg *(imipramine hydrochloride)* SKF 322	**SK-Pramine 50 mg** *(imipramine hydrochloride)* SKF 323	**Elavil 10 mg** *(amitriptyline hydrochloride)* MSD 23	**Triavil 2-10** MSD 914
Amytal 65 mg *(amobarbital sodium)* Schedule II Lilly F23	**Amytal 200 mg** *(amobarbital sodium)* Schedule II Lilly F33	**Navane 10 mg** *(thiothixene)* Roerig 574	**Levothroid 0.175 mg** *(levothyroxine sodium)* Armour LP
Statobex *(phendimetrazine tartrate)* Schedule III Lemmon 7171	**Buticaps 30 mg** *(butabarbital sodium)* Schedule III McNeil	**Levothroid 0.15 mg** *(levothyroxine sodium)* Armour LN	**Haldol 10 mg** *(haloperidol)* McNeil
Centrax 10 mg *(prazepam)* Schedule IV Parke-Davis 553	**Butisol 30 mg** *(butabarbital sodium)* Schedule III McNeil	**Synthroid 0.3 mg** *(levothyroxine sodium)* Flint	**Norgesic Forte** Riker
Zactirin Wyeth 30	**SK-Amitriptyline 25 mg** *(amitriptyline hydrochloride)* SKF 121	**Donnatal Extentab** Robins	**Norgesic** Riker
Libritabs 5 mg *(chlordiazepoxide)* Schedule IV Roche 13	**Libritabs 10 mg** *(chlordiazepoxide)* Schedule IV Roche 14	**Libritabs 25 mg** *(chlordiazepoxide)* Schedule IV Roche 15	**SK-Amitriptyline 75 mg** *(amitriptyline hydrochloride)* SKF 124

DRUGS THAT CAN BE ABUSED

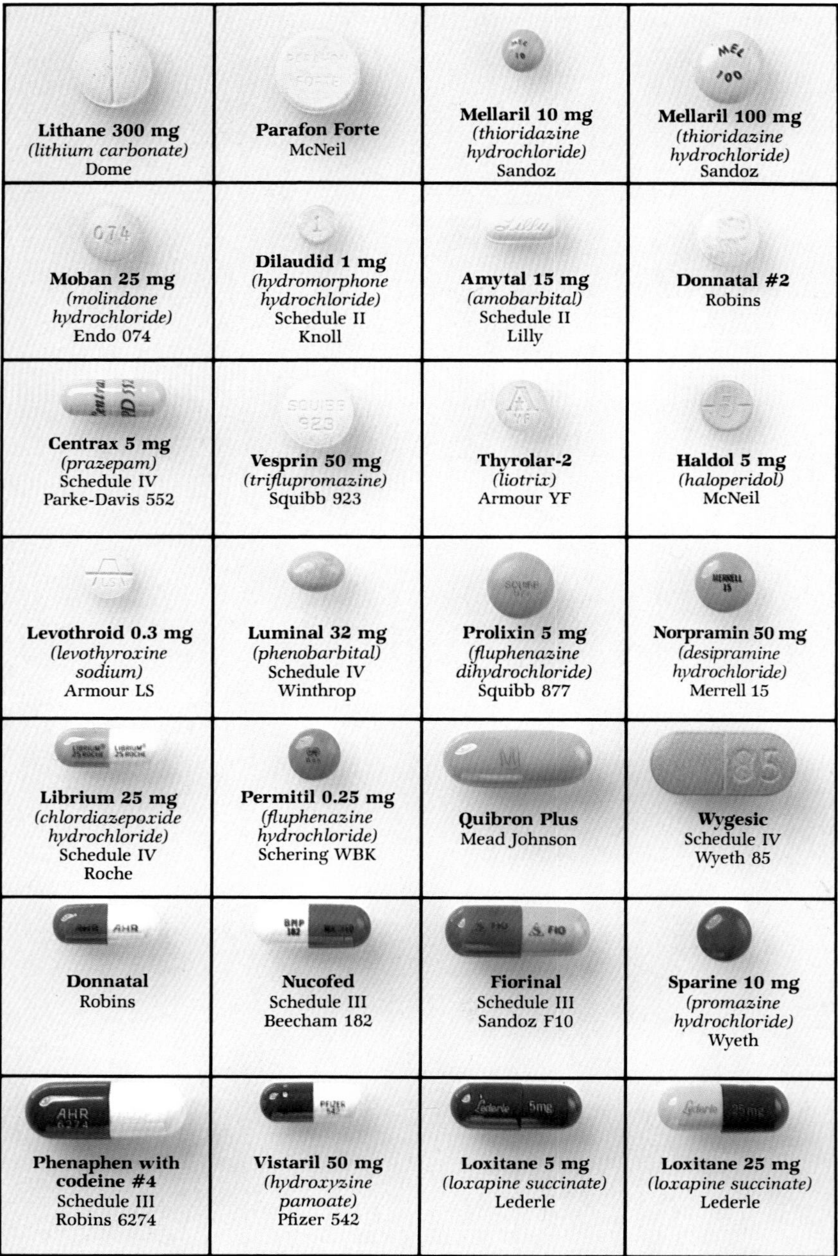

Lithane 300 mg *(lithium carbonate)* Dome	**Parafon Forte** McNeil	**Mellaril 10 mg** *(thioridazine hydrochloride)* Sandoz	**Mellaril 100 mg** *(thioridazine hydrochloride)* Sandoz
Moban 25 mg *(molindone hydrochloride)* Endo 074	**Dilaudid 1 mg** *(hydromorphone hydrochloride)* Schedule II Knoll	**Amytal 15 mg** *(amobarbital)* Schedule II Lilly	**Donnatal #2** Robins
Centrax 5 mg *(prazepam)* Schedule IV Parke-Davis 552	**Vesprin 50 mg** *(triflupromazine)* Squibb 923	**Thyrolar-2** *(liotrix)* Armour YF	**Haldol 5 mg** *(haloperidol)* McNeil
Levothroid 0.3 mg *(levothyroxine sodium)* Armour LS	**Luminal 32 mg** *(phenobarbital)* Schedule IV Winthrop	**Prolixin 5 mg** *(fluphenazine dihydrochloride)* Squibb 877	**Norpramin 50 mg** *(desipramine hydrochloride)* Merrell 15
Librium 25 mg *(chlordiazepoxide hydrochloride)* Schedule IV Roche	**Permitil 0.25 mg** *(fluphenazine hydrochloride)* Schering WBK	**Quibron Plus** Mead Johnson	**Wygesic** Schedule IV Wyeth 85
Donnatal Robins	**Nucofed** Schedule III Beecham 182	**Fiorinal** Schedule III Sandoz F10	**Sparine 10 mg** *(promazine hydrochloride)* Wyeth
Phenaphen with codeine #4 Schedule III Robins 6274	**Vistaril 50 mg** *(hydroxyzine pamoate)* Pfizer 542	**Loxitane 5 mg** *(loxapine succinate)* Lederle	**Loxitane 25 mg** *(loxapine succinate)* Lederle

DRUGS THAT CAN BE ABUSED

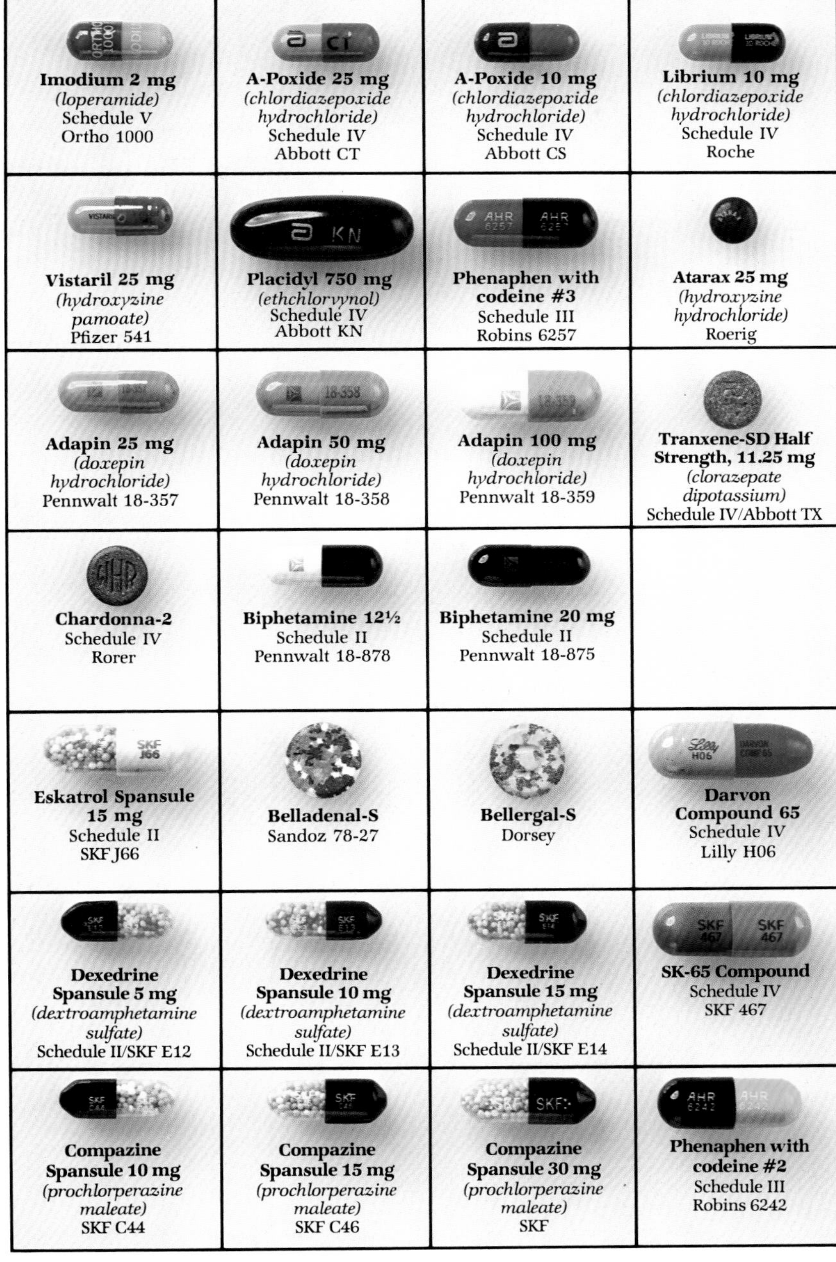
Imodium 2 mg *(loperamide)* Schedule V Ortho 1000
A-Poxide 25 mg *(chlordiazepoxide hydrochloride)* Schedule IV Abbott CT
A-Poxide 10 mg *(chlordiazepoxide hydrochloride)* Schedule IV Abbott CS
Librium 10 mg *(chlordiazepoxide hydrochloride)* Schedule IV Roche
Vistaril 25 mg *(hydroxyzine pamoate)* Pfizer 541
Placidyl 750 mg *(ethchlorvynol)* Schedule IV Abbott KN
Phenaphen with codeine #3 Schedule III Robins 6257
Atarax 25 mg *(hydroxyzine hydrochloride)* Roerig
Adapin 25 mg *(doxepin hydrochloride)* Pennwalt 18-357
Adapin 50 mg *(doxepin hydrochloride)* Pennwalt 18-358
Adapin 100 mg *(doxepin hydrochloride)* Pennwalt 18-359
Tranxene-SD Half Strength, 11.25 mg *(clorazepate dipotassium)* Schedule IV/Abbott TX
Chardonna-2 Schedule IV Rorer
Biphetamine 12½ Schedule II Pennwalt 18-878
Biphetamine 20 mg Schedule II Pennwalt 18-875
Eskatrol Spansule 15 mg Schedule II SKF J66
Belladenal-S Sandoz 78-27
Bellergal-S Dorsey
Darvon Compound 65 Schedule IV Lilly H06
Dexedrine Spansule 5 mg *(dextroamphetamine sulfate)* Schedule II/SKF E12
Dexedrine Spansule 10 mg *(dextroamphetamine sulfate)* Schedule II/SKF E13
Dexedrine Spansule 15 mg *(dextroamphetamine sulfate)* Schedule II/SKF E14
SK-65 Compound Schedule IV SKF 467
Compazine Spansule 10 mg *(prochlorperazine maleate)* SKF C44
Compazine Spansule 15 mg *(prochlorperazine maleate)* SKF C46
Compazine Spansule 30 mg *(prochlorperazine maleate)* SKF
Phenaphen with codeine #2 Schedule III Robins 6242

DRUGS THAT CAN BE ABUSED

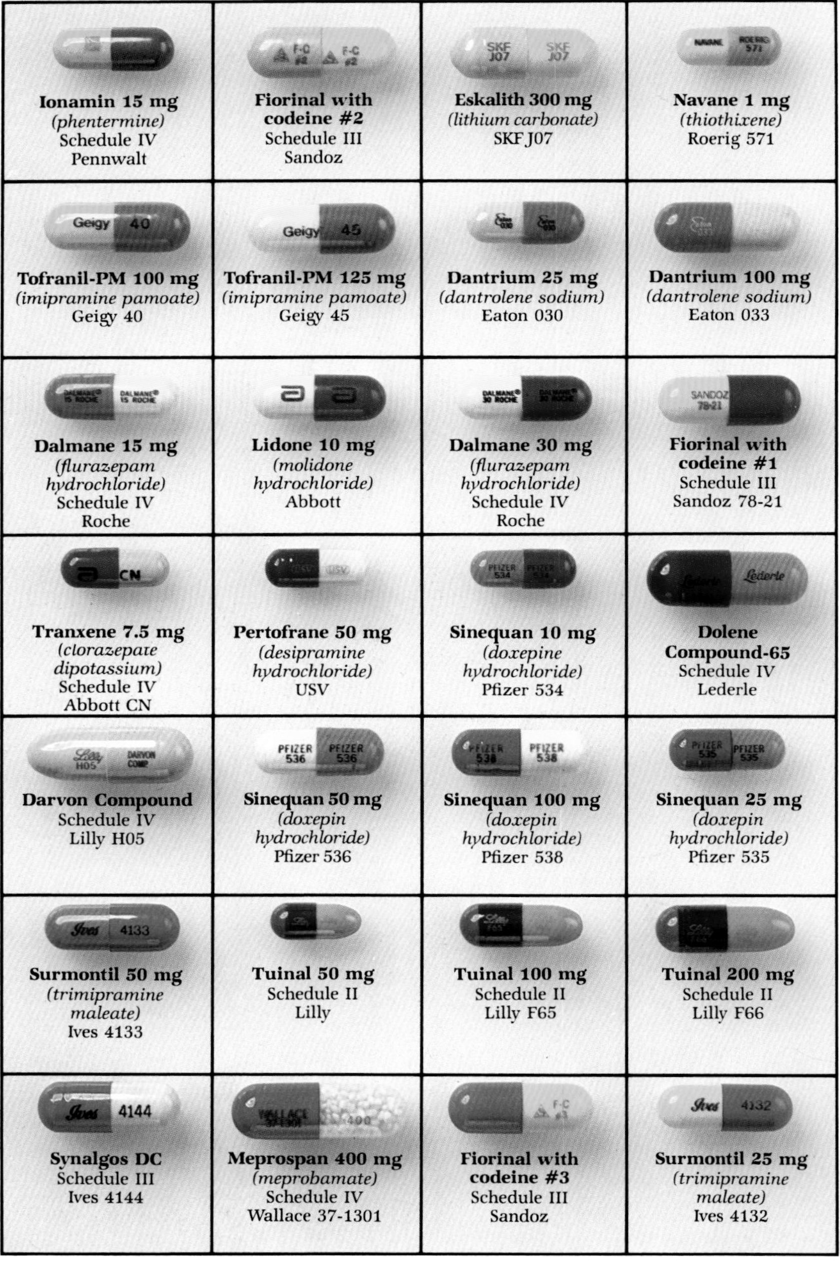

Ionamin 15 mg *(phentermine)* Schedule IV Pennwalt	**Fiorinal with codeine #2** Schedule III Sandoz	**Eskalith 300 mg** *(lithium carbonate)* SKF J07	**Navane 1 mg** *(thiothixene)* Roerig 571
Tofranil-PM 100 mg *(imipramine pamoate)* Geigy 40	**Tofranil-PM 125 mg** *(imipramine pamoate)* Geigy 45	**Dantrium 25 mg** *(dantrolene sodium)* Eaton 030	**Dantrium 100 mg** *(dantrolene sodium)* Eaton 033
Dalmane 15 mg *(flurazepam hydrochloride)* Schedule IV Roche	**Lidone 10 mg** *(molidone hydrochloride)* Abbott	**Dalmane 30 mg** *(flurazepam hydrochloride)* Schedule IV Roche	**Fiorinal with codeine #1** Schedule III Sandoz 78-21
Tranxene 7.5 mg *(clorazepate dipotassium)* Schedule IV Abbott CN	**Pertofrane 50 mg** *(desipramine hydrochloride)* USV	**Sinequan 10 mg** *(doxepine hydrochloride)* Pfizer 534	**Dolene Compound-65** Schedule IV Lederle
Darvon Compound Schedule IV Lilly H05	**Sinequan 50 mg** *(doxepin hydrochloride)* Pfizer 536	**Sinequan 100 mg** *(doxepin hydrochloride)* Pfizer 538	**Sinequan 25 mg** *(doxepin hydrochloride)* Pfizer 535
Surmontil 50 mg *(trimipramine maleate)* Ives 4133	**Tuinal 50 mg** Schedule II Lilly	**Tuinal 100 mg** Schedule II Lilly F65	**Tuinal 200 mg** Schedule II Lilly F66
Synalgos DC Schedule III Ives 4144	**Meprospan 400 mg** *(meprobamate)* Schedule IV Wallace 37-1301	**Fiorinal with codeine #3** Schedule III Sandoz	**Surmontil 25 mg** *(trimipramine maleate)* Ives 4132

DRUGS THAT CAN BE ABUSED

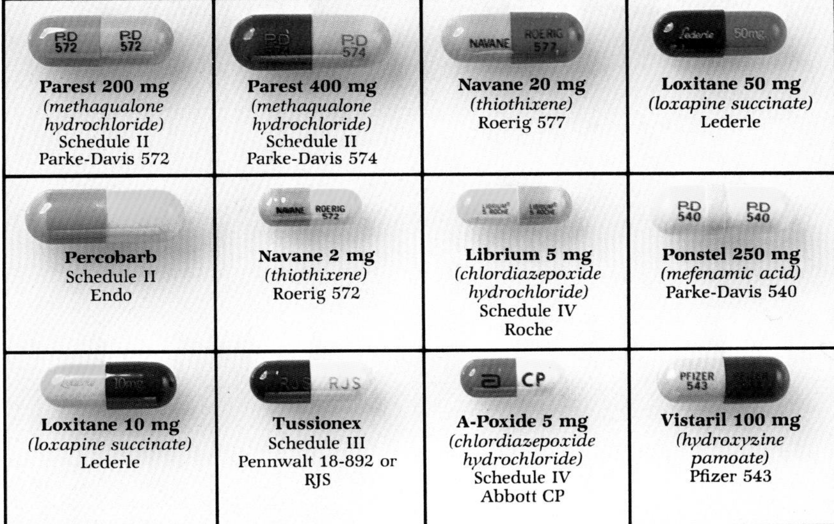

Parest 200 mg
(methaqualone hydrochloride)
Schedule II
Parke-Davis 572

Parest 400 mg
(methaqualone hydrochloride)
Schedule II
Parke-Davis 574

Navane 20 mg
(thiothixene)
Roerig 577

Loxitane 50 mg
(loxapine succinate)
Lederle

Percobarb
Schedule II
Endo

Navane 2 mg
(thiothixene)
Roerig 572

Librium 5 mg
(chlordiazepoxide hydrochloride)
Schedule IV
Roche

Ponstel 250 mg
(mefenamic acid)
Parke-Davis 540

Loxitane 10 mg
(loxapine succinate)
Lederle

Tussionex
Schedule III
Pennwalt 18-892 or RJS

A-Poxide 5 mg
(chlordiazepoxide hydrochloride)
Schedule IV
Abbott CP

Vistaril 100 mg
(hydroxyzine pamoate)
Pfizer 543

MANAGING DRUG OVERDOSE EMERGENCIES

In a drug overdose emergency, proper respiratory management and quick treatment of complications are essential. Follow these guidelines:

- To establish ventilation and maintain an open airway, extend the patient's head and pull his lower jaw forward. Then clear his airway of foreign material. If necessary, use suctioning to clear the airway of mucus or secretions.
- Insert an oral airway. If the patient's level of consciousness is high and he's having no apparent respiratory problems, place him in semi-Fowler's position and keep him under close observation. You may administer oxygen by nasal cannula.
- When ordered, administer a narcotic antagonist to reverse drug-induced respiratory depression. Onset of antagonism and reversal of narcotic depression is rapid, generally occurring within 2 to 3 minutes. Observe the patient closely for several hours for relapse of narcosis symptoms. Repeat administration of an antagonist may be necessary, depending on the amount, route of administration, and type of narcotic being antagonized. Be alert for withdrawal symptoms following administration of a narcotic antagonist.

If respiratory depression is severe and persistent (patient's gag and cough reflexes remain absent and respiratory rate is inadequate), an endotracheal tube may be inserted and a respirator used to achieve adequate ventilation. You may draw samples for arterial blood gas analysis to assess respiratory status, blood pH, and acid-base balance.

When the patient's respiratory status is stable, ingested drugs should be removed from his stomach as soon as possible. Therapies for this vary according to the type of drug taken. See APPENDIX, *Drug Toxicities,* for specific guidelines.

After the acute toxic emergency phase of the overdose has passed, continue maintenance and stabilization of the patient. Close observation of vital signs and level of consciousness is essential. Monitoring techniques and support therapy vary according to patient condition and the type of substance that produced the overdose. Be alert for withdrawal symptoms, especially if the patient is a narcotic abuser or addict.

OVER-THE-COUNTER DRUGS THAT CAN BE ABUSED
with major active ingredients listed

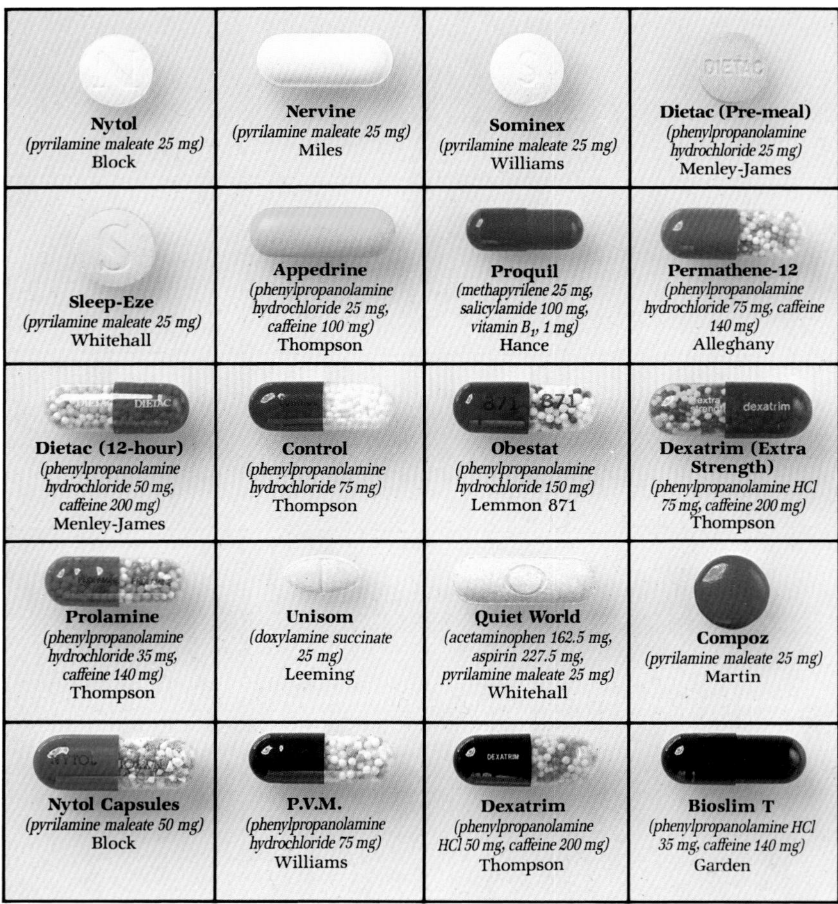

A FINAL CAUTION ON DRUG IDENTIFICATION

As a health-care professional, you're probably aware of the many look-alike products available today. In emergency situations, identification has to be accurate because overdose treatments for controlled substances are different from those for look-alike drugs.

As long as these drugs are properly labeled—that is, comply with current labeling requirements—they can be legally sold and are easily available in drugstores. The same drugs might be sold on the street, however—repackaged without proper labeling. Street buyers might take several of these look-alike tablets or capsules without much effect. At another time, they might get the authentic controlled substance and unknowingly take an overdose.

The federal government has begun to enforce postal regulations to curtail direct-mail advertising of look-alikes, and many states are enacting legislation to strictly curb deceptive marketing of these substances. The Drug Enforcement Agency (DEA) is recommending a model state law against drugs that may mislead consumers either by dosage-unit appearance or by misrepresentations about the drugs.

STREET NAMES TO KNOW

DRUG	STREET NAMES
Amphetamines, amphetamine (Benzedrine), methamphetamine (Desoxyn, Methedrine), dextroamphetamine (Dexedrine)	Beans, bennies, black beauties, black mollies, copilots, crank, crossroads, crystal, dexies, double cross, hearts, love drug, meth, minibennies, peaches, pep pills, speed, rosas, roses, thrusters, truck drivers, uppers, wake-ups, whites
Barbiturates, amobarbital (Amytal), pentobarbital (Nembutal), phenobarbital (Luminal), secobarbital (Seconal)	Barbs, blockbusters, bluebirds, blue devils, blues, Christmas trees, downers, green dragons, Mexican reds, pink ladies, pinks, rainbows, red and blues, redbirds, red devils, reds, sleeping pills, yellow jackets, yellow
Camphorated tincture of opium (Paregoric)	"Blue velvet" when mixed with pyribenzamine and taken I.V.
Cannabis (marijuana)	Acapulco gold, Colombian, grass, hash, herb, J, jay, joint, Mary Jane, Panama red, pot, reefer, smoke, tea, weed
Cocaine	Blow, C, coca, coke, flake, girl, heaven, dust, lady, mujer, nose candy, paradise, perico, rock, snow, stardust, upper, white
Diacetylmorphine (heroin)	Big H, boy, brown, brown sugar, crap, estuffa, H, heroina, hombre, horse, junk, Mexican mud, scag, smack, stuff, thing
Dimethyltryptamine (DMT)	Businessman's special
Lysergic acid diethylamide (LSD)	Acid, big D, blotter acid, brown dot, California sunshine, cubes, haze, microdots, paper acid, purple haze, sugar, sunshine, trips
Merperidine (Demerol)	Dollies
Methadone (Dolophine)	Dollies
Methaqualone (Quaalude)	Ludes, quads, quas, soapers, sopes, sopor
Methylphenidate (Ritalin)	California sunshine
Morphine	Cube, first line, goma, morf, morfina, morpho
Pentazocine (Talwin)	Dollies
Phenycyclidine (PCP, Sernylan)	Angel dust, crystal, crystal joint, cyclone, elephant, hog, KJs, peace pill, rocket fuel
3, 4, 5-trimethoxyphenethylamine (Mescaline, Peyote)	Big chief, buttons, cactus, mesc, mescal, mescal buttons
2, 5-dimethoxy-4, α-dimethylphenthylamine (STP, DOM)	Serenity-tranquility-peace pill
3-(2-dimethylaminoethyl) Indol-4-y1 dihydrogen phosphate (Psilocybin)	Silly putty, the mushrooms, magic Mexican mushrooms

ADDITIONAL RESOURCES

For a list of drug abuse treatment centers, see APPENDIX, p.1330.

In communities without local treatment facilities, narcotic addicts can be referred to the U.S. District Attorney, who will arrange for civil commitment under provision of the Federal Narcotic Addict Rehabilitation Act. Eligible patients will be treated in federal facilities and returned to their home communities for supervised aftercare.

For further information on drug abuse, contact the National Clearinghouse for Drug Abuse Information, P.O. Box 416, Kensington, Md. 20795, (301) 443-6500.

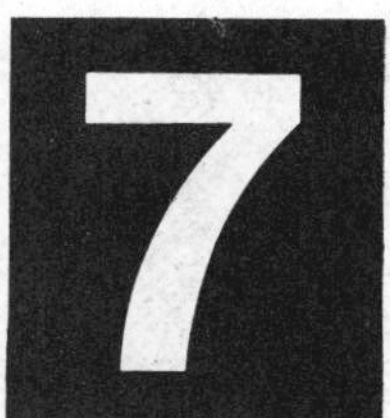

Parenteral and enteral nutrition therapy

Nutritional support therapy has significantly decreased the morbidity and mortality of serious illnesses that preclude normal nutrition and metabolism. In a debilitated patient who is unable to ingest enough nutrients orally but whose gastrointestinal (GI) system is still functioning, *enteral* tube feeding is the preferred treatment. In a patient with GI dysfunction and increased metabolic demands, however, *parenteral* nutritional supplementation may be necessary to restore anabolism.

Nutritional assessment

Although no single test or measurement can identify and classify malnutrition, a comprehensive profile of pertinent subjective and objective data allows prevention and early recognition of nutritional depletion. Nutritional therapy and repletion of body stores minimize the harmful effects of poor nutrition, such as indolent wound healing, increased incidence of infection and complications, and prolonged hospitalization.

During the initial evaluation of the patient, obtain a dietary history to determine recent changes in appetite, food intake, and body weight. Note medical conditions that impair nutrient intake and absorption. A thorough and complete physical assessment—including inspection, palpation, percussion, and auscultation of each body system—reveals other signs and symptoms of malnutrition.

Additional objective data commonly gathered for nutritional assessment include anthropometric measurements (height, weight, triceps skinfold, midarm circumference), biochemical determinations (serum concentrations of albumin, transferrin, prealbumin, and retinol-binding protein; total lymphocyte count; and 24-hour urinary excretion of urea and creatinine), and recall antigen skin test results.

Fat, skeletal muscle protein, and visceral protein are the three major energy reserves of the patient with a catabolic disorder. Adipose (fat) tissue—the body's primary calorie reserve—is assessed by measuring the triceps skinfold, which includes the subcutaneous fat layer. Skeletal muscle mass can be estimated by determining midarm muscle circumference as well as the creatinine-height index. Visceral protein depletion is quantified by serum albumin and serum transferrin concentrations, and the status of the cellular immune response, as manifested by total lymphocyte count and recall antigen skin testing.

Critical analysis of these energy reserves is essential to determine the severity and classification of malnutrition. *Marasmus*—the severe depletion of both protein and calories—results in growth retardation in children, weight loss without edema, muscular atrophy, and decreased subcutaneous tissue. The acute protein loss or deprivation known as *kwashiorkor* produces generalized edema, skin lesions, hair changes, and fatty infiltration of the liver. In many

HOW TO TAKE ANTHROPOMETRIC MEASUREMENTS

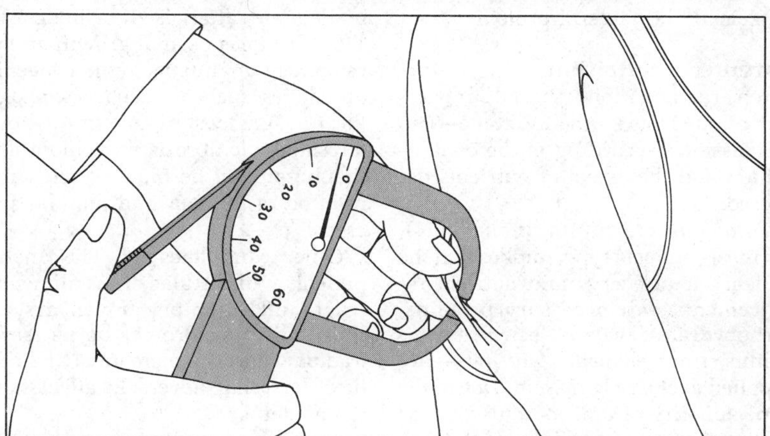

Anthropometric measurements help you assess your patient's nutritional status. Body height and weight, skinfold thickness, and midarm muscle circumference measurements allow you to identify body fat, muscle mass, and protein and caloric adequacy.

Follow these techniques for accurate anthropometric measurements:

• Weigh your patient around the same time every day; use the same scale, and have him wear the same amount of clothing. It's the easiest and least expensive way to assess nutritional status quickly.

• Record the patient's height and weight. Compare actual weight to ideal body weight. For some patients, you may need to determine the basal energy requirement. This will give an approximation of the number of calories needed daily to maintain the body at rest. An easy method of doing this is to multiply 10 times the ideal body weight in pounds. For example, if ideal body weight for your patient is 120 lb, then 120 × 10 equals 1,200 calories, the amount needed to maintain basal metabolism.

• Measure, record, and compare with standard values the *triceps skinfold thickness,* measured by skinfold calipers like the ones shown here.

You can also compare with standard values the *subscapular and abdominal skinfold thickness,* although these measurements are not as accurate.

• Measure, record, and compare with standard values the *mid–upper-arm circumference* to estimate the size of the triceps muscles. This represents the muscle mass.

• Make sure the following laboratory values are recorded since such data may indicate potential nutritional problems before clinical signs develop.

LABORATORY VALUES	PURPOSE
Serum albumin and serum transferrin	To measure visceral protein stores
Total lymphocyte counts	To measure immune competence
Skin tests using common recall antigens such as *Candida,* mumps, and trichophyton*	To measure immune competence
24-hour urine specimens	To calculate both the creatinine clearance and height indices (a measure of skeletal or somatic protein stores) and urine urea nitrogen (a measure of nitrogen balance).

*Make sure skin tests are read at 24 and 48 hours.

hospitalized patients both conditions are present concurrently, and are thus characterized by depletion of fat and of skeletal and visceral protein.

Parenteral nutrition

Parenteral nutrition—the administration of nutrients by the I.V. route—can be classified according to the concentration and the extent of nutrients delivered.

Total parenteral nutrition (TPN), the most complete type, implies that the patient's total energy and nutrient requirements—all necessary proteins, carbohydrates, water, electrolytes, vitamins, trace elements, and fats—are supplied exclusively by vein. Due to the hypertonicity of amino acid–glucose solutions, they must be infused through a central vein; fat emulsion, however, may be infused centrally or peripherally. The average adult patient who receives TPN for longer than several months will develop essential fatty acid deficiency unless I.V. fat emulsion is added to the total nutrient regimen.

Peripheral parenteral nutrition is a more limited form of nutritional therapy. It provides fewer nonprotein calories but greater volume than TPN; peripheral veins cannot tolerate the concentrated hypertonic glucose solution used in TPN. For this reason, peripheral parenteral nutrition is considered less complete than TPN, and significant weight gain rarely occurs in patients receiving this type of treatment. Therefore, it's used only for periods of less than 3 weeks in patients who don't need to gain weight, yet need to maintain their current basal metabolic needs.

Other forms of parenteral nutrition include protein-sparing therapy and standard I.V. therapy. See the chart on pp. 102 to 103 for more information and a comparison of the four types of parenteral nutrition.

Since most patients who require parenteral nutritional therapy receive TPN, only this method is discussed in detail here.

Indications

TPN is indicated when use of the GI tract for nutritional replenishment is inadequate, ill advised, or impossible. TPN promotes normal growth and development in infants with congenital anomalies such as tracheoesophageal fistula, gastroschisis, small-bowel atresia, cystic fibrosis, meconium ileus, diaphragmatic hernia, volvulus, malrotation of the gut, and annular pancreas.

Other candidates for TPN include patients with fistulas of the alimentary tract, inflammatory bowel disease, short-bowel syndrome, burns, severe trauma, cancer, pancreatitis, and other disorders that adversely affect nutritional status.

Specially prepared formulas have been devised for patients with renal and hepatic failure.

Solution components

TPN solutions are quite hypertonic, with an osmolarity of 1,800 to 2,400 mOsm/liter. These solutions are admixed in the pharmacy under laminar-flow, filtered-air hoods (see illustration on p. 75). Usually, 500 ml of 50% dextrose are mixed with 500 ml of 8.5% crystalline amino acid solution, or 350 ml of 50% dextrose are mixed with 750 ml of 5% to 10% protein hydrolysate solution. Electrolytes, vitamins, and trace elements must be added to the base solution in sufficient amounts to satisfy daily requirements. Pertinent details of TPN solution components may be summarized as follows:

1. *Dextrose.* The number of nonprotein calories needed to promote positive nitrogen balance depends on the severity of the patient's illness. Maximum energy expenditure occurs in multiple trauma, severe sepsis, long bone fractures, and burns. A patient who weighs 60 kg (132 lb) requires 1,800 to 3,000 nonprotein calories/day (usually 30 to 50 calories/kg/day).

In the absence of adequate exogenous calories, energy is generated primarily by lipolysis and glyconeogenesis. Research has confirmed that approximately 50 g/day of dextrose can have a significant nitrogen-sparing effect; infusions of greater quantities result in only minor increases in nitrogen sparing. In fact, if the amount of dextrose provided greatly exceeds the energy expended, excess glycogen and fat can be deposited in the liver, with subsequent hepatomegaly, upper right quadrant tenderness or pain, and disordered hepatic function. For the average patient, a ratio of 150 to 200 calories per gram of nitrogen administered seems best.

2. *Protein.* The recommended dietary allowance of protein for a healthy adult is approximately 0.9 g/kg of body weight. Protein requirements in patients with malnutrition are substantially higher. Determination of nitrogen balance is probably the best way to accurately assess individual protein requirements. The typical patient on TPN receives approximately 18 g of nitrogen daily in the form of amino acids, the building blocks of new muscles and protein.

Protein hydrolysate solutions, the earliest form of parenteral nitrogen, are formulated by acid hydrolysis of animal fibrin or casein; such solutions are not the best sources of nitrogen and amino acids. They contain peptides of minimal biologic value; they don't have ideal amino acid patterns; and occasionally, they may cause sensitivity reactions. These disadvantages have been overcome by the more recently developed crystalline amino acid solutions.

3. *Electrolytes.* Electrolytes are added exogenously to the TPN solution. Apparently, potassium, phosphorus, and magnesium depletion parallel the protein depletion in patients with catabolic conditions. Additions to the base solution include sodium (acetate, lactate, chloride, or bicarbonate), potassium (acetate, lactate, chloride, acid phosphate), magnesium (sulfate), phosphate (potassium acid salt), and calcium (gluconate).

NURSING TIPS

NOTE INSULIN ADSORPTION TO I.V. CONTAINERS

Insulin adsorbs onto I.V. glass bottles and polyvinylchloride infusion sets, resulting in a loss of insulin (2 to 40 units/1,500 ml of normal saline solution).

The addition of small amounts of human serum albumin to the solution lessens insulin adsorption.

Therefore, if your patient is receiving insulin I.V., be aware of the loss through adsorption and monitor your patient's response to therapy. The insulin dose may have to be adjusted.

4. *Vitamins.* Vitamins must be administered daily to ensure normal body functions and optimal utilization of the nutrient substrates. A mixture of fat- and water-soluble vitamins, biotin, and folic acid (MVI-12) is added to any single unit of a daily regimen. Because the vitamins in MVI-12 are generally in the therapeutic dosage range, administering more than one ampul daily for the adult patient is neither necessary nor advisable, as hypervitaminosis A or D can occur within several days or weeks. In addition, the patient should receive vitamin K supplementation to maintain normal blood coagulation.

5. *Trace elements.* Trace elements are found as contaminants in nutrient solutions. If parenteral nutrition therapy lasts longer than 2 weeks, additional trace elements may be needed. Commercial solutions contain zinc, copper, chromium, and manganese; however, many hospitals compound their own solutions.

Zinc is an essential component of approximately 70 enzymes in humans. It functions in the metabolism of DNA, protein, and mucopolysaccharides. Zinc

COMPARING TYPES OF PARENTERAL NUTRITION

TYPE	SOLUTION COMPONENTS/LITER
Total parenteral nutrition (TPN) (via central venous line)	• Dextrose 20% to 25% (1 liter dextrose 25% = 850 nonprotein calories) • Crystalline amino acids 2.5% to 5% • Electrolytes, vitamins, trace elements, insulin, and heparin as ordered • Fat emulsion 10% to 20% (usually infused as a separate solution; can be given peripherally or centrally)
Peripheral parenteral nutrition	• Dextrose 5% to 10% • Crystalline amino acids 2.75% to 4.25% • Electrolytes, trace elements, and vitamins as ordered • Fat emulsion 10% or 20% (1 liter dextrose 10% and amino acids 3.5% infused at same time with liter fat emulsion = 1,440 nonprotein calories: 340 from dextrose and 1,100 from fat emulsion) • Heparin or hydrocortisone as ordered
Protein-sparing therapy	• Crystalline amino acids in same amounts as TPN • Electrolytes, vitamins, and minerals as ordered
Standard I.V. therapy	• Dextrose, water, and electrolytes in varying amounts *Examples of frequently used parenteral fluids:* D_5W = 170 calories/liter $D_{10}W$ = 340 calories/liter 0.9% NaCl (normal saline solution) = 0 calories • Vitamins as ordered

USES	SPECIAL CONSIDERATIONS
• 3 weeks or more (long term) • For patients with large caloric and nutrient needs • Provides needed calories; restores nitrogen balance; replaces essential vitamins, electrolytes, minerals, and trace elements • Promotes tissue synthesis, wound healing, normal metabolic function • Allows bowel rest and healing; reduces activity in the gallbladder, pancreas, and small intestine • Improves tolerance to surgery	**Basic solution** • Nutritionally complete • Requires minor surgical procedure for central line insertion (can be done at bedside by doctor) • Delivers hypertonic solutions • May cause metabolic complications (glucose intolerance, electrolyte imbalances, essential fatty acid deficiency) **I.V. fat emulsion** • May not be utilized effectively in severely stressed patients (especially burn patients) • May interfere with immune mechanisms • Irritates peripheral vein in long-term use
• 3 weeks or less • Maintains nutritional state in patients who can tolerate relatively high fluid volume; those who usually resume bowel function and oral feedings in a few days; and those who are susceptible to catheter-related infections of central venous TPN	**Basic solution** • Nutritionally complete for a short term • Can't be used in nutritionally depleted patients • Can't be used in volume-restricted patients since higher volumes of solution needed than with central venous TPN • Doesn't cause patient to gain weight • Avoids insertion and maintenance of central catheter, but patient must have good veins; I.V. site should be changed every 48 hours • Doesn't require surgery for peripheral line insertion • Delivers less hypertonic solutions than central venous TPN • May cause phlebitis • Less chance of metabolic complications than central venous TPN **I.V. fat emulsion** • As effective as dextrose for caloric source • Diminishes phlebitis if infused at same time as basic nutrient solution • Irritates vein in long-term use
• 2 weeks or less • May preserve body protein in a stable patient • Augments oral or tube feedings	• Nutritionally incomplete • Requires little mixing • May be initiated or stopped at any point in a patient's hospital stay • Other I.V. fluids, medications, and blood byproducts may be given through same I.V. line • Not as likely to cause phlebitis as peripheral TPN • Adds a major expense, with limited benefits
• Less than 1 week as nutrition source • Maintains hydration (main function) • Facilitates and maintains normal metabolic function	• Nutritionally incomplete; does not administer sufficient calories to maintain adequate nutritional status

deficiency is characterized by anorexia, alopecia, impaired wound healing, hypogeusia (diminished sense of taste), hypogonadism, intractable diarrhea, and vesicular dermatitis.

Copper, together with albumin, is transported to the liver, where it's incorporated into ceruloplasmin. Copper deficiency results in anemia that doesn't respond to treatment with iron.

Chromium deficiency may result in glucose intolerance, since this element is important in the action of insulin.

6. *Insulin.* Most patients receiving TPN don't require exogenous insulin unless glucose intolerance is secondary to diabetes mellitus, pancreatitis, or sepsis. Crystalline insulin preferably is added to the I.V. bag or bottle in initial doses of 5 to 10 units/liter of TPN solution when urine and serum glucose levels exceed 200 mg/100 ml. Thereafter, the insulin dosage can be increased gradually until the desired serum glucose level is achieved. Although some of the crystalline insulin will adhere to the sides of an infusion bag or bottle, only a negligible quantity of insulin is lost in this manner. Moreover, I.V. insulin administration is preferable to subcutaneous injection, because rebound insulin shock is less likely to result if the infusion is stopped abruptly due to mechanical problems.

NURSING TIPS

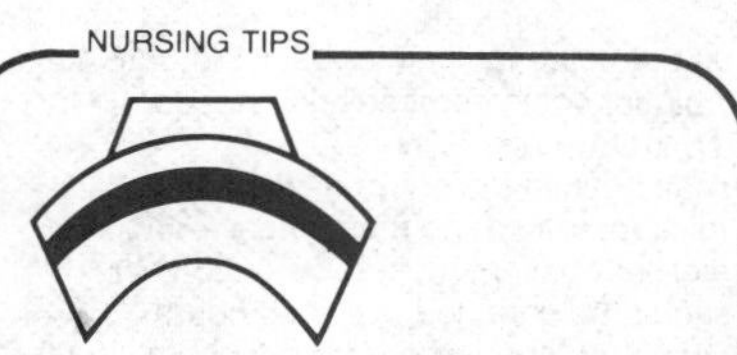

ADMINISTERING I.V. FAT EMULSIONS

Administer I.V. fat emulsions *slowly* (1 ml/minute or less) for the first 30 minutes. Observe the patient carefully for any adverse or allergic reactions. Watch for such signs as fever, diaphoresis, flushing, and/or dyspnea. Remember:

- Don't shake the container of fat emulsion, since this may impair the solution's stability.
- Don't add anything to the I.V. container of fat emulsion.
- Don't place a filter on a line intended for I.V. fat infusion.
- Piggyback the fat emulsion below or downstream of the filter if another solution is being infused simultaneously and requires a filter.
- Monitor the patient's serum triglyceride levels and liver function studies for signs of fat overload, such as headache, irritability, abdominal pain, nausea, coagulopathy, hepatomegaly, or splenomegaly. The doctor may order heparin I.V. to help clear lipids from your patient's plasma if fat overload occurs.

7. *Fat emulsions.* Three types of fat emulsions are currently available in the United States: Intralipid 10%, a soybean oil emulsion with 1.1 calories/ml; Intralipid 20%, a soybean oil emulsion with 2.2 calories/ml; and Liposyn 10%, a safflower oil emulsion with 1.1 calories/ml. To minimize the possibility of fat overload or fat embolism, no more than 3 g/kg/day should be administered to an adult.

Ordinarily, two or three 500-ml infusions of a 10% or 20% fat emulsion are administered twice weekly to prevent essential fatty acid deficiency in adults. Signs of essential fatty acid deficiency include desquamating dermatitis, alopecia, poor wound healing, and growth retardation in children.

The isotonicity of fat emulsions permits peripheral administration. Occasionally, piggybacking the emulsion into the TPN tubing is preferable. A 0.22-micron cellulose membrane filter cannot be used when fat is also being infused, because the fat particles are larger than the pores of the filter.

Ensuring the stability and sterility of the lipid emulsion before and during administration is an important nursing priority. Never shake the lipid container excessively or use the emulsion if there's any inconsistency in texture or color. During the initial infusion of fat, monitor the patient's vital signs as baseline indices. The flow rate should not exceed 1 ml/minute for the first 30 minutes. During this time, observe for fever, chills, flushing, diaphoresis, dyspnea, and allergic reactions. The patient's fat tolerance can be monitored biochemically by routine measurement of serum triglyceride levels and by liver function studies. Fat overload may be accompanied by headache, irritability, low-grade fever, abdominal pain, nausea, coagulopathy, hepatomegaly, and splenomegaly. I.V. heparin solution is the drug of choice to help clear lipids from the patient's plasma.

Administration
Because TPN fluid has approximately six times the solute concentration of blood, peripheral administration results in sclerosis and thrombosis. To ensure optimal dilution, the superior vena cava—a wide-bore, high-flow vein—is catheterized. In central venous access, the catheter tip must never be advanced into the right atrium because of the risk of cardiac perforation and arrhythmias.

There are several types of TPN catheters. In adults and in children who weigh more than 4.5 kg (10 lb), subclavian venipuncture has been the most commonly used technique for catheterization of the superior vena cava. After local infiltration of an anesthetic, a 14G or 16G needle, with a syringe attached, is inserted percutaneously beneath the medial one third of the clavicle and toward the suprasternal notch. When a venous return of blood is obtained, the syringe is detached and a subclavian catheter is threaded into the vein. The needle is withdrawn, and a plastic clamp is placed over the bevel to prevent inadvertent catheter severing. Complications are minimal when meticulous attention is given to anatomic details, proper insertion technique, and asepsis. Subclavian catheters typically remain in place 30 days or longer.

When cannulation is necessary for longer than 2 months, implantation of a silicone rubber, Dacron-cuffed catheter is preferable. The catheter is inserted into the jugular, subclavian, cephalic, thyroid, or facial vein, and is then tunneled so the catheter exit site is lateral to the xiphoid process. Firm tissue ingrowth into the Dacron cuff, with secondary catheter fixation, occurs in 2 to 3 weeks; the cuff then serves as a mechanical barrier against bacterial and fungal invasion. Many implanted catheters have remained in place longer than 5 years. The location of the catheter exit site enables the knowledgeable and capable patient to care for his own catheter.

Occasionally, the catheter is inserted into the brachial vein in the antecubital fossa or into one of the internal or external jugular veins. However, the catheter tip is always positioned in the superior vena cava.

Equipment
Equipment for administration includes a TPN *reservoir* (bag or bottle), I.V. *tubing*, a 0.22-micron *filter* (optional), and an *infusion pump*. The infusion apparatus must be a closed system to preserve the sterility of the catheter.

A volumetric infusion pump ensures an accurate, constant flow of TPN fluid. A controller device is not recommended, because the viscosity of the nutrient fluid makes consistent flow a problem.

There are several types of volumetric pumps, with various pumping mechanisms: peristaltic, rotary, linear, and cylinder and piston.

Most volumetric infusion devices have both visible and audible alarms equipped with a circuit outlet to connect the pump into a nurse call system. If the pump has only one alarm, the nurse must systematically determine the reason for the warning and correct whatever malfunction may exist. More complex infusion pumps include alarms for air in the I.V. tubing, low battery power, occlusion, and completion or near-completion of the infusion.

Selection of the most appropriate model should be based on a thorough evaluation of existing pumps. Evaluation criteria include cost, size, weight, availability, and service agreements.

Complications of TPN therapy
Major complications of TPN therapy may be insertion-related, septic, metabolic, or mechanical.

1. *Catheter insertion complications.* To minimize or obviate complications of central venous catheterization, ensure that skin preparation before insertion is adequate. During the insertion procedure, you serve as a quality control assistant to maintain strict sterile technique. In subclavian insertion, place the patient in Trendelenburg position to promote maximal dilatation and filling of the subclavian vein and to minimize the risk of inadvertent puncture of the lung pleura. Just before the doctor inserts the central venous catheter, he will tell the patient to take a deep breath, close his mouth, and bear down as if he were having a bowel movement. This procedure is called the Valsalva maneuver. Performing the Valsalva maneuver increases intrathoracic pressure and central venous pressure, and prevents air from entering the vein (air embolus). This procedure may be done whenever a new container is hung.

After catheter insertion, a container of 5% dextrose in water is hung temporarily until a chest X-ray is taken to check catheter tip position. Proper catheter tip positioning in the middle of the superior vena cava is necessary before TPN solution can be infused.

Complications associated with insertion of a central line into the subclavian vein include pneumothorax, tension pneumothorax, hemothorax, hydrothorax, subcutaneous emphysema, subclavian hematoma, thoracic duct injury, hydromediastinum, air embolism, catheter embolism, brachial plexus injury, arteriovenous fistula, endocarditis, venobronchial fistulization, and osteomyelitis of the clavicle. Report symptoms of these complications immediately for prompt intervention. (See chart opposite for symptoms and nursing interventions.)

2. *Sepsis.* The most feared and serious complication of TPN is sepsis. Defects in normal defense mechanisms make the patient with malnutrition prone to infections. Furthermore, hyperglycemia, administration of steroids or immunosuppressives, chemotherapy, and radiation therapy increase the likelihood of infection secondary to common skin bacteria such as *Staphylococcus epidermidis* and *Staphylococcus aureus.* Increased incidence of candidiasis has been reported in patients receiving antibiotics and those with hypophosphatemia.

Catheter-related sepsis is a potentially lethal complication; prevention depends on meticulous and consistent catheter care. Follow these guidelines:

- Provide catheter care at least three times weekly and whenever the sterile occlusive dressing becomes wet, nonocclusive, or soiled. First, clean the skin surface with an organic solvent to remove oil and residual surface debris. Then, using an iodine-containing antiseptic solution, cleanse the insertion site for at least 5 minutes. Next, apply antimicrobial or antibiotic ointment prophylactically to the skin at the exit site, and cover it with an occlusive, perhaps waterproof, covering (dressing) and adhesive tape.
- The same nurse should routinely change the catheter dressing to report comparative changes in skin appearance. Local erythema, inflammation, purulence, and tenderness suggest catheter contamination.
- Refrigerate the TPN solution until 30 minutes before the infusion.
- Don't manipulate the catheter unnecessarily, or use it for measuring central venous pressure or infusing medication. This may increase the risk of sepsis. Discourage the use of the central venous line catheter and delivery mechanism for any purpose other than supplying parenteral nutrients.

A peripheral venous route is recommended for infusion of blood or blood products, for intermittent or continuous injection of bolus medication, and for administration of additional solutions during TPN therapy. Unless an emergency arises, don't use the cath-

RECOGNIZING TPN COMPLICATIONS

COMPLICATIONS	SYMPTOMS	TREATMENT
Catheter-related		
Pneumothorax and hydrothorax	Dyspnea, chest pain, cyanosis, decreased breath sounds	Suction; insert chest tube.
Brachial plexus injury	Tingling and numbness along arm in peripheral TPN catheters	Remove catheter.
Air embolism	Dyspnea, chest pain, tachycardia, "mill wheel churning," murmur over precordium	Clamp catheter. Place patient in Trendelenburg position on left side.
Sepsis	Fever, chills, leukocytosis, erythema or pus at insertion site	Remove catheter and culture tip. Start appropriate antibiotics.
Metabolic		
Hyperglycemia	Polyuria, dehydration, elevated blood and urine glucose levels	Start insulin therapy or adjust flow rate.
Hyperosmolar, hyperglycemic nonketotic coma	Confusion, lethargy, seizures, coma, hyperglycemia, dehydration, glucosuria	Stop dextrose. Give insulin and 0.45% NaCl to rehydrate.
Hypokalemia	Muscle weakness, paralysis, paresthesias, arrhythmias	Increase potassium supplementation.
Hypomagnesemia	Tingling around mouth, paresthesias in fingers, mental changes, hyperreflexia	Increase magnesium supplementation.
Hypophosphatemia	Irritability, weakness, paresthesias, coma, respiratory arrest	Increase phosphate supplementation.
Hypocalcemia	Paresthesias, twitching, positive Chvostek's sign	Increase calcium supplementation.
Metabolic acidosis	Increased serum chloride level, decreased serum bicarbonate level	Use acetate or lactate salts of Na^+ or H^+.
Hepatic dysfunction	Increased serum transaminases, LDH, and bilirubin levels	Change to cyclical schedule. Decrease carbohydrate, add I.V. fats.
Hypoglycemia	Sweating, shaking, irritability when infusion is stopped	Infuse with 5% dextrose.
Mechanical		
Obliteration of catheter lumen	Interrupted flow rate	Reposition catheter. Attempt to aspirate clot.
Air embolism	Apprehension, chest pain, tachycardia, hypotension, cyanosis, seizure, loss of consciousness, possible cardiopulmonary arrest	Place patient in supine or Trendelenburg position on left side. Have patient perform the Valsalva maneuver. Tape tubing junctions securely.
Thrombosis	Erythema and edema at puncture site; ipsilateral swelling of arm, neck, or face; pain along vein; malaise; fever; tachycardia	Remove catheter promptly. Administer anticoagulant doses of heparin.
Fluid extravasation	Swelling of neck and shoulder area on affected side; pain	Observe patient for cardiopulmonary abnormalities by assessment and chest X-ray.

eter for obtaining aliquot portions of venous blood. Never incorporate a three-way stopcock into the infusion line or mix additives with the TPN solution after pharmacy preparation. The risk of contamination is too great.

• Don't automatically stop nutritional therapy if your patient suddenly develops a fever. Temporarily replace the TPN solution with 10% dextrose in water. Change the catheter dressing and tubing, and culture the TPN solution container, the administration tubing, and a sample of peripheral blood. If the patient becomes afebrile 4 to 6 hours later, a positive culture may identify the source of the fever. Negative cultures indicate a nonspecific pyrogenic response.

However, if the patient's temperature remains elevated or his condition deteriorates, peripheral blood is cultured a second time; blood from the catheter is withdrawn for fungal, and aerobic and anaerobic bacterial culture; and a sepsis workup is completed. Whenever the catheter must be removed, it is cultured for bacteria and fungi. If the catheter is the source of the fever, the patient's adverse reaction usually subsides in 12 to 24 hours. Systemic antibiotic or antifungal medication is not required unless the patient fails to respond to catheter removal and develops septic shock.

In most cases, a new feeding catheter is not inserted until all blood cultures are negative; however, if interruption of nutrient delivery is life-threatening, a new catheter can be inserted immediately and changed every 48 to 72 hours.

3. *Metabolic abnormalities.* The most common and serious metabolic complications are glucose intolerance and imbalances of potassium, phosphate, and magnesium. (For symptoms of these complications and nursing interventions, see the chart on the previous page.)

Here are the pertinent details you should know about these metabolic complications:

• *Glucose intolerance and hyperglycemia.* Endogenous insulin output increases gradually after the start of TPN therapy. The average adult tolerates 1 liter of TPN solution during the first 24 hours, then progresses to 1 liter every 12 hours for at least 2 consecutive days. Within the first 3 to 5 days, the typical adult can accommodate a daily ration of 3 liters of TPN solution or 500 mg/kg/hour of glucose without suffering adverse effects. This infusion schedule permits pancreatic islet cells sufficient opportunity to adapt to the continuous dextrose load by increasing insulin output.

Hyperglycemia can occur when the total dextrose load is excessive, the delivery rate is too rapid, or glucose tolerance is lowered. In a patient with normal renal function, desirable glucose tolerance is verified by routinely measuring fractional urine and ketone concentrations every 6 hours. If your patient is receiving cephalosporins, methyldopa, aspirin, or vitamin C, don't use reagent tablets to analyze the urine since they produce false-positive readings. Glycosuria is one of the first signs of sepsis when the infusion rate has not been altered. In addition, a high serum glucose level increases serum osmolality, causing a fluid shift from the intracellular space to the extracellular space. The expanded plasma volume dilutes the serum sodium and bicarbonate concentrations, producing hyponatremia with hypertonic metabolic acidosis. This alteration in the body fluid compartment results in osmotic diuresis with both intracellular and extracellular dehydration.

Other symptoms of hypoglycemia include nausea, vomiting, diarrhea, confusion, headache, and lethargy. Untreated hyperosmolar hyperglycemic dehydration can lead to convulsions, coma, and death.

Although most patients receiving between 2,000 and 3,000 calories/day tolerate sudden termination of the TPN infusion without incident, others experience profound reactive hypogly-

NURSING TIPS

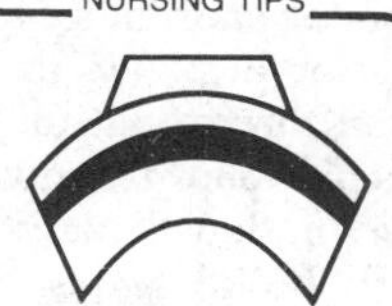

AN ALTERNATIVE TO CONTINUOUS PARENTERAL FEEDINGS—CYCLICAL TPN

Cyclical TPN is a scheduled parenteral nutrition plan whereby a patient receives 1,000 to 2,000 calories parenterally overnight and the rest of his nutritional requirements orally during the day.

Cyclical TPN allows your patient freedom while receiving parenteral therapy. Instead of continuous feedings, he receives parenteral feedings of I.V. dextrose and amino acids for 12 to 16 hours. Then, during the remaining 8 to 12 hours, depending on the patient's particular therapy regimen, he may receive I.V. fluids without glucose,* no I.V. fluids, and/or restricted enteral feedings.

Who receives cyclical TPN?

- A patient who is being weaned from TPN to enteral feedings.
- A patient on home TPN. Parenteral feedings overnight allow your patient to follow a routine life-style during the day.

Tips for stopping the TPN solution

When your patient stops continuous TPN and starts cyclical TPN, his blood sugar level must adjust to the new therapy. Stopping the TPN solution shouldn't cause a hypoglycemic episode in a patient with normal endocrine function if you follow this procedure:

- Reduce the flow rate to one half its normal rate 1 hour before TPN is discontinued.
- Stop the infusion after 1 hour at this slower rate.
- Observe the patient closely for hypoglycemic symptoms (tachycardia, sweating, tremors, weakness, and hunger) for the first 2 hours after the infusion is stopped.
- Draw a blood sample 1 hour after the infusion is stopped, to measure blood sugar level. Rarely will patients develop symptoms or have blood sugar levels below 60 to 70 mg/100 ml.
- To maintain patency, flush the I.V. line with heparin periodically during the 8-to-12-hour period the patient is off TPN. Follow your hospital's guidelines for heparin concentration and flushing of the central line.

*When no parenteral glucose is given, insulin levels fall, allowing the normal process of lipolysis of essential fatty acids and transport of nonessential fats from the liver to occur.

cemia. This disorder is commonly manifested by muscle weakness, mental confusion, anxiety, restlessness, diaphoresis, pallor, tremors, and palpitations. Therefore, taper the TPN solution dosage gradually over 24 to 48 hours. More rapid weaning is safe when the patient is ingesting sufficient carbohydrates or when peripheral I.V. infusion of 10% dextrose in water is begun.

- *Hypokalemia.* Severe hypokalemia can develop quickly since, during TPN-induced anabolism, potassium is transported into the cells. This intracellular flow is augmented by the hypertonic glucose-insulin solution.

Hypokalemia is suggested by muscle cramps and weakness, nausea, vomiting, paresthesias, and electrocardiographic aberrations. Catastrophic myocardial dysfunction and arrhythmias with ventricular asystole or fibrillation occur when serum potassium levels fall below 2 mEq/liter. A patient with severe cachexia may require as much as 60 to 100 mEq of potassium/1,000 calories to achieve potassium equilibrium. As anabolism progresses and metabolism stabilizes, protein turnover slows, and potassium requirements are reduced commensurately.

- *Hypophosphatemia.* Phosphorus depletion parallels potassium and protein depletion in the patient with malnutrition; some hypothesize that the mechanism for phosphorus loss is similar to that for potassium. Although high phosphate concentrations are found in bone, phosphate is not sufficiently labile or available for rapid redistribution throughout the body. If exogenous phosphorus is not provided in the TPN solution (usually 10 to 15 mEq/liter), blood levels may fall below 0.5 mg/dl. Neurologic and hematologic dysfunctions occur, exhibited by paresthesias, weakness, lethargy, and respiratory difficulty. Low serum phosphate levels are associated with impaired platelet function and decreased phagocytic and bactericidal activity of granulocytes.

• *Hypocalcemia.* Calcium levels must be monitored closely because of the relationship between calcium and phosphorus. Calcium deficiency increases neuronal membrane permeability and allows sodium to enter the cell more easily than usual, thus facilitating spontaneous depolarization. The central and the peripheral nervous systems can be affected, causing nausea, vomiting, diarrhea, hyperactive reflexes, muscular irritability, arrhythmias, diminished cardiac contractility, and bleeding due to abnormal clotting. Usually, 4.8 to 9.6 mEq/day of calcium gluconate prevents hypocalcemia in the patient receiving TPN therapy.

• *Hypomagnesemia.* Magnesium concentrations are much higher in the intracellular compartment than in the extracellular compartment, and loss of body cell mass probably results in relative magnesium deficiency. This may be manifested by muscle weakness, tremors, spasms, confusion, delirium, and seizures. Diuretics and cisplatin administered concurrently with TPN solution make the patient even more prone to hypomagnesemia. Usually, 10 to 15 mEq of magnesium sulfate/liter of TPN solution is sufficient to maintain normal blood levels.

4. *Mechanical complications.* The most common mechanical complications of the feeding catheter are obliteration of the catheter lumen, air embolism, thrombosis, and fluid extravasation.

• *Obliteration of the catheter lumen.* This mechanical difficulty may be caused by kinking of the catheter. Repositioning the catheter and replacing the suture can resolve the problem. Unless the catheter is heparinized, any interruption in the continuous infusion of I.V. solution, such as catheter kinking, can precipitate clot formation as well as occlusion of the catheter.

To restore catheter patency, attempt to aspirate the clot by applying slightly negative pressure to the barrel of a sterile syringe fixed snugly into the hub of the catheter. If this is ineffective, consult the doctor, who may elect to replace the occluded catheter, to *gently* irrigate the catheter with normal saline solution, or to instill streptokinase for lysis of the clot. The recommended technique is to instill 250,000 units of streptokinase that has been reconstituted in sterile sodium chloride solution into the entire length of the catheter over 20 minutes. Then the streptokinase-filled catheter is clamped for 2 hours while the nurse observes the patient for urticaria, flushing, fever, and other allergic reactions. The entire contents of the catheter must be extracted before fluid is introduced into the catheter. Since this is a specialized procedure, the doctor has to assess the patient's ability to tolerate the procedure without untoward reactions.

• *Air embolism.* To prevent this potentially lethal complication, make sure the patient is in supine or Trendelenburg position before disconnecting the catheter from the infusion line and exposing its open hub to the atmosphere. An additional precaution is to instruct the patient to perform the Valsalva maneuver or to hold his breath after deep inspiration.

Secure any I.V. tubing junctions with tape, and replace tubing if a hairline crack develops.

A significant air embolism with sudden vascular collapse may be accompanied by apprehension, chest pain, tachycardia, hypotension, cyanosis, seizure, loss of consciousness, and cardiopulmonary arrest. Emergency nursing intervention includes immediate action to stop air infiltration into the bloodstream. The patient is then positioned on his left side, with his head down. Air can thus be dissipated slowly by way of the pulmonary outflow tract as normal circulation returns. Several minutes can elapse before the patient becomes asymptomatic.

• *Thrombosis.* Thromboses of the subclavian or jugular vein or of the superior vena cava—although rare—are often associated with sepsis or a malpositioned catheter. Potential for this complication is lessened by optimal nursing care of the catheter exit site, by chest X-ray confirmation of proper catheter position, and by securing the catheter to the skin.

Evidence of thrombosis includes erythema and edema of the catheter insertion site; ipsilateral swelling of the arm, neck, or face; pain along the course of the vein; and systemic manifestations, such as malaise, fever, and tachycardia. When thrombosis or thrombophlebitis occurs, the catheter must be removed properly and the patient given anticoagulant doses of heparin to prevent thrombus propagation. With prompt action, the signs and symptoms of venous obstruction usually subside within several days.

• *Fluid extravasation.* If the feeding catheter ruptures or comes out of the vein, close observation for pulmonary and cardiac abnormalities, in conjunction with radiography, is critical. Because of the proximity of the catheter tract to the thoracic cavity, this complication is serious.

Furthermore, infusion of TPN solution into subcutaneous tissue can produce tissue necrosis, with sequential sloughing of the epidermal and dermal layers.

Enteral nutrition

Although tube feeding has long been used in patients who can't take adequate nourishment by mouth, recent advances in formulas and methods of administration have made widespread application more feasible. Some of the problems and complications historically associated with tube feeding have been resolved.

Indications

Generally, the ideal candidate for tube feeding is a patient with a functional GI system who can't ingest sufficient food and nutrients for energy. Conditions that warrant tube feeding include anorexia, coma (with caution to prevent aspiration), head and neck surgery, physical impairment (such as fractured jaw, obstructive lesions of the esophagus, and stroke), and hypermetabolic states.

Tube feeding is usually contraindicated in patients with adynamic ileus, intestinal obstruction, intractable vomiting, abnormal gastric emptying, and proximal high-output enterocutaneous or enteroenteric fistulas.

Administration routes

Tube feeding can be administered by the following GI routes, each of which indicates the site of insertion and final tube-tip placement: nasogastric, nasoduodenal, nasojejunal, esophagostomy, gastrostomy, and jejunostomy. The latter three, tube feeding ostomies, require surgical insertion of the feeding tube.

A cervical esophagostomy is created as a skin-lined canal, starting at the lower neck border and extending immediately below the cervical esophagus. The feeding tube is passed through this opening to the stomach for each feeding and then is removed after the feeding.

Since the surgical opening in gastrostomy and jejunostomy penetrates the peritoneum, excoriation and infection are potential complications of these methods.

Transnasal tube placement

Transnasal (nasogastric, nasoduodenal, nasojejunal) tube placement is a relatively safe and simple procedure commonly performed by qualified

COMPOSITION OF COMMONLY USED ENTERAL PRODUCTS

PRODUCT AND TYPE	PERCENT COMPOSITION Carbo-hydrate	Protein*	Fat	MAJOR COMPONENTS†	CALORIE CONTENT
Compleat-B Blenderized tube feeding	48	16	36	Pureed beef, green beans, peas, peaches, maltodextrin, nonfat dry milk, corn oil, sucrose, orange juice	1,070/liter
Ensure Tube feeding	54.5	14	31.5	Sodium and calcium caseinate, soy protein isolate, corn oil, corn syrup solids, sucrose	1,060/liter
Ensure Plus Tube feeding	53.3	14.6	31.9	Sodium and calcium caseinate, soy protein isolate, corn oil, corn syrup solids, sucrose	1,500/liter
Flexical Low-residue, elemental feeding	61	9	30	Casein hydrolysate, essential amino acids, MCT, soy oil, corn syrup solids, sucrose	250/2 oz
Isocal Tube feeding	50	13	37	Corn syrup solids, soy oil, sodium and calcium caseinate, MCT oil, protein isolate	250/8 oz
Meritene High-protein feeding	46	24	30	Sweet skim milk, corn syrup, vegetable oil, sodium caseinate, sucrose	1,200/750 ml
Precision LR Low-residue feeding	84	8.2	0.3	Egg white solids, maltodextrin, sugar, vegetable oil	1,900/18 oz
Sustacal High-protein tube feeding	55	24	21	Skim milk, sodium caseinate, soy, corn syrup, sugar	360/12 oz
Vivonex Low-residue, elemental feeding	90.8	8.5	0.7	Amino acids, safflower oil, glucose, and glucose oligosaccharides	1,000/liter
Vivonex HN Low-residue, high nitrogen, elemental feeding	81.34	18.26	0.4	Amino acids, safflower oil, glucose, and glucose oligosaccharides	1,000/liter

*Protein or protein equivalent
†Vitamins and minerals are also added.

Note: The composition of enteral products are subject to change

nurses. These are the steps to follow:

- After thoroughly explaining the procedure to the patient, you and he should agree on a hand signal he can use in case he experiences respiratory distress or discomfort.
- Examine the tubing for mechanical flaws, such as rough or sharp distal edges and closed or clogged outlet holes.
- After examining the nasal passages to rule out possible obstruction and to determine the more patent nostril, position the patient comfortably at a 90° angle.
- Lubricate the distal 10 cm of the tube, using a water-soluble lubricant. Ease the tube gently through the nostril, while aiming down and back toward the ear. The approximate depth of insertion has been defined by Hansen as the midway point between the 50-cm mark on the tube and the traditional distance from the tip of the nose to the earlobe to the xiphoid process.
- When the tube reaches the nasopharynx, rotate it 180°, and instruct the patient to swallow. Sipping water, if permissible, may facilitate swallowing. To initiate reflex swallowing in an unconscious patient, stimulate the throat.

Using a wire or gelatin stylet or a #16 French Levin tube as a carrier facilitates tube passage. Of course, when nasoenteric placement is desired, additional tubing must be passed. Some feeding tubes (Dobbhoff, Keofeed, Nutriflex) are weighted with a mercury bolus to allow the tube to pass spontaneously from the stomach into the intestine and to help anchor the tube after placement.

- Remove the enteral feeding catheter promptly if coughing, choking, gasping, cyanosis, or inability to vocalize occurs.
- Tube placement is verified by aspiration of gastric contents (contents may be checked with litmus paper for acidity), by auscultation of the gastric air bubble when 20 cc of air are injected in the distal lumen, and/or by chest X-ray.

In your daily nursing care of patients receiving enteral nutrition, pay special attention to oral hygiene and care of the nostrils. Promote patient comfort by using a cotton-tipped applicator moistened with warm water to remove dried secretions.

Handle enteral solutions carefully during preparation, storage, and administration to avoid contamination. Change the tubing every 48 to 72 hours to prevent introduction and proliferation of bacterial contamination.

If the patient has a gastrostomy or jejunostomy, clean the skin around the tube exit site daily with soap and warm water, and protect it with a small sterile gauze pad. During dressing changes, examine the skin to detect erythema, purulent drainage, or skin excoriation secondary to leaking gastric or intestinal contents.

Administration methods

Enteral solutions may be administered by bolus, gravity drip, or continuous drip methods.

- *Bolus.* In this method, 50 to 250 ml of solution are infused over a 20-minute period every 3 to 4 hours, and the tube is flushed with water afterward.
- *Gravity drip.* The enteral formula is delivered by gravity over 1 hour.
- *Continuous drip.* Because the bolus and gravity methods may cause a high residual volume and increased diarrhea, the continuous drip method provides the optimal schedule. The feeding is infused over 24 hours. An infusion pump may be used to administer this type of feeding.

Continuous feeding procedures

The volume and concentration of enteral formula delivered by tube feeding are individually tailored to the patient. History of oral intake and current medical condition, the infusion site, and type of formula are considered.

Feedings delivered into the duodenum and proximal jejunum are usually given by continuous pump infusion to prevent dumping syndrome. Since the duodenum and jejunum are more sensitive to volume and osmolality, isotonic formulas are more easily tolerated and don't require the dilution necessary with hypertonic solutions.

Usually, a half-strength formula is initiated at 50 ml/hour. If the patient tolerates the half-strength feeding without glycosuria, diarrhea, or nausea, the rate is increased 25 ml/hour every 8 hours. The strength is changed to full concentration when the final desired rate has been achieved.

During feedings, check urine every 4 hours for the presence of glucose and acetone until results are negative for 48 hours.

Keep the head of the bed elevated at least 30° at all times to prevent aspiration. Also, verify proper tube location at least every 4 hours, and check gastric residual every 4 hours. If more than 150 ml are aspirated, stop the infusion for 1 hour.

Complications

The major complications of tube feeding are fluid and electrolyte imbalance, aspiration pneumonia, diarrhea, constipation, and GI upset.

- *Fluid and electrolyte disturbances.* Dehydration can result from excessive diarrhea, excessive protein intake, and osmotic diuresis. Tube-feeding syndrome may result from excessive protein intake accompanied by inadequate fluid intake. Symptoms include confusion, decreased level of consciousness, dehydration, hypernatremia, hyperchloremia, and azotemia. Monitor serum electrolyte and glucose levels, blood urea nitrogen, and hematocrit daily until stable, then once or twice weekly. You can also use intake and output records and daily weights to monitor fluid status.
- *Aspiration pneumonia.* This life-threatening complication requires special precautions. Elevate the head of the bed at least 30° when using continuous drip, or elevate the head for at least 30 minutes after bolus or gravity drip. Proper tube selection and placement are also important. Large-bore feeding tubes diminish gastroesophageal sphincter competency, increasing the possibility of gastric reflux. When the risk of aspiration is high—as in the patient who is severely debilitated, moribund, or comatose—nasoenteric, gastrostomy, or jejunostomy feedings are preferred.
- *Diarrhea.* Diarrhea is the most common complication of tube feeding. Introducing a hyperosmolar solution into the intestinal lumen may alone cause diarrhea. This condition may be alleviated by delivering the solution by 24-hour continuous drip, initially diluting hyperosmolar solutions, and gradually increasing concentration as tolerated. However, diarrhea can also be secondary to bacterial contamination, lactose intolerance, low serum albumin, and concurrent drug therapy.
- *Constipation.* Constipation has been reported in patients on long-term tube feeding. Since many commercial feeding solutions are low in residue, decreased frequency of bowel movements is to be expected. If constipation is painful to the patient, adding bulk to the diet may be necessary. This may be done by changing the formula to include more residue.
- *Other GI upsets.* Nausea, distention, and abdominal cramping are usually prevented by a continuous feeding schedule. Nausea may be alleviated by temporarily stopping the feeding or slowing the drip rate. If nausea results from gastric distention, ambulation may help, when possible. Discontinue enteral feedings in the event of vomiting, decreased gastric motility, or obstruction.

Home nutritional support

Recent advances in the methods and techniques of long-term nutritional support have enabled patients to be discharged from the hospital while receiving TPN or enteral nutrition therapy. A more normal life-style is possible

PATIENT PREPARATION

BRIEFING PATIENTS ON HOME NUTRITIONAL SUPPORT: A NURSE'S CHECKLIST

If your patient no longer requires hospital care but still needs parenteral therapy, he can now receive treatment at home. To promote successful home nutritional therapy ask your patient if he understands:

☐ how to perform all necessary procedures, before he leaves the hospital
☐ how to obtain the best possible results from his therapy at home
☐ what complications can arise
☐ when to seek medical assistance
☐ how to respond to an emergency.

Check that you've thoroughly explained each of these specific points:

Care of the catheter site*

☐ Sterile techniques
☐ Dressing care
☐ Catheter exit site complications
☐ Heparinization procedures
☐ What to do if the catheter becomes damaged or dislodged

Pump operation

☐ How to use the pump
☐ What can be infused with the I.V. solution
☐ How to set the infusion rate
☐ How to run the infusion

Disconnecting the infusion

☐ The importance of running a slow infusion for the last hour
☐ Catheter clamping procedure
☐ Final catheter heparinization

Before your patient goes home, remind him to:

☐ check the I.V. container under light for cracks in the glass (if bottle is used instead of bag) and make certain the I.V. solution is clear.
☐ inspect the product label for correct fluid contents and valid expiration date.
☐ follow the manufacturer's instructions on all administration equipment.
☐ use new, sterile I.V. tubing, pump cassette, and filter each day to prevent infection.

*The catheter is surgically implanted into the superior vena cava or right atrium before the patient leaves the hospital.

when a patient receives his nutrient requirements at night for 8 to 10 hours. The implanted TPN catheter can be heparinized, allowing patient mobility without the infusion apparatus.

When your patient is selected for home nutritional support, formulate an individualized teaching plan that is well organized, sequenced, and designed to meet his learning needs. Base the teaching plan on a thorough assessment of your patient and others involved in his care.

Instructional materials such as patient manuals, audiovisual aids, and mannequins can facilitate learning. Before discharge, critically evaluate your patient's competence in catheter care.

The accompanying nurse's checklist may help you prepare your patient for home nutritional support. You may also copy the troubleshooting guide on the next page for your patient's use at home.

The patient on home nutritional support requires close follow-up after discharge; at least one member of the health-care team must be available 24 hours a day in case of a crisis.

ALAN W. HOPEFL, PharmD
DEANN M. ENGLERT, RN, MSN

PATIENT-TEACHING AID

TROUBLESHOOTING HOME HYPERALIMENTATION

Dear Patient:

Complications, although rare, may develop while you're undergoing home hyperalimentation. Here are signs and symptoms to watch for, and what to do about them:

PROBLEM	WHAT TO WATCH FOR	WHAT TO DO
Infiltration	Swelling of tissues around catheter insertion site (shoulder, neck, or arm), discomfort, pain in shoulder or arm on catheter side; swollen tissues cooler than rest of body tissues	• Call the doctor immediately if you think the catheter has come out of the vein or has ruptured. • Slow the flow rate if you can't reach the doctor immediately.
Cloudy solution or sediment in solution	Solution cloudy or showing undissolved particles	• Don't use. Solution may be contaminated. Return solution container to pharmacy at once for exchange. • If you're mixing your own solution, take extra care with preparation, and don't prepare more than 24 hours' worth of solution at a time.
Too rapid infusion	Nausea, headache, lassitude	• Check to be sure solution is flowing at the rate ordered by your doctor. If you're using an infusion pump, check for mechanical problems. • If the flow rate is correct and symptoms persist, contact your doctor.
Catheter dislodgment	Catheter pulled out of vein	• Place a sterile gauze pad on insertion site, and apply pressure. • Notify your doctor.
Crack or break in catheter tubing	Fluid leaking out through crack or break in tubing	• Apply padded hemostat above break, to prevent entry of air. • Call your doctor at once.
Clotted catheter	Solution flow stops and doesn't enter the vein	• Notify doctor. He may instill streptokinase or heparin into the catheter to try to dissolve clot.
Hyperglycemia (high blood sugar)	Fatigue, restlessness, confusion, anxiety, weakness, urine tests positive for sugar, and in severe cases, possibly delirium and/or coma	• Notify doctor at once.

PROBLEM	WHAT TO WATCH FOR	WHAT TO DO
Phlebitis	Pain, tenderness, skin redness and warmth	• Rest, and apply gentle heat to the site. Elevate your arm if the catheter is inserted in your arm. • Relief should occur within 24 to 72 hours, and condition should subside within 3 to 5 days. • Notify your doctor immediately. He may want to examine you or give you additional care instructions.
Infection	Fever (body temperature above 37.8° C. [100° F.]), redness and/or pus at insertion site.	• Notify your doctor so he can determine the fever's source. • If infection is present, the doctor will remove the catheter to have the tip cultured.
Thrombosis	Redness and swelling around catheter entrance site; swelling of catheterized arm and of neck or face on catheter's side of body, pain at insertion site and along vein, rapid heart beat, fever	• Notify your doctor at once. He will evaluate the catheter for removal. • These symptoms usually indicate blood clot formation around the catheter, a problem that requires prompt medical and nursing treatment.
Air embolism	Apprehension, chest pain, rapid heart beat, low blood pressure resulting in dizziness and fainting, bluish appearance; problem caused by air entering catheter, usually during bottle changes	• Call your doctor immediately. If symptoms are severe, go to hospital emergency department at once. • Lie on your left side, with your head slightly lower than the rest of your body.

Note: Complications from home hyperalimentation are uncommon if proper technique is maintained. Despite the possibility of these problems, home hyperalimentation results in decreased hospitalization and significant cost savings for you. In addition, this therapy lets you maintain a more normal life-style.

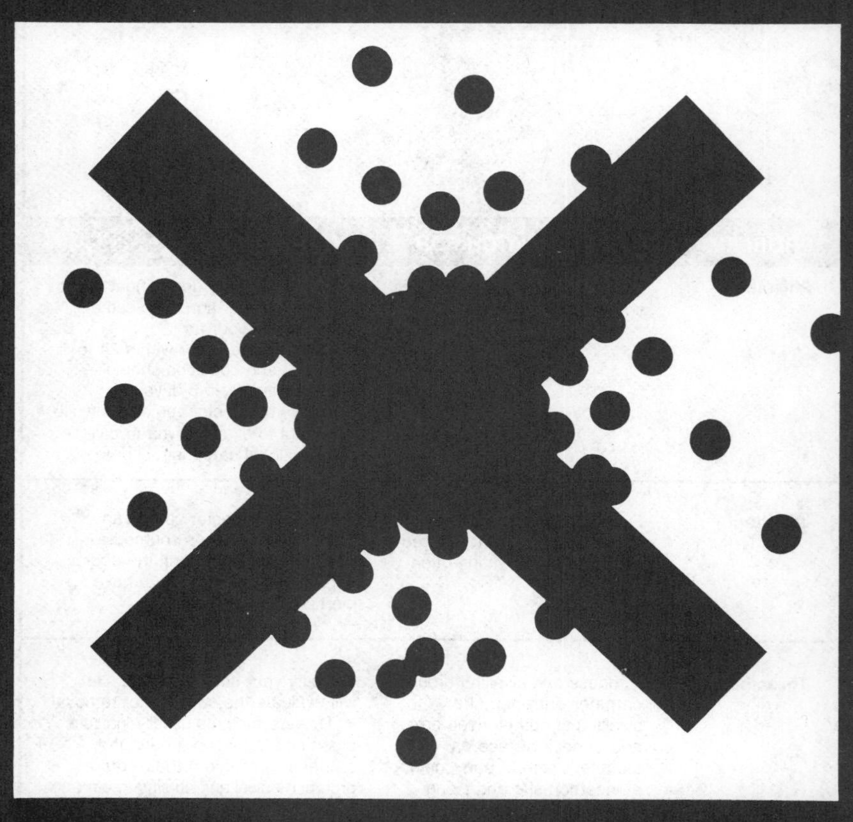

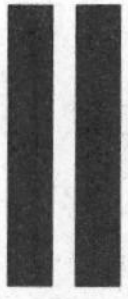

Antimicrobial and Antiparasitic Agents

8 Amebicides and trichomonacides

carbarsone
chloroquine hydrochloride
chloroquine phosphate
diiodohydroxyquin
emetine hydrochloride
metronidazole
oxamniquine
paromomycin sulfate

Amebicides and trichomonacides cure or control diseases caused by amebic or trichomonal infection, such as amebiasis, primary amebic meningoencephalitis, and trichomoniasis. Amebiasis, or amebic dysentery, is an intestinal disorder caused by the parasite *Entamoeba histolytica.* The condition is now being reported more often than it was in the past, particularly among homosexual males.

Primary amebic meningoencephalitis, commonly transmitted through infected swimming pools, is caused by the ameba *Naegleria monocytogenes* and is almost always fatal.

Trichomoniasis is a relatively common vaginal infection caused by *Trichomonas vaginalis.* The infection spreads through sexual activity; infected males and about 70% of infected females are usually asymptomatic.

Major uses

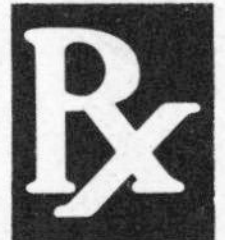

• Metronidazole is the drug of choice for amebic dysentery and trichomonal infections; it may also be useful in treating gram-negative anaerobic infections. Alternate drugs are usually administered in combination with at least one other drug and are not always efficacious.

• The drug of choice for amebic meningoencephalitis is amphotericin B. (See Chapter 10, ANTIFUNGALS, for complete information about amphotericin B.)

Mechanism of action

• Carbarsone is an organic arsenic derivative with amebicidal activity in the intestinal lumen, possibly due to inhibition of sulfhydryl enzymes.

• Chloroquine is mainly an antimalarial. Its mechanism of action as an amebicide is unknown, but it's useful in treating extraintestinal amebiasis.

• Diiodohydroxyquin is an iodine derivative with amebicidal activity in the intestinal lumen. Its precise mechanism of action is unknown.

• Emetine kills *E. histolytica* by indirectly inhibiting protein synthesis.

• Metronidazole is a direct-acting trichomonacide and amebicide that works at both intestinal and extraintestinal sites.

• Oxamniquine reduces the egg load of *Schistosoma mansoni,* but its exact mechanism of action is unknown.

• Paromomycin is an aminoglycoside antibiotic that acts as an amebicide in intestinal sites, effective in the presence or absence of bacteria. Its specific mechanism of action is unknown.

Absorption, distribution, metabolism, and excretion

• Carbarsone is readily absorbed from

the gastrointestinal (GI) tract after oral and rectal administration but is excreted slowly in urine. The drug may accumulate, causing toxicity.

- Chloroquine is almost completely absorbed in the small intestine after oral administration. About 55% of the drug is bound to plasma proteins, and high concentrations are found in body tissues. It is excreted slowly in urine; small amounts are detectable after therapy is stopped—sometimes even years later.
- Diiodohydroxyquin is poorly absorbed from the GI tract; most of it is eliminated in the stool.
- Emetine is absorbed from parenteral sites, slowly detoxified by the liver, and excreted primarily by the kidneys. Detectable in urine 40 to 60 days after treatment, emetine concentrates in the liver, kidneys, and spleen.
- Metronidazole is well absorbed after oral administration, primarily in the small intestine. Limited data suggest wide distribution, with significant concentration in abscesses, bile, cerebrospinal fluid, and many tissues. From 60% to 70% is excreted in the urine unchanged; the remainder is metabolized in the liver.
- Oxamniquine, well absorbed when administered orally, is metabolized to inactive metabolites and excreted in the urine.
- Paromomycin is poorly absorbed from the GI tract after oral administration; almost all the drug is eliminated unchanged in the stool.

Onset and duration

- Chloroquine: Daily doses of 50 mg result in peak blood levels of 125 mcg/ml within 2 to 4 hours; half-life is about 3 days.
- Diiodohydroxyquin, emetine, and paromomycin: Onset is generally within 4 to 8 hours; effects can last 4 to 7 days.
- Metronidazole: Single oral doses of 750 mg cause peak blood levels of 10 to 15 mcg/ml within 2 to 4 hours; half-life is 6 to 12 hours.
- Oxamniquine: After doses of 12 to 15 mg/kg, blood levels peak in 1 to 1½ hours; half-life is 1 to 2½ hours.

Combination products

None.

PREVENTING AMEBIASIS

Amebic invasion of intestinal mucosa occurs most commonly in the cecum and rectosigmoid area, causing diarrhea and possibly abdominal pain, moderate leukocytosis, dehydration, or intermittent fever. After being carried into the bloodstream, the amebic infection may affect other parts of the body. For example, passage through the diaphragm may result in secondary pulmonary abscess formation.

To avoid contracting the infection, all nurses and visitors in contact with the patient with amebiasis must wear a gown and gloves, and wash their hands on entering and leaving the room. Private rooms are necessary only for children or confused patients. Masks are not needed at all.

Remember to disinfect or discard articles contaminated with the patient's urine and feces. Be extremely cautious in handling and disposing of stool specimens.

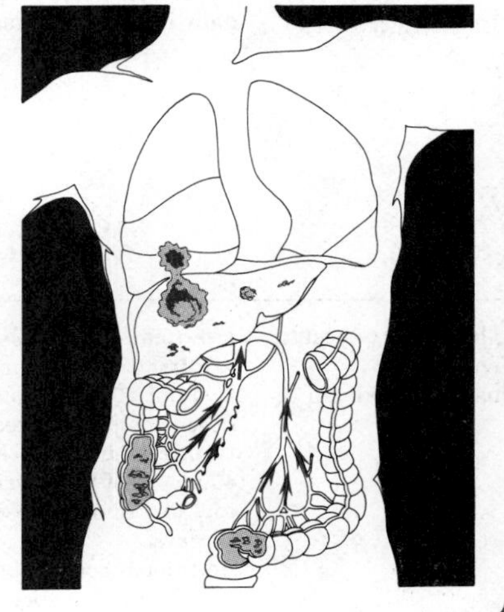

NAME	INDICATIONS & DOSAGE	SIDE EFFECTS
carbarsone	*Intestinal amebiasis*— **Adults:** 250 mg P.O. b.i.d. or t.i.d. for 10 days. Rectal (as retention enema): 2 g dissolved in 200 ml warm 2% sodium bicarbonate solution, every other night for 5 doses. Discontinue oral therapy when enema is given. **Children:** average total dose is 75 mg/kg P.O. daily in 3 divided doses over 10-day period. Recommended total varies according to age—2 to 4 years, 2 g total; 5 to 8 years, 3 g total; 9 to 12 years, 4 g total; and over 12 years, 5 g total.	**Blood:** *agranulocytosis.* **CNS:** neuritis, convulsions, *hemorrhagic encephalitis.* **EENT:** sore throat, retinal edema, visual disturbances. **GI:** epigastric pain and burning, irritation, *nausea, vomiting,* diarrhea, anorexia, constipation, increased motility, abdominal cramps. **GU:** polyuria, albuminuria, kidney damage. **Hepatic:** hepatomegaly, jaundice, hepatitis. **Skin:** eruptions, *exfoliative dermatitis,* pruritus. **Other:** edema of wrists, ankles, and knees; weight loss; splenomegaly.
chloroquine hydrochloride Aralen HCl **chloroquine phosphate** Aralen Phosphate♦, Chlorocon, Roquine	*Extraintestinal amebiasis*— **Adults:** 160 to 200 mg chloroquine (hydrochloride) base I.M. daily for no more than 10 or 12 days. As soon as possible, substitute 1 g (600 mg base) chloroquine phosphate P.O. daily for 2 days; then 500 mg (300 mg base) daily for at least 2 to 3 weeks. Treatment is usually combined with an effective intestinal amebicide. *Rheumatoid arthritis*— 250 mg chloroquine phosphate daily with evening meal.	**Blood:** *agranulocytosis.* **CNS:** mild and transient headache, neuromyopathy, psychic stimulation, fatigue, irritability, nightmares, convulsions, dizziness. **EENT:** *visual disturbances* (blurred vision; difficulty in focusing; reversible corneal changes; generally irreversible, sometimes progressive or delayed retinal changes, e.g., narrowing of arterioles; macular lesions; pallor of optic disk; optic atrophy; patchy retinal pigmentation, often leading to blindness), ototoxicity, nerve deafness, vertigo, tinnitus. **GI:** anorexia, abdominal cramps, diarrhea, nausea, vomiting. **Skin:** pruritus, lichen planus-like eruptions, skin and mucosal pigmentary changes, pleomorphic skin eruptions.
diiodohydroxyquin Gynovules♦♦, Inserfem, Yodoxin	*Intestinal amebiasis*— **Adults:** 630 to 650 mg P.O. t.i.d. for 20 days. Total daily dose should not exceed 2 g. **Children:** usual dose: 30 to 40 mg/kg of body weight daily in 2 to 3 divided doses for 20 days. Additional courses of diiodohy-	**Blood:** *agranulocytosis.* **CNS:** neurotoxicity, dysesthesia, weakness, vertigo, malaise, headache, agitation, retrograde amnesia, ataxia, peripheral neuropathy. **EENT:** optic neuritis, optic atrophy, loss of vision. **GI:** anorexia, nausea, vomiting, abdominal cramps, diarrhea, in-

INTERACTIONS	NURSING CONSIDERATIONS
None significant.	• Contraindicated as initial treatment in patients with hepatic or renal disease; in patients with contracted visual or color fields; and in patients with known hypersensitivity or intolerance to any arsenical treatment. • Don't exceed recommended dose; toxicity may result. If second treatment is needed, allow at least 10 days between courses. • Divide carbarsone capsule to obtain required dose. Give in ½ glass orange juice or milk, in small amount of 1% sodium bicarbonate solution, or in jelly or other food. • Discontinue at first sign of intolerance or toxicity. Fatal exfoliative dermatitis has been reported. • Tell patient to report any unusual symptoms, even post-treatment. • Liver function studies should precede therapy. Careful inspection of skin, vision testing, and palpation of liver and spleen should be repeated regularly. • Monitor intake/output. Notify doctor of number, frequency, and character of stools. • Give a cleansing enema before giving carbarsone enema. • Deliver stool specimen to laboratory promptly; movements of parasites are seen only when stool is warm. Amebic cysts in stool indicate need for additional therapy. Stool specimen should be studied 1 week after stopping therapy and monthly for 1 year. To help prevent reinfestation, instruct patient in proper hygiene.
None significant.	• Contraindicated in patients with retinal or visual field changes, porphyria. Use with extreme caution in presence of severe GI, neurologic, or blood disorders. Drug concentrates in liver; use cautiously in patients with hepatic disease or alcoholism. Use with caution in patients with G-6-PD deficiency or psoriasis; drug may exacerbate these conditions. • Complete blood cell counts and liver function studies should be made periodically during prolonged therapy; if severe disorder appears that is not attributable to disease under treatment, drug may need to be discontinued. • Overdosage can quickly lead to toxic symptoms: headache, drowsiness, visual disturbances, cardiovascular collapse, and convulsions, followed by respiratory and cardiac arrest. Children are extremely susceptible to toxicity; avoid long-term treatment. • Baseline and periodic ophthalmologic examinations needed. Report blurred vision, increased sensitivity to light, or muscle weakness. Check periodically for muscle weakness after long-term use. Audiometric examinations recommended before, during, and after therapy, especially if long term. • To prevent exacerbated drug-induced dermatoses, warn patient to avoid excessive exposure to sun. • Each ml parenteral solution containing 50 mg dihydrochloride salt = 40 mg chloroquine base; each 500 mg tablet phosphate = 300 mg chloroquine base.
None significant.	• Contraindicated in patients with known hypersensitivity to 8-hydroxyquinoline derivatives or iodine-containing preparations. Diiodohydroxyquin causes hepatic damage in such patients. Also contraindicated in patients with hepatic or renal disease, or preexisting optic neuropathy. • Patient should have periodic ophthalmologic examinations during treatment. • Give after meals. Crush tablets and mix with applesauce or chocolate syrup.

(continued on following page)

NAME	INDICATIONS & DOSAGE	SIDE EFFECTS
diiodohydroxyquin *(continued)*	droxyquin therapy should not be repeated before a resting interval of 2 to 3 weeks.	creased motility, constipation, epigastric burning and pain, gastritis, anal irritation and itching. **Skin:** pruritus, hives, papular and pustular eruptions, urticaria, discoloration of hair and nails. **Other:** thyroid enlargement, fever, chills, generalized furunculosis, hair loss.
emetine hydrochloride	*Acute fulminating amebic dysentery*— **Adults:** 1 mg/kg daily up to 65 mg daily (1 or 2 doses) deep S.C. or I.M. 3 to 5 days to control symptoms. Give another antiamebic drug simultaneously. **Children over 8 years:** no more than 20 mg daily deep S.C. or I.M. for 3 to 5 days. **Children under 8 years:** no more than 10 mg daily for 3 to 5 days. *Amebic hepatitis and abscess*— **Adults:** 65 mg daily (1 or 2 doses) deep S.C. or I.M. for 10 days. **Children over 8 years:** no more than 20 mg daily for 10 days. **Children under 8 years:** no more than 10 mg daily for 10 days.	**CNS:** dizziness, headache, mild sensory disturbances, central or peripheral nerve function changes, neuromuscular symptoms (weakness, aching, stiffness, tenderness, pain, tremors). **CV:** *acute toxicity*—can occur at any dose (hypotension, tachycardia, precordial pain, dyspnea, *EKG abnormalities,* gallop rhythm, cardiac dilatation, severe acute degenerative myocarditis, pericarditis, congestive failure). **GI:** *nausea, vomiting, diarrhea,* abdominal cramps, loss of sense of taste. **Metabolic:** decreased serum potassium levels. **Skin:** eczematous, urticarial purpuric lesions. **Local:** skeletal muscle stiffness, aching, tenderness, muscle weakness at injection site. **Other:** edema.
metronidazole Flagyl♦, Neo-Tric♦♦, Novonidazol♦♦, Trikacide♦♦	*Amebic hepatic abscess*— **Adults:** 500 to 750 mg P.O. t.i.d. for 5 to 10 days. **Children:** 35 to 50 mg/kg daily (in 3 doses) for 10 days. *Intestinal amebiasis*— **Adults:** 750 mg P.O. t.i.d. for 5 to 10 days. **Children:** 35 to 50 mg/kg daily (in 3 doses) for 10 days. Follow this therapy with oral	**Blood:** leukopenia, neutropenia. **CNS:** vertigo, headache, ataxia, incoordination, confusion, irritability, depression, restlessness, weakness, fatigue, drowsiness, insomnia, sensory neuropathy, paresthesias of extremities, psychic stimulation, neuromyopathy. **CV:** EKG change (flattened T wave). **EENT:** blurred vision, difficulty

♦ Available in U.S. and Canada. ♦♦ Available in Canada only. All other products (no symbol) available in U.S. only. Italicized side effects are common or life-threatening.

INTERACTIONS	NURSING CONSIDERATIONS
	• Record intake/output and color and amount of stool. Send warm specimens to laboratory frequently. • Watch for diarrhea during the first 2 to 3 days of treatment. Notify doctor if it continues past 3 days. • Advise patient not to discontinue the medication prematurely. Tell him to notify doctor if skin rash occurs.
None significant.	• Contraindicated in patients with cardiac or renal disease, except those with amebic abscess or hepatitis not controlled by chloroquine; patients who have received a course of emetine less than 6 to 8 weeks previously; children, except for severe dysentery unresponsive to other amebicides; and in those with polyneuropathy or muscle disease. Use with caution in aged or debilitated patients, patients with hypotension, or those about to undergo surgery. • Record pulse rate and blood pressure 2 to 3 times daily. Discontinue use if drug produces tachycardia, precipitous fall in blood pressure, neuromuscular symptoms, marked gastrointestinal effects, or considerable weakness. Weakness and muscle symptoms usually precede more serious symptoms and serve as a guide for avoiding toxicity. • Don't exceed recommended dose or extend therapy beyond 10 days. Patient confined to bed during treatment and for several days thereafter. • Drug may alter EKG tracings for 6 weeks. EKG should be taken before therapy, after fifth dose, upon completion, and 1 week after therapy. Patterns can resemble those of myocardial infarction. First and most consistent change is T wave inversion. • Deep S.C. administration is preferred; I.M. acceptable, but I.V. route is dangerous and contraindicated. Injections cause necrosis and edema. Rotate sites and apply warm soaks. • Record intake/output; odor and consistency of stools; and presence of mucus, blood, or other foreign matter. Send warm specimens to laboratory frequently. Repeat fecal examinations at 3-month intervals to ensure elimination of amebae. Patients with acute amebic dysentery commonly become asymptomatic carriers. Check family members and suspected contacts. • Suspect emetine-induced reaction if stools increase in number following initial relief of diarrhea. • To help prevent reinfection, instruct patient in proper hygiene. • Drug is very irritating. Avoid contact with eyes and mucous membranes. • Restoration of body fluids and nutrients is an important adjunct to therapy.
Alcohol: disulfiram-like reaction (nausea, vomiting, headache, cramps, flushing). Don't use together. *Disulfiram:* acute psychoses and confusional states. Don't use together.	*Warning:* This drug has been shown to be carcinogenic in mice and possibly rats. Unnecessary use should be avoided. • Contraindicated in patients with a history of blood dyscrasia or CNS disorder, and in patients with retinal or visual field changes. Use with caution in patients with hepatic disease or alcoholism; in conjunction with known hepatotoxic drugs. • Tell patients to avoid alcohol or alcohol-containing medications. • Give with meals to minimize GI distress. • Tell patients metallic taste and dark or red-brown urine are possible. • Record number and character of stools when used in the treatment

(continued on following page)

NAME	INDICATIONS & DOSAGE	SIDE EFFECTS
metronidazole *(continued)*	diiodohydroxyquin. *Trichomoniasis—* **Adults (both male and female):** 250 mg P.O. t.i.d. for 7 days or 2 g P.O. in single dose; 4 to 6 weeks should elapse between courses of therapy. *Refractory trichomoniasis—* **Women:** 250 mg P.O. b.i.d. for 10 days.	in focusing, nasal congestion. **GI:** abdominal cramping, stomatitis, *nausea, vomiting, anorexia,* diarrhea, constipation, proctitis, dry mouth. **GU:** darkened urine, polyuria, dysuria, pyuria, incontinence, cystitis, decreased libido, dyspareunia, dryness of vagina and vulva, sense of pelvic pressure. **Skin:** pruritus, flushing. **Other:** overgrowth of nonsusceptible organisms, especially *Candida* (glossitis, furry tongue), metallic taste, fever.
oxamniquine Vansil	*Treatment of schistosomiasis caused by* Schistosoma mansoni— **Adults:** 12 to 15 mg/kg given as a single oral dose. **Children (under 30 kg):** 20 mg/kg given in 2 equally divided oral doses at 2- to 8-hour intervals.	**CNS:** *convulsions, dizziness, drowsiness,* headache. **GI:** nausea, vomiting, abdominal pain, anorexia. **Skin:** urticaria.
paromomycin sulfate Humatin	*Intestinal amebiasis, acute and chronic—* **Adults and children:** 25 to 35 mg/kg daily P.O. in 3 doses for 5 to 10 days after meals.	**Blood:** eosinophilia. **CNS:** headache, vertigo. **EENT:** ototoxicity. **GI:** anorexia, nausea, vomiting, epigastric pain and burning, abdominal cramps, diarrhea, constipation, increased motility, steatorrhea, pruritus ani, malabsorption syndrome. **GU:** hematuria, nephrotoxicity. **Skin:** rash, exanthema, pruritus. **Other:** overgrowth of nonsusceptible organisms.

OBTAINING UNAPPROVED AMEBICIDAL DRUGS

The doctor may ask you to obtain an amebicidal drug that is not commercially available. What should you do?

Call the Center for Disease Control to secure one of these *investigational* drugs. With a doctor's order, you can contact:

Parasitic Disease Drug Service
Center for Infectious Diseases
Center for Disease Control
Atlanta, Ga. 30333
(404) 329-3670

Here's a list of investigational amebicides and the infections they're used to treat:

INTERACTIONS	NURSING CONSIDERATIONS
	of amebiasis. Metronidazole should be used only after *Trichomonas vaginalis* has been confirmed by wet smear or culture or *Entamoeba histolytica* has been identified. Asymptomatic sexual partners of patients being treated for *T. vaginalis* infection should be treated simultaneously to avoid reinfection. Instruct patient in proper hygiene. • Has been used to treat anaerobic infections.
None significant	• Use cautiously in patients with a history of convulsive conditions. Epileptiform convulsions have rarely been observed within the first few hours after ingestion. Patients with history of convulsions should be kept under medical supervision. • Instruct patient to avoid driving and other hazardous activities if he's dizzy or drowsy. • GI tolerance is improved if given after meals. • Although *S. mansoni* infection is rare in the U.S. and Canada, travelers or immigrants from such areas as Puerto Rico, Latin America, and Africa may have contracted it from contaminated water.
None significant.	• Contraindicated in patients with impaired renal function or intestinal obstruction. Use with caution in patients with ulcerative lesions of the bowel to avoid inadvertent absorption and resulting renal toxicity. Poorly absorbed orally but accumulates with renal impairment or ulcerative lesions. • Ask about history of sensitivity to drug before giving first dose. • Administer after meals. • Emphasize personal hygiene, particularly handwashing before eating and after defecation. • Criterion of cure is absence of amebae in stools examined weekly for 6 weeks after treatment and at monthly intervals for 2 years. Examine feces of family members or suspected contacts. • Avoid high doses or prolonged therapy. • Watch for signs of superinfection (continued fever and other signs of new infections, especially monilial infections).

INVESTIGATIONAL DRUG	AMEBIC INFECTION
bithionol	Sheep liver fluke infection
cycloguanil pamoate	Leishmaniasis
dehydroemetine	Amebiasis
diloxanide furoate	Amebiasis
melarsoprol	African trypanosomiasis
metrifonate	Schistosomiasis
niclosamide	Tapeworm infection
pentamidine isethionate	*Pneumocystis carinii*
sodium antimony dimercaptosuccinate	Schistosomiasis
stibogluconate sodium	Leishmaniasis
suramin	African trypanosomiasis

Anthelmintics

antimony potassium tartrate
diethylcarbamazine citrate
gentian violet
mebendazole
piperazine adipate
piperazine citrate
piperazine phosphate
piperazine tartrate
pyrantel pamoate
pyrvinium pamoate
quinacrine hydrochloride
thiabendazole

Anthelmintics rid the body of helminths, or parasitic worms. Although helmintic infections are usually confined to the intestines, dissemination to the genitalia, peritoneum, and hematopoietic system may occur.

Major uses

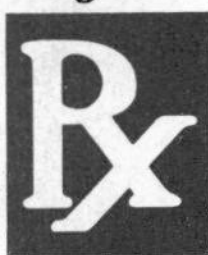

Anthelmintics eradicate various helminths, including tapeworms, pinworms, hookworms, roundworms, and schistosomes.

Mechanism of action

- Antimony potassium tartrate inhibits phosphofructokinase, and therefore glucose utilization, in schistosomes.
- Diethylcarbamazine appears to sensitize the worms to phagocytosis by the reticuloendothelial system.
- Mebendazole appears to selectively and irreversibly inhibit uptake of glucose and other nutrients in susceptible helminths.
- Piperazine and pyrantel block neuromuscular action, paralyzing the worm and causing its expulsion by normal peristalsis.
- Pyrvinium, a cyanine dye, appears to destroy parasites by preventing them from using exogenous carbohydrates.
- Quinacrine inhibits deoxyribonucleic acid metabolism.
- Mechanism of action of gentian violet and thiabendazole is unknown.

Absorption, distribution, metabolism, and excretion

- Antimony potassium tartrate is extensively bound within erythrocytes after parenteral administration. Excretion is primarily by the kidneys.
- Diethylcarbamazine is readily absorbed from the gastrointestinal (GI) tract, distributed to all body tissues except fat, and excreted in the urine.
- Piperazine is readily absorbed from the GI tract. Some piperazine is metabolized in the liver; the remainder is excreted unchanged in the urine.
- Pyrantel is poorly absorbed from the GI tract. It is metabolized primarily in the liver, and the rest is eliminated unchanged in the urine and feces. The rate of excretion varies greatly among patients.
- Quinacrine is readily absorbed from the GI tract and is highly concentrated in the liver. Its metabolism and excretion are unknown.
- Thiabendazole is rapidly absorbed from the GI tract; it's metabolized, then excreted in the urine.
- Other anthelmintics—gentian vi-

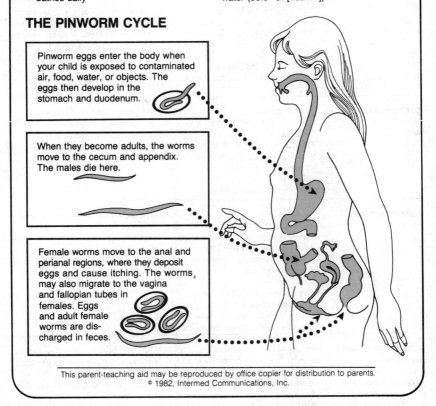

HOW TO PREVENT AND CONTROL PINWORMS

Dear Parents:

Pinworms are small, threadlike worms, ⅓″ to ⅔″ (0.8 to 1.7 cm) long. They're found throughout the world, most frequently in preschool age and school-age children. The infection usually spreads to other family members.

To help prevent and control pinworms, make sure your child:

- washes his hands carefully after using lavatory facilities and before handling food
- avoids nail-biting
- bathes daily
- changes his underwear daily.

If you suspect a household member has pinworms, have the doctor examine and treat the whole family at the same time. Have all family members avoid bathing in or drinking water that may be contaminated. Also, observe these precautions:

- Cook meat thoroughly to kill any infectious larvae.
- During pinworm treatment, disinfect clothing and bed linens by washing in hot water (55.5° C. [132° F.]).

THE PINWORM CYCLE

Pinworm eggs enter the body when your child is exposed to contaminated air, food, water, or objects. The eggs then develop in the stomach and duodenum.

When they become adults, the worms move to the cecum and appendix. The males die here.

Female worms move to the anal and perianal regions, where they deposit eggs and cause itching. The worms may also migrate to the vagina and fallopian tubes in females. Eggs and adult female worms are discharged in feces.

olet, mebandazole, and pyrvinium—are poorly absorbed from the GI tract and are mainly eliminated in the feces.

Onset and duration

Anthelmintics have a rapid onset and short duration.

NAME	INDICATIONS & DOSAGE	SIDE EFFECTS
antimony potassium tartrate (not commercially available; must be compounded)	Schistosoma japonicum *infection*— **Adults:** initially, 8 ml of 0.5% solution in sterile water for injection or 5% dextrose solution given slow I.V. Increase each subsequent dose 4 ml until 11th day, when 28 ml are given. Give 28 ml on alternate days until a total of 360 ml (1.8 g) is given.	**Blood:** thrombocytopenia. **CV:** hypotension, syncope, bradycardia, EKG changes. **GI:** nausea, vomiting, diarrhea, colic. **Hepatic:** jaundice, *hepatic necrosis.* **Local:** pain at I.V. injection site. **Other:** dyspnea, severe arthralgia, albuminuria, fever, dermatitis.
diethylcarbamazine citrate Hetrazan	*Ascariasis (roundworm)*— **Adults:** 13 mg/kg P.O. daily for 7 days. **Children:** 6 to 10 mg/kg P.O. t.i.d. for 7 to 10 days. *Loiasis, dipetalonemiasis, onchocerciasis, Bancroftian or Malayan filariasis*— **Adults and children:** 2 mg/kg P.O. t.i.d. for 3 to 4 weeks. Repeat if necessary. *Tropical (pulmonary) eosinophilia*— **Adults and children:** 13 mg/kg P.O. daily for 4 to 7 days.	**Blood:** leukocytosis, eosinophilia. **CNS:** *headache, malaise, weakness,* lassitude, syncope. **CV:** tachycardia, tachypnea, hypotension. **GI:** anorexia, nausea, vomiting. **Skin:** pruritus, dermatitis, bullous eruptions. **Other:** arthralgia, myalgia, joint pain, swelling and edema of face, severe pedal edema, fever, lymphadenitis, sweating, cough.
gentian violet Jayne's P-W Vermifuge	*Pinworms*— **Adults:** 60 mg P.O. t.i.d. 7 to 10 days. **Children:** 2 mg/kg P.O. daily in 2 to 3 doses for 8 to 10 days, not to exceed 90 mg/day. Discontinue treatment after 7 to 10 days. Resume if needed.	**CNS:** headache, dizziness, lassitude. **GI:** nausea, diarrhea, vomiting (purple), abdominal cramps.
mebendazole Vermox♦	*Pinworms*— **Adults, and children over 2 years:** 100 mg P.O. as a single dose. If infection persists 3 weeks later, repeat treatment. *Roundworm, whipworm, hookworm*— **Adults, and children over 2 years:** 100 mg P.O. b.i.d. for 3 days. If infection persists 3 weeks later, repeat treatment.	**GI:** occasional, transient abdominal pain and diarrhea in massive infection and expulsion of worms.
piperazine adipate Entacyl♦♦ **piperazine citrate** Antepar♦, Bryrel, Pin-Tega Tabs, Pipril, Ta-Verm, Vermazine	*Pinworms*— **Adults and children:** 65 mg/kg P.O. daily 7 to 8 days. Maximum daily dose is 2.5 g. *Roundworm*— **Adults:** 3.5 g P.O. in single doses for 2 consecutive days.	**CNS:** ataxia, tremors, choreiform movements, muscular weakness, myoclonus, hyporeflexia, paresthesias, convulsions, sense of detachment, EEG abnormalities, memory defect, headache, vertigo. **EENT:** nystagmus, blurred vision,

♦ Available in U.S. and Canada. ♦♦ Available in Canada only. All other products (no symbol) available in U.S. only. Italicized side effects are common or life-threatening.

INTERACTIONS	NURSING CONSIDERATIONS
None significant.	• Treatment of choice for *S. japonicum*. • Not for use in other worm infections; toxicity with this agent is high. • Solutions must be fresh (within 12 hours of pharmacy's preparation). • Doses should be given 2 hours after a light meal. • Patient should lie down for 1 hour after treatment. • Antiemetics should not be given, since they mask nausea and vomiting, which are signs of hepatic toxicity. • Extravasation may cause painful cellulitis. • Avoid rapid injection. May lead to severe coughing, vomiting, or even death.
None significant.	• Use with caution in patients with hypertension; severe hepatic, renal, or cardiac disease; and in children under 1 year of age. Treat patients with recent history of malaria with an antimalarial agent first to prevent relapse in asymptomatic malarial infections. • Administer carefully to avoid or control allergic or other untoward reactions. Minimize allergic reactions by giving with corticosteroids, antihistamines, or aspirin. • Inform patient that side effects will usually be minor and transient. • Instruct patient in good hygiene. • Give immediately after meals. Drug has sweet but unpleasant taste.
None significant.	• Use with caution in patients with cardiac, hepatic, renal, or GI disease. • Tablets must be taken whole with water. Give with meals. • Patient should abstain from alcohol during treatment. • If nausea and vomiting occur, stop treatment for 1 to 2 days; resume at reduced dosage and notify doctor. Warn that skin, clothing, vomitus, and feces will be stained purple. • Instruct patient in good hygiene. Treat all family members.
None significant.	• Tablets may be chewed, swallowed whole, or crushed and mixed with food. • No dietary restrictions, laxatives, or enemas necessary. • To avoid reinfection, wash perianal area daily. Change undergarments and bedclothes daily. Wash hands and clean fingernails after bowel movements and before meals. Treat all family members.
None significant.	• Contraindicated in patients with hepatic and/or renal impairment, or convulsive disorders. Use with caution in patients with severe malnutrition or anemia. • Discontinue if CNS or significant GI reactions occur. • Because of potential neurotoxicity, avoid prolonged or repeated treatment, especially in children. • No dietary restrictions, laxatives, or enemas necessary.

(continued on following page)

NAME	INDICATIONS & DOSAGE	SIDE EFFECTS
piperazine *(continued)* **piperazine phosphate** Antepar Phosphate, Piperaval **piperazine tartrate** Razine Tartrate	**Children:** 75 mg/kg P.O. daily in single dose for 2 consecutive days. Maximum daily dose: 3.5 g.	paralytic strabismus, cataracts with visual impairment, lacrimation, difficulty in focusing, rhinorrhea. **GI:** *nausea, vomiting,* diarrhea, abdominal cramps. **Skin:** urticaria, photodermatitis, *erythema multiforme,* purpura, eczematous skin reactions. **Other:** arthralgia, fever, bronchospasm.
pyrantel pamoate Antiminth, Combantrin♦♦	*Roundworm and pinworm—* **Adults, and children over 2 years:** single dose of 11 mg/kg P.O. Maximum dose 1 g. For pinworm, dose should be repeated in 2 weeks.	**CNS:** headache, dizziness, drowsiness, insomnia. **GI:** anorexia, nausea, vomiting, gastralgia, cramps, diarrhea, tenesmus. **Hepatic:** transient elevation of SGOT. **Skin:** rashes. **Other:** fever, weakness.
pyrvinium pamoate Pamovin♦♦, Povan, Pyr-Pam♦♦, Vanquin♦♦	*Pinworm—* **Adults and children:** 5 mg/kg P.O. single dose (maximum 350 mg). Repeat in 2 weeks if needed.	**GI:** nausea, vomiting, cramping, diarrhea (vomiting more common with suspension than with tablets). **Skin:** photosensitivity, *erythema multiforme.*
quinacrine hydrochloride Atabrine	*Treatment of giardiasis—* **Adults:** 100 mg P.O. for 5 to 7 days. **Children:** 7 mg/kg/day P.O. given in 3 divided doses after meals for 5 days. Maximum 300 mg/day. If necessary, the dosage may be repeated in 2 weeks. *Treatment of tapeworm—* **Adults, and children over 14 years:** Administer a cleansing enema. Then administer 4 doses of 200 mg P.O. every 10 minutes (total 800 mg). **Children 11 to 14 years:** Total 600 mg P.O. in 3 to 4 doses at 10-minute intervals. **Children 5 to 10 years:** Total 400 mg P.O. in 3 to 4 doses at 10-minute intervals.	**CNS:** *headache, dizziness,* nervousness, vertigo, mood shifts, nightmares. **GI:** *diarrhea, anorexia, nausea, abdominal cramps,* vomiting. **Skin:** pleomorphic skin eruptions.
thiabendazole Mintezol♦	*Systemic infection with pinworm, roundworm, threadworm, whipworm, cutaneous larva migrans, and*	**CNS:** impaired mental alertness, impaired physical coordination, *drowsiness, giddiness,* headache, dizziness.

♦ Available in U.S. and Canada. ♦♦ Available in Canada only. All other products (no symbol) available in U.S. only. Italicized side effects are common or life-threatening.

INTERACTIONS	NURSING CONSIDERATIONS
	• May be taken with food. • To avoid reinfection, wash perianal area daily. Change undergarments and bedclothes daily. Wash hands and clean fingernails before meals and after bowel movements. Treat all family members. • Protect drug from air, light, and moisture.
None significant.	• Use cautiously in severe malnutrition or anemia, or in hepatic dysfunction. Treat for anemia, dehydration, or malnutrition before giving drug. • No dietary restrictions, laxatives, or enemas necessary. • May be taken with food. Shake well before pouring. • To avoid reinfection, wash perianal area daily. Change undergarments and bedclothes daily. Wash hands and clean fingernails before meals and after bowel movements. Treat all family members. • Protect drug from light. Store below 30° C. (86° F.).
None significant.	• Safe use in children who weigh less than 36 kg not established. • Swallow tablets whole to avoid staining teeth. May be taken with food. • Warn that drug stains fabrics, skin, vomitus, and stools bright red. • No dietary restrictions, laxatives, or enemas necessary. • To avoid reinfection, wash perianal area daily. Change undergarments and bedclothes daily. Wash hands and clean fingernails before meals and after bowel movements. Treat all family members. • Protect drug from light.
None significant	• Contraindicated if primaquine is being given concurrently since primaquine toxicity could be increased. • Use with extreme caution in patients with porphyria or psoriasis; may exacerbate these conditions. • Use with caution in patients with hepatic disease, alcoholism, severe renal or cardiac disease, psychosis, G-6-PD deficiency, and in those over 60 years or under 1 year. • Saline cathartic is necessary after treatment to dispel worms. • Give after meals with large glass of water, tea, or fruit juice to reduce GI irritation. Bitter taste may be diguised by jam or honey. • Nausea and vomiting after large doses may be lessened by taking sodium bicarbonate with each dose. • Collect all of stool after treatment. Don't put toilet paper in bedpan. Look for the scolex (attachment organ), which will be stained yellow from drug. • Warn patients about temporary yellow color of skin and urine; it is not jaundice. • Patient should be on a bland, nonfat, semisolid diet for 24 hours, and should fast after the evening meal before treatment. • Keep out of reach of children; drug is highly toxic. • Induce emesis for overdose.
None significant.	• Use with caution in patients with hepatic or renal dysfunction, severe malnutrition, anemia, and in patients who are vomiting. Supportive therapy indicated for anemic, dehydrated, or malnourished patients. In children under 15 kg, weigh benefits against risks.

(continued on following page)

NAME	INDICATIONS & DOSAGE	SIDE EFFECTS
thiabendazole *(continued)*	*trichinosis—* **Adults or children over 70 kg:** 1.5 g P.O. **Adults or children under 70 kg:** 25 mg/kg P.O. in two doses daily. Maximum dose is 3 g daily. *Cutaneous infestations with larva migrans (creeping eruption)—* **Adults and children:** dose depends on patient's weight—70 kg or over, 1.5 g P.O./dose; under 70 kg, 4.6 mg/kg/dose. Two doses daily for 2 successive days. If active lesions still present 2 days after therapy, give second course. *Pinworms*—two doses daily for 1 day; repeat in 7 days. *Roundworms, threadworms, whipworms*—two doses daily for 2 successive days. *Trichinosis*—two doses daily for 2 to 4 successive days.	**GI:** anorexia, nausea, vomiting, diarrhea, epigastric distress. **Skin:** rash, pruritus, *erythema multiforme.* **Other:** lymphadenopathy, fever, flushing, chills.

BASIC FACTS ABOUT COMMON HELMINTH INFECTIONS

CONDITION	CAUSE	SOURCE OF INFECTION
Tapeworm infection	Tapeworm *(Hymenolepis nana, Taenia saginata, Taenia solium, Diphyllobothrium latum)*	Poorly cooked or infected beef, pork, or fish
Enterobiasis	Pinworm *(Enterobius vermicularis)*	Eggs from contaminated objects (books, clothes, toys, wooden objects)
Hookworm infection	Hookworm *(Necator americanus, Ancylostoma duodenale)*	Contaminated feces
Roundworm infection	Roundworm *(Ascaris lumbricoides)*	Contaminated feces
Schistosomiasis	Schistosome *(Schistosoma japonicum, Schistosoma mansoni, Schistosoma haematobium)*	Infested water containing larvae from snail vector

INTERACTIONS	NURSING CONSIDERATIONS
	• Warn that medication may cause drowsiness and dizziness. • Give after meals. Shake suspension before measuring; chew tablets before swallowing. • Laxatives, enemas, and diet restrictions not needed. • To avoid reinfection, wash perianal area daily. Change undergarments and bedclothes daily. Wash hands and clean fingernails before meals and after bowel movements. Treat all family members.

ENTRY SITE	SYMPTOMS	DRUG
Mouth	• Diarrhea • Abdominal discomfort • Dizziness • Anemia	quinacrine
Mouth (embryonated eggs)	• Perianal pruritus • Perineal irritation, superinfection, and vulvovaginitis • Salpingitis and abdominal pain (females)	pyrvinium, gentian violet, mebendazole, piperazine, pyrantel, thiabendazole
Feet, mouth, skin (filariform larvae)	• Iron deficiency anemia • Abdominal pain • Diarrhea • Urticaria	mebendazole
Mouth (embryonated eggs)	• Colicky abdominal pain • Nausea and vomiting • Malnutrition	piperazine, diethylcarbamazine citrate, mebendazole, pyrantel, thiabendazole
Skin (cercariae)	• Dermatitis, urticaria • Abdominal pain, bloody diarrhea, hematuria • Lymphadenopathy • Hepatomegaly • Fever • Cough	antimony potassium tartrate, oxamniquine

10 Antifungals

amphotericin B
flucytosine
griseofulvin microsize
griseofulvin ultramicrosize
miconazole
nystatin

Fungi resist most antibiotics at therapeutic levels; only the antifungals are currently effective against them. Amphotericin B has been the most widely used antifungal, although others have recently been developed. The new drug ketoconazole (Nizoral) shows great promise (see *Know the Advantages of Ketoconazole,* p. 143, and APPENDIX, *New Drugs*).

Much of the recent increase in systemic fungal infections is related to cancer chemotherapy's compromise of the immune system.

Major uses

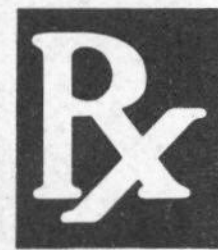

Besides systemic fungal infections, antifungals are effective against meningitis, severe fungal infections caused by *Candida* and *Cryptococcus* organisms, and yeast infections.

• Amphotericin B is useful in the treatment of central nervous system (CNS), pulmonary, cardiac, renal, and other systemic fungal infections. It is effective against blastomycosis, histoplasmosis, cryptococcosis, candidiasis, sporotrichosis, aspergillosis, phycomycosis (mucormycosis), and coccidioidomycosis. It is of no value in treatment of topical fungal infections.

• Flucytosine is effective when used alone in the treatment of systemic candidiasis, cryptococcosis, and aspergillosis. However, the best results are achieved when this drug is used with amphotericin B.

• Griseofulvin is used systemically in the treatment of tinea capitis and other tinea infections that don't respond to topical agents.

• Miconazole is given intravenously to treat systemic coccidioidomycosis, candidiasis, cryptococcosis, and paracoccidioidomycosis. It is usually less effective than amphotericin B.

• Nystatin is used topically to treat superficial candidal infections of the oral mucosa and esophagus.

Mechanism of action

• Amphotericin B and nystatin probably act by binding to sterols in the fungal cell membrane, altering cell permeability and allowing leakage of intracellular components. They may also inhibit glycolysis and protein synthesis.

• Flucytosine appears to penetrate fungal cells, where it is converted to fluorouracil, a known metabolic antagonist. Flucytosine is incorporated into fungal ribonucleic acid (RNA) and causes defective protein synthesis.

• Griseofulvin arrests fungal cell activity by disrupting its mitotic spindle structure.

• Miconazole inhibits purine transport, and deoxyribonucleic acid, RNA, and protein synthesis; and it increases cell-wall permeability, making the fungus more susceptible to osmotic pressure.

Absorption, distribution, metabolism, and excretion

• Amphotericin B is poorly absorbed from the gastrointestinal (GI) tract, so it's generally administered by I.V. infusion. It is 90% bound to plasma proteins. Amphotericin B diffuses poorly into body cavities, eyes, and cerebrospinal fluid, and is slowly excreted by the kidneys.

• Flucytosine is rapidly absorbed from the GI tract, reaching peak levels in about 6 hours. About 90% is excreted unchanged in the urine. The drug is well distributed to all body tissues and to the CNS.

• Griseofulvin, although almost completely absorbed through the duodenum in ultramicrosize formulation, is absorbed unpredictably in microsize formulation. Administration with a high-fat meal, however, may enhance absorption.

The drug concentrates in skin, hair, nails, liver, fat, and skeletal muscles. The highest concentration is found in the outermost horny layer of the skin; the lowest, in the deep layers.

Metabolized in the liver, griseofulvin is eliminated in urine, feces, and perspiration, mostly as inactive metabolite and unchanged drug.

• Miconazole is poorly absorbed from the GI tract, rapidly metabolized in the liver, and excreted mainly as inactive metabolites. Miconazole penetrates joints but not the CNS.

• Nystatin's oral absorption is negligible. The drug is not absorbed through intact skin or mucous membranes, and blood levels are not measurable at therapeutic doses. The drug is eliminated unchanged in the stool.

Onset and duration

• Amphotericin B has an average peak blood level of 1 mcg/ml after I.V. infusion of 30 mg. Immediately after infusion, no more than 10% of the dose appears in blood; the half-life is 24 hours.

Amphotericin B can be detected in blood and urine 4 weeks after therapy is discontinued.

• Flucytosine is well absorbed from the GI tract. It reaches peak blood levels of 30 to 45 mcg/ml within 6 hours of a single 2-g oral dose in patients with normal renal function.

The dose must be altered, however, for patients with renal impairment. Flucytosine has a half-life of 6 hours and is eliminated unchanged, primarily in the urine.

• Griseofulvin blood levels peak in 4 hours. It is undetectable in skin 2 days—and in blood 4 days—after drug is discontinued. Drug concentrations in skin are highest in warm climates.

• Miconazole, with I.V. infusion of 9 mg/kg, reaches blood levels of at least 1 mcg/ml, but they fall rapidly within 30 minutes. The half-life of miconazole is unchanged in patients with renal impairment.

• Nystatin products vary in onset and duration.

Combination products

ACHROSTATIN-V: nystatin 250,000 units and tetracycline HCl 250 mg.
DECLOSTATIN CAPS: nystatin 250,000 units and demeclocycline HCl 150 mg.
DECLOSTATIN TABS: nystatin 500,000 units and demeclocycline HCl 300 mg.
MYSTECLIN-F CAPS: tetracycline HCl 250 mg and amphotericin B 50 mg buffered with potassium metaphosphate.
MYSTECLIN-F CAPS: tetracycline HCl 125 mg and amphotericin B 25 mg buffered with potassium metaphosphate.
MYSTECLIN-F SYRUP:tetracycline HCl 125 mg and amphotericin B 25 mg per 5 ml buffered with potassium metaphosphate.
TERRASTATIN CAPS: nystatin 250,000 units and oxytetracycline 250 mg.
TETRASTATIN CAPS: nystatin 250,000 units and tetracycline HCl 250 mg.

NAME	INDICATIONS & DOSAGE	SIDE EFFECTS
amphotericin B Fungizone♦	*Systemic fungal infections (histoplasmosis, coccidioidomycosis, blastomycosis, cryptococcosis, disseminated moniliasis, aspergillosis, phycomycosis), meningitis—* **Adults and children:** initially, 1 mg in 250 ml of 5% dextrose in water infused over 2 to 4 hours; or 0.25 mg/kg daily by slow infusion over 6 hours. Increase gradually as patient tolerance develops to maximum 1 mg/kg daily. Therapy must not exceed 1.5 mg/kg. If drug is discontinued for a week or more, administration must resume with initial dose and again increase gradually. *Topical* (3% cream, lotion, ointment): apply liberally and rub well into affected area b.i.d. to q.i.d. *Intrathecal:* 25 mcg/0.1 ml diluted with 10 to 20 ml of cerebrospinal fluid and administered by barbotage 2 or 3 times weekly. Initial dose should not exceed 50 mcg. *Coccidioidal arthritis—* **Adults:** 5 to 15 mg into joint spaces.	**Blood:** normochromic, normocytic anemia. **CNS:** headache, peripheral neuropathy; with intrathecal administration—peripheral nerve pain, paresthesias. **GI:** anorexia, weight loss, nausea, vomiting, dyspepsia, diarrhea, epigastric cramps. **GU:** abnormal renal function with *hypokalemia, azotemia, hyposthenuria,* renal tubular acidosis, nephrocalcinosis; with large doses—permanent renal impairment, anuria, oliguria. **Local:** burning, stinging, irritation, tissue damage with extravasation, *thrombophlebitis,* pain at site of injection. **Other:** arthralgia, myalgia, muscle weakness secondary to hypokalemia, *fever, chills,* malaise, generalized pain.
flucytosine Ancobon, Ancotil♦♦	*For severe fungal infections caused by susceptible strains of* Candida *(including septicemia, endocarditis, urinary-tract and pulmonary infections) and* Cryptococcus *(meningitis, pulmonary infection, and possible urinary-tract infections)—* **Adults, and children weighing more than 50 kg:** 50 to 150 mg/kg daily q 6 hours P.O. **Children weighing less than 50 kg:** 1.5 to 4.5 g/m²/day in 4 divided doses P.O.	**Blood:** anemia, leukopenia, bone marrow depression, thrombocytopenia. **CNS:** dizziness, drowsiness, confusion, headache. **GI:** *nausea, vomiting, diarrhea,* abdominal bloating. **Hepatic:** elevated SGOT, SGPT. **Metabolic:** elevated serum alkaline phosphatase, BUN, serum creatinine. **Skin:** occasional rash.

♦ Available in U.S. and Canada. ♦♦ Available in Canada only. All other products (no symbol) available in U.S. only. Italicized side effects are common or life-threatening.

INTERACTIONS	NURSING CONSIDERATIONS
None significant.	• Use cautiously in patients with impaired renal function. • Use parenterally only in hospitalized patients, under close supervision, when diagnosis of potentially fatal fungal infection has been confirmed. • Monitor vital signs; fever may appear 1 to 2 hours after start of I.V. infusion and should subside within 4 hours of discontinuation. • Monitor intake/output; report change in urine appearance or volume. Renal damage usually reversible if drug is stopped with first sign of dysfunction. • Obtain liver and renal function studies weekly. If BUN exceeds 40 mg/100 ml, or if serum creatinine exceeds 3 mg/100 ml, doctor may reduce or stop drug until renal function improves. Monitor CBC weekly. Stop drug if Bromsulphalein, alkaline phosphatase, or bilirubin levels become elevated. • Monitor potassium levels closely. Report any signs of hypokalemia. Check calcium and magnesium levels periodically. • In the dry state, store at 2° to 8° C. (35.6° to 46.4° F.). Protect from light. Expires 2 years after date of manufacture. Reconstitute with 10 ml sterile water only. Mixing with solutions containing sodium chloride, other electrolytes, or bacteriostatic agents such as benzyl alcohol causes precipitation. Do not use if solution contains precipitate or foreign matter. Use aseptic technique. • Appears to be compatible with limited amounts of heparin sodium, hydrocortisone sodium succinate, and methylprednisolone sodium succinate. • Reconstituted solution is stable for 1 week under refrigeration or 24 hours at room temperature. Protect from light. Wrap bottle in aluminum foil. • Recommended infusion solution is 10 mg/100 ml of 5% dextrose in water. • Severity of some side effects can be reduced by premedication with aspirin, antihistamines, antiemetics, or small doses of corticosteroids; addition of phosphate buffer and heparin to the solution; and alternate-day dose schedule. For severe reactions, drug may have to be stopped. See *Preventing Amphotericin B Toxicity*, p. 142. • For I.V. infusion, an in-line membrane with mean pore diameter larger than 1 micron can be used. Infuse very slowly; rapid infusion may result in cardiovascular collapse. Warn patient of discomfort at infusion site and other potential side effects. Advise patient that several months of therapy may be needed to assure adequate response. • Antibiotics should be given separately; don't mix or piggyback with amphotericin B. • Topical preparations may stain clothing.
None significant.	• Use with extreme caution in patients with impaired hepatic or renal function, or bone marrow depression. • Hematologic tests and renal and liver function studies should precede therapy and should be repeated at frequent intervals thereafter. Before treatment, susceptibility tests should establish that organism is flucytosine-sensitive. Tests should be repeated weekly to monitor drug resistance. • Well absorbed from the GI tract. Nausea, vomiting, stomach upset are reduced if capsules given a few at a time over a 15-minute period. • Monitor intake and output; report any marked change. • If possible, blood level assays of drug should be performed regularly to maintain flucytosine at therapeutic level (25 to 120 mcg/ml). • Drug is often combined with amphotericin B; use may be synergistic, but may increase toxic effects.

(continued on following page)

NAME	INDICATIONS & DOSAGE	SIDE EFFECTS
flucytosine *(continued)*	Severe infections such as meningitis may require doses up to 250 mg/kg.	
griseofulvin microsize Fulvicin U/F♦, Grifulvin V, Grisactin, Grisovin-FP♦♦, Grisowen **griseofulvin ultramicrosize** Fulvicin P/G, Gris-PEG	*Ringworm infections of skin, hair, nails (tinea corporis, tinea pedis, tinea cruris, tinea barbae, tinea capitis, and tinea unguium) when caused by* Trichophyton, Microsporum, *or* Epidermophyton— **Adults:** 500 mg (microsize) P.O. daily in single or divided doses. Severe infections may require up to 1 g daily. **Children over 22 kg:** 250 to 500 mg P.O. daily. **Children 13 to 22 kg:** 125 to 250 mg P.O. daily. **Adults:** 125 mg tablet (ultramicrosize) P.O. b.i.d. or 250 mg daily. Resistant fungal infections of tinea pedis and tinea unguium may require divided daily dose of 500 mg. **Children over 22 kg:** 125 mg to 250 mg P.O. daily. **Children 13 to 22 kg:** 62.5 mg to 125 mg P.O. daily.	**Blood:** leukopenia, *granulocytopenia (requires discontinuation of drug).* **CNS:** headaches (in early stages of treatment), fatigue with large doses, occasional mental confusion, impaired performance of routine activities, psychotic symptoms. **GI:** nausea, vomiting, excessive thirst, flatulence, diarrhea. **Metabolic:** porphyria. **Skin:** rash, urticaria, photosensitive reactions (may aggravate lupus erythematosus). **Other:** estrogen-like effects in children, oral thrush.
miconazole Monistat I.V.	*Treatment of systemic fungal infections (coccidioidomycosis, candidiasis, cryptococcosis, paracoccidioidomycosis), chronic mucocutaneous candidiasis—* **Adults:** 200 to 3,600 mg per day. Doses may vary with diagnosis and with infective agent. May divide daily dose over 3 infusions, 200 to 1,200 mg per infusion. Repeated courses may be needed due to relapse or reinfection. **Children:** 20 to 40 mg/kg per day. Do not exceed 15 mg/kg per infusion.	**Blood:** transient decreases in hematocrit, thrombocytopenia. **CNS:** dizziness, drowsiness. **GI:** *nausea, vomiting,* diarrhea. **Metabolic:** *transient decrease in serum sodium.* **Skin:** *pruritic rash.* **Local:** *phlebitis at injection site.*
nystatin Mycostatin♦, Nadostine♦♦, Nilstat♦, O-V Statin	*Gastrointestinal infections—* **Adults:** 500,000 to 1,000,000 units as oral tablets, t.i.d. *Treatment of oral, vaginal, and intestinal infections caused by* Candida albicans (Monilia) *and other* Candida *species—* **Adults:** 400,000 to 600,000 units oral suspension q.i.d. for oral candidiasis.	**GI:** transient nausea, vomiting, diarrhea (usually with large oral dosage).

♦ Available in U.S. and Canada. ♦♦ Available in Canada only. All other products (no symbol) available in U.S. only. Italicized side effects are common or life-threatening.

INTERACTIONS	NURSING CONSIDERATIONS
	• Store in light-resistant containers. • Inform patient that adequate response may take weeks or months.
Barbiturates: decreased griseofulvin absorption. Divide into 3 doses of griseofulvin per day.	• Contraindicated in patients with porphyria or hepatocellular failure. Since griseofulvin is a penicillin derivative, cross-sensitivity is possible. Use cautiously in penicillin-sensitive patients. Use only when topical treatment fails to arrest mycotic disease. • CBC should be repeated regularly. • Advise patient that prolonged treatment may be needed to control infection and prevent relapse, even if symptoms abate in first few days of therapy. Tell patient to keep skin clean and dry and to maintain good hygiene. Caution him to avoid intense sunlight. • Most effectively absorbed and causes least GI distress when given after high-fat meal. • Effective treatment of tinea pedis may require concomitant use of topical agent. • Diagnosis of infecting organism should be verified in laboratory. Continue drug until clinical and laboratory examinations confirm complete eradication. • Because griseofulvin ultramicrosize is dispersed in polyethylene glycol (PEG), it is absorbed more rapidly and completely than microsize preparations and is effective at one half the usual griseofulvin dose.
None significant.	• Rapid injection of undiluted miconazole may produce arrhythmia. • Premedication with antiemetic may lessen nausea and vomiting. • Avoid administration at mealtime in order to lessen GI side effects. • Lesser incidence and severity of side effects with this drug may offer a significant advantage over other antifungals. • In treatment of fungal meningitis and urinary bladder infections, must be supplemented with intrathecal administration and bladder irrigation, respectively. • I.V. infusion should be given over 30 to 60 minutes. • Inform patient that adequate response may take weeks or months. • Monitor levels of hemoglobin, hematocrit, electrolytes, and lipids regularly. Transient elevations in serum cholesterol and triglycerides may be due to castor oil vehicle.
None significant.	• Nystatin is virtually nontoxic and nonsensitizing when used orally, vaginally, or topically; but advise patient to report redness, swelling, or irritation. • Vaginal tablets can be used by pregnant women up to 6 weeks before term to prevent thrush in newborn. Continue therapy during menstruation. Instruct patient to wash applicator thoroughly after each use. • Explain that use of antibiotics, oral contraceptives, and corticosteroids; diabetes; reinfection by sexual partner; and tight-fitting panty hose are predisposing factors of vaginal infection.

(continued on following page)

NAME	INDICATIONS & DOSAGE	SIDE EFFECTS
nystatin *(continued)*	**Children, and infants over 3 months:** 250,000 to 500,000 units oral suspension q.i.d. **Newborn and premature infants:** 100,000 units oral suspension q.i.d. *Vaginal infections—* **Adults:** 100,000 units, as vaginal tablets, inserted high into vagina, daily or b.i.d. for 14 days.	

DRUG ALERT

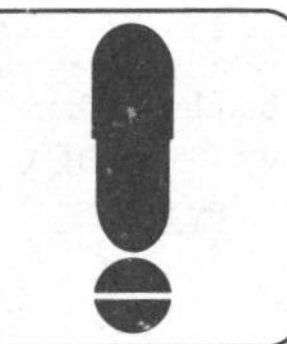

PREVENTING AMPHOTERICIN B TOXICITY

Amphotericin B (Fungizone) is usually prescribed for progressive and life-threatening fungal infections. But the drug can have toxic side effects:

- Fever, chills, nausea, vomiting, and headache commonly occur within minutes after the infusion begins. Prevent or minimize side effects by giving the patient 600 to 900 mg of aspirin or acetaminophen and 50 mg of diphenhydramine 1 hour before the infusion. Repeat doses every 3 to 4 hours, if necessary. Adding hydrocortisone to the infusion may also reduce these side effects.
- Thrombophlebitis develops at the I.V. site in about 70% of patients receiving amphotericin B. Report signs of thrombophlebitis to the doctor so he can order heparin or hydrocortisone added to the infusion to control inflammation.
- Hypokalemia is serious and possibly life-threatening, especially to patients taking digitalis. Watch closely for neuromuscular disturbances, such as weakness, decreased reflexes, or tingling in fingers and toes; EKG abnormalities, such as flat T waves, depressed ST segments, or widened QRS complexes; GI symptoms, such as nausea or paralytic ileus; and CNS symptoms, such as irritability and stupor.

  Hypokalemia can be corrected with potassium supplements, but large amounts may be needed.
- Renal tubular acidosis results from decreased renal excretion of acids after several weeks of amphotericin B therapy. The drug may also decrease the patient's glomerular filtration rate and may possibly precipitate azotemia. Be sure to monitor your patient's serum creatinine and BUN frequently.

  If the renal function indicators are too high (serum creatinine greater than 3 mg/100 ml and BUN greater than 40 mg/100 ml), the drug usually must be stopped to prevent permanent renal damage.

INTERACTIONS	NURSING CONSIDERATIONS
	• For treatment of oral candidiasis (thrush): Be sure the mouth is clean of food debris before drug administration, then tell patient to hold suspension in mouth for several minutes before swallowing. For treatment of infants, swab medication on oral mucosa. Instruct patient in good oral hygiene techniques. Tell patient overuse of mouthwash or poorly fitting dentures, especially in older patients, may alter flora and promote infection. • Advise patient to continue medication for 1 to 2 weeks after symptomatic improvement to ensure against reinfection. Consult doctor for exact length of therapy. • Immunosuppressed patients sometimes take vaginal tablets (100,000 units) by mouth as this provides prolonged contact with *Candida*-infected oral mucosa. • Instruct patient in careful hygiene for affected areas. • Store in tightly closed, light-resistant containers in cool place. • Not effective against systemic infections.

DRUG ADVANCES

KNOW THE ADVANTAGES OF KETOCONAZOLE— A NEW ORAL ANTIFUNGAL

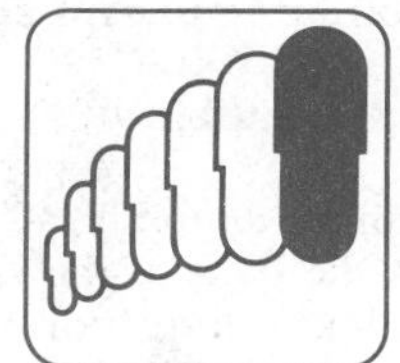

Ketoconazole (Nizoral) represents an important advance in antifungal drug development because it:

- shows none of the serious side effects that usually occur with other antifungal drugs.
- shows impressive cure rates for fungal infections previously resistant to other drugs.
- provides new therapeutic options for long-term treatment and maintenance of severe fungal infections, as well as for prophylaxis in high-risk patients.
- can be administered orally with a once-daily dosage. (This should encourage patient compliance.)
- is effective for a broad range of acute and chronic fungal infections.

Like other antifungals, ketoconazole is particularly useful in treating deep systemic fungal infections and lesions affecting subcutaneous tissue layers. It's also highly effective in treating oral and genitourinary monilial infections, particularly in patients with cancer since chemotherapeutic drugs make them vulnerable to such infections.

Ketoconazole effectively combats these other infections as well:

- systemic candidiasis
- chronic mucocutaneous candidiasis
- oral thrush
- candiduria
- coccidioidomycosis
- histoplasmosis
- chromomycosis
- paracoccidioidomycosis.

Side effects of ketoconazole include headache, dizziness, constipation, diarrhea, somnolence, and nervousness.

Note: Ketoconazole should not be used for fungal meningitis because it penetrates poorly into the cerebrospinal fluid. For complete information on ketoconazole, see APPENDIX, *New Drugs*.

11 Antimalarials

amodiaquine hydrochloride
chloroquine hydrochloride
chloroquine phosphate
hydroxychloroquine sulfate
primaquine phosphate
pyrimethamine
quinine sulfate

Quinine—the bitter alkaloid obtained from the bark of the cinchona tree—the 4-aminoquinoline derivatives (amodiaquine, chloroquine, and hydroxychloroquine), and related drugs are used in prophylaxis and treatment of malaria infections.

In many areas of the world, malaria is a common infectious disease with a high mortality. Transmitted by the bite of the anopheles mosquito, malaria is most commonly contracted in Asia, Africa, and Latin America. In the United States, however, malarial infections are usually nonepidemic.

Major uses

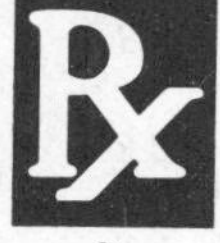

• Amodiaquine, chloroquine, hydroxychloroquine, primaquine, and pyrimethamine suppress susceptible strains of *Plasmodium—P. vivax, P. malariae, P. ovale,* and *P. falciparum.*

• Chloroquine and hydroxychloroquine are also used in the treatment of systemic lupus erythematosus and rheumatoid arthritis. Chloroquine is used in combination with emetine to treat amebic hepatic abscesses as well as certain fluke infections.

• Quinine may relieve nocturnal leg cramps.

• Pyrimethamine is used in combination with sulfonamides to treat toxoplasmosis.

Mechanism of action

• The 4-aminoquinoline compounds bind to, and alter the properties of, both microbial and mammalian deoxyribonucleic acid.

• Primaquine phosphate is a gametocidal drug that destroys exoerythrocytic forms and prevents delayed primary attack. Its precise mechanism of action is unknown.

• Pyrimethamine inhibits the enzyme dihydrofolate reductase, thereby impeding reduction of folic acid.

• Quinine's exact mechanism of action is unknown, but the drug is often referred to as a generalized protoplasmic poison.

Absorption, distribution, metabolism, and excretion

All the antimalarials are rapidly absorbed from the gastrointestinal tract.

• The 4-aminoquinoline compounds, bound to plasma proteins, achieve very high levels in the liver, spleen, kidneys, and lungs. They are metabolized in the liver and slowly excreted in the urine for months after treatment.

• Primaquine is rapidly metabolized in the liver. Only a small amount of unchanged drug is excreted in the urine; the rest is excreted as metabolite.

• Pyrimethamine is metabolized in

the liver and excreted in the urine.

• Quinine, highly protein-bound, is excreted in the urine—mostly as inactive metabolite.

Onset and duration

• The 4-aminoquinolines and primaquine reach peak blood concentrations 6 hours after oral administration. Levels fall rapidly; only very small quantities are detectable after 24 hours. Minute amounts may still, however, be detectable in the urine months after therapy ends.

• Pyrimethamine is eliminated slowly and has a half-life of 4 days. Therapeutic concentrations may remain in the blood for as long as 2 weeks.

• Quinine sulfate achieves peak blood levels within 1 to 3 hours; only a negligible concentration can be measured 24 hours after therapy ends.

Combination products

ARALEN PHOSPHATE WITH PRIMAQUINE PHOSPHATE: chloroquine phosphate 500 mg (300 mg base) and primaquine phosphate 79 mg (45 mg base).

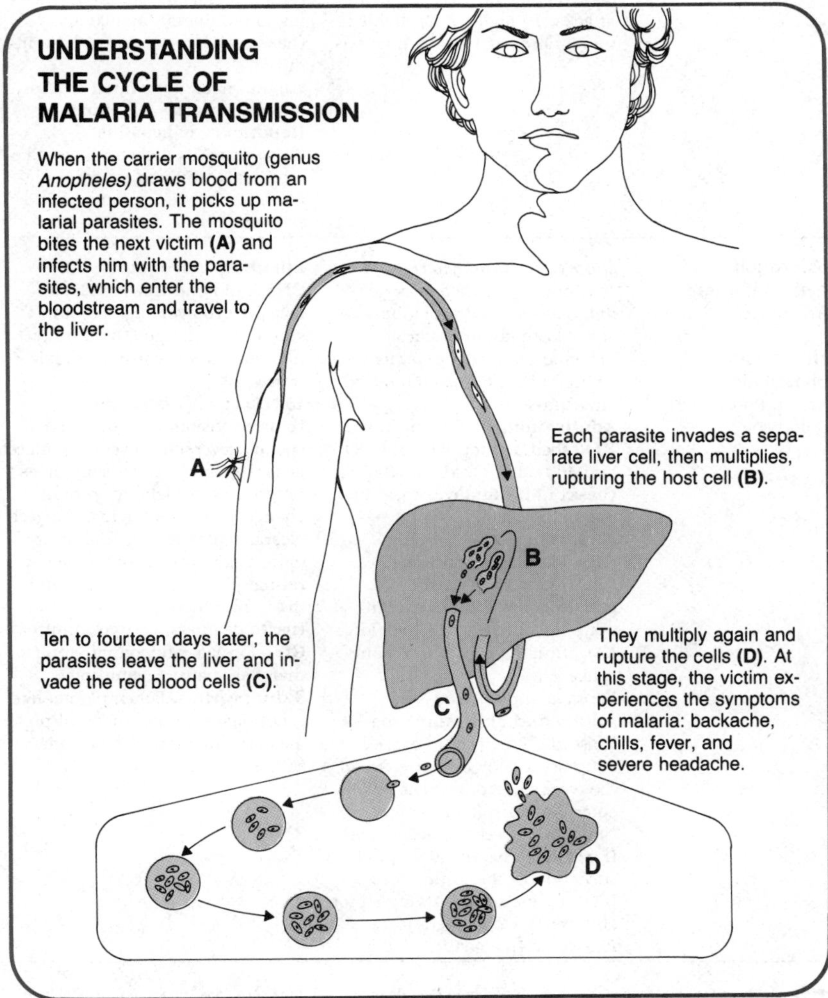

UNDERSTANDING THE CYCLE OF MALARIA TRANSMISSION
When the carrier mosquito (genus *Anopheles*) draws blood from an infected person, it picks up malarial parasites. The mosquito bites the next victim **(A)** and infects him with the parasites, which enter the bloodstream and travel to the liver.
Each parasite invades a separate liver cell, then multiplies, rupturing the host cell **(B)**.
Ten to fourteen days later, the parasites leave the liver and invade the red blood cells **(C)**.
They multiply again and rupture the cells **(D)**. At this stage, the victim experiences the symptoms of malaria: backache, chills, fever, and severe headache.
A
B
C
D

NAME	INDICATIONS & DOSAGE	SIDE EFFECTS
amodiaquine hydrochloride Camoquin HCl	*Suppressive prophylaxis and treatment of acute attacks of malaria due to* Plasmodium vivax, Plasmodium malariae, Plasmodium ovale, *and susceptible strains of* Plasmodium falciparum— **Adults:** for suppression, single dose of 300 to 600 mg P.O. weekly, preferably on same day of week; for acute attacks, 600 mg P.O. initially, then 300 mg at 6, 24, and 48 hours. **Children:** for suppression, 5 mg/kg P.O. weekly, preferably on same day of week; for acute attacks, 10 mg/kg P.O. divided into 3 doses at 12-hour intervals.	**Blood:** *agranulocytosis, leukopenia, pancytopenia.* **CNS:** mild and transient headache, neuromyopathy, polyneuritis, psychic stimulation, fatigue, irritability, nightmares, convulsions, dizziness, toxic psychosis. **EENT:** visual disturbances (blurred vision; difficulty in focusing; reversible corneal changes; generally irreversible, sometimes progressive or delayed, retinal changes, e.g., narrowing of arterioles; macular lesions; pallor of optic disk; optic atrophy; patchy retinal pigmentation, often leading to blindness), ototoxicity (nerve deafness, tinnitus, labyrinthitis). **GI:** anorexia, abdominal cramps, diarrhea, nausea, vomiting. **Hepatic:** toxic hepatitis. **Skin:** pruritus, lichen planus-like eruptions, skin and mucosal pigmentary changes, pleomorphic skin eruptions.
chloroquine hydrochloride Aralen HCl, Roquine **chloroquine phosphate** Aralen Phosphate♦, Chlorocon	*Suppressive prophylaxis and treatment of acute attacks of malaria due to* Plasmodium vivax, Plasmodium malariae, Plasmodium ovale, *and susceptible strains of* Plasmodium falciparum— **Adults:** initially, 600 mg (base) P.O., then 300 mg P.O. at 6, 24, and 48 hours. Or 160 to 200 mg (base) I.M. initially; repeat in 6 hours if needed. **Children:** initially, 10 mg (base)/kg P.O., then 5 mg (base)/kg dose P.O. at 6, 24, and 48 hours (do not exceed adult dose). Or 5 mg (base)/kg I.M. initially; repeat in 6 hours if needed. *Malaria suppression*— **Adults and children:** 5 mg (base)/kg P.O. (not to exceed 300 mg) weekly on same day of the week (begin 2 weeks before entering endemic area and continue for 8 weeks after leaving). If treatment begins after exposure, double the initial dose (600 mg for adults, 10 mg/kg for children) in 2 divided doses, P.O. 6 hours apart.	**Blood:** *agranulocytosis.* **CNS:** mild and transient headache, neuromyopathy, psychic stimulation, fatigue, irritability, nightmares, convulsions, dizziness. **EENT:** *visual disturbances* (blurred vision; difficulty in focusing; reversible corneal changes; generally irreversible, sometimes progressive or delayed, retinal changes, e.g., narrowing of arterioles; macular lesions; pallor of optic disk; optic atrophy; patchy retinal pigmentation, often leading to blindness), ototoxicity (nerve deafness, vertigo, tinnitus). **GI:** anorexia, abdominal cramps, diarrhea, nausea, vomiting. **Skin:** pruritus, lichen planus-like eruptions, skin and mucosal pigmentary changes, pleomorphic skin eruptions.

INTERACTIONS	NURSING CONSIDERATIONS
None significant.	• Contraindicated in patients with retinal or visual field changes, porphyria, severe hepatic disease. Use with extreme caution in presence of severe GI, neurologic, or blood disorders. Use with caution in patients with G-6-PD deficiency or psoriasis; drug may exacerbate these conditions. • Complete blood cell counts and liver function studies should be made periodically during prolonged therapy; if severe blood disorder appears that is not attributable to disease under treatment, drug may need to be discontinued. • Overdosage can quickly lead to toxic symptoms: headache, drowsiness, visual disturbances, cardiovascular collapse and convulsions, followed by respiratory and cardiac arrest. Children are extremely susceptible to toxicity; avoid long-term treatment. • Baseline and periodic ophthalmologic examinations needed. Report blurred vision, increased sensitivity to light, or muscle weakness. Check periodically for ocular muscle weakness after long-term use. Audiometric examinations recommended before, during, and after therapy, especially if long term. • Give immediately before or after meals on same day each week. • To avoid exacerbated drug-induced dermatoses, warn patient to avoid excessive exposure to sun.
None significant.	• Contraindicated in patients with retinal or visual field changes, porphyria. Use with extreme caution in presence of severe GI, neurologic, or blood disorders. Drug concentrates in liver; use cautiously in patients with hepatic disease or alcoholism. Use with caution in patients with G-6-PD deficiency or psoriasis; drug may exacerbate these conditions. • Complete blood cell counts and liver function studies should be made periodically during prolonged therapy; if severe blood disorder appears that is not attributable to disease under treatment, drug may need to be discontinued. • Overdosage can quickly lead to toxic symptoms: headache, drowsiness, visual disturbances, cardiovascular collapse and convulsions, followed by respiratory and cardiac arrest. Children are extremely susceptible to toxicity; avoid long-term treatment. • Baseline and periodic ophthalmologic examinations needed. Report blurred vision, increased sensitivity to light, or muscle weakness. Check periodically for ocular muscle weakness after long-term use. Audiometric examinations recommended before, during, and after therapy, especially if long term. • Give drug immediately before or after meals on same day each week. • To avoid exacerbated drug-induced dermatoses, warn patient to avoid excessive exposure to sun. • Each ml parenteral solution containing 50 mg dihydrochloride salt = 40 mg chloroquine base; each 500 mg tablet phosphate = 300 mg chloroquine base. • Patients should be switched from intramuscular to oral therapy as soon as possible.

NAME	INDICATIONS & DOSAGE	SIDE EFFECTS
hydroxychloroquine sulfate Plaquenil Sulfate♦	*Suppressive prophylaxis of attacks of malaria due to* Plasmodium vivax, Plasmodium malariae, Plasmodium ovale, *and susceptible strains of* Plasmodium falciparum— **Adults and children:** for suppression: 5 mg (base)/kg body weight P.O. (not to exceed 310 mg) weekly on same day of the week (begin 2 weeks prior to entering endemic area and continue for 8 weeks after leaving area). If not started prior to exposure, double initial dose (620 mg for adults, 10 mg/kg for children) in 2 divided doses P.O. 6 hours apart. *Treatment of acute malarial attacks*— **Adults, and children over 15 years:** initially, 800 mg (sulfate) P.O., then 400 mg after 6 to 8 hours, then 400 mg daily for 2 days (total 2 g sulfate salt). **Children 11 to 15 years:** 600 mg (sulfate) P.O. stat, then 200 mg 8 hours later, then 200 mg 24 hours later (total 1 g sulfate salt). **Children 6 to 10 years:** 400 mg (sulfate) P.O. stat, then 2 doses of 200 mg at 8-hour intervals (total 800 mg sulfate salt). **Children 2 to 5 years:** 400 mg (sulfate) P.O. stat, then 200 mg 8 hours later (total 600 mg sulfate salt). **Children under 1 year:** 100 mg (sulfate) P.O. stat; then 3 doses of 100 mg 6 to 9 hours apart (total 400 mg sulfate salt). *Lupus erythematosus (chronic discoid and systemic)*— **Adults:** 400 mg P.O. daily or b.i.d., continued for several weeks or months, depending on response. Prolonged maintenance—200 to 400 mg P.O. daily. *Rheumatoid arthritis*— **Adults:** initially, 400 to 600 mg P.O. daily. When good response occurs (usually in 4 to 12 weeks), cut dosage in half.	**Blood:** *agranulocytosis, leukopenia,* thrombocytopenia, *aplastic anemia.* **CNS:** irritability, nightmares, ataxia, convulsions, psychic stimulation, toxic psychosis, vertigo, tinnitus, nystagmus, lassitude, fatigue, dizziness, hypoactive deep-tendon reflexes, skeletal muscle weakness. **EENT:** visual disturbances (blurred vision; difficulty in focusing; reversible corneal changes; generally irreversible, sometimes progressive or delayed, retinal changes, e.g., narrowing of arterioles; macular lesions; pallor of optic disk; optic atrophy; visual field defects; patchy retinal pigmentation, often leading to blindness), ototoxicity (irreversible nerve deafness, tinnitus, labyrinthitis). **GI:** anorexia, abdominal cramps, diarrhea, nausea, vomiting. **Skin:** pruritus, lichen planus-like eruptions, skin and mucosal pigmentary changes, pleomorphic skin eruptions. **Other:** weight loss, bleaching of hair.

INTERACTIONS	NURSING CONSIDERATIONS
None significant.	• Contraindicated in patients with retinal or visual field changes, or porphyria. Use with extreme caution in presence of severe GI, neurologic, or blood disorders. Drug concentrates in the liver; use cautiously in patients with hepatic disease or alcoholism. Use with caution in patients with G-6-PD deficiency or psoriasis; drug may exacerbate these conditions. • Complete blood cell counts and liver function studies should be made periodically during prolonged therapy; if severe blood disorder appears that is not attributable to disease under treatment, consider discontinuing. • Overdosage can quickly lead to toxic symptoms: headache, drowsiness, visual disturbances, cardiovascular collapse and convulsions, followed by respiratory and cardiac arrest. Children are extremely susceptible to toxicity; avoid long-term treatment. • Baseline and periodic ophthalmologic examinations needed. Report blurred vision, increased sensitivity to light, or muscle weakness. Check periodically for ocular muscle weakness after long-term use. Audiometric examinations recommended before, during, and after therapy, especially if long term. • Give drug immediately before or after meals on same day of each week. • 100 mg sulfate salt = 77.5 mg hydroxychloroquine base.

NAME	INDICATIONS & DOSAGE	SIDE EFFECTS
primaquine phosphate	*Radical cure of relapsing vivax malaria, eliminating symptoms and infection completely; prevention of relapse—* **Adults:** 15 to 30 mg (base) P.O. daily for 14 days. (26.3 mg tablet = 15 mg of base.)	**Blood:** leukopenia, hemolytic anemia in G-6-PD deficiency, methemoglobinemia in NADH methemoglobin reductase deficiency, leukocytosis, acute intravascular hemolysis, mild anemia, *granulocytopenia, agranulocytosis.* **EENT:** disturbances of visual accommodation. **GI:** nausea, vomiting, epigastric distress, abdominal cramps. **Skin:** urticaria.
pyrimethamine Daraprim♦	*Malaria prophylaxis and transmission control—* **Adults, and children over 10 years:** 25 mg P.O. weekly. **Children 4 to 10 years:** 12.5 mg P.O. weekly. **Children under 4 years:** 6.25 mg P.O. weekly. Continue in all age-groups at least 10 weeks after leaving endemic areas. *Acute attacks of malaria—* not recommended alone in nonimmune persons; use with faster-acting antimalarials, such as chloroquine, for 2 days to initiate transmission control and suppressive cure. **Adults, and children over 15 years:** 25 mg P.O. daily for 2 days. **Children under 15 years:** 12.5 mg P.O. daily for 2 days. *Toxoplasmosis—* **Adults:** initially, 100 mg P.O., then 25 mg P.O. daily for 4 to 5 weeks; during same time give 1 g sulfadiazine P.O. q 6 hours. **Children:** initially, 1 mg/kg P.O., then 0.25 mg/kg daily for 4 to 5 weeks, along with 100 mg sulfadiazine/kg P.O. daily, divided q 6 hours.	**Blood:** megaloblastic anemia, bone marrow suppression, leukopenia, thrombocytopenia, pancytopenia. **CNS:** stimulation and convulsions (acute toxicity). **GI:** anorexia, vomiting, diarrhea, atrophic glossitis. **Skin:** rashes.

♦ Available in U.S. and Canada. ♦♦ Available in Canada only. All other products (no symbol) available in U.S. only. Italicized side effects are common or life-threatening.

INTERACTIONS	NURSING CONSIDERATIONS
None significant.	• Contraindicated in patients with lupus erythematosus and rheumatoid arthritis; in patients taking bone marrow suppressants and potentially hemolytic drugs. • Use with a fast-acting blood schizonticide, such as amodiaquine or chloroquine. Use full dose to reduce possibility of drug-resistant strains. • Caucasians taking more than 30 mg daily, dark-skinned patients taking more than 15 mg (base) daily, and patients with severe anemia or suspected sensitivity should have frequent blood studies and urine examinations. Sudden fall in hemoglobin concentration, erythrocyte or leukocyte count, or marked darkening of the urine suggests impending hemolytic reactions. • Observe closely for tolerance in patients with previous idiosyncrasy (manifested by hemolytic anemia, methemoglobinemia, or leukopenia); family or personal history of favism; erythrocytic G-6-PD deficiency or NADH methemoglobin reductase deficiency. • Administer drug with meals or with antacids.
Folic acid and para-aminobenzoic acid: decreased antitoxoplasmic effects. May require dosage adjustment.	• Contraindicated in chloroguanide-resistant malaria. Use cautiously in patients with convulsive disorders; smaller doses may be needed. Also use cautiously following treatment with chloroguanide. • Dosages required to treat toxoplasmosis approach toxic levels. Twice-weekly blood counts, including platelets, are required. If signs of folic or folinic acid deficiency develop, dosage should be reduced or discontinued while patient receives parenteral folinic acid (leucovorin) until blood counts become normal. • Do not exceed recommended dosage. • Give with meals to minimize GI distress.

NAME	INDICATIONS & DOSAGE	SIDE EFFECTS
quinine sulfate Coco-Quinine	*Malaria due to* Plasmodium falciparum *(chloroquine-resistant)*— **Adults:** 650 mg P.O. q 8 hours for 10 days, with 25 mg pyrimethamine q 12 hours for 3 days, and with 500 mg sulfadiazine q.i.d. for 5 days.	**Blood:** hemolytic anemia, thrombocytopenia, agranulocytosis, hypoprothrombinemia. **CNS:** severe headache, apprehension, excitement, confusion, delirium, syncope, hypothermia, convulsions (with toxic doses). **CV:** hypotension, cardiovascular collapse with overdosage or rapid I.V. administration. **EENT:** altered color perception, photophobia, blurred vision, night blindness, amblyopia, scotoma, diplopia, mydriasis, optic atrophy, tinnitus, impaired hearing. **GI:** epigastric distress, diarrhea, nausea, vomiting. **GU:** renal tubular damage, anuria. **Skin:** rashes, pruritus. **Local:** thrombosis at infusion site. **Other:** asthma, flushing.

INTERACTIONS	NURSING CONSIDERATIONS
Sodium bicarbonate: elevates quinine levels by decreasing quinine excretion. Use together cautiously.	• Contraindicated in patients with G-6-PD deficiency. Use with caution in patients with cardiovascular conditions. • Discontinue if any signs of idiosyncrasy or toxicity occur. • I.V. therapy must be used cautiously, as marked fall in blood pressure often follows. Monitor blood pressure frequently. • I.V. route is preferred to I.M. route. Avoid extravasation. • Has been used as a treatment for nocturnal leg cramps. • Quinine is no longer used for acute attacks of malaria due to *Plasmodium vivax* or for suppression of malaria due to organism resistance. • Administer after meals to minimize GI distress. • May interfere with laboratory determinations of urine catecholamines and steroids.

BASIC FACTS ABOUT MALARIA

Malaria is uncommon outside of Asia, Africa, and South America, but you can't rule out the possibility of dealing with it in one of your patients. Here are some facts to bring your knowledge about malaria up to date.

Cause:	Protozoa are introduced into the human body through the bite of an infected anopheles mosquito, transfusion of blood from an infected donor, or use of a common syringe by drug addicts.
Incubation:	This period usually lasts 10 to 35 days, followed by a 2- to 3-day prodrome of irregular low-grade fever, malaise, headache, and myalgia.
Symptoms:	Clinical effects include periodic attacks of chills and fever without apparent cause, especially with spleen enlargement, in a person who has been in a malarious area within the year, as well as headache, nausea, and vomiting.
Diagnosis:	A blood smear is obtained to check for hepatosplenomegaly cells and Kupffer's cells distended with parasites. (Since intensity of the parasites may vary, more than one blood smear is required.)
Prevention:	Because malarial parasites have shown increasing resistance to antimalarial drugs, these preventive measures are important: control of mosquito breeding places; use of residual insecticide sprays in homes and public buildings, screens on windows and doors, and mosquito netting where screens are unsuitable; personal use of mosquito repellents; and sufficient clothing, particularly after sundown, to protect as much skin as possible.
Nursing consideration:	Disqualify from blood donation for 3 years persons on suppressive antimalarial therapy and those exposed to malaria (anyone who has visited a region where malaria is prevalent).

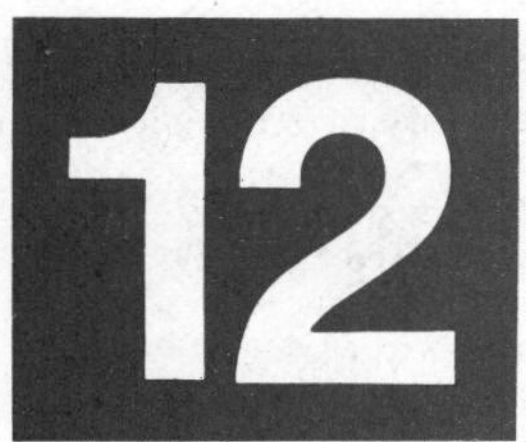

Antituberculars and antileprotics

capreomycin sulfate
cycloserine
dapsone
ethambutol hydrochloride
ethionamide
isoniazid (INH)
para-aminosalicylic acid
sodium aminosalicylate
pyrazinamide
rifampin
streptomycin sulfate
sulfoxone sodium

Antitubercular agents combat the different types of tuberculosis. Once known as the "white plague" or "consumption," tuberculosis is an infectious disease that can attack any body organ but most commonly compromises the lungs.

Although this disease was usually fatal in the past, medical progress over the last few decades has rendered tuberculosis both controllable and curable. Becoming less prevalent in the United States, tuberculosis nevertheless remains a significant disease among alcoholics; in thickly populated, impoverished communities; on southwestern Indian reservations; and in parts of Asia, Africa, and Europe.

Antileprotics (dapsone and sulfoxone sodium) are therapeutically effective against leprosy (Hansen's disease), a chronic, intracellular, nonfatal disease unique to humans. Uncommon in the United States (overall incidence of reported cases is about 0.06/100,000 population), leprosy claims an estimated 12 to 15 million victims in the world today. Lepers may become severely disfigured and be isolated from the rest of society. Although the precise mechanism and routes of transmission are unknown, leprosy is thought to be transmitted directly from person to person.

Major uses

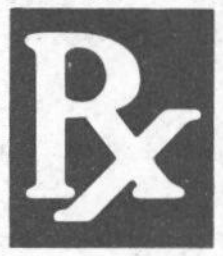

- Dapsone and sulfoxone are used to treat all forms of leprosy.
- Ethambutol, isoniazid, para-aminosalicylic acid, rifampin, and streptomycin are first-line drugs in the treatment of all forms of tuberculosis.
- Capreomycin, cycloserine, ethionamide, and pyrazinamide are second-line antitubercular agents, used in cases of drug resistance or in retreatment programs.
- Isoniazid is used prophylactically in susceptible persons exposed to tuberculosis.
- Rifampin is used prophylactically in meningococcal infections and *Hemophilus influenzae* meningitis. (It may be used with dapsone or sulfoxone in the initial management of lepromatous leprosy.)

Mechanism of action

- Cycloserine and isoniazid inhibit cell wall biosynthesis by a mechanism that's not well understood.
- Dapsone and sulfoxone are thought to inhibit folic acid biosynthesis.

• The aminosalicylates inhibit the enzymes responsible for folic acid biosynthesis.
• Rifampin inhibits DNA-dependent RNA polymerase, thus impairing ribonucleic acid synthesis.
• Streptomycin inhibits protein synthesis by binding to 30S ribosomal subunits.
• The mechanism of action of capreomycin, ethambutol, ethionamide, and pyrazinamide is not known.

Absorption, distribution, metabolism, and excretion

• Capreomycin sulfate is not significantly absorbed when given orally. Given I.M., it quickly reaches peak blood levels and is excreted in the urine essentially unchanged.
• Cycloserine is rapidly absorbed when given orally. It is distributed throughout body fluids and tissues, including the cerebrospinal fluid (CSF). It is partially metabolized in the liver and excreted in the urine.
• Dapsone is almost completely absorbed orally; it is metabolized in the liver and slowly excreted in the urine. Sulfoxone sodium is hydrolyzed and absorbed mainly as its parent compound, dapsone.
• Ethambutol is well absorbed from the gastrointestinal (GI) tract (75% to 80%). Distribution is unknown, but the drug is detoxified in the liver. Most is recovered unchanged from the urine and as much as 25% from the feces.
• Ethionamide is rapidly absorbed when given orally and widely distributed; significant levels appear in CSF. Most of the drug is metabolized slowly in the liver and is subsequently excreted in the urine.
• Isoniazid is readily absorbed when given orally or I.M., diffusing into all body fluids and tissues. About half the drug is metabolized in the liver and is excreted, together with unchanged drug (about 40%), in the urine.
• Pyrazinamide is well absorbed from the GI tract.

It is widely distributed, detoxified in the liver, and excreted in the urine.
• Rifampin is well absorbed and widely distributed. Partially metabolized in the liver, rifampin is eliminated as both metabolite and unchanged drug in urine and feces.
• The aminosalicylates are readily absorbed from the GI tract, distributed throughout most body fluids and tissues, and excreted in the urine as both metabolite and free acid.
• Streptomycin is well absorbed and widely distributed in most body tissues after I.M. injection. It is rapidly excreted, mostly unchanged, in the urine.

Onset and duration

• Capreomycin sulfate reaches peak blood levels in 1 to 2 hours; duration is about 24 hours.
• Cycloserine reaches peak blood levels in 4 to 8 hours; duration is about 12 hours.
• Dapsone produces peak levels within 1 to 3 hours; duration is 8 to 12 days.
• Ethambutol reaches peak levels in 2 to 4 hours; duration is about 24 hours.
• Ethionamide produces peak levels in 3 hours; since it's metabolized slowly, blood levels are prolonged.
• Isoniazid reaches peak levels within 1 to 2 hours; levels decline to about 50% within either 50 minutes (rapid acetylators) or 3 hours (slow acetylators).
• The aminosalicylates reach peak levels within 1 hour; duration is about 10 to 12 hours.
• Pyrazinamide levels peak in 2 hours; duration is about 15 hours.
• Rifampin produces peak levels within 1½ to 4 hours; duration is 24 hours.
• Streptomycin's peak level occurs within 30 minutes to 2 hours; duration is about 8 to 12 hours.
• Sulfoxone sodium levels peak rapidly (15 to 30 minutes); duration is about 8 hours.

Combination products

RIFAMATE: isoniazid 150 mg and rifampin 300 mg.
TEEBACONIN AND VITAMIN B_6: isoniazid 100 mg and pyridoxine HCl 10 mg.

NAME	INDICATIONS & DOSAGE	SIDE EFFECTS
capreomycin sulfate Capastat Sulfate	*Adjunctive treatment in pulmonary tuberculosis—* **Adults:** 15 mg/kg/day up to 1 g I.M. daily injected deeply into large muscle mass for 60 to 120 days; then 1 g 2 to 3 times weekly for a period of 18 to 24 months. Maximum dose should not exceed 20 mg/kg daily. Must be given in conjunction with another antitubercular drug.	**Blood:** eosinophilia, leukocytosis, leukopenia. **CNS:** headache. **EENT:** *ototoxicity* (tinnitus, vertigo, hearing loss). **GU:** *nephrotoxicity* (elevated BUN and nonprotein nitrogen, proteinuria, casts, red blood cells, leukocytes; tubular necrosis, decreased creatinine clearance). **Local:** pain, induration, excessive bleeding and sterile abscesses at injection site.
cycloserine Seromycin	*Adjunctive treatment in pulmonary or extrapulmonary tuberculosis—* **Adults:** initially, 250 mg P.O. every 12 hours for 2 weeks; then, if blood levels are below 25 to 30 mcg/ml and there are no clinical signs of toxicity, dose is increased to 250 mg P.O. q 8 hours for 2 weeks. If optimum blood levels are still not achieved, and there are no signs of clinical toxicity, then dose is increased to 250 mg P.O. q 6 hours. Maximum dose 1 g/day. If CNS toxicity occurs, drug is discontinued for 1 week, then resumed at 250 mg daily for 2 weeks. If no serious toxic effects occur, dose is increased by 250 mg increments every 10 days until blood level of 25 to 30 mcg/ml is obtained.	**CNS:** drowsiness, headache, tremor, dysarthria, vertigo, confusion, loss of memory, *possible suicidal tendencies and other psychotic symptoms, nervousness,* hyperirritability, paresthesias, paresis, hyperreflexia. **Other:** hypersensitivity (allergic dermatitis).
dapsone Avlosulfon♦	*Lepromatous leprosy—* **Adults:** weeks 1 to 4: 25 mg P.O. 2 times a week; weeks 5 to 8: 50 mg 2 times a week; weeks 9 to 12: 75 mg 2 times a week; weeks 13 to 16: 100 mg 2 times a week; weeks 17 to 20: 100 mg 3 times a week; weeks 21 to 24: 100 mg 4 times a week. **Children:** reduced dosage, but not necessarily by body weight; usually approximately ½ of adult dose using same schedule. *Tuberculoid leprosy—* **Adults:** same as for *lepromatous leprosy* in adults, but maximum dosage is 200 mg P.O. weekly (i.e., 100 mg 2 times a week).	**Blood:** anemia, especially hemolytic; methemoglobinemia; possible leukopenia. **CNS:** psychosis, headache, dizziness, lethargy, severe malaise, paresthesias. **EENT:** tinnitus, allergic rhinitis. **GI:** anorexia, abdominal pain, nausea, vomiting. **Hepatic:** hepatitis. **Skin:** allergic dermatitis (generalized or fixed maculopapular rash).

INTERACTIONS	NURSING CONSIDERATIONS
None significant.	• Contraindicated in patients receiving other ototoxic or nephrotoxic drugs. Use cautiously in patients with impaired renal function, history of allergies, or hearing impairment. • Considered a second-line drug in the treatment of tuberculosis. • Drug is never given I.V.; may cause neuromuscular blockade. • Evaluate patient's hearing before and during therapy. Notify doctor if patient complains of tinnitus, vertigo, hearing impairment. • Monitor renal function (output, specific gravity, urinalysis, BUN, serum creatinine) before and during therapy; notify doctor of decreasing renal function. Dose must be reduced in renal impairment. • Monitor serum potassium levels and hepatic function periodically. • Reconstituted solutions can be stored for 48 hours at room temperature or 14 days if refrigerated. Straw- or dark-colored solution does not indicate a loss in potency.
Isoniazid: monitor for CNS toxicity (dizziness or drowsiness).	• Contraindicated in patients with seizure disorders, depression or severe anxiety, severe renal insufficiency, or chronic alcoholism. Use cautiously in patients with impaired renal function; reduced dosage required. • Considered a second-line drug in the treatment of tuberculosis. • Obtain specimen for culture and sensitivity tests before therapy begins and periodically thereafter to detect possible resistance. • Toxic reactions may occur with blood levels above 30 mcg/ml. • Pyridoxine, anticonvulsants, tranquilizers, or sedatives may help to relieve side effects. • Observe for personality changes. • Monitor hematologic tests, and kidney and liver function studies. • Instruct patient to take drug exactly as prescribed; warn against discontinuing use without doctor's consent.
Probenecid: elevates levels of dapsone. Use together with extreme caution.	• Contraindicated in renal amyloidosis. Use cautiously in chronic renal, hepatic, or cardiovascular disease; refractory types of anemia. • Therapy should be interrupted if generalized, diffuse dermatitis occurs. • Dapsone dosage should be reduced or temporarily discontinued if hemoglobin falls below 9 g/dl; if leukocyte count falls below 5,000/mm³; if erythrocyte count falls below 2.5 million/mm³ or remains low. • Patient should receive hematinics during dapsone therapy. • Antihistamines may help to combat dapsone-induced allergic dermatitis. • Erythema nodosum type of lepra reaction may occur during therapy as a result of *Mycobacterium leprae* bacilli (malaise, fever, painful inflammatory induration in the skin and mucosa, iritis, neuritis). In severe cases, therapy should be stopped and glucocorticoids given cautiously. • Twice-a-week dosage schedule reduces toxic effects. • Obtain CBC before treatment; monitor frequently during therapy (weekly for first month, monthly for 6 months, then semiannually).

(continued on following page)

NAME	INDICATIONS & DOSAGE	SIDE EFFECTS
dapsone *(continued)*	*Alternate dosage schedule—* **Adults:** 10 to 15 mg P.O. daily for 6 days a week, slowly increased to 62.5 mg daily for 6 days a week over a 6-month period.	
ethambutol hydrochloride Etibi♦♦, Myambutol♦	*Adjunctive treatment in pulmonary tuberculosis—* **Adults, and children over 13 years:** initial treatment for patients who have not received previous antitubercular therapy 15 mg/kg P.O. daily single dose. Re-treatment: 25 mg/kg P.O. daily single dose for 60 days with at least 1 other antitubercular drug; then decrease to 15 mg/kg P.O. daily single dose.	**CNS:** headache, dizziness, mental confusion, possible hallucinations, peripheral neuritis (numbness and tingling of extremities). **EENT:** optic neuritis (vision loss and loss of color discrimination, especially red and green). **GI:** anorexia, nausea, vomiting, abdominal pain. **Metabolic:** elevated uric acid. **Skin:** dermatitis, pruritus. **Other:** anaphylactoid reactions, joint pain, fever, malaise, bloody sputum.
ethionamide Trecator SC	*Adjunctive treatment in pulmonary or extrapulmonary tuberculosis (when primary therapy with streptomycin, isoniazid, and para-aminosalicylic acid cannot be used or has failed)—* **Adults:** 500 mg to 1 g P.O. daily in divided doses. Concomitant administration of other effective antitubercular drugs and pyridoxine recommended. **Children:** 12 to 15 mg/kg P.O. daily in 3 to 4 doses. Maximum dose 750 mg.	**Blood:** thrombocytopenia. **CNS:** *peripheral neuritis,* psychic disturbances (especially mental depression). **CV:** postural hypotension. **GI:** *anorexia,* metallic taste in mouth, nausea, vomiting, sialorrhea, *epigastric distress,* diarrhea, stomatitis, weight loss. **Hepatic:** jaundice, hepatitis, elevated SGOT and SGPT. **Skin:** rash, *exfoliative dermatitis.*
isoniazid (INH) Hyzyd, Isotamine♦♦, Laniazid, Niconyl, Nydrazid, Rimifon♦♦, Rolazid, Teebaconin	*Primary treatment against actively growing tubercle bacilli—* **Adults:** 5 mg/kg P.O. or I.M. daily single dose, up to 300 mg/day, continued for 18 months to 2 years. **Infants and children:** 10 to 20 mg/kg P.O. or I.M. daily single dose, up to 300 to 500 mg/day, continued for 18 months to 2 years. Concomitant administration of at least one other effective antitubercular drug is recommended. *Preventive therapy against tubercle bacilli of those closely exposed or those with positive skin tests whose chest X-rays and bacteriologic studies are consistent with nonprogressive tuberculous disease—*	**Blood:** *agranulocytosis,* hemolytic anemia, *aplastic anemia,* eosinophilia, leukopenia, neutropenia, thrombocytopenia, methemoglobinemia, pyridoxine-responsive hypochromic anemia. **CNS:** *peripheral neuropathy* (especially in the malnourished, alcoholics, diabetics, and slow acetylators), usually preceded by paresthesias of hands and feet. **GI:** nausea, vomiting, epigastric distress, constipation, dryness of the mouth. **Hepatic:** *hepatitis, occasionally severe and sometimes fatal, especially in the elderly.* **Metabolic:** hyperglycemia, metabolic acidosis. **Local:** irritation at injection site. **Other:** rheumatic syndrome and

♦ Available in U.S. and Canada. ♦♦ Available in Canada only. All other products (no symbol) available in U.S. only. Italicized side effects are common or life-threatening.

INTERACTIONS	NURSING CONSIDERATIONS
None significant.	• Contraindicated in patients with optic neuritis and in children under 13 years. Use cautiously in patients with impaired renal function, cataracts, recurrent eye inflammations, gout, and diabetic retinopathy. • Dose must be reduced in renal impairment. • Perform visual acuity and color discrimination tests before and during therapy. • Always monitor serum uric acid; monitor renal, hematopoietic, and hepatic functions in long-term use. • Observe patient for symptoms of gout. • Instruct patient to take this drug exactly as prescribed; warn against discontinuing use without doctor's consent.
None significant.	• Contraindicated in patients with severe hepatic damage. Use cautiously in patients with diabetes mellitus. • Culture and sensitivity tests should be performed before starting therapy. Stop drug if skin rash occurs; may progress to exfoliative dermatitis. • Monitor hepatic, hematopoietic, and renal functions. • Give with meals or antacids to minimize GI effects. Patient may require antiemetic. • Pyridoxine may be ordered to prevent neuropathy. • Instruct patient to take this drug exactly as prescribed; warn against discontinuing drug without doctor's consent. • Warn patient to avoid excess alcohol ingestion because it may make him more vulnerable to hepatic damage.
Aluminum-containing antacids and laxatives: may decrease the rate and amount of isoniazid absorbed. Give isoniazid at least 1 hour before antacid or laxative. *Disulfiram:* neurologic symptoms, including changes in behavior and coordination, may develop with concomitant isoniazid use. Avoid concomitant use.	• Contraindicated in patients with acute hepatic disease, or isoniazid-associated hepatic damage. Use cautiously in patients with chronic non–isoniazid-associated hepatic disease, seizure disorder (especially those taking phenytoin), severe renal impairment, chronic alcoholism; in elderly patients; in slow acetylator phenotypes (approximately 50% of Blacks and Caucasians). • Monitor hepatic function if clinical signs of hepatic dysfunction occur during therapy. Tell patient to notify doctor immediately if symptoms of hepatic impairment occur (loss of appetite, fatigue, malaise, jaundice, dark urine). • Alcohol may be associated with increased incidence of isoniazid-related hepatitis. Discourage use. • Pyridoxine may be given to prevent peripheral neuropathy, especially in malnourished patients. • Instruct patient to take this drug exactly as prescribed; warn against discontinuing drug without doctor's consent. • Store drug at room temperature. • Advise patient to avoid cheese, which may precipitate hypertensive crisis, and avoid excessive laxative use. • Inform patient to take with food if GI irritation occurs.

(continued on following page)

NAME	INDICATIONS & DOSAGE	SIDE EFFECTS
isoniazid (INH) *(continued)*	**Adults:** 300 mg P.O. daily single dose, continued for 1 year. **Infants and children:** 10 mg/kg P.O. daily single dose, up to 300 mg/day, continued for 1 year.	systemic lupus erythematosus–like syndrome; hypersensitivity (fever, rash, lymphadenopathy, vasculitis).
para-aminosalicylic acid PAS, Nemasol Sodium♦♦ **sodium aminosalicylate** Parasal Sodium, Pasdium, Teebacin	*Treatment of tuberculosis—* **Adults:** 10 to 12 g P.O. daily, divided in 2 or 3 doses. **Children:** 200 to 300 mg/kg P.O. daily, divided in 3 or 4 doses. *Treatment of tuberculosis—* **Adults:** 14 to 16 g P.O. daily, divided in 3 or 4 doses. **Children:** 200 to 300 mg/kg P.O. daily, divided in 3 or 4 doses.	**Blood:** *leukopenia, agranulocytosis,* eosinophilia, thrombocytopenia, hemolytic anemia. **CNS:** encephalopathy. **CV:** vasculitis. **GI:** *nausea, vomiting,* diarrhea, abdominal pain. **GU:** albuminuria, hematuria, crystalluria. **Hepatic:** *jaundice, hepatitis.* **Metabolic:** goiter, with or without myxedema; acidosis; hypokalemia. **Skin:** rash. **Other:** infectious mononucleosis-like syndrome, fever, lymphadenopathy.
pyrazinamide Tebrazid♦♦	*Hospitalized patients seriously ill with tuberculosis (when primary and secondary antitubercular drugs cannot be used or have failed)—* **Adults:** 20 to 35 mg/kg P.O. daily, divided in 3 to 4 doses. Maximum dose 3 g daily.	**Blood:** hemolytic anemia, possible bleeding tendency due to altered clotting mechanism or vascular integrity. **GI:** anorexia, nausea, vomiting. **GU:** dysuria. **Hepatic:** *hepatitis.* **Metabolic:** interference with control in diabetes mellitus, hyperuricemia. **Other:** malaise, fever, arthralgia.
rifampin Rifadin♦, Rimactane♦	*Primary treatment in pulmonary tuberculosis—* **Adults:** 600 mg P.O. daily single dose 1 hour before or 2 hours after meals. **Children over 5 years:** 10 to 20 mg/kg P.O. daily single dose 1 hour before or 2 hours after meals. Maximum dose 600 mg daily.	**Blood:** eosinophilia, thrombocytopenia, transient leukopenia, hemolytic anemia, decreased hemoglobin. **CNS:** headache, fatigue, *drowsiness,* ataxia, dizziness, mental confusion, generalized numbness. **EENT:** visual disturbances, exudative conjunctivitis. **GI:** epigastric distress, anorexia,

♦ Available in U.S. and Canada. ♦♦ Available in Canada only. All other products (no symbol) available in U.S. only. Italicized side effects are common or life-threatening.

INTERACTIONS	NURSING CONSIDERATIONS
Ascorbic acid, ammonium chloride: acidify urine, increasing possibility of para-aminosalicylic acid crystalluria. Avoid if possible. *Probenecid:* may increase levels of para-aminosalicylic acid. Use together cautiously. *Rifampin:* para-aminosalicylic acid may interfere with absorption of rifampin. Give these drugs 8 to 12 hours apart. *Diphenhydramine:* inhibits para-aminosalicylic acid absorption. Monitor for decreased para-aminosalicylic acid effect.	• Use cautiously in patients with impaired renal function, decreased hepatic function, and gastric ulcers. • Sodium aminosalicylate should not be given to patients on sodium-restricted diets. A 15-g dose provides 1.6 g sodium. • Give with meals or antacid to reduce gastrointestinal distress. Tell patient to swallow enteric-coated tablets whole and not with antacids. • Monitor renal, hematopoietic, hepatic functions, and serum electrolytes. • Tell patient to notify doctor at once if symptoms of hepatic impairment (loss of appetite, fatigue, malaise, jaundice, dark urine), fever, sore throat, or skin rash occurs. • Instruct patient to take any of these drugs exactly as prescribed; warn against discontinuing drug without doctor's consent. • Protect from water, heat, and sun; don't use if drug turns brown or purple. • Concomitant administration of at least one other effective antitubercular drug is recommended.
None significant.	• Contraindicated in patients with severe hepatic disease. Use cautiously in patients with diabetes mellitus or gout. • Nearly 100% excreted in urine; reduced dose needed in patients with renal impairment. • Perform liver function studies and examination for jaundice, liver tenderness or enlargement before and frequently during therapy. • Watch closely for signs of gout and of hepatic impairment (loss of appetite, fatigue, malaise, jaundice, dark urine, liver tenderness). Call doctor at once. • Monitor hematopoietic studies and serum uric acid levels. • Due to serious hepatotoxic effects, this drug is not recommended for initial therapy or long-term use. • When used with surgical management of tuberculosis, start pyrazinamide 1 to 2 weeks before surgery and continue for 4 to 6 weeks postoperatively.
Para-aminosalicylic acid: may interfere with absorption of rifampin. Give these drugs 8 to 12 hours apart. *Probenecid:* may increase rifampin levels. Use cautiously.	• Use cautiously in patients with hepatic disease or in those receiving other hepatotoxic drugs. • Monitor hepatic function, hematopoietic studies, and serum uric acid levels. • Warn patient about drowsiness and the possibility of red-orange discoloration of urine, feces, saliva, sweat, sputum, and tears. Soft contact lenses may be permanently stained. • Tell patient to take this drug exactly as prescribed and to report side effects. Warn against discontinuing use without doctor's consent. • Give 1 hour before or 2 hours after meals for optimal absorption.

(continued on following page)

NAME	INDICATIONS & DOSAGE	SIDE EFFECTS
rifampin *(continued)*	Concomitant administration of other effective antitubercular drugs is recommended. *Meningococcal carriers*— **Adults:** 600 mg P.O. daily for 2 days. **Children over 5 years:** 10 to 20 mg/kg/day P.O., not to exceed 600 mg/day.	nausea, vomiting, abdominal pain, diarrhea, flatulence, sore mouth and tongue. **GU:** menstrual disturbances. **Metabolic:** hyperuricemia. **Hepatic:** *serious hepatotoxicity as well as transient abnormalities in liver function tests.* **Skin:** pruritus, urticaria, rash.
streptomycin sulfate	*Primary treatment in tuberculosis*— **Adults:** with normal renal function, 1 g I.M. daily for 2 to 3 months, then 1 g 2 or 3 times a week. Inject deeply into upper outer quadrant of buttocks. **Children:** with normal renal function, 20 mg/kg daily in divided doses injected deeply into large muscle mass. Give concurrently with other antitubercular agents. Continue until sputum specimen becomes negative.	**Blood:** eosinophilia, leukopenia, neutropenia, pancytopenia, hemolytic anemia. **CNS:** *transient paresthesias,* especially circumoral; lassitude; muscle weakness. **CV:** myocarditis. **EENT:** *ototoxicity* (damage to vestibular and auditory portions of 8th cranial nerve, severe headache, *nausea, vomiting, vertigo,* ataxia, *tinnitus, roaring and sense of fullness in the ears,* hearing loss), optic nerve dysfunction (blurred vision, amblyopia). **GI:** stomatitis. **GU:** *nephrotoxicity* (transient proteinuria, increase in BUN and serum creatinine levels); nephrotoxicity less common than with other aminoglycosides. **Local:** pain, irritation at injection site. **Other:** respiratory depression, muscle weakness, systemic lupus erythematosus syndrome, *hypersensitivity* (rash, fever, urticaria, pruritus, angioneurotic edema).
sulfoxone sodium Diasone Sodium♦	*Lepromatous and tuberculoid leprosy*— **Adults:** weeks 1 and 2: 330 mg P.O. 2 times a week; weeks 3 and 4: 330 mg 4 times a week; week 5 and following weeks: 330 mg daily for 6 days, skip a day and continue. **Children (4 years and older):** give ½ the adult dose.	**Blood:** possible leukopenia, *anemia, especially hemolytic;* methemoglobinemia. **CNS:** psychosis, headache, dizziness, lethargy, severe malaise, paresthesias. **EENT:** tinnitus, allergic rhinitis. **GI:** anorexia, *abdominal pain,* nausea, vomiting. **Skin:** allergic dermatitis (generalized or fixed maculopapular rash). **Other:** hepatitis, drug fever, lepra reaction.

INTERACTIONS	NURSING CONSIDERATIONS
	• Increases enzyme activity of liver; may require increased doses of warfarin, corticosteroids, oral contraceptives, and oral hypoglycemics. See each drug entry for specific drug interactions.
Other aminoglycosides, methoxyflurane: may increase streptomycin's ototoxic and nephrotoxic effects. Use cautiously. *Ethacrynic acid, furosemide:* may increase streptomycin's ototoxic effects. Monitor carefully. *Dimenhydrinate:* may mask symptoms of ototoxicity. Use together cautiously.	• Contraindicated in patients with labyrinthine disease; hypersensitivity to any of the aminoglycosides; or those receiving other ototoxic or nephrotoxic drugs, neuromuscular blocking agents, and general anesthetics. Use cautiously in elderly patients and in those with impaired renal function. • Monitor renal function studies. Reduce dose in renal impairment. • Test patient's hearing before, during, and 6 months after therapy. Notify doctor if patient complains of tinnitus, roaring noises, fullness in ears. • Observe patient for respiratory depression. • To minimize renal damage, patient should be well hydrated. • Watch for signs of superinfection (continued fever and other signs of new infections, especially of the upper respiratory tract). • Very sensitizing topically. Protect hands when preparing drug. • In primary treatment of tuberculosis, streptomycin is discontinued when sputum becomes negative.
None significant.	• Contraindicated in renal amyloidosis. Use cautiously in chronic renal, hepatic, or cardiovascular disease, or refractory anemias. • Therapy should be interrupted if generalized, diffuse dermatitis occurs. Antihistamines may help sulfoxone sodium-induced allergic dermatitis. • Drug should be reduced or temporarily discontinued if hemoglobin falls below 9 g/dl; if leukocyte count falls below 5,000/mm³; erythrocyte count falls below 2.5 million/mm³ or stays low. • Patient should receive hematinics during sulfoxone sodium therapy. • Erythema nodosum type of lepra reaction may occur during sulfoxone sodium therapy as a result of circulating antigens caused by disintegrating *Mycobacterium leprae* bacilli (malaise, fever, painful areas of inflammatory induration in the skin and mucosa, iritis, neuritis). In severe cases, therapy should be interrupted and glucocorticoids given cautiously. • Monitor CBC frequently. • With severe or frequent drug fever, interrupt therapy or cut dose. • To minimize stomach upset, give drug with meals. • Protect drug from light.

13 Aminoglycosides

amikacin sulfate
gentamicin sulfate
kanamycin sulfate
neomycin sulfate
streptomycin sulfate
tobramycin sulfate

Aminoglycosides are broad-spectrum antibiotics that act against both gram-positive and gram-negative bacteria as well as some strains of mycobacteria. Because of the risk of serious nephrotoxicity and ototoxicity (auditory and vestibular effects), their systemic use is generally reserved for infections caused by gram-negative organisms resistant to less toxic agents.

WATCH FOR OTOTOXICITY

Ototoxicity, a significant adverse reaction to aminoglycosides, causes damage to the vestibular and the cochlear portions of the auditory nerve. Watch for these symptoms: headache, vertigo, nausea and vomiting with motion, tinnitus, and high-frequency hearing loss. (*Note:* Patients scheduled for aminoglycoside therapy should have a baseline audiogram as well as testing for high-frequency hearing loss during therapy.)

Ototoxicity occurs most often when peak blood levels of aminoglycosides are in the toxic range. This usually happens when the aminoglycoside is administered I.V. too rapidly; in elderly patients; and in patients with impaired renal function, prior aminoglycoside therapy, concurrent therapy using other ototoxic drugs, abnormal baseline audiogram, history of excessive noise exposure, or history of ear infections.

Major uses

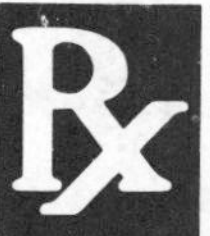

Aminoglycosides combat serious bacterial infection and provide presurgical bacteriostatic and bactericidal action in the intestine.

All aminoglycosides (except neomycin) may be used alone or in combination with penicillin to treat infections caused by group D streptococcus (enterococcus).

- Amikacin, gentamicin, kanamycin, and tobramycin may be used to treat serious infections caused by susceptible strains of *Escherichia coli, Klebsiella, Proteus, Enterobacter,* and *Pseudomonas aeruginosa.* They may also be used in combination with other antibiotics in serious infections when the organism has not been identified.
- Neomycin may be administered orally as adjunctive treatment in hepatic encephalopathy. It may also be used as an antimicrobial irrigating agent of the urinary tract or peritoneum.
- Neomycin and kanamycin may be used orally to promote bowel sterility before gastrointestinal surgical procedures.

Mechanism of action

Aminoglycosides act directly on the ribosomes of susceptible organisms. By binding directly to the 30S ribosomal subunit, they inhibit protein synthesis.

PREVENT NEPHROTOXICITY IN AMINOGLYCOSIDE THERAPY

Since aminoglycosides are excreted unchanged in urine, renal tissue is exposed to high concentrations of these drugs.

Impaired renal function, or nephrotoxicity, may result. Fortunately, it can be reversed if it's detected early and the dosage is immediately decreased.

To help prevent this adverse effect, watch your patient's renal status closely and follow these guidelines:

- Weigh the patient, and be sure baseline renal function studies are performed before therapy begins. By assessing the patient's daily weight in terms of fluid retention, you'll know if his renal function changes.
- During therapy, monitor blood urea nitrogen (BUN) and serum creatinine levels regularly.
- Encourage the patient to drink plenty of fluids.
- Regularly monitor and record urinary output in milliliters instead of vague measures such as "urine quantity sufficient (q.s.)."

Notify the doctor immediately if you notice:

- cells or casts in urine
- oliguria
- proteinuria
- decreased creatinine clearance (or elevated serum creatinine)
- elevated BUN.

Of the currently available aminoglycosides, streptomycin is thought to be the least nephrotoxic. But streptomycin is not very effective in treating gram-negative bacterial infections such as those caused by *Pseudomonas*. Tobramycin, amikacin, and gentamicin are the most effective of these drugs against such organisms. Studies show that of these three, tobramycin is probably the least nephrotoxic (see the illustration below).

New aminoglycosides that will have even less nephrotoxicity than these drugs may soon be available.

When administering the most nephrotoxic drugs, carefully observe patients with a history of renal disease or concurrent renal disease not induced by aminoglycosides.

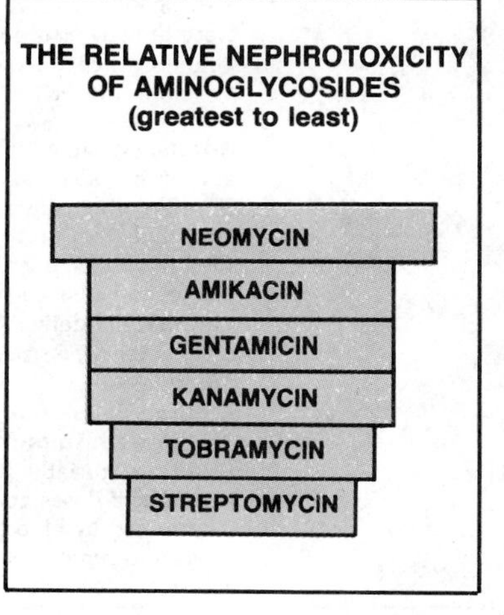

THE RELATIVE NEPHROTOXICITY OF AMINOGLYCOSIDES
(greatest to least)
NEOMYCIN
AMIKACIN
GENTAMICIN
KANAMYCIN
TOBRAMYCIN
STREPTOMYCIN

Generally, they are bactericidal in high concentrations and bacteriostatic in low concentrations.

Absorption, distribution, metabolism, and excretion

Aminoglycosides are not well absorbed from the gastrointestinal tract, so they must be given parenterally for systemic effect. Given orally, they produce only a local effect (bowel sterilization).

They are distributed uniformly to most body fluids and tissues; penetration into cerebrospinal fluid, however, is inadequate.

Since aminoglycosides accumulate in the kidneys, nephrotoxicity is possible. (See chart above.)

All aminoglycosides are rapidly excreted, mostly unchanged, in the urine by normal kidneys.

Onset and duration

Aminoglycoside blood levels peak within 30 minutes after I.V. infusion and within 60 minutes after I.M. injection.

The half-life of all aminoglycosides is from 2 to 4 hours but is significantly prolonged in patients with impaired renal function.

Combination products

None.

NAME	INDICATIONS & DOSAGE	SIDE EFFECTS
amikacin sulfate Amikin♦	*Serious infections caused by sensitive* Pseudomonas aeruginosa, Escherichia coli, Proteus, Klebsiella, Serratia, Enterobacter, Acinetobacter, Providencia, Citrobacter, Staphylococcus— **Adults and children with normal renal function:** 15 mg/kg/day divided q 8 to 12 hours I.M. or I.V. infusion (in 100 to 200 ml 5% dextrose in water run in over 30 to 60 minutes). May be given by direct I.V. push if necessary. **Neonates with normal renal function:** initially, 10 mg/kg I.M. or I.V. infusion (in 5% dextrose in water run in over 1 to 2 hours), then 7.5 mg/kg q 12 hours I.M. or I.V. infusion. *Meningitis—* **Adults:** systemic therapy as above; may also use up to 4 mg intrathecally or intraventricularly daily. **Children:** systemic therapy as above; may also use 1 to 2 mg intrathecally daily. *Serious urinary tract infections—* **Adults:** 250 mg I.M. b.i.d. **Adults with impaired renal function:** initially, 7.5 mg/kg. Subsequent doses and frequency determined by blood amikacin levels and renal function studies.	**CNS:** headache, lethargy. **EENT:** *ototoxicity (tinnitus, vertigo, hearing loss).* **GI:** nausea, vomiting. **GU:** *nephrotoxicity (cells or casts in urine, oliguria, proteinuria, decreased creatinine clearance, increased BUN and serum creatinine levels).* **Skin:** rash, urticaria.
gentamicin sulfate Cidomycin♦♦, Garamycin♦, U-Gencin	*Serious infections caused by sensitive* Pseudomonas aeruginosa, Escherichia coli, Proteus, Klebsiella, Serratia, Enterobacter, Citrobacter, Staphylococcus— **Adults with normal renal function:** 3 mg/kg/day in divided doses q 8 hours I.M. or I.V. infusion (in 50 to 200 ml of normal saline solution or 5% dextrose in water infused over 30 minutes to 2 hours). May be given by direct I.V. push if necessary. For life-threatening infections, patient may receive up to 5 mg/kg/day in 3 to 4 divided doses. **Children with normal renal function:** 2 to 2.5 mg/kg I.M.	**CNS:** headache, lethargy. **EENT:** *ototoxicity (tinnitus, vertigo, hearing loss).* **GI:** nausea, vomiting. **GU:** *nephrotoxicity (casts or protein in the urine, oliguria, proteinuria, decreased creatinine clearance, increased BUN, nonprotein nitrogen, and serum creatinine levels).* **Skin:** rash, urticaria.

♦ Available in U.S. and Canada. ♦♦ Available in Canada only. All other products (no symbol) available in U.S. only. Italicized side effects are common or life-threatening.

INTERACTIONS	NURSING CONSIDERATIONS
I.V. ethacrynic acid, I.V. furosemide: increase ototoxicity. Use cautiously. *Dimenhydrinate:* may mask symptoms of ototoxicity. Use with caution. *Carbenicillin:* amikacin antagonism. Don't mix together in I.V. Schedule 1 hour apart. *Other aminoglycosides, methoxyflurane:* increase ototoxicity and nephrotoxicity. Use together cautiously.	• Use cautiously in patients with impaired renal function; in neonates and infants, elderly patients. • Obtain specimen for culture and sensitivity before first dose. Therapy may begin pending test results. • Weigh patient and obtain baseline renal function studies before therapy begins. • Monitor renal function (output, specific gravity, urinalysis, BUN, creatinine levels, and creatinine clearance). Notify doctor of signs of decreasing renal function. • Patient should be well hydrated while taking this drug to minimize chemical irritation of the renal tubules. • Evaluate patient's hearing before and during therapy. Notify doctor if patient complains of tinnitus, vertigo, hearing loss. • Watch for superinfection (continued fever and other signs of new infections, especially of upper respiratory tract). • Usual duration of therapy is 7 to 10 days. If no response after 3 to 5 days, therapy should be stopped and new specimens obtained for culture and sensitivity. • Peak blood levels above 35 mcg/ml are associated with higher incidence of toxicity. • After I.V. infusion, flush line with normal saline solution. • Amikacin is usually reserved for gentamicin-resistant organisms.
I.V. ethacrynic acid, I.V. furosemide: increase ototoxicity. Use cautiously. *Dimenhydrinate:* may mask symptoms of ototoxicity. Use with caution. *Carbenicillin:* gentamicin antagonism. Don't mix together in I.V. Schedule 1 hour apart. *Cephalosporins:* increase nephrotoxicity. Use together cautiously. *Other aminoglycosides, methoxyflurane:* increase	• Use cautiously in patients with impaired renal function, and in neonates, infants, and elderly patients. • Obtain specimen for culture and sensitivity before first dose. Therapy may begin pending test results. • Weigh patient and obtain baseline renal function studies before therapy begins. • Monitor renal function (output, specific gravity, urinalysis, BUN, creatinine levels, and creatinine clearance). Notify doctor of signs of decreasing renal function. • Patient should be well hydrated while taking this drug to minimize chemical irritation of the renal tubules. • After completing I.V. infusion, flush the line with normal saline solution. • Evaluate patient's hearing before and during therapy. Notify doctor if patient complains of tinnitus, vertigo, hearing loss. • Watch for superinfection (continued fever and other signs of new infections, especially of upper respiratory tract). • Usual duration of therapy is 7 to 10 days. If no response in 3 to 5 days, therapy should be stopped and new specimens obtained for culture and sensitivity.

(continued on following page)

NAME	INDICATIONS & DOSAGE	SIDE EFFECTS
gentamicin sulfate *(continued)*	or I.V. infusion q 8 hours. **Infants and neonates over 1 week with normal renal function:** 2.5 mg/kg q 8 hours I.M. or I.V. infusion. **Neonates under 1 week:** 2.5 mg/kg I.V. q 12 hours. For I.V. infusion, dilute in normal saline solution or 5% dextrose in water and infuse over 30 minutes to 2 hours. *Meningitis—* **Adults:** systemic therapy as above; may also use 4 to 8 mg intrathecally daily. **Children:** systemic therapy as above; may also use 1 to 2 mg intrathecally daily. *Endocarditis prophylaxis for GI or GU procedure or surgery—* **Adults:** 1.5 mg/kg I.M. or I.V. 30 to 60 minutes before procedure or surgery and q 8 hours after, for 2 doses. Given with aqueous penicillin G or ampicillin. **Children:** 2 mg/kg I.M. or I.V. 30 to 60 minutes before procedure or surgery and q 8 hours after, for 2 doses. Given with aqueous penicillin G or ampicillin. **Patients with impaired renal function:** initial dose is same as for those with normal renal function. Subsequent doses and frequency determined by renal function studies. *Posthemodialysis to maintain therapeutic blood levels—* **Adults:** 1 to 1.7 mg/kg I.M. or I.V. infusion after each dialysis. **Children:** 2 mg/kg I.M. or I.V. infusion after each dialysis.	
kanamycin sulfate Kantrex♦, Klebcil	*Serious infections caused by sensitive* Escherichia coli, Proteus, Enterobacter aerogenes, Klebsiella pneumoniae, Serratia marcescens, Acinetobacter— **Adults and children with normal renal function:** 15 mg/kg/day divided q 8 to 12 hours deep I.M. into upper outer quadrant of buttocks or I.V. infusion (diluted 500 mg/200 ml of normal saline solution or 5% dextrose in water infused at 60 to 80 drops/minute). Maxi-	**CNS:** headache, lethargy. **EENT:** *ototoxicity (tinnitus, vertigo, hearing loss).* **GI:** nausea, vomiting. **GU:** *nephrotoxicity (cells or casts in the urine, oliguria, proteinuria, decreased creatinine clearance, increased BUN and serum creatinine levels).* **Skin:** rash, urticaria.

♦ Available in U.S. and Canada. ♦♦ Available in Canada only. All other products (no symbol) available in U.S. only. Italicized side effects are common or life-threatening.

INTERACTIONS	NURSING CONSIDERATIONS
ototoxicity and nephrotoxicity. Use together cautiously.	• Peak blood levels above 12 mcg/ml and trough levels (those drawn just before next dose) above 2 mcg/ml are associated with higher incidence of toxicity. • Draw blood for peak gentamicin level 1 hour after I.M. injection and 1 hour after I.V. infusion begins; for trough levels, draw blood just before next dose. • Hemodialysis (8 hours) removes up to 50% of drug from blood. • Endocarditis prophylaxis is recommended for all patients with rheumatic or congenital heart disease or prosthetic heart valve. • Intrathecal form (without preservatives) should be used when intrathecal administration is indicated.
Ethacrynic acid, furosemide: increase ototoxicity. Use cautiously. *Dimenhydrinate:* may mask symptoms of ototoxicity. Use with caution. *Other aminoglycosides, methoxyflurane:* increase ototoxicity and nephrotoxicity. Don't use together.	• Oral use contraindicated in patients with intestinal obstruction; in treatment of systemic infection. Use cautiously in patients with impaired renal function and in the elderly. • Obtain specimen for culture and sensitivity before first dose. Therapy may begin pending test results. • Weigh patient and obtain baseline renal function studies before therapy begins. • Monitor renal function (output, specific gravity, urinalysis, BUN, creatinine levels, and creatinine clearance). Notify doctor of signs of decreasing renal function. • Patient should be well hydrated while taking this drug to minimize chemical irritation of the renal tubules. • Evaluate patient's hearing before and during therapy. Notify doctor if patient complains of tinnitus, vertigo, hearing loss.

(continued on following page)

NAME	INDICATIONS & DOSAGE	SIDE EFFECTS
kanamycin sulfate *(continued)*	mum daily dose 1.5 g. **Neonates:** 15 mg/kg/day I.M. or I.V. divided q 12 hours. *Adjunctive treatment in hepatic coma—* **Adults:** 8 to 12 g/day P.O. in divided doses. *Preoperative bowel sterilization—* **Adults:** 1 g P.O. q hour for 4 doses, then q 4 hours for 4 doses; or 1 g P.O. q hour for 4 doses, then q 6 hours for 36 to 72 hours. *Intraperitoneal irrigation—* 500 mg in 20 ml sterile distilled water instilled via catheter into wound after patient fully recovered from anesthetic and neuromuscular blocking agent effects. *Wound irrigation*—up to 2.5 mg/ml in normal saline irrigation solution.	
neomycin sulfate Mycifradin Sulfate♦, Neobiotic	*Infectious diarrhea caused by enteropathogenic* Escherichia coli— **Adults:** 50 mg/kg/day P.O. in 4 divided doses for 2 to 3 days. **Children:** 50 to 100 mg/kg/day P.O. divided q 4 to 6 hours for 2 to 3 days. *Suppression of intestinal bacteria preoperatively—* **Adults:** 1 g P.O. q hour for 4 doses, then 1 g q 4 hours for the balance of the 24 hours. **Children:** 40 to 100 mg/kg/day P.O. divided q 4 to 6 hours. First dose should be preceded by saline cathartic. *Adjunctive treatment in hepatic coma—* **Adults:** 1 to 3 g P.O. q.i.d. for 5 to 6 days; or 200 ml of 1% or 100 ml of 2% solution as enema retained for 20 to 60 minutes q 6 hours.	**CNS:** headache, lethargy. **EENT:** *ototoxicity (tinnitus, vertigo, hearing loss).* **GI:** nausea, vomiting. **GU:** *nephrotoxicity (cells or casts in the urine, oliguria, proteinuria, decreased creatinine clearance, increased BUN and serum creatinine levels).* **Skin:** rash, urticaria.
streptomycin sulfate	*Nonhemolytic streptococcal endocarditis—* **Adults:** 1 g I.M. deep into upper outer quadrant of buttocks q 12 hours for 1 week, then 500 mg I.M. q 12 hours for 1 week with penicillin.	**EENT:** *ototoxicity (tinnitus, vertigo, hearing loss).* **GU:** some nephrotoxicity (not nearly as frequent as with other aminoglycosides). **Skin:** *exfoliative dermatitis.* **Local:** pain, irritation, and sterile

♦ Available in U.S. and Canada. ♦♦ Available in Canada only. All other products (no symbol) available in U.S. only. Italicized side effects are common or life-threatening.

INTERACTIONS	NURSING CONSIDERATIONS
	• Watch for superinfection (continued fever and other signs of new infection, especially of upper respiratory tract). • If no response in 3 to 5 days, therapy should be stopped and new specimens obtained for culture and sensitivity. • Peak blood levels over 30 mcg/ml are associated with increased incidence of toxicity.
Ethacrynic acid, furosemide: increase ototoxicity. Use cautiously. *Dimenhydrinate:* may mask symptoms of ototoxicity. Use with caution. *Other aminoglycosides, methoxyflurane:* increase ototoxicity and nephrotoxicity. Use together cautiously.	• Contraindicated in patients with intestinal obstruction. Use cautiously in patients with impaired renal function, ulcerative bowel lesions, and in elderly patients. • Oral therapy not recommended for systemic infection; parenteral dosage form available for I.M. use but not recommended because of extreme ototoxicity and nephrotoxicity. • Weigh patient and obtain baseline renal function studies before therapy begins. • Monitor renal function (output, specific gravity, urinalysis, BUN, creatinine levels, and creatinine clearance). Notify doctor of signs of decreasing renal function. • Patient should be well hydrated while taking this drug to minimize chemical irritation of the renal tubules. • Watch for respiratory depression in patients with renal disease, hypocalcemia, or neuromuscular diseases such as myasthenia gravis. • Evaluate hearing of patient with hepatic or renal disease before and during prolonged therapy. Notify doctor if patient complains of tinnitus, vertigo, hearing loss. Onset of deafness may occur several weeks after drug is stopped. • Watch for superinfection (continued fever and other signs of new infections, especially of upper respiratory tract). • Sometimes used in the treatment of high blood cholesterol. • Nonabsorbable at recommended dosage. However, more than 4 g of neomycin per day may be systemically absorbed and lead to nephrotoxicity.
Dimenhydrinate: may mask symptoms of streptomycin-induced ototoxicity. Use together cautiously. *Ethacrynic acid, furosemide:* increase	• Contraindicated in labyrinthine disease. Use cautiously in patients with impaired renal function and in the elderly. • Obtain specimen for culture and sensitivity before first dose except when treating tuberculosis. Therapy may begin pending test results. • Patient should be well hydrated while taking this drug to minimize chemical irritation of the renal tubules. • Evaluate patient's hearing before, during, and 6 months after ther-

(continued on following page)

NAME	INDICATIONS & DOSAGE	SIDE EFFECTS
streptomycin sulfate *(continued)*	*Treatment of tuberculosis*— **Adults:** initially, 0.75 to 1 g I.M. daily for 60 to 90 days, then 1 g 2 to 3 times weekly. *Endocarditis prophylaxis for dental and upper respiratory tract procedures*— **Adults:** 1 g I.M. 30 to 60 minutes before procedure. Used with penicillin. **Children:** 20 mg/kg I.M. 30 to 60 minutes before procedure. Used with penicillin. *Endocarditis prophylaxis for GI or GU procedures or surgery*— **Adults:** 1 g I.M. 30 to 60 minutes before procedure and q 12 hours for 2 doses after. Used with penicillin or ampicillin. **Children:** 20 mg/kg I.M. 30 to 60 minutes before procedure and q 12 hours for 2 doses after. Used with penicillin or ampicillin. **Patients with impaired renal function:** initial dose is same as for those with normal renal function. Subsequent doses and frequency determined by renal function study results. *Enterococcal endocarditis*— **Adults:** 1 g I.M. q 12 hours for 2 weeks, then 500 mg I.M. q 12 hours for 4 weeks with penicillin. *Tularemia*— **Adults:** 1 to 2 g I.M. daily in divided doses injected deep into upper outer quadrant of buttocks. Continue until patient is afebrile for 5 to 7 days.	abscesses at injection site. **Other:** *hypersensitivity* (rash, fever, urticaria, and angioneurotic edema).
tobramycin sulfate Nebcin♦	*Serious infections caused by sensitive strains of* Escherichia coli, Proteus, Klebsiella, Enterobacter, Serratia, Staphylococcus aureus, Pseudomonas, Citrobacter, Providencia— **Adults and children with normal renal function:** 3 mg/kg I.M. or I.V. daily divided q 8 hours. Up to 5 mg/kg I.M. or I.V. daily divided q 6 to 8 hours for life-threatening infections. **Neonates under 1 week:** up to 4 mg/kg I.M. or I.V. daily divided q 12 hours. For I.V. use, dilute in 50 to 100 ml normal saline solution or 5% dextrose	**CNS:** headache, lethargy. **EENT:** *ototoxicity (tinnitus, vertigo, hearing loss).* **GI:** nausea, vomiting. **GU:** *nephrotoxicity (cells or casts in the urine, oliguria, proteinuria, decreased creatinine clearance, increased BUN and serum creatinine levels).* **Skin:** rash, urticaria.

INTERACTIONS	NURSING CONSIDERATIONS
ototoxicity. Use cautiously. *Other aminoglycosides, methoxyflurane:* may increase streptomycin's ototoxic and nephrotoxic effects. Use cautiously.	apy. Notify doctor if patient complains of tinnitus, roaring noises, or fullness in ears. • Watch for superinfection (continued fever and other signs of new infections, especially of upper respiratory tract) and respiratory depression. • Peak blood concentrations over 25 mcg/ml are associated with increased incidence of toxicity. • Endocarditis prophylaxis is recommended for all patients with rheumatic or congenital heart disease or with prosthetic heart valve. Patients should receive prophylactic antibiotics during GI or GU procedures or surgery, or during upper respiratory tract procedures.
I.V. ethacrynic acid, I.V. furosemide: increase ototoxicity. Use cautiously. *Dimenhydrinate:* may mask symptoms of ototoxicity. Use with caution. *Carbenicillin:* tobramycin antagonism. Don't mix together in I.V. Schedule 1 hour apart. *Cephalosporins:* increase nephrotoxicity. Use together cautiously.	• Use cautiously in patients with impaired renal function and in the elderly. • Obtain specimen for culture and sensitivity before first dose. Therapy may begin pending test results. • Weigh patient and obtain baseline renal function studies before starting therapy. • Usual duration of therapy is 7 to 10 days. • Monitor renal function (output, specific gravity, urinalysis, BUN, creatinine, and creatinine clearance). Notify doctor of signs of decreasing renal function. • Patient should be well hydrated while taking this drug to minimize chemical irritation of the renal tubules. • Evaluate patient's hearing before and during therapy. Notify doctor if patient complains of tinnitus, vertigo, hearing loss. • Watch for superinfection (continued fever and other signs of new infections, especially of upper respiratory tract). • Draw blood for peak tobramycin level 1 hour after I.M. injection

(continued on following page)

NAME	INDICATIONS & DOSAGE	SIDE EFFECTS
tobramycin sulfate *(continued)*	in water for adults and less volume for children. Infuse over 20 to 60 minutes. **Patients with impaired renal function:** initial dose is same as for those with normal renal function. Subsequent doses and frequency determined by renal function study results.	

NURSING TIPS

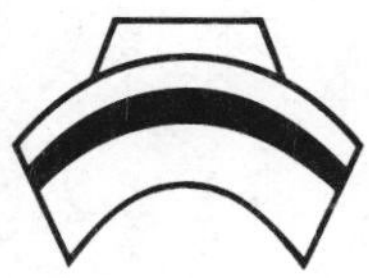

GETTING RELIABLE BLOOD LEVEL MEASUREMENTS

You need *accurate* data on your patient's aminoglycoside blood levels to ensure that he's getting enough—but not too much—of the drug. Keep these points in mind:

- The doctor may order blood samples drawn to determine peak-and-trough (valley) aminoglycoside blood levels. To measure the peak level, the sample is obtained shortly after the drug is administered.
- However, you may misinterpret the blood levels if the sample is collected too soon; if it is collected before the blood level achieves equilibrium, test results may show artificially elevated peak levels.
- To make sure your information is reliable, collect the sample 15 to 30 minutes after the end of a 30-minute I.V. infusion (or about 1 hour after the infusion begins). To measure the trough level, collect the sample *immediately before* the next dose.

INTERACTIONS	NURSING CONSIDERATIONS
Other aminoglycosides, methoxyflurane: increase ototoxicity and nephrotoxicity. Use together cautiously.	and 1 hour after I.V. infusion begins; draw blood for trough level just before next dose. • Peak blood levels over 12 mcg/ml are associated with increased incidence of toxicity. • After I.V. infusion, flush line with normal saline solution. • Recent studies indicate tobramycin is less nephrotoxic than gentamicin.

DRUG ERROR

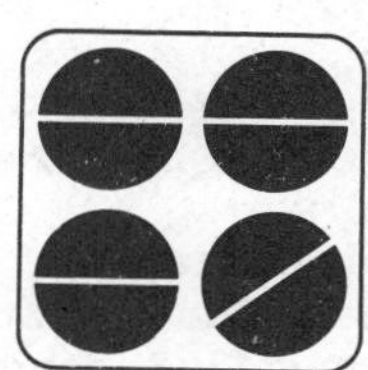

KNOW WHY A DRUG HAS BEEN PRESCRIBED

Do you always know *why* a drug has been prescribed before administering it? This knowledge may help you prevent medication errors. Here's an example:

A surgeon wrote this order for a woman being prepared for bowel resection: kanamycin 1 g every hour × 4, then 1 g every 6 hours until surgery.

The surgeon didn't specify the route of administration. The nurse who transcribed the order usually administered kanamycin parenterally. So without checking with the doctor or finding out why the drug had been prescribed, she took 1 g of kanamycin sulfate injection from the floor stock and administered it I.M.

But an I.M. injection is worthless before bowel surgery because the drug is rapidly absorbed and eventually excreted unchanged by the kidneys.

Clearly, the surgeon was at fault. But the nurse should have known that because oral kanamycin sulfate is poorly absorbed and remains in the bowel, it's ideal for reducing intestinal flora locally before bowel surgery. And she should have checked with him before administering even one dose, since there was no route of administration specified. Had she taken the time to find out why the drug had been prescribed, she could have prevented this error.

14 Penicillins

amoxicillin trihydrate
ampicillin
ampicillin sodium
carbenicillin disodium
carbenicillin indanyl sodium
cloxacillin sodium
cyclacillin
dicloxacillin sodium
hetacillin
hetacillin potassium
methicillin sodium
nafcillin sodium
oxacillin sodium
penicillin G benzathine
penicillin G potassium
penicillin G procaine
penicillin G sodium
penicillin V
penicillin V potassium
ticarcillin disodium

For information on bacampicillin and mezlocillin sodium, see APPENDIX, *New Drugs*.

More than 5 decades after their discovery, penicillins remain the most popular class of antibiotic in clinical use. Chemical modifications of the original penicillin molecule have enhanced its activity against most gram-positive and gram-negative organisms.

Major uses

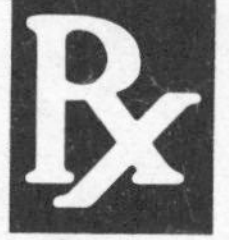

Penicillins are highly effective against infections due to gram-positive cocci, such as *Streptococcus pneumoniae* and nonpenicillinase-producing staphylococci; they are also effective against some gram-negative cocci, such as *Neisseria meningitidis* and *Neisseria gonorrhoeae*.

They're effective in varying degrees against *Bacillus anthracis*, *Bacteroides* species, *Clostridium perfringens*, *Treponema pallidum*, *Actinomyces*, and *Corynebacterium diphtheriae*.

Penicillins are *not* effective against viruses, mycobacteria, yeasts, plasmodia, fungi, or rickettsiae.

- Amoxicillin, ampicillin, cyclacillin, and hetacillin are also active against strains of *Escherichia coli*, *Hemophilus influenzae*, *Proteus mirabilis*, *Salmonella* species, and *Shigella* species.
- Carbenicillin and ticarcillin have a broader activity than other penicillins against strains of *E. coli*, *Proteus* species, and *Pseudomonas aeruginosa*.
- Cloxacillin, dicloxacillin, methicillin, nafcillin, and oxacillin are resistant to penicillinase and thus are extremely useful in the treatment of infections due to *Staphylococcus aureus*. They may be used prophylactically before orthopedic and cardiac surgery.

Mechanism of action

Penicillins are thought to be bactericidal against microorganisms by inhibiting cell-wall synthesis during active multiplication. They inhibit dipeptidoglycan, a substance necessary for cell-wall rigidity. Penicillins are more effective against young, rapidly dividing organisms than against mature resting cells that are not in the process of cell-wall formation.

Bacteria resist penicillin by producing penicillinases—enzymes that convert penicillin to inactive penicilloic acid. The penicillinase-resistant penicillins (cloxacillin, dicloxacillin, methicillin, nafcillin, and oxacillin) resist these enzymes.

Absorption, distribution, metabolism, and excretion

Oral absorption occurs primarily in the duodenum; a small percentage of penicillin is absorbed in the stomach. Penicillins are widely distributed in body fluids and in such tissues as kidneys, liver, lungs, heart, spleen, skin, and intestine. Adequate penetration into cerebrospinal fluid and the brain occurs only with meningeal inflammation.

Penicillins except nafcillin are excreted mostly unchanged in urine (nafcillin is extensively metabolized in the liver). Excretion is delayed in infants, elderly patients, and persons with impaired renal function.

- Ampicillin, cloxacillin, dicloxacillin, hetacillin, nafcillin, oxacillin, penicillin G, and penicillin V are all acid-labile, that is, broken down by gastric and duodenal acid. Therefore, they are best taken on an empty stomach 30 to 60 minutes before or 2 hours after meals. Parenteral administration results in higher but more transient blood levels.
- Carbenicillin disodium, methicillin, nafcillin, and ticarcillin disodium are very poorly absorbed orally and should be reserved for parenteral use.
- Penicillin G benzathine is slowly absorbed from I.M. injection sites, and therapeutic levels for certain organisms (pneumococcus, *T. pallidum*) may be observed as long as 30 days after a dose.
- Penicillin G procaine is more rapidly absorbed than penicillin G benzathine, but therapeutic levels may be observed as long as 24 hours after administration.
- Carbenicillin indanyl sodium given orally reaches therapeutic levels only in the urine, so it can't be used for systemic infections.

Onset and duration

- Peak blood level for oral penicillins is usually reached within 1 to 2 hours. Because the half-lives of all penicillins are very short (30 to 60 minutes), frequent doses are necessary.
- After parenteral administration, ampicillin, carbenicillin, methicillin, nafcillin, oxacillin, and penicillin G rapidly reach peak blood levels (immediately with I.V. infusion). The more insoluble procaine and benzathine salts of penicillin G are slowly absorbed from I.M. injection sites.
- Duration of action is generally 3 to 6 hours in patients with normal renal function.

In patients with impaired renal function, the drug may remain in the blood as long as 24 hours after administration.

Combination products

None.

DRUG ERROR

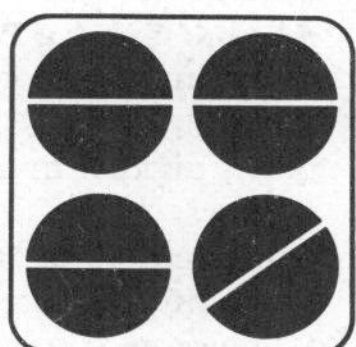

ADMINISTERING SUSPENSIONS

Be sure to follow basic techniques for administering suspensions. Otherwise, you may give patients supernatant fluid that doesn't contain any medication.

This happened to one inexperienced nurse: After several days of administering penicillin G procaine, she went to the pharmacy for a new vial. While there, she complained about the "icky stuff" at the bottom of the old vial.

Obviously, she hadn't read the vial's label that said to shake well before using. As a result, her patient hadn't received any of the penicillin G procaine prescribed.

If you see two distinct colors or viscosities, the preparation is probably a suspension and should be shaken vigorously.

NAME	INDICATIONS & DOSAGE	SIDE EFFECTS
amoxicillin trihydrate Amoxil♦, Larotid, Polymox♦, Robamox, Sumox, Trimox, Utimox	*Systemic infections caused by susceptible strains of gram-positive and gram-negative organisms—* **Adults:** 750 mg to 1.5 g P.O. daily, divided into doses given q 8 hours. **Children:** 20 to 40 mg/kg P.O. daily, divided into doses given q 8 hours. *Uncomplicated gonorrhea—* **Adults:** 3 g P.O. with 1 g probenecid given as a single dose.	**Blood:** anemia, thrombocytopenia, thrombocytopenic purpura, eosinophilia, leukopenia. **GI:** *nausea,* vomiting, *diarrhea.* **Other:** *hypersensitivity (erythematous maculopapular rash, urticaria, anaphylaxis),* overgrowth of nonsusceptible organisms.
ampicillin Amcill♦, Ampilean♦♦, Omnipen, Penbritin♦, Pensyn, Pfizerpen A, Roampicillin **ampicillin sodium** Amcill-S, Omnipen-N, Pen A/N, Penbritin-S, Polycillin-N, Principen/N, Totacillin-N	*Systemic infections caused by susceptible strains of gram-positive and gram-negative organisms—* **Adults:** 1 to 4 g P.O. daily, divided into doses given q 6 hours; 2 to 12 g I.M. or I.V. daily, divided into doses given q 6 hours. **Children:** 50 to 100 mg/kg P.O. daily, divided into doses given q 6 hours; or 100 to 200 mg/kg I.M. or I.V. daily, divided into doses given q 6 hours. *Meningitis—* **Adults:** 8 to 14 g I.V. daily for 3 days, then I.M. divided q 3 to 4 hours. **Children:** up to 300 mg/kg I.V. daily for 3 days, then I.M. divided q 4 hours. *Uncomplicated gonorrhea—* **Adults:** 3.5 g P.O. with 1 g probenecid given as a single dose.	**Blood:** anemia, thrombocytopenia, thrombocytopenic purpura, eosinophilia, leukopenia. **GI:** *nausea,* vomiting, *diarrhea,* glossitis, stomatitis. **Local:** pain at injection site, vein irritation, thrombophlebitis. **Other:** *hypersensitivity (erythematous maculopapular rash, urticaria, anaphylaxis),* overgrowth of nonsusceptible organisms.

INTERACTIONS	NURSING CONSIDERATIONS
Probenecid: increases blood levels of penicillin. Probenecid is often used for this purpose. *Chloramphenicol, erythromycin, tetracyclines:* antibiotic antagonism. Give penicillins at least 1 hour before bacteriostatic antibiotics.	• Use cautiously in patients with other drug allergies, especially to cephalosporins (possible cross-allergenicity); and in patients with mononucleosis—high incidence of maculopapular rash in those receiving amoxicillin. • Obtain cultures for sensitivity tests before first dose. Unnecessary to wait for results before beginning therapy. • Before giving penicillin, ask patient if he's had any allergic reactions to this drug. However, a negative history of penicillin allergy is no guarantee against a future allergic reaction. • Tell patient to take medication exactly as prescribed, even after he feels better. Entire quantity prescribed should be taken. • Give with food to prevent GI distress. • Large doses may cause increased yeast growths. Report symptoms to doctor. • With prolonged therapy, bacterial and fungal superinfection may occur, especially in the elderly, debilitated, or those with low resistance to infection due to immunosuppressives or irradiation. Close observation essential. • Check expiration date. Warn patient never to use leftover penicillin for a new illness or to share penicillin with family and friends. • Tell patient to call the doctor if rash, fever, or chills develop. A rash is the most common allergic reaction. • Amoxicillin and ampicillin have similar clinical applications. • For treatment of anaphylaxis, see inside front cover.
Probenecid: increases blood levels of penicillin. Probenecid is often used for this purpose. *Chloramphenicol, erythromycin, tetracyclines:* antibiotic antagonism. Give penicillins at least 1 hour before bacteriostatic antibiotics.	• Use cautiously in patients with other drug allergies, especially to cephalosporins (possible cross-allergenicity); and in patients with mononucleosis—high incidence of maculopapular rash in those receiving ampicillin. • Obtain cultures for sensitivity tests before first dose. Unnecessary to wait for results before beginning therapy. • Before giving penicillin, ask patient if he's had any allergic reactions to this drug. However, a negative history of penicillin allergy is no guarantee against a future allergic reaction. • Tell patient to take medication exactly as prescribed, even after he feels better. Entire quantity prescribed should be taken. • Tell the patient to call the doctor if rash, fever, or chills develop. A rash is the most common allergic reaction. • When given orally, drug may cause GI disturbances. Food may interfere with absorption, so give 1 to 2 hours before meals or 2 to 3 hours after. • Don't give I.M. or I.V. unless infection is severe or patient can't take oral dose. • Dosage should be altered in patients with impaired hepatic and renal functions. • When giving I.V., mix with 5% dextrose in water or a saline solution. Don't mix with other drugs or solutions: they might be incompatible. • Give I.V. intermittently to prevent vein irritation. Change site every 48 hours. • Large doses may cause increased yeast growths. Report symptoms to doctor. • With prolonged therapy, bacterial or fungal superinfection may occur, especially in the elderly, debilitated, or those with low resistance to infection due to immunosuppressives or irradiation. Close observation is essential. • Check expiration date. Warn patient never to use leftover penicillin for a new illness or to share penicillin with family and friends.

(continued on following page)

NAME	INDICATIONS & DOSAGE	SIDE EFFECTS
ampicillin *(continued)*		
carbenicillin disodium Geopen, Pyopen♦	*Systemic infections caused by susceptible strains of gram-positive and especially gram-negative organisms* (Proteus, Pseudomonas aeruginosa)— **Adults:** 30 to 40 g daily I.V. infusion, divided into doses given q 4 to 6 hours. **Children:** 300 to 500 mg/kg daily I.V. infusion, divided into doses given q 4 to 6 hours. *Urinary tract infections*— **Adults:** 200 mg/kg daily I.M. or I.V. infusion, divided into doses given q 4 to 6 hours. **Children:** 50 to 200 mg/kg daily I.M. or I.V. infusion, divided into doses given q 4 to 6 hours.	**Blood:** *bleeding with high doses,* neutropenia, eosinophilia, leukopenia, *thrombocytopenia.* **CNS:** *convulsions,* neuromuscular irritability. **GI:** nausea. **Local:** pain at injection site, vein irritation, phlebitis. **Metabolic:** *hypokalemia.* **Other:** *hypersensitivity (edema, fever, chills, rash, pruritus, urticaria, anaphylaxis),* overgrowth of nonsusceptible organisms.
carbenicillin indanyl sodium Geocillin, Geopen Oral♦♦	*Urinary tract infection and prostatitis caused by susceptible strains of gram-negative organisms*— **Adults:** 382 to 764 mg P.O. q.i.d. Not recommended for children.	**Blood:** leukopenia, neutropenia, eosinophilia, anemia, thrombocytopenia. **GI:** *nausea,* vomiting, *diarrhea, flatulence, abdominal cramps, unpleasant taste.* **Other:** *hypersensitivity (rash, chills, fever, urticaria, pruritus, anaphylaxis),* overgrowth of nonsusceptible organisms.

♦ Available in U.S. and Canada. ♦♦ Available in Canada only. All other products (no symbol) available in U.S. only. Italicized side effects are common or life-threatening.

INTERACTIONS	NURSING CONSIDERATIONS
	• Initial dilution in vial is stable for 1 hour. Follow manufacturer's direction for stability data when ampicillin is further diluted for I.V. infusion. • For treatment of anaphylaxis, see inside front cover.
Probenecid: increases blood levels of penicillin. Probenecid is often used for this purpose. *Gentamicin, tobramycin:* chemically incompatible. Don't mix together in I.V. Give 1 hour apart. *Chloramphenicol, erythromycin, tetracyclines:* antibiotic antagonism. Give penicillins at least 1 hour before bacteriostatic antibiotics.	• Use cautiously in patients with other drug allergies, especially to cephalosporins (possible cross-allergenicity); and in those with bleeding tendencies, uremia, hypokalemia. Use cautiously in patients on sodium-restricted diets; contains 4.7 mEq sodium/g. • Obtain cultures for sensitivity tests before first dose. Unnecessary to wait for test results before beginning therapy. • Before giving penicillin, ask patient if he's had any allergic reactions to this drug. However, a negative history of penicillin allergy is no guarantee against a future allergic reaction. • Dosage should be altered in patients with impaired hepatic and renal function. Patients with impaired renal function are susceptible to nephrotoxicity. Monitor intake and output. • Check CBC frequently. Drug may cause thrombocytopenia. • Monitor serum potassium. Patients may develop hypokalemia due to large amount of sodium in the preparation. • If patient has high blood level of this drug, he may have convulsions. Be prepared by keeping side rails up on bed. • When giving I.V., mix with 5% dextrose in water or other suitable I.V. fluids. • Give I.V intermittently to prevent vein irritation. Change site every 48 hours. • Almost always used with another antibiotic, such as gentamicin. • Large doses may cause increased yeast growths. Report symptoms to doctor. • With prolonged therapy, other superinfections may occur, especially in the elderly, debilitated, or those with low resistance to infection due to immunosuppressives or irradiation. Close observation is essential. • Check expiration date; do not use any penicillin that is outdated. • For treatment of anaphylaxis, see inside front cover.
None significant.	• Use cautiously in patients with other drug allergies, especially to cephalosporins (possible cross-allergenicity). • Obtain cultures for sensitivity tests before first dose. Unnecessary to wait for test results before starting therapy. • Before giving penicillin, ask patient if he's had any allergic reactions to this drug. However, a negative history of penicillin allergy is no guarantee against a future allergic reaction. • Tell patient to take medication exactly as prescribed, even after he feels better. Entire quantity prescribed should be taken. • Tell patient to call the doctor if he develops rash, fever, or chills. A rash is the most common allergic reaction. • When given orally, drug may cause GI disturbances. Food may interfere with absorption, so give 1 to 2 hours before meals or 2 to 3 hours after. • Large doses may cause increased yeast growths. Report symptoms to doctor. • With prolonged therapy, other superinfections may occur, especially in the elderly, debilitated, or those with low resistance to infection due to immunosuppressives or irradiation. Close observation is essential. • Check expiration date. Warn patient never to use leftover penicillin for a new illness or to share penicillin with family and friends.

(continued on following page)

NAME	INDICATIONS & DOSAGE	SIDE EFFECTS
carbenicillin indanyl sodium *(continued)*		
cloxacillin sodium Bactopen♦♦, Cloxapen♦, Novocloxin♦♦, Orbenin♦♦, Tegopen♦	*Systemic infections caused by penicillinase-producing staphylococci—* **Adults:** 2 to 4 g P.O. daily, divided into doses given q 6 hours. **Children:** 50 to 100 mg/kg P.O. daily, divided into doses given q 6 hours.	**Blood:** eosinophilia. **GI:** *nausea,* vomiting, *epigastric distress, diarrhea.* **Other:** *hypersensitivity (rash, urticaria, chills, fever, sneezing, wheezing, anaphylaxis),* overgrowth of nonsusceptible organisms.
cyclacillin Cyclapen	*Systemic and urinary tract infections caused by susceptible strains of gram-positive and gram-negative organisms—* **Adults:** 250 to 500 mg P.O. q.i.d. in equally spaced doses. **Children:** 50 to 100 mg/kg/day P.O. in equally divided doses.	**Blood:** anemia, thrombocytopenia, thrombocytopenic purpura, leukopenia, neutropenia, eosinophilia. **GI:** *nausea,* vomiting, *diarrhea.* **Other:** *hypersensitivity (edema, fever, chills, rash, pruritus, urticaria, anaphylaxis),* overgrowth of nonsusceptible organisms.
dicloxacillin sodium Dycill, Dynapen♦, Pathocil, Veracillin	*Systemic infections caused by penicillinase-producing staphylococci—* **Adults:** 1 to 2 g daily P.O. or	**Blood:** eosinophilia. **GI:** *nausea,* vomiting, *epigastric distress,* flatulence, *diarrhea.* **Other:** *hypersensitivity (pruritus,*

♦ Available in U.S. and Canada. ♦♦ Available in Canada only. All other products (no symbol) available in U.S. only. Italicized side effects are common or life-threatening.

INTERACTIONS	NURSING CONSIDERATIONS
	• Use only in patients whose creatinine clearance is 10 ml/minute or more. • Excellent treatment for *Pseudomonas* urinary tract infections in ambulatory patients. • May be useful in treatment of cystitis, but not pyelonephritis. • Not effective for any systemic infection because blood levels are nil. • For treatment of anaphylaxis, see inside front cover.
Probenecid: increases blood levels of penicillin. Probenecid is often used for this purpose. *Chloramphenicol, erythromycin, tetracyclines:* antibiotic antagonism. Give penicillins at least 1 hour before bacteriostatic antibiotics.	• Use with caution in patients with other drug allergies, especially to cephalosporins (possible cross-allergenicity). • Obtain cultures for sensitivity tests before first dose. Unnecessary to wait for test results before starting therapy. • Before giving penicillin, ask patient if he's had any allergic reactions to this drug. However, a negative history of penicillin allergy is no guarantee against a future allergic reaction. • Tell patient to take medication exactly as prescribed, even if he feels better. Entire quantity prescribed should be taken. • Tell patient to call the doctor if rash, fever, or chills develop. A rash is the most common allergic reaction. • May cause GI disturbances. Food may interfere with absorption, so give 1 to 2 hours before meals or 2 to 3 hours after. • Large doses may cause increased yeast growths. Report symptoms to doctor. • With prolonged therapy, other superinfections may occur, especially in the elderly, debilitated, or those with low resistance to infection due to immunosuppressives or irradiation. Close observation is essential. • Check expiration date. Warn patient never to use leftover penicillin for a new illness or to share penicillin with family and friends. • For treatment of anaphylaxis, see inside front cover.
Probenecid: increases blood levels of penicillin. Probenecid is often used for this purpose. *Chloramphenicol, erythromycin, tetracyclines:* antibiotic antagonism. Give penicillins at least 1 hour before bacteriostatic antibiotics.	• Contraindicated in patients allergic to other penicillins. • Obtain cultures for sensitivity tests before first dose. Unnecessary to wait for test results before starting therapy. • Before giving penicillin, ask patient if he's had any hypersensitive reactions to it. However, a negative history of penicillin allergy is no guarantee against a future allergic reaction. • Tell patient he must take all medication exactly as prescribed, for as long as ordered, even after he feels better. • Patients with renal insufficiency should receive less drug in accordance with their creatinine clearance level. • Large doses of penicillin may cause increased yeast growths. Watch for signs and symptoms, and report to doctor. • With prolonged therapy, bacterial and fungal superinfection may occur, especially in the elderly, debilitated, or those with low resistance to infection due to immunosuppressives or irradiation. Close observation is essential. • Check expiration date before giving this drug. Warn patient never to use leftover penicillin for a new illness or to share his penicillin with family and friends. • Tell patient to call the doctor if he develops rash, fever, chills. A rash is the most common allergic reaction. • For treatment of anaphylaxis, see inside front cover.
Chloramphenicol, erythromycin, tetracyclines: antibiotic antagonism. Give	• Use cautiously in patients allergic to cephalosporins (possible cross-allergenicity). • Obtain cultures for sensitivity tests before first dose. Unnecessary to wait for test results before starting therapy.

(continued on following page)

NAME	INDICATIONS & DOSAGE	SIDE EFFECTS
dicloxacillin sodium *(continued)*	I.M., divided into doses given q 6 hours. **Children:** 25 to 50 mg/kg P.O. or I.M. daily, divided into doses given q 6 hours.	*urticaria, rash, anaphylaxis),* overgrowth of nonsusceptible organisms.
hetacillin Versapen **hetacillin potassium** Versapen K	*Systemic infections caused by susceptible strains of gram-positive and gram-negative organisms—* **Adults:** 225 to 450 mg P.O. q.i.d. **Children:** 22.5 to 45 mg/kg P.O. daily, divided into doses given q 6 hours.	**Blood:** thrombocytopenia, thrombocytopenic purpura, eosinophilia, leukopenia. **GI:** vomiting, *nausea, epigastric distress, diarrhea,* glossitis, stomatitis. **Local:** pain at injection site, vein irritation, phlebitis. **Other:** *hypersensitivity (chills, fever, anaphylaxis, maculopapular rash, urticaria),* overgrowth of nonsusceptible organisms.
methicillin sodium Azapen, Celbenin, Staphcillin♦	*Systemic infections caused by penicillinase-producing staphylococci—* **Adults:** 4 to 12 g I.M. or I.V. daily, divided into doses given q 4 to 6 hours. **Children:** 100 to 200 mg/kg I.M. or I.V. daily, divided into	**Blood:** *eosinophilia,* hemolytic anemia, transient neutropenia. **CNS:** neuropathy, convulsions with high doses. **GI:** glossitis, stomatitis. **GU:** interstitial nephritis. **Local:** *vein irritation, thrombophlebitis.*

♦ Available in U.S. and Canada. ♦♦ Available in Canada only. All other products (no symbol) available in U.S. only. Italicized side effects are common or life-threatening.

INTERACTIONS	NURSING CONSIDERATIONS
penicillins at least 1 hour before bacteriostatic antibiotics. *Probenecid:* increases blood levels of penicillin. Probenecid is often used for this purpose.	• Before giving penicillin, ask patient if he's had any allergic reactions to this drug. However, a negative history of penicillin allergy is no guarantee against a future allergic reaction. • Tell patient to take medication exactly as prescribed, even if he feels better. Entire quantity prescribed should be taken. • Tell patient to call the doctor if rash, fever, or chills develop. A rash is the most common allergic reaction. • When given orally, drug may cause GI disturbances. Food may interfere with absorption, so give 1 to 2 hours before meals or 2 to 3 hours after. • Don't give I.M. unless infection is severe or patient can't take oral dose. • Large doses may cause increased yeast growths. Report symptoms to doctor. • With prolonged therapy, other superinfections may occur, especially in the elderly, debilitated, or those with low resistance to infection due to immunosuppressives or irradiation. Close observation is essential. • Periodic assessments of renal, hepatic, and hematopoietic function should be made when therapy is prolonged. • Check expiration date. Warn patient never to use leftover penicillin for a new illness or to share penicillin with family and friends. • For treatment of anaphylaxis, see inside front cover.
Chloramphenicol, erythromycin, tetracyclines: antibiotic antagonism. Give penicillins at least 1 hour before bacteriostatic antibiotics. *Probenecid:* increased blood levels of penicillin. Probenecid is often used for this purpose.	• Contraindicated in patients with mononucleosis. Use cautiously in patients with other drug allergies, especially to cephalosporins (possible cross-allergenicity), or with GI disturbances. • Obtain cultures for sensitivity tests before first dose. Unnecessary to wait for test results before beginning therapy. • Before giving penicillin, ask patient if he's had any allergic reactions to this drug. However, a negative history of penicillin allergy is no guarantee against a future allergic reaction. • Tell patient to take medication exactly as prescribed, even if he feels better. Entire quantity prescribed should be taken. • Tell patient to call the doctor if rash, fever, or chills develop. A rash is the most common allergic reaction. • When given orally, drug may cause GI disturbances. Food may interfere with absorption, so give 1 to 2 hours before meals or 2 to 3 hours after. • Large doses may cause increased yeast growths. Report symptoms to doctor. • With prolonged therapy, other superinfections may occur, especially in the elderly, debilitated, or those with low resistance to infection due to immunosuppressives or irradiation. Close observation is essential. • Check expiration date. Warn patient never to use leftover penicillin for a new illness or to share penicillin with family and friends. • Very similar to ampicillin. • For treatment of anaphylaxis, see inside front cover.
Chloramphenicol, erythromycin, tetracyclines: antibiotic antagonism. Give penicillins at least 1 hour before bacteriostatic antibiotics. *Probenecid:* increases	• Use cautiously in patients with other drug allergies, especially to cephalosporins (possible cross-allergenicity), and in infants. • Obtain cultures for sensitivity tests before first dose. Unnecessary to wait for test results before starting therapy. • Before giving penicillin, ask patient if he's had any allergic reactions to this drug. However, a negative history of penicillin allergy is no guarantee against a future allergic reaction. • Urinalysis should be done frequently to monitor renal function.

(continued on following page)

NAME	INDICATIONS & DOSAGE	SIDE EFFECTS
methicillin sodium *(continued)*	doses given q 4 to 6 hours.	**Other:** *hypersensitivity (chills, fever, edema, rash, urticaria, anaphylaxis),* overgrowth of nonsusceptible organisms.
nafcillin sodium Nafcil, Unipen♦	*Systemic infections caused by penicillinase-producing staphylococci—* **Adults:** 2 to 4 g P.O. daily, divided into doses given q 6 hours; 2 to 12 g I.M. or I.V. daily, divided into doses given q 4 to 6 hours. **Children:** 50 to 100 mg/kg P.O. daily, divided into doses given q 4 to 6 hours; or 100 to 200 mg/kg I.M. or I.V. daily, divided into doses given q 4 to 6 hours.	**Blood:** transient leukopenia, neutropenia, granulocytopenia, thrombocytopenia with high doses. **GI:** *nausea,* vomiting, diarrhea. **Local:** *vein irritation, thrombophlebitis.* **Other:** *hypersensitivity (chills, fever, rash, pruritus, urticaria, anaphylaxis).*
oxacillin sodium Bactocill, Prostaphilin♦	*Systemic infections caused by penicillinase-producing staphylococci—* **Adults:** 2 to 4 g P.O. daily,	**Blood:** granulocytopenia, thrombocytopenia, eosinophilia, hemolytic anemia, transient neutropenia.

♦ Available in U.S. and Canada. ♦♦ Available in Canada only. All other products (no symbol) available in U.S. only. Italicized side effects are common or life-threatening.

INTERACTIONS	NURSING CONSIDERATIONS
blood levels of penicillin. Probenecid is often used for this purpose.	• If ordered 4 times a day, be sure to give every 6 hours—even during the night. • If patient has high blood level of this drug, he may have convulsions. Be prepared by keeping side rails up on bed. • Dosage should be altered in patients with impaired hepatic and renal functions. • When giving I.V., mix with a normal saline solution. Don't mix with others because methicillin may be inactivated. Initial dilution must be made with sterile water for injection. • Give I.V. intermittently to prevent vein irritation. Change site every 48 hours. • Large doses may cause increased yeast growths. Report symptoms to doctor. • With prolonged therapy, other superinfections may occur, especially in the elderly, debilitated, or those with low resistance to infection due to immunosuppressives or irradiation. Close observation is essential. • Periodic assessment of hepatic, renal, and hematopoietic function required during prolonged therapy. • Check expiration date. • For treatment of anaphylaxis, see inside front cover.
Chloramphenicol, erythromycin, tetracyclines: antibiotic antagonism. Give penicillins at least 1 hour before bacteriostatic antibiotics. *Probenecid:* increases blood levels of penicillin. Probenecid is often used for this purpose.	• Use cautiously in patients with drug allergies, especially to cephalosporins (possible cross-allergenicity), and in those with GI distress. • Obtain cultures for sensitivity tests before first dose. Unnecessary to wait for test results before starting therapy. • Before giving penicillin, ask patient if he's had any allergic reactions to this drug. However, a negative history of penicillin allergy is no guarantee against a future allergic reaction. • Tell patient to take medication exactly as prescribed, even if he feels better. Entire quantity prescribed should be taken. • Tell patient to call the doctor if rash, fever, or chills develop. A rash is the most common allergic reaction. • When given orally, drug may cause GI disturbances. Food may interfere with absorption, so give 1 to 2 hours before meals or 2 to 3 hours after. • Don't give I.M. or I.V. unless infection is severe or patient can't take oral dose. • When giving I.V., mix with 5% dextrose in water or a saline solution. See Chapter 6, UNDERSTANDING INTRAVENOUS SOLUTION COMPATIBILITY. • Give I.V. intermittently to prevent vein irritation. Change site every 48 hours. • Large doses may increase yeast growths. Report symptoms to doctor. • With prolonged therapy, other superinfections may occur, especially in the elderly, debilitated, or those with low resistance to infection due to immunosuppressives or irradiation. Close observation is essential. • Check expiration date. Warn patient never to use leftover penicillin for a new illness or to share penicillin with family and friends. • For treatment of anaphylaxis, see inside front cover.
Probenecid: increases blood levels of penicillin. Probenecid is often used for this	• Use cautiously in patients with other drug allergies, especially to cephalosporins (possible cross-allergenicity), in premature newborns, and in infants. • Obtain cultures for sensitivity tests before first dose. Unnecessary

(continued on following page)

NAME	INDICATIONS & DOSAGE	SIDE EFFECTS
oxacillin sodium *(continued)*	divided into doses given q 6 hours; 2 to 12 g I.M. or I.V. daily, divided into doses given q 4 to 6 hours. **Children:** 50 to 100 mg/kg P.O. daily, divided into doses given q 6 hours; 100 to 200 mg/kg I.M. or I.V. daily, divided into doses given q 4 to 6 hours.	**CNS:** neuropathy. **GI:** oral lesions. **GU:** interstitial nephritis. **Hepatic:** hepatitis. **Local:** *thrombophlebitis.* **Other:** *hypersensitivity (fever, chills, rash, urticaria, anaphylaxis),* overgrowth of nonsusceptible organisms.
penicillin G benzathine Bicillin L-A♦, Megacillin Suspension♦♦, Permapen	*Congenital syphilis—* **Children under age 2:** 50,000 units/kg I.M. as a single dose. *Group A streptococcal upper respiratory tract infections—* **Adults:** 1.2 million units I.M. in a single injection. **Children over 27 kg:** 900,000 units I.M. in a single injection. **Children under 27 kg:** 300,000 to 600,000 units I.M. in a single injection. *Prophylaxis of poststreptococcal rheumatic fever or glomerulonephritis—* **Adults and children:** 1.2 million units I.M. once a month or 600,000 units twice a month. *Syphilis of less than 1 year's duration—* **Adults:** 2.4 million units I.M. in a single dose. *Syphilis of more than 1 year's duration—* **Adults:** 2.4 million units I.M. weekly for 3 successive weeks.	**Blood:** eosinophilia, hemolytic anemia, thrombocytopenia, leukopenia. **CNS:** neuropathy, convulsions with high doses. **Local:** pain and sterile abscess at injection site. **Other:** *hypersensitivity (maculopapular and exfoliative dermatitis, chills, fever, edema, anaphylaxis).*
penicillin G potassium Arcocillin, Biotic-T,	*Moderate to severe systemic infections—* **Adults:** 1.6 to 3.2 million units	**Blood:** hemolytic anemia, leukopenia, thrombocytopenia. **CNS:** neuropathy, convulsions

♦ Available in U.S. and Canada. ♦♦ Available in Canada only. All other products (no symbol) available in U.S. only. Italicized side effects are common or life-threatening.

INTERACTIONS	NURSING CONSIDERATIONS
purpose. *Sulfamethoxypyridazine:* decreases blood levels of oxacillin. Avoid if possible. *Chloramphenicol, erythromycin, tetracyclines:* antibiotic antagonism. Give penicillins at least 1 hour before bacteriostatic antibiotics.	to wait for test results before starting therapy. • Before giving penicillin, ask patient if he's had any allergic reactions to this drug. However, a negative history of penicillin allergy is no guarantee against a future allergic reaction. • Tell the patient to take medication exactly as prescribed, even if he feels better. The entire quantity prescribed should be taken. • Tell patient to call the doctor if rash, fever, or chills develop. A rash is the most common allergic reaction. • When given orally, drug may cause GI disturbances. Food may interfere with absorption, so give 1 to 2 hours before meals or 2 to 3 hours after. • Don't give I.M. or I.V. unless infection is severe or patient can't take oral dose. • Periodic liver function studies are indicated; watch for elevated SGOT and SGPT. • When giving I.V., mix with 5% dextrose in water or a saline solution. See Chapter 6, UNDERSTANDING INTRAVENOUS SOLUTION COMPATIBILITY. • Give I.V. intermittently to prevent vein irritation. Change site every 48 hours. • Large doses may increase yeast growths. Report symptoms to doctor. • With prolonged therapy, other superinfections may occur, especially in the elderly, debilitated, or those who have had immunosuppressives or irradiation. Close observation is essential. • Check expiration date. Warn patient never to use leftover penicillin for a new illness or to share penicillin with family and friends. • For treatment of anaphylaxis, see inside front cover.
Chloramphenicol, erythromycin, tetracyclines: antibiotic antagonism. Give penicillins at least 1 hour before bacteriostatic antibiotics. *Probenecid:* increases blood levels of penicillin. Probenecid is often used for this purpose.	• Use cautiously in patients with other drug allergies, especially to cephalosporins (possible cross-allergenicity). • Obtain cultures for sensitivity tests before first dose. Unnecessary to wait for test results before beginning therapy. • Before giving penicillin, ask patient if he's had any allergic reactions to this drug. However, a negative history of penicillin allergy is no guarantee against a future allergic reaction. • Tell patient to call the doctor if rash, fever, or chills develop. Fever and eosinophilia are the most common allergic reactions. • Shake medication well before injection. • Never give I.V. Inadvertent I.V. administration has caused cardiac arrest and death. • Very slow absorption time makes allergic reactions difficult to treat. • Inject deeply into upper outer quadrant of buttocks in adults; in midlateral thigh in infants and small children. • Check expiration date. • For treatment of anaphylaxis, see inside front cover.
Chloramphenicol, erythromycin, tetracyclines: antibiotic	• Use cautiously in patients with other drug allergies, especially to cephalosporins (possible cross-allergenicity). • Obtain cultures for sensitivity tests before first dose. Unnecessary

(continued on following page)

NAME	INDICATIONS & DOSAGE	SIDE EFFECTS
penicillin G potassium *(continued)* Burcillin-G, Cryspen, Deltapen, Falapen♦♦, G-Recillin-T, Hyasorb, Hylenta♦♦, K-Cillin, K-Pen, Ka-Pen♦♦, Lanacillin, Megacillin♦♦, Novopen-G♦, Palocillin, Parcillin, Pensorb, Pentids, P-50♦♦, Pfizerpen	P.O. daily, divided into doses given q 6 hours (1 mg = 1,600 units); 1.2 to 24 million units I.M. or I.V. daily, divided into doses given q 4 hours. **Children:** 25,000 to 100,000 units/kg P.O. daily, divided into doses given q 6 hours; or 25,000 to 300,000 units/kg I.M. or I.V. daily, divided into doses given q 4 hours.	with high doses. **Metabolic:** possible severe potassium poisoning with high doses (hyperreflexia, convulsions, coma). **Local:** *thrombophlebitis, pain at injection site.* **Other:** *hypersensitivity (rash, urticaria, maculopapular eruptions, exfoliative dermatitis, chills, fever, edema, anaphylaxis),* overgrowth of nonsusceptible organisms.
penicillin G procaine Ayercillin♦♦, Crysticillin A.S., Duracillin A.S., Pfizerpen A.S., Tu-Cillin, Wycillin♦	*Moderate to severe systemic infections—* **Adults:** 600,000 to 1.2 million units I.M. daily given as a single dose. **Children:** 300,000 units I.M. daily given as a single dose. *Uncomplicated gonorrhea—* **Adults, and children over 12 years:** give 1 g probenecid; then 30 minutes later give 4.8 million units of penicillin G procaine I.M., divided into 2 injection sites. *Pneumococcal pneumonia—* **Adults, and children over 12 years:** 300,000 to 600,000 units I.M. daily q 6 to 12 hours.	**Blood:** thrombocytopenia, hemolytic anemia, leukopenia. **CNS:** arthralgia, convulsions. **Other:** *hypersensitivity (rash, urticaria, chills, fever, edema, prostration, anaphylaxis),* overgrowth of nonsusceptible organisms.

♦ Available in U.S. and Canada. ♦♦ Available in Canada only. All other products (no symbol) available in U.S. only. Italicized side effects are common or life-threatening.

INTERACTIONS	NURSING CONSIDERATIONS
antagonism. Give penicillins at least 1 hour before bacteriostatic antibiotics. *Probenecid:* increases blood levels of penicillin. Probenecid is often used for this purpose.	to wait for results before beginning therapy. • Before giving penicillin, ask patient if he's had any allergic reactions to this drug. However, a negative history of penicillin allergy is no guarantee against a future allergic reaction. • Tell patient to take medication exactly as prescribed, even if he feels better. • Tell patient to call the doctor if rash, fever, or chills develop. A rash is the most common allergic reaction. • When given orally, drug may cause GI disturbances. Food may interfere with absorption, so give 1 to 2 hours before meals or 2 to 3 hours after. • Don't give I.M. or I.V. unless infection is severe or patient can't take oral dose. Extremely painful when given I.M. Inject deep into large muscle. • If patient has high blood level of this drug, he may have convulsions. Be prepared by keeping side rails up on bed. • When giving I.V., mix with 5% dextrose in water or a saline solution. See Chapter 6, UNDERSTANDING INTRAVENOUS SOLUTION COMPATIBILITY. • Give I.V. intermittently to prevent vein irritation. Change site every 48 hours. • Large doses may increase yeast growths. Report symptoms to doctor. • With prolonged therapy, other superinfections may occur, especially in the elderly, debilitated, or those who have had immunosuppressives or irradiation. Close observation is essential. • Check expiration date. Warn patient never to use leftover penicillin for a new illness or to share penicillin with family and friends. • For treatment of anaphylaxis, see inside front cover.
Chloramphenicol, erythromycin, tetracyclines: antibiotic antagonism. Give penicillins at least 1 hour before bacteriostatic antibiotics. *Probenecid:* increases blood levels of penicillin. Probenecid is often used for this purpose.	• Contraindicated in patients with hypersensitivity to procaine. Use cautiously in patients with other drug allergies, especially to cephalosporins (possible cross-allergenicity). • Obtain cultures for sensitivity tests before first dose. Unnecessary to wait for test results before beginning therapy. • Before giving penicillin, ask patient if he's had any allergic reactions to this drug. However, a negative history of penicillin allergy is no guarantee against a future allergic reaction. • Tell patient to call doctor if rash, fever, or chills develop. A rash is the most common allergic reaction. • Give deep I.M. in upper outer quadrant of buttocks in adults; in midlateral thigh in small children. Do not give subcutaneously. • Never give I.V. Inadvertent I.V. administration has caused death due to CNS toxicity from procaine. • Large doses may cause increased yeast growths. Report symptoms to doctor. • Due to slow absorption rate, allergic reactions are hard to treat. • With prolonged therapy, other superinfections may occur, especially in the elderly, debilitated, or those with low resistance to infection due to immunosuppressives or irradiation. Close observation is essential. • Periodic evaluations of renal and hematopoietic function are recommended. • Check expiration date. • For treatment of anaphylaxis, see inside front cover.

NAME	INDICATIONS & DOSAGE	SIDE EFFECTS
penicillin G sodium Crystapen♦♦	*Moderate to severe systemic infections—* **Adults:** 1.2 to 24 million units daily I.M. or I.V., divided into doses given q 4 hours. **Children:** 25,000 to 300,000 units/kg daily I.M. or I.V., divided into doses given q 4 hours.	**Blood:** hemolytic anemia, leukopenia, thrombocytopenia. **CNS:** arthralgia, neuropathy, convulsions. **CV:** *congestive heart failure with high doses.* **Local:** *vein irritation, pain at injection site, thrombophlebitis.* **Other:** *hypersensitivity (chills, fever, edema, maculopapular rash, exfoliative dermatitis, urticaria, anaphylaxis),* overgrowth of nonsusceptible organisms.
penicillin V Biotic Powder, Compocillin-V, Ledercillin VK♦, Pfizerpen VK♦, Robicillin-VK, SK-Penicillin VK, Uticillin VK, V-Cillin Drops, V-Pen **penicillin V potassium** Betapen VK, Biotic-V-Powder, Bopen V-K, Cocillin V-K, Compocillin-VK, Dowpen VK, Lanacillin VK, Ledercillin VK♦, LV, Nadopen-V♦♦, Novopen-V♦♦, Penapar VK, Penbec-V♦♦, Pen-Vee-K♦, Pfizerpen VK, PVF K♦♦, Repen-VK, Uticillin VK, V-Cillin K♦	*Mild to moderate systemic infections—* **Adults:** 250 to 500 mg (400,000 to 800,000 units) P.O. q 6 hours. **Children:** 15 to 50 mg/kg (25,000 to 90,000 units/kg) P.O. daily, divided into doses given q 6 to 8 hours.	**Blood:** eosinophilia, hemolytic anemia, leukopenia, thrombocytopenia. **CNS:** neuropathy. **GI:** *epigastric distress,* vomiting, diarrhea, *nausea.* **Other:** *hypersensitivity (rash, urticaria, chills, fever, edema, anaphylaxis),* overgrowth of nonsusceptible organisms.
ticarcillin disodium Ticar	*Severe systemic infections caused by susceptible strains of gram-positive and especially gram-negative organisms* (Pseu-	**Blood:** leukopenia, neutropenia, eosinophilia, *thrombocytopenia,* hemolytic anemia. **CNS:** convulsions, neuromuscular

♦ Available in U.S. and Canada. ♦♦ Available in Canada only. All other products (no symbol) available in U.S. only. Italicized side effects are common or life-threatening.

INTERACTIONS	NURSING CONSIDERATIONS
Chloramphenicol, erythromycin, tetracyclines: antibiotic antagonism. Give penicillins at least 1 hour before bacteriostatic antibiotics. *Probenecid:* increases blood levels of penicillin. Probenecid is often used for this purpose.	• Contraindicated in patients on sodium restriction. Use cautiously in patients with other drug allergies, especially to cephalosporins (possible cross-allergenicity). • Obtain cultures for sensitivity tests before first dose. Unnecessary to wait for test results before beginning therapy. • Before giving penicillin, ask patient if he's had any allergic reactions to this drug. However, a negative history of penicillin allergy is no guarantee against a future allergic reaction. • If patient has high blood level of this drug, he may have convulsions. Be prepared by keeping side rails up on bed. • When giving I.V., mix with 5% dextrose in water or a saline solution. See Chapter 6, UNDERSTANDING INTRAVENOUS SOLUTION COMPATIBILITY. • Give I.V. intermittently to prevent vein irritation. Change site every 48 hours. • Large doses may increase yeast growths. Report symptoms to doctor. • With prolonged therapy, other superinfections may occur, especially in the elderly, debilitated, or those with low resistance to infection due to immunosuppressives or irradiation. Close observation is essential. • Monitor vital signs frequently. • Monitor serum sodium. • Check expiration date. • For treatment of anaphylaxis, see inside front cover.
Chloramphenicol, erythromycin, tetracyclines: antibiotic antagonism. Give penicillins at least 1 hour before bacteriostatic antibiotics. *Neomycin:* decreases absorption of penicillin. Give penicillin by injection. *Probenecid:* increases blood levels of penicillin. Probenecid is often used for this purpose.	• Use cautiously in patients with other drug allergies, especially to cephalosporins (possible cross-allergenicity), and GI disturbances. • Obtain cultures for sensitivity tests before first dose. Unnecessary to wait for test results before beginning therapy. • Before giving penicillin, ask patient if he's had any allergic reactions to this drug. However, a negative history of penicillin allergy is no guarantee against a future allergic reaction. • Tell patient to take medication exactly as prescribed, even if he feels better. Entire quantity prescribed should be taken. • Tell patient to call the doctor if rash, fever, or chills develop. A rash is the most common allergic reaction. • May cause GI disturbances. Food may interfere with absorption, so give 1 to 2 hours before meals or 2 to 3 hours after. • Large doses may cause increased yeast growths. Report symptoms to doctor. • With prolonged therapy, other superinfections may occur, especially in the elderly, debilitated, or those with low resistance to infection due to immunosuppressives or irradiation. Close observation is essential. • Periodic renal and hematopoietic function studies are recommended in patients receiving prolonged therapy. • Check expiration date. Warn patient never to use leftover penicillin for a new illness or to share penicillin with family and friends. • For treatment of anaphylaxis, see inside front cover.
Chloramphenicol, erythromycin, tetracyclines: antibiotic antagonism. Give	• Use cautiously in patients with other drug allergies, especially to cephalosporins (possible cross-allergenicity); and in patients with impaired renal function, hemorrhagic conditions, hypokalemia, or sodium restrictions (contains 5.2 mEq sodium/g).

(continued on following page)

NAME	INDICATIONS & DOSAGE	SIDE EFFECTS
ticarcillin disodium *(continued)*	domonas, Proteus)— **Adults:** 18 g I.V. or I.M. daily, divided into doses given q 4 to 6 hours. **Children:** 200 to 300 mg/kg I.V. or I.M. daily, divided into doses given q 4 to 6 hours.	excitability. **GI:** nausea. **Metabolic:** *hypokalemia.* **Local:** pain at injection site, vein irritation, phlebitis. **Other:** *hypersensitivity (rash, pruritus, urticaria, chills, fever, edema, anaphylaxis),* overgrowth of nonsusceptible organisms.

♦ Available in U.S. and Canada. ♦♦ Available in Canada only. All other products (no symbol) available in U.S. only. Italicized side effects are common or life-threatening.

TESTING FOR PENICILLIN ALLERGY

To test for penicillin allergy:

- Make a scratch on the inner surface of the patient's forearm, but don't make it deep enough to bleed.
- Place a drop of reagent (commercially available as Pre-Pen) on the scratch and gently rub it in. A positive reaction shows a wheal, with or without erythema, and itching occurs in 15 to 20 minutes. (*Note:* Wipe the solution off immediately if a positive reaction occurs.)
- If the scratch test is negative, inject 0.01 to 0.02 ml of reagent into the intradermal layer of the inner aspect of the patient's forearm so that a small bleb is raised. If this test is also negative, the patient is not allergic to the drug at this time.

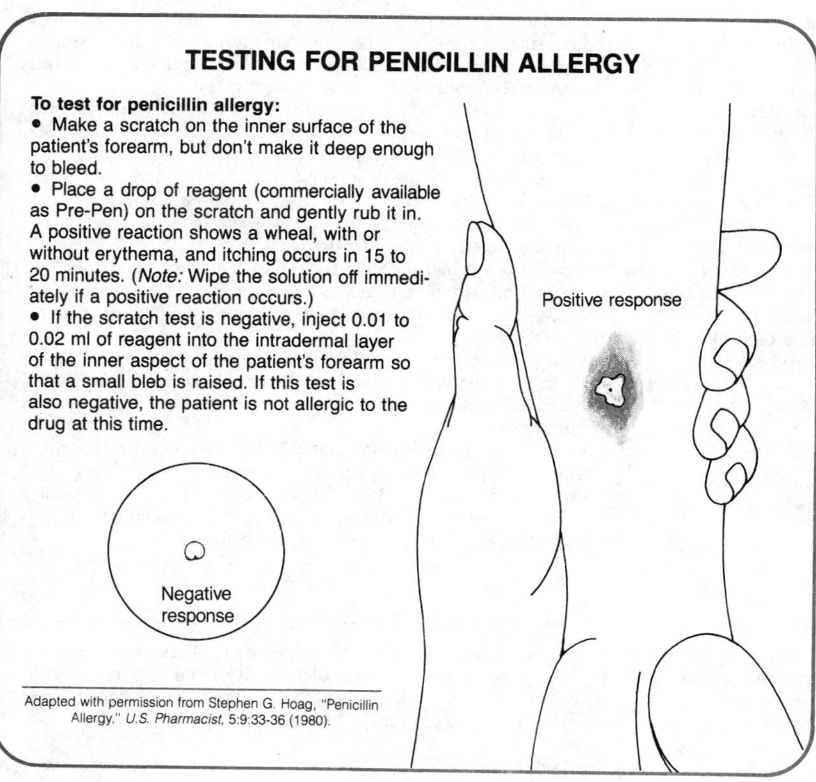

Adapted with permission from Stephen G. Hoag, "Penicillin Allergy," *U.S. Pharmacist,* 5:9:33-36 (1980).

INTERACTIONS	NURSING CONSIDERATIONS
Chloramphenicol, erythromycin, tetracyclines: antibiotic antagonism. Give penicillins at least 1 hour before bacteriostatic antibiotics. *Probenecid:* increases blood levels of penicillin. Probenecid is often used for this purpose. *Gentamicin, tobramycin:* chemically incompatible. Don't mix together in I.V. Give 1 hour apart.	• Obtain cultures for sensitivity tests before first dose. Unnecessary to wait for test results before beginning therapy. • Before giving penicillin, ask patient if he's had any allergic reactions to this drug. However, a negative history of penicillin allergy is no guarantee against a future allergic reaction. • Dosage should be decreased in patients with impaired hepatic and renal functions. • Check CBC frequently. Drug may cause thrombocytopenia. • If patient has high blood level of this drug, he may develop convulsions. Be prepared by keeping side rails up on bed. • When giving I.V., mix with 5% dextrose in water or other suitable I.V. fluids. • Give I.V. intermittently to prevent vein irritation. Change site every 48 hours. • Administer deep I.M. into large muscle. • Large doses may increase yeast growths. Report symptoms to doctor. • Almost always used with another antibiotic such as gentamicin. • With prolonged therapy, other superinfections may occur, especially in the elderly, debilitated, or those who have had immunosuppressives or irradiation. Close observation is essential. • Monitor serum potassium. • Check expiration date. • For treatment of anaphylaxis, see inside front cover.

DESENSITIZING PATIENTS WITH PENICILLIN ALLERGIES

If no other antibiotic will help the patient who's allergic to penicillin, an allergist may desensitize him. (*Note:* If an allergist isn't available and the patient's life depends on penicillin treatment, another doctor can perform the procedure.

Desensitization should always be performed in your hospital's intensive care unit and should begin early in the morning, when the unit's fully staffed. Before the doctor starts:

• Establish an I.V. line so medications can be given if necessary.

• Have emergency drugs, such as epinephrine, aminophylline, and theophylline, at bedside. Don't give antihistamines during desensitization. They could mask the beginning of an allergic reaction.

Although your hospital may use a slightly different desensitization procedure, this is how it's done at the University of Texas Health Sciences Center in Dallas:

To desensitize the patient, the doctor administers 17 doses of penicillin during a 4-hour period. He gives the first 13 doses orally, using a pediatric suspension of penicillin G. Then the doctor doubles each successive dose.

After the last oral dose, the doctor halves the dosage and begins giving penicillin subcutaneously. (Halving the dose compensates for bypassing the gastrointestinal tract.) He administers two more subcutaneous doses, each time doubling the previous dose.

After the last subcutaneous dose, the doctor administers the final dose by intramuscular injection. If the patient hasn't had an adverse reaction, he's ready to undergo full I.V. therapy.

Studies suggest that after patients are desensitized, they could probably receive penicillin by any route, but so far all desensitized patients have needed I.V. penicillin. Also, therapy does not have to be continued with the same penicillin; any of the beta-lactam antibiotics can be used. But the antibiotic *must* be given on schedule. Researchers don't know exactly how long it takes for sensitivity to return, but they're sure it does.

Everyone involved with such a procedure should understand the potential danger and agree the situation warrants the risk. Have consent forms signed, as a permanent part of the patient's chart.

Adapted with permission from "Penicillin Allergies Undone," *Emergency Medicine,* 12:59-61, September 30, 1980.

15 Cephalosporins

cefaclor
cefadroxil monohydrate
cefamandole naftate
cefazolin sodium
cefoxitin sodium
cephalexin monohydrate
cephaloglycin dihydrate
cephaloridine
cephalothin sodium
cephapirin sodium
cephradine

Structurally related to penicillins, cephalosporins are broad-spectrum antibiotics active against a variety of aerobic gram-positive and gram-negative microorganisms. They all contain 7-aminocephalosporanic acid (beta-lactam ring).

"Third generation" cephalosporins have recently been introduced. Cefotaxime and moxalactam, the first of these, are discussed in the APPENDIX, *New Drugs*. These agents have expanded utility against gram-negative microorganisms.

Major uses

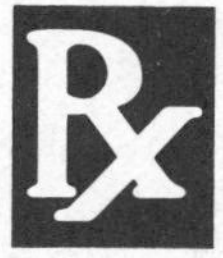

Cephalosporins are used to treat infections caused by gram-positive cocci (except enterococci), penicillinase-producing staphylococci, and some gram-negative bacilli, including *Pseudomonas, Escherichia coli, Proteus mirabilis,* and *Klebsiella*. Although these drugs may be used for patients allergic to penicillin, a small percentage of such patients subsequently develop allergies to cephalosporins.

As penicillin alternatives, parenteral and oral cephalosporins combat infec-

DRUG ALERT

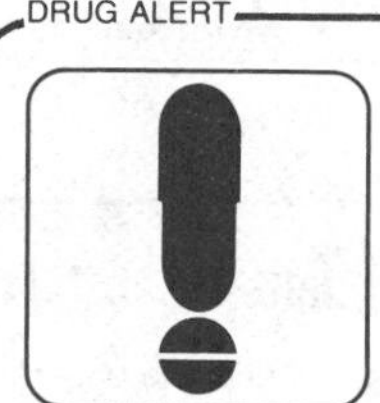

WATCH FOR CEPHALOSPORIN AND PENICILLIN CROSS-SENSITIVITY

Before administering a cephalosporin, ask your patient whether he's allergic to penicillin. If he is, be wary. Allergic reactions to cephalosporins are about five times more common in patients with a history of penicillin allergy than in other patients.

Why? Cephalosporins and penicillins are similar in structure. This may explain why cephalosporins are capable of forming an antigenic complex resembling the one formed by penicillin.

Avoid administering cephalosporins to a patient who has recently experienced a severe, immediate reaction to penicillin. And when you do administer a cephalosporin, make sure you have all the necessary supplies to deal with an adverse reaction immediately.

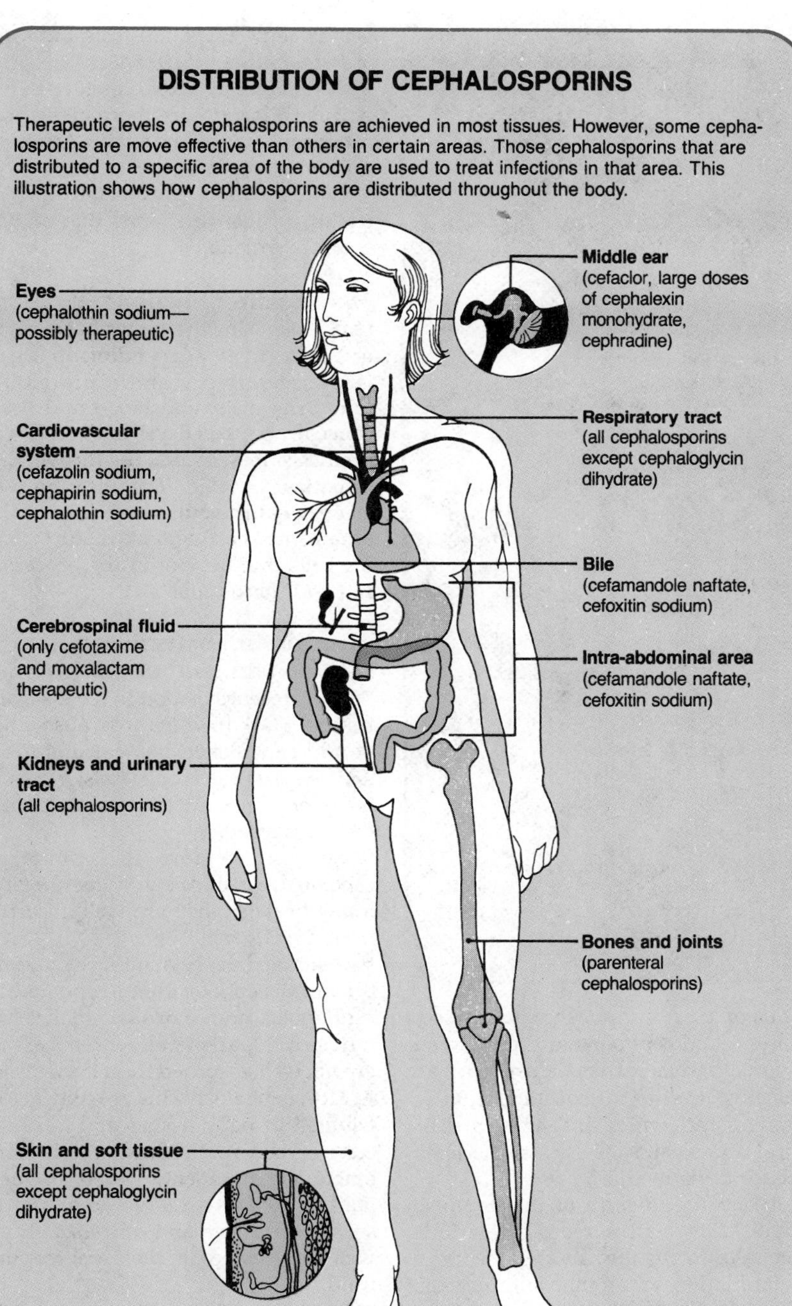
DISTRIBUTION OF CEPHALOSPORINS
Therapeutic levels of cephalosporins are achieved in most tissues. However, some cephalosporins are move effective than others in certain areas. Those cephalosporins that are distributed to a specific area of the body are used to treat infections in that area. This illustration shows how cephalosporins are distributed throughout the body.
Eyes (cephalothin sodium—possibly therapeutic)
Middle ear (cefaclor, large doses of cephalexin monohydrate, cephradine)
Respiratory tract (all cephalosporins except cephaloglycin dihydrate)
Cardiovascular system (cefazolin sodium, cephapirin sodium, cephalothin sodium)
Bile (cefamandole naftate, cefoxitin sodium)
Cerebrospinal fluid (only cefotaxime and moxalactam therapeutic)
Intra-abdominal area (cefamandole naftate, cefoxitin sodium)
Kidneys and urinary tract (all cephalosporins)
Bones and joints (parenteral cephalosporins)
Skin and soft tissue (all cephalosporins except cephaloglycin dihydrate)

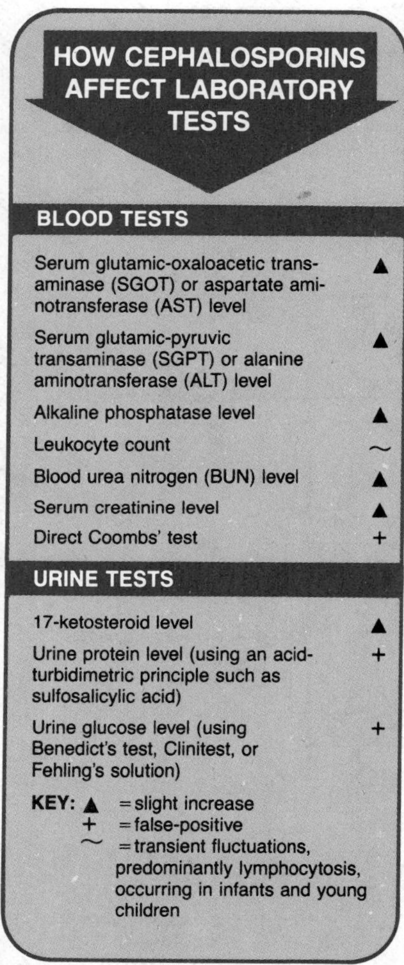

HOW CEPHALOSPORINS AFFECT LABORATORY TESTS

BLOOD TESTS	
Serum glutamic-oxaloacetic transaminase (SGOT) or aspartate aminotransferase (AST) level	▲
Serum glutamic-pyruvic transaminase (SGPT) or alanine aminotransferase (ALT) level	▲
Alkaline phosphatase level	▲
Leukocyte count	~
Blood urea nitrogen (BUN) level	▲
Serum creatinine level	▲
Direct Coombs' test	+
URINE TESTS	
17-ketosteroid level	▲
Urine protein level (using an acid-turbidimetric principle such as sulfosalicylic acid)	+
Urine glucose level (using Benedict's test, Clinitest, or Fehling's solution)	+

KEY: ▲ = slight increase
+ = false-positive
~ = transient fluctuations, predominantly lymphocytosis, occurring in infants and young children

tions of the respiratory tract, skin, soft tissues, and genitourinary tract. In addition, parenteral cephalosporins are effective against osteoarticular infections, septicemia, and endocarditis. Oral cephalosporins are also therapeutic for otitis media.

When the identity of the organism is unknown in serious infections, cephalosporins may be therapeutic in combination with other antimicrobial drugs (aminoglycosides, for example).

Cephalosporins may be used prophylactically before orthopedic, cardiac, bowel, and gynecologic surgery.

- Cefamandole and cefaclor are active against some ampicillin-resistant strains of *Hemophilus influenzae.*
- Cefamandole, cefotaxime, cefoxitin, and moxalactam are more active than other cephalosporins against strains of the Enterobacteriaceae.
- Cefoxitin and moxalactam may be useful against infections due to *Bacteroides fragilis.*

Mechanism of action

Cephalosporins are either bactericidal or bacteriostatic, depending on organism susceptibility and reproduction rate, drug dose, and blood and tissue concentrations. They inhibit cell-wall synthesis, thereby making the wall less osmotically stable. They are more effective against young, rapidly dividing organisms than against mature, resting cells that are not in the process of cell-wall formation.

Absorption, distribution, metabolism, and excretion

- The presence of food in the gastrointestinal (GI) tract retards absorption of oral cephalosporins, causing lower and delayed peak blood levels; it doesn't, however, diminish the total amount of drug absorbed.
- Cefaclor, cefadroxil, cephalexin, cephaloglycin, and cephradine are given orally because they are well absorbed from the GI tract.
- Cefamandole, cefazolin, cefotaxime, cefoxitin, cephaloridine, cephalothin, cephapirin and moxalactam are administered parenterally because they are not well absorbed from the GI tract.
- Most cephalosporins are widely distributed in body tissues and fluid but enter cerebrospinal fluid in only small amounts. Therapeutic levels of these antibiotics are achieved in most tissues. Cefotaxime and moxalactam are well distributed in the cerebrospinal fluid.
- Cefaclor, cefadroxil, cefamandole, cefazolin, cefoxitin, cephalexin, cephaloridine, cephradine, and moxalactam are excreted unchanged in the urine and accumulate in patients with renal insuf-

THERAPEUTIC ACTIVITY

THERAPEUTIC ACTIVITY OF CEPHALOSPORINS

DRUG	ROUTE	PEAK	HALF-LIFE *
cefaclor	P.O.	30 to 60 min	36 to 54 min
cefadroxil monohydrate	P.O.	90 to 120 min	72 to 90 min
cefamandole naftate	I.M.	30 to 120 min	30 to 72 min
	I.V.	end of infusion	30 to 72 min
cefazolin sodium	I.M.	60 min	108 min
	I.V.	end of infusion	108 min
cefotaxime sodium	I.M.	30 min	60 min
	I.V.	end of infusion	60 min
cefoxitin sodium	I.M.	30 min	42 to 60 min
	I.V.	end of infusion	42 to 60 min
cephalexin monohydrate	P.O.	60 min	36 to 54 min
cephaloglycin dihydrate	P.O.	(blood levels not significant	90 min
cephaloridine	I.M.	30 min	90 min
cephalothin sodium	I.V.	end of infusion	30 to 48 min
cephapirin sodium	I.M.	60 min	30 to 36 min
	I.V.	end of infusion	30 to 36 min
cephradine	I.M.	48 to 120 min	48 to 78 min
	I.V.	end of infusion	48 to 78 min
	P.O.	60 min	48 to 78 min
moxalactam	I.M.	30 to 60 min	120 to 180 min
	I.V.	end of infusion	120 to 180 min

*Based on normal renal function. Renal impairment prolongs half-life, so doses should be adjusted.

ficiency.

• Cefotaxime, cephaloglycin, cephalothin, and cephapirin are partially metabolized in the liver.

Onset and duration

Onset and duration depend on route of administration and the patient's renal function.

• After oral administration, peak blood levels occur within 1 to 2 hours.

• Peak levels after I.V. administration depend on the rate of infusion; they occur when the infusion is finished.

• Blood levels reach a peak between 30 minutes and 2 hours after I.M. administration.

For additional details, see the chart above.

Combination products

None.

NAME	INDICATIONS & DOSAGE	SIDE EFFECTS
cefaclor Ceclor	*Treatment of infections of respiratory or urinary tract, skin, and soft tissue; and otitis media due to* Hemophilus influenzae, Streptococcus pneumoniae, Streptococcus pyogenes, Escherichia coli, Proteus mirabilis, Klebsiella *species, and staphylococci—* **Adults:** 250 to 500 mg P.O. q 8 hours. Total daily dose should not exceed 4 g. **Children:** 20 mg/kg/day P.O. in divided doses q 8 hours. In more serious infections, 40 mg/kg/day are recommended, not to exceed 1 g per day.	**Blood:** transient leukopenia, lymphocytosis, anemia, eosinophilia. **CNS:** dizziness, headache, somnolence. **GI:** *nausea,* vomiting, diarrhea, anorexia. **GU:** red and white cells in urine, vaginal moniliasis, vaginitis. **Skin:** *maculopapular rash,* dermatitis. **Other:** hypersensitivity, fever.
cefadroxil monohydrate Duricef	*Treatment of urinary tract infections caused by* Escherichia coli, Proteus mirabilis, *and* Klebsiella *species; infections of skin and soft tissue; and streptococcal pharyngitis—* **Adults:** 500 mg to 2 g P.O. per day, depending on the infection being treated. Usually given in once-daily or b.i.d. dosage. **Children:** 30 mg/kg/day in 2 divided doses.	**Blood:** transient neutropenia, eosinophilia, leukopenia, anemia. **CNS:** dizziness, headache, malaise, paresthesias. **GI:** *nausea,* anorexia, vomiting, *diarrhea,* glossitis, *dyspepsia,* abdominal cramps, anal pruritus, tenesmus, oral candidiasis (thrush). **GU:** genital pruritus, moniliasis. **Skin:** *maculopapular and erythematous rashes.* **Other:** dyspnea.
cefamandole naftate Mandol	*Treatment of serious infections of respiratory or genitourinary tract, skin and soft-tissue infections, bone and joint infections, septicemia, and peritonitis due to* Escherichia coli *and other coliform bacteria,* Staphylococcus aureus *(penicillinase- and nonpenicillinase-producing),* Staphyloccus epidermidis, *group A beta-hemolytic streptococci,* Klebsiella, Hemophilus influenzae, Proteus mirabilis, *and* Enterobacter *species—* **Adults:** 500 mg to 1 g q 4 to 8 hours. In life-threatening infections, up to 2 g q 4 hours may be needed. **Infants and children:** 50 to 100 mg/kg/day in equally divided doses q 4 to 8 hours. May	**Blood:** transient neutropenia, eosinophilia, hemolytic anemia. **CNS:** headache, malaise, paresthesias, dizziness. **GI:** nausea, anorexia, vomiting, diarrhea, glossitis, dyspepsia, abdominal cramps, tenesmus, anal pruritus, oral candidiasis (thrush). **GU:** nephrotoxicity, genital pruritus and moniliasis. **Skin:** *maculopapular and erythematous rashes, urticaria.* **Local:** *at injection site—pain, induration, sterile abscesses,* temperature elevation, tissue sloughing; *phlebitis and thrombophlebitis with I.V. injection.* **Other:** *hypersensitivity,* dyspnea.

♦ Available in U.S. and Canada. ♦♦ Available in Canada only. All other products (no symbol) available in U.S. only. Italicized side effects are common or life-threatening.

INTERACTIONS	NURSING CONSIDERATIONS
Probenecid: may inhibit excretion and increase blood levels of cefaclor. Use together cautiously.	• Contraindicated in hypersensitivity to other cephalosporins. Use cautiously in patients with impaired renal status and in those with history of sensitivity to penicillin. Ask patient if he's had any reaction to previous cephalosporin or penicillin therapy before administering first dose. • Prolonged use may result in overgrowth of nonsusceptible organisms. Careful observation of patient for superinfection is essential. • Obtain cultures for sensitivity tests before first dose, but therapy may begin pending test results. • Major clinical use appears to be in treating otitis media caused by *H. influenzae* when resistant to ampicillin or amoxicillin. • Mostly used in ambulatory setting. • Tell patient to take medication exactly as prescribed, even after he feels better. • Call doctor if skin rash develops. • Store reconstituted suspension in refrigerator. Stable for 14 days if refrigerated. Shake well before using. • Drug may be taken with meals. • Cefaclor is a relatively expensive antibiotic and should be used only when the organism is resistant to other agents.
Probenecid: may inhibit excretion and increase blood levels of cefadroxil. Use together cautiously.	• Contraindicated in hypersensitivity to other cephalosporins. Use cautiously in patients with impaired renal status and in those with history of sensitivity to penicillin. Ask patient if he's had any reaction to previous cephalosporin or penicillin therapy before administering first dose. • Prolonged use may result in overgrowth of nonsusceptible organisms. Careful observation of patient for superinfection is essential. • Obtain cultures for sensitivity tests before first dose, but therapy may begin pending test results. • If creatinine clearance is below 50 ml/minute, dosage interval should be lengthened so drug doesn't accumulate. • Tell patient to take medication exactly as prescribed, even after he feels better. • Call doctor if skin rash develops. • Absorption not delayed by presence of food. • Longer half-life permits twice-daily dosing.
Probenecid: may inhibit excretion and increase blood levels of cefamandole. Use together cautiously.	• Contraindicated in hypersensitivity to other cephalosporins. Use cautiously in patients with impaired renal status and in those with history of sensitivity to penicillin. Ask patient if he's had any reaction to previous cephalosporin or penicillin therapy before administering first dose. • Prolonged use may result in overgrowth of nonsusceptible organisms. Careful observation of patient for superinfection is essential. • Obtain cultures for sensitivity tests before first dose, but therapy may begin pending test results. • Cephalosporin of choice for treatment of *Enterobacter* sepsis. • Not as effective as cefoxitin in treating anaerobic infections. • For most cephalosporin-sensitive organisms, cefamandole offers little advantage over previously available agents. • For I.V. use, reconstitute 1 g with 10 ml of sterile water for injection, 5% dextrose or 0.9% sodium chloride for injection. May be combined with the following intravenous fluids: 0.9% sodium chloride injection, 5% dextrose injection, 10% dextrose injection, 5% dextrose and 0.9% sodium chloride injection, 5% dextrose and 0.45% sodium chloride injection, 5% dextrose and 0.2% sodium chloride injection, or sodium lactate injection. • I.M. cefamandole is not as painful as cefoxitin. Does not require

(continued on following page)

NAME	INDICATIONS & DOSAGE	SIDE EFFECTS
cefamandole naftate *(continued)*	be increased to total daily dose of 150 mg/kg (not to exceed maximum adult dose) for severe infections. Total daily dosage is same for I.M. or I.V. administration and depends on susceptibility of organism and severity of infection. In patients with impaired renal function, doses or frequency of administration must be modified according to degree of renal impairment, severity of infection, susceptibility of organism, and blood levels of drug. Should be injected deep I.M. into a large muscle mass, such as gluteus or vastus lateralis.	
cefazolin sodium Ancef♦, Kefzol♦	*Treatment of serious infections of respiratory and genitourinary tracts, skin and soft-tissue infections, bone and joint infections, septicemia, and endocarditis due to* Escherichia coli, *Enterobacteriaceae, gonococci,* Hemophilus influenzae, Klebsiella, Proteus mirabilis, Staphylococcus aureus, Streptococcus pneumoniae, *and group A beta-hemolytic streptococci; prophylaxis before, during, and after surgery—* **Adults:** 250 mg I.M. or I.V. q 8 hours to 1 g q 6 hours. **Children over 1 month:** 8 to 16 mg/kg I.M. or I.V. q 8 hours, or 6 to 12 mg/kg q 6 hours. Total daily dosage is same for I.M. or I.V. administration and depends on susceptibility of organism and severity of infection. In patients with impaired renal function, doses or frequency of administration must be modified according to degree of renal impairment, severity of infection, susceptibility of organism, and serum levels of drug. Should be injected deep I.M. into a large muscle mass, such as gluteus or vastus lateralis.	**Blood:** transient neutropenia, leukopenia, eosinophilia, anemia. **CNS:** dizziness, headache, malaise, paresthesias. **GI:** nausea, anorexia, vomiting, diarrhea, glossitis, dyspepsia, abdominal cramps, anal pruritus, tenesmus, oral candidiasis (thrush). **GU:** nephrotoxicity, genital pruritus and moniliasis, vaginitis. **Skin:** *maculopapular and erythematous rashes, urticaria.* **Local:** *at injection site—pain, induration, sterile abscesses,* tissue sloughing; *phlebitis and thrombophlebitis with I.V. injection.* **Other:** *hypersensitivity,* dyspnea.
cefoxitin sodium Mefoxin	*Treatment of serious infection of respiratory and genitourinary tracts, skin and soft-tissue infections, bone and joint infec-*	**Blood:** transient neutropenia, eosinophilia, hemolytic anemia. **CNS:** headache, malaise, paresthesias, dizziness.

♦ Available in U.S. and Canada. ♦♦ Available in Canada only. All other products (no symbol) available in U.S. only. Italicized side effects are common or life-threatening.

INTERACTIONS	NURSING CONSIDERATIONS
	addition of lidocaine. • After reconstitution, remains stable for 24 hours at room temperature or 96 hours under refrigeration.
Probenecid: may increase blood levels of cephalosporins. Use together cautiously.	• Use cautiously in patients with impaired renal status and in those with history of sensitivity to penicillin. Ask patient if he's ever had any reaction to cephalosporin or penicillin therapy before administering first dose. • Avoid doses greater than 4 g daily in patients with severe renal impairment. • Prolonged use may result in overgrowth of nonsusceptible organisms. Watch carefully for superinfection. • Obtain cultures for sensitivity tests before first dose, but therapy may begin pending test results. • Because of long duration of effect, most infections can be treated with a single dose q 8 hours. • For I.M. administration, reconstitute with sterile water, bacteriostatic water, or 0.9% sodium chloride solution as follows: 2 ml to 250-mg vial; 2 ml to 500-mg vial; 2.5 ml to 1-g vial. Shake well until dissolved. Resultant concentration: 125 mg/ml, 225 mg/ml, 330 mg/ml, respectively. • Not as painful as other cephalosporins when given I.M. • Alternate injection sites if I.V. therapy lasts longer than 3 days. Use of small I.V. needles in the larger available veins may be preferable. • For I.V. administration, reconstituted cefazolin sodium is diluted in 50 to 100 ml of 0.9% sodium chloride injection, 5% or 10% dextrose injection, 5% dextrose in lactated Ringer's, 5% dextrose and 0.9% sodium chloride, 5% dextrose and 0.45% or 0.2% sodium chloride, lactated Ringer's injection, Normosol-M in 5% dextrose in water, Ionosol B with 5% dextrose, or Plasma-Lyte with 5% dextrose. • Reconstituted cefazolin sodium is stable for 24 hours at room temperature, for 96 hours under refrigeration. • About 40% to 75% of patients receiving cephalosporins show a false-positive direct Coombs' test; only a few of these indicate hemolytic anemia. • Urine glucose tests with Benedict's Qualitative Reagent, Clinitest, or Fehling's solution may cause false-positive reaction during cephalosporin therapy. Clinistix, Diastix, and Tes-Tape are not affected.
Probenecid: may inhibit excretion and increase blood levels of cefoxitin. Use to-	• Contraindicated in hypersensitivity to other cephalosporins. Use cautiously in patients with impaired renal status and in those with history of sensitivity to penicillin. Ask patient if he's had any reaction to previous cephalosporin or penicillin therapy before administering

(continued on following page)

NAME	INDICATIONS & DOSAGE	SIDE EFFECTS
cefoxitin sodium *(continued)*	*tions, bloodstream and intra-abdominal infections due to* Escherichia coli *and other coliform bacteria,* Staphylococcus aureus *(penicillinase- and nonpenicillinase-producing),* Staphylococcus epidermidis, *streptococci,* Klebsiella, Hemophilus influenzae, *and* Bacteroides *species, including* B. fragilis— **Adults:** 1 to 2 g q 6 to 8 hours for uncomplicated forms of infection. Up to 12 g/day in life-threatening infections. **Children:** 80 to 160 mg/kg/day. Total daily dosage is same for I.M. or I.V. administration and depends on susceptibility of organism and severity of infection. In patients with impaired renal function, doses or frequency of administration must be modified according to degree of renal impairment, severity of infection, susceptibility of organism, and blood levels of drug. Should be injected deep I.M. into a large muscle mass, such as gluteus or vastus lateralis.	**GI:** nausea, anorexia, vomiting, diarrhea, glossitis, dyspepsia, abdominal cramps, tenesmus, anal pruritus, oral candidiasis (thrush). **GU:** nephrotoxicity, genital pruritus and moniliasis. **Skin:** *maculopapular and erythematous rashes, urticaria.* **Local:** *at injection site—pain, induration, sterile abscesses, tissue sloughing; phlebitis and thrombophlebitis with I.V. injection.* **Other:** *hypersensitivity,* dyspnea, elevated temperature.
cephalexin monohydrate Ceporex♦♦, Keflex♦	*Treatment of infections of respiratory or genitourinary tract, skin and soft-tissue infections, bone and joint infections, and otitis media due to* Escherichia coli *and other coliform bacteria, group A beta-hemolytic streptococci,* Hemophilus influenzae, Klebsiella, Proteus mirabilis, Streptococcus pneumoniae, *and staphylococci—* **Adults:** 250 mg to 1 g P.O. q 6 hours. **Children:** 6 to 12 mg/kg P.O. q 6 hours. Maximum 25 mg/kg q 6 hours.	**Blood:** transient neutropenia, eosinophilia, anemia. **CNS:** dizziness, headache, malaise, paresthesias. **GI:** *nausea, anorexia,* vomiting, *diarrhea,* glossitis, dyspepsia, abdominal cramps, anal pruritus, tenesmus, oral candidiasis (thrush). **GU:** genital pruritus and moniliasis, vaginitis. **Skin:** *maculopapular and erythematous rashes, urticaria.* **Other:** *hypersensitivity,* dyspnea.
cephaloglycin dihydrate Kafocin	*Treatment of acute and chronic urinary tract infections, including cystitis, pyelitis, pyelonephritis, and asymptomatic*	**Blood:** transient neutropenia, eosinophilia, anemia. **CNS:** dizziness, headache, malaise, paresthesias.

♦ Available in U.S. and Canada. ♦♦ Available in Canada only. All other products (no symbol) available in U.S. only. Italicized side effects are common or life-threatening.

INTERACTIONS	NURSING CONSIDERATIONS
gether cautiously.	first dose. • Prolonged use may result in overgrowth of nonsusceptible organisms. Observe patient for superinfection. • Obtain cultures for sensitivity tests before first dose, but therapy may begin pending test results. • A very useful cephalosporin when anaerobic or mixed aerobic-anaerobic infection is suspected, especially *B. fragilis.* • For most cephalosporin-sensitive organisms, cefoxitin offers little advantage over previously available agents. • For I.V. use, reconstitute 1 g with at least 10 ml of sterile water for injection, and 2 g with 10 to 20 ml. Solutions of 5% dextrose and 0.9% sodium chloride for injection can also be used. These primary solutions can be further diluted with the following solutions: Ringer's injection, lactated Ringer's injection, 5% dextrose in lactated Ringer's injection, 5% or 10% invert sugar in water, 10% invert sugar in saline solution, 5% sodium bicarbonate injection, Aminosol 5% solution, Normosol-M in 5% dextrose in water, Ionosol B with 5% dextrose, Polyonic M 56 in 5% dextrose. • I.M. injection can be reconstituted with 0.5% or 1% lidocaine HCl (without epinephrine) to minimize pain. • May cause false-positive result for urine glucose with Clinitest tablets. • May be useful in the treatment of resistant gonorrhea. • After reconstitution, remains stable for 24 hours at room temperature or 1 week under refrigeration.
Probenecid: may increase blood levels of cephalosporins. Use together cautiously.	• Use cautiously in patients with impaired renal status and in those with history of sensitivity to penicillin. Ask patient if he's had any reaction to previous cephalosporin or penicillin therapy before administering first dose. • Prolonged use may result in overgrowth of nonsusceptible organisms. Watch closely for superinfection. • Obtain cultures for sensitivity tests before first dose, but therapy may begin pending test results. • Tell patient to take medication exactly as prescribed, even after he feels better. Group A beta-hemolytic streptococcal infections should be treated for a minimum of 10 days. • Call doctor if skin rash develops. • Preparation of oral suspension: add required amount of water to powder in two portions. Shake well after each addition. After mixing, store in refrigerator. Stable for 14 days without significant loss of potency. Keep tightly closed and shake well before using. • About 40% to 75% of patients receiving cephalosporins show a false-positive direct Coombs' test, but only a few indicate anemia. • Urine glucose tests with Benedict's Qualitative Reagent, Clinitest, or Fehling's solution may give false-positive results during cephalosporin therapy. Clinistix, Diastix, and Tes-Tape are not affected.
Probenecid: may increase blood levels of cephalosporins. Use together cautiously.	• Use cautiously in patients with impaired renal function and in those with history of sensitivity to penicillin. Ask patient if he's had any reaction to previous cephalosporin or penicillin therapy before administering first dose.

(continued on following page)

NAME	INDICATIONS & DOSAGE	SIDE EFFECTS
cephaloglycin dihydrate *(continued)*	*bacteriuria when due to susceptible strains of* Escherichia coli, Klebsiella, Enterobacter, Proteus, *staphylococci, and enterococci—* **Adults:** 250 to 500 mg P.O. q 6 hours.	**GI:** *nausea, anorexia, vomiting, diarrhea,* glossitis, dyspepsia, abdominal cramps, anal pruritus, tenesmus, oral candidiasis (thrush). **GU:** genital pruritus and moniliasis, vaginitis. **Skin:** *maculopapular and erythematous rashes, urticaria.* **Other:** *hypersensitivity,* dyspnea.
cephaloridine Ceporan♦♦, Loridine♦	*Treatment of serious infections of respiratory tract, central nervous system, genitourinary tract, bones and joints, bloodstream, skin, and soft tissue due to* Escherichia coli *and other coliform bacteria, gonococci,* Hemophilus influenzae, Klebsiella, Proteus mirabilis, *pneumococci, staphylococci (coagulase-positive and coagulase-negative), beta-hemolytic and other streptococci; also, gonorrhea and early syphilis when penicillin is contraindicated—* **Adults:** 250 mg to 1 g I.M. or I.V. q 6 to 12 hours. Not to exceed 4 g daily. **Children:** 7 to 12 mg/kg I.M. or I.V. q 6 hours. *Severe infections*—up to 25 mg/kg q 6 hours. Not recommended for children under 1 month or for premature infants. Total daily dosage is same for I.M. or I.V. administration and depends on susceptibility of organism and severity of infection. Initial loading dose (usually 500 mg) recommended. In patients with impaired renal function, doses and frequency of administration must be modified according to degree of renal impairment, severity of infection, susceptibility of causative organism, and blood levels of drug. Should be injected deep I.M. into large muscle mass, such as gluteus or vastus lateralis. I.V. administration is preferable in severe or life-threatening infections.	**Blood:** transient neutropenia, eosinophilia, anemia. **CNS:** headache, malaise, paresthesias. **GI:** nausea, anorexia, vomiting, diarrhea, glossitis, dyspepsia, abdominal cramps, tenesmus, anal pruritus, oral candidiasis (thrush). **GU:** *nephrotoxicity (especially in doses greater than 4 g daily or in patients with renal impairment),* genital pruritus and moniliasis. **Skin:** *maculopapular and erythematous rashes, urticaria.* **Local:** at injection site—pain, induration, sterile abscesses, tissue sloughing; phlebitis and thrombophlebitis with I.V. injection. **Other:** *hypersensitivity,* dyspnea.

INTERACTIONS	NURSING CONSIDERATIONS
	• Cephaloglycin blood levels are low; used only for urinary tract infections. • Prolonged use may result in overgrowth of nonsusceptible organisms. Watch for superinfection. • Obtain cultures for sensitivity tests before first dose, but therapy may begin pending test results. • Tell patient to take exactly as prescribed, even after he feels better. • About 40% to 75% of patients receiving cephalosporins show a false-positive direct Coombs' test, but only a few indicate anemia. • Urine glucose tests with Benedict's Qualitative Reagent, Clinitest, or Fehling's solution may give false-positive results during cephalosporin therapy. Clinistix, Diastix, and Tes-Tape are not affected.
Probenecid: may increase blood levels of cephalosporins. Use together cautiously. *Ethacrynic acid, furosemide:* may enhance nephrotoxicity of cephaloridine. Use cautiously.	• Contraindicated in patients with renal impairment, since drug causes a relatively high incidence of dose-related nephrotoxicity. Use cautiously in patient with history of sensitivity to penicillin. Ask patient if he's had any reaction to previous cephalosporin or penicillin therapy before administering first dose. Safe use not established in patients with proteinuria, declining urinary output, rising BUN or serum creatinine, decreasing creatinine clearance, and those receiving other antibiotics with nephrotoxic potential. • Prolonged use may result in overgrowth of nonsusceptible organisms. Watch for superinfection. • Obtain cultures for sensitivity tests before first dose, but therapy may begin pending test results. • Drug causes relatively little pain when given I.M. • Good CNS penetration makes cephaloridine useful in treating meningitis. • When giving this drug I.V., check frequently for vein irritation and phlebitis. Alternate injection sites if I.V. therapy lasts longer than 3 days. Use of small I.V. needles in the larger available veins may be preferable. • Excreted in urine. Monitor renal function carefully. Watch for signs of impairment: casts in urine, proteinuria, decreased creatinine clearance/serum creatinine ratio. Avoid doses greater than 4 g daily. • About 40% to 75% of patients receiving cephalosporins show a false-positive direct Coombs' test, but only a few indicate hemolytic anemia. • Urine glucose tests with Benedict's Qualitative Reagent, Clinitest, or Fehling's solution may give false-positive results during cephalosporin therapy. Clinistix, Diastix, and Tes-Tape are not affected.

NAME	INDICATIONS & DOSAGE	SIDE EFFECTS
cephalothin sodium Keflin Neutral♦	*Treatment of serious infections of respiratory, genitourinary, or gastrointestinal tract; skin and soft-tissue infections (including peritonitis); bone and joint infections; septicemia; endocarditis; and meningitis due to* Escherichia coli *and other coliform bacteria, Enterobacteriaceae, enterococci, gonococci, group A beta-hemolytic streptococci,* Hemophilus influenzae, Klebsiella, Proteus mirabilis, Salmonella, Staphylococcus aureus, Shigella, Streptococcus pneumoniae, *staphylococci, and* Streptococcus viridans— **Adults:** 500 mg to 1 g I.M. or I.V. (or intraperitoneally) q 4 to 6 hours; in life-threatening infections, up to 2 g q 4 hours. **Children:** 14 to 27 mg/kg I.V. q 4 hours, or 20 to 40 mg/kg q 6 hours; dose should be proportionately less in accordance with age, weight, and severity of infection. Dosage schedule is determined by degree of renal impairment, severity of infection, and susceptibility of causative organism. Should be injected deep I.M. into a large muscle mass, such as gluteus or vastus lateralis. I.V. route is preferable in severe or life-threatening infections.	**Blood:** transient neutropenia, eosinophilia, hemolytic anemia. **CNS:** headache, malaise, paresthesias, dizziness. **GI:** nausea, anorexia, vomiting, diarrhea, glossitis, dyspepsia, abdominal cramps, tenesmus, anal pruritus, oral candidiasis (thrush). **GU:** nephrotoxicity, genital pruritus and moniliasis. **Skin:** maculopapular and erythematous rashes, urticaria. **Local:** *at injection site—pain, induration, sterile abscesses, tissue sloughing; phlebitis and thrombophlebitis with I.V. injection.* **Other:** *hypersensitivity,* dyspnea, temperature elevation.
cephapirin sodium Cefadyl♦	*Serious infections of respiratory, genitourinary, or gastrointestinal tract; skin and soft-tissue infections; bone and joint infections (including osteomyelitis); septicemia; endocarditis due to* Streptococcus pneumoniae, Escherichia coli, *group A beta-hemolytic streptococci,* Hemophilus influenzae, Klebsiella, Proteus mirabilis, Staphylococcus aureus, *and* Streptococcus viridans— **Adults:** 500 mg to 1 g I.V. or I.M. q 4 to 6 hours up to 12 g daily. **Children over 3 months:** 10 to 20 mg/kg I.V. or I.M. q 6 hours; dose depends on age, weight,	**Blood:** transient neutropenia, eosinophilia, anemia. **CNS:** dizziness, headache, malaise, paresthesias. **GI:** nausea, anorexia, vomiting, diarrhea, glossitis, dyspepsia, abdominal cramps, tenesmus, anal pruritus, oral candidiasis (thrush). **GU:** nephrotoxicity, genital pruritus and moniliasis, vaginitis. **Skin:** *maculopapular and erythematous rashes, urticaria.* **Local:** *at injection site—pain, induration, sterile abscesses, tissue sloughing; phlebitis and thrombophlebitis with I.V. injection.* **Other:** *hypersensitivity,* dyspnea.

INTERACTIONS	NURSING CONSIDERATIONS
Probenecid: may increase blood levels of cephalosporins. Use together cautiously.	• Use cautiously in patients with impaired renal function and in those with history of sensitivity to penicillin. Ask patient if he's had any reaction to previous cephalosporin or penicillin therapy before administering first dose. • Obtain cultures for sensitivity tests before first dose, but therapy may begin pending test results. • Prolonged use may result in overgrowth of nonsusceptible organisms. Watch for superinfection. • Drug causes severe pain when administered I.M.; avoid this route if possible. • When giving this drug I.V., check frequently for vein irritation and phlebitis. Alternate injection sites if I.V. therapy lasts longer than 3 days. Use of small I.V. needle in the larger available veins may be preferable. Addition of a small concentration of heparin (100 units) may reduce incidence of phlebitis. • For I.M. administration, reconstitute each gram of cephalothin sodium with 4 ml of sterile water for injection, providing 500 mg in each 2.2 ml. If vial contents do not dissolve completely, add an additional 0.2 to 0.4 ml of diluent, and warm contents slightly. • For I.V. administration, dilute contents of 4-g vial with at least 20 ml of sterile water for injection, 5% dextrose injection, or 0.9% sodium chloride injection and add to one of following I.V. solutions: acetated Ringer's injection, 5% dextrose injection, 5% dextrose in lactated Ringer's injection, Ionosol B in 5% dextrose in water, lactated Ringer's injection, Normosol-N in 5% dextrose in water, Plasma-Lyte injection, Plasma-Lyte-N injection in 5% dextrose, Ringer's injection, or 0.9% sodium chloride injection. Choose solution and fluid volume according to patient's fluid and electrolyte status. • About 40% to 75% of patients receiving cephalosporins show a false-positive direct Coombs' test; only a few of these indicate hemolytic anemia. • Urine glucose tests with Benedict's Qualitative Reagent, Clinitest, or Fehling's solution may give false-positive results during cephalosporin therapy. Clinistix, Diastix, and Tes-Tape are not affected.
Probenecid: may increase blood levels of cephalosporins. Use together cautiously.	• Use cautiously in patients with impaired renal function and in those with a history of sensitivity to penicillin. Ask patient if he's had any reaction to previous cephalosporin or penicillin therapy before administering first dose. • Prolonged use may result in overgrowth of nonsusceptible organisms. Watch for superinfection. • Obtain cultures for sensitivity tests before first dose, but therapy may begin pending test results. • For I.M. administration, reconstitute 1-g vial with 2 ml of sterile water for injection or bacteriostatic water for injection so that 1.2 ml contains 500 mg of cephapirin. I.M. injection is painful; prepare patient for this. • When giving this drug I.V., check frequently for vein irritation and phlebitis. Alternate injection sites if I.V. therapy lasts longer than 3 days. Use of small I.V. needles in the larger available veins may be preferable. • Prepare I.V. infusion using dextrose injection, sodium chloride injection, or bacteriostatic water for injection as diluent: 20 ml yields 1 g per 10 ml; 50 ml yields 1 g per 25 ml; 100 ml yields 1 g per 50 ml.

(continued on following page)

NAME	INDICATIONS & DOSAGE	SIDE EFFECTS
cephapirin sodium *(continued)*	and severity of infection. Should be injected deep I.M. into a large muscle mass, such as gluteus or vastus lateralis. Depending on causative organism and severity of infection, patients with reduced renal function may be treated adequately with a lower dose (7.5 to 15 mg/kg q 12 hours). Patients with severely reduced renal function and who are to be dialyzed should receive same dose just before dialysis and q 12 hours thereafter.	
cephradine Anspor, Velosef♦	*Serious infection of respiratory, genitourinary, or gastrointestinal tract; skin and soft-tissue infections; bone and joint infections; septicemia; endocarditis; and otitis media due to* Escherichia coli *and other coliform bacteria, group A beta-hemolytic streptococci,* Hemophilus influenzae, Klebsiella, Proteus mirabilis, Staphylococcus aureus, Streptococcus pneumoniae, *staphylococci, and* Streptococcus viridans— **Adults:** 500 mg to 1 g I.M. or I.V. 2 to 4 times daily; do not exceed 8 g daily. Or 250 to 500 mg P.O. q 6 hours. Severe or chronic infections may require larger and/or more frequent doses (up to 1 g P.O. q 6 hours). **Children over 1 year:** 6 to 12 mg/kg P.O. q 6 hours. 12 to 25 mg/kg I.M. or I.V. q 6 hours. *Otitis media*—19 to 25 mg/kg P.O. q 6 hours. Do not exceed 4 g daily. **All patients, regardless of age and weight:** larger doses (up to 1 g q.i.d.) may be given for severe or chronic infections. Parenteral therapy may be followed by oral. Injections should be given deep I.M. into a large muscle mass, such as gluteus or vastus lateralis.	**Blood:** transient neutropenia, eosinophilia. **CNS:** dizziness, headache, malaise, paresthesias. **GI:** *nausea, anorexia,* vomiting, heartburn, glossitis, dyspepsia, abdominal cramping, *diarrhea,* tenesmus, anal pruritus, oral candidiasis (thrush). **GU:** genital pruritus and moniliasis, vaginitis. **Skin:** *maculopapular and erythematous rashes, urticaria.* **Local:** *at injection site—pain, induration, sterile abscesses, tissue sloughing; phlebitis and thrombophlebitis with I.V. injection.* **Other:** *hypersensitivity,* dyspnea.

♦ Available in U.S. and Canada. ♦♦ Available in Canada only. All other products (no symbol) available in U.S. only. Italicized side effects are common or life-threatening.

INTERACTIONS	NURSING CONSIDERATIONS
	• I.V. infusion with Y-tubing: during infusion of cephapirin solution, it is desirable to stop other solution. Check volume of cephapirin solution carefully so that calculated dose is infused. When Y-tubing is used, dilute 4-g vial with 40 ml of diluent. • Compatible with following infusion solutions: sodium chloride injection, 5% dextrose in water, sodium lactate injection, 5% dextrose in normal saline solution, 10% invert sugar in normal saline solution, 10% invert sugar in water, 5% dextrose and 0.2% sodium chloride injection, lactated Ringer's with 5% dextrose, 5% dextrose and 0.45% sodium chloride injection, Ringer's injection, lactated Ringer's injection, 10% dextrose injection, sterile water for injection, 20% dextrose injection, 5% sodium chloride in water, and 5% dextrose in Ringer's injection. • Reconstituted cephapirin is stable and compatible for 10 days under refrigeration and for 24 hours at room temperature. • About 40% to 75% of patients receiving cephalosporins show a false-positive direct Coombs' test, but only a few indicate anemia. • Urine glucose tests with Benedict's Qualitative Reagent, Clinitest, or Fehling's solution may give false-positive results during cephalosporin therapy. Clinistix, Diastix, and Tes-Tape are not affected.
Probenecid: may increase blood levels of cephalosporins. Use together cautiously.	• Use cautiously in patients with impaired renal function and in those with a history of sensitivity to penicillin. Ask patient if he's had any reaction to previous cephalosporin or penicillin therapy before administering first dose. • Obtain cultures for sensitivity tests before first dose, but therapy may begin pending test results. • Prolonged use may result in overgrowth of nonsusceptible organisms. Watch for superinfection. • When giving this drug I.V., check frequently for vein irritation and phlebitis. Alternate injection sites if I.V. therapy lasts longer than 3 days. Use of small I.V. needle in the larger available veins may be preferable. • Tell patient to take medication exactly as prescribed, even after he feels better. Group A beta-hemolytic streptococcal infections should be treated for a minimum of 10 days. • I.M. injection is painful; prepare patient for this. • For I.M. administration, reconstitute with sterile water for injection or with bacteriostatic water for injection as follows: 1.2 ml to 250-mg vial; 2 ml to 500-mg vial; 4 ml to 1-g vial. I.M. solutions must be used within 2 hours if kept at room temperature and within 24 hours if refrigerated. Solutions may vary in color from light straw to yellow without affecting potency. • When preparing cephradine for intravenous administration, when available, use preparation specifically supplied for infusion. Follow specific product directions carefully when reconstituting. • About 40% to 75% of patients receiving cephalosporins show a false-positive direct Coombs' test, but only a few indicate anemia. • Urine glucose tests with Benedict's Qualitative Reagent, Clinitest, or Fehling's solution may give false-positive results during cephalosporin therapy. Clinistix, Diastix, and Tes-Tape are not affected.

16 Tetracyclines

demeclocycline hydrochloride
doxycycline hyclate
methacycline hydrochloride
minocycline hydrochloride
oxytetracycline hydrochloride
tetracycline hydrochloride
tetracycline phosphate complex

The tetracyclines are bacteriostatic antibiotics with broad activity against gram-positive and gram-negative bacteria, *Mycoplasma, Chlamydia,* and *Rickettsia.* Since chlortetracycline was first isolated in 1948, the pharmacologic and microbiologic effects of tetracyclines have been modified. However, because of widespread microbial resistance (*Proteus* and *Pseudomonas* infection, for example), the tetracyclines are the drugs of choice in only a few clinical situations.

Major uses

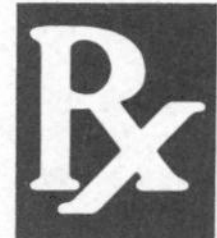

The tetracyclines are used in prophylaxis and therapy of numerous bacterial diseases, especially of the mixed type, such as chronic bronchitis and peritonitis. They're drugs of choice in treatment of bubonic plague, brucellosis, cholera, mycoplasmosis, trachoma, lymphogranuloma venereum, and Rocky Mountain spotted fever.

They're alternative therapeutic agents for syphilis, gonorrhea, anthrax, nocardiosis, and *Hemophilus influenzae* respiratory infections.

They're effective against uncomplicated urinary tract infections from susceptible strains of *Escherichia coli, Klebsiella, Enterobacter,* and *Citrobacter* and in exacerbations of chronic bronchitis.

- Tetracyclines may also be useful as single-dose therapy for shigellosis.
- Oral or topical tetracyclines are therapeutic against acne vulgaris.
- Minocycline is prophylactic in meningococcal infections when rifampin is contraindicated.
- Demeclocycline is a useful adjunct for treating syndrome of inappropriate antidiuretic hormone (SIADH).

Mechanism of action

Tetracyclines are thought to exert bacteriostatic effect by binding to the 30S ribosomal subunit of microorganisms, thus inhibiting protein synthesis.

Absorption, distribution, metabolism, and excretion

- Tetracyclines are readily absorbed after oral administration—some better than others. (See chart opposite.)
- I.M. administration produces lower blood levels than oral administration. Local anesthetic agents are added to I.M. preparations; be sure patient has no hypersensitivity to these agents before administering.
- I.V. administration may produce rapid, high blood levels. Be sure to dilute the dose and give it slowly: phlebitis of the injected vein is common. Avoid extravasation.
- Tetracyclines are widely distributed in most body fluids, including bile,

sinus secretions, and synovial, pleural, and ascitic fluids. Cerebrospinal fluid levels vary, but the drugs tend to diffuse well when the meninges are inflamed; the drugs accumulate in bones, liver, spleen, and teeth.

• Doxycycline and minocycline are partially metabolized by the liver; their elimination routes are unclear. The rest of the tetracyclines are eliminated unchanged in the feces (through the bile) and urine.

Onset and duration

• Blood levels after oral administration peak in 2 to 4 hours.

• Blood levels of 1 to 3 mcg/ml persist for 6 or more hours. (Doxycycline and minocycline give the most prolonged blood levels.)

• Peak levels occur 1 hour after I.M. administration; drug is detectable in the blood for as long as 12 hours.

• Half-lives—hence blood levels—of all tetracyclines except doxycycline are prolonged in patients with severe renal impairment (see chart below).

Combination products

MYSTECLIN-F CAPS: tetracycline HCl 125 mg and amphotericin B 25 mg buffered with potassium metaphosphate.

MYSTECLIN-F CAPS: tetracycline HCl 250 mg and amphotericin B 50 mg buffered with potassium metaphosphate.

MYSTECLIN-F SYRUP: tetracycline HCl 125 mg and amphotericin B 25 mg per 5 ml, buffered with potassium metaphosphate.

For more combinations, see Chapter 18.

HALF-LIFE AND ABSORPTION OF TETRACYCLINES

DRUG	HALF-LIFE Normal Kidneys	Severe Renal Failure	% ABSORBED*
demeclocycline	15 hr	50 hr	66
doxycycline	15 hr†	15 hr†	93
methacycline	12 hr	44 hr	80
minocycline	19 hr	24 hr	100
oxytetracycline	9 hr	55 hr	58
tetracycline	10 hr	75 hr	77

*On an empty stomach. The administration of tetracyclines with food, iron, calcium, phosphates, or antacids significantly impairs absorption.

†The elimination route for this drug is unclear, but independent of the kidneys.

Note: Since tetracyclines accumulate in the teeth and bones, avoid using them in children younger than 8 years.

NAME	INDICATIONS & DOSAGE	SIDE EFFECTS
demeclocycline hydrochloride Declomycin♦, Ledermycin	*Infections caused by susceptible gram-negative and gram-positive organisms, trachoma, amebiasis—* **Adults:** 150 mg P.O. q 6 hours or 300 mg P.O. q 12 hours. **Children over 8 years:** 6 to 12 mg/kg P.O. daily, divided q 6 to 12 hours. *Gonorrhea—* **Adults:** 600 mg P.O. initially, then 300 mg P.O. q 12 hours for 4 days (total 3 g). *Syndrome of inappropriate ADH (hyposmolarity)—* **Adults:** 600 to 1,200 mg P.O. daily in divided doses.	**Blood:** neutropenia, eosinophilia. **CV:** pericarditis. **EENT:** dysphagia, glossitis. **GI:** anorexia, *nausea, vomiting, diarrhea,* enterocolitis, anogenital inflammation. **Metabolic:** *increased BUN,* diabetes insipidus syndrome (polyuria, polydipsia, weakness). **Skin:** *maculopapular and erythematous rashes, photosensitivity, increased pigmentation, urticaria.* **Other:** hypersensitivity.
doxycycline hyclate Doxychel, Vibramycin♦, Vibra Tabs	*Infections caused by sensitive gram-negative and gram-positive organisms, trachoma, amebiasis—* **Adults:** 100 mg P.O. q 12 hours on first day, then 100 mg P.O. daily; or 200 mg I.V. on first day in 1 or 2 infusions, then 100 to 200 mg I.V. daily. **Children over 8 years (under 45 kg):** 4.4 mg/kg P.O. or I.V. daily, divided q 12 hours first day, then 2.2 to 4.4 mg/kg daily. Over 45 kg, same as adults. Give I.V. infusion slowly (minimum time 1 hour). Infusion must be completed within 12 hours (within 6 hours in lactated Ringer's solution or 5% dextrose in lactated Ringer's solution). *Gonorrhea in patients allergic to penicillin—* **Adults:** 200 mg P.O. initially, followed by 100 mg P.O. at bedtime, and 100 mg P.O. b.i.d. for 3 days; or 300 mg P.O. initially and repeat dose in 1 hour. *Primary or secondary syphilis in patients allergic to penicillin—* **Adults:** 300 mg P.O. daily in divided doses for 10 days.	**Blood:** neutropenia, eosinophilia. **CNS:** benign intracranial hypertension. **CV:** pericarditis. **EENT:** sore throat, glossitis, dysphagia. **GI:** anorexia, *epigastric distress, nausea,* vomiting, *diarrhea,* enterocolitis, anogenital inflammation. **Skin:** *maculopapular and erythematous rashes, photosensitivity, increased pigmentation, urticaria.* **Local:** thrombophlebitis. **Other:** hypersensitivity.

INTERACTIONS	NURSING CONSIDERATIONS
Antacids (including $NaHCO_3$) and laxatives containing aluminum, calcium, and magnesium; food, milk, or other dairy products: decrease antibiotic absorption. Give antibiotic 1 hour before or 2 hours after any of the above. *Ferrous sulfate and other iron products, zinc:* decrease antibiotic absorption. Give demeclocycline 3 hours after or 2 hours before iron administration. *Methoxyflurane:* may cause nephrotoxicity with tetracyclines. Monitor carefully.	• Use with extreme caution in impaired renal or hepatic function. Use of these drugs during last half of pregnancy and in children younger than 8 years may cause permanent discoloration of teeth, enamel defects, and retardation of bone growth. • Obtain cultures before starting therapy. • Check expiration date. Outdated or deteriorated demeclocycline may cause nephrotoxicity. • Do not expose these drugs to light or heat; store in tight container. • Watch for overgrowth of nonsusceptible organisms. Check patient's tongue for signs of monilia infection. Stress good oral hygiene. If superinfection occurs, drug should be discontinued. • Diarrhea may result, due to local irritation or superinfection. • May cause false-positive reading of Clinitest; false-negative reading of Clinistix or Tes-Tape. • Warn patient to avoid direct sunlight and ultraviolet light. A sunscreen may help prevent photosensitivity reactions. Photosensitivity persists for some time after discontinuation of drug. • Effectiveness is reduced when taken with milk or other dairy products, food, antacids, or iron products. Explain this to patient. Tell patient to take each dose with a full glass of water on an empty stomach, at least 1 hour before meals or 2 hours afterward. Give at least 1 hour before bedtime to prevent esophagitis. • Instruct patient to take medication for as long as prescribed, exactly as prescribed, even after he feels better. Treat streptococcal infections for at least 10 days.
Antacids (including $NaHCO_3$) and laxatives containing aluminum, magnesium, or calcium: decrease antibiotic absorption. Give antibiotic 1 hour before or 2 hours after any of the above. *Ferrous sulfate and other iron products, zinc:* decrease antibiotic absorption. Give doxycycline 3 hours after or 2 hours before iron administration. *Phenobarbital, carbamazepine, alcohol:* decrease antibiotic effect. Avoid if possible.	• Use of these drugs during last half of pregnancy and in children younger than 8 years may cause permanent discoloration of teeth, enamel defects, and retardation of bone growth. • Patient may develop thrombophlebitis with I.V. administration. • Obtain cultures before starting therapy. • Check expiration date. • Don't expose drug to light or heat. Protect from sunlight during infusion. • Watch for overgrowth of nonsusceptible organisms. Check patient's tongue for signs of monilia infection. Stress good oral hygiene. If superinfection occurs, drug should be discontinued. • Observe patient for diarrhea, which may result from local irritation or superinfection. • May be taken with milk or food if GI side effects develop. • Do not give with antacids. • Tell patient to take medication exactly as prescribed, even after he feels better. Treat streptococcal infections for at least 10 days. • Reconstitute powder for injection with sterile water for injection. Use 10 ml in 100-mg vial, 20 ml in 200-mg vial. Dilute solution to 100 to 1,000 ml before giving. Don't infuse solutions more concentrated than 1 mg/ml. See Chapter 6, UNDERSTANDING INTRAVENOUS SOLUTION COMPATIBILITY. • Reconstituted solution is stable for 72 hours refrigerated. • Doxycycline may be used in patients with renal impairment; does not accumulate or cause a significant rise in BUN. • May cause false-positive reading of Clinitest; false-negative reading of Clinistix or Tes-Tape. • Should not be taken within 1 hour of bedtime because of increased incidence of dysphagia.

NAME	INDICATIONS & DOSAGE	SIDE EFFECTS
methacycline hydrochloride Rondomycin	*Infections caused by sensitive gram-negative and gram-positive organisms, trachoma, amebiasis—* **Adults:** 150 mg P.O. q 6 hours or 300 mg q 12 hours. **Children over 8 years:** 6 to 12 mg/kg P.O. daily, divided q 6 hours to q 12 hours. *Gonorrhea in patients sensitive to penicillin—* **Adults:** 900 mg P.O. initially, then 300 mg P.O. q.i.d. for total of 5.4 g. *Syphilis in patients sensitive to penicillin—* **Adults:** total dose of 18 to 24 g in equally divided doses over 10 to 15 days.	**Blood:** neutropenia, eosinophilia. **CV:** pericarditis. **EENT:** dysphagia, glossitis. **GI:** anorexia, *epigastric distress, nausea,* vomiting, *diarrhea,* enterocolitis, anogenital inflammation. **Metabolic:** increased BUN. **Skin:** *maculopapular and erythematous rashes, photosensitivity, urticaria.* **Other:** hypersensitivity.
minocycline hydrochloride Minocin♦, Ultramycin♦♦, Vectrin	*Infections caused by sensitive gram-negative and gram-positive organisms, trachoma, amebiasis—* **Adults:** initially, 200 mg P.O., I.V.; then 100 mg q 12 hours or 50 mg P.O. q 6 hours. **Children over 8 years:** initially, 4 mg/kg P.O., I.V.; then 4 mg/kg P.O. daily, divided q 12 hours. Give I.V. in 500 to 1,000 ml solution without calcium over 6 hours. *Gonorrhea in patients sensitive to penicillin—* **Adults:** initially, 200 mg, then 100 mg q 12 hours for 4 days. *Syphilis in patients sensitive to penicillin—* **Adults:** initially, 200 mg, then 100 mg q 12 hours for 10 to 15 days. *Meningococcal carrier state—* 100 mg P.O. q 12 hours for 5 days.	**Blood:** neutropenia, eosinophilia. **CNS:** *light-headedness, dizziness from vestibular toxicity.* **CV:** pericarditis. **EENT:** dysphagia, glossitis. **GI:** *anorexia,* epigastric distress, *nausea,* vomiting, *diarrhea,* enterocolitis, inflammatory lesions in anogenital region. **Metabolic:** increased BUN. **Skin:** *maculopapular and erythematous rashes, photosensitivity, increased pigmentation, urticaria.* **Local:** *thrombophlebitis.* **Other:** hypersensitivity.
oxytetracycline hydrochloride Dalimycin, Oxlopar, Oxy-Kesso-Tetra, Oxytetrachlor, Terramycin♦, Uri-tet	*Infections caused by sensitive gram-negative and gram-positive organisms, trachoma, amebiasis—* **Adults:** 250 mg P.O. q 6 hours; 100 mg I.M. q 8 to 12 hours; 250 mg I.M. q 12 hours; or	**Blood:** neutropenia, eosinophilia. **CNS:** benign intracranial hypertension. **CV:** pericarditis. **EENT:** dysphagia, glossitis. **GI:** *anorexia, nausea,* vomiting, *diarrhea,* enterocolitis, anogenital

♦ Available in U.S. and Canada. ♦♦ Available in Canada only. All other products (no symbol) available in U.S. only. Italicized side effects are common or life-threatening.

INTERACTIONS	NURSING CONSIDERATIONS
Antacids (including $NaHCO_3$) and laxatives containing aluminum, magnesium, or calcium; food, milk, or other dairy products: decrease antibiotic absorption. Give antibiotic 1 hour before or 2 hours after any of the above. *Ferrous sulfate and other iron products, zinc:* decrease antibiotic absorption. Give tetracyclines 3 hours after or 2 hours before iron administration.	• Use with extreme caution in patients with impaired renal or hepatic function. Use during last half of pregnancy and in children younger than 8 years may cause permanent discoloration of teeth, enamel defects, and retardation of bone growth. • Obtain cultures before starting therapy. • Check expiration date. Outdated or deteriorated methacycline may cause nephrotoxicity. • Do not expose these drugs to light or heat. • Watch for overgrowth of nonsusceptible organisms. Check patient's tongue for signs of monilia infection. Stress good oral hygiene. If superinfection occurs, drug should be discontinued. • Observe patient for diarrhea, which may result from local irritation or superinfection. • Warn patient to avoid direct sunlight and ultraviolet light. A sunscreen may help prevent photosensitivity reactions. Photosensitivity persists for considerable time after discontinuation of drug. • Effectiveness is reduced when taken with milk or other dairy products, food, antacids, or iron products. Explain this to patient. Tell patient to take each dose with a full glass of water on an empty stomach, at least 1 hour before meals or 2 hours afterward. Give at least 1 hour before bedtime to prevent esophagitis. • Instruct patient to take medication exactly as prescribed, even after he feels better. Treat streptococcal infections for at least 10 days. • May cause false-positive reading of Clinitest; false-negative reading of Clinistix or Tes-Tape.
Antacids (including $NaHCO_3$) or laxatives containing aluminum, magnesium, or calcium: decrease antibiotic absorption. Give antibiotic 1 hour before or 2 hours after any of the above. *Ferrous sulfate or other iron products, zinc:* decrease antibiotic absorption. Tetracyclines should be given 3 hours after or 2 hours before iron administration. *Methoxyflurane:* may cause severe nephrotoxicity with tetracyclines. Monitor carefully.	• Use with extreme caution in patients with impaired renal or hepatic function. Use during last half of pregnancy and in children younger than 8 years may cause permanent discoloration of teeth, enamel defects, and retardation of bone growth. • Patient may develop thrombophlebitis with I.V. administration of this drug. Avoid extravasation. • Obtain cultures before starting therapy. • Check expiration date. • Do not expose these drugs to light or heat. Keep cap tightly closed. • Watch for overgrowth of nonsusceptible organisms. Check patient's tongue for signs of monilia infection. Stress good oral hygiene. If superinfection occurs, drug should be discontinued. • Observe patient for diarrhea, which may result from local irritation or superinfection. • May be taken with food. Tell patient to take medication exactly as prescribed, even after he feels better. Treat streptococcal infections for at least 10 days, syphilis for 10 to 15 days, gonorrhea for at least 4 days, and meningococcal carriers for 5 days. • Reconstitute 100 mg powder with 5 ml sterile water for injection, with further dilution of 100 to 1,000 ml for I.V. infusion. Stable for 24 hours at room temperature. See Chapter 6, UNDERSTANDING INTRAVENOUS SOLUTION COMPATIBILITY. • May cause false-positive reading of Clinitest; false-negative reading of Clinistix or Tes-Tape. • Vestibular toxicity resulting in dizziness may commonly occur.
Antacids (including $NaHCO_3$) and laxatives containing aluminum, magnesium, or calcium; food, milk, or other dairy products: decrease	• Use with extreme caution in patients with impaired renal or hepatic function. Use during last half of pregnancy and in children younger than 8 years may cause permanent discoloration of teeth, enamel defects, and retardation of bone growth. • Patient may develop thrombophlebitis with I.V. administration. Avoid extravasation. • Obtain cultures before starting therapy.

(continued on following page)

NAME	INDICATIONS & DOSAGE	SIDE EFFECTS
oxytetracycline hydrochloride *(continued)*	250 to 500 mg I.V. q 6 to 12 hours. **Children over 8 years:** 25 to 50 mg/kg P.O. daily, divided q 6 hours; 15 to 25 mg/kg I.M. daily, divided q 8 to 12 hours; or 10 to 20 mg/kg I.V. daily, divided q 12 hours. *Brucellosis*— **Adults:** 500 mg P.O. q.i.d. for 3 weeks with streptomycin 1 g I.M. q 12 hours first week, once daily second week. *Syphilis in patients sensitive to penicillin*— **Adults:** 30 to 40 g total dose P.O., divided equally over 10 to 15 days. *Gonorrhea in patients sensitive to penicillin*— **Adults:** initially, 1.5 g P.O., followed by 0.5 g q.i.d. for a total of 9 g.	inflammation. **Metabolic:** *increased BUN.* **Skin:** *maculopapular and erythematous rashes, urticaria, photosensitivity, increased pigmentation.* **Local:** *irritation after I.M. injection, thrombophlebitis.* **Other:** hypersensitivity.
tetracycline hydrochloride Achromycin♦, Amer-Tet, Bicycline, Cefracycline♦♦, Centet-250, Cycline, Cyclopar, Maso-Cycline, Medicycline♦♦, Neo-Tetrine♦♦, Nor-Tet 500, Novotetra♦♦, Paltet 250, Panmycin, Partrex, Piracaps, Retet, Robitet, Sarocycline, Scotrex, SK-Tetracycline, Sumycin♦, T-125, T-250, Tet-Cy, Tetra-C, Tetrachel, Tetraclor, Tetra-Co, Tetracrine♦♦, Tetracyn♦, Tetralan, Tetralean♦♦, Tetram, Tetram S, Tetramax, Trexin, Triacycline♦♦ **tetracycline phosphate complex** Tetrex♦	*Infections caused by sensitive gram-negative and gram-positive organisms, trachoma, amebiasis,* Mycoplasma, Rickettsia, *and* Chlamydia— **Adults:** 250 to 500 mg P.O. q 6 hours; 250 mg I.M. daily or 150 mg I.M. q 12 hours; or 250 to 500 mg I.V. q 8 to 12 hours (I.M. and I.V. hydrochloride salt only). **Children over 8 years:** 25 to 50 mg/kg P.O. daily, divided q 6 hours; 15 to 25 mg/kg/day (maximum 250 mg) I.M. single dose or divided q 8 to 12 hours; or 10 to 20 mg/kg I.V. daily, divided q 12 hours. *Brucellosis*— **Adults:** 500 mg P.O. q 6 hours for 3 weeks with streptomycin 1 g I.M. q 12 hours week 1 and daily week 2. *Gonorrhea in patients sensitive to penicillin*— **Adults:** initially, 1.5 g P.O., then 500 mg q 6 hours for total of 9 g. *Syphilis in patients sensitive to*	**Blood:** neutropenia, eosinophilia. **CNS:** dizziness, headache. **CV:** pericarditis. **EENT:** sore throat, glossitis, dysphagia. **GI:** anorexia, *epigastric distress, nausea,* vomiting, *diarrhea,* stomatitis, enterocolitis, inflammatory lesions in anogenital region. **Hepatic:** hepatotoxicity with doses given I.V. **Metabolic:** *increased BUN.* **Skin:** *maculopapular and erythematous rashes, urticaria, photosensitivity, increased pigmentation.* **Local:** *irritation after I.M. injection, thrombophlebitis.*

INTERACTIONS	NURSING CONSIDERATIONS
antibiotic absorption. Give antibiotic 1 hour before or 2 hours after any of the above. *Ferrous sulfate and other iron products, zinc:* decrease antibiotic absorption. Give tetracyclines 3 hours after or 2 hours before iron administration. *Methoxyflurane:* may cause severe nephrotoxicity with tetracyclines. Monitor carefully.	• Check expiration date. Outdated or deteriorated oxytetracycline may cause nephrotoxicity. • Do not expose these drugs to light or heat. • Inject I.M. dose deeply. Warn that it may be painful. Rotate sites. I.M. preparations contain a local anesthetic; ask patient about hypersensitivity to local anesthetics. • Watch for overgrowth of nonsusceptible organisms. Check patient's tongue for signs of monilia infection. Stress good oral hygiene. If superinfection occurs, drug should be discontinued. • Observe patient for diarrhea, which may result from local irritation or superinfection. • Warn patient to avoid direct sunlight and ultraviolet light. A sunscreen may help prevent photosensitivity reactions. Photosensitivity persists for considerable time after discontinuation of drug. • Effectiveness is reduced when taken with milk or other dairy products, food, antacids, or iron products. Explain this to patient. Tell patient to take each dose with a full glass of water on an empty stomach, at least 1 hour before meals or 2 hours afterward. Give at least 1 hour before bedtime to prevent esophagitis. • Tell patient to take medication exactly as prescribed, even after he feels better. • For I.V. use, reconstitute 250 mg and 500 mg powder for injection with 10 ml sterile water. Dilute to at least 100 ml in 5% dextrose in water, normal saline solution, or Ringer's solution. Do not mix with any other drug. See Chapter 6, UNDERSTANDING INTRAVENOUS SOLUTION COMPATIBILITY. • Store reconstituted solutions in refrigerator. Stable for 48 hours. • May cause false-positive reading of Clinitest; false-negative reading of Clinistix or Tes-Tape.
Antacids (including $NaHCO_3$) and laxatives containing aluminum, magnesium, or calcium; food, milk, or other dairy products: decrease antibiotic absorption. Give antibiotic 1 hour before or 2 hours after any of the above. *Ferrous sulfate and other iron products, zinc:* decrease antibiotic absorption. Give tetracyclines 3 hours after or 2 hours before iron administration. *Methoxyflurane:* may cause severe nephrotoxicity with tetracyclines. Monitor carefully.	• Use with extreme caution in patients with impaired renal or hepatic function. Use during last half of pregnancy and in children younger than 8 years may cause permanent discoloration of teeth, enamel defects, and retardation of bone growth. • Obtain cultures before starting therapy. • Effectiveness reduced when taken with milk or other dairy products, food, antacids, or iron products. Explain this to patient. Tell patient to take each dose with a full glass of water on an empty stomach, at least 1 hour before meals or 2 hours afterward. Give at least 1 hour before bedtime to prevent esophagitis. • Patient may develop thrombophlebitis with I.V. administration. Avoid extravasation. • Check expiration date. Outdated or deteriorated tetracycline may cause nephrotoxicity. • Discard I.M. solutions after 24 hours because they deteriorate. Exception: discard Achromycin solution in 12 hours. • Do not expose these drugs to light or heat. • Inject I.M. dose deeply. Warn patient that it may be painful. Rotate sites. I.M. preparations often contain a local anesthetic; ask patient about hypersensitivity to local anesthetics. • Watch for overgrowth of nonsusceptible organisms. Check patient's tongue for signs of monilia infection. Stress good oral hygiene. If superinfection occurs, drug should be discontinued. • Observe patient for diarrhea, which may result from local irritation or superinfection. • Warn patient to avoid direct sunlight and ultraviolet light. A sunscreen may help prevent photosensitivity reactions. Photosensitivity persists for some time after discontinuation of drug. • Tell patient to take medication exactly as prescribed, even after he

(continued on following page)

NAME	INDICATIONS & DOSAGE	SIDE EFFECTS
tetracycline *(continued)*	*penicillin—* **Adults:** 30 to 40 g total in equally divided doses over 10 to 15 days. *Acne—* **Adults and adolescents:** initially, 250 mg P.O. q 6 hours, then 125 to 500 mg P.O. daily or every other day. *Shigellosis—* **Adults:** 2.5 g P.O. in 1 dose.	

NURSING TIPS

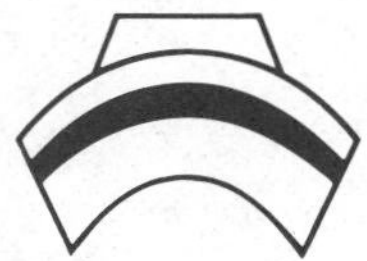

DON'T MIX CALCIUM AND TETRACYCLINES

If your patient complains of gastrointestinal disturbances during tetracycline therapy, don't take the seemingly logical step of administering these drugs with milk or antacids. And advise *him* not to take dairy products, antacids, or even sodium bicarbonate for his distress.

Why? Taking dairy products and antacids simultaneously with tetracyclines has been shown to significantly reduce blood levels of the drugs. The calcium, magnesium, and aluminum in milk products and antacids form insoluble tetracycline complexes that are not absorbed well by the body.

Sodium bicarbonate impairs tetracycline absorption as well, although the reasons have not been established. It may inhibit a tetracycline's solubility by increasing its pH.

Tetracyclines may differ, however, in their susceptibility to dairy-product and antacid interaction. And, according to some studies, certain tetracyclines (doxycycline and minocycline, for example) are less susceptible to such interaction.

What you should do

In general, follow these guidelines to help your patient:

- Administer all tetracyclines *without dairy products* and resort to *nondairy* snacks if you have to.
- If your patient is very uncomfortable, administer tetracyclines *with food.* But be sure that the food product contains *no* calcium or magnesium, such as crackers. Keep in mind, though, that absorption is decreased slightly when tetracycline is taken with food. You'll be trading off some of the drug's effectiveness for your patient's comfort.
- Consult the doctor about substituting another antibiotic. Although tetracycline may be the preferred treatment, another drug may be effective and might not cause gastrointestinal upset.

INTERACTIONS	NURSING CONSIDERATIONS
	feels better. Treat streptococcal infections for at least 10 days. • For I.V. use, reconstitute 100 mg and 250 mg powder for injection with 5 ml sterile water; with 10 ml for 500 mg. Dilute in 100 to 1,000 ml volume of 5% dextrose in 0.9% saline solution. Refrigerate diluted solution for I.V. use and use within 24 hours. Exception: use Achromycin solution immediately. • Do not mix tetracycline solution with any other I.V. additive. See Chapter 6, UNDERSTANDING INTRAVENOUS SOLUTION COMPATIBILITY. • For I.M. use, reconstitute 100 mg powder for injection with 2 ml sterile water for injection. Concentration will be 50 mg/ml. Amount of diluent for 250-mg injection varies according to brand. Check with pharmacy or follow manufacturer's instructions. • May cause false-positive reading of Clinitest; false-negative reading of Clinistix or Tes-Tape.

HOW TETRACYCLINES AFFECT LABORATORY TESTS

BLOOD TESTS

Test	Effect
Serum amylase level	▲
Indirect Coombs' test	+
Lupus erythematosus cell preparation	+
Hemoglobin value	▼
Platelet count	▼
Serum glucose level	ALT

URINE TESTS

Test	Effect
Serum creatinine level	▲
Urine protein level	▲
Urea nitrogen level	▲
Urine glucose level	ALT
Urine catecholamine level	▲

LIVER FUNCTION TESTS

Test	Effect
Blood ammonia level	▼
Bilirubin level	▲
Alkaline phosphatase level	▲
Serum glutamic-oxaloacetic transaminase (SGOT) or aspartate aminotransferase (AST) level	▲
Serum glutamic-pyruvic transaminase (SGPT) or alanine aminotransferase (ALT) level	▲
Lactic dehydrogenase (LDH) level	▲

KEY: ▲ = increased
\+ = false positive
▼ = decreased
ALT = altered laboratory findings

17 Sulfonamides

co-trimoxazole
sulfachlorpyridazine
sulfacytine
sulfadiazine
sulfamerazine
sulfameter
sulfamethizole
sulfamethoxazole
sulfamethoxypyridazine
sulfapyridine
sulfasalazine
sulfisoxazole

Sulfonamides were the first drugs to be used systemically for the treatment of bacterial infections in humans. First used clinically in the mid-1930s, they significantly reduced incidence of morbidity and mortality of the treatable infectious diseases.

Major uses

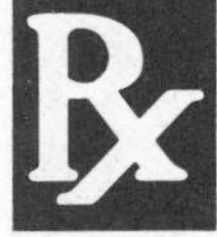

Although increased microbial resistance in recent years has limited their utility, sulfonamides are still the drugs of choice for urinary tract infections, otitis media, conjunctivitis, toxoplasmosis, and trachoma.

- Co-trimoxazole is a primary prophylactic and therapeutic drug for acute and chronic urinary tract infections. It is therapeutic for bacterial prostatitis, shigellosis, otitis media, and *Pneumocystis carinii* pneumonia. It may also combat infections caused by organisms resistant to the simple sulfonamides (*Escherichia coli,* for example, which is resistant to sulfisoxazole).
- Sulfachlorpyridazine, sulfacytine, sulfadiazine, sulfamerazine, sulfamethizole, sulfamethoxazole, and sulfisoxazole are useful in the treatment of cystitis and pyelonephritis caused by susceptible strains of *E. coli, Klebsiella, Staphylococcus aureus,* and *Proteus mirabilis.* They are also indicated in the treatment of chancroid, trachoma, and nocardiosis. They are effective against *Hemophilus influenzae* otitis media when combined with penicillin, and against toxoplasmosis when combined with pyrimethamine.
- Sulfadiazine may be prophylactic for rheumatic heart disease in patients allergic to penicillin.
- Sulfameter and sulfamethoxypyridazine are restricted to treatment of urinary tract and soft-tissue infections caused by susceptible organisms.
- Sulfapyridine is therapeutic for dermatitis herpetiformis.
- Sulfasalazine is useful in the treatment of mild to moderate cases of ulcerative colitis.

Mechanism of action

Sulfonamides have a broad spectrum of antibacterial action and are bacteriostatic. Chemically similar to para-aminobenzoic acid (PABA), these drugs competitively inhibit dihydropteroate synthetase, a bacterial enzyme responsible for incorporation of PABA into dihydrofolic acid (folic acid). This mechanism blocks folic acid synthesis. Hence, nucleic acids—essential building blocks of the bacterial cell—cannot be synthesized. Susceptible bacteria are those that must synthesize their own folic acid.

Absorption, distribution, metabolism, and excretion

These drugs are rapidly and adequately absorbed from the gastrointestinal tract, except for sulfasalazine, which is designed to produce a local effect in the bowel and is absorbed at a rate of only 10% to 15%.

All sulfonamides are readily distributed throughout the body, largely metabolized in the liver, and excreted in the urine (excretion rate increases with alkaline urine).

Onset and duration

Peak blood levels of the sulfonamides usually appear 2 to 8 hours after oral administration and within minutes after I.V. administration.

- Co-trimoxazole and sulfamethoxazole have half-lives of 12 hours and may be administered twice daily.
- Sulfachlorpyridazine, sulfacytine, sulfadiazine, sulfamerazine, sulfamethizole, sulfapyridine, and sulfisoxazole have half-lives of 4 to 6 hours and are usually administered four times daily.
- Sulfameter and sulfamethoxypyridazine have very long half-lives and may be administered once daily or once every other day.
- Sulfasalazine, usually administered several times daily, has a half-life of 4 to 10 hours.

DRUG ALERT

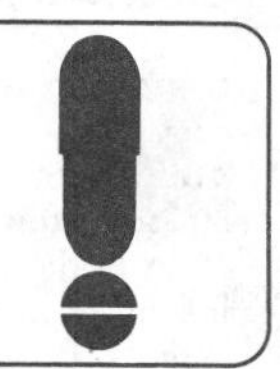

BE PREPARED FOR STEVENS-JOHNSON SYNDROME

One side effect of sulfonamides is Stevens-Johnson syndrome, the most common serious skin disorder in hospitalized patients. Onset may be sudden; symptoms include lesions on the skin and mucous membranes, severe pain in mucosal areas (accompanied by secondary photophobia), fever, malaise, and inability to eat and drink.

The characteristic bullous lesions of Stevens-Johnson syndrome produce a thick hemorrhagic crusting on the lips. The patient's eyelids and genitalia may also erode. His temperature may hover around 39° C. (102.2° F.), then begin to fall after 7 to 9 days, as the lesions dry and heal. However, the disease sometimes becomes life-threatening, and large areas of the skin may slough off. Stevens-Johnson syndrome has a mortality of 15% to 20%.

To care for the patient with Stevens-Johnson syndrome:

- Obtain daily skin and blood cultures.
- Watch for fluid and electrolyte imbalance. If this occurs, notify the doctor. He may order appropriate I.V. therapy.
- Give aspirin or acetaminophen, if ordered, to suppress fever.
- Sponge the denuded areas of the skin four times a day with a 1:1 mixture of povidone-iodine skin cleanser in water.
- If ordered, give prednisone P.O. or prednisolone I.M. to help decrease inflammation.

Combination products

AZO GANTANOL: sulfamethoxazole 500 mg and phenazopyridine hydrochloride 100 mg.

AZO GANTRISIN: sulfisoxazole 500 mg and phenazopyridine hydrochloride 50 mg.

AZOTREX: sulfamethizole 250 mg, tetracycline phosphate complex equivalent to 125 mg tetracycline HCl activity, and phenazopyridine hydrochloride 50 mg.

SULADYNE: sulfamethizole 125 mg, sulfadiazine 125 mg, and phenazopyridine hydrochloride 75 mg.

THIOSULFIL-A: sulfamethizole 250 mg and phenazopyridine hydrochloride 50 mg.

TRIPLE SULFA: sulfadiazine 167 mg, sulfamerazine 167 mg, and sulfamethazine 167 mg.

UROBIOTIC-250: sulfamethizole 250 mg, oxytetracycline 250 mg, and phenazopyridine hydrochloride 50 mg.

NAME	INDICATIONS & DOSAGE	SIDE EFFECTS
co-trimoxazole (sulfamethoxazole-trimethoprim) Bactrim♦, Bactrim DS♦, Septra♦, Septra DS♦	*Urinary tract infections and shigellosis*— **Adults:** 160 mg trimethoprim/ 800 mg sulfa q 12 hours for 10 to 14 days in urinary tract infections and for 5 days in shigellosis. **Children:** 8 mg/kg trimethoprim/40 mg/kg sulfa per 24 hours, in 2 divided doses q 12 hours (10 days for urinary tract infections; for 5 days in shigellosis). *Otitis media*— **Children:** 8 mg/kg trimethoprim/40 mg/kg sulfa per 24 hours, in 2 divided doses q 12 hours for 10 days. Pneumocystis carinii *pneumonitis*— **Adults:** 20 mg/kg trimethoprim/ 100 mg/kg sulfa per 24 hours, in equally divided doses q 6 hours for 14 days. **Children up to 36 kg:** 160 mg trimethoprim/800 mg sulfa q 6 hours for 14 days. *Chronic bronchitis*— **Adults:** 160 mg trimethoprim/ 800 mg sulfa q 12 hours for 10 to 14 days. Not recommended for infants less than 2 months old. Available as tablets or suspension only.	**Blood:** *agranulocytosis, aplastic anemia,* megaloblastic anemia, thrombocytopenia, leukopenia, hemolytic anemia. **CNS:** headache, mental depression, convulsions, hallucinations. **GI:** *nausea, vomiting, diarrhea,* abdominal pain, anorexia, stomatitis. **GU:** toxic nephrosis with oliguria and anuria, crystalluria, hematuria. **Hepatic:** jaundice. **Skin:** *erythema multiforme (Stevens-Johnson syndrome), generalized skin eruption, epidermal necrolysis, exfoliative dermatitis,* photosensitivity, urticaria, pruritus. **Other:** *hypersensitivity, serum sickness, drug fever, anaphylaxis.*
sulfachlorpyridazine Cosulid, Sonilyn, Vetisulid	*Urinary tract infections and some systemic infections*— **Adults:** 2 to 4 g P.O. initially, then 500 mg to 1 g P.O. q 6 hours. **Children over 2 months:** 75 mg/kg P.O. initially, then 150 mg/kg daily, divided into doses given q 6 hours. Maximum daily dose 6 g.	**Blood:** *agranulocytosis, aplastic anemia,* megaloblastic anemia, thrombocytopenia, leukopenia, hemolytic anemia. **CNS:** headache, mental depression, convulsions, hallucinations. **GI:** *nausea, vomiting, diarrhea,* abdominal pain, anorexia, stomatitis. **GU:** toxic nephrosis with oliguria and anuria, crystalluria, hematuria. **Hepatic:** jaundice. **Skin:** *erythema multiforme (Stevens-Johnson syndrome), generalized skin eruption, epidermal necrolysis, exfoliative dermatitis,* photosensitivity, urticaria, pruritus. **Other:** *hypersensitivity, serum sickness, drug fever, anaphylaxis.*

♦ Available in U.S. and Canada. ♦♦ Available in Canada only. All other products (no symbol) available in U.S. only. Italicized side effects are common or life-threatening.

INTERACTIONS	NURSING CONSIDERATIONS
Ammonium chloride, ascorbic acid, paraldehyde: doses sufficient to acidify urine may cause precipitation of sulfonamide and crystalluria. Don't use together. *PABA-containing local anesthetics and other PABA drugs:* inhibit antibacterial action. Don't use together.	• Contraindicated in patients with porphyria. Use cautiously and in reduced dosages in patients with impaired hepatic or renal function and in those with severe allergy or bronchial asthma, G-6-PD deficiency, blood dyscrasias. • Tell patient to drink a full glass of water with each dose and to drink plenty of water during the day to prevent crystalluria. Monitor fluid intake and urinary output. • This combination is often used in extremely ill immunosuppressed patients when prescribed for treatment of *Pneumocystis* pneumonia. • I.V. form now available. • Oral suspension available for patients who cannot swallow large tablets. • Note that the "DS" product means "double strength." • Promptly report skin rash, sore throat, fever, or mouth sores—early signs of blood dyscrasias. • Tell patient to take 1 hour before or 2 hours after meals for best absorption. • Used effectively for treatment of chronic bacterial prostatitis. • Used prophylactically for recurrent urinary-tract infections in women. • Most side effects develop within 2 weeks of onset of therapy. • For treatment of anaphylaxis, see inside front cover.
Ammonium chloride, ascorbic acid, paraldehyde: doses sufficient to acidify urine may cause precipitation of sulfonamide and crystalluria. Don't use together. *PABA-containing local anesthetics and other PABA drugs:* inhibit antibacterial action. Don't use together.	• Contraindicated in porphyria. Use cautiously and in reduced dosages in patients with impaired hepatic or renal function, asthma or blood dyscrasias, G-6-PD deficiency, history of multiple allergies. • Tell patient to drink a full glass of water with each dose and to drink plenty of water throughout the day to prevent crystalluria. Monitor fluid intake and urinary output. Intake should be sufficient to produce output of 1,500 ml daily (between 3,000 and 4,000 ml daily for adults). • To aid in prevention of crystalluria, sodium bicarbonate may be administered to alkalinize urine. Monitor urine pH daily. • Tell patient to take medication for as long as prescribed, even after he feels better. • Monitor urine cultures, CBCs, and urinalyses before and during therapy. • Tell patient to report early signs of blood dyscrasias (sore throat, fever, pallor) immediately and to stop taking drug. Warn patient to avoid direct sunlight and ultraviolet light to prevent photosensitivity reaction. • For treatment of anaphylaxis, see inside front cover.

NAME	INDICATIONS & DOSAGE	SIDE EFFECTS
sulfacytine Renoquid	*Urinary tract infections—* **Adults:** initially, 500 mg P.O., then 250 mg P.O. q.i.d. for 10 days.	**Blood:** *agranulocytosis, aplastic anemia,* megaloblastic anemia, thrombocytopenia, leukopenia, hemolytic anemia. **CNS:** headache, mental depression, convulsions, hallucinations. **GI:** *nausea, vomiting, diarrhea,* abdominal pain, anorexia, stomatitis. **GU:** toxic nephrosis with oliguria and anuria, crystalluria, hematuria. **Hepatic:** jaundice. **Skin:** *erythema multiforme (Stevens-Johnson syndrome), generalized skin eruption, epidermal necrolysis, exfoliative dermatitis,* photosensitivity, urticaria, pruritus. **Other:** *hypersensitivity, serum sickness, drug fever, anaphylaxis.*
sulfadiazine Microsulfon, Neo-Quinette	*Urinary tract infections—* **Adults:** initially, 2 to 4 g P.O., then 500 mg to 1 g P.O. q 6 hours. **Children:** initially, 75 mg/kg or 2 g/m² P.O., then 150 mg/kg or 4 g/m² P.O. in 4 to 6 divided doses daily. Maximum daily dose 6 g. *Rheumatic fever prophylaxis, as an alternative to penicillin—* **Children over 30 kg:** 1 g P.O. daily. **Children under 30 kg:** 500 mg P.O. daily. *Adjunctive treatment in toxoplasmosis—* **Adults:** 4 g P.O. in divided doses q 6 hours for 3 to 4 weeks, discontinued for 1 week, then repeated; given with pyrimethamine 75 mg P.O. daily for 1 to 3 days, then 25 mg P.O. daily for 3 to 4 weeks, discontinued for 1 week, then repeated using 25 mg P.O. daily. **Children:** 100 mg/kg P.O. in divided doses q 6 hours for 3 to 4 weeks, discontinued for 1 week, then repeated; given with pyrimethamine, 1 mg/kg P.O. daily for 1 to 3 days, then 0.5 mg/kg P.O. daily for 3 to 4 weeks, discontinued for 1 week, then repeated using 0.5 mg/kg P.O. daily.	**Blood:** *agranulocytosis, aplastic anemia,* megaloblastic anemia, thrombocytopenia, leukopenia, hemolytic anemia. **CNS:** headache, mental depression, convulsions, hallucinations. **GI:** *nausea, vomiting, diarrhea,* abdominal pain, anorexia, stomatitis. **GU:** toxic nephrosis with oliguria and anuria, crystalluria, hematuria. **Hepatic:** jaundice. **Skin:** *erythema multiforme (Stevens-Johnson syndrome), generalized skin eruption, epidermal necrolysis, exfoliative dermatitis,* photosensitivity, urticaria, pruritus. **Local:** irritation, extravasation. **Other:** *hypersensitivity, serum sickness, drug fever, anaphylaxis.*

INTERACTIONS	NURSING CONSIDERATIONS
Ammonium chloride, ascorbic acid, paraldehyde: doses sufficient to acidify urine may cause precipitation of sulfonamide and crystalluria. Don't use together. *PABA-containing local anesthetics and other PABA drugs:* inhibit antibacterial action. Don't use together.	• Contraindicated in porphyria. Use cautiously and in reduced dosages in patients with impaired hepatic or renal function, bronchial asthma, history of multiple allergies, G-6-PD deficiency, blood dyscrasias. • Tell patient to drink a full glass of water with each dose and to drink plenty of water throughout the day to prevent crystalluria. Monitor fluid intake and urinary output. Intake should be sufficient to produce output of 1,500 ml daily (between 3,000 and 4,000 ml daily for adults). • To aid in prevention of crystalluria, sodium bicarbonate may be administered to alkalinize urine. Monitor urine pH daily. • Tell patient to take medication for as long as prescribed, even after he feels better. Warn patient to avoid direct sunlight and ultraviolet light to prevent photosensitivity reaction. • Monitor urine cultures, CBCs, and urinalyses before and during therapy. • Tell patient to report early signs of blood dyscrasias (sore throat, fever, pallor) immediately and to stop taking drug. • For treatment of anaphylaxis, see inside front cover.
Ammonium chloride, ascorbic acid, paraldehyde: doses sufficient to acidify urine may cause precipitation of sulfonamide and crystalluria. Don't use together. *PABA-containing local anesthetics and other PABA drugs:* inhibit antibacterial action. Don't use together.	• Contraindicated in patients with porphyria or in infants younger than 2 months (except in congenital toxoplasmosis). Use cautiously and in reduced dosages in patients with impaired hepatic or renal function, bronchial asthma, history of multiple allergies, G-6-PD deficiency, blood dyscrasias. • Tell patient to drink a full glass of water with each dose and to drink plenty of water throughout the day to prevent crystalluria. Monitor fluid intake and urinary output. Intake should be sufficient to produce output of 1,500 ml daily (between 3,000 and 4,000 ml daily for adults). To aid in prevention of crystalluria, sodium bicarbonate may be administered to alkalinize urine. Monitor urine pH daily. • Tell patient to take medication for as long as prescribed, even if he feels better. Warn patient to avoid direct sunlight and ultraviolet light to prevent photosensitivity reaction. • Give drug on schedule to maintain constant blood level. • Watch for signs of blood dyscrasias (purpura, ecchymosis, sore throat, fever, pallor). Report them immediately. • When giving I.V., make sure drug is well diluted. Infuse I.V. dosages slowly. If extravasation occurs, stop infusion and notify the doctor. Restart an I.V. at another site. • Monitor urine cultures, CBCs, and urinalyses before and during therapy. • Mix with 5% dextrose in normal saline or Ringer's solution for I.V. infusion; acidic solution (especially with pH below 9.0) causes precipitation. Use diluent cautiously. Discard solution if precipitation occurs. See Chapter 6, UNDERSTANDING INTRAVENOUS SOLUTION COMPATIBILITY. • Sulfadiazine with pyrimethamine for treatment of toxoplasmosis may be continued for life. Therapy controls but does not cure toxoplasmosis. • Folic or folinic acid may be used during rest periods in toxoplasmosis therapy to reverse hematopoietic depression and/or anemia associated with pyrimethamine and sulfadiazine. • Protect drug from light. • For treatment of anaphylaxis, see inside front cover.

NAME	INDICATIONS & DOSAGE	SIDE EFFECTS
sulfamerazine	*Antibacterial (rarely used alone)*— **Adults:** initially, 2 to 4 g P.O., then 500 mg to 1 g P.O. q 6 hours. **Children over 2 months:** initially, 75 mg/kg or 2 g/m², then 150 mg/kg or 4 g/m² P.O. daily in 4 to 6 equally divided doses. Maximum daily dose 6 g.	**Blood:** *agranulocytosis, aplastic anemia,* megaloblastic anemia, thrombocytopenia, leukopenia, hemolytic anemia. **CNS:** headache, mental depression, convulsions, hallucinations. **GI:** *nausea, vomiting, diarrhea,* abdominal pain, anorexia, stomatitis. **GU:** toxic nephrosis with oliguria and anuria, crystalluria, hematuria. **Hepatic:** jaundice. **Skin:** *erythema multiforme (Stevens-Johnson syndrome), generalized skin eruption, epidermal necrolysis, exfoliative dermatitis,* photosensitivity, urticaria, pruritus. **Other:** *hypersensitivity, serum sickness, drug fever, anaphylaxis.*
sulfameter Sulla♦	*Urinary tract infections only*— **Adults, and children over 12 years:** initially, 1.5 g P.O., then 500 mg daily.	**Blood:** *agranulocytosis, aplastic anemia,* megaloblastic anemia, thrombocytopenia, leukopenia, hemolytic anemia. **CNS:** headache, mental depression, convulsions, hallucinations. **GI:** *nausea, vomiting, diarrhea,* abdominal pain, anorexia, stomatitis. **GU:** toxic nephrosis with oliguria and anuria, crystalluria, hematuria. **Hepatic:** jaundice. **Skin:** *erythema multiforme (Stevens-Johnson syndrome), generalized skin eruption, epidermal necrolysis, exfoliative dermatitis,* photosensitivity, urticaria, pruritus. **Other:** *hypersensitivity, serum sickness, drug fever, anaphylaxis.*
sulfamethizole Bursul, Microsul, Proklar-M, Sulfasol, Sulfstat, Sulfurine, Thiosulfil♦, Unisul, Uri-Pak, Urifon, Utrasul	*Urinary tract infections only*— **Adults:** 500 mg to 1 g P.O. t.i.d. to q.i.d. **Children over 2 months:** 30 to 45 mg/kg P.O. daily, divided into doses given q 6 hours.	**Blood:** *agranulocytosis, aplastic anemia,* megaloblastic anemia, thrombocytopenia, leukopenia, hemolytic anemia. **CNS:** headache, mental depression, convulsions, hallucinations. **GI:** *nausea, vomiting, diarrhea,* abdominal pain, anorexia, stomatitis. **GU:** toxic nephrosis with oliguria and anuria, crystalluria,

♦ Available in U.S. and Canada. ♦♦ Available in Canada only. All other products (no symbol) available in U.S. only. Italicized side effects are common or life-threatening.

INTERACTIONS	NURSING CONSIDERATIONS
Ammonium chloride, ascorbic acid, paraldehyde: doses sufficient to acidify urine may cause precipitation of sulfonamide and crystalluria. Don't use together. *PABA-containing local anesthetics and other PABA drugs:* inhibit antibacterial action. Don't use together.	• Contraindicated in infants younger than 2 months (except in congenital toxoplasmosis) and in patients with porphyria. Use cautiously in impaired hepatic or renal function, asthma, blood dyscrasias, G-6-PD deficiency, history of multiple allergies. • Although drug has low incidence of crystalluria, tell patient to drink a full glass of water with each dose and to drink plenty of water throughout the day to prevent crystalluria. Monitor fluid intake and urinary output. Intake should be sufficient to produce output of 1,500 ml daily (between 3,000 to 4,000 ml daily for adults). To aid in prevention of crystalluria, sodium bicarbonate may be administered to alkalinize urine. Monitor urine pH daily. • Tell patient to take medication for as long as prescribed, even after he feels better. Warn patient to avoid direct sunlight and ultraviolet light to prevent photosensitivity reaction. Instruct patient to report early signs of blood dyscrasias (sore throat, fever, pallor) immediately and to stop taking drug. • Monitor urine cultures, CBCs, and urinalyses before and during therapy. • Used in sulfonamide combination preparations such as Triple Sulfa along with pyrimethamine to treat toxoplasmosis. • Watch for signs of GI superinfection during long-term therapy. • When given preoperatively, the patient should receive a low-residue diet and a minimal number of enemas and cathartics. • For treatment of anaphylaxis, see inside front cover.
Ammonium chloride, ascorbic acid, paraldehyde: doses sufficient to acidify urine may cause precipitation of sulfonamide and crystalluria. Don't use together. *PABA-containing local anesthetics and other PABA drugs:* inhibit antibacterial action. Don't use together.	• Contraindicated in patients weighing less than 45 kg (100 lb); porphyria. Use cautiously and in reduced dosages in patients with impaired hepatic or renal function; those receiving oral hypoglycemic agents (sulfonylureas); in early pregnancy, blood dyscrasias, G-6-PD deficiency, asthma; and in patients with history of multiple allergies. • Tell patient to drink a full glass of water with each dose and to drink plenty of water throughout the day to prevent crystalluria. Monitor fluid intake and urinary output. Intake should be sufficient to produce output of 1,500 ml daily (between 3,000 and 4,000 ml daily for adults). To aid in prevention of crystalluria, sodium bicarbonate may be administered to alkalinize urine. Monitor urine pH daily. • Tell patient to take medication for as long as prescribed, even after he feels better. Warn patient to avoid direct sunlight and ultraviolet light to prevent photosensitivity reaction. Instruct patient to report early signs of blood dyscrasias (sore throat, fever, pallor) immediately and to stop taking drug. • Monitor urine cultures, CBCs, and urinalyses before and during therapy. • Long-acting sulfonamide; never use in place of short-acting sulfonamides to treat systemic infections. • For treatment of anaphylaxis, see inside front cover.
Ammonium chloride, ascorbic acid, paraldehyde: doses sufficient to acidify urine may cause precipitation of sulfonamide and crystalluria. Don't use together. *PABA-containing local anesthetics and other PABA drugs:*	• Contraindicated in porphyria. Use cautiously and in reduced dosages in patients with impaired hepatic or renal function, blood dyscrasias, G-6-PD deficiency, asthma, history of multiple allergies. • Tell patient to drink a full glass of water with each dose and to drink plenty of water throughout the day to prevent crystalluria. Monitor fluid intake and urinary output. Intake should be sufficient to produce output of 1,500 ml daily (between 3,000 and 4,000 ml daily for adults). To aid in prevention of crystalluria, sodium bicarbonate may be administered to alkalinize urine. Monitor urine pH daily. • Tell patient to take medication for as long as prescribed, even after he feels better. Warn patient to avoid direct sunlight and ultraviolet

(continued on following page)

NAME	INDICATIONS & DOSAGE	SIDE EFFECTS
sulfamethizole *(continued)*		hematuria. **Hepatic:** jaundice. **Skin:** *erythema multiforme (Stevens-Johnson syndrome), generalized skin eruption, epidermal necrolysis, exfoliative dermatitis,* photosensitivity, urticaria, pruritus. **Other:** *hypersensitivity, serum sickness, drug fever, anaphylaxis.*
sulfamethoxazole Gantanol♦	*Urinary tract and systemic infections—* **Adults:** initially, 2 g P.O., then 1 g P.O. b.i.d. up to t.i.d. for severe infections. **Children and infants over 2 months:** initially, 50 to 60 mg/kg P.O., then 25 to 30 mg/kg b.i.d. Maximum dose should not exceed 75 mg/kg daily.	**Blood:** *agranulocytosis, aplastic anemia,* megaloblastic anemia, thrombocytopenia, leukopenia, hemolytic anemia. **CNS:** headache, mental depression, convulsions, hallucinations. **GI:** *nausea, vomiting, diarrhea,* abdominal pain, anorexia, stomatitis. **GU:** toxic nephrosis with oliguria and anuria, crystalluria, hematuria. **Hepatic:** jaundice. **Skin:** *erythema multiforme (Stevens-Johnson syndrome), generalized skin eruption, epidermal necrolysis, exfoliative dermatitis,* photosensitivity, urticaria, pruritus. **Other:** *hypersensitivity, serum sickness, drug fever, anaphylaxis.*
sulfamethoxypyridazine Midicel	*Urinary tract and systemic infections—* **Adults over 60 kg:** initially, 1 g P.O. followed by 500 mg daily or 1 g every other day. For severe infection, initially, 2 g P.O. followed by 500 mg daily. **Adults under 60 kg:** initially, 1 g P.O. followed by 250 mg P.O. daily. **Children over 2 months:** initially, 30 mg/kg P.O. followed by 15 mg/kg P.O. daily. Maximum initial dose 1 g and 500 mg thereafter.	**Blood:** *agranulocytosis, aplastic anemia,* megaloblastic anemia, thrombocytopenia, leukopenia, hemolytic anemia. **CNS:** headache, mental depression, convulsions, hallucinations. **GI:** *nausea, vomiting, diarrhea,* abdominal pain, anorexia, stomatitis. **GU:** toxic nephrosis with oliguria and anuria, crystalluria, hematuria. **Hepatic:** jaundice. **Skin:** *erythema multiforme (Stevens-Johnson syndrome), generalized skin eruption, epidermal necrolysis, exfoliative dermatitis,* photosensitivity, urticaria, pruritus. **Other:** *hypersensitivity, serum sickness, drug fever, anaphylaxis.*

INTERACTIONS	NURSING CONSIDERATIONS
inhibit antibacterial action. Don't use together.	light to prevent photosensitivity reaction. Instruct patient to report early signs of blood dyscrasias (sore throat, fever, pallor) immediately and to stop taking drug. • Monitor urine cultures, CBCs, and urinalyses before and during therapy. • For treatment of anaphylaxis, see inside front cover.
Ammonium chloride, ascorbic acid, paraldehyde: doses sufficient to acidify urine may cause precipitation of sulfonamide and crystalluria. Don't use together. *PABA-containing local anesthetics and other PABA drugs:* inhibit antibacterial action. Don't use together.	• Contraindicated in patients with porphyria or in infants younger than 2 months (except in congenital toxoplasmosis). Use cautiously and in reduced dosages in patients with impaired hepatic or renal function and in those with severe allergy or bronchial asthma, G-6-PD deficiency, blood dyscrasias. • Tell patient to drink a full glass of water with each dose and to drink plenty of water during the day to prevent crystalluria. Monitor fluid intake/urinary output. Intake should be sufficient to produce output of 1,500 ml daily (between 3,000 and 4,000 ml daily for adults). To aid in prevention of crystalluria, sodium bicarbonate may be administered to alkalinize urine. Monitor urine pH daily. • Tell patient to take medication for as long as prescribed, even after he feels better. Warn patient to avoid direct sunlight and ultraviolet light to prevent photosensitivity reaction. • Monitor urine cultures, CBCs, and urinalyses before and during therapy. • Sulfamethoxazole is also used in adjunctive therapy for treatment of toxoplasmosis following therapy with other first-line agents. • Instruct patient to report early signs of blood dyscrasias (sore throat, fever, pallor) immediately and to stop taking the drug. • For treatment of anaphylaxis, see inside front cover.
Ammonium chloride, ascorbic acid, paraldehyde: doses sufficient to acidify urine may cause precipitation of sulfonamide and crystalluria. Don't use together. *PABA-containing local anesthetics and other PABA drugs:* inhibit antibacterial action. Don't use together.	• Contraindicated in porphyria. Use cautiously and in reduced dosages in patients with impaired hepatic or renal function, asthma, blood dyscrasias, G-6-PD deficiency, history of multiple allergies. • Administer immediately after meals. • Watch for signs of Stevens-Johnson syndrome (high fever, rash, severe headache, stomatitis, conjunctivitis). Stop drug immediately if these occur. • Tell patient to drink a full glass of water with each dose and to drink plenty of water during the day to prevent crystalluria. Monitor fluid intake/urinary output. Intake should be sufficient to produce output of 1,500 ml daily (between 3,000 and 4,000 ml daily for adults). To aid in prevention of crystalluria, sodium bicarbonate may be administered to alkalinize urine. Monitor urine pH daily. • Tell patient to take medication for as long as prescribed, even after he feels better. Warn patient to avoid direct sunlight and ultraviolet light to prevent photosensitivity reaction. • Monitor urine cultures, CBCs, and urinalyses before and during therapy. • Sulfamethoxypyridazine is a long-acting sulfonamide and should not be used in place of short-acting sulfonamides to treat systemic infections. • For treatment of anaphylaxis, see inside front cover.

NAME	INDICATIONS & DOSAGE	SIDE EFFECTS
sulfapyridine Dagenan♦♦	*Dermatitis herpetiformis*— **Adults:** 500 mg P.O. q.i.d. until improvement noted, then decrease dose by 500 mg every 3 days until minimum effective maintenance dose achieved.	**Blood:** *agranulocytosis, aplastic anemia,* megaloblastic anemia, thrombocytopenia, leukopenia, hemolytic anemia. **CNS:** headache, mental depression, convulsions, hallucinations. **GI:** *nausea, vomiting, diarrhea,* abdominal pain, anorexia, stomatitis. **GU:** toxic nephrosis with oliguria and anuria, crystalluria, hematuria. **Hepatic:** jaundice. **Skin:** *erythema multiforme (Stevens-Johnson syndrome), generalized skin eruption, epidermal necrolysis, exfoliative dermatitis,* photosensitivity, urticaria, pruritus. **Other:** *hypersensitivity, serum sickness, drug fever, anaphylaxis.*
sulfasalazine Azulfidine, Azulfidine En-Tabs, SAS-500	*Mild to moderate ulcerative colitis, adjunctive therapy in severe ulcerative colitis*— **Adults:** initially, 3 to 4 g P.O. daily in evenly divided doses; usual maintenance dose is 1.5 to 2 g P.O. daily in divided doses q 6 hours. May need to start with 1 to 2 g initially, with a gradual increase in dose to minimize side effects. **Children over 2 years:** initially, 40 to 60 mg/kg P.O. daily, divided into 3 to 6 doses; then 30 mg/kg daily in 4 doses. May need to start at lower dose if gastrointestinal intolerance occurs.	**Blood:** *agranulocytosis, aplastic anemia,* megaloblastic anemia, thrombocytopenia, leukopenia, hemolytic anemia. **CNS:** headache, mental depression, convulsions, hallucinations. **GI:** *nausea, vomiting, diarrhea,* abdominal pain, anorexia, stomatitis. **GU:** toxic nephrosis with oliguria and anuria, crystalluria, hematuria. **Hepatic:** jaundice. **Skin:** *erythema multiforme (Stevens-Johnson syndrome), generalized skin eruption, epidermal necrolysis, exfoliative dermatitis,* photosensitivity, urticaria, pruritus. **Other:** *hypersensitivity, serum sickness, drug fever, anaphylaxis.*
sulfisoxazole Barazole, Gantrisin♦, G-Sox, J-Sul, Lipo Gantrisin, Novosoxazole♦♦, Rosoxol, SK-Soxazole, Sosol, Soxa, Soxomide, Sulfagan, Sulfalar, Sulfizin, Sulfizole♦♦, Urisoxin, Urizole, Velmatrol	*Urinary tract and systemic infections*— **Adults:** initially, 2 to 4 g P.O., then 1 to 2 g P.O. q.i.d.; extended-release suspension 4 to 5 g P.O. q 12 hours. **Children over 2 months:** initially, 75 mg/kg P.O. daily or 2 g/m² P.O. daily in divided doses q 6 hours, then 150 mg/kg or 4 g/m² P.O. daily in divided doses q 6 hours; extended-release suspension 60 to 70 mg/kg P.O. q 12 hours.	**Blood:** *agranulocytosis, aplastic anemia,* megaloblastic anemia, thrombocytopenia, leukopenia, hemolytic anemia. **CNS:** headache, mental depression, convulsions, hallucinations. **GI:** *nausea, vomiting, diarrhea,* abdominal pain, anorexia, stomatitis. **GU:** toxic nephrosis with oliguria and anuria, crystalluria, hematuria. **Hepatic:** jaundice. **Skin:** *erythema multiforme*

♦ Available in U.S. and Canada. ♦♦ Available in Canada only. All other products (no symbol) available in U.S. only. Italicized side effects are common or life-threatening.

INTERACTIONS	NURSING CONSIDERATIONS
Ammonium chloride, ascorbic acid, paraldehyde: doses sufficient to acidify urine may cause precipitation of sulfonamide and crystalluria. Don't use together. *PABA-containing local anesthetics and other PABA drugs:* inhibit antibacterial action. Don't use together.	• Contraindicated in porphyria. Use cautiously and in reduced dosages in patients with impaired hepatic or renal function, G-6-PD deficiency, history of multiple allergies, asthma, blood dyscrasias. • Tell patient to drink a full glass of water with each dose and to drink plenty of water during the day to prevent crystalluria. Monitor fluid intake/urinary output. Intake should be sufficient to produce output of 1,500 ml daily (between 3,000 and 4,000 ml daily for adults). • Alkalinization of the urine may decrease the danger of crystalluria but may greatly increase renal tubular reabsorption of the drug, sustained blood levels, and risk of toxicity. • Tell patient to take medication for as long as prescribed, even after he feels better. Warn patient to avoid direct sunlight and ultraviolet light to prevent photosensitivity reaction. • Monitor urine cultures, CBCs, and urinalyses before and during therapy. • Sulfapyridine is an intermediate-acting sulfonamide with a high potential for toxicity; its use is restricted to treatment of dermatitis herpetiformis when sulfone therapy is contraindicated. • Tell patient to report any side effects at once and to stop drug. • For treatment of anaphylaxis, see inside front cover.
Ammonium chloride, ascorbic acid, paraldehyde: doses sufficient to acidify urine may cause precipitation of sulfonamide and crystalluria. Don't use together. *PABA-containing local anesthetics and other PABA drugs:* inhibit antibacterial action. Don't use together.	• Contraindicated in porphyria. Use cautiously and in reduced dosages in patients with impaired hepatic or renal function and in those with severe allergy or bronchial asthma, G-6-PD deficiency. • Tell patient to drink a full glass of water with each dose and to drink plenty of water during the day to prevent crystalluria. Monitor fluid intake/urinary output. Intake should be sufficient to produce output of 1,500 ml daily (between 3,000 and 4,000 ml daily for adults). • Instruct patient to take medication for as long as prescribed, even after he feels better. Warn patient to avoid direct sunlight and ultraviolet light to prevent photosensitivity reaction. • Monitor CBCs and urinalyses before and during therapy. • Colors alkaline urine orange-yellow. • Side effects are usually those affecting GI tract. Minimize symptoms by spacing doses evenly and administering after food intake. • For treatment of anaphylaxis, see inside front cover.
PABA-containing local anesthetics and other PABA drugs: inhibit antibacterial action. Don't use together. *Ammonium chloride, ascorbic acid, paraldehyde:* doses sufficient to acidify urine may cause crystalluria and precipitation of sulfonamide. Don't use together.	• Contraindicated in patients with porphyria and in infants younger than 2 months (except in congenital toxoplasmosis). Use cautiously in patients with impaired hepatic or renal function, severe allergy or bronchial asthma, G-6-PD deficiency. • Tell patient to drink a full glass of water with each dose and to drink plenty of water throughout the day to prevent crystalluria. Monitor fluid intake and urinary output. Intake should be sufficient to produce output of 1,500 ml daily (between 3,000 and 4,000 ml daily for adults). To aid in prevention of crystalluria, sodium bicarbonate may be administered to alkalinize urine. Monitor urine pH daily. • Tell patient to take medication for as long as prescribed, even after he feels better. Warn patient to avoid direct sunlight and ultraviolet light to prevent photosensitivity reaction. • Monitor urine cultures and CBCs before and during therapy.

(continued on following page)

NAME	INDICATIONS & DOSAGE	SIDE EFFECTS
sulfisoxazole *(continued)*	**Adults, and children over 2 months:** parenteral dosages (sulfisoxazole diolamine) initially, 50 mg/kg or 1.125 g/m² by slow I.V. injection, then 100 mg/kg daily or 2.25 g/m² daily in divided doses q 6 hours by slow I.V. injection. 40% solution must be diluted to a concentration of 5% for I.V. use.	*(Stevens-Johnson syndrome), generalized skin eruption, epidermal necrolysis, exfoliative dermatitis,* photosensitivity, urticaria, pruritus. **Other:** *hypersensitivity, serum sickness, drug fever, anaphylaxis.*

INTERACTIONS	NURSING CONSIDERATIONS
	• Parenteral form can be given I.M. or subcutaneously but is discouraged. Administration of this form with parenteral fluids is not recommended. Diluents other than sterile distilled water may cause precipitation. See Chapter 6, UNDERSTANDING INTRAVENOUS SOLUTION COMPATIBILITY. • Gantrisin suspension and Lipo Gantrisin suspension cannot be interchanged, since the latter is an extended-release preparation. • Sulfisoxazole/pyrimethamine combination is used to treat toxoplasmosis. • Tell patient to report early signs of blood dyscrasias (sore throat, fever, pallor) immediately and to stop taking drug. • Watch for signs of GI superinfection during long-term therapy. • When given preoperatively, the patient should receive a low-residue diet and a minimal number of enemas and cathartics. • Although often given, initial loading dose is not pharmacologically necessary. • For treatment of anaphylaxis, see inside front cover.

CO-TRIMOXAZOLE: A SULFONAMIDE WITH "SOMETHING EXTRA"

Co-trimoxazole (Bactrim, Septra) is a fixed-combination drug that contains the sulfonamide sulfamethoxazole and another antibiotic, trimethoprim. Together, these drugs work *synergistically* to treat infections that would be resistant to either drug alone.

Co-trimoxazole thus provides a double-barreled effect on bacteria: it interferes with nucleic acid synthesis by *two* different mechanisms. First, sulfamethoxazole interferes with the conversion of para-aminobenzoic acid (PABA) to folic acid by competitively inhibiting the enzyme dihydropteroate synthetase. Because of this inhibition, only a small amount of folic acid forms. Then, trimethoprim comes into play; by inactivating the enzyme dihydrofolate reductase, it blocks the remaining folic acid's conversion to tetrahydrofolic acid.

As a result, no tetrahydrofolic acid is formed, so no nucleic acid can be synthesized. Without nucleic acid, the bacteria can't sustain themselves.

Note: Recently, both Bactrim and Septra have been marketed in double-strength (DS) tablets, so when you see Bactrim DS or Septra DS on a medication order sheet, be sure to administer the double-strength dose.

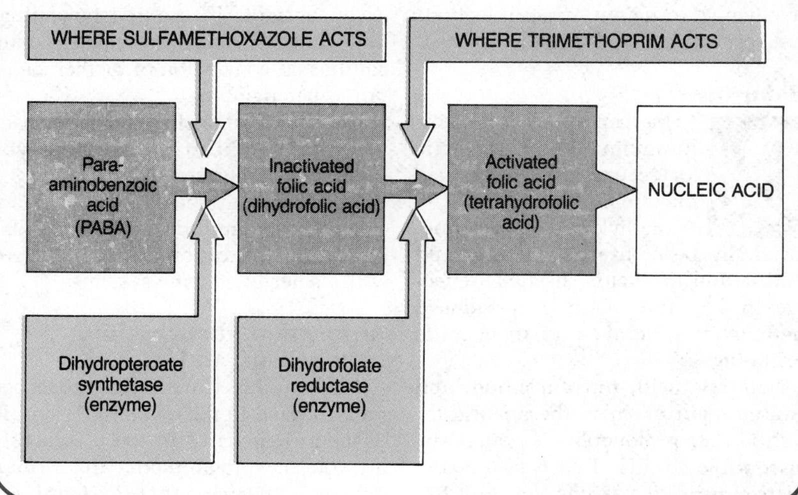

18 Urinary tract antiseptics

methenamine hippurate
methenamine mandelate
methenamine sulfosalicylate
methylene blue
nalidixic acid
nitrofurantoin
nitrofurantoin macrocrystals
oxolinic acid

For information on cinoxacin, see APPENDIX, *New Drugs*.

Urinary tract antiseptics concentrate in the renal parenchyma, including the uriniferous tubules and bladder. Because they don't achieve blood levels high enough to treat systemic infections, they act only locally for urinary tract infections. Although rarely used except with other agents, these drugs cause few adverse reactions. They can be effective in urinary tract infections that resist other modes of therapy.

Major uses

Rx

• Methenamine and nitrofurantoin are prophylactic for recurrent urinary tract infections.

• Methylene blue may occasionally be of use in treating mild cystitis and urethritis. It is also effective in idiopathic and drug-induced methemoglobinemia and in cyanide poisoning.

• Nalidixic acid, nitrofurantion, and oxolinic acid are also therapeutic for cystitis and pyelonephritis caused by susceptible strains of *Escherichia coli, Proteus mirabilis, Klebsiella,* and *Enterobacter*. Nalidixic and oxolinic acids also are effective against *Proteus vulgaris;* nitrofurantoin is effective against *Staphylococcus aureus* and enterococci.

Mechanism of action

• In acid urine, methenamines are hydrolyzed to ammonia and to formaldehyde, which is responsible for antibacterial action against gram-positive and gram-negative organisms. Mandelic and hippuric acids, with which methenamines are combined, are also antibacterial.

Methylene blue is a mildly antiseptic dye. High concentrations convert the ferrous iron of reduced hemoglobin to ferric iron to form methemoglobin. This mechanism is the basis for its use as an antidote in cyanide poisoning. Low concentrations of methylene blue can hasten conversion of methemoglobin to hemoglobin.

• Nalidixic and oxolinic acids are bacteriostatic, inhibiting DNA biosynthesis in microorganisms.

• Nitrofurantoin's bacteriostatic in low concentration and may be bactericidal in high concentration. It may interfere with bacterial enzyme systems.

Absorption, distribution, metabolism, and excretion

• Methenamines are rapidly absorbed and excreted in the urine (90% within 24 hours). Inactive in the blood, they are converted to ammonia and formaldehyde in the urine (at pH 5.5 or less).

• Methylene blue is poorly absorbed orally, but once in the tissues it is rapidly metabolized. It slowly passes into the bile and urine.
• Nalidixic and oxolinic acids are readily absorbed after oral administration, partially metabolized in the liver, and rapidly excreted by the kidneys.
• Nitrofurantoin is usually well absorbed from the gastrointestinal tract in either crystalline or macrocrystalline form. Various products may not be bioequivalent. Rapidly metabolized, the drug reaches therapeutic concentration only in the urine, where it is excreted.

Onset and duration

• With methenamine, methylene blue, and nitrofurantoin, antibacterial activity begins within 30 minutes; nalidixic and oxolinic acids begin to act within 4 hours.
• Antibacterial levels are sustained with twice-daily dosing of methenamine hippurate and oxolinic acid. The other urinary tract antiseptics require more frequent dosing.

Combination products

AZO GANTANOL: sulfamethoxazole 500 mg and phenazopyridine HCl 100 mg.
AZO GANTRISIN: sulfisoxazole 500 mg and phenazopyridine HCl 50 mg.
AZO-MANDELAMINE: methenamine mandelate 500 mg and phenazopyridine HCl 50 mg.
AZOTREX: tetracycline phosphate complex equivalent to 125 mg tetracycline HCl activity, sulfamethizole 250 mg, and phenazopyridine HCl 50 mg.
CYSTEX: methenamine 162 mg, salicylamide 65 mg, sodium salicylate 97 mg, and benzoic acid 32 mg.
CYSTISED IMPROVED: methenamine 40.8 mg, phenyl salicylate 18.1 mg, atropine sulfate 0.03 mg, hyoscyamine 0.03 mg, benzoic acid 4.5 mg, methylene blue 5.4 mg, and gelsemium 6.1 mg.
HEXALOL: methenamine 40.8 mg, phenyl salicylate 18.1 mg, atropine sulfate 0.03 mg, hyoscyamine 0.03 mg, benzoic acid 4.5 mg, and methylene blue 5.4 mg.
METHENAMINE AND SODIUM BIPHOSPHATE: methenamine 325 mg and sodium biphosphate 325 mg.
PROSED: methylene blue 5.4 mg, methenamine 40.8 mg, phenyl salicylate 18.1 mg, atropine sulfate 0.03 mg, hyoscyamine 0.03 mg, and benzoic acid 4.5 mg.
SULADYNE: sulfamethizole 125 mg, sulfadiazine 125 mg, and phenazopyridine HCl 75 mg.
THIOSULFIL-A: sulfamethizole 250 mg and phenazopyridine HCl 50 mg.
URO-PHOSPHATE: methenamine 300 mg and sodium acid phosphate 500 mg. Sugar coated.
UROQID-ACID: methenamine mandelate 350 mg and sodium acid phosphate 200 mg.

QUESTIONS & ANSWERS

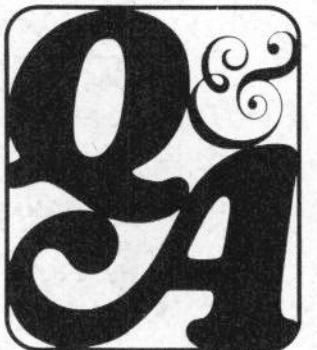

COPING WITH NITROFURANTOIN NAUSEA

What can you do to minimize gastrointestinal upset in a patient taking nitrofurantoin?

You have several alternatives:
• Report your patient's nausea and vomiting to the doctor. He may want to reduce the dose, especially in small persons. But keep in mind that the minimum effective dose of nitrofurantoin is 5 mg/kg/day.
• Suggest the macrocrystalline form of the drug (Macrodantin). You'll find it's better tolerated by your patient because it's absorbed more slowly than the crystalline form. Although effective urine concentrations may be delayed, this doesn't hinder macrocrystalline nitrofurantoin treatment. Your patient will experience fewer side effects with this form as well.
• Administer with milk or meals. This also slows drug absorption, reducing nausea.
• Notify the doctor, who may substitute another drug to treat the infecting organism.

NAME	INDICATIONS & DOSAGE	SIDE EFFECTS
methenamine hippurate Hiprex, Hip-Rex♦♦, Urex **methenamine mandelate** Mandacon, Mandelamine♦, Mandelets, Mandelurine♦♦, Methandine♦♦, Prov-U-Sep, Renelate, Sterine♦♦ **methenamine sulfosalicylate** Hexalet	*Long-term prophylaxis or suppression of chronic urinary tract infections—* **Adults, and children over 12 years:** 1 g P.O. q 12 hours. **Children 6 to 12 years:** 500 mg to 1 g P.O. q 12 hours. *Urinary tract infections, infected residual urine in patients with neurogenic bladder—* **Adults:** 1 g P.O. q.i.d. after meals. **Children 6 to 12 years:** 500 mg P.O. q.i.d. after meals. **Children under 6 years:** 50 mg/kg divided in 4 doses after meals. *Long-term prophylaxis or suppression of chronic urinary tract infections—* **Adults, and children over 12 years:** 1 g P.O. q.i.d. after meals with ½ glass of water. **Children 6 to 12 years:** 500 mg P.O. q.i.d. after meals with ½ glass water.	**GI:** *nausea.* **GU:** with high doses, urinary tract irritation, dysuria, frequency, albuminuria, hematuria. **Hepatic:** elevated liver enzymes. **Skin:** rashes.
methylene blue M-B Tabs, MG-Blue, Urolene Blue, Wright's Stain	*Cystitis, urethritis—* **Adults:** 65 mg P.O. b.i.d. or t.i.d. after meals with glass of water. *Methemoglobinemia and cyanide poisoning—* **Adults and children:** 1 to 2 mg/kg of 1% sterile solution slow I.V.	**Blood:** anemia (long-term use). **GI:** nausea, vomiting, diarrhea. **GU:** dysuria, bladder irritation. **Other:** fever (large doses).
nalidixic acid NegGram♦	*Acute and chronic urinary tract infections caused by susceptible gram-negative organisms* (Proteus, Klebsiella, Enterobacter, *and* Escherichia coli)— **Adults:** 1 g P.O. q.i.d. for 7 to 14 days; 2 g daily for long-term use. **Children over 3 months:** 55 mg/kg P.O. daily divided q.i.d. for 7 to 14 days; 33 mg/kg/day for long-term use.	**Blood:** eosinophilia. **CNS:** drowsiness, weakness, headache, dizziness, vertigo, convulsions in epileptics. **EENT:** sensitivity to light, change in color perception, diplopia, blurred vision. **GI:** *abdominal pain, nausea, vomiting,* diarrhea. **Skin:** pruritus, photosensitivity, urticaria, rash. **Other:** angioedema, fever, chills, increased intracranial pressure and bulging fontanelles in infants and children.
nitrofurantoin Cyantin, Furadantin, Furalan, Furatine♦♦,	*Pyelonephritis, pyelitis, and cystitis due to susceptible* Escherichia coli, Staphylococcus	**Blood:** hemolysis in patients with G-6-PD deficiency (reversed after stopping drug).

♦ Available in U.S. and Canada. ♦♦ Available in Canada only. All other products (no symbol) available in U.S. only. Italicized side effects are common or life-threatening.

INTERACTIONS	NURSING CONSIDERATIONS
Alkalinizing agents: inhibit methenamine action. Don't use together. *Acetazolamide:* antagonizes methenamine effect. Use together cautiously.	• Contraindicated in patients with renal insufficiency, severe hepatic disease, or severe dehydration. • Ineffective against *Candida* infection. • Oral suspension contains vegetable oil. Administer cautiously to elderly or debilitated patients because aspiration could cause lipid pneumonia. • Monitor intake and output. Intake should be at least 1,500 to 2,000 ml/day. • Obtain a clean-catch urine specimen for culture and sensitivity tests before starting therapy, and repeat p.r.n. • Limit intake of alkaline foods, such as vegetables, milk, peanuts, fruits, and fruit juices, except cranberry, plum, and prune juices. These juices or ascorbic acid may be used to acidify urine. • Warn patient not to take antacids, including Alka-Seltzer and sodium bicarbonate. • Maintain urine pH at 5.5 or less. Use Nitrazine paper to check pH. • *Proteus* and *Pseudomonas* tend to raise urine pH; urinary acidifiers are usually necessary when treating these infections. • Obtain liver function studies periodically during long-term therapy. • Administer after meals to minimize GI upset. • If rash appears, hold dose and contact doctor.
None significant.	• Contraindicated in patients with renal insufficiency. • Monitor intake and output carefully. Intake should be at least 2,000 ml/day. • Monitor hemoglobin; possibility of anemia from accelerated destruction of erythrocytes. • Turns urine and stool blue-green. • Seldom used as urinary tract antiseptic. • I.V. form has been used to treat nitrite intoxication.
Nitrofurantoin: may antagonize nalidixic acid effect. Use together cautiously.	• Contraindicated in patients with convulsive disorders. Use with caution in impaired liver or kidney function, or severe cerebral arteriosclerosis. • Not effective against *Pseudomonas*. • Tell the patient to report visual disturbances; these usually disappear with reduced dose. • Obtain clean-catch urine specimen for culture and sensitivity tests before starting therapy and repeat p.r.n. • Obtain CBC, kidney and liver function studies during long-term therapy. • Resistant bacteria may emerge within the first 48 hours of therapy. • May cause a false-positive Clinitest reaction. Use Clinistix or Tes-Tape to monitor urine glucose. Also gives false elevations in urine vanillylmandelic acid (VMA) and 17-ketosteroids. Repeat tests after therapy completed. • Avoid undue exposure to sunlight due to photosensitivity, which may continue for as long as 3 months after drug is stopped.
None significant.	• Contraindicated in patients with moderate to severe renal impairment, anuria, oliguria, creatinine clearance under 40 ml/minute; in patients with G-6-PD deficiency.

(continued on following page)

NAME	INDICATIONS & DOSAGE	SIDE EFFECTS
nitrofurantoin *(continued)* Furantoin, Ivadantin, J-Dantin, Nephronex♦♦, Nifuran♦♦, Nitrex, Novofuran♦♦, Parfuran, Sarodant **nitrofurantoin macrocrystals** Macrodantin♦	aureus, *enterococci; certain strains of* Klebsiella, Proteus, *and* Enterobacter— **Adults, and children over 12 years:** 50 to 100 mg P.O. q.i.d. with meals. Or, 180 mg I.M. or I.V. b.i.d. in patients over 55 kg; 5 to 7 mg/kg daily I.M. or I.V. in patients under 55 kg. **Children 1 month to 12 years:** 5 to 7 mg/kg P.O. daily, divided q.i.d.	**CNS:** peripheral neuropathy, headache, dizziness, drowsiness, ascending polyneuropathy with high doses or renal impairment. **GI:** anorexia, *nausea, vomiting,* abdominal pain, *diarrhea.* **Hepatic:** hepatitis. **Skin:** maculopapular, erythematous, or eczematous eruption; pruritus; urticaria. **Other:** asthmatic attacks in patients with history of asthma; *anaphylaxis;* drug fever; overgrowth of nonsusceptible organisms in the urinary tract; *pulmonary sensitivity reactions (cough, chest pains, fever, chills, dyspnea).*
oxolinic acid Utibid	*Cystitis, urethritis, pyelonephritis, pyelitis caused by susceptible gram-negative organisms* (Proteus, Klebsiella, Escherichia coli, *and* Enterobacter)— **Adults:** 1 tablet (750 mg) P.O. b.i.d. for 2 weeks.	**Blood:** transient leukopenia. **CNS:** *insomnia, dizziness, nervousness,* drowsiness, headache, impaired alertness, impaired physical coordination, weakness. **GI:** *nausea,* abdominal cramps, anorexia, vomiting, diarrhea, constipation.

♦ Available in U.S. and Canada. ♦♦ Available in Canada only. All other products (no symbol) available in U.S. only. Italicized side effects are common or life-threatening.

INTERACTIONS	NURSING CONSIDERATIONS
	• Obtain a clean-catch urine specimen for culture and sensitivity tests before starting therapy and repeat p.r.n. • Give with food or milk to minimize GI distress. • I.M. route painful and should not be used for more than 5 days. • Dilute I.V. nitrofurantoin to 500 ml of suitable I.V. solution before administering. Constitute in sterile water without preservatives. See Chapter 6, UNDERSTANDING INTRAVENOUS SOLUTION COMPATIBILITY. • Monitor intake/output carefully. May turn urine brown or darker. • Store in amber container. Keep away from metals other than stainless steel or aluminum to avoid precipitate formation. Warn patients not to use pillboxes made of these materials. • Continue treatment for 3 days after sterile urine specimens have been obtained. • Monitor pulmonary status. • May cause false-positive results with urine sugar test using copper sulfate reduction method (Clinitest) but not with glucose oxidase tests (Tes-Tape, Diastix, Clinistix). • For treatment of anaphylaxis, see inside front cover.
Nitrofurantoin: decreases response to oxolinic acid. Avoid if possible.	• Contraindicated in patients with convulsive disorders. Use cautiously in patients with impaired renal function; in older patients, as the drug may cause CNS stimulation. • Safety of taking concurrently with other CNS stimulants has not been established. • Before and during therapy, monitor for development of resistant organisms by obtaining urine specimens for culture and sensitivity. • Warn patient that drug may cause dizziness. • Monitor intake/output. • If treatment continues for more than 2 weeks, periodically obtain CBC, kidney and liver function studies.

DRUG ALERT

WATCH FOR PULMONARY REACTIONS IN PATIENTS TAKING NITROFURANTOIN

Nitrofurantoin can cause both acute and chronic pulmonary reactions in your patients.

If your patient complains of dyspnea, coughing, pleuritic pain, hemoptysis, fever, or chills while taking nitrofurantoin, make sure the medication is discontinued immediately. Onset of pulmonary complications is generally quick and severe in these cases, especially after a second exposure to the drug.

19 Miscellaneous anti-infectives

amantadine hydrochloride
bacitracin
chloramphenicol
chloramphenicol palmitate
chloramphenicol sodium succinate
clindamycin hydrochloride
clindamycin palmitate hydrochloride
clindamycin phosphate
colistimethate sodium
erythromycin base
erythromycin estolate
erythromycin ethylsuccinate
erythromycin gluceptate
erythromycin lactobionate
erythromycin stearate
furazolidone
lincomycin hydrochloride
novobiocin calcium
novobiocin sodium
polymyxin B sulfate
spectinomycin dihydrochloride
trimethoprim
troleandomycin phosphate
vancomycin hydrochloride
vidarabine monohydrate

By inhibiting or destroying bacteria or viruses, these miscellaneous anti-infectives provide broad protection against several infectious diseases.

Major uses

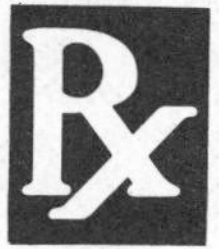

- Amantadine is prophylactic in epidemic influenza A viral infections.
- Bacitracin is occasionally used parenterally to treat infants with staphylococcal pneumonia when it's resistant to other drugs. As a bladder irrigating agent, bacitracin protects against gram-positive bacteria.
- Chloramphenicol has broad activity against rickettsia and many gram-positive and gram-negative bacteria. It's the drug of choice in both salmonella infections and infections caused by ampicillin-resistant strains of *Hemophilus influenzae.*
- Clindamycin and lincomycin are effective against respiratory tract, skin, and soft-tissue infections caused by susceptible strains of staphylococci, streptococci, and pneumococci.
- Parenteral colistimethate may be used to treat serious infections caused by susceptible strains of *Pseudomonas aeruginosa, Escherichia coli,* and *Klebsiella pneumoniae.* Oral preparations are occasionally used to treat infants with diarrhea due to enterotoxigenic strains of *E. coli.*
- Erythromycins are the drugs of choice in Legionnaires' disease, *Mycoplasma pneumoniae* pneumonia, *Campylobacter fetus* enteritis, and acute diphtheria and its carrier state. As alternatives to penicillin, they're therapeutic in streptococcal, pneumococcal, staphylococcal, gonococcal, and syphilitic diseases, and prophylactic in rheumatic fever. They may also be used for chronic bronchitis, otitis media, and nongonococcal urethritis.
- Furazolidone is now used rarely for intestinal infections caused by susceptible strains of *E. coli, Staphylococcus*

THE ROLE OF ORAL VANCOMYCIN IN PSEUDOMEMBRANOUS ENTEROCOLITIS

Pseudomembranous enterocolitis is a serious and possibly fatal disease. It occurs when long-term, high-dose antibiotic therapy (such as with clindamycin) kills most normal bowel flora, causing *Clostridium difficile* to overgrow and produce an endotoxin that damages the bowel wall. Once the bowel wall is damaged, a pseudomembrane composed of creamy white or yellow fibrous patches, fibrin debris, and white cells forms over the damaged area (see illustration).

Symptoms of pseudomembranous enterocolitis include severe diarrhea, fever, chills, abdominal distention with crampy pain, and loss of appetite. Patients with this disorder also have clostridial toxin in the stool and lesions in the bowel wall.

If these symptoms appear, your patient will probably be treated with oral vancomycin for 7 to 14 days. Given orally, vancomycin reaches high levels in the stool, decreasing toxin concentrations there and gradually alleviating diarrhea. Because vancomycin's not absorbed systemically, it probably won't cause unpleasant side effects.

After receiving oral vancomycin therapy, relapse is unlikely but if it occurs, is responsive to retreatment. Because pseudomembranous enterocolitis has responded to retreatment, researchers believe that relapse isn't due to the development of a resistant strain.

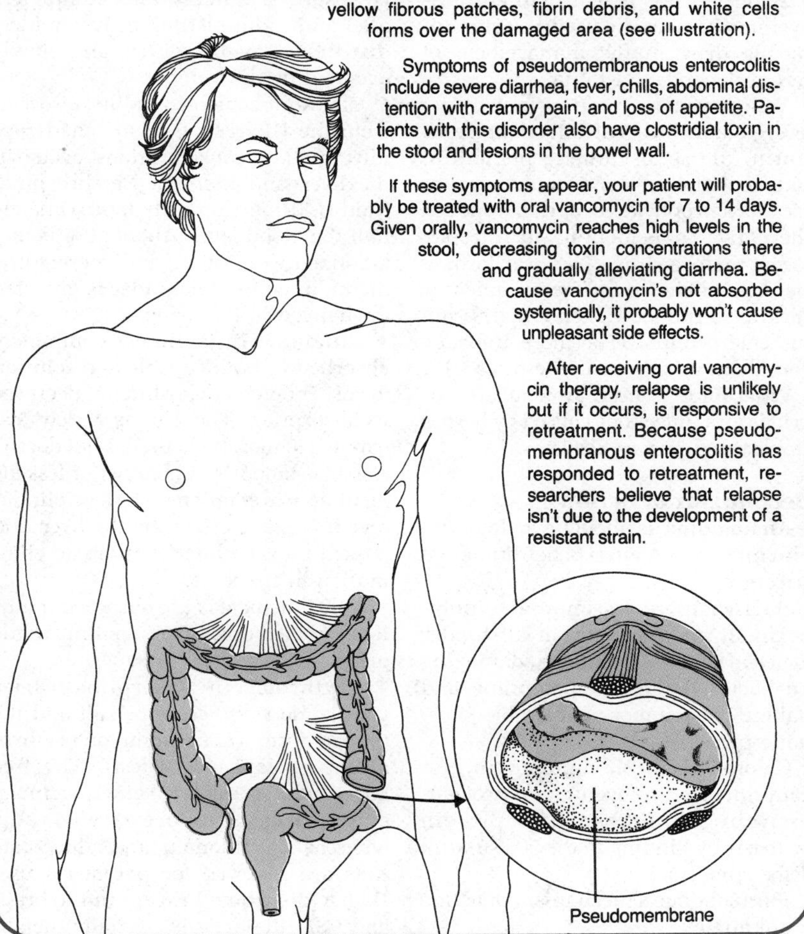

aureus, *Proteus*, and *Giardia lamblia*.

- Novobiocin is used rarely in the treatment of serious infections caused by strains of *S. aureus* and *Proteus* that resist other antibiotics.
- Polymyxin B is usually combined with bacitracin or neomycin in topical creams and ointments and in bladder-irrigating solutions to protect against *P. aeruginosa*, *E. coli*, *Enterobacter*, and *Klebsiella*. It is rarely used systemically for serious infections caused by *P. aeruginosa*.
- Spectinomycin is used in the treatment of penicillin-resistant strains of gonorrhea.
- Trimethoprim is most commonly combined with sulfamethoxazole. It is

also therapeutic when used alone for urinary tract infections caused by susceptible strains of *E. coli, Enterobacter,* and *K. pneumoniae.*

• Troleandomycin may be used to treat infections caused by *Streptococcus pyogenes* and *Streptococcus pneumoniae,* but it's less potent than erythromycin. It may also be used as a steroid-sparing drug in the management of steroid-dependent asthma.

• Vancomycin is used primarily for severe staphylococcal infections resistant to the semisynthetic penicillins and cephalosporins. It may also be used as a prophylactic and therapeutic alternative to penicillins for streptococcal endocarditis. The oral form is the drug of choice for the treatment of antibiotic-induced pseudomembranous enterocolitis. (For more information about this disease, see p. 243.)

• Vidarabine is used systemically for serious viral infections caused by herpes simplex and herpes zoster.

Mechanism of action

• Amantadine is thought to interfere with influenza A virus penetration into susceptible cells.

• Bacitracin, colistimethate, polymyxin B, and vancomycin all hinder bacterial cell-wall synthesis, damaging the bacterial plasma membrane and making the cell more vulnerable to osmotic pressure.

• Chloramphenicol, clindamycin, lincomycin, erythromycin, and troleandomycin inhibit bacterial protein synthesis by binding to the 50S subunit of the ribosome.

• Furazolidone's mechanism of action is unknown.

• Novobiocin interferes with bacterial cell-wall, protein, and nucleic acid synthesis.

• Trimethoprim interferes with the action of dihydrofolate reductase, inhibiting bacterial synthesis of folic acid.

• Vidarabine, as its phosphorylated metabolite, becomes incorporated into viral deoxyribonucleic acid and inhibits viral multiplication.

Absorption, distribution, metabolism, and excretion

• Amantadine is well absorbed from the gastrointestinal (GI) tract. More than 90% is excreted unchanged in the urine within 4 days.

• Bacitracin is not absorbed orally but is absorbed quickly and completely after I.M. administration. It is widely distributed to the tissues and slowly excreted by the kidneys.

• Chloramphenicol, readily absorbed from the GI tract, is distributed rapidly; highest concentrations occur in the liver and kidneys. Cerebrospinal fluid (CSF) levels reach approximately half the blood level. About 90% is metabolized in the liver and excreted by the kidneys; the remainder is excreted unchanged in the urine.

• Clindamycin is almost completely absorbed in both capsule and solution forms. Food can delay but not decrease its absorption. The drug is widely distributed to most body tissues but doesn't cross the blood-brain barrier unless the meninges are inflamed. Most clindamycin is metabolized by the liver and passed into the bile for ultimate elimination in the feces.

• Colistimethate is not absorbed orally. It is excreted unchanged, mainly in the urine.

• Erythromycin absorption varies greatly, depending on the salt and the dosage form (absorption of erythromycin estolate is greatest). The free base and the estolate, ethylsuccinate, and stearate salts are given orally, whereas lactobionate and gluceptate salts are reserved for parenteral use. Widely distributed except in the brain and CSF, the drug is partially metabolized in the liver and passed into the bile for elimination in the feces.

• Furazolidone, when given orally, is poorly absorbed and doesn't reach therapeutic blood levels. About 5% is excreted in the urine.

• Lincomycin absorption is impaired by food; patients in the fasting state, however, may absorb as much as 30%. Widely distributed except in CSF, it is partly metabolized by the liver and passed into the bile for elimination primarily in the feces.

- Novobiocin diffuses well into pleural, joint, and ascitic fluids but poorly or not at all into CSF, unless the meninges are inflamed; the drug is eliminated in bile, urine, and feces.
- Polymyxin B is not absorbed from the GI tract; blood levels are low, as the drug loses 50% of its activity in blood. It diffuses poorly into tissues and is excreted slowly by the kidneys.
- Spectinomycin is not absorbed from the GI tract but is well absorbed after I.M. administration. It is widely distributed and excreted unchanged by the kidneys.
- Trimethoprim is well absorbed after oral administration. It is widely distributed to most body tissues, except the central nervous system. About 50% is excreted unchanged by the kidneys; the rest is metabolized to inactive compounds and excreted in the urine.
- Troleandomycin is more readily absorbed orally than is erythromycin; 18% to 24% is excreted in the urine, 60% to 70% in the bile.
- Vancomycin is not absorbed orally. After I.V. administration, it is widely distributed, except in CSF, and excreted in urine virtually unchanged.
- Vidarabine is poorly absorbed from the GI tract. It is extensively metabolized to the active metabolite arabinosylhypoxanthine, which is widely distributed in all tissues, including the CSF. It is excreted by the kidneys over 24 hours.

DRUG ERROR

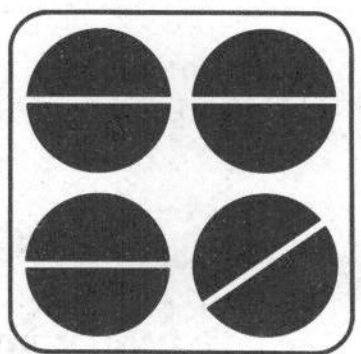

DOUBLE-CHECK NEW MEDICATION LABELS

To avoid dosing errors, always read medication labels carefully, *especially when new labels appear on familiar products.* Here's what happened to a nurse who misinterpreted a new label:

On a vial of chloramphenicol, the new label stated that 1 ml of the reconstituted drug contained 100 mg of chloramphenicol, but it didn't state the total amount of drug in the vial. (The old labels on chloramphenicol vials had clearly stated 1 g as the total amount in the vials.)

The nurse needed 2 g of chloramphenicol. She glanced at the new label and thought the vial contained only 100 mg. So she reconstituted 20 1-g vials and administered the drug. Her patient died of an overdose 11 hours later.

You may think this error was due to unusual carelessness. Yet, in 1975, at least five patients were accidently given ten times the intended dose of chloramphenicol. As a result, the manufacturer redesigned the label, clarifying the contents.

Since a label can easily be misinterpreted, read it three times before you administer any medication. Make sure you understand exactly how much drug a vial contains. And before you administer a dose of more than one or two units (capsules, tablets, vials, or ampuls), check with your pharmacist.

Onset and duration

- Orally administered drugs (amantadine, chloramphenicol, clindamycin, erythromycin, lincomycin, novobiocin, trimethoprim, and troleandomycin) give peak blood levels usually within 2 hours.
- Drugs given I.M. (bacitracin, clindamycin, colistimethate, lincomycin, novobiocin, polymyxin B, and spectinomycin) give peak blood levels usually within 1 hour.
- Drugs given I.V. give peak blood levels almost immediately, so they should be given by this route in acute, life-threatening situations.
- Duration of effect varies from 2 to 6 hours for most of these drugs. The effects of amantadine, novobiocin, polymyxin B, and vancomycin last up to 24 hours; trimethoprim is active for about 12 hours.

Combination products

None.

NAME	INDICATIONS & DOSAGE	SIDE EFFECTS
amantadine hydrochloride Symmetrel♦	*Prophylaxis or symptomatic treatment of influenza type A virus, respiratory tract illnesses—* **Adults, and children over 9 years:** 200 mg P.O. daily in a single dose or divided b.i.d. **Children 1 to 9 years:** 4.4 to 8.8 mg/kg P.O. daily, divided b.i.d. or t.i.d. Don't exceed 150 mg daily. Treatment should continue for 24 to 48 hours after symptoms disappear. Prophylaxis should start as soon as possible after initial exposure and continue for at least 10 days after exposure. Continue prophylaxis up to 90 days for repeated or suspected exposures if influenza vaccine unavailable. If used with influenza vaccine, continue dose for 2 to 3 weeks until protection from vaccine develops.	**CNS:** depression, fatigue, confusion, dizziness, psychosis, hallucinations, anxiety, irritability, ataxia, insomnia, weakness, headache. **CV:** peripheral edema, orthostatic hypotension, congestive heart failure. **GI:** anorexia, nausea, constipation, vomiting, dry mouth. **GU:** urinary retention.
bacitracin	*Pneumonia or empyema caused by susceptible staphylococci—* **Infants over 2.5 kg:** 1,000 units/kg I.M. daily, divided q 8 to 12 hours. **Infants under 2.5 kg:** 900 units/kg I.M. daily, divided q 8 to 12 hours. Although the FDA approves the use of bacitracin in infants only, adults with susceptible staphylococcal infections may receive 10,000 to 25,000 units I.M. q 6 hours (maximum 25,000 units/dose, 100,000 units/day).	**Blood:** blood dyscrasias, eosinophilia. **GI:** nausea, vomiting, anorexia, diarrhea, rectal itching or burning. **GU:** nephrotoxicity *(albuminuria,* cylindruria, oliguria, anuria, increased BUN, tubular and glomerular necrosis). **Skin:** urticaria, rash. **Local:** *pain at injection site.* **Other:** superinfection, fever, *anaphylaxis.*
chloramphenicol **chloramphenicol palmitate** **chloramphenicol sodium succinate** Chloromycetin♦, Mychel, Novochlorocap♦♦	Hemophilus influenzae *meningitis, acute* Salmonella typhi *infection, severe infections caused by sensitive* Salmonella *species,* Rickettsia, *lymphogranuloma, psittacosis, various sensitive gram-negative organisms causing meningitis, bacteremia, or other serious infections—* **Adults and children:** 50 to 100 mg/kg P.O. or I.V. daily, divided q 6 hours. Maximum dose is 100 mg/kg/day.	**Blood:** *aplastic anemia,* hypoplastic anemia, *granulocytopenia,* thrombocytopenia. **CNS:** headache, mild depression, confusion, delirium, peripheral neuropathy with prolonged therapy. **EENT:** optic neuritis (in patients with cystic fibrosis), glossitis, decreased visual acuity. **GI:** nausea, vomiting, stomatitis, diarrhea, enterocolitis. **Other:** infections by nonsuscepti-

♦ Available in U.S. and Canada. ♦♦ Available in Canada only. All other products (no symbol) available in U.S. only. Italicized side effects are common or life-threatening.

INTERACTIONS	NURSING CONSIDERATIONS
None significant.	• Use cautiously in patients with history of epilepsy, congestive heart failure, peripheral edema, hepatic disease, mental illness, eczematoid rash, renal impairment, orthostatic hypotension, cardiovascular disease, and in elderly patients. • For best absorption, drug should be taken after meals. • Instruct patient to report side effects to the doctor, especially dizziness, depression, anxiety, nausea, and urinary retention. • Monitor electrolyte balance and urinary output. • If orthostatic hypotension occurs, instruct patient not to stand or change positions too quickly. • If insomnia occurs, dose should be taken several hours before bedtime. • Prophylactic use recommended for patients who can't receive influenza virus vaccine.
None significant.	• Contraindicated in patients with impaired renal function. Use cautiously in superinfections or neuromuscular disease. • Do culture and sensitivity tests before treatment and p.r.n. • For I.M. use only. Give deep I.M.; injection may be painful; dilute in solution containing sodium chloride and 2% procaine hydrochloride. Don't give to those sensitive to procaine or PABA derivatives. • Maintain adequate fluid intake, and monitor urinary output closely. If intake or output decreases, notify the doctor. • Obtain baseline renal function studies before starting therapy. Monitor renal function (BUN, serum creatinine, creatinine clearance, urinalysis) daily during therapy. Notify doctor of any change. • Drug concentration should be between 5,000 and 10,000 units/ml. Keep refrigerated. Drug is inactivated at room temperature. • May be used with neomycin as a bowel preparation, or in solution as a wound irrigating agent. • Urine pH should be kept above 6.0. • Prolonged therapy may result in overgrowth of nonsusceptible organisms, especially *Candida albicans*. • For treatment of anaphylaxis, see inside front cover.
Penicillins: antagonize antibacterial effect. Give penicillin at least 1 hour before. *Acetaminophen:* elevates chloramphenicol levels. Monitor for chloramphenicol toxicity.	• Use cautiously in patients with impaired hepatic or renal function, and with other drugs causing bone marrow depression or blood disorders. *Don't use for infections caused by organisms susceptible to other agents or for trivial infections such as colds; use only when clearly indicated for severe infection.* • Culture and sensitivity test may be done concurrently with first dose and p.r.n. • Monitor CBC, platelets, serum iron, and reticulocytes before and every 2 days during therapy. Stop drug immediately if anemia, reticulocytopenia, leukopenia, or thrombocytopenia develops. • Instruct patient to report side effects to the doctor, especially nausea, vomiting, diarrhea, fever, confusion, sore throat, or mouth sores. • Watch for evidence of superinfection by nonsusceptible organisms.

(continued on following page)

NAME	INDICATIONS & DOSAGE	SIDE EFFECTS
chloramphenicol *(continued)*	**Premature infants and neonates (2 weeks or younger):** 25 mg/kg P.O. or I.V. daily, divided q 6 hours. I.V. route must be used to treat meningitis.	ble organisms, hypersensitivity reaction (fever, rash, urticaria, *anaphylaxis), gray baby syndrome in premature infants and neonates (abdominal distention, gray cyanosis, vasomotor collapse, respiratory distress, death within a few hours of onset of symptoms).*
clindamycin hydrochloride **clindamycin palmitate hydrochloride** **clindamycin phosphate** Cleocin, Dalacin C♦♦	*Infections caused by sensitive staphylococci, streptococci, pneumococci,* Bacteroides, Fusobacterium, Clostridium perfringens, *and other sensitive aerobic and anaerobic organisms*— **Adults:** 150 to 450 mg P.O. q 6 hours; or 300 mg I.M. or I.V. q 6, 8, or 12 hours. Up to 2,700 mg I.M. or I.V. daily, divided q 6, 8, or 12 hours. May be used for severe infections. **Children over 1 month:** 8 to 25 mg/kg P.O. daily, divided q 6 to 8 hours; or 15 to 40 mg/kg I.M. or I.V. daily, divided q 6 hours.	**Blood:** transient leukopenia, eosinophilia, thrombocytopenia. **GI:** *nausea,* vomiting, abdominal pain, *diarrhea, pseudomembranous enterocolitis,* esophagitis, flatulence, anorexia, *bloody or tarry stools.* **Hepatic:** elevated SGOT, alkaline phosphatase, bilirubin. **Skin:** maculopapular rash, urticaria. **Local:** *pain,* induration, *sterile abscess with I.M. injection;* thrombophlebitis, erythema, and pain after I.V. administration. **Other:** unpleasant or bitter taste, *anaphylaxis.*
colistimethate sodium Colistin Sulfate, Coly-Mycin M♦, Coly-Mycin S Oral	*Enterocolitis caused by sensitive* Escherichia coli, *sensitive* Shigella, *gastroenteritis*— **Infants and children:** 5 to 15 mg/kg P.O. daily, divided q 6 to 8 hours. *Severe infections, especially of urinary tract, caused by sensitive* Pseudomonas, Enterobacter, E. coli, *and* Klebsiella— **Adults and children:** 2.5 to 5 mg/kg I.M. or I.V. daily, divided q 6 to 12 hours. Maximum daily dose not to exceed 5 mg/kg/day in patients with normal renal function.	**CNS:** *circumoral and lingual paresthesias;* paresthesias of extremities; neuromuscular blockage with respiratory arrest, especially in patients with impaired renal function; dizziness; slurring of speech. **GI:** nausea, vomiting, discomfort. **GU:** *nephrotoxicity* (decreased urinary output, increased BUN and serum creatinine). **Skin:** pruritus, urticaria. **Local:** pain at I.M. site. **Other:** "drug fever," overgrowth of nonsusceptible organisms.
erythromycin base E-Mycin♦,	*Acute pelvic inflammatory disease caused by* Neisseria	**EENT:** hearing loss with high doses I.V.

♦ Available in U.S. and Canada. ♦♦ Available in Canada only. All other products (no symbol) available in U.S. only. Italicized side effects are common or life-threatening.

INTERACTIONS	NURSING CONSIDERATIONS
	• Tell patient to take medication for as long as prescribed, exactly as directed, even after he feels better. • Give I.V. slowly over 1 minute. Check injection site daily for phlebitis and irritation. • Reconstitute 1-g vial of powder for injection with 10 ml of sterile water for injection. Concentration will be 100 mg/ml. Stable for 30 days at room temperature, but refrigeration recommended. Do not use cloudy solutions. • For treatment of anaphylaxis, see inside front cover.
Erythromycin: antagonist that may block access of clindamycin to its site of action; don't use together.	• Contraindicated in patients with known hypersensitivity to the antibiotic congener lincomycin; also in patients with history of GI disease, especially colitis. Use cautiously in newborns and patients with renal or hepatic disease, asthma, or significant allergies. • Monitor renal, hepatic, and hematopoietic functions during prolonged therapy. • Do culture and sensitivity tests before treatment and p.r.n. • Don't refrigerate reconstituted oral solution, as it will thicken. Drug is stable for 2 weeks at room temperature. • Instruct patient to report side effects to the doctor, especially diarrhea. Warn patient not to treat such diarrhea himself. • Don't give diphenoxylate compound (Lomotil) to treat drug-induced diarrhea. May prolong and worsen diarrhea. • Give deep I.M. Rotate sites. Warn that I.M. injection may be painful. Doses greater than 600 mg per injection are not recommended. • When giving I.V., check site daily for phlebitis and irritation. For I.V. infusion, dilute each 300 mg in 50 ml solution; give no faster than 30 mg/minute. Several drugs are incompatible with clindamycin; see Chapter 6, UNDERSTANDING INTRAVENOUS SOLUTION COMPATIBILITY. • I.M. injection may cause CPK levels to rise due to muscle irritation. • Topical form is now available to treat acne. • For treatment of anaphylaxis, see inside front cover.
None significant.	• Contraindicated in patients with known hypersensitivity to the antibiotic congener polymyxin B. Use cautiously in renal impairment. • Give deep I.M. Rotate sites. Warn that I.M. injection may be painful. • Use sterile water for injection to reconstitute. When mixing, swirl solution gently to avoid frothing. Always prepare I.V. infusion fresh. Use within 24 hours. • When giving I.V., check site daily for phlebitis and irritation. For direct I.V. administration, inject ½ daily dose over 3 to 5 minutes at 12-hour intervals. • For continuous I.V. infusion, directly inject ½ daily dose over 3 to 5 minutes. Add the remaining ½ to 5% dextrose, 5% dextrose in 0.9% sodium chloride, 5% dextrose in 0.45% sodium chloride, 5% dextrose in 0.225% sodium chloride, 10% invert sugar, lactated Ringer's injection, or 0.9% sodium chloride solution; then infuse 1 to 2 hours later at rate of 5 mg/hour. • Monitor renal function closely (BUN, creatinine clearance, urinary output). Discontinue if BUN increases and urinary output decreases. • Report side effects immediately, especially speech impairment or paresthesias. Watch for signs of superinfection. • Store reconstituted oral suspension at 2° to 15° C. (35.6° to 59° F.), and use within 7 days.
Clindamycin, lincomycin: may be antag-	• Erythromycin estolate contraindicated in hepatic disease. Use other erythromycin salts cautiously in impaired hepatic function.

(continued on following page)

NAME	INDICATIONS & DOSAGE	SIDE EFFECTS
erythromycin base *(continued)* Erythromid♦♦, Ethril 500, Ilotycin♦, Novorythro♦♦, Robimycin♦, Staticin **erythromycin estolate** Ilosone♦, Novorythro♦♦ **erythromycin ethylsuccinate** E.E.S., Erythrocin♦, Pediamycin, Wyamycin Liquid **erythromycin gluceptate** Ilotycin♦ **erythromycin lactobionate** Erythrocin♦ **erythromycin stearate** Bristamycin, E-Biotic, Ethril, Erypar, Erythrocin♦, Novorythro♦♦, Pfizer E, Romycin, SK-Erythromycin, Wintrocin, Wyamycin	gonorrhoeae— **Women:** 500 mg I.V. (erythromycin gluceptate, lactobionate) q 6 hours for 3 days, then 250 mg (erythromycin base, estolate, stearate) or 400 mg (erythromycin ethylsuccinate) P.O. q 6 hours for 7 days. *Endocarditis prophylaxis for dental procedures*— **Adults:** 1 g (erythromycin base, estolate, stearate) P.O. before procedure, then 250 mg P.O. q 6 hours for 8 doses; or 1,200 mg (erythromycin ethylsuccinate) P.O. before procedure, then 400 mg P.O. q 6 hours for 8 doses. **Children:** 20 mg/kg (oral erythromycin salts) P.O. 1½ to 2 hours before procedure, then 10 mg/kg q 6 hours for 8 doses. *Intestinal amebiasis*— **Adults:** 250 mg (erythromycin base, estolate, stearate) P.O. q 6 hours for 10 to 14 days. **Children:** 30 to 50 mg/kg (erythromycin base, estolate, stearate) P.O. daily, divided q 6 hours for 10 to 14 days. *Mild-to-moderately severe respiratory tract, skin, and soft-tissue infections caused by sensitive group A beta-hemolytic streptococci,* Diplococcus pneumoniae, Mycoplasma pneumoniae, Corynebacterium diphtheriae, Bordetella pertussis, Listeria monocytogenes— **Adults:** 250 to 500 mg (erythromycin base, estolate, stearate) P.O. q 6 hours; or 400 to 800 mg (erythromycin ethylsuccinate) P.O. q 6 hours; or 15 to 20 mg/kg I.V. daily, as continuous infusion or divided q 6 hours. **Children:** 30 mg/kg to 50 mg/kg (oral erythromycin salts) P.O. or 15 to 20 mg/kg I.V. daily, divided q 4 to 6 hours. *Syphilis*— **Adults:** 500 mg (erythromycin base, estolate, stearate) P.O. q.i.d. for 15 days.	**GI:** *abdominal pain and cramping, nausea, vomiting, diarrhea.* **Hepatic:** cholestatic jaundice (with erythromycin estolate). **Skin:** urticaria, rashes. **Local:** *venous irritation, thrombophlebitis following I.V. injection.* **Other:** overgrowth of nonsusceptible bacteria or fungi; *anaphylaxis;* fever.
furazolidone Furoxone	*Gastroenteritis, adjunctive therapy in cholera*— **Adults:** 100 mg P.O. q.i.d.	**Blood:** hemolytic anemia in infants under 1 month and patients with G-6-PD deficiency; *agranulo-*

♦ Available in U.S. and Canada. ♦♦ Available in Canada only. All other products (no symbol) available in U.S. only. Italicized side effects are common or life-threatening.

INTERACTIONS	NURSING CONSIDERATIONS
onistic. Don't use together. *Penicillins:* antagonize antibacterial effect. Give penicillin at least 1 hour before.	• Culture and sensitivity tests should be performed before starting treatment and p.r.n. • For best absorption, instruct patient to take oral form of drug with a full glass of water 1 hour before or 2 hours after meals. If tablets are coated, they may be taken with meals. Tell patient not to drink fruit juice with medication. Chewable erythromycin tablets should not be swallowed whole. • When administering suspension, be sure to note the concentration. • May cause overgrowth of nonsusceptible bacteria or fungi. Watch for signs and symptoms of superinfection. • Tell patient to take medication for as long as prescribed, exactly as directed, even after he feels better. Treat streptococcal infections for 10 days. • Report side effects, especially nausea, abdominal pain, or fever. • Erythromycin estolate may cause serious hepatotoxicity in adults (reversible cholestatic jaundice). Monitor hepatic function (increased levels of bilirubin, SGOT, SGPT, alkaline phosphatase may occur). Other erythromycin salts cause hepatotoxicity to a lesser degree. • I.V. dose should be administered over 20 to 60 minutes. Reconstitute according to manufacturer's directions and dilute each 250 mg in at least 100 ml 0.9% normal saline solution. • Erythromycin lactobionate should not be administered with other drugs. See Chapter 6, UNDERSTANDING INTRAVENOUS SOLUTION COMPATIBILITY. • Has been used successfully in treatment of Legionnaires' disease. • Topical form now available to treat acne. • For treatment of anaphylaxis, see inside front cover.

Sympathomimetics: hypertensive crisis. Don't use together.	• Tell patient to take medication exactly as directed, even after he feels better. • Report side effects , especially fever, rash, abdominal pain.

(continued on following page)

NAME	INDICATIONS & DOSAGE	SIDE EFFECTS
furazolidone *(continued)*	**Children 5 to 12 years:** 25 to 50 mg P.O. q.i.d. **Children 1 to 4 years:** 17 to 25 mg P.O. q.i.d. **Infants (1 month to 1 year):** 8 to 17 mg P.O. q.i.d. Dosage based on 5 mg/kg daily; maximum dose 8.8 mg/kg daily.	*cytosis.* **CNS:** headache, malaise. **GI:** nausea, vomiting, abdominal pain, diarrhea. **Other:** hypersensitivity reaction (arthralgia, fever, hypotension, rash, urticaria, angioedema), hypoglycemia.
lincomycin hydrochloride Lincocin♦	*Respiratory tract, skin and soft-tissue, and urinary tract infections; osteomyelitis, septicemia, caused by sensitive group A beta-hemolytic streptococci, pneumococci, and staphylococci—* **Adults:** 500 mg P.O. q 6 to 8 hours (not to exceed 8 g daily); or 600 mg I.M. daily or q 12 hours; or 600 mg to 1 g I.V. q 8 to 12 hours (not to exceed 8 g daily). **Children over 1 month:** 30 to 60 mg/kg P.O. daily, divided q 6 to 8 hours; or 10 mg/kg I.M. daily or divided q 12 hours; or 10 to 20 mg/kg I.V. daily, divided q 6 to 8 hours. For I.V. infusion, dilute to 100 ml; infuse over 1 hour to avoid hypotension.	**Blood:** *neutropenia, leukopenia,* thrombocytopenia, purpura. **CNS:** dizziness, headache. **CV:** hypotension with rapid I.V. infusion. **EENT:** glossitis, tinnitus. **GI:** nausea, vomiting, *persistent diarrhea,* abdominal cramps, enterocolitis, stomatitis, pruritus ani. **GU:** vaginitis. **Hepatic:** cholestatic jaundice. **Skin:** rashes, urticaria. **Local:** pain at injection site. **Other:** hypersensitivity, angioedema.
novobiocin calcium **novobiocin sodium** Albamycin	*Serious infections from sensitive* Staphylococcus aureus *and* Proteus *when other antibiotics are contraindicated—* **Adults:** 250 to 500 mg P.O. q 6 hours, or 500 mg to 1 g q 12 hours (not to exceed 2 g daily). **Children:** 15 to 45 mg/kg P.O. daily, divided q 6 hours.	**Blood:** pancytopenia, *leukopenia, agranulocytosis,* anemia, thrombocytopenia, eosinophilia. **GI:** nausea, vomiting, anorexia, diarrhea, intestinal hemorrhage. **Hepatic:** jaundice, hepatitis. **Skin:** urticaria, *maculopapular dermatitis.* **Local:** pain at injection site. **Other:** *erythema multiforme,* fever in hypersensitivity reactions, swollen joints, overgrowth of nonsusceptible organisms.
polymyxin B sulfate Aerosporin♦	*Acute urinary tract infections or septicemia caused by sensitive* Pseudomonas aeruginosa, *or when other antibiotics are ineffective or contraindicated; bac-*	**CNS:** irritability, drowsiness, facial flushing, weakness, ataxia, respiratory paralysis, headache and meningeal irritation with intrathecal administration, periph-

♦ Available in U.S. and Canada. ♦♦ Available in Canada only. All other products (no symbol) available in U.S. only. Italicized side effects are common or life-threatening.

INTERACTIONS	NURSING CONSIDERATIONS
	• Store medication in dark place at 2° to 15° C. (36.5° to 59° F.). • Warn patient not to use over-the-counter nasal sprays or cold and hay fever products. • Drug may turn urine brown. Flushing, nausea, sweating, tachycardia, dyspnea may occur following ethanol ingestion. Tell patient not to drink alcohol or use alcohol-containing medication. • If patient is taking drug for more than 5 days, instruct him not to eat broad beans, cheese, pickled herring, chicken livers, yeast extracts, or fermented products. Drug is similar to monoamine oxidase inhibitor. • May cause false-positive urine glucose with Benedict's reagent. • Blood and urine studies should be performed frequently on patients with G-6-PD deficiency to detect hemolysis.
Antidiarrheal medication (kaolin, pectin, attapulgite): reduce oral absorption of lincomycin by as much as 90%. Antidiarrheals should be avoided or given at least 2 hours before lincomycin.	• Contraindicated in known hypersensitivity to clindamycin. Use cautiously in patients with history of GI disorders (especially colitis); asthma or significant allergies; hepatic or renal disease; and endocrine or metabolic disorders. • Culture and sensitivity tests should be done before starting treatment and p.r.n. • For best absorption, instruct patient to take drug with a full glass of water 1 hour before or 2 hours after meals. • Tell patient to take medication exactly as directed, even after he feels better. • Tell patient to report side effects to doctor, especially diarrhea. Warn him not to treat diarrhea himself. Watch for signs of superinfection, especially when therapy exceeds 10 days. • Never treat drug-induced diarrhea with diphenoxylate compound (Lomotil); it may prolong or worsen diarrhea. • Give deep I.M. Rotate sites. Warn that I.M. injection may be painful. • When giving I.V., check site daily for phlebitis and irritation. • Monitor blood pressure in patients receiving the drug parenterally. • Monitor hepatic function (increased levels of alkaline phosphatase, SGOT, SGPT, bilirubin may occur). • Monitor CBC and platelets. Stop drug immediately if neutropenia, leukopenia, or other blood disorders develop.
None significant.	• Use cautiously in patients with hepatic disease or blood disorders. Do not use in infants, as it may cause kernicterus. • Culture and sensitivity tests should be done before starting treatment and p.r.n. • For best absorption, instruct patient to take drug with a full glass of water 1 hour before or 2 hours after meals. • Tell patient to take medication for as long as prescribed exactly as directed, even after he feels better. • Report side effects, especially skin rash, fever, jaundice, or GI distress. Stop drug immediately and notify the doctor. • Monitor hepatic function (bilirubin, SGOT, SGPT, and alkaline phosphatase). • Monitor CBC, and platelet, reticulocyte counts before and during therapy.
None significant.	• Use cautiously in patients with impaired renal function or myasthenia gravis. • Give only to hospitalized patients under constant medical supervision. • For meningitis, must give intrathecally to achieve adequate cerebrospinal fluid levels.

(continued on following page)

NAME	INDICATIONS & DOSAGE	SIDE EFFECTS
polymyxin B sulfate *(continued)*	*teremia caused by sensitive* Enterobacter aerogenes *and* Klebsiella pneumoniae, *or acute urinary tract infections caused by* Escherichia coli— **Adults and children:** 15,000 to 25,000 units/kg/day I.V. infusion, divided q 12 hours; or 25,000 to 30,000 units/kg/day, divided q 4 to 8 hours. I.M. not advised. *Meningitis caused by sensitive* P. aeruginosa *or* Hemophilus influenzae *when other antibiotics ineffective or contraindicated*— **Adults, and children over 2 years:** 50,000 units intrathecally once daily for 3 to 4 days, then 50,000 units every other day for at least 2 weeks after cerebrospinal fluid tests are negative and cerebrospinal fluid sugar is normal. **Children under 2 years:** 20,000 units intrathecally once daily for 3 to 4 days, then 25,000 units every other day for at least 2 weeks after cerebrospinal fluid tests are negative and cerebrospinal fluid sugar is normal.	eral and perioral paresthesias, convulsions, *coma.* **EENT:** blurred vision. **GU:** nephrotoxicity (albuminuria, cylindruria, hematuria, proteinuria, decreased urine output, increased BUN). **Skin:** urticaria. **Local:** *pain at I.M. injection site.* **Other:** hypersensitivity reactions with fever, *anaphylaxis.*
spectinomycin dihydrochloride Trobicin♦	*Gonorrhea*— **Adults:** 2 to 4 g I.M. single dose injected deeply into the upper outer quadrant of the buttock.	**CNS:** insomnia, dizziness. **GI:** nausea. **GU:** decreased urine output. **Skin:** urticaria. **Local:** pain at injection site. **Other:** fever, chills (may mask or delay symptoms of incubating syphilis).
trimethoprim Proloprim, Trimpex	*Treatment of uncomplicated urinary tract infections caused by susceptible strains of* Escherichia coli, Proteus mirabilis, Klebsiella, *and* Enterobacter *species*— **Adults:** 100 mg P.O. every 12 hours for 10 days. Not recommended for children under 12 years.	**Blood:** thrombocytopenia, leukopenia, megaloblastic anemia, methemoglobinemia. **GI:** epigastric distress, nausea, vomiting, glossitis. **Skin:** *rash, pruritus, exfoliative dermatitis.* **Other:** fever.
troleandomycin phosphate Tao	*Sensitive pneumococcal pneumonia or group A beta-hemolytic streptococcal respiratory tract infection*— **Adults:** 250 to 500 mg P.O. q	**GI:** *nausea,* vomiting, diarrhea, discomfort. **Hepatic:** cholestatic jaundice. **Skin:** urticaria and rashes in hypersensitivity reactions.

♦ Available in U.S. and Canada. ♦♦ Available in Canada only. All other products (no symbol) available in U.S. only. Italicized side effects are common or life-threatening.

INTERACTIONS	NURSING CONSIDERATIONS
	• Give deep I.M. Warn that injection may be painful. If patient isn't allergic to procaine, use 1% procaine as diluent to decrease pain. Rotate sites. • Don't give solution containing local anesthetics I.V. or intrathecally. • When giving I.V., check site daily for phlebitis and irritation. Dilute each 500,000 units in 300 to 500 ml of 5% dextrose in water; infuse over 60 to 90 minutes. • Parenteral solutions should be refrigerated and used within 72 hours. • Monitor renal function (BUN, serum creatinine, creatinine clearance, urinary output) before and during therapy. Intake should be sufficient to maintain output at 1,500 ml/day (between 3,000 and 4,000 ml/day for adults). • Discontinue therapy if BUN increases and urinary output decreases. • Notify doctor immediately if patient develops fever, CNS side effects, rash, or symptoms of nephrotoxicity. • If patient is scheduled for surgery, notify anesthesiologist of preoperative treatment with this drug since neuromuscular blockade can occur. • For treatment of anaphylaxis, see inside front cover.
None significant.	• Not effective in the treatment of syphilis. • Serologic test for syphilis should be done before treatment dose and 3 months after. • Use 20G needle to administer drug. The 4-g dose (10 ml) should be divided into two 5-ml injections—one in each buttock. • Shake vial vigorously after reconstitution and before withdrawing dose. Store at room temperature after reconstitution and use within 24 hours. • Should be reserved for penicillin-resistant strains of gonorrhea.
None significant.	• Contraindicated in documented megaloblastic anemia due to folate deficiency. • Clinical signs such as sore throat, fever, pallor, or purpura may be early indications of serious blood disorders. Monitor CBC routinely. Prolonged use of trimethoprim at high doses may cause bone marrow depression. • Dose should be decreased in patients with severely impaired renal function. Give cautiously to patients with impaired hepatic function. • To be of benefit, full course of therapy must be completed.
None significant.	• Use cautiously in patients with hepatic impairment. • Drug is not recommended for routine use. • For best absorption, instruct patient to take drug with a full glass of water 1 hour before or 2 hours after meals. • Tell patient to take medication for as long as prescribed, exactly as

(continued on following page)

NAME	INDICATIONS & DOSAGE	SIDE EFFECTS
troleandomycin phosphate *(continued)*	6 hours. **Children:** 6.6 to 11 mg/kg P.O. daily, q 6 hours.	**Other:** *anaphylaxis.*
vancomycin hydrochloride Vancocin♦	*Severe staphylococcal infections when other antibiotics ineffective or contraindicated—* **Adults:** 500 mg I.V. q 6 hours, or 1 g q 12 hours. **Children:** 44 mg/kg I.V. daily, divided q 6 hours. **Neonates:** 10 mg/kg I.V. daily, divided q 6 to 12 hours. *Antibiotic-associated pseudomembranous and staphylococcal enterocolitis—* **Adults:** 500 mg P.O. in 30 ml of water q 6 hours. **Children:** 44 mg/kg P.O. daily, divided q 6 hours with 30 ml of water.	**Blood:** transient eosinophilia. **EENT:** tinnitus, ototoxicity (deafness). **GI:** nausea. **GU:** nephrotoxicity (hyaline casts in urine, albuminuria, increased BUN). **Local:** *pain or thrombophlebitis with I.V. administration, necrosis.* **Other:** chills, fever, *anaphylaxis,* overgrowth of nonsusceptible organisms.
vidarabine monohydrate Vira-A	*Herpes simplex virus encephalitis—* **Adults:** 15 mg/kg/day for 10 days. Slowly infuse the total daily dose by I.V. infusion at a constant rate over 12- to 24-hour period. Avoid rapid or bolus injection.	**Blood:** anemia, neutropenia, thrombocytopenia. **CNS:** tremor, dizziness, hallucinations, confusion, psychosis, ataxia. **GI:** *anorexia, nausea,* vomiting, diarrhea. **Hepatic:** elevated SGOT, bilirubin. **Skin:** pruritus, rash. **Local:** pain at injection site. **Other:** weight loss.

♦ Available in U.S. and Canada. ♦♦ Available in Canada only. All other products (no symbol) available in U.S. only. Italicized side effects are common or life-threatening.

INTERACTIONS	NURSING CONSIDERATIONS
	directed, even after he feels better. Treat streptococcal infections at least 10 days. • Monitor hepatic function (bilirubin, SGOT, SGPT, and alkaline phosphatase). • Report side effects, especially abdominal pain, nausea, or jaundice. • For treatment of anaphylaxis, see inside front cover.
Oral contraceptives: cholestatic jaundice. Monitor bilirubin values.	• Contraindicated in patients receiving other neurotoxic, nephrotoxic, or ototoxic drugs. Use cautiously in patients with impaired hepatic or renal function; in patients with existing hearing loss; in patients over age 60; in patients with allergies to other antibiotics. • Tell patient to take medication exactly as directed, even after he feels better. Treat staphylococcal endocarditis for at least 4 weeks. • Patients should receive auditory function tests before and during therapy. • Tell patient to report side effects at once, especially dizziness, fullness or ringing in ears. Stop drug immediately if these occur. • Do not give drug I.M. • For I.V. infusion, dilute in 200 ml of sodium chloride injection or 5% glucose solution and infuse over 20 to 30 minutes. Check site daily for phlebitis and irritation. Report pain at infusion site. Avoid extravasation. Severe irritation and necrosis can result. • Refrigerate I.V. solution after reconstitution and use within 96 hours. • Monitor renal function (BUN, serum creatinine, urinalysis, creatinine clearance, urinary output) before and during therapy. Watch for signs of superinfection. • Oral preparation stable for 2 weeks if refrigerated. • Has been used recently to treat pseudomembranous enterocolitis caused by clindamycin. • For treatment of anaphylaxis, see inside front cover.
None significant.	• Will reduce mortality caused by herpes simplex virus encephalitis from 70% to 28%. No evidence that vidarabine is effective in encephalitis due to other viruses. • Don't give I.M. or subcutaneously because of low solubility and poor absorption. • Monitor hematologic tests such as hemoglobin, hematocrit, WBC, and platelets during therapy. Also monitor kidney and liver function studies. • Patient with impaired renal function may need dosage adjustment. • Once in solution, vidarabine is stable at room temperature for at least 2 weeks. • Use with an I.V. filter. • Must be diluted to a concentration of less than 0.5 mg/ml. • Any I.V. solution is suitable as a diluent.

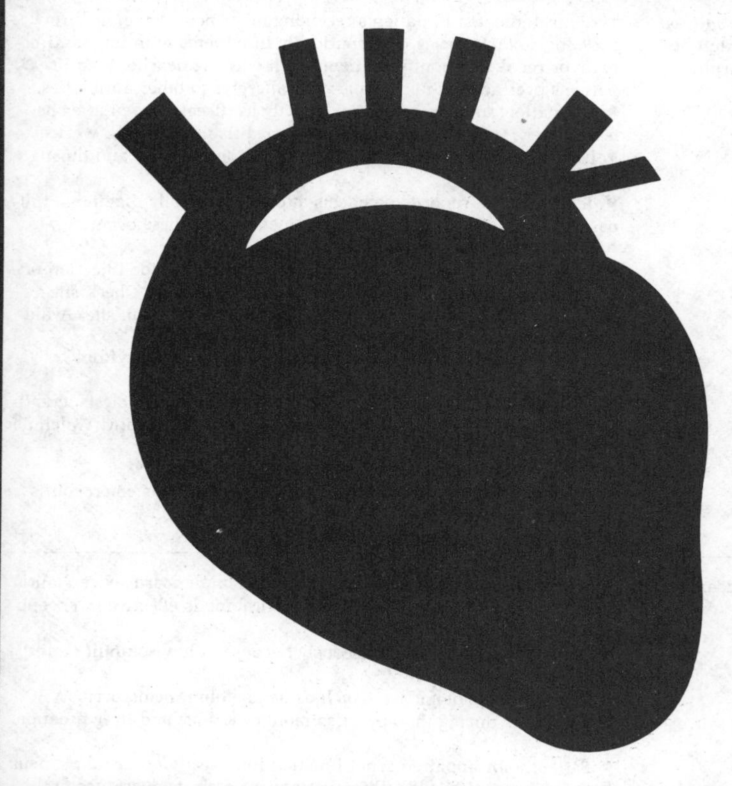

Cardiovascular System Drugs

20 Cardiotonic glycosides

deslanoside
digitalis leaf
digitoxin
digoxin
gitalin
lanatoside C
ouabain

The cardiotonic (cardiac or digitalis) glycosides, which are extracted from plants of the genus *Digitalis* or chemically synthesized from the plant extract, are used to treat congestive heart failure and tachyarrhythmias. All the cardiotonic glycosides act similarly on the cardiovascular system; however, they differ in extent of absorption, metabolism, and excretion.

The range between therapeutic and toxic doses is extremely narrow. Toxicity may be due to altered absorption, serum electrolyte concentrations, renal or hepatic dysfunction, drug interactions, or other factors. The choice of cardiotonic glycoside and route of administration depend on the disorder

THERAPEUTIC ACTIVITY

THERAPEUTIC ACTIVITY OF CARDIOTONIC GLYCOSIDES

DRUG	ONSET	PEAK	HALF-LIFE	DURATION
deslanoside	10 to 30 min	1 to 2 hr	1½ days	2 to 5 days
digitalis leaf	15 to 120 min	4 to 12 hr	5 to 7 days	2 to 3 wk
digitoxin	30 to 120 min	4 to 12 hr	5 to 7 days	2 to 3 wk
digoxin	15 to 30 min	1½ to 5 hr	1½ days	2 to 3 days
gitalin	30 to 120 min	12 to 20 hr	8 to 12 days	10 to 12 days
lanatoside C	15 to 30 min	1½ to 5 hr	1½ days	2 to 3 days
ouabain	5 to 10 min	½ to 2 hr	21 hr	1 to 2½ days

PATIENT-TEACHING AID

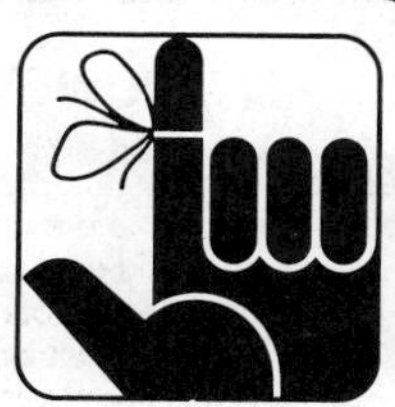

WHAT YOU SHOULD KNOW ABOUT DIGITALIS

Dear Patient:

Digitalis strengthens your heart so it can pump blood through your body more efficiently. For your therapy to be most effective, please follow these guidelines:

1. Check your pulse rate and rhythm for a full minute before taking your digitalis. If you notice sudden spurts of rapid pulse rate, skipped beats, or irregular rhythm, of if your pulse rate is not within the range the doctor set for you, call him before taking your digitalis.

2. Eat properly. Avoiding salt helps prevent water retention, and eating foods rich in potassium helps protect against digitalis-induced arrhythmias (variations in rhythm). The dietitian can help you plan specific menus before you leave the hospital.

3. Don't take any other medications—including antacids, cold remedies, and nose drops—without first asking the doctor. Many medications either increase or decrease sensitivity to digitalis.

4. Contact the doctor if you:
- gain weight
- feel your shoes and rings getting tight
- experience fatigue and tire too easily when exercising
- lose your appetite
- are nauseated or vomit
- have blurred vision, or see flickering lights or yellow borders around dark objects
- are frequently confused or have headaches.

and the desired onset of activity.

Major uses

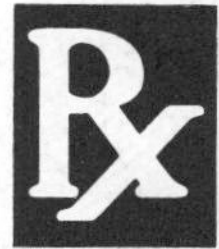

Cardiotonic glycosides increase cardiac output in acute or chronic congestive heart failure (CHF). They control the rate of ventricular contraction in atrial flutter or fibrillation. They're also used to prevent or treat paroxysmal atrial tachycardia and angina associated with CHF.
- Ouabain, a fast-acting cardiotonic glycoside for I.V. use only, is effective in emergencies such as acute left-sided heart failure with pulmonary edema, cardiogenic shock, or atrial arrhythmias.

Mechanism of action

- Cardiotonic glycosides act directly on the myocardium to increase the force of contraction (produce a positive inotropic effect) by two mechanisms:

They promote movement of calcium from extracellular to intracellular cytoplasm. The force of contraction is directly related to the concentration of calcium in the myocardial cytoplasm.

They also inhibit adenosinetriphosphatase (ATPase), the enzyme that regulates potassium and sodium electrolyte concentrations in myocardial cells. Inhibition of ATPase increases intracellular sodium concentration, which in turn increases the force of contraction.
- They decrease conduction velocity through the atrioventricular (AV) node to slow heart rate.
- They prolong the effective refractory period of the AV node by both direct and sympatholytic effects on the sinoatrial (SA) node.

Absorption, distribution, metabolism, and excretion

- Deslanoside is given I.V. or I.M. only

HOW TO RECOGNIZE DIGITALIS TOXICITY

Digitalis reduces the myocardium's resting membrane potential, which in turn reduces its action potential and causes increased excitability and slower conduction. Automaticity is increased, and sodium and potassium pumps are inhibited.

These digitalis effects produce classic EKG changes, such as a sagging S-T segment (a gradual downward sloping effect) and a prolonged P-R interval (> 0.2 second).

Digitalis toxicity occurs when toxic amounts of this drug stimulate ectopic ventricular foci to discharge, producing arrhythmias. The most common toxic effects are ectopic beats and atrioventricular (AV) heart block. Toxicity is enhanced by hypercalcemia.

Examples of digitalis toxicity in EKG tracings appear below. If it is ascertained that the toxicity is caused by digitalis, the digitalis should be immediately discontinued. *Remember:* Although these are commonly seen in digitalis toxicity, they may also be caused by other factors, such as myocardial infarction, heart failure, cardiac ischemia, electrolyte imbalances, toxic effects of other drugs, or various disease states. In these instances, treatment is symptomatic.

PREMATURE VENTRICULAR CONTRACTION (PVC)

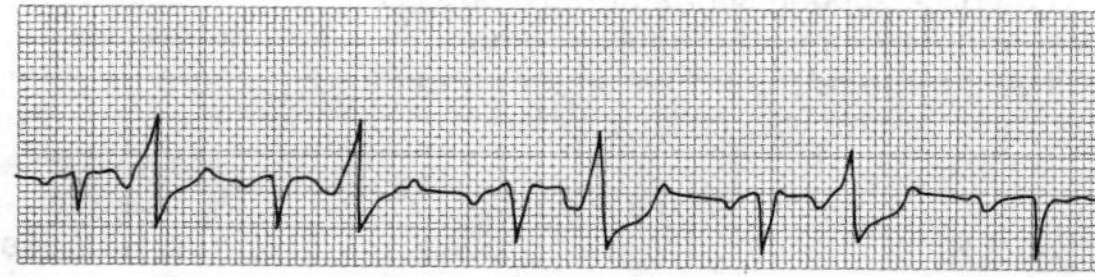

Description and treatment
Beat occurs prematurely, usually followed by a complete compensatory pause after PVC; pulse is irregular. QRS complex is wide and distorted. It can occur singly, in pairs, or in threes, and can alternate with normal beats. Focus can be made from one or more sites. PVCs are most ominous when clustered, multifocal, with R wave on T pattern. To correct, use a lidocaine I.V. bolus and drip infusion, and procainamide I.V. If induced by digitalis, stop this drug. If induced by hypokalemia, give potassium chloride I.V.

NODAL RHYTHM (AV JUNCTIONAL RHYTHM)

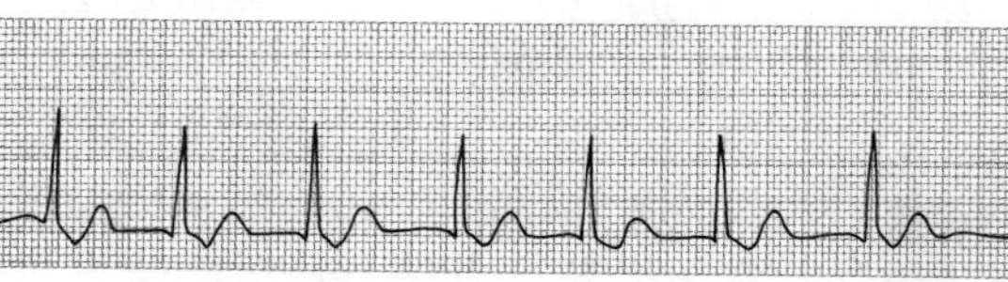

Description and treatment
Ventricular rate is usually 40 to 60 beats per minute (60 to 100 beats per minute is accelerated junctional rhythm). P waves may precede, be hidden within (absent), or follow QRS; if visible, they're altered. QRS duration is normal, except in aberrant conduction. The patient may be asymptomatic unless ventricular rate is very slow. To correct, stop digitalis. Atropine may be given.

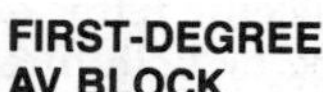

FIRST-DEGREE AV BLOCK

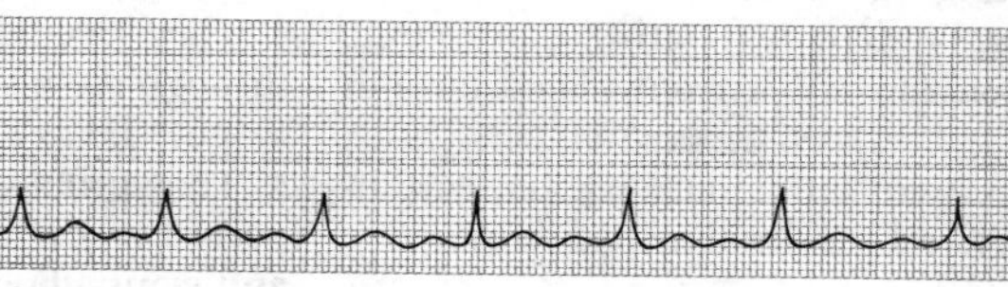

Description and treatment
P-R interval prolonged > 0.2 second QRS complex normal. If patient is taking digitalis, don't discontinue. Correct any underlying cause. However, be alert for increasing AV block that may necessitate digitalis discontinuation.

DRUG ALERT

MONITOR FOR DIGOXIN-QUINIDINE INTERACTION

Research has recently shown that digoxin toxicity may result when quinidine is given to the digoxin-stabilized patient. Since these two drugs are often used concurrently to treat arrhythmias, remember to watch for this potential problem.

Several studies have shown that, in more than 90% of patients who had steady blood levels of digoxin, the addition of quinidine significantly elevated the digoxin concentration.

How does this happen? Two major mechanisms have been proposed:

- Quinidine reduces the amount of digoxin excreted by inhibiting both its renal and nonrenal elimination from the body.
- Quinidine reduces digoxin's volume of distribution by displacing it from binding sites in muscle.

Together, all these effects produce digoxin blood levels up to *twice* as high as digoxin levels *before* quinidine was given. Incidentally, this result may occur from just a single dose of quinidine—and within the first hour of quinidine administration!

What's the clinical significance? Doctors are still not sure. Some decrease digoxin dosage by one half when they prescribe quinidine; others feel that although digoxin blood levels are almost always elevated after quinidine is begun, there's no added risk of life-threatening digoxin toxicity. This is because quinidine may also displace digoxin from the heart muscle's (myocardium's) binding sites. Therefore, the heart is "protected" from increased digoxin blood levels.

However, you should still monitor your patient carefully if he's just had quinidine prescribed. Be sure to:

- remind the doctor to order an analysis of digoxin blood levels within a few days.
- pay careful attention to the clinical symptoms of digoxin toxicity (see APPENDIX, *Drug Toxicities.*) while your patient's being given both drugs concurrently.

because absorption from the gastrointestinal (GI) tract is erratic or incomplete. It is primarily excreted unchanged in the urine. Use with caution in patients with renal dysfunction.

- Digitalis leaf, when given orally, is 20% to 40% absorbed. It's hydrolyzed in the GI tract to form several cardiotonic glycosides, including digitoxin.
- Digitoxin is 90% to 100% absorbed after oral administration. Passing through the enterohepatic circulation, the drug is extensively metabolized in the liver to inactive metabolites and is excreted by the kidneys. Neither the drug nor its metabolites accumulate in the renal parenchyma when renal function is impaired, since biliary and fecal elimination increase.
- Digoxin is 60% to 85% absorbed after oral administration. (Absorption varies with manufacturer.) Although 80% is absorbed after I.M. administration, this route may cause pain and irritation at the injection site.

Digoxin is excreted primarily unchanged in the urine. Use with caution in patients with renal dysfunction.

- Gitalin is a combination of various cardiotonic glycosides. It is well absorbed after oral administration and excreted primarily in the urine.
- Lanatoside C is converted to digoxin by acid and bacterial hydrolysis in the GI tract.
- Oubain is a fast-acting cardiotonic glycoside for I.V. use only. It is not metabolized but is eliminated as unchanged drug in urine and feces.
- None of the cardiotonic glycosides are distributed to adipose tissues. In obese patients, dosage should be based on ideal body weight.

Onset and duration

See table on p. 260.

NAME	INDICATIONS & DOSAGE	SIDE EFFECTS
deslanoside Cedilanid-D	*Congestive heart failure, paroxysmal atrial tachycardia, atrial fibrillation and flutter—* **Adults:** loading dose 1.2 to 1.6 mg I.M. or I.V. in 2 divided doses over 24 hours; for maintenance, use another glycoside. Not recommended for children.	*The following are signs of toxicity that may occur with all cardiotonic glycosides:* **CNS:** *fatigue, generalized muscle weakness, agitation, hallucinations,* headache, malaise, dizziness, vertigo, stupor, paresthesias. **CV:** *increased severity of congestive heart failure, arrhythmias (most commonly conduction disturbances with or without AV block, premature ventricular contractions, and supraventricular arrhythmias),* hypotension. *Toxic effects on heart may be life-threatening and require immediate attention.* **EENT:** *yellow-green halos around visual images, blurred vision,* light flashes, photophobia, diplopia. **GI:** *anorexia, nausea,* vomiting, diarrhea.
digitalis leaf Digifortis, Pil-Digis	*Congestive heart failure, paroxysmal atrial tachycardia, atrial fibrillation and flutter—* **Adults:** loading dose 1.2 to 1.8 g P.O. in divided doses over 24 hours; usual maintenance 100 mg P.O. daily. Not recommended for children.	*The following are signs of toxicity that may occur with all cardiotonic glycosides:* **CNS:** *fatigue, generalized muscle weakness, agitation, hallucinations,* headache, malaise, dizziness, vertigo, stupor, paresthesias. **CV:** *increased severity of congestive heart failure, arrhythmias (most commonly conduction disturbances with or without AV block, premature ventricular contractions, and supraventricular arrhythmias),* hypotension. *Toxic effects on heart may be life-threatening and require immediate attention.* **EENT:** *yellow-green halos around visual images, blurred vision,* light flashes, photophobia, diplopia. **GI:** *anorexia, nausea,* vomiting, diarrhea.

♦ Available in U.S. and Canada. ♦♦ Available in Canada only. All other products (no symbol) available in U.S. only. Italicized side effects are common or life-threatening.

INTERACTIONS	NURSING CONSIDERATIONS
Amphotericin B, carbenicillin, ticarcillin, corticosteroids, and diuretics, including chlorthalidone, ethacrynic acid, furosemide, metolazone, and thiazides: hypokalemia, predisposing patient to digitalis toxicity. Monitor serum potassium. *Parenteral calcium, thiazides:* hypercalcemia and hypomagnesemia, predisposing patient to digitalis toxicity. Monitor serum calcium and serum magnesium.	• Contraindicated in presence of any digitalis-induced toxicity; ventricular fibrillation; ventricular tachycardia unless caused by congestive heart failure. Administering calcium salts to digitalized patient is contraindicated. Calcium affects cardiac contractility and excitability in much the same way that glycosides do and may lead to serious arrhythmias in digitalized patient. Use with extreme caution in patients with acute myocardial infarction, incomplete AV block, chronic constrictive pericarditis, idiopathic hypertrophic subaortic stenosis, renal insufficiency, severe pulmonary disease, hypothyroidism; and in the elderly. • Hypothyroid patients are very sensitive to cardiotonic glycosides; hyperthyroid patients may need larger doses. • Obtain baseline data (heart rate and rhythm, blood pressure, electrolytes, BUN, serum creatinine) before giving first dose. • Question patient about recent use of cardiotonic glycosides (within the previous 2 to 3 weeks) before administering a loading dose. Always divide loading dose over first 24 hours unless clinical situation indicates otherwise. • Use only for rapid digitalization, not maintenance. • Dose is adjusted to patient's clinical condition and is monitored by serum levels of cardiotonic glycoside, calcium, potassium, magnesium, and by EKG. • Take apical-radial pulse for a full minute. Record and report to doctor any significant changes (sudden increase or decrease in rate, pulse deficit, irregular beats, and particularly regularization of a previously irregular rhythm). Check blood pressure and obtain 12-lead EKG with these changes. • Observe eating pattern. Ask patient about nausea, vomiting, anorexia, visual disturbances, and other symptoms of toxicity. • I.M. injection is painful; give I.V. if possible. • Monitor serum potassium carefully. Take corrective action *before* hypokalemia occurs. • For toxicity, see APPENDIX, *Drug Toxicities.*
Para-aminosalicylic acid, antacids, cholestyramine, kaolin-pectin, neomycin, colestipol: decreased absorption of digitoxin, the main active component of the digitalis leaf. Schedule doses as far as possible from administration of digitalis leaf. *Amphotericin B, carbenicillin, ticarcillin, corticosteroids, and diuretics, including chlorthalidone, ethacrynic acid, furosemide, metolazone, and thiazides:* hypokalemia, predisposing patient to digitalis toxicity. Monitor serum	• Contraindicated in presence of any digitalis-induced toxicity; ventricular fibrillation; ventricular tachycardia unless caused by congestive heart failure. Administering calcium salts to digitalized patient is contraindicated. Calcium affects cardiac contractility and excitability in much the same way that glycosides do and may lead to serious arrhythmias in digitalized patient. Use with extreme caution in patients with acute myocardial infarction, incomplete AV block, chronic constrictive pericarditis, idiopathic hypertrophic subaortic stenosis, renal insufficiency, severe pulmonary disease, hypothyroidism; and in the elderly. • Hypothyroid patients are very sensitive to cardiotonic glycosides; hyperthyroid patients may need larger doses. • Obtain baseline data (heart rate and rhythm, blood pressure, electrolytes, BUN, serum creatinine) before giving first dose. • Question patient about recent use of cardiotonic glycosides (within the previous 2 to 3 weeks) before administering a loading dose. Always divide loading dose over first 24 hours unless clinical situation indicates otherwise. • Dose is adjusted to patient's clinical condition and is monitored by serum levels of cardiotonic glycoside, calcium, potassium, magnesium, and by EKG. • Take apical-radial pulse for a full minute. Record and report to doctor any significant changes (sudden increase or decrease in rate, pulse deficit, irregular beats, and particularly regularization of a

(continued on following page)

NAME	INDICATIONS & DOSAGE	SIDE EFFECTS
digitalis leaf *(continued)*		
digitoxin Crystodigin, De-Tone, Purodigin♦	*Congestive heart failure, paroxysmal atrial tachycardia, atrial fibrillation and flutter—* **Adults:** loading dose 1.2 to 1.6 mg I.V. or P.O. in divided doses over 24 hours; maintenance 0.1 mg daily. **Children 2 to 12 years:** loading dose 0.03 mg/kg or 0.75 mg/m² I.M., I.V., or P.O. in divided doses over 24 hours; maintenance $^1/_{10}$ loading dose or 0.003 mg/kg or 0.075 mg/m² daily. Monitor closely for toxicity. **Children 1 to 2 years:** loading dose 0.04 mg/kg over 24 hours in divided doses; maintenance 0.004 mg/kg daily. Monitor closely for toxicity. **Infants 2 weeks to 1 year:** loading dose 0.045 mg/kg I.M., I.V., or P.O. in divided doses over 24 hours; maintenance 0.0045 mg/kg daily. Monitor closely for toxicity. **Premature infants, neonates, severely ill older infants:** loading dose 0.022 mg/kg I.M., I.V., or P.O. in divided doses over 24 hours; maintenance 0.0022 mg/kg daily. Monitor closely for toxicity.	*The following are signs of toxicity that may occur with all cardiotonic glycosides:* **CNS:** *fatigue, generalized muscle weakness, agitation, hallucinations,* headache, malaise, dizziness, vertigo, stupor, paresthesias. **CV:** *increased severity of congestive heart failure, arrhythmias (most commonly conduction disturbances with or without AV block, premature ventricular contractions, and supraventricular arrhythmias),* hypotension. *Toxic effects on heart may be life-threatening and require immediate attention.* **EENT:** *yellow-green halos around visual images, blurred vision,* light flashes, photophobia, diplopia. **GI:** *anorexia, nausea,* vomiting, diarrhea.

♦ Available in U.S. and Canada. ♦♦ Available in Canada only. All other products (no symbol) available in U.S. only. Italicized side effects are common or life-threatening.

INTERACTIONS	NURSING CONSIDERATIONS
potassium. *Parenteral calcium, thiazides:* hypercalcemia and hypomagnesemia, predisposing patient to digitalis toxicity. Monitor serum calcium and serum magnesium. *Phenylbutazone, phenobarbital, phenytoin, rifampin:* faster metabolism and shorter duration of action of digitoxin. Observe for underdigitalization.	previously irregular rhythm). Check blood pressure and obtain 12-lead EKG with these changes. • Observe eating pattern. Ask patient about nausea, vomiting, anorexia, visual disturbances, and other symptoms of toxicity. • Monitor serum potassium carefully. Take corrective action *before* hypokalemia occurs. • Digitalis leaf is a long-acting drug; watch for cumulative effects. • Withhold for 1 to 2 days before elective electrocardioversion. Adjust dosage after cardioversion. • Instruct patient and responsible family member about drug action, dosage regimen, how to take pulse, reportable signs, and follow-up plans. • Therapeutic blood levels of digitoxin (the active agent in the leaf) range from 25 to 35 ng/ml. • For more information on digitalis toxicity, see p. 262 and APPENDIX, *Drug Toxicities*.
Para-aminosalicylic acid, antacids, cholestyramine, colestipol, kaolin-pectin, neomycin: decreased absorption of oral digitoxin. Schedule doses as far as possible from oral digitoxin administration. *Amphotericin B, carbenicillin, ticarcillin, corticosteroids, and diuretics, including chlorthalidone, ethacrynic acid, furosemide, metolazone, and thiazides:* hypokalemia, predisposing patient to digitalis toxicity. Monitor serum potassium. *Parenteral calcium, thiazides:* hypercalcemia and hypomagnesemia, predisposing patient to digitalis toxicity. Monitor serum calcium and serum magnesium. *Phenylbutazone, phenobarbital, phenytoin, rifampin:* faster metabolism and shorter duration of digitoxin. Observe	• Contraindicated in presence of any digitalis-induced toxicity; ventricular fibrillation; ventricular tachycardia unless caused by congestive heart failure. Administering calcium salts to digitalized patient is contraindicated. Calcium affects cardiac contractility and excitability in much the same way that glycosides do and may lead to serious arrhythmias in digitalized patient. Use with extreme caution in patients with acute myocardial infarction, incomplete AV block, chronic constrictive pericarditis, idiopathic hypertrophic subaortic stenosis, renal insufficiency, severe pulmonary disease, hypothyroidism; and in the elderly. • Hypothyroid patients are very sensitive to cardiotonic glycosides; hyperthyroid patients may need larger doses. • Obtain baseline data (heart rate and rhythm, blood pressure, electrolytes, BUN, serum creatinine) before giving first dose. • Question patient about recent use of cardiotonic glycosides (within the previous 2 to 3 weeks) before administering a loading dose. Always divide loading dose over first 24 hours unless clinical situation indicates otherwise. • Dose is adjusted to patient's clinical condition and is monitored by serum levels of cardiotonic glycoside, calcium, potassium, magnesium, and by EKG. • Take apical-radial pulse for a full minute. Record and report to doctor any significant changes (sudden increase or decrease in rate, pulse deficit, irregular beats, and particularly regularization of a previously irregular rhythm). Check blood pressure and obtain 12-lead EKG with these changes. • Observe eating pattern. Ask patient about nausea, vomiting, anorexia, visual disturbances, and other symptoms of toxicity. • Watch closely for signs of toxicity, especially in children and the elderly. • Monitor serum potassium carefully. Take corrective action *before* hypokalemia occurs. • I.M. injection is painful; give I.V. if parenteral route is necessary. • Digitoxin is a long-acting drug; watch for cumulative effects. • Withhold for 1 to 2 days before elective electrocardioversion. Adjust dose after cardioversion. • Protect solution from light. • Instruct patient and responsible family member about drug action,

(continued on following page)

NAME	INDICATIONS & DOSAGE	SIDE EFFECTS
digitoxin *(continued)*		
digoxin Lanoxin♦, Masoxin, SK-Digoxin	*Congestive heart failure, atrial fibrillation and flutter, paroxysmal atrial tachycardia—* **Adults:** loading dose 0.5 to 1 mg I.V. or P.O. in divided doses over 24 hours; maintenance 0.125 to 0.5 mg I.V. or P.O. daily (average 0.25 mg). Larger doses are often needed for treatment of arrhythmias, depending on patient response. **Children over 2 years:** loading dose 0.04 to 0.06 mg/kg P.O. divided q 8 hours over 24 hours; I.V. loading dose 0.025 to 0.04 mg/kg; maintenance 0.02 mg/kg P.O. daily divided q 12 hours. **Infants 1 month to 2 years:** loading dose 0.06 to 0.075 mg/kg P.O. divided into three doses over 24 hours; I.V. loading dose 0.035 to 0.05 mg/kg; maintenance 0.02 to 0.025 mg/kg P.O. daily divided q 12 hours. **Neonates under 1 month:** loading dose 0.05 mg/kg P.O. divided q 8 hours over 24 hours; I.V. loading dose 0.015 to 0.04 mg/kg; maintenance 0.0167 mg/kg P.O. daily divided q 12 hours. **Premature infants:** loading dose 0.04 mg/kg I.V. divided into 3 doses over 24 hours; maintenance 0.0133 mg/kg I.V. daily divided q 12 hours.	*The following are signs of toxicity that may occur with all cardiotonic glycosides:* **CNS:** *fatigue, generalized muscle weakness, agitation, hallucinations,* headache, malaise, dizziness, vertigo, stupor, paresthesias. **CV:** *increased severity of congestive heart failure, arrhythmias (most commonly conduction disturbances with or without AV block, premature ventricular contractions, and supraventricular arrhythmias),* hypotension. *Toxic effects on heart may be life-threatening and require immediate attention.* **EENT:** *yellow-green halos around visual images, blurred vision,* light flashes, photophobia, diplopia. **GI:** *anorexia, nausea,* vomiting, diarrhea.
gitalin Gitaligin	*Congestive heart failure, atrial fibrillation and flutter, paroxysmal atrial tachycardia—* **Adults:** loading dose 2.5 mg P.O. initially, then 0.75 mg q 6 hours until therapeutic effect is attained (not to exceed 6 mg total in 24 hours); maintenance 0.25 to 1.25 mg daily. Not recommended for children.	*The following are signs of toxicity that may occur with all cardiotonic glycosides:* **CNS:** *fatigue, generalized muscle weakness, agitation, hallucinations,* headache, malaise, dizziness, vertigo, stupor, paresthesias. **CV:** *increased severity of congestive heart failure, arrhythmias (most commonly conduction disturbances with or without AV block, premature ventricular contractions, and supraventricular*

♦ Available in U.S. and Canada. ♦♦ Available in Canada only. All other products (no symbol) available in U.S. only. Italicized side effects are common or life-threatening.

INTERACTIONS	NURSING CONSIDERATIONS
for underdigitalization.	dosage regimen, how to take pulse, reportable signs, and follow-up plans. • Do not substitute one brand for another. • Therapeutic blood levels of digitoxin range from 25 to 35 ng/ml. • For toxicity, see APPENDIX, *Drug Toxicities.*
Para-aminosalicylic acid, antacids, cholestyramine, colestipol, kaolin-pectin, neomycin: decreased absorption of oral digoxin. Schedule doses as far as possible from oral digoxin administration. *Quinidine:* increased digoxin blood levels. Monitor for toxicity. *Amphotericin B, carbenicillin, ticarcillin, corticosteroids, and diuretics, including chlorthalidone, ethacrynic acid, furosemide, metolazone, and thiazides:* hypokalemia, predisposing patient to digitalis toxicity. Monitor serum potassium. *Parenteral calcium, thiazides:* hypercalcemia and hypomagnesemia, predisposing patient to digitalis toxicity. Monitor serum calcium and serum magnesium.	• Contraindicated in presence of any digitalis-induced toxicity; ventricular fibrillation; ventricular tachycardia unless caused by congestive heart failure. Administering calcium salts to digitalized patient is contraindicated. Calcium affects cardiac contractility and excitability in much the same way that glycosides do and may lead to serious arrhythmias in digitalized patient. Use with extreme caution in patients with acute myocardial infarction, incomplete AV block, chronic constrictive pericarditis, idiopathic hypertrophic subaortic stenosis, renal insufficiency, severe pulmonary disease, hypothyroidism; and in the elderly. Dose must be reduced in renal impairment. • Hypothyroid patients are very sensitive to cardiotonic glycosides; hyperthyroid patients may need larger doses. • Obtain baseline data (heart rate and rhythm, blood pressure, electrolytes, BUN, serum creatinine) before giving first dose. • Question patient about recent use of cardiotonic glycosides (within the previous 2 to 3 weeks) before administering a loading dose. Always divide loading dose over first 24 hours unless clinical situation indicates otherwise. • Dose is adjusted to patient's clinical condition and is monitored by serum levels of cardiotonic glycoside, calcium, potassium, magnesium, and by EKG. • Take apical-radial pulse for a full minute. Record and report to doctor any significant changes (sudden increase or decrease in rate, pulse deficit, irregular beats, and particularly regularization of a previously irregular rhythm). Check blood pressure and obtain 12-lead EKG with these changes. • Observe eating pattern. Ask patient about nausea, vomiting, anorexia, visual disturbances, and other symptoms of toxicity. • Monitor serum potassium carefully. Take corrective action *before* hypokalemia occurs. • Withhold for 1 to 2 days before elective electrocardioversion. Adjust dose after cardioversion. • Instruct patient and responsible family member about drug action, dosage regimen, how to take pulse, reportable signs, and follow-up plans. • Don't substitute one brand for another. • Therapeutic blood levels of digoxin range from 0.5 to 2.5 ng/ml. • For toxicity, see APPENDIX, *Drug Toxicities.*
Para-aminosalicylic acid, antacids, cholestyramine, colestipol, kaolin-pectin, neomycin: decreased absorption of oral gitalin. Schedule doses as far as possible from oral gitalin administration. *Amphotericin B, carbenicillin, ticarcillin, corticosteroids, and*	• Contraindicated in presence of any digitalis-induced toxicity; ventricular fibrillation; ventricular tachycardia unless caused by congestive heart failure. Administering calcium salts to digitalized patient is contraindicated. Calcium affects cardiac contractility and excitability in much the same way that glycosides do and may lead to serious arrhythmias in digitalized patient. Use with extreme caution in patients with acute myocardial infarction, incomplete AV block, chronic constrictive pericarditis, idiopathic hypertrophic subaortic stenosis, renal insufficiency, severe pulmonary disease, hypothyroidism; and in the elderly. • Hypothyroid patients are very sensitive to cardiotonic glycosides; hyperthyroid patients may need larger doses. • Obtain baseline data (heart rate and rhythm, blood pressure, elec-

(continued on following page)

NAME	INDICATIONS & DOSAGE	SIDE EFFECTS
gitalin *(continued)*		*arrhythmias),* hypotension. *Toxic effects on heart may be life-threatening and require immediate attention.* **EENT:** *yellow-green halos around visual images, blurred vision,* light flashes, photophobia, diplopia. **GI:** *anorexia, nausea,* vomiting, diarrhea.
lanatoside C Cedilanid♦	*Congestive heart failure, atrial fibrillation and flutter, paroxysmal atrial tachycardia—* **Adults:** average total dose for digitalization is 10 mg P.O. given as follows: loading dose. First day, 3.5 mg; second day, 2.5 mg; third day, 2 mg; thereafter 1.5 mg per day until digitalization obtained; maintenance 0.5 to 1.5 mg daily. Not recommended for children.	*The following are signs of toxicity that may occur with all cardiotonic glycosides:* **CNS:** *fatigue, generalized muscle weakness, agitation, hallucinations,* headache, malaise, dizziness, vertigo, stupor, paresthesias. **CV:** *increased severity of congestive heart failure, arrhythmias (most commonly conduction disturbances with or without AV block, premature ventricular contractions, and supraventricular arrhythmias),* hypotension. *Toxic effects on heart may be life-threatening and require immediate attention.* **EENT:** *yellow-green halos around visual images, blurred vision,* light flashes, photophobia, diplopia. **GI:** *anorexia, nausea,* vomiting, diarrhea.

♦ Available in U.S. and Canada. ♦♦ Available in Canada only. All other products (no symbol) available in U.S. only. Italicized side effects are common or life-threatening.

INTERACTIONS	NURSING CONSIDERATIONS
diuretics, including chlorthalidone, ethacrynic acid, furosemide, metolazone, and thiazides: hypokalemia, predisposing patient to digitalis toxicity. Monitor serum potassium. *Parenteral calcium, thiazides:* hypercalcemia and hypomagnesemia, predisposing patient to digitalis toxicity. Monitor serum calcium and serum magnesium.	trolytes, BUN, serum creatinine) before giving first dose. • Question patient about recent use of cardiotonic glycosides (within the previous 2 to 3 weeks) before administering a loading dose. Always divide loading dose over first 24 hours unless clinical situation indicates otherwise. • Dose is adjusted to patient's clinical condition and is monitored by serum levels of cardiotonic glycoside, calcium, potassium, magnesium, and by EKG. • Take apical-radial pulse for a full minute. Record and report to doctor any significant changes (sudden increase or decrease in rate, pulse deficit, irregular beats, and particularly regularization of a previously irregular rhythm). Check blood pressure and obtain 12-lead EKG with these changes. • Observe eating pattern. Ask patient about nausea, vomiting, anorexia, visual disturbances, and other symptoms of toxicity. • Monitor serum potassium carefully. Take corrective action *before* hypokalemia occurs. • Gitalin is a long-acting drug; watch for cumulative effects. • Withhold for 1 to 2 days before elective electrocardioversion. Adjust dose after cardioversion. • Instruct patient and responsible family member about drug action, dosage regimen, how to take pulse, reportable signs, and follow-up plans. • For toxicity, see APPENDIX, *Drug Toxicities.*
Para-aminosalicylic acid, antacids, cholestyramine, kaolin-pectin, neomycin, colestipol: decreased absorption of digoxin formed in stomach from lanatoside C. Schedule doses as far as possible from lanatoside C administration. *Amphotericin B, carbenicillin, ticarcillin, corticosteroids, and diuretics, including chlorthalidone, ethacrynic acid, furosemide, metolazone, and thiazides:* hypokalemia, predisposing patient to digitalis toxicity. Monitor serum potassium. *Parenteral calcium, thiazides:* hypercalcemia and hypomagnesemia, predisposing patient to digitalis toxicity. Monitor serum cal-	• Contraindicated in presence of any digitalis-induced toxicity; ventricular fibrillation; ventricular tachycardia unless caused by congestive heart failure. Administering calcium salts to digitalized patient is contraindicated. Calcium affects cardiac contractility and excitability in much the same way that glycosides do and may lead to serious arrhythmias in digitalized patient. Use with extreme caution in patients with acute myocardial infarction, incomplete AV block, chronic constrictive pericarditis, idiopathic hypertrophic subaortic stenosis, renal insufficiency, severe pulmonary disease, hypothyroidism; and in the elderly. Dose should be reduced in renal impairment. • Hypothyroid patients are very sensitive to cardiotonic glycosides; hyperthyroid patients may need larger doses. • Obtain baseline data (heart rate and rhythm, blood pressure, electrolytes, BUN, serum creatinine) before giving first dose. • Question patient about recent use of cardiotonic glycosides (within the previous 2 to 3 weeks) before administering a loading dose. Always divide loading dose over first 24 hours unless clinical situation indicates otherwise. • Dose is adjusted to patient's clinical condition and is monitored by serum levels of cardiotonic glycoside, calcium, potassium, magnesium, and by EKG. • Take apical-radial pulse for a full minute. Record and report to doctor any significant changes (sudden increase or decrease in rate, pulse deficit, irregular beats, and particularly regularization of a previously irregular rhythm). Check blood pressure and obtain 12-lead EKG with these changes. • Observe eating pattern. Ask patient about nausea, vomiting, anorexia, visual disturbances, and other symptoms of toxicity. • Monitor serum potassium carefully. Take corrective action *before* hypokalemia occurs. • Withhold for 1 to 2 days before elective electrocardioversion. Adjust dose after cardioversion.

(continued on following page)

NAME	INDICATIONS & DOSAGE	SIDE EFFECTS
lanatoside C *(continued)*		
ouabain	*Congestive heart failure, atrial fibrillation and flutter, paroxysmal atrial tachycardia—* **Adults:** loading dose 0.25 to 0.5 mg by slow I.V. injection. Additional 0.1 mg doses may be given every hour until a therapeutic effect is achieved or a total of 1 mg is given. For maintenance, use another glycoside. Not recommended for children.	*The following are signs of toxicity that may occur with all cardiotonic glycosides:* **CNS:** *fatigue, generalized muscle weakness, agitation, hallucinations,* headache, malaise, dizziness, vertigo, stupor, paresthesias. **CV:** *increased severity of congestive heart failure, arrhythmias (most commonly conduction disturbances with or without AV block, premature ventricular contractions, and supraventricular arrhythmias),* hypotension. *Toxic effects on heart may be life-threatening and require immediate attention.* **EENT:** *yellow-green halos around visual images, blurred vision,* light flashes, photophobia, diplopia. **GI:** *anorexia, nausea,* vomiting, diarrhea.

◆ Available in U.S. and Canada. ◆◆ Available in Canada only. All other products (no symbol) available in U.S. only. Italicized side effects are common or life-threatening.

INTERACTIONS	NURSING CONSIDERATIONS
cium and serum magnesium.	• Instruct patient and responsible family member about drug action, dosage regimen, how to take pulse, reportable signs, and follow-up plans. • For toxicity, see APPENDIX, *Drug Toxicities.*
Amphotericin B, carbenicillin, ticarcillin, corticosteroids, and diuretics, including chlorthalidone, ethacrynic acid, furosemide, metolazone, and thiazides: hypokalemia, predisposing patient to toxicity. Monitor serum potassium. *Parenteral calcium, thiazides:* hypercalcemia and hypomagnesemia, predisposing patient to toxicity. Monitor serum calcium and serum magnesium.	• Contraindicated in presence of any digitalis-induced toxicity; ventricular fibrillation; ventricular tachycardia unless caused by congestive heart failure. Administering calcium salts to digitalized patient is contraindicated. Calcium affects cardiac contractility and excitability in much the same way that glycosides do and may lead to serious arrhythmias in digitalized patient. Use with extreme caution in patients with acute myocardial infarction, incomplete AV block, chronic constrictive pericarditis, idiopathic hypertrophic subaortic stenosis, renal insufficiency, severe pulmonary disease, hypothyroidism; and in the elderly. Dose should be reduced in renal impairment. • Hypothyroid patients are very sensitive to cardiotonic glycosides; hyperthyroid patients may need larger doses. • Obtain baseline data (heart rate and rhythm, blood pressure, electrolytes, BUN, serum creatinine) before giving first dose. • Question patient about recent use of cardiotonic glycosides (within the previous 2 to 3 weeks) before administering a loading dose. Always divide loading dose over first 24 hours unless clinical situation indicates otherwise. • Use only for rapid digitalization, not maintenance. • Dose is adjusted to patient's clinical condition and is monitored by serum levels of cardiotonic glycoside, calcium, potassium, magnesium, and by EKG. • Take apical-radial pulse for a full minute. Record and report to doctor any significant changes (sudden increase or decrease in rate, pulse deficit, irregular beats, and particularly regularization of a previously irregular rhythm). Check blood pressure and obtain 12-lead EKG with these changes. • Observe eating pattern. Ask patient about nausea, vomiting, anorexia, visual disturbances, and other symptoms of toxicity. • I.M. route is painful; absorption is unpredictable. Not recommended. • Monitor serum potassium carefully. Take corrective action *before* hypokalemia occurs. • For toxicity, see APPENDIX, *Drug Toxicities.*

21 Antiarrhythmics

atropine sulfate
bretylium tosylate
disopyramide
disopyramide phosphate
lidocaine hydrochloride
phenytoin
phenytoin sodium
procainamide hydrochloride
propranolol hydrochloride
quinidine bisulfate
quinidine gluconate
quinidine polygalacturonate
quinidine sulfate
verapamil

For information on nifedipine, see APPENDIX, *New Drugs*.

Antiarrhythmics are used to prevent or treat atrial and ventricular arrhythmias, including those secondary to myocardial infarction (MI) or digitalis toxicity.

Bradycardia can be due to decreased generation of atrial impulses or to conduction of fewer atrial impulses to the ventricles. Similarly, ventricular tachycardia can develop from an increased number of impulses from either atrial or ventricular areas.

As a group, the antiarrhythmics have a narrow therapeutic index (the toxic dose is not much greater than the therapeutic dose). Careful monitoring of therapy is imperative, since side effects of these drugs are usually serious.

Before therapy begins, underlying conditions, such as electrolyte imbalances should be corrected.

If drug therapy fails, synchronized cardioversion and electrical pacemakers are effective antiarrhythmic alternatives.

Major uses

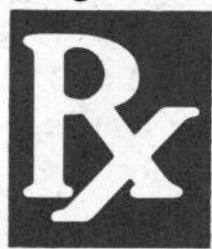

Antiarrhythmics are therapeutic for atrial and ventricular arrhythmias of various causes. They're both prophylactic and therapeutic for post-MI arrhythmias.

Verapamil represents a new class of antiarrhythmic agents called *calcium antagonists* or slow channel blockers. Verapamil is effective in managing supraventricular arrhythmias, premature ventricular beats, and Prinzmetal's angina. The overall incidence of side effects has been lower with the calcium antagonists than with conventional antiarrhythmics.

Mechanism of action

• Group I drugs (disopyramide, procainamide, and quinidine) decrease sodium transport through cardiac tissues, slowing conduction through the atrioventricular (AV) node. These drugs also prolong the effective refractory period and decrease automaticity.

• Group II drugs (lidocaine and phenytoin) increase conduction block against reentry impulses, but have little effect on conduction velocity. They stabilize reentry ventricular arrhythmias associated with MI; phenytoin may also combat arrhythmias due to digitalis toxicity.

• Group III drugs (beta blockers) decrease conduction of impulses through

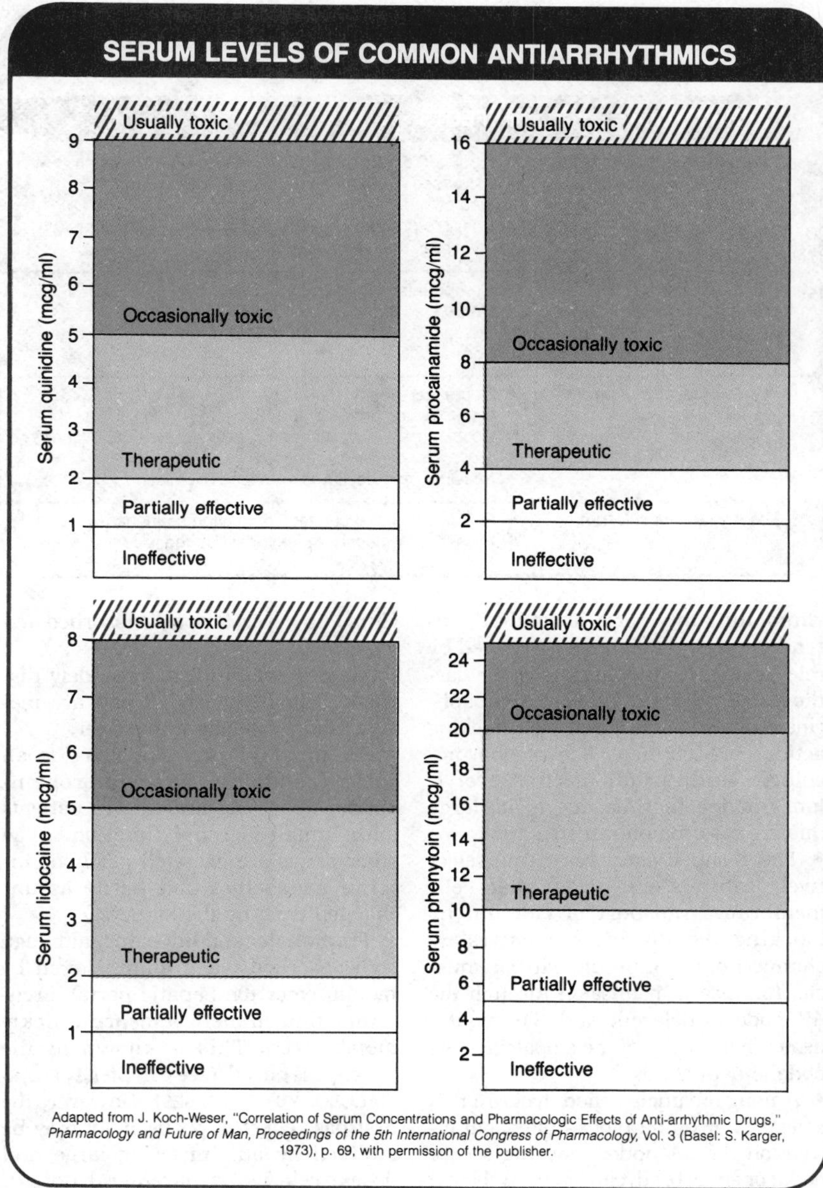

Adapted from J. Koch-Weser, "Correlation of Serum Concentrations and Pharmacologic Effects of Anti-arrhythmic Drugs," *Pharmacology and Future of Man, Proceedings of the 5th International Congress of Pharmacology,* Vol. 3 (Basel: S. Karger, 1973), p. 69, with permission of the publisher.

the AV node and increase the effective refractory period. In addition to their beta blockade, group III drugs also have reentry blocking effects similar to those of group II. Propranolol, the only beta blocker approved for use as an antiarrhythmic, is effective for supraventricular arrhythmias and, to a lesser extent, for ventricular arrhythmias.

• The group IV drug bretylium was originally thought to act as an antiadrenergic agent whose action is mediated through the sympathetic division of the autonomic nervous system. Bret-

HOW ARRHYTHMIAS AFFECT THE CARDIOVASCULAR SYSTEM

ARRHYTHMIA	EFFECTS
Paroxysmal tachycardia	• Reduced cardiac output, with associated symptoms • Increased oxygen demands on myocardium • Decreased coronary blood supply • Possible progression to atrial fibrillation, ventricular tachycardia, and ventricular fibrillation
Atrial fibrillation with rapid ventricular response	• Compromised cardiac output • Decreased coronary blood supply • Increased oxygen consumption • Loss of "atrial kick"
Ventricular tachycardia	• Decreased ventricular filling • Rapid fall in cardiac output • Development of dyspnea, angina, hypotension, oliguria, syncope • Possible progression to ventricular fibrillation
Ventricular fibrillation	• Failure of normal cardiac contraction sequence • Loss of consciousness, seizures, apnea, death

ylium initially exerts short-lived adrenergic stimulatory effects (caused by release of norepinephrine) on the cardiovascular system. When norepinephrine is depleted, the adrenergic blocking actions predominate. Recent pharmacologic studies indicate that bretylium's action may be due to its large quaternary ammonium structure.

• The group V agent verapamil selectively inhibits the myocardial cell-membrane transport of calcium by blocking the inward current (slow channel) of calcium into cardiac muscle. Impulse transmission through the AV node is delayed, and the spontaneous rhythmicity of the sinoatrial (SA) node is depressed.

• Among the unclassified drugs in this category, atropine blocks the vagal effects on the SA node, relieving severe nodal or sinus bradycardia, or AV block. Increased conduction through the AV node speeds heart rate.

Absorption, distribution, metabolism, and excretion

After oral administration, most antiarrhythmic drugs are well absorbed from the gastrointestinal tract. Bretylium, however, is poorly absorbed and must be given parenterally.

All antiarrhythmics are widely distributed in body tissues and are metabolized primarily in the liver.

• Procainamide is metabolized to an active metabolite, N-acetylprocainamide, which accumulates in patients with impaired renal function. (The other drugs are excreted partly as inactive metabolites and partly as unchanged drug by the kidneys.)

• Propranolol and lidocaine, although well absorbed when administered by mouth, enter the hepatic portal circulation immediately and are quickly metabolized. This is known as the "first-pass effect" (see Chapter 1, PHARMACOLOGY FOR NURSES). However, the first-pass effect of propranolol may be nullified by administering large oral doses (relative to parenteral doses). Therefore, propranolol is commonly used both orally and parenterally.

Onset and duration

See chart on opposite page.

Combination products

None.

THERAPEUTIC ACTIVITY

THERAPEUTIC ACTIVITY OF ANTIARRHYTHMICS

DRUG	ROUTE OF ADMINIS-TRATION	ONSET	PEAK	DURATION	THERA-PEUTIC BLOOD LEVELS
atropine	I.V.	immediate	within minutes	4 to 6 hr	†
bretylium	I.M.	up to 2 hr	6 to 9 hr	up to 10 hr	†
	I.V.	within minutes	within 20 min	up to 10 hr	†
disopyramide	P.O.	30 min	2 hr	6 to 8 hr	3 to 8 mcg/ml
lidocaine	I.M.	5 to 15 min	20 to 30 min	60 to 90 min	2 to 5 mcg/ml
	I.V.	immediate	immediate (after I.V. bolus)	10 to 20 min	2 to 5 mcg/ml
phenytoin	I.V.	immediate	immediate	up to 24 hr	10 to 20 mcg/ml
	P.O.	2 hr	6 hr	up to 24 hr	10 to 20 mcg/ml
procainamide	I.V.	immediate	25 to 60 min	3 to 4 hr	4 to 8 mcg/ml*
	P.O.	30 min	1 hr	3 to 4 hr	4 to 8 mcg/ml*
propranolol	I.V.	immediate	2 to 4 hr	3 to 6 hr	†
	P.O.	30 min	60 to 90 min	3 to 6 hr	†
quinidine	I.M.	30 min	30 to 90 min	6 to 8 hr	2 to 5 mcg/ml
	I.V.	30 min	immediate	6 to 8 hr	2 to 5 mcg/ml
	P.O.	30 min	1 to 3 hr	6 to 8 hr	2 to 5 mcg/ml
verapamil	I.V.	immediate	3 to 5 min	10 to 20 min	†

*N-acetylprocainamide (active metabolite of procainamide): 2 to 8 mcg/ml
† Not established

NAME	INDICATIONS & DOSAGE	SIDE EFFECTS
atropine sulfate	*Bradycardia, bradyarrhythmia (junctional or escape rhythm)*— **Adults:** usually 0.5 to 1 mg I.V. push; repeat q 5 minutes, to maximum 2 mg. Lower doses (less than 0.5 mg) can cause bradycardia. **Children:** 0.01 mg/kg dose up to maximum 0.4 mg; or 0.3 mg/m² dose; may repeat q 4 to 6 hours.	**Blood:** leukocytosis. **CNS:** *with doses greater than 5 mg— headache, restlessness,* ataxia, disorientation, hallucinations, delirium, coma, *insomnia, dizziness.* **CV:** *1 to 2 mg—tachycardia, palpitations; greater than 2 mg—extreme tachycardia, angina.* **EENT:** *1 mg—slight mydriasis,* photophobia; *2 mg—blurred vision, mydriasis.* **GI:** *dry mouth (common even at low doses),* thirst, *constipation,* nausea, vomiting. **GU:** *urinary retention.* **Skin:** 2 mg—flushed, dry skin; 5 mg or more—hot, dry, reddened skin.
bretylium tosylate Bretylol	*Ventricular fibrillation*— **Adults:** 5 mg/kg by rapid I.V. injection. If necessary, increase dose to 10 mg/kg and repeat q 15 to 30 minutes until 30 mg/kg have been given. *Other ventricular arrhythmias*— **Adults:** initially, 500 mg diluted to 50 ml with 5% dextrose in water or normal saline solution and infused I.V. over more than 8 minutes at 5 to 10 mg/kg. Dose may be repeated in 1 to 2 hours. Thereafter, dose q 6 to 8 hours. *I.V. maintenance*— **Adults:** infused in diluted solution of 500 ml 5% dextrose in water or normal saline solution at 1 to 2 mg/minute. *I.M. injection*— **Adults:** 5 to 10 mg/kg undiluted. Repeat in 1 to 2 hours if needed. Thereafter, repeat q 6 to 8 hours. Not recommended for children.	**CNS:** *vertigo, dizziness, lightheadedness, syncope* (usually secondary to hypotension). **CV:** *severe hypotension (especially orthostatic), bradycardia,* anginal pain. **GI:** severe nausea, vomiting (with rapid infusion).
disopyramide Rythmodan♦ **disopyramide phosphate** Norpace♦	*Premature ventricular contractions (unifocal, multifocal, or coupled); ventricular tachycardia not severe enough to require electrocardioversion*— **Adults:** Usual maintenance dose 150 to 200 mg P.O. q 6 hours; for patients who weigh less than 50 kg or those with renal, hepatic, or cardiac impairment—100 mg P.O. q 6 hours.	**CNS:** dizziness, fatigue, muscle weakness, syncope. **CV:** *hypotension, congestive heart failure, heart block.* **EENT:** *blurred vision, dry eyes, dry nose.* **GI:** nausea, vomiting, anorexia, bloating, abdominal pain, *constipation, dry mouth.* **GU:** *urinary retention, hesitancy.* **Hepatic:** cholestatic jaundice.

INTERACTIONS	NURSING CONSIDERATIONS
Methotrimeprazine: may produce extrapyramidal symptoms. Monitor patient carefully.	• Side effects vary considerably with dose. Most common are dry mouth (which can be treated with pilocarpine syrup) and thirst. Recommend sucking sour hard candy. • Watch for tachycardia in cardiac patients; report to doctor. • Antidote for atropine overdose is physostigmine salicylate. • Other anticholinergic drugs may increase vagal blockage. • For toxicity, see APPENDIX, *Drug Toxicities*.
All antihypertensives: may potentiate hypotension. Monitor blood pressure.	• Contraindicated in digitalis-induced arrhythmias. Use cautiously in patients with fixed cardiac output, aortic stenosis, and pulmonary hypertension to avoid severe and sudden drop in blood pressure. • Monitor blood pressure, heart rate and rhythm frequently. Notify doctor immediately of any change. If supine systolic blood pressure falls below 75 mm Hg, notify doctor, who may order norepinephrine or dopamine, or volume expansion to raise blood pressure. • Keep patient supine until tolerance to hypotension develops. • Follow dosage directions carefully to avoid nausea and vomiting. • Give I.V. injections for ventricular fibrillation as rapidly as possible. Do not dilute. • Rotate I.M. injection sites to prevent tissue damage, and don't exceed 5-ml volume. • To be used with other cardioresuscitative measures. • Avoid subtherapeutic doses (less than 5 mg/kg), since such doses may cause hypotension. • Ventricular tachycardia and other ventricular arrhythmias respond less rapidly to treatment than ventricular fibrillation does. • Dosage should be decreased in renal impairment. • Monitor carefully if pressor amines (sympathomimetics) are given to correct hypotension, as bretylium potentiates pressor amines. • Not first-line therapy; used for refractory arrhythmias only. Ineffective treatment for atrial arrhythmias. • Has been used investigationally to treat hypertension. • Observe for increased anginal pain in susceptible patients. • Observe patient for side effects and notify doctor if any occur.
None significant.	• Contraindicated in cardiogenic shock or second- or third-degree heart block with no pacemaker. Use cautiously in congestive heart failure, underlying conduction abnormalities, urinary tract diseases (especially prostatic hypertrophy), hepatic or renal impairment, myasthenia gravis, narrow-angle glaucoma. Adjust dosage in renal insufficiency. • Discontinue if heart block develops, if QRS complex widens by more than 25%, or if Q-T interval lengthens by more than 25% above baseline. • Correct any underlying electrolyte abnormalities before use. • Watch for recurrence of arrhythmias; check for side effects; notify

(continued on following page)

NAME	INDICATIONS & DOSAGE	SIDE EFFECTS
disopyramide *(continued)*	**Recommended doses in advanced renal insufficiency: Creatinine clearance 15 to 40 ml/ minute: 100 mg q 10 hours; creatinine clearance 5 to 15 ml/ minute: 100 mg q 20 hours; creatinine clearance 1 to 5 ml/minute: 100 mg q 30 hours.**	**Skin:** rash in 1% to 3% of patients.
lidocaine hydrochloride Lido Pen Auto-Injector, Xylocaine♦	*Ventricular arrhythmias from myocardial infarction, cardiac manipulation, or cardiotonic glycosides; ventricular tachycardia*— **Adults:** 50 to 100 mg (1 to 1.5 mg/ kg) I.V. bolus at 25 to 50 mg/minute. Give half this amount to elderly or lightweight patients, and to those with congestive heart failure or hepatic disease. Repeat bolus q 3 to 5 minutes until arrhythmias subside or side effects develop. Don't exceed 300 mg total bolus in a 1-hour period. Simultaneously, begin constant infusion: 1 to 4 mg/minute. Use lower dose in elderly patients, those with congestive heart failure or hepatic disease, or patients who weigh less than 50 kg. After single bolus is given, repeat smaller bolus 15 to 20 minutes after start of infusion to maintain therapeutic serum level. After 24 hours continuous infusion, decrease rate by half. *I.M. administration:* 200 to 300 mg in deltoid muscle only.	**CNS:** *confusion, tremors,* lethargy, *stupor, restlessness,* slurred speech, euphoria, depression, *light-headedness,* muscle twitching, convulsions, coma. **CV:** *hypotension,* bradycardia, further arrhythmias. **EENT:** *tinnitus, blurred or double vision.* **Other:** *anaphylaxis,* soreness at injection site.
phenytoin Dilantin Infatab♦, Dilantin Pediatric **phenytoin sodium** Dantoin♦♦, Dihycon, Dilantin♦, Di-Phen, Diphenylan Sodium, EKKO, Toin Unicelles	*Ventricular arrhythmias unresponsive to lidocaine or procainamide; supraventricular and ventricular arrhythmias induced by cardiotonic glycosides*— **Adults:** loading dose 1 g P.O. divided over first 24 hours, followed by 500 mg daily for 2 days, then maintenance dose 300 mg P.O. daily; 250 mg I.V. over 5 minutes until arrhythmias subside, side effects develop, or 1 g has been given. Infusion rate should never exceed 50 mg/minute (slow I.V. push). *Alternate method:* 100 mg I.V. q 15 minutes until side effects develop, arrhythmias are controlled, or 1 g has been given. I.M. dose not recommended because of pain and erratic ab-	**Blood:** thrombocytopenia, leukopenia, *agranulocytosis, pancytopenia, lymphadenopathy,* megaloblastic anemia. **CNS:** *ataxia,* slurred speech, insomnia, headache, muscle twitching, *lethargy.* **CV:** *severe hypotension, vascular collapse (with rapid I.V. infusions greater than 50 mg/minute),* vasodilation, asystole, ventricular fibrillation, AV block. **EENT:** *nystagmus, diplopia,* blurred vision. **GI:** *gingival hyperplasia, nausea, vomiting,* constipation. **Metabolic:** hyperglycemia. **Skin:** rash (*morbilliform* most common), dermatitis (bullous, *exfoliative,* purpuric), lupus erythematosus, Stevens-Johnson

♦ Available in U.S. and Canada. ♦♦ Available in Canada only. All other products (no symbol) available in U.S. only. Italicized side effects are common or life-threatening.

INTERACTIONS	NURSING CONSIDERATIONS
	doctor. • Check apical pulse rate before administering. Notify doctor if rate is less than 60 beats per minute or more than 120 beats per minute. • Teach patient the importance of taking drug on time, exactly as prescribed. He may need to set an alarm clock for night doses. • Relieve discomfort of dry mouth by chewing gum or hard candy. • Manage constipation with proper diet or bulk laxatives. • Use of disopyramide with other antiarrhythmics may cause further myocardial depression.
Barbiturates: may decrease patient's response to lidocaine. Adjust dose. *Phenytoin:* additive cardiac depressant effects. Monitor carefully. *Procainamide:* may increase neurologic side effects. Monitor carefully.	• Contraindicated in complete or second-degree heart block. Use of lidocaine with epinephrine (for local anesthesia) to treat arrhythmias contraindicated. Use with caution in elderly patients, those with congestive heart failure, renal or hepatic disease, or patients who weigh less than 50 kg. Such patients will need a reduced dose. • Serum levels of 5 mcg/ml can indicate toxicity. • If toxic signs (dizziness) occur, stop drug at once and notify doctor. Continued infusion could lead to convulsions and coma. Give oxygen via nasal cannula, if not contraindicated. Keep oxygen and CPR equipment handy. • Patients receiving infusions must be *attended at all times.* Use an infusion pump or a microdrip system and timer for monitoring infusion precisely. Never exceed an infusion rate of 4 mg/minute, if possible. A faster rate greatly increases risk of toxicity. • Monitor patient's response, especially blood pressure, serum electrolytes, BUN, and creatinine. Notify doctor promptly if abnormalities develop. • A bolus dose not followed by infusion will have a short-lived effect. • A patient who has received lidocaine I.M. will show a sevenfold increase in serum CPK level. Such CPK originates in the skeletal muscle, not the heart. Test isoenzymes if using I.M. route. • Used investigationally to treat refractory status epilepticus. • For treatment of anaphylaxis, see inside front cover.
Alcohol, barbiturates, folic acid, loxapine succinate: monitor for decreased phenytoin activity. *Oral anticoagulants, antihistamines, chloramphenicol, diazepam, diazoxide, disulfiram, isoniazid, phenylbutazone, phenyramidol, salicylates, sulfamethizole, valproate:* monitor for increased phenytoin activity.	• Contraindicated in heart block, sinus bradycardia, Stokes-Adams attacks. Use cautiously in congestive heart failure, hepatic or renal dysfunction, elderly or debilitated patients, hypotension, myocardial insufficiency, respiratory depression. Cardiac patients on thyroid replacement therapy should be given I.V. phenytoin cautiously to prevent supraventricular tachycardia. • Administer drug slow I.V. push, not to exceed 50 mg/minute in adults. • Monitor blood pressure and EKG. Notify doctor if side effects occur. • Don't mix with 5% dextrose I.V. fluids, as crystallization will occur. Flush I.V. line with saline solution before and after administration. See Chapter 6, UNDERSTANDING INTRAVENOUS SOLUTION COMPATIBILITY. • Watch patients on phenytoin and other antiarrhythmics (disopyramide, quinidine, procainamide, propranolol) closely for signs of additive cardiac depression. • Phenytoin can be diluted in normal saline solution and infused without precipitation. Such infusions should not take longer than 1 hour. • Shake oral suspensions well to make dosage uniform. After giving suspension by nasogastric tube, flush tube with water to facilitate passage to stomach. • Avoid I.M. route of administration.

(continued on following page)

NAME	INDICATIONS & DOSAGE	SIDE EFFECTS
phenytoin *(continued)*	sorption. **Children:** 3 to 8 mg/kg P.O. or slow I.V. daily or 250 mg/m^2 daily given as single dose or divided in 2 doses.	syndrome.
procainamide hydrochloride Procan SR, Pronestyl♦, Sub-Quin	*Premature ventricular contractions, ventricular tachycardia, atrial arrhythmias unresponsive to quinidine, paroxysmal atrial tachycardia—* **Adults:** 100 mg q 5 minutes slow I.V. push, no faster than 25 to 50 mg/minute until arrhythmias disappear, side effects develop, or 1 g has been given. When arrhythmias disappear, give continuous infusion of 2 to 6 mg/minute. Usual effective dose 500 to 600 mg. If arrhythmias recur, repeat bolus as above and increase infusion rate; 0.5 to 1 g I.M. q 4 to 8 hours until oral therapy begins. *Loading dose for atrial fibrillation or paroxysmal atrial tachycardia—* **Adults:** 1 to 1.25 g P.O. If arrhythmias persist after 1 hour, give additional 750 mg. If no change occurs, give 500 mg to 1 g q 2 hours until arrhythmias disappear or side effects occur. Maintenance 0.5 to 1 g q 4 to 6 hours. *Loading dose for ventricular tachycardia—* **Adults:** 1 g P.O. Maintenance 50 mg/kg daily given at 3-hour intervals; average 250 to 500 mg q 3 hours. *Note:* Sustained-release tablet may be used for maintenance dosing in ventricular tachycardia, atrial fibrillation, and paroxysmal atrial tachycardia. Dose is 500 mg to 1 g q 6 hours.	**Blood:** thrombocytopenia, *agranulocytosis,* hemolytic anemia, *increased ANA titer.* **CNS:** hallucinations, confusion, convulsions, depression. **CV:** *severe hypotension, bradycardia,* AV block, ventricular fibrillation (after parenteral use). **GI:** *nausea, vomiting, anorexia, diarrhea, bitter taste.* **Skin:** *maculopapular rash.* **Other:** *fever, lupus erythematosus syndrome (especially after prolonged administration),* myalgia.
propranolol hydrochloride Inderal♦	*Supraventricular, ventricular, and atrial arrhythmias; tachyarrhythmias due to excessive catecholamine action during anesthesia, hyperthyroidism, and*	**CNS:** *fatigue, lethargy,* vivid dreams, hallucinations. **CV:** *bradycardia, hypotension, congestive heart failure,* peripheral vascular disease.

♦ Available in U.S. and Canada. ♦♦ Available in Canada only. All other products (no symbol) available in U.S. only. Italicized side effects are common or life-threatening.

INTERACTIONS	NURSING CONSIDERATIONS
	• Dose should be decreased in hepatic dysfunction. • Blood levels greater than 20 mcg/ml may be toxic. The difference between therapeutic and toxic levels of phenytoin in the blood is very slight. If toxic symptoms occur, draw blood to determine drug level. • Patients with uremia may require dose adjustment for stabilization. • Patients concurrently on digitoxin and phenytoin may need larger doses. • Warn patient not to drink alcohol as he may lose control of previously stable antiarrhythmic effects.
None significant.	• Contraindicated in patients with hypersensitivity to procaine and related drugs; with complete, second-, or third-degree heart block unassisted by electrical pacemaker; or with myasthenia gravis. Use with caution in congestive heart failure or other conduction disturbances, such as bundle branch block or cardiotonic glycoside intoxication, or with hepatic or renal insufficiency. • Patients receiving infusions must be *attended at all times.* Use an infusion pump or a microdrip system and timer to monitor the infusion precisely. • Monitor blood pressure and EKG continuously during I.V. administration. Watch for prolonged Q-T and Q-R intervals, heart block, or increased arrhythmias. If these occur, withhold drug, obtain rhythm strip, and notify doctor immediately. • Keep patient in supine position for I.V. administration. • Watch closely for side effects and notify doctor if they occur. Instruct patient to report fever, rash, muscle pain, diarrhea, or pleuritic chest pain. • Decrease dose in hepatic and renal dysfunction, and give over 6 hours. Half-life of procainamide is increased as much as threefold in these states. • Patient with congestive heart failure has a lower volume of distribution and can be treated with lower doses. • Positive antinuclear antibody titer common in about 60% of patients who don't have symptoms of lupus erythematosus syndrome. This response seems related to prolonged use, not dosage. • After long-standing atrial fibrillation, restoration of normal rhythm may result in thromboembolism, due to dislodgment of thrombi from atrial wall. Anticoagulation usually advised before restoration of normal sinus rhythm. • Stress importance of taking drug exactly as prescribed. Patient may need to set an alarm clock for night doses. • Serum levels of 8 mcg/ml can indicate toxicity.
Insulin, hypoglycemic drugs (oral): can alter requirements for these drugs in previously stabilized dia-	• Contraindicated in asthma or allergic rhinitis; during ethyl ether anesthesia; in sinus bradycardia and in heart block greater than first degree; in cardiogenic shock; in right ventricular failure secondary to pulmonary hypertension. Use with caution in patients with congestive heart failure, diabetes mellitus, or respiratory disease.

(continued on following page)

NAME	INDICATIONS & DOSAGE	SIDE EFFECTS
propranolol hydrochloride *(continued)*	*pheochromocytoma; angina*— **Adults:** 1 to 3 mg I.V. diluted in 50 ml 5% dextrose in water or normal saline solution infused slowly, not to exceed 1 mg/minute. After 3 mg have been infused, another dose may be given in 2 minutes; subsequent doses no sooner than q 4 hours. Maintenance 10 to 80 mg P.O. t.i.d. or q.i.d.	**GI:** nausea, vomiting, diarrhea. **Metabolic:** hypoglycemia without tachycardia. **Skin:** rash. **Other:** *increased airway resistance,* fever.
quinidine bisulfate (66% quinidine base) Biquin Durules♦♦ **quinidine gluconate** (62% quinidine base) Duraquin, Quinaglute Dura-Tabs♦, Quinate♦♦ **quinidine polygalacturonate** (60.5% quinidine base) Cardioquin♦ **quinidine sulfate** (83% quinidine base) CinQuin, Quine, Quinidex Extentabs♦, Quinora, SK-Quinidine Sulfate	*Atrial flutter or fibrillation*— **Adults:** 200 mg quinidine sulfate or equivalent base P.O. q 2 to 3 hours for 5 to 8 doses with subsequent daily increases until sinus rhythm is restored or toxic effects develop. Administer quinidine only after digitalization to avoid increasing AV block. Maximum 3 to 4 g daily. *Paroxysmal supraventricular tachycardia*— **Adults:** 400 to 600 mg I.M. gluconate q 2 to 3 hours until toxic side effects develop or arrhythmia subsides. *Premature atrial and ventricular contractions; paroxysmal atrioventricular junctional rhythm; paroxysmal atrial tachycardia; paroxysmal ventricular tachycardia; maintenance after cardioversion of atrial fibrillation or flutter*— **Adults:** test dose 50 to 200 mg P.O., then monitor vital signs before beginning therapy. Quinidine sulfate or equivalent base 200 to 400 mg P.O. q 4 to 6 hours; or initially, quinidine gluconate 600 mg I.M., then up to 400 mg q 2 hours, p.r.n.; or quinidine gluconate 800 mg I.V. diluted in 40 ml 5% dextrose in water, infused at 1 mg/minute. **Children:** test dose 2 mg/kg; 3 to 6 mg/kg q 2 to 3 hours for 5 doses P.O. daily.	**Blood:** *hemolytic anemia, thrombocytopenia, agranulocytosis.* **CNS:** *vertigo, headache, lightheadedness,* confusion, restlessness, cold sweat, pallor, fainting. **CV:** *premature ventricular contractions; severe hypotension; SA and AV block; ventricular fibrillation, tachycardia; aggravated congestive heart failure; EKG changes (particularly widening of QRS complex, notched P waves, widened Q-T interval, ST segment depression).* **EENT:** *tinnitus,* excessive salivation, blurred vision. **GI:** *diarrhea, nausea, vomiting,* anorexia, abdominal pains. **Skin:** rash, petechial hemorrhage of buccal mucosa, pruritus. **Other:** angioedema, acute asthmatic attack, respiratory arrest, *fever, cinchonism.*

♦ Available in U.S. and Canada. ♦♦ Available in Canada only. All other products (no symbol) available in U.S. only. Italicized side effects are common or life-threatening.

INTERACTIONS	NURSING CONSIDERATIONS
betics. Monitor for hypoglycemia. *Cardiotonic glycosides:* cause excessive bradycardia and increased depressant effect on myocardium. Use together cautiously. *Aminophylline:* antagonizes beta-blocking effects of propranolol. Use together cautiously. *Isoproterenol, glucagon:* antagonizes propranolol effect. May be used therapeutically and in emergencies.	• Always withdraw drug slowly. Abrupt withdrawal might precipitate myocardial infarction or aggravate angina, thyrotoxicosis, pheochromocytoma. Abrupt withdrawal in thyrotoxicosis may exacerbate hyperthyroidism or precipitate thyroid storm. In thyrotoxicosis, propranolol may mask clinical signs of hyperthyroidism. • *Don't discontinue before surgery for pheochromocytoma.* Before any surgery, notify anesthesiologist that patient's taking propranolol. • Double-check dose and route. I.V. doses much smaller than P.O. • Check apical pulse rate and blood pressure before giving drug. If you detect extremes in pulse rate, withhold drug and notify doctor at once. Severe bradycardia may be treated with atropine 0.25 to 1 mg I.V. • After long-standing atrial fibrillation, restoration of normal sinus rhythm may result in thromboembolism due to dislodgment of thrombi from atrial wall. Anticoagulation often advised before restoration of normal atrial rhythm. • Monitor blood pressure, EKG, heart rate and rhythm frequently, especially during I.V. administration. When used with other antihypertensives, monitor patient's sitting and standing blood pressures. • Auscultate patient's lungs for rales and his heart for gallop rhythm or for third or fourth heart sounds. If these develop, notify doctor at once.
Acetazolamide, antacids, sodium bicarbonate: may increase quinidine blood levels due to alkaline urine. Monitor for increased effect. *Barbiturates, phenytoin:* may antagonize quinidine activity. Monitor for decreased quinidine effect.	• Contraindicated in cardiotonic glycoside toxicity when AV conduction is grossly impaired; complete AV block with AV nodal or idioventricular pacemaker. Use with caution in myasthenia gravis. Anticholinergic drug doses may have to be increased. • May increase toxicity of digitalis derivatives. Use with caution in patients previously digitalized. Monitor digoxin levels. • Dosage varies—some patients may require drug q 4 hours, others q 6 hours. Titrate dose by both clinical response and blood levels. • When changing route of administration, alter dosage to compensate for variations in quinidine base content. • Dose should be decreased in congestive heart failure and hepatic disease. • Check apical pulse rate and blood pressure before starting therapy. If you detect extremes in pulse rate, withhold drug and notify doctor at once. • Lidocaine may be effective in treating quinidine-induced arrhythmias, since it increases AV conduction. • GI side effects, especially diarrhea, are signs of toxicity. Notify doctor. Check quinidine blood levels, which can be toxic when greater than 8 mcg/ml. GI symptoms may be decreased by giving with meals. Monitor drug response carefully. • Instruct patient to notify doctor if skin rash, fever, unusual bleeding, bruising, ringing in ears, or visual disturbance occurs. • After long-standing atrial fibrillation, restoration of normal sinus rhythm may result in thromboembolism due to dislodgment of thrombi from atrial wall. Anticoagulation often advised before restoration of normal atrial rhythm. • Never use discolored (brownish) quinidine solution.

NAME	INDICATIONS & DOSAGE	SIDE EFFECTS
verapamil Calan, Isoptin	*Treatment of atrial arrhythmias—* **Adults:** 0.075 to 0.15 mg/kg (5 to 10 mg) I.V. push over 60 seconds with EKG and blood pressure monitoring. Repeat dose in 30 minutes if no response. Follow bolus injection with maintenance infusion of 0.005 mg/kg/minute.	**CNS:** *dizziness, headache.* **CV:** *transient hypotension, heart failure,* bradycardia, AV block, ventricular asystole. **GI:** *constipation.*

♦ Available in U.S. and Canada. ♦♦ Available in Canada only. All other products (no symbol) available in U.S. only. Italicized side effects are common or life-threatening.

CALCIUM BLOCKERS: CARDIAC BREAKTHROUGH?

Verapamil and nifedipine, and the even newer diltiazem and lidoflazine, belong to the new breed of cardiac drugs—the calcium blockers. Used for several years, these drugs prevent calcium transport across the cell membrane so the cardiac muscle and the smooth muscle of the coronary arteries won't contract as forcefully.

1. Under normal conditions, a protein complex prevents muscle contraction by keeping actin and myosin (the contractile proteins) apart. Actin and myosin must interact for a muscle to contract. When the muscle cell is stimulated, calcium ions enter the cell.

This influx of calcium releases more calcium from the sarcoplasmic reticulum inside the muscle cell.

2. When enough calcium is released, it binds with the protein complex. Hence, the actin and myosin can interact and the muscle contracts.

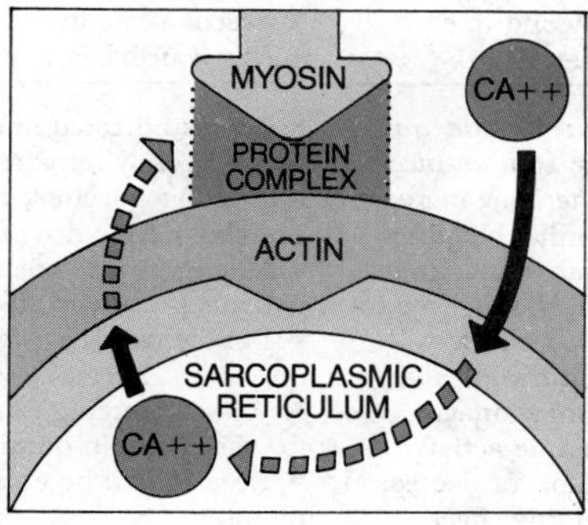

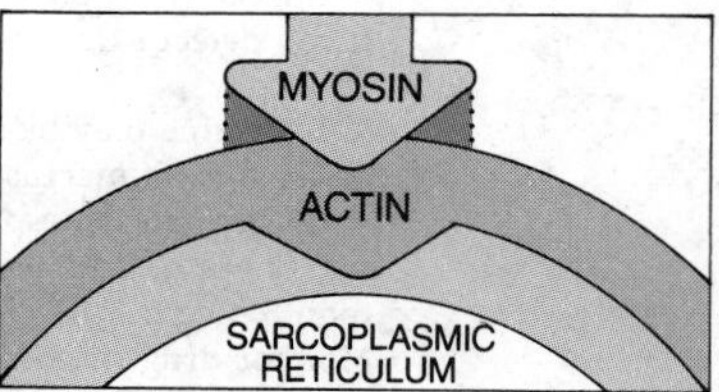

INTERACTIONS	NURSING CONSIDERATIONS
Propranolol (and other beta blockers) and disopyramide: may cause heart failure. Use together cautiously.	• Contraindicated in patients with advanced heart failure, AV block, cardiogenic shock, sinus node disease, and severe hypotension. • Use cautiously in patients with myocardial infarction followed by coronary occlusion, sick sinus syndrome, impaired AV conduction, and heart failure with atrial tachyarrhythmia. • Patients with severely compromised cardiac function or those receiving beta blockers should receive lower doses of verapamil. Monitor these patients very closely. • A new and very effective drug for treatment of supraventricular arrhythmias. Not very effective for ventricular arrhythmias. • Oral form of verapamil is investigational. Being used in treatment of both Prinzmetal's (variant) angina and classic angina pectoris.

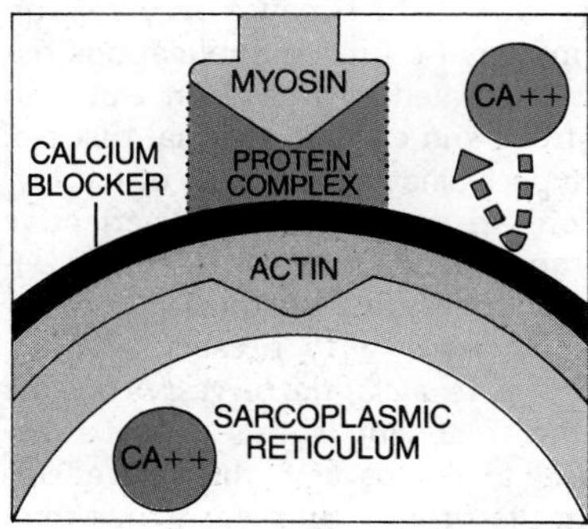

3. Calcium blockers prevent calcium from entering the cell, thereby preventing calcium release from the sarcoplasmic reticulum.

Although all the calcium blockers exert this effect on cardiac muscle, one compound may prove to be more effective for a specific heart condition than another. In general, however, calcium blockers can:

- *reduce electrical excitation and mechanical contraction of the heart.* Arrhythmias, especially those of atrial origin, can be relieved and perhaps even prevented.
- *relieve excruciating anginal pain* caused by spasms of the coronary arteries.
- *allow more rest for damaged tissue.*
- *reduce peripheral arterial resistance and myocardial oxygen demand.*

In addition, calcium blockers *present relatively mild side effects;* headache, dizziness, and constipation are the most common. Unlike beta blockers, these drugs can be used by patients with asthma and those with congestive heart failure that's not too severe.

Some researchers believe calcium blockers have several exciting potential uses, and are speculating that these drugs may eventually be used to treat high blood pressure, prevent recurrent heart attacks, limit damage from attacks, and delay or even eliminate the need for coronary bypass operations. The research continues.

22 Antihypertensives

Sympatholytics
alkavervir
alseroxylon
captopril
clonidine hydrochloride
cryptenamine acetate
cryptenamine tannate
deserpidine
guanethidine sulfate
mecamylamine hydrochloride
methyldopa
metoprolol tartrate
metyrosine
nadolol
pargyline hydrochloride
phenoxybenzamine hydrochloride
phentolamine hydrochloride
phentolamine methanesulfonate
propranolol hydrochloride
rauwolfia serpentina
rescinnamine
reserpine
trimethaphan camsylate

Vasodilators
diazoxide
hydralazine hydrochloride
minoxidil
nitroprusside sodium
prazosin hydrochloride

(All drugs are listed in alphabetical order in the tables that follow. For information on atenolol and timolol, see APPENDIX, *New Drugs*.)

Antihypertensives are used to lower blood pressure in patients whose diastolic blood pressure averages 90 to 95 mm Hg or more. To control blood pressure effectively with minimal side effects, two or more antihypertensive agents—with different modes of action—may be needed.

About 15% of adults are hypertensive. About half these people don't realize they're ill because they remain asymptomatic until complications occur. Untreated hypertension can lead to stroke and cardiac or renal disease.

Hypertension is now one of the few chronic diseases for which effective therapy exists. However, treatment depends on accurate diagnosis.

Compliance with prescribed drug regimens is one of the biggest problems in the treatment of this disorder because, to the patient, the side effects from the drugs may seem worse than the disease.

Major uses

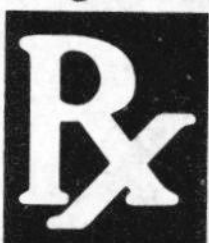

Antihypertensives are used primarily to treat mild-to-severe essential hypertension (about 90% of all cases of hypertension). Virtually all parenteral drugs are reserved for treatment of hypertensive emergencies such as hypertensive encephalopathy or malignant hypertension.

Antihypertensives can also be used to control hypertension in the 10% of patients who have secondary hypertension until a surgical cure can be obtained.

• Two alpha-blockers—phenoxybenzamine and phentolamine—and the tyrosine hydroxylase inhibitor metyrosine can be used to diagnose and manage pheochromocytoma until surgery, if feasible, can be performed.

HOW ANTIHYPERTENSIVES WORK

Sympatholytics
As their name suggests, the sympatholytics dampen the actions of the sympathetic (adrenergic) branch of the autonomic nervous system. Whereas the parasympathetic (cholinergic) system controls the body's daily functions through its chemical mediator, acetylcholine, emergency functions are taken over by the sympathetic system mediated by norepinephrine. These functions include the "fight or flight" reactions—pallor, hair standing on end, dilated pupils and bronchi, decreased gastrointestinal secretions, and conversion of glycogen to glucose, as well as increased heart rate and blood pressure.

Direct-acting vasodilators
Vasodilating drugs dilate the peripheral arterioles, which primarily control peripheral resistance. The drugs act directly on the vessel musculature, enlarging the container, so to speak, and reducing the pressure within it.

Because all vasodilators produce varying degrees of sodium and water retention, a diuretic should be given at the same time. The cardiac-stimulating effect of vasodilators may be minimized by a beta-adrenergic blocking agent, such as propranolol (Inderal).

Diuretics
Diuretics reduce blood volume by causing the excretion of fluid through the kidneys. Their main use in treating hypertension is to prevent the sodium and water retention caused by other hypotensive drugs, thereby potentiating their effect.

(For more information on these drugs, see Chapter 63, DIURETICS.)

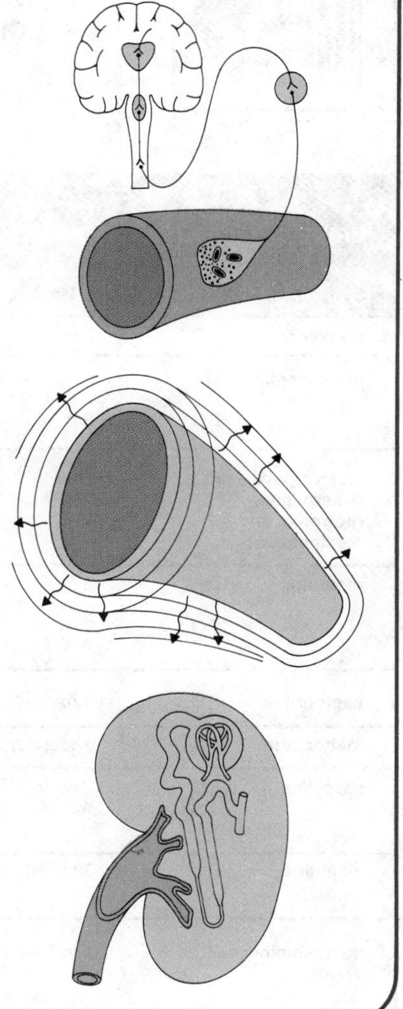

• Some vasodilating antihypertensives can also be used in chronic refractory congestive heart failure (CHF) to decrease the arterial resistance (afterload) that the heart must pump against. This decrease in arterial impedance causes an increase in cardiac output. Minoxidil and hydralazine affect mainly the arterial bed, whereas prazosin and nitroprusside affect both the arterial and venous sides.

A vasodilator affecting the arterial bed (afterload) may be used alone or in combination with a nitrate affecting the venous bed (preload) to treat refractory CHF. Preload and afterload agents are used in combination with standard therapy for CHF (salt reduc-

THERAPEUTIC ACTIVITY

THERAPEUTIC ACTIVITY OF ANTIHYPERTENSIVES

DRUG	ROUTE	ONSET	DURATION	SITE AND MECHANISM OF ACTION
Sympatholytics				
alkavervir	P.O.	2 hr	4 to 6 hr	Veratrum alkaloids; alkavervir and cryptenamine stimulate pressor receptors in the heart and the carotid sinus.
cryptenamine	I.M. I.V. P.O.	30 to 40 min 2 to 3 min 2 hr	3 to 6 hr 1 to 2 hr 4 to 6 hr	
alseroxylon, deserpidine, rauwolfia, and rescinnamine	P.O.	days to weeks	days	Peripherally acting antihypertensives; they deplete stores of norepinephrine by inhibiting its uptake.
reserpine	I.M. I.V. P.O.	2 hr 4 to 60 min days to weeks	10 to 12 hr 6 to 8 hr days	
captopril	P.O.	1 hr	6 to 12 hr	Enzyme inhibitors; captopril inhibits angiotensin-converting enzyme and prevents conversion of angiotensin I to angiotensin II in the lungs: metyrosine inhibits tyrosine hydroxylase; and pargyline inhibits monoamine oxidase.
metyrosine	P.O.	1 to 2 days	3 to 4 days	
pargyline	P.O.	days to weeks	weeks	
clonidine	P.O.	30 to 60 min	8 hr	Centrally acting drug: decreases central sympathetic outflow.
guanethidine	P.O.	1 to 3 wk	1 to 3 wk	Peripherally acting drug; directly inhibits release of norepinephrine and depletes stores of norepinephrine in adrenergic nerve endings.
mecamylamine	P.O.	½ to 2 hr	6 to 12 hr	Ganglionic blockers; mecamylamine competes with acetylcholine for cholinergic receptors; trimethanphan stabilizes postsynaptic membranes.
trimethaphan	I.V.	immediate	10 min after infusion is stopped	

DRUG	ROUTE	ONSET	DURATION	SITE AND MECHANISM OF ACTION
methyldopa	I.V. P.O.	4 to 6 hr 12 to 24 hr	24 to 48 hr 24 to 48 hr	Centrally acting drug; activates inhibitory alpha-adrenergic receptors, reducing central sympathetic output.
metoprolol	P.O.	days to weeks*	12 to 24 hr	Beta blockers: all three drugs block response to beta stimulation; they also depress renin output.
nadolol	P.O.	days to weeks*	24 to 36 hr	
propranolol	I.V. P.O.	1 to 5 min days to weeks*	4 to 6 hr 12 to 24 hr	
phenoxybenzamine	P.O.	up to 4 days*	24 to 36 hr	Alpha blockers; both drugs competitively inhibit alpha-adrenergic receptors.
phentolamine	I.M. I.V. P.O.	2 to 5 min 30 to 60 sec up to 4 days*	30 to 45 min 15 to 30 min 24 to 36 hr	
Vasodilators				
diazoxide	I.V.	5 min	3 to 12 hr	Directly relaxes arteriolar smooth muscle.
hydralazine	I.M. I.V. P.O.	10 to 30 min 5 to 20 min 20 to 30 min	2 to 6 hr 2 to 6 hr 3 to 8 hr†	
minoxidil	P.O.	30 min	24 hr	Directly relaxes arteriolar smooth muscle.
nitroprusside	I.V.	immediate	1 to 10 min after infusion is stopped (effect dissipates rapidly)	Relaxes both arteriolar and venous smooth muscle.
prazosin	P.O.	2 hr	less than 24 hr	Relaxes both arteriolar and venous smooth muscle.

* Depending on dosage
† Depending on acetylator status

NURSING TIPS

ADMINISTERING DRUGS FOR HYPERTENSIVE CRISIS: TWO RULES

When administering antihypertensives, keep in mind these basic rules:

1. Before giving a drug, check its *dosage.* Then, check the patient's *blood pressure.* Even if you've checked the pressure routinely 5 minutes before, check it again *immediately* before giving the medication.

Also check blood pressure after giving the drug—how often depends on the drug used. For example, with nitroprusside sodium (Nipride) or trimethaphan camsylate (Arfonad), check blood pressure every 5 to 10 minutes; with hydralazine hydrochloride (Apresoline) or methyldopa (Aldomet), check less frequently, say every hour.

2. Watch I.V. infusions of antihypertensive medications. Be sure the I.V. site is always patent. Letting an I.V. infiltrate for even a short time can have disastrous effects, especially when you're using drugs with rapid onset, such as Nipride.

When using an infusion pump, be sure it's operating optimally at all times. Its failure can either give the patient a bolus of the drug—risking hypotension—or prevent him from receiving the dosage he needs.

tion, diuretics, and digoxin) to achieve maximal results. For further discussion of this type of treatment, see Chapter 23, VASODILATORS.

Mechanism of action

The chart on pp. 290 to 291 summarizes the neuromuscular and enzymatic mechanisms of the major classes of antihypertensive agents. (See Chapter 63, DIURETICS, for more information on the diuretic effects of the antihypertensives.)

Absorption, distribution, metabolism, and excretion

Given orally, most antihypertensives are rapidly absorbed from the gastrointestinal (GI) tract. Alkavervir and methyldopa, however, are erratically absorbed.

All antihypertensives are widely distributed in body tissues, and most are excreted predominately through the kidneys. Prazosin, however, is eliminated through bile and feces.

• Captopril: This drug is well absorbed from the GI tract, distributed to most body tissues, and partially metabolized in the liver. Both metabolite and unchanged drug are excreted in the urine.

• Hydralazine: Some patients acetylate (metabolize) hydralazine at a faster rate than others (see chart). Since acetylation inactivates the drug, rapid acetylators may require doses up to 60% larger than the usual dose to control their blood pressure.

• Methyldopa: The extent of methyldopa absorption varies in patients from day to day but averages 50% of the administered dose. The drug's onset is delayed about 12 to 24 hours after an oral dose because methyldopa is biotransformed in the liver to the metabolite alpha-methylnorepinephrine, which produces the antihypertensive effect.

Onset and duration

The chart on pp. 290 to 291 describes the onset and duration of antihypertensives.

Combination products

ALDOCLOR-150: chlorothiazide 150 mg and methyldopa 250 mg.
ALDOCLOR-250: chlorothiazide 250 mg and methyldopa 250 mg.
ALDORIL-15♦: hydrochlorothiazide 15 mg and methyldopa 250 mg.
ALDORIL-25♦: hydrochlorothiazide 25 mg and methyldopa 250 mg.
ALDORIL D30: hydrochlorothiazide 30 mg and methyldopa 500 mg.
ALDORIL D50: hydrochlorothiazide 50 mg and methyldopa 500 mg.
APRESAZIDE 25/25: hydrochlorothiazide 25 mg and hydralazine HCl 25 mg.
APRESAZIDE 50/50: hydrochlorothiazide 50 mg and hydralazine HCl 50 mg.
APRESAZIDE 100/50: hydrochlorothia-

zide 50 mg and hydralazine HCl 100 mg.
APRESOLINE-ESIDRIX: hydrochlorothiazide 15 mg and hydralazine HCl 25 mg.
COMBIPRES 0.1♦: chlorthalidone 15 mg and clonidine HCl 0.1 mg.
COMBIPRES 0.2: chlorthalidone 15 mg and clonidine HCl 0.2 mg.
DEMI-REGROTON: chlorthalidone 25 mg and reserpine 0.125 mg.
DIUPRES-250♦: chlorothiazide 250 mg and reserpine 0.125 mg.
DIUPRES-500: chlorothiazide 500 mg and reserpine 0.125 mg.
DIUTENSEN: methyclothiazide 2.5 mg and cryptenamine 2 mg (as tannate).
DIUTENSEN-R: methyclothiazide 2.5 mg and reserpine 0.1 mg.
ENDURONYL: methyclothiazide 5 mg and deserpidine 0.25 mg.
ENDURONYL-FORTE: methyclothiazide 5 mg and deserpidine 0.5 mg.
ESIMIL: hydrochlorothiazide 25 mg and guanethidine monosulfate 10 mg.
EUTRON FILMTABS: methyclothiazide 5 mg and pargyline HCl 25 mg.
EXNA-R TABLETS: benzthiazide 50 mg and reserpine 0.125 mg.
HYDROMOX-R: quinethazone 50 mg and reserpine 0.125 mg.
HYDROPRES-25♦: hydrochlorothiazide 25 mg and reserpine 0.125 mg.
HYDROPRES-50♦: hydrochlorothiazide 50 mg and reserpine 0.125 mg.
HYDROSERP: hydrochlorothiazide 50 mg and reserpine 0.125 mg.
HYDROTENSIN-25 TABS: hydrochlorothiazide 25 mg and reserpine 0.125 mg.
HYDROTENSIN-50: hydrochlorothiazide 50 mg and reserpine 0.125 mg.
HYSTON TABLETS: hydrochlorothiazide 15 mg and hydralazine 25 mg.
INDERIDE 40/25: propranolol HCl 40 mg and hydrochlorothiazide 25 mg.
INDERIDE 80/25: propranolol HCl 80 mg and hydrochlorothiazide 25 mg.
METATENSIN TABLETS: trichlormethiazide 2 or 4 mg and reserpine 0.1 mg.
NAQUIVAL: trichlormethiazide 4 mg and reserpine 0.1 mg.
NATURETIN W/K 2.5 mg♦: bendroflumethiazide 2.5 mg and potassium chloride 500 mg.
NATURETIN W/K 5 mg♦: bendroflumethiazide 5 mg and potassium chloride 500 mg.
ORETICYL FORTE: hydrochlorothiazide 25 mg and deserpidine 0.25 mg.
ORETICYL 25: hydrochlorothiazide 25 mg and deserpidine 0.125 mg.
ORETICYL 50: hydrochlorothiazide 50 mg and deserpidine 0.125 mg.
RAUTRAX: flumethiazide 400 mg, potassium chloride 400 mg, and powdered rauwolfia serpentina 50 mg.
RAUTRAX-N: bendroflumethiazide 4 mg, powdered rauwolfia serpentina 50 mg,

QUESTIONS & ANSWERS

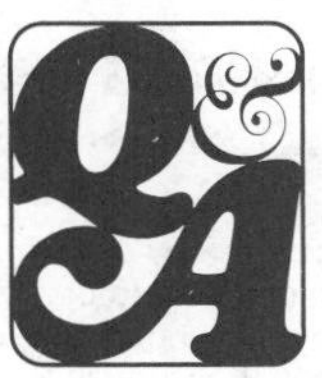

NADOLOL: A BETA BLOCKER THAT MAY INCREASE PATIENT COMPLIANCE

How will my patient benefit from nadolol?

The major advantage of nadolol is its longer half-life and duration of action. Because of this, it can be taken once a day, which may help noncompliant patients stick to their schedules. The usual starting dose is 40 mg/day; this can be increased to 320 mg/day or higher, depending on the patient's need. Nadolol is available as a 40-, 80-, or 120-mg tablet. It has no parenteral form at this time.

Is it safer than propranolol?

Most experts would *not* agree that nadolol is safer than propranolol. Basically, these drugs share the same side effects and precautions, including the contraindication for patients with asthma (since the drugs block the beta receptors of the bronchi and the myocardium). And both drugs must be used cautiously in patients with diabetes or congestive heart failure.

Nadolol's long half-life may present an added problem—drug toxicity. Your first indication of toxicity is the development of bradycardia. Be especially watchful of patients with poor renal function; nadolol is excreted unchanged by the kidneys.

UNDERSTANDING THE STEPPED-CARE APPROACH TO ANTIHYPERTENSIVE THERAPY

In this cumulative drug therapy plan, you'll see progression from one step to the next when the already prescribed drug or drugs don't lower blood pressure sufficiently. Before proceeding to the next step, however, reasons other than drug failure must be ruled out. These include:

- poor patient compliance
- excessive sodium intake or retention
- use of vasoconstricting drugs, including those in some cold remedies
- secondary hypertension.

SUMMARY OF THE STEPPED-CARE APPROACH

Step 1
Therapy should be initiated with less than the maximum dose of a thiazide-type diuretic and increased to the maximum dose, as required.

Step 2
If blood pressure isn't controlled with the diuretic alone, a sympathetic inhibitor is added. The drug chosen should be administered in small doses and increased gradually until the therapeutic effect has been achieved, the maximum dose has been reached, or side effects appear.

Step 3
If a third drug is needed, hydralazine—an effective peripheral vasodilator—may be added. It is used in combination with the sympathetic inhibitor (step 2) and the diuretic (step 1).

Step 4
If the first three steps of the stepped-care plan are ineffective and reasons other than drug failure have been ruled out, guanethidine, minoxidil, or captopril may be added in increasing doses as needed or substituted for one of the drugs in step 2 or step 3.

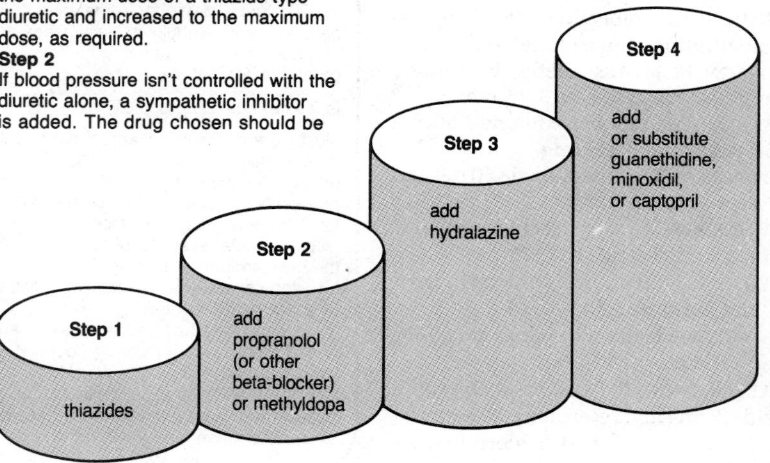

Adapted with permission from Sydney Kofman, *The Nurse's Role in the Care of Patients with Primary Hypertension, Book II: A Programmed Learning Course on Treatment and Compliance* (Northfield, Ill.: SPAN Publications, Inc., 1978).

and potassium chloride 400 mg.
RAUTRAX-N MODIFIED: bendroflumethiazide 5 mg, potassium chloride 40 mg and powdered rauwolfia serpentina 50 mg.
RAUZIDE: bendroflumethiazide 4 mg and powdered rauwolfia serpentina 50 mg.
REGROTON: chlorthalidone 50 mg and reserpine 0.25 mg.
RENESE-R: polythiazide 2 mg and reserpine 0.25 mg.
SALUTENSIN♦: hydroflumethiazide 50 mg and reserpine 0.125 mg.
SALUTENSIN DEMI: hydroflumethiazide 25 mg and reserpine 0.125 mg.
SER-AP-ES♦: hydrochlorothiazide 15 mg, reserpine 0.1 mg, and hydral-

NURSING TIPS

CHECKING FOR HYPERTENSION? FOLLOW THESE NEW RECOMMENDATIONS

You'll probably be performing more blood pressure checks and seeing more drug therapy for patients with mild hypertension.

Why? Doctors are beginning to implement 1980 recommendations of the National Institutes of Health (NIH) Joint National Committee on Detection, Evaluation, and Treatment of High Blood Pressure. These recommendations update those issued in 1977. Since then, NIH received results of a massive clinical study showing that early detection and treatment of mild hypertension can reduce mortality and morbidity.

According to the 1977 recommendations, hypertension therapy was indicated only for patients with diastolic blood pressures of 105 mm Hg or higher. *The new recommendations indicate that all adults with diastolic blood pressure of 95 mm Hg or higher on first screening should have the elevation confirmed promptly.* (For office-based nurses, "promptly" means within 1 month.)

A hospitalized patient with a diastolic blood pressure of 90 to 95 mm Hg should be periodically checked until he's discharged. Within 3 months after discharge, the patient's blood pressure should be checked again during an office visit.

According to NIH recommendations, *a diastolic reading of 115 mm Hg or higher warrants immediate referral.* This contrasts with the 1977 reading of 120 mm Hg.

The earlier recommendations didn't mention nondrug hypertension therapies. However, the update suggests that dietary management—weight control and sodium restriction—be used as an adjunct to drug therapy.

azine HCl 25 mg.
SERPASIL-APRESOLINE #1: reserpine 0.1 mg and hydralazine HCl 25 mg.
SERPASIL-APRESOLINE #2♦: reserpine 0.2 mg and hydralazine HCl 50 mg.
SERPASIL-ESIDRIX #1♦: hydrochlorothiazide 25 mg and reserpine 0.1 mg (called Serpasil-Esidrix 25 in Canada).
SERPASIL-ESIDRIX #2♦: hydrochlorothiazide 50 mg and reserpine 0.1 mg (called Serpasil-Esidrix 50 in Canada).
THIASERP-250: chlorothiazide 250 mg and reserpine 0.125 mg.
UNIPRES: hydrochlorothiazide 15 mg, reserpine 0.1 mg, and hydralazine HCl 25 mg.

NAME	INDICATIONS & DOSAGE	SIDE EFFECTS
alkavervir Veriloid	*Essential, renal, or malignant hypertension; toxemia of pregnancy*— **Adults:** 3 to 5 mg P.O. daily, given in 3 to 4 divided doses not less than 4 hours apart. Give after meals. Initial recommended dose is 8 to 9 mg. No dosing recommendations for children.	**CNS:** mental confusion. **CV:** *orthostatic hypotension,* cardiac arrhythmias, *bradycardia.* **EENT:** blurred vision, excessive salivation, unpleasant taste. **GI:** *nausea, vomiting,* epigastric burning, hiccups. **Other:** respiratory depression, bronchial constriction, sweating.
alseroxylon Raudolfin, Rauwiloid	*Mild, labile hypertension*— **Adults:** initially, 4 mg P.O. daily as a single dose or divided in 2 doses for 1 to 3 weeks. Maintenance dose: 2 mg or less daily. No dosing recommendations for children.	**CNS:** mental confusion, *depression, drowsiness, nervousness, anxiety,* insomnia, *nightmares,* sedation. **CV:** *orthostatic hypotension, bradycardia.* **EENT:** *mouth dryness, nasal stuffiness,* glaucoma. **GI:** *hypersecretion of gastric acid, nausea, vomiting,* gastrointestinal bleeding. **Skin:** pruritus, rash. **Other:** *impotence, weight gain.*
captopril Capoten	*Treatment of severe hypertension*— **Adults:** 25 mg t.i.d. initially. If blood pressure isn't satisfactorily controlled in 1 to 2 weeks, dose may be increased to 50 mg t.i.d. If not satisfactorily controlled after another 1 to 2 weeks, a diuretic should be added to regimen. If further blood pressure reduction is necessary, dose may be raised to as high as	**Blood:** *leukopenia, agranulocytosis, pancytopenia.* **CNS:** dizziness, fainting. **CV:** *tachycardia,* hypotension, angina pectoris, congestive heart failure. **EENT:** *loss of taste (dysgeusia).* **GI:** anorexia. **GU:** *proteinuria, nephrotic syndrome, membranous glomerulopathy, renal failure,* urinary frequency.

♦ Available in U.S. and Canada. ♦♦ Available in Canada only. All other products (no symbol) available in U.S. only. Italicized side effects are common or life-threatening.

INTERACTIONS	NURSING CONSIDERATIONS
Anesthetic agents: may cause additive hypotensive effect. Observe patient carefully. *Tricyclic antidepressants:* may diminish hypotensive response. Avoid if possible.	• Contraindicated in patients with pheochromocytoma. Use cautiously in patients with angina, cerebrovascular disease, or bronchial asthma, or in those receiving other antihypertensive drugs. • Rarely used to treat hypertension because of unsatisfactory response and high incidence of side effects. • The range between therapeutic and toxic doses of this drug is narrow. Call the doctor immediately if side effects develop. • Monitor blood pressure and pulse rate closely. Keep phenylephrine or ephedrine handy in case severe hypotension develops. If patient develops bradycardia, he may require atropine. • Teach patient about his disease and therapy. Explain why it's important to take this drug exactly as prescribed, even when he's feeling well. Tell outpatient not to stop this drug suddenly, but to call the doctor if unpleasant side effects develop. • Inform patient that orthostatic hypotension can be minimized by rising slowly and avoiding sudden position changes. Unpleasant taste can be relieved with sugarless chewing gum, sour hard candy, or ice chips; nausea and vomiting can be prevented by not eating for at least 4 hours after each dose. • In very hot weather, patient may require smaller doses. • Give this drug after meals.
MAO inhibitors: may cause excitability and hypertension. Avoid if possible.	• Use cautiously in patients with severe cardiac or cerebrovascular disease, peptic ulcer, ulcerative colitis, renal disease, gallstones, or mental depressive disorders, or in those undergoing surgery. • Use cautiously in patients taking other antihypertensive drugs. • Monitor patient's blood pressure and pulse rate frequently. • Teach patient about his disease and therapy. Explain why it's important to take this drug exactly as prescribed, even when he's feeling well. Tell outpatient not to discontinue this drug suddenly, but to call the doctor if unpleasant side effects, such as mental depression, nightmares, or insomnia, develop. Watch patient closely for signs of mental depression. • Effect of drug may last for 10 days after discontinuation. • Warn patient that this drug can cause drowsiness. • Warn female patient to notify doctor if she becomes pregnant. • Inform patient that orthostatic hypotension can be minimized by rising slowly and avoiding sudden position changes. Mouth dryness can be relieved with sugarless chewing gum, sour hard candy, or ice chips. • Tell patient to contact doctor if relief is needed for nasal stuffiness. • Give this drug with meals. • Patient should weigh himself daily and notify doctor of any weight gain. • One mg of alseroxylon is approximately equal to 0.1 mg of reserpine.
None significant.	• Use cautiously in patients with impaired renal function or serious autoimmune disease (particularly systemic lupus erythematosus), or those who have been exposed to other drugs known to affect white cell counts or immune response. • Proteinuria and nephrotic syndrome may occur in patients who are on captopril therapy. Those who develop persistent proteinuria or proteinuria that exceeds 1 g/day should have their captopril therapy reevaluated. • Monitor patient's blood pressure and pulse rate frequently. • Perform WBC and differential counts before starting treatment, every 2 weeks for the first 3 months of therapy, and periodically thereafter.

(continued on following page)

NAME	INDICATIONS & DOSAGE	SIDE EFFECTS
captopril *(continued)*	150 mg t.i.d. while continuing the diuretic. Maximum dose is 450 mg/day.	**Skin:** *urticarial rash, maculopapular rash,* pruritus. **Other:** fever, angioedema of face and extremities, transient increases in liver enzymes.
clonidine hydrochloride Catapres♦	*Essential, renal, and malignant hypertension—* **Adults:** initially, 0.1 mg P.O. b.i.d. Then increase by 0.1 to 0.2 mg daily on a weekly basis. Usual dose range: 0.2 to 0.8 mg daily in divided doses. Infrequently, doses as high as 2.4 mg daily. No dosing recommendations for children.	**CNS:** *drowsiness,* dizziness, fatigue, sedation, nervousness, headache. **CV:** orthostatic hypotension, bradycardia. **EENT:** *mouth dryness.* **GI:** *constipation.* **GU:** urinary retention. **Other:** impotence.
cryptenamine acetate Unitensen Aqueous **cryptenamine tannate** Unitensen, Unitensyl♦♦	*Mild to moderate hypertension, toxemia—* **Adults:** initially, 2 mg P.O. b.i.d., increased at weekly intervals, depending on response. Total daily dose not to exceed 12 mg daily. I.V. (for hypertensive crises and convulsive toxemia)—0.5 ml (130 CSR units) diluted to 20 ml with 5% dextrose in water. Administer at infusion rate of 1 ml/minute. When giving this drug I.V., record blood pressure approximately every minute.	**CNS:** mental confusion. **CV:** *orthostatic hypotension,* cardiac arrhythmias, *bradycardia.* **EENT:** blurred vision, excessive salivation, unpleasant taste. **GI:** *nausea, vomiting,* epigastric burning, hiccups. **Other:** respiratory depression, bronchial constriction.
deserpidine Harmonyl	*Mild essential hypertension—* **Adults:** 0.25 mg P.O. t.i.d. to	**CNS:** mental confusion, *depression, drowsiness, nervousness,*

♦ Available in U.S. and Canada. ♦♦ Available in Canada only. All other products (no symbol) available in U.S. only. Italicized side effects are common or life-threatening.

INTERACTIONS	NURSING CONSIDERATIONS
	• Advise patients to report any sign of infection (sore throat, fever). • Because captopril may cause serious side effects, it should be reserved for those patients who have developed undesirable side effects from or failed to respond to other antihypertensive drugs. Commonly used in patients who fail to respond to "triple-drug therapy" (a diuretic, a beta-blocker, and a vasodilator). • Although captopril can be used alone, its beneficial effects are increased when a thiazide diuretic is added. • May cause dizziness or fainting; advise patients to avoid sudden postural changes. • Question patient about impaired taste sensation. • Should be taken 1 hour before meals since food in the GI tract may reduce absorption.
Tricyclic antidepressants and MAO inhibitors: may decrease antihypertensive effect. Use together cautiously.	• Use cautiously in patients with severe coronary insufficiency, myocardial infarction, cerebral vascular disease, chronic renal failure, or history of depression, or in those taking other antihypertensives. • Monitor blood pressure and pulse rate frequently. Dosage is usually adjusted to patient's blood pressure and tolerance. • Reduce dose gradually over 2 to 4 days. If discontinued abruptly, this drug may cause severe hypertension. • Teach patient about his disease and therapy. Explain why it's important to take this drug exactly as prescribed, even when he's feeling well. Tell outpatient not to discontinue this drug suddenly, but to call the doctor if unpleasant side effects develop. Warn that this drug can cause drowsiness. • Inform patient that orthostatic hypotension can be minimized by rising slowly and avoiding sudden position changes. Mouth dryness can be relieved with sugarless chewing gum, sour hard candy, or ice chips. • Last dose should be taken immediately before retiring. • Has been used investigationally to decrease the subjective symptoms of opiate withdrawal, migraine headache prophylaxis, and dysmenorrhea.
Anesthetic agents: may cause additive hypotensive effect. Observe patient carefully. *Tricyclic antidepressants:* may diminish hypotensive response. Avoid if possible.	• Contraindicated in patients with pheochromocytoma. Use cautiously in patients with angina, cerebrovascular disease, bronchial asthma, or renal insufficiency, or in those taking other antihypertensives. • Monitor blood pressure and pulse rate closely. If severe hypotension develops, stop infusion and notify doctor, as he may use phenylephrine or ephedrine to counteract effect. Hypotension should dissipate in 60 to 90 minutes. If patient develops bradycardia, he may require atropine. Notify doctor promptly. • The range between therapeutic and toxic doses of this drug is narrow. Call doctor immediately if side effects develop. • Teach patient about his disease and therapy. Explain why it's important to take this drug exactly as prescribed, even when he's feeling well. Tell outpatient not to discontinue this drug suddenly, but to call the doctor if unpleasant side effects develop. • Inform patient that orthostatic hypotension can be minimized by rising slowly and avoiding sudden position changes. Unpleasant taste can be relieved with sugarless chewing gum, sour hard candy, or ice chips.
MAO inhibitors: may cause excitability and	• Contraindicated in patients with mental depression. Use cautiously in patients with severe cardiac or cerebrovascular disease, peptic ul-

(continued on following page)

NAME	INDICATIONS & DOSAGE	SIDE EFFECTS
deserpidine *(continued)*	q.i.d. for up to 2 weeks, then maintenance dose of 0.25 mg once daily may be adequate. No dosing recommendations for children.	anxiety, nightmares, sedation. **CV:** bradycardia. **EENT:** *mouth dryness, nasal stuffiness,* glaucoma. **GI:** *hypersecretion of gastric acid, nausea, vomiting,* gastrointestinal bleeding. **Skin:** pruritus, rash. **Other:** *impotence, weight gain.*
diazoxide Hyperstat♦ (I.V. only)	*Hypertensive crisis—* **Adults:** 300 mg I.V. bolus push, administered in 30 seconds or less into peripheral vein. Repeat at intervals of 4 to 24 hours, p.r.n. Mini-boluses of 1 to 3 mg/kg repeated at intervals of 5 to 15 minutes or infusions of 15 mg/minute are equally effective. Switch to therapy with oral antihypertensives as soon as possible. **Children:** 5 mg/kg I.V. rapid bolus push.	**CNS:** *headaches,* dizziness, lightheadedness, euphoria. **CV:** *sodium and water retention, orthostatic hypotension,* sweating, flushing, warmth, angina, myocardial ischemia, arrhythmias, EKG changes. **GI:** *nausea, vomiting,* abdominal discomfort. **Metabolic:** *hyperglycemia,* hyperuricemia. **Local:** inflammation and pain from extravasation.
guanethidine sulfate Ismelin♦	*For moderate to severe hypertension; usually used in combination with other antihypertensives—* **Adults:** initially, 10 mg P.O. daily. Increase by 10 mg at weekly to monthly intervals, p.r.n. Usual dose is 25 to 50 mg daily. Some patients may require up to 300 mg. **Children:** initially, 200 mcg/kg P.O. daily. Increase gradually every 1 to 3 weeks to maximum of 8 times initial dose.	**CNS:** *dizziness, weakness, syncope.* **CV:** *orthostatic hypotension, bradycardia,* congestive heart failure, arrhythmias. **EENT:** *nasal stuffiness,* mouth dryness. **GI:** *diarrhea.* **Other:** *edema, weight gain, inhibition of ejaculation.*

INTERACTIONS	**NURSING CONSIDERATIONS**
hypertension. Avoid if possible.	cer, ulcerative colitis, gallstones, or mental depressive disorders; in patients undergoing surgery; and in patients taking other antihypertensives or anticonvulsants. • Monitor patient's blood pressure and pulse rate frequently. • Teach patient about his disease and therapy. Explain why it's important to take this drug exactly as prescribed, even when he's feeling well. Tell outpatient not to discontinue this drug suddenly, but to call the doctor if unpleasant side effects, such as mental depression, insomnia, or loss of appetite, develop. Warn that drug can cause drowsiness. • Watch patient closely for signs of mental depression. Warn him to notify doctor promptly if he starts having nightmares. • Tell patient to avoid alcohol and to follow prescribed diet. • Mouth dryness can be relieved with chewing gum, sour hard candy, or ice chips. Tell patient to contact doctor if relief is needed for nasal stuffiness. • Give this drug with meals to increase absorption. • Patient should weigh himself daily and notify doctor of any weight gain. • The 0.1-mg dosage strength contains tartrazine dye, which may produce allergic reactions in susceptible patients.
Hydralazine: may cause severe hypotension. Use together cautiously. *Thiazide diuretics:* may increase the effects of diazoxide. Use together cautiously.	• Use cautiously in patients with impaired cerebral or cardiac function, diabetes, or uremia, or in those taking other antihypertensives. • Monitor blood pressure frequently. Notify doctor immediately if severe hypotension develops. Keep levarterenol available. • Monitor patient's intake and output carefully. If fluid or sodium retention develops, doctor may want to order furosemide. • Take care to avoid extravasation. • This drug may alter requirements for insulin, diet, or oral hypoglycemic drugs in previously controlled diabetics. Monitor blood glucose daily. • Weigh patient daily. Notify doctor of any weight increase. • Watch diabetics closely for signs of severe hyperglycemia or hyperosmolar nonketotic coma. Insulin may be needed. • Check patient's uric acid levels frequently. Report abnormalities to doctor. • Inform patient that orthostatic hypotension can be minimized by rising slowly and avoiding sudden position changes. Instruct patient to remain supine for 30 minutes after injection. • Infusion of diazoxide has been shown to be as effective as a bolus in some patients.
Levodopa, alcohol: may increase hypotensive effect of guanethidine. Use together cautiously. *MAO inhibitors, ephedrine, levarterenol, methylphenidate, tricyclic antidepressants, amphetamines, phenothiazines:* may inhibit the antihypertensive effect of gua-	• Contraindicated in patients with pheochromocytoma. Use cautiously in patients with severe cardiac disease, recent MI, cerebrovascular disease, peptic ulcer, impaired renal function, or bronchial asthma, or in those taking other antihypertensives. • Discontinue drug 2 to 3 weeks before elective surgery to reduce the possibility of vascular collapse and cardiac arrest during anesthesia. • Teach patient about his disease and therapy. Explain why it's important to take this drug exactly as prescribed, even when he's feeling well. Tell patient not to discontinue this drug suddenly, but to call the doctor if unpleasant side effects develop. • Inform patient that orthostatic hypotension can be minimized by rising slowly and avoiding sudden position changes. Mouth dryness can be relieved with sugarless chewing gum, sour hard candy, or ice chips.

(continued on following page)

NAME	INDICATIONS & DOSAGE	SIDE EFFECTS
guanethidine sulfate *(continued)*		
hydralazine hydrochloride Apresoline♦, Dralzine, Hydralyn, Nor-Pres 25, Rolazine	*Essential hypertension (oral, alone or in combination with other antihypertensives); to reduce afterload in severe congestive heart failure (with nitrates); and severe essential hypertension (parenteral to lower blood pressure quickly)*— **Adults:** initially, 10 mg P.O. q.i.d.; gradually increased to 50 mg q.i.d. Maximum recommended dosage is 200 mg daily, but some patients may require 300 to 400 mg daily. I.V.—20 to 40 mg given slowly and repeated as necessary, generally q 4 to 6 hours. Switch to oral antihypertensives as soon as possible. I.M.—20 to 40 mg repeated as necessary, generally q 4 to 6 hours. Switch to oral antihypertensives as soon as possible. **Children:** initially, 0.75 mg/kg P.O. daily in 4 divided doses (25 mg/m² daily). May increase gradually to 10 times this dose, if necessary. I.V.—give slowly 1.7 to 3.5 mg/kg daily or 50 to 100 mg/m² daily in 4 to 6 divided doses. I.M.—1.7 to 3.5 mg/kg daily or 50 to 100 mg/m² daily in 4 to 6 divided doses.	**CNS:** peripheral neuritis, *headache,* dizziness. **CV:** orthostatic hypotension, *tachycardia,* arrhythmias, *angina, palpitations, sodium retention.* **GI:** *nausea, vomiting, diarrhea, anorexia.* **Skin:** rash. **Other:** *lupus erythematosus-like syndrome, weight gain.*
mecamylamine hydrochloride Inversine	*For moderate to severe essential hypertension and uncomplicated malignant hypertension*— **Adults:** initially, 2.5 mg P.O. b.i.d. Increase by 2.5 mg daily every 2 days. Average daily dose 25 mg given in 3 divided doses. No dosing recommendations for children.	**CNS:** *paresthesias,* sedation, *fatigue, tremor, choreiform movements,* convulsions, psychic changes, dizziness, *weakness, headaches.* **CV:** *orthostatic hypotension.* **EENT:** *mouth dryness,* glossitis, dilated pupils, *blurred vision.* **GI:** *anorexia, nausea, vomiting, constipation, adynamic ileus, diarrhea.* **GU:** urinary retention. **Other:** decreased libido, impotence.

INTERACTIONS	NURSING CONSIDERATIONS
nethidine. Adjust dose accordingly.	• Tell outpatient to avoid strenuous exercise. • Give this drug with meals to increase absorption. • If patient develops diarrhea, doctor may prescribe atropine or paregoric.
Diazoxide: may cause severe hypotension. Use together cautiously.	• Use cautiously in patients with cardiac disease or in those taking other antihypertensives. • Monitor patient's blood pressure and pulse rate frequently. • Watch patient closely for signs of lupus erythematosus-like syndrome (sore throat, fever, muscle and joint aches, skin rash). Call doctor immediately if any of these develop. • Teach patient about his disease and therapy. Explain why it's important to take this drug exactly as prescribed, even when he's feeling well. Tell outpatient not to discontinue this drug suddenly, but to call the doctor if unpleasant side effects develop. • Inform patient that orthostatic hypotension can be minimized by rising slowly and avoiding sudden position changes. • Give this drug with meals to increase absorption. • Compliance may be improved by administering this drug b.i.d. Check with doctor. • Complete blood count, LE cell preparation, and antinuclear antibody titer determinations should be done before therapy and periodically during long-term therapy.
Sodium bicarbonate and acetazolamide: may increase effect of mecamylamine. Use together cautiously. Watch for increased hypotensive effects and toxicity.	• Contraindicated in patients with recent MI, or uremia, chronic pyelonephritis. Use cautiously in patients with lower urinary tract pathology, renal insufficiency, glaucoma, pyloric stenosis, coronary insufficiency, or cerebrovascular insufficiency, or in those taking other antihypertensives. • Effects of this drug are increased by high environmental temperature, fever, stress, or severe illness. • Don't withdraw this drug suddenly; rebound hypertension may occur. Tell outpatient to call the doctor if unpleasant side effects develop. • Monitor patient's blood pressure frequently while he's standing. • Give with meals for better absorption. Don't restrict sodium intake. • If patient develops constipation from this drug, the doctor may want him to take milk of magnesia. Instruct patient to avoid bulk laxatives. • Teach the patient about his disease and therapy. Explain why it's important to take this drug exactly as prescribed, even when he's feeling well. • Inform patient that orthostatic hypotension can be minimized by

(continued on following page)

NAME	INDICATIONS & DOSAGE	SIDE EFFECTS
mecamylamine hydrochloride *(continued)*		
methyldopa Aldomet♦, Dopamet♦♦, Medimet-250♦♦, Novomedopa♦♦	*For sustained mild to severe hypertension; should not be used for acute treatment of hypertensive emergencies—* **Adults:** initially, 250 mg P.O. b.i.d. to t.i.d. in first 48 hours. Then increase as needed every 2 days. Dosages may need adjustment if other antihypertensive drugs are added to or deleted from therapy. Maintenance dosages—500 mg to 2 g daily in 2 to 4 divided doses. Maximum recommended daily dose is 3 g. I.V.—500 mg to 1 g q 6 hours, diluted in 5% dextrose in water, and administered over 30 to 60 minutes. Switch to oral antihypertensives as soon as possible. **Children:** initially, 10 mg/kg/day P.O. in 2 to 3 divided doses; or 20 to 40 mg/kg/day I.V. in 4 divided doses. Increase dose daily until desired response occurs. Maximum daily dose 65 mg/kg.	**Blood:** *hemolytic anemia,* reversible granulocytopenia, thrombocytopenia. **CNS:** *sedation,* headache, asthenia, weakness, dizziness, *decreased mental acuity,* involuntary choreoathetotic movements, psychic disturbances, depression. **CV:** bradycardia, *orthostatic hypotension,* aggravated angina, myocarditis, *edema and weight gain.* **EENT:** *dry mouth, nasal stuffiness.* **GI:** diarrhea. **Hepatic:** *hepatic necrosis.* **Other:** gynecomastia, lactation, skin rash, drug-induced fever, impotence.
metoprolol tartrate Betaloc♦♦, Lopresor♦♦, Lopressor	*For hypertension; may be used alone or in combination with other antihypertensives—* **Adults:** 50 mg b.i.d. P.O. initially. Up to 200 to 400 mg daily in 2 to 3 divided doses. No dosage recommendations for children.	**CNS:** *fatigue, lethargy,* vivid dreams, hallucinations. **CV:** *bradycardia, hypotension, congestive heart failure,* peripheral vascular disease. **GI:** nausea, vomiting, diarrhea. **Metabolic:** hypoglycemia without tachycardia. **Skin:** rash. **Other:** *increased airway resistance,* fever.
metyrosine Demser	*Preoperative preparation of patients with pheochromocytoma; management of such patients when surgery is contraindicated; to control or prevent hypertension before or during pheochromocytomectomy—* **Adults, and children over 12 years:** 250 mg P.O. q.i.d. May be increased by 250 to	**CNS:** *sedation,* extrapyramidal symptoms such as speech difficulty and tremors, disorientation. **GI:** *diarrhea,* nausea, vomiting, abdominal pain. **GU:** *crystalluria,* hematuria. **Other:** impotence, hypersensitivity.

INTERACTIONS	NURSING CONSIDERATIONS
	rising slowly and avoiding sudden position changes. Mouth dryness can be relieved with sugarless chewing gum, sour hard candy, or ice chips.
Norepinephrine, phenothiazines, tricyclic antidepressants, amphetamines: possible hypertensive effects. Monitor carefully.	• Use cautiously in patients receiving other antihypertensives or MAO inhibitors. Monitor blood pressure and pulse rate frequently. • Observe patient for side effects, particularly unexplained fever. Report side effects to doctor. • If patient requires blood transfusion, make sure he gets direct and indirect Coombs' tests to avoid cross-matching problems. • Monitor blood studies (complete blood count) before and during therapy. • If patient has been on this drug for several months, positive reaction to direct Coombs' test indicates hemolytic anemia. • Weigh patient daily. Notify doctor of any weight increase. Salt and water retention may occur but can be relieved with diuretics. • Tell patient that urine may turn dark in toilet bowls treated with bleach. • Teach patient about his disease and therapy. Explain why it's important to take this drug exactly as prescribed, even when he's feeling well. Tell outpatient not to stop this drug suddenly, but to call the doctor if unpleasant side effects develop. Once-daily dosage administered at bedtime will minimize drowsiness during daytime. Check with doctor. • Inform patient that orthostatic hypotension can be minimized by rising slowly and avoiding sudden position changes. Mouth dryness can be relieved with sugarless chewing gum, sour hard candy, or ice chips.
Insulin, hypoglycemic drugs (oral): can alter dosage requirements in previously stabilized diabetics. Observe patient carefully. *Cardiotonic glycosides:* excessive bradycardia and increased depressant effect on myocardium. Use together cautiously.	• Use cautiously in patients with heart block, congestive heart failure, diabetes, or respiratory disease, or in those taking other antihypertensives. Always check patient's apical pulse rate before giving this drug. If it's slower than 60 beats/minute, hold drug and call doctor immediately. • Monitor blood pressure frequently. If patient develops severe hypotension, administer a vasopressor as ordered. • Teach patient about his disease and therapy. Explain why it's important to take this drug, even when he's feeling well. Tell outpatient not to discontinue this drug suddenly; abrupt discontinuation can exacerbate angina and MI. Instruct patient to call doctor if unpleasant side effects develop. • Food may increase absorption of metoprolol. Give consistently with meals.
Phenothiazines and haloperidol: increased inhibition of catecholamine synthesis may result in extrapyramidal symptoms. Use cautiously.	• During surgery, monitor blood pressure and EKG continuously. If a serious arrhythmia occurs during anesthesia and surgery, treatment with a beta-blocking drug or lidocaine may be necessary. • Warn patient that sedation almost always occurs in those treated with metyrosine. Sedation usually subsides after several days' treatment. • Instruct patient to increase daily fluid intake to prevent crystalluria. Daily urine volume should be 2,000 ml or more. • Tell patient to notify doctor if any of the listed side effects occur. • Insomnia may occur when metyrosine is stopped.

(continued on following page)

NAME	INDICATIONS & DOSAGE	SIDE EFFECTS
metyrosine *(continued)*	500 mg q day to a maximum of 4 g/day in divided doses. When used for preoperative preparation, optimally effective dosage should be given for at least 5 to 7 days.	
minoxidil Loniten	*Treatment of severe hypertension*— **Adults:** 5 mg P.O. initially as a single dose. Effective dosage range is usually 10 to 40 mg/day. Maximum dose 100 mg/day. **Children (under 12 years):** 0.2 mg/kg as a single daily dose. Effective dosage range usually 0.25 to 1.0 mg/kg/day. Maximum dose is 50 mg.	**CV:** *edema, tachycardia, pericardial effusion and tamponade, congestive heart failure,* EKG changes. **Other:** *hypertrichosis* (elongation, thickening, and enhanced pigmentation of fine body hair), breast tenderness.
nadolol Corgard♦	*Treatment of hypertension*— **Adults:** 40 mg P.O. once daily, initially. Dosage may be increased in 40- to 80-mg increments until optimum response occurs. Usual maintenance dosage range: 80 to 320 mg once daily. Doses of 640 mg may be necessary in rare cases. *Long-term management of angina pectoris*— **Adults:** 40 mg P.O. once daily, initially. Dosage may be increased in 40- to 80-mg increments until optimum response occurs. Usual maintenance dosage range: 80 to 240 mg once daily.	**CNS:** *fatigue, lethargy,* vivid dreams, hallucinations. **CV:** *bradycardia, hypotension, congestive heart failure,* peripheral vascular disease. **GI:** nausea, vomiting, diarrhea. **Metabolic:** hypoglycemia without tachycardia. **Skin:** rash. **Other:** *increased airway resistance,* fever.
nitroprusside sodium Nipride♦	*To lower blood pressure quickly in hypertensive emergencies; to control hypotension during anesthesia; to reduce preload and afterload in cardiac pump failure or cardiogenic shock; may be used with or without dopamine*— **Adults:** 50-mg vial diluted with 2 to 3 ml of 5% dextrose in water I.V. and then added to 250, 500, or 1,000 ml 5% dextrose in water. Infuse at 0.5 to 10 mcg/kg/minute. Average dose: 3 mcg/kg/minute.	*The following effects generally indicate overdosage:* **CNS:** *headache, dizziness,* ataxia, loss of consciousness, coma, weak pulse, absent reflexes, widely dilated pupils, *restlessness, muscle twitching, diaphoresis.* **CV:** distant heart sounds, palpitations, dyspnea, shallow breathing. **GI:** *vomiting, nausea, abdominal pain.* **Metabolic:** acidosis. **Skin:** pink color. **Local:** *tissue sloughing and necrosis with extravasation.*

♦ Available in U.S. and Canada. ♦♦ Available in Canada only. All other products (no symbol) available in U.S. only. Italicized side effects are common or life-threatening.

INTERACTIONS	NURSING CONSIDERATIONS
	• If patient's hypertension is not adequately controlled by metyrosine, an alpha-adrenergic blocking agent, such as phenoxybenzamine, should be added to the regimen. • Available as 250-mg capsules.
Guanethidine: severe orthostatic hypotension. Advise patient to stand up slowly.	• Contraindicated in patients with pheochromocytoma. • A potent vasodilator: Use only when other antihypertensives have failed. • About 8 out of 10 patients will experience hypertrichosis within 3 to 6 weeks of beginning treatment. Unwanted hair can be controlled with a depilatory or shaving. Assure patient that extra hair will disappear within 1 to 6 months of stopping minoxidil. Advise patient, however, not to discontinue drug without doctor's consent. • Drug is usually prescribed with a beta-blocking drug to control tachycardia and a diuretic to counteract fluid retention. Make sure patient complies with total treatment regimen. • A patient package insert (PPI) has been prepared by the manufacturer of minoxidil, describing in layman's terms the drug and its side effects. Be sure your patient receives this insert and reads it thoroughly. Provide an oral explanation also. • Available as a 2.5-mg and 10-mg tablet.
Insulin, hypoglycemic drugs (oral): can alter dosage requirements in previously stabilized diabetics. Observe patient carefully. *Cardiotonic glycosides:* excessive bradycardia and increased depressant effect on myocardium. Use together cautiously.	• Contraindicated in patients with bronchial asthma, sinus bradycardia and greater than first degree conduction block, and cardiogenic shock. • Use cautiously in patients with heart failure, chronic bronchitis, and emphysema. • Always check patient's apical pulse before giving this drug. If slower than 60 beats/minute, hold drug and call doctor. • Monitor blood pressure frequently. If patient develops severe hypotension, administer a vasopressor as ordered. • Don't discontinue abruptly: can exacerbate angina and MI. • Teach patient about his disease and therapy. Explain why it's important to take this drug, even when he's feeling well. Tell outpatient not to discontinue drug suddenly, but to call doctor if unpleasant side effects develop. • This drug masks common signs of shock and hypoglycemia.
None significant.	• Use cautiously in patients with hypothyroidism or hepatic or renal disease, or in those receiving other antihypertensives. • Due to light sensitivity, wrap I.V. solution in foil. It's not necessary to wrap the tubing in foil. Fresh solution should have faint brownish tint. Discard after 4 hours. • Obtain baseline vital signs before giving this drug, and find out what parameters the doctor wants to achieve. • Check blood pressure every 5 minutes at start of infusion and every 15 minutes thereafter. If severe hypotension occurs, turn off I.V. nitroprusside—effects of drug quickly reversed. Notify doctor. If possible, an arterial pressure line should be started. Regulate drug flow to specified level. • Don't use bacteriostatic water for injection or sterile saline solution for reconstitution. • Infuse with automatic infusion pump.

(continued on following page)

NAME	INDICATIONS & DOSAGE	SIDE EFFECTS
nitroprusside sodium *(continued)*	Maximum infusion rate: 10 mcg/kg/minute. Patients taking other antihypertensive drugs along with nitroprusside are very sensitive to this drug. Adjust dosage accordingly.	
pargyline hydrochloride Eutonyl	*For moderate to severe hypertension, usually given in combination with other drugs—* **Adults:** initially, 25 to 50 mg P.O. once daily, if not receiving any other antihypertensive drugs. Then increase dosage by 10 mg daily at weekly intervals. Maximum daily dosage 200 mg. Usual daily dose for patients over 65 years or those who've had sympathectomy: 10 to 25 mg. When used in combination with other drugs, total daily dose of pargyline should not exceed 25 mg. No dosage recommendations for children.	**CNS:** *tremors,* convulsions, choreiform movements, psychic changes, *nightmares, hyperexcitability, sweating,* dizziness, fainting, drowsiness. **CV:** palpitations, *orthostatic hypotension,* fluid retention. **EENT:** *mouth dryness,* optic damage. **GI:** *nausea, vomiting, increased appetite, constipation.* **Other:** impotence.
phenoxybenzamine hydrochloride Dibenzyline	*To control hypertension and sweating secondary to pheochromocytoma; may be used in combination with propranolol to control excessive tachycardia—* **Adults:** initially, 10 mg P.O. daily. Increase by 10 mg daily every 4 days. Maintenance dose: 20 to 60 mg daily. **Children:** initially, 0.2 mg/kg or 6 mg/m² P.O. daily in a single dose. Maintenance dose: 12 to 36 mg/m² daily as a single dose or in divided doses.	**CNS:** lethargy, drowsiness. **CV:** *orthostatic hypotension, tachycardia,* shock. **EENT:** *nasal stuffiness, dry mouth, miosis.* **GI:** vomiting, abdominal distress. **Other:** *impotence.*

◆ Available in U.S. and Canada. ◆◆ Available in Canada only. All other products (no symbol) available in U.S. only. Italicized side effects are common or life-threatening.

INTERACTIONS	NURSING CONSIDERATIONS
	• This drug is best run piggyback through a peripheral line with no other medication. Don't adjust rate of main I.V. line while drug is running. Even small bolus of nitroprusside can cause severe hypotension. • This drug can cause cyanide toxicity, so check serum thiocyanate levels every 72 hours. Watch for signs of thiocyanate toxicity: profound hypotension, metabolic acidosis, dyspnea, headache, loss of consciousness, ataxia, vomiting. If these occur, discontinue drug immediately and notify doctor. • Extravasation can cause tissue irritation.
Amphetamines, ephedrine, levodopa, metaraminol, methotrimeprazine, methylphenidate, phenylephrine, phenylpropanolamine, pseudoephedrine: enhanced pressor effects. Use together cautiously. *Alcohol, barbiturates, and other sedatives; tranquilizers; narcotics; dextromethorphan; tricyclic antidepressants:* unpredictable interactions. Should be used with caution and in reduced dosage.	• Contraindicated in patients with advanced renal failure, pheochromocytoma, hyperthyroidism, or Parkinson's disease; in patients who are hyperactive and hyperexcitable. Use cautiously in patients who are receiving other antihypertensives, or who have hepatic disease. • Discontinue this drug at least 2 weeks before elective surgery. • Hypotensive effects of this drug are increased by high temperatures, fever, stress, or severe illness. If patient develops severe hypotension, counteract with ephedrine or phenylephrine. • Monitor blood pressure and pulse rate frequently. Take blood pressure while patient is standing. • Patient should have periodic ophthalmic evaluations during therapy. • If patient is scheduled for surgery and has been taking this drug, be sure narcotic dosages are reduced. • This drug may require up to several weeks to reach optimal effect. • Warn patient not to take any other medications, including over-the-counter cold remedies, without first asking doctor. • This drug is an MAO inhibitor. Tell patient not to eat foods with high tyramine content: for example, aged cheese, Chianti wine, sour cream, canned figs, raisins, chicken livers, yeast extract, chocolate, pickled herring, caffeine, cola drinks. • Teach patient about his disease and therapy. Explain why it's important to take this drug exactly as prescribed, even when he's feeling well. Tell outpatient not to discontinue this drug suddenly, but to call the doctor if unpleasant side effects develop. • Inform patient that orthostatic hypotension can be minimized by rising slowly and avoiding sudden position changes. Mouth dryness can be relieved with sugarless chewing gum, sour hard candy, or ice chips.
None significant.	• Use cautiously in patients with cerebrovascular or coronary insufficiency, advanced renal disease, respiratory disease. • Watch patient closely for side effects, and call doctor promptly if they occur. If severe hypotension develops, patient may require levarterenol to counteract effect. • Nasal congestion, miosis, and impotence usually decrease with continued therapy. • Patient with tachycardia may require concurrent propranolol therapy. • Monitor patient's heart rate and blood pressure frequently. • This drug may take several weeks to achieve optimal effect. • Monitor respiratory status carefully. This drug may aggravate symptoms of pneumonia and asthma. • Teach patient about his disease and therapy. Explain why it's important to take this drug exactly as prescribed, even when he's feeling well. Tell outpatient not to discontinue this drug suddenly, but to call the doctor if unpleasant side effects develop.

(continued on following page)

NAME	INDICATIONS & DOSAGE	SIDE EFFECTS
phenoxybenzamine hydrochloride *(continued)*		
phentolamine hydrochloride Regitine **phentolamine methanesulfonate** Regitine, Rogitine♦♦	*To aid in diagnosis of pheochromocytoma; to control or prevent hypertension before or during pheochromocytomectomy—* **Adults:** P.O. therapeutic dose: 50 mg q.i.d. I.V. diagnostic dose: 5 mg, with close monitoring of blood pressure. Before surgical removal of tumor, give 2 to 5 mg I.M. or I.V. During surgery, patient may need small I.V. doses (1 mg) or small I.M. doses (3 mg). **Children:** P.O. therapeutic dose: 5 mg/kg daily or 150 mg/m² daily in 4 to 6 divided doses. I.V. diagnostic dose: 0.1 mg/kg or 3 mg/m² as single dose, with close monitoring of blood pressure. Before surgical removal of tumor give 1 mg I.V. or 3 mg I.M. During surgery, patient may need small I.V. doses (1 mg).	**CNS:** *dizziness, weakness, flushing.* **CV:** *hypotension,* shock, *arrhythmias,* palpitations, *tachycardia,* angina pectoris. **GI:** *diarrhea,* abdominal pain, *nausea, vomiting,* hyperperistalsis. **Other:** *nasal stuffiness,* hypoglycemia.
prazosin hydrochloride Minipress♦	*For mild to moderate hypertension; used alone or in combination with a diuretic or other antihypertensive drugs; also used to decrease afterload in severe chronic congestive heart failure—* **Adults:** P.O. test dose: 1 mg given before bedtime to prevent "first-dose syncope." Initial dose: 1 mg t.i.d. Increase dosage slowly. Maximum daily dose 20 mg. Maintenance dose: 3 to 20 mg daily in 3 divided doses. A few patients have required dosages larger than this (up to 40 mg daily). If other antihypertensive drugs or diuretics are added to this drug, decrease prazosin dosage to 1 to 2 mg t.i.d. and retitrate.	**CNS:** *dizziness,* headache, drowsiness, weakness, *"first-dose syncope,"* depression. **CV:** orthostatic hypotension, *palpitations.* **EENT:** blurred vision, dry mouth. **GI:** vomiting, diarrhea, abdominal cramps, constipation, *nausea.* **GU:** priapism.

♦ Available in U.S. and Canada. ♦♦ Available in Canada only. All other products (no symbol) available in U.S. only. Italicized side effects are common or life-threatening.

INTERACTIONS	NURSING CONSIDERATIONS
	• Inform patient that orthostatic hypotension can be minimized by rising slowly and avoiding sudden position changes. Mouth dryness can be relieved with sugarless chewing gum, sour hard candy, or ice chips. • Used investigationally to treat chronic urinary retention. • Small initial doses are increased gradually until desired effect is obtained. Patient should be observed at each dose for at least 4 days.
None significant.	• Contraindicated in patients with angina, coronary artery disease, and history of MI. Use cautiously in patients with gastritis or peptic ulcer and in those receiving other antihypertensives. • When this drug is given for diagnostic test, check patient's blood pressure first. Make frequent blood pressure checks during administration. • Diagnosis positive for pheochromocytoma if severe hypotension results from I.V. test dose. • Administer levarterenol to counteract severe hypotensive effect of this drug. Don't administer epinephrine to raise blood pressure, as this may cause further drop. • Don't give sedatives or narcotics 24 hours before diagnostic test.
None significant.	• Use cautiously in patients receiving other antihypertensive drugs. • Monitor patient's blood pressure and pulse rate frequently. • If initial dose is greater than 1 mg, patient may develop severe syncope with loss of consciousness (first-dose syncope). Increase dosage slowly. Instruct patient to sit or lie down if he experiences dizziness. • Teach patient about his disease and therapy. Explain why it's important to take this drug exactly as prescribed, even when he's feeling well. Tell outpatient not to discontinue this drug suddenly, but to call the doctor if unpleasant side effects develop. • Inform patient that orthostatic hypotension can be minimized by rising slowly and avoiding sudden position changes. Mouth dryness can be relieved with sugarless chewing gum, sour hard candy, or ice chips. • Compliance *may* be improved by giving this drug once a day. Check with doctor.

NAME	INDICATIONS & DOSAGE	SIDE EFFECTS
propranolol hydrochloride Inderal♦	*Hypertension (usually used with thiazide diuretics)—* **Adults:** initial treatment of hypertension: 80 mg P.O. daily in 2 to 4 divided doses. Increase at 3- to 7-day intervals to maximum daily dose of 640 mg. Usual maintenance dose for hypertension: 160 to 480 mg daily. No dosing recommendations for children.	**CNS:** *fatigue, lethargy,* vivid dreams, hallucinations. **CV:** *bradycardia, hypotension, congestive heart failure,* peripheral vascular disease. **GI:** nausea, vomiting, diarrhea. **Metabolic:** hypoglycemia without tachycardia. **Skin:** rash. **Other:** *increased airway resistance,* fever.
rauwolfia serpentina HBP, Hiwolfia, Hyper-Rauw, Hywolfia, Rau, Raudixin♦, Rauja, Raumason, Rauneed, Raupoid, Rauserpa, Rauserpin, Rausertina, Rauval, Rauwoldin, Rawfola, Ru-Hy-T, Serfia, Serfolia, T-Rau, Wolfina	*Mild to moderate hypertension—* **Adults:** initially and for 1 to 3 weeks thereafter, 200 to 400 mg P.O. daily as a single dose or in 2 divided doses. Maintenance dose: 50 to 300 mg/day. No dosing recommendations for children.	**CNS:** mental confusion, *depression, drowsiness, nervousness,* anxiety, nightmares, sedation, headache. **CV:** *orthostatic hypotension, bradycardia, syncope.* **EENT:** *mouth dryness, nasal stuffiness,* glaucoma. **GI:** *hypersecretion of gastric acid, nausea, vomiting,* gastrointestinal bleeding. **Skin:** pruritus, rash. **Other:** *impotence, weight gain.*
rescinnamine Anaprel, Cinnasil, Moderil	*For mild to moderate hypertension; may be used alone or in combination with other antihypertensives—* **Adults:** initially, 0.5 mg b.i.d. Maintenance dose: 0.25 to 0.5 mg daily. No dosing recommendations for children.	**CNS:** mental confusion, *depression, drowsiness, nervousness, anxiety, nightmares,* sedation, parkinsonism. **CV:** *orthostatic hypotension, bradycardia, syncope.* **EENT:** *mouth dryness, nasal stuffiness,* glaucoma. **GI:** *hypersecretion of gastric acid,*

INTERACTIONS	NURSING CONSIDERATIONS
Insulin, hypoglycemic drugs (oral): can alter requirements for these drugs in previously stabilized diabetics. Monitor for hypoglycemia. *Cardiotonic glycosides:* excessive bradycardia and increased depressant effect on myocardium. Use together cautiously. *Aminophylline:* antagonized beta-blocking effects of propranolol. Use together cautiously. *Isoproterenol, glucagon:* antagonized propranolol effect. May be used therapeutically and in emergencies.	• Contraindicated in diabetes mellitus, asthma, allergic rhinitis; during ethyl ether anesthesia; in sinus bradycardia and heart block greater than first degree; in cardiogenic shock; in right ventricular failure secondary to pulmonary hypertension. Use with caution in patients with congestive heart failure or respiratory disease, and in patients taking other antihypertensive drugs. • Always check patient's apical pulse rate before giving this drug. If you detect extremes in pulse rates, hold medication and call the doctor immediately. • Monitor blood pressure frequently. If patient develops severe hypotension, notify doctor. He may prescribe a vasopressor. • Teach patient about his disease and therapy. Explain why it's important to take this drug exactly as prescribed, even when he's feeling well. Tell outpatient not to discontinue this drug suddenly; abrupt discontinuation can exacerbate angina and MI. Tell patient to call doctor if unpleasant side effects develop. • This drug masks common signs of shock and hypoglycemia. • Food may increase the absorption of propranolol. Give consistently with meals. • Compliance may be improved by administering this drug on a twice-daily basis. Check with doctor.
MAO inhibitors: may cause excitability and hypertension. Use together cautiously.	• Contraindicated in patients with depression. Use cautiously in patients with severe cardiac or cerebrovascular disease, impaired renal function, peptic ulcer, ulcerative colitis, gallstones; in those undergoing surgery; and in those taking other antihypertensives or tricyclic antidepressants. • Monitor patient's blood pressure and pulse rate frequently. • Teach patient about his disease and therapy. Explain why it's important to take this drug exactly as prescribed, even when he's feeling well. Tell outpatient not to discontinue this drug suddenly, but to call the doctor if unpleasant side effects develop. Warn that this drug can cause drowsiness. • Watch patient closely for signs of mental depression. Warn him to notify doctor promptly if he starts having nightmares. • Inform patient that orthostatic hypotension can be minimized by rising slowly and avoiding sudden position changes. Mouth dryness can be relieved with sugarless chewing gum, sour hard candy, or ice chips. Tell patient to contact doctor if relief is needed for nasal stuffiness. • Give this drug with meals. • Patient should weigh himself daily and notify doctor of any weight gain. • Effects of this drug may last for 10 days after it's discontinued.
MAO inhibitors: may cause excitability and hypertension. Use together cautiously.	• Contraindicated in patients with depression. Use cautiously in patients with severe cardiac or cerebrovascular disease, peptic ulcer, ulcerative colitis, gallstones, or in those undergoing surgery. Also use cautiously in patients taking other antihypertensives. • Monitor patient's blood pressure and pulse rate frequently. • Teach patient about his disease and therapy. Explain why it's important to take this drug exactly as prescribed, even when he's feeling well. Tell outpatient not to discontinue this drug suddenly, but to call the doctor if unpleasant side effects develop. Warn that this drug can

(continued on following page)

NAME	INDICATIONS & DOSAGE	SIDE EFFECTS
rescinnamine *(continued)*		*nausea, vomiting,* gastrointestinal bleeding. **Skin:** pruritus, rash. **Other:** *impotence, weight gain.*
reserpine Alkarau, Arcum R-S, Bonapene, Broserpine, De Serpa, Elserpine, Geneserp #2, Hiserpia, Hyperine, Lemiserp, Maso-Serpine, Neo-Serp♦♦, Rauloydin, Raurine, Rau-Sed, Rauserpin, Releserp-5, Reserfia♦♦Reserjen, Reserpanca♦♦, Reserpaneed, Reserpoid, Rolserp, Sandril, Serp, Serpalan, Serpanray, Serpasil♦, Serpate, Serpena, Sertabs, Sertina, Tensin, Tri-Serp, T-Serp, Vio-Serpine, Zepine	*Mild to moderate essential hypertension (oral); hypertensive emergencies (parenteral)—* **Adults:** initially, 0.5 mg P.O. daily for 1 to 2 weeks. Maintenance dose: 0.1 to 0.5 mg daily. I.M—initially, 0.5 to 1 mg, followed by doses of 2 to 4 mg at 2-hour intervals. Maximum recommended dose 4 mg. **Children:** 0.07 mg/kg or 2 mg/m^2 with hydralazine I.M. every 12 to 24 hours.	**CNS:** mental confusion, *depression, drowsiness, nervousness, anxiety, nightmares,* sedation. **CV:** *orthostatic hypotension, bradycardia, syncope.* **EENT:** *mouth dryness, nasal stuffiness,* glaucoma. **GI:** *hyperacidity, nausea, vomiting,* gastrointestinal bleeding. **Skin:** pruritus, rash. **Other:** *impotence, weight gain.*
trimethaphan camsylate Arfonad♦	*To lower blood pressure quickly in hypertensive emergencies; for controlled hypotension during surgery—* **Adults:** 500 mg (10 ml) diluted in 500 ml dextrose 5% in water to yield concentration of 1 mg/ml I.V. Start I.V. drip at 1 to 2 mg/minute and titrate to achieve desired hypotensive response. Range: 0.3 mg to 6 mg/minute.	**CNS:** dilated pupils, *extreme weakness.* **CV:** *severe orthostatic hypotension, tachycardia.* **GI:** anorexia, *nausea, vomiting, dry mouth.* **GU:** *urinary retention.* **Other:** respiratory depression.

♦ Available in U.S. and Canada. ♦♦ Available in Canada only. All other products (no symbol) available in U.S. only. Italicized side effects are common or life-threatening.

INTERACTIONS	NURSING CONSIDERATIONS
	cause drowsiness. • Watch patient closely for signs of mental depression. Warn him to notify doctor promptly if he starts having nightmares. • Inform patient that orthostatic hypotension can be minimized by rising slowly and avoiding sudden position changes. Mouth dryness can be relieved with sugarless chewing gum, sour hard candy, or ice chips. Tell patient to contact doctor if relief is needed for nasal stuffiness. • Give this drug with meals. • Patient should weigh himself daily and notify doctor of any weight gain. • Effects of this drug may last for 10 days after it's discontinued.
MAO inhibitors: may cause excitability and hypertension. Use together cautiously.	• Contraindicated in patients with depression. Use cautiously in patients with severe cardiac or cerebrovascular disease, peptic ulcer, ulcerative colitis, gallstones, mental depressive disorders; in those undergoing surgery; and in those taking other antihypertensive drugs. • Monitor patient's blood pressure and pulse rate frequently. • Teach patient about his disease and therapy. Explain why it's important to take this drug exactly as prescribed, even when he's feeling well. Tell outpatient not to discontinue this drug suddenly, but to call doctor if unpleasant side effects develop. Warn that this drug can cause drowsiness. • Warn female patient to notify doctor if she becomes pregnant. • Watch patient closely for signs of mental depression. Warn him to notify doctor promptly if he starts having nightmares. • Inform patient that orthostatic hypotension can be minimized by rising slowly and avoiding sudden position changes. Mouth dryness can be relieved with sugarless chewing gum, sour hard candy, or ice chips. Tell patient to contact doctor if relief is needed for nasal stuffiness. • Give this drug with meals. • Patient should weigh himself daily and notify doctor of any weight gain. • Effects of this drug may last for 10 days after it's discontinued. • Parenteral form erratically absorbed; commonly replaced by other antihypertensives for hypertensive emergencies.
None significant.	• Contraindicated in patients with anemia, respiratory insufficiency. Use cautiously in patients with arteriosclerosis; cardiac, hepatic, or renal disease; degenerative CNS disorders; Addison's disease; diabetes. Also use cautiously in patients receiving glucocorticoids; or in those receiving other antihypertensives. • Monitor patient's blood pressure and vital signs frequently. • If extreme hypotension occurs, discontinue drug and call doctor. Use phenylephrine or mephentermine to counteract hypotension. • Watch closely for respiratory distress, especially if large doses are used. • Use infusion pump to administer this drug slowly. • Discontinue drug before wound closure in surgery to allow blood pressure to return to normal. • Position patient to avoid cerebral anoxia. • Patient should receive oxygen therapy during use of this agent.

23 Vasodilators

amyl nitrite
cyclandelate
dioxyline phosphate
dipyridamole
erythrityl tetranitrate
ethaverine hydrochloride
isosorbide dinitrate
isoxsuprine hydrochloride
mannitol hexanitrate
nicotinyl alcohol
nitroglycerin
nylidrin hydrochloride
papaverine hydrochloride
pentaerythritol tetranitrate
tolazoline hydrochloride

Vasodilators can be grouped into two categories: peripheral vasodilators and coronary vasodilators.

Peripheral vasodilators include cyclandelate, dioxyline, ethaverine, isoxsuprine, nicotinyl alcohol, nylidrin, papaverine, and tolazoline. Although these drugs have limited clinical value in patients with obstructive vascular disease, they may be useful in patients with minimal organic involvement. Studies in healthy persons indicate that the peripheral vasodilators increase blood flow to vascular areas. Although we lack evidence of their vasodilating effect in diseased vascular areas, these drugs are still widely used.

The *coronary vasodilators,* or antianginal agents, include drugs that abort acute angina episodes (amyl nitrite, isosorbide dinitrate, and nitroglycerin) and long-term prophylactic drugs (erythrityl tetranitrate, isosorbide dinitrate, mannitol hexanitrate, nitroglycerin, and pentaerythritol tetranitrate).

Major uses

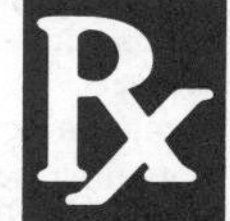

Peripheral vasodilators are used to treat symptoms of peripheral vascular and vasospastic conditions as well as cerebrovascular disease.

Coronary vasodilators combat acute episodes of angina or furnish long-term anginal prophylaxis.

- Dipyridamole (in combination with aspirin or warfarin) inhibits platelet aggregation to reduce risk of thrombus formation.
- Isosorbide dinitrate and nitroglycerin act as therapeutic adjuncts in chronic congestive heart failure.

Mechanism of action

- Some peripheral vasodilators directly relax smooth muscle. This effect may be due to the inhibition of phosphodiesterase, resulting in increased concentrations of cyclic adenosine monophosphate, which causes the vasodilation.
- Other peripheral vasodilators have a different mechanism of action. Tolazoline blocks alpha receptors; isoxsuprine and nylidrin stimulate beta receptors. Although isoxsuprine originally was thought only to stimulate beta receptors, newer evidence indicates that it may also be a direct-acting peripheral vasodilator.
- Coronary vasodilation occurs in

THERAPEUTIC ACTIVITY OF SELECTED VASODILATORS

DRUG	FORM	ONSET	DURATION
amyl nitrite	inhalant	instantaneous	4 to 8 min
erythrityl tetranitrate	chewable	5 min	2 hr
	oral	30 min	3 to 4 hr
	sublingual	5 to 10 min	3 to 4 hr
isosorbide dinitrate	chewable	2 to 5 min	1 to 2 hr
	oral	30 min	4 hr
	sublingual	2 min	1 to 2 hr
mannitol hexanitrate	oral	15 to 30 min	4 to 6 hr
nitroglycerin	oral (extended-release)	1 hr	4 to 6 hr
	sublingual	1 to 2 min	30 min
	topical	15 to 30 min	4 to 6 hr
pentaerythritol tetranitrate	oral	1 hr	4 to 5 hr

normal but not in diseased arteries. Thus, the assumption that coronary vasodilators relieve angina by dilating coronary arteries is only partly correct. Coronary vasodilators cause a pooling of venous blood, which decreases the heart's work load by lowering ventricular diastolic pressure and reducing the stretching of myocardial fibers.

• Dipyridamole, originally classified as a coronary vasodilator, has no value in treating acute attacks of angina. In fact, we lack evidence that its long-term use is beneficial in preventing chronic angina. It does, however, inhibit platelet adhesion.

• Nitrates are effective in chronic congestive heart failure refractory to standard therapy. The dilating effect of nitrates on venous circulation ultimately produces more efficient contraction.

Absorption, distribution, metabolism, and excretion

Vasodilators are well absorbed, widely distributed in body tissues, metabolized in the liver, and excreted mainly in the urine.

Onset and duration

Onset and duration of vasodilators depend on the drug used, form selected, and route of administration. The accompanying chart shows the range of onset and duration for these drugs.

PATIENT-TEACHING AID

HOW TO USE NITROGLYCERIN OINTMENT

Dear Patient:

The doctor has prescribed your nitroglycerin as an ointment. In this form, nitroglycerin is continuously absorbed through the skin into the circulation; it's effective for about 4 hours.

To get the most from your therapy, follow these instructions carefully:

1. Apply ointment to a hairless or shaved area of skin (chest, arm, thigh, abdomen, forehead, ankle, or back) to promote uniform absorption. Choose a new site each time you apply a new dose to prevent minor skin irritations. Remove any traces of ointment left from previous application.
2. Use the ruled applicator paper that comes with the ointment to measure your dose accurately.
3. Use the applicator paper to apply the ointment in a thin, uniform layer over an area of about 7.5 to 15 cm (3″ to 6″). Leave the applicator paper on the site.
4. Cover the applicator paper with plastic wrap and secure it with tape. This will protect your clothing and ensure maximum absorption.

Call your doctor immediately if you experience headache, feel dizzy or faint, or notice any redness or irritation at the application site. He may want to adjust your dosage or check the application site.

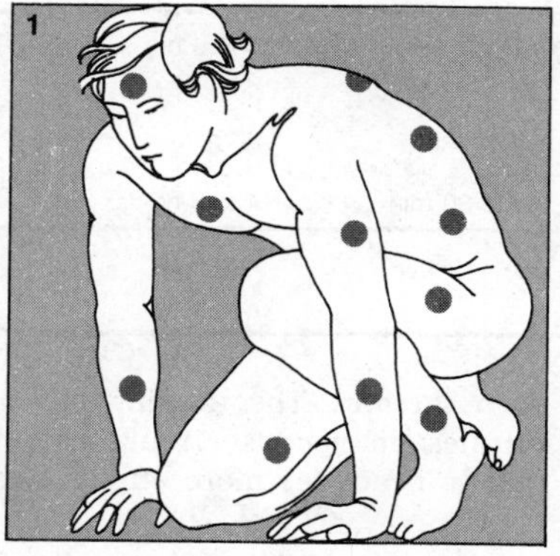

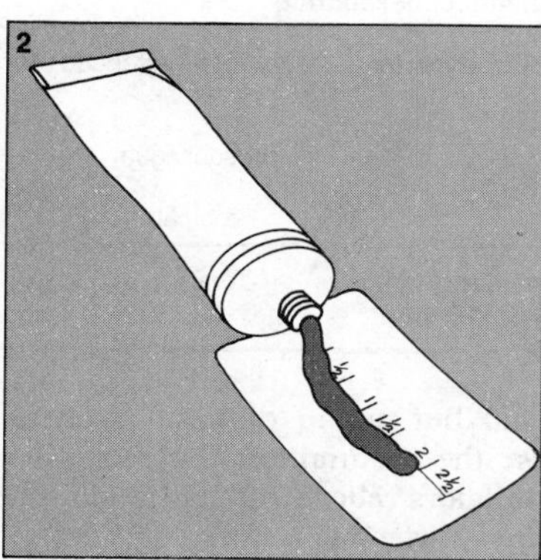

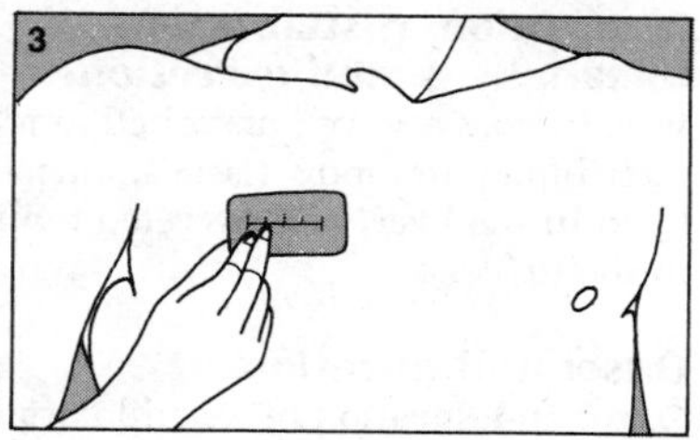

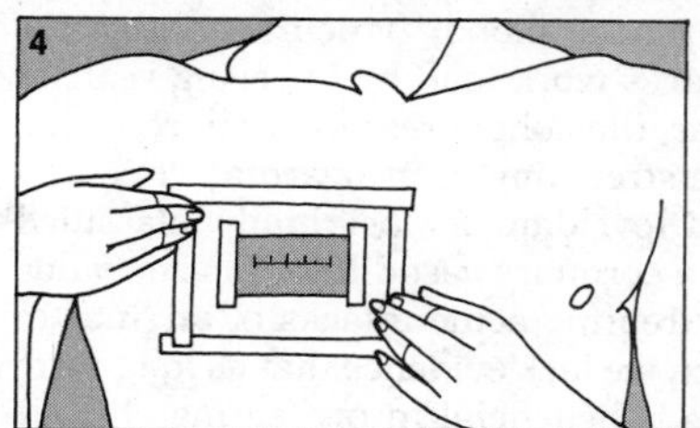

This patient-teaching aid may be reproduced by office copier for distribution to patients.

PATIENT-TEACHING AID

HOW TO TAKE SUBLINGUAL NITROGLYCERIN TABLETS

Dear Patient:

Nitroglycerin relieves anginal pain by temporarily dilating veins and arteries. This brings more blood and oxygen to the heart so it doesn't have to work as hard.

To get the most from your therapy, follow these instructions carefully:

- When you experience anginal pain, lie down and put a tablet under your tongue. Let it dissolve completely, and hold the saliva in your mouth for 1 or 2 minutes before swallowing. Don't stand up until you've swallowed the saliva or you may become dizzy. If you feel headachy or your face flushes after taking your tablet, don't worry. These effects are only temporary.
- Take up to three tablets—one every 4 to 5 minutes—if necessary. Record each dose. If the pain doesn't go away after 30 minutes, call the doctor at once or go to the hospital emergency department.
- Don't stop taking your tablets altogether without asking the doctor. But don't worry about taking them as often as you need; they aren't habit-forming.
- Keep your tablets in their original container, but remove the cotton. They will lose their strength if they're exposed to light, moisture, or heat, or if they're more than 3 months old. Fresh tablets produce a slight burning sensation under your tongue.

Call the doctor immediately if you notice unusually severe or prolonged pain, fainting, or dizziness.

Always have a supply of tablets with you when you go out. Keep a bottle in your car, at work, and at home if you can. Nitroglycerin is available in different strengths, so don't lend tablets or borrow them from anyone else taking this medication.

Combination products

CARDILATE-P: erythrityl tetranitrate 10 mg and phenobarbital 15 mg.

CARTRAX-10: pentaerythritol tetranitrate 10 mg and hydroxyzine HCl 10 mg.

CARTRAX-20: pentaerythritol tetranitrate 20 mg together with hydroxyzine HCl 10 mg.

COROVAS TYMCAPS: pentaerythritol tetranitrate 30 mg and secobarbital 50 mg.

DEAPRIL-ST: dihydroergocornine mesylate 0.167 mg, dihydroergocristine mesylate 0.167 mg, and dihydroergocryptine mesylate 0.167 mg.

EQUANITRATE 10: pentaerythritol tetranitrate 10 mg and meprobamate 200 mg.

EQUANITRATE 20: pentaerythritol tetranitrate 20 mg and meprobamate 200 mg.

HYDERGINE: dihydroergocornine mesylate 0.167 mg, dihydroergocristine mesylate 0.167 mg, and dihydroergocryptine mesylate 0.167 mg.

ISORIL WITH PHENOBARBITAL: isosorbide dinitrate 10 mg and phenobarbital 15 mg.

MILTRATE-10: pentaerythritol tetranitrate 10 mg and meprobamate 200 mg.

MILTRATE-20: pentaerythritol tetranitrate 20 mg and meprobamate 200 mg.

PAPAVATRAL L.A. CAPSULES: pentaerythritol tetranitrate 50 mg and ethaverine HCl 30 mg.

PERITRATE WITH PHENOBARBITAL: pentaerythritol tetranitrate 10 mg and phenobarbital 15 mg.

PERITRATE WITH PHENOBARBITAL: pentaerythritol tetranitrate 20 mg and phenobarbital 15 mg.

NAME	INDICATIONS & DOSAGE	SIDE EFFECTS
amyl nitrite	*Antidote for cyanide poisoning*— 0.2 or 0.3 ml by inhalation for 30 to 60 seconds q 5 minutes until conscious. *Relief of angina pectoris, bronchospasm, biliary spasm*— **Adults and children:** 0.2 to 0.3 ml by inhalation (1 glass ampul inhaler), p.r.n.	**Blood:** methemoglobinemia. **CNS:** *headache, sometimes with throbbing;* dizziness; weakness. **CV:** *orthostatic hypotension, tachycardia,* flushing, palpitations, fainting. **GI:** nausea, vomiting. **Skin:** cutaneous vasodilation. **Other:** hypersensitivity reactions.
cyclandelate Cyclanfor, Cyclospasmol♦	*Adjunct in intermittent claudication, arteriosclerosis obliterans, vasospasm and muscular ischemia associated with thrombophlebitis, nocturnal leg cramps, Raynaud's phenomenon, selected cases of ischemic cerebrovascular disease*— **Adults:** initially, 200 mg P.O. q.i.d. (before meals and h.s.); maximum 400 mg P.O. q.i.d. When clinical response is noted, decrease dosage gradually until maintenance dosage is reached. Maintenance dose 400 to 800 mg daily in divided doses.	**CNS:** *headache, tingling of the extremities, dizziness.* **CV:** *mild flushing,* tachycardia. **GI:** pyrosis, eructation, nausea, heartburn. **Other:** *sweating.*
dioxyline phosphate Paveril Phosphate♦	*Treatment of angina pectoris and conditions in which there is reflex spasm of blood vessels in arms, legs, or lungs; smooth-muscle spasm*— **Adults:** 100 to 400 mg 3 to 4 times daily, as required.	**CNS:** dizziness, sedation. **CV:** sweating, flushing, hypotension. **GI:** nausea, abdominal cramps.
dipyridamole Persantine♦	*Long-term therapy for chronic angina pectoris, prevention of recurrent transient ischemic attack*— **Adults:** 50 mg P.O. t.i.d. at least 1 hour before meals, to maximum of 400 mg daily. *Inhibition of platelet adhesion in patients with prosthetic heart valves, in combination with warfarin*— **Adults:** 100 to 400 mg P.O. daily. *Transient ischemic attack*— **Adults:** 100 mg P.O. daily as a single dose.	**CNS:** *headache, dizziness,* weakness. **CV:** flushing, fainting, *hypotension.* **GI:** *nausea,* vomiting, diarrhea. **Skin:** rash.

♦ Available in U.S. and Canada. ♦♦ Available in Canada only. All other products (no symbol) available in U.S. only. Italicized side effects are common or life-threatening.

INTERACTIONS	NURSING CONSIDERATIONS
None significant.	• Contraindicated in hypersensitivity to nitrites. Use with caution in cerebral hemorrhage, hypotension, head injury, and glaucoma. • Watch for orthostatic hypotension. Have patient sit down and avoid rapid position changes while inhaling drug. • Extinguish all cigarettes before using or ampul may ignite. • Wrap ampul in cloth and crush. Hold near patient's nose and mouth so vapor is inhaled. • Effective within 30 seconds but has a short duration of action (4 to 8 minutes). • Keeping the head low, deep breathing, and movement of extremities may help relieve dizziness, syncope, or weakness from postural hypotension. • Drug is often abused. Claimed to have aphrodisiac benefits. Sometimes called "Amy."
None significant.	• Use with extreme caution in severe obliterative coronary artery or cerebrovascular disease, since circulation to these diseased areas may be compromised by vasodilatory effects of the drug elsewhere (coronary steal syndrome). Use with caution in patients with glaucoma, hypotension. • Give with food or antacids to lessen GI distress. • Use in conjunction with, not as a substitute for, appropriate medical or surgical therapy for peripheral or cerebrovascular disease. • Short-term therapy of little benefit. Instruct patient to expect long-term treatment and to continue to take medication. • Side effects usually disappear after several weeks of therapy.
None significant.	• Alert patient to possible side effects.
None significant.	• Use with caution in hypotension, anticoagulant therapy. • Observe for side effects, especially with large doses. Monitor blood pressure. • Administer 1 hour before meals. • Watch for signs of bleeding, prolonged bleeding time (large doses, long-term). • Clinical response to antianginal therapy may not be evident before second or third month. Tell patient to continue drug despite lack of observable response.

NAME	INDICATIONS & DOSAGE	SIDE EFFECTS
erythrityl tetranitrate Anginar, Cardilate♦	*Prophylaxis and long-term management of frequent or recurrent anginal pain, reduced exercise tolerance associated with angina pectoris—* **Adults:** 5 mg sublingually or buccally t.i.d. or 10 mg P.O., a.c. chewed t.i.d., increasing in 2 to 3 days if needed.	**CNS:** *headache, sometimes with throbbing; dizziness;* weakness. **CV:** *orthostatic hypotension, tachycardia, flushing, palpitations,* fainting. **GI:** nausea, vomiting. **Local:** sublingual burning. **Skin:** cutaneous vasodilation. **Other:** hypersensitivity reactions.
ethaverine hydrochloride Cebral, Circubid, Etalent, Ethaquin, Ethatab, Ethavex, Isovex, Laverin, Myoquin, Neopavrin, Pavaspan, Roldiol, Spasodil	*Long-term treatment of peripheral and cerebrovascular insufficiency associated with arterial spasm; spastic conditions of gastrointestinal and genitourinary tracts—* **Adults:** 100 to 200 mg P.O. t.i.d. or 150 mg of sustained-release preparation P.O. q 12 hours.	**CNS:** *headache,* drowsiness. **CV:** *hypotension, flushing,* sweating, vertigo, cardiac depression, arrhythmias. **GI:** *nausea; anorexia; abdominal distress; dryness of throat;* constipation; diarrhea. **Hepatic:** jaundice, altered liver function studies. **Skin:** rash. **Other:** respiratory depression, malaise, lassitude.
isosorbide dinitrate Angidil, Coronex♦♦, Iso-Bid, Iso-D, Isordil♦, Isosorb, Isotrate, Neo-Corovas-80, Onset, Sorate, Sorbitrate, Sorquad, Vasotrate	*Treatment of acute anginal attacks (sublingual and chewable only); prophylaxis in situations likely to cause attacks; treatment of chronic ischemic heart disease (by preload reduction); adjunct with other vasodilators, such as hydralazine and prazosin, in treatment of severe chronic congestive heart failure—*	**CNS:** *headache, sometimes with throbbing; dizziness;* weakness. **CV:** *orthostatic hypotension, tachycardia, palpitations,* fainting. **GI:** nausea, vomiting. **Local:** sublingual burning. **Skin:** cutaneous vasodilation, *flushing.* **Other:** hypersensitivity reactions.

♦ Available in U.S. and Canada. ♦♦ Available in Canada only. All other products (no symbol) available in U.S. only. Italicized side effects are common or life-threatening.

INTERACTIONS	NURSING CONSIDERATIONS
None significant.	• Contraindicated in hypersensitivity to nitrites, head trauma, cerebral hemorrhage, severe anemia. Use with caution in hypotension. • Monitor blood pressure, and intensity and duration of response to drug. • May cause headaches, especially at first. Treat headache with aspirin or acetaminophen. Dosage may need to be reduced temporarily, but tolerance usually develops. • Tell patient to take medication regularly, even long-term, if ordered, and to keep it easily accessible at all times. Physiologically necessary but not habit-forming. • Additional dose may be taken before anticipated stress or at bedtime if angina is nocturnal. • Advise patient to avoid alcoholic beverages; they may produce unpleasant disulfiram-like side effects. • May cause orthostatic hypotension. Patient should get out of bed, go up and down stairs, and change position slowly; he should lie down at first sign of dizziness. • Teach patient to take sublingual tablet at first sign of attack. He should wet the tablet with saliva, place it under the tongue until completely absorbed, and sit down and rest. Burning sensation indicates potency. Dose may be repeated every 10 to 15 minutes for a maximum of three doses. If no relief, patient should call doctor or go to hospital emergency room. If patient complains of tingling sensation with drug placed sublingually, he may try holding tablet in buccal pouch. • Teach patient to take oral tablet on empty stomach, either ½ hour before or 1 to 2 hours after meals; to swallow oral tablets whole; and chew chewable tablets thoroughly before swallowing. • Drug should not be discontinued abruptly—coronary vasospasm may occur. • Store medication in cool place, in tightly closed container, away from light. To assure freshness, replace supply every 3 months. Remove cotton from container, since it absorbs drug.
None significant.	• Contraindicated in complete AV dissociation and in severe hepatic disease. Use with caution in women who are pregnant or of childbearing age, and in patients with glaucoma or pulmonary embolus; may precipitate arrhythmias. • Hold dose and call doctor if signs of hepatic hypersensitivity develop (gastrointestinal symptoms, altered liver function studies, jaundice, eosinophilia). • Monitor and record vital signs during therapy. • FDA has announced this drug may not be effective for disease states indicated.
None significant.	• Contraindicated in hypersensitivity to nitrites, head trauma, cerebral hemorrhage, severe anemia. Use with caution in hypotension. • Monitor blood pressure, and intensity and duration of response to drug. • May cause headaches, especially at first. Treat headache with aspirin or acetaminophen. Dosage may need to be reduced temporarily, but tolerance usually develops. • Tell patient to take medication regularly, even long-term, if ordered, and to keep it easily accessible at all times. Physiologically necessary but not habit-forming. • May cause orthostatic hypotension. Patient should get out of bed,

(continued on following page)

NAME	INDICATIONS & DOSAGE	SIDE EFFECTS
isosorbide dinitrate *(continued)*	**Adults:** *Sublingual form*—2.5 to 10 mg under the tongue for prompt relief of anginal pain, repeated q 2 to 3 hours during acute phase, or q 4 to 6 hours for prophylaxis. *Chewable form*—5 to 10 mg, p.r.n., for acute attack or q 2 to 3 hours for prophylaxis but only after initial test dose of 5 mg to determine risk of severe hypotension. *Oral form*—5 to 30 mg P.O. q.i.d. for prophylaxis only (use smallest effective dose); sustained-release forms 40 mg P.O. q 6 to 12 hours.	
isoxsuprine hydrochloride Rolisox, Vasodilan♦, Vasoprine	*Adjunct for relief of symptoms associated with cerebrovascular insufficiency, peripheral vascular diseases (such as arteriosclerosis obliterans, thromboangiitis obliterans, Raynaud's disease)*— **Adults:** 10 to 20 mg P.O. t.i.d. or q.i.d.; initially, 5 to 10 mg I.M. b.i.d. or t.i.d. in severe or acute conditions, to maximum of 10 mg. Intramuscular doses greater than 10 mg may be associated with hypotension and tachycardia and are not recommended.	**CNS:** *dizziness,* nervousness, weakness, trembling, *lightheadedness.* **CV:** *hypotension, tachycardia, transient palpitations.* **GI:** vomiting, abdominal distress, intestinal distention. **Skin:** severe rash.
mannitol hexanitrate Mannex, Vascunitol	*Chronic prophylaxis against attacks of angina pectoris*— **Adults:** 15 to 60 mg P.O. q 4 to 6 hours.	**CNS:** *headache, sometimes with throbbing; dizziness;* weakness, increased intracranial pressure. **CV:** *orthostatic hypotension, tachycardia, flushing, palpitations,* fainting. **EENT:** rise in intraocular tension. **GI:** nausea, vomiting. **Skin:** cutaneous vasodilation. **Local:** sublingual burning. **Other:** hypersensitivity.

INTERACTIONS	NURSING CONSIDERATIONS
	go up and down stairs, and change position slowly; he should lie down at first sign of dizziness. • Additional dose may be taken before anticipated stress or at bedtime if angina is nocturnal. • Advise patient to avoid alcoholic beverages; they may produce unpleasant disulfiram-like side effects. • Teach patient to take sublingual tablet at first sign of attack. He should wet the tablet with saliva, place it under the tongue until completely absorbed, and sit down and rest. Burning sensation indicates potency. Dose may be repeated every 10 to 15 minutes for a maximum of three doses. If no relief, patient should call doctor or go to hospital emergency room. If patient complains of tingling sensation with drug placed sublingually, he may try holding tablet in buccal pouch. • Warn patient not to confuse sublingual with oral form. • Teach patient to take oral tablet on empty stomach, either ½ hour before or 1 to 2 hours after meals; to swallow oral tablets whole; and to chew chewable tablets thoroughly before swallowing. • Drug should not be discontinued abruptly—coronary vasospasm may occur. • Store in cool place, in tightly closed container, away from light. • Has been used investigationally in treatment of congestive heart failure.
None significant.	• Contraindicated in immediate postpartum period, arterial bleeding; I.M. contraindicated in hypotension or tachycardia. • Safe use in pregnancy and lactation not established, although drug has been used to inhibit contractions in premature labor. • Do not give intravenously. • Observe for hypotension and tachycardia with parenteral use. Monitor blood pressure and pulse rate. • Discontinue if rash develops.
None significant.	• Contraindicated in head trauma, cerebral hemorrhage, severe anemia. Use with caution in hypotension. • Monitor blood pressure, and intensity and duration of response to drug. • Medication may cause headaches, especially at first. Treat headache with aspirin or acetaminophen. Dosage may need to be reduced temporarily, but tolerance usually develops. • Tell patient to take medication regularly, even long-term, if ordered. Physiologically necessary but not habit-forming. • Additional doses may be taken before anticipated stress or at bedtime if angina is nocturnal. • Alcoholic beverages should be avoided, since they may produce unpleasant disulfiram-like side effects. • Medication may cause orthostatic hypotension. Patient should get out of bed, go up and down stairs, or change position slowly; he should lie down at first sign of dizziness. • Store medication in cool dark place in tightly covered container. • Effective within 15 to 30 minutes; duration 4 to 6 hours.

NAME	INDICATIONS & DOSAGE	SIDE EFFECTS
nicotinyl alcohol Roniacol♦	*Treatment of conditions of deficient circulation such as peripheral vascular disease, vascular spasm, varicose ulcers, decubital ulcers, Ménière's syndrome, vertigo—* **Adults:** 50 to 100 mg regular tablets P.O. b.i.d. or t.i.d. (may increase to 150 to 200 mg P.O. t.i.d. or q.i.d.); 150 to 300 mg sustained-release tablets P.O. b.i.d.; 5 to 10 ml of elixir P.O. t.i.d.	**CNS:** paresthesias. **CV:** *transient flushing.* **GI:** *gastric irritation.* **Skin:** minor rashes. **Other:** allergic reactions.
nitroglycerin Ang-O-Span, Cardabid, Corobid, Glyceryl Trinitrate, Gly-Trate, Nitrine, Nitrobid, Nitrocap, Nitrocels, Nitro-Dial, Nitrodisc, Nitro-Dur, Nitroglyn, Nitrol♦, Nitro-Lyn, Nitrong♦, Nitrospan, Nitrostabilin♦♦, Nitrostat♦, Nitro-TD, Nitrotym, Nitrozem, Nyglycon, Transderm-Nitro-Trates, Vasoglyn	*Prophylaxis against chronic anginal attacks—* **Adults:** 1 sustained-release capsule q 8 to 12 hours; or 2% ointment: Start with ½" of ointment, increasing with ½"-increments until headache occurs, then decreasing to previous dose. Range of dosage with ointment 2" to 5". Usual dose 1" to 2". Alternatively, transdermal disc or pad may be applied to hairless site once daily. *Relief of acute angina pectoris, prophylaxis to prevent or minimize anginal attacks when taken immediately prior to stressful events—* **Adults:** 1 sublingual tablet (gr $^1/_{400}$, $^1/_{200}$, $^1/_{150}$, $^1/_{100}$) dissolved under the tongue or in the buccal pouch immediately on indication of anginal attack. May repeat q 5 minutes for 15 minutes.	**CNS:** *headache, sometimes with throbbing; dizziness;* weakness. **CV:** *orthostatic hypotension, tachycardia, flushing, palpitations,* fainting. **GI:** nausea, vomiting. **Skin:** cutaneous vasodilation. **Local:** sublingual burning. **Other:** hypersensitivity reactions.
nylidrin hydrochloride Arlidin♦, Pervadil♦♦, Rolidrin	*To increase blood supply in vasospastic disorders (arteriosclerosis obliterans, thromboangiitis obliterans, diabetic vascular disease, night leg cramps, Ray-*	**CNS:** trembling, *nervousness,* weakness, *dizziness (not associated with labyrinth artery insufficiency).* **CV:** *palpitations, hypotension,*

♦ Available in U.S. and Canada. ♦♦ Available in Canada only. All other products (no symbol) available in U.S. only. Italicized side effects are common or life-threatening.

INTERACTIONS	NURSING CONSIDERATIONS
Clonidine: may inhibit vasodilation. Observe for lack of response.	• Contraindicated in active peptic ulcer or gastritis. • Tolerance to side effects develops with continued therapy.
None significant.	• Contraindicated in hypersensitivity to nitrites, head trauma, cerebral hemorrhage, severe anemia. Use with caution in hypotension. • Monitor blood pressure, and intensity and duration of response to drug. • May cause headaches, especially at first. Treat headache with aspirin or acetaminophen. Dosage may need to be reduced temporarily, but tolerance usually develops. • Tell patient to take medication regularly, even long-term, if ordered, and to keep it easily accessible at all times. Physiologically necessary but not habit-forming. • Additional dose may be taken before anticipated stress or at bedtime if angina is nocturnal. • Advise patient to avoid alcoholic beverages; they may produce unpleasant disulfiram-like side effects. • May cause orthostatic hypotension. Patient should get out of bed, go up and down stairs, and change position slowly; he should lie down at first sign of dizziness. • Teach patient to take sublingual tablet at first sign of attack. He should wet the tablet with saliva; place it under the tongue until completely absorbed and sit down and rest. Burning sensation indicates potency. Dose may be repeated every 5 to 15 minutes for a maximum of three doses. If no relief, patient should call doctor or go to hospital emergency room. If patient complains of tingling sensation with drug placed sublingually, he may try holding tablet in buccal pouch. • Teach patient to take oral tablet on empty stomach, either ½ hour before or 1 to 2 hours after meals; to swallow oral tablets whole; and to chew chewable tablets thoroughly before swallowing. • Store in cool dark place, in tightly closed container. To assure freshness, replace supply every 3 months. Remove cotton from container, since it absorbs drug. • To apply ointment, spread in uniform thin layer on any nonhairy area. Do not rub in. Cover with plastic film to aid absorption and to protect clothing. • Doctor may prescribe nitroglycerin by its chemical name, glyceryl trinitrate (GTN).
None significant.	• Contraindicated in acute myocardial infarction, paroxysmal tachycardia, angina pectoris, thyrotoxicosis. Use with caution in uncompensated heart disease or peptic ulcer.

(continued on following page)

NAME	INDICATIONS & DOSAGE	SIDE EFFECTS
nylidrin hydrochloride *(continued)*	*naud's phenomenon and disease, ischemic ulcer, frostbite, acrocyanosis, acroparesthesia, sequelae of thrombophlebitis); and in circulatory disturbances of the middle ear (primary cochlear ischemia, cochlear striae, vascular ischemia, macular or ampullar ischemia); other disturbances due to labyrinth artery spasm or obstruction—* **Adults:** 3 to 12 mg P.O. t.i.d. or q.i.d.	flushing. **GI:** *nausea, vomiting.*
papaverine hydrochloride Blupav, BP-Papaverine, Cerebid, Cerespan, Cirbed, Delapav, DiPav, J-Pav, Kavrin, Lapay, Myobid, Papacon, Papalease, Papital T.R., PapKaps-150, Meta-Kaps, P-A-V, Pavabid, Pavacap, Pavacen, Pavaclor, Pavacron, Pavadel, Pavadur, Pavadyl, Pavakey S.A., Pava-lyn, Pava-Par, Pava-Rx, Pavasule, Pavatime, Pavatran T.D., Pava-Wol, Paverolan, Pavex, PT-300, Ro-Papav, S.M.R.-Kaps, Sustaverine, Vasal, Vasocap, Vasospan, Vazosan	*Relief of cerebral and peripheral ischemia associated with arterial spasm and myocardial ischemia; treatment of smooth-muscle spasm (coronary occlusion, angina pectoris, sequelae of peripheral and pulmonary embolism, certain cerebral angiospastic states); and visceral spasms (biliary, ureteral, or gastrointestinal colic)—* **Adults:** 60 to 300 mg P.O. 1 to 5 times daily, or 150 to 300 mg sustained-release preparations q 8 to 12 hours; 30 to 120 mg I.M. or I.V. q 3 hours, as indicated.	**CNS:** *headache.* **CV:** *increased heart rate, increased blood pressure* (with parenteral use), depressed AV and intraventricular conduction, arrhythmias. **GI:** constipation, *nausea.* **Other:** *sweating, flushing,* malaise, increased depth of respiration.
pentaerythritol tetranitrate Angijen Green, Angitrate, Antora, Arcotrate Nos. 1 & 2, Baritrate, Blaintrate, Desatrate 30, Desatrate 50, Dilar, Dinate, Duotrate, El-PETN, Kaytrate, Maso-Trol, Naptrate, Nitrin, Penta-Cap-No. 1, Penta-E., Penta-E. S.A., Pentaforte-T, Penta-Tal No. 1 & 2,	*Prophylaxis against angina pectoris—* **Adults:** 10 to 20 mg P.O. q.i.d.; may be titrated upward to 40 mg P.O. q.i.d. ½ hour before or 1 hour after meals and h.s.; 80 mg sustained-release preparations P.O. b.i.d.	**CNS:** *headache, sometimes with throbbing; dizziness;* weakness. **CV:** *orthostatic hypotension, tachycardia, flushing, palpitations,* fainting. **GI:** nausea, vomiting. **Skin:** cutaneous vasodilation. **Other:** hypersensitivity reactions.

INTERACTIONS	NURSING CONSIDERATIONS
None significant.	• Contraindicated for I.V. use in complete AV block. Use with caution in glaucoma. • Monitor blood pressure, heart rate and rhythm, especially in cardiac disease. Hold dose and notify doctor immediately if changes occur. • Not often used parenterally, except when immediate effect is desired. • Give I.V. slowly (over 1 to 2 minutes) to avoid side effects. • Most effective when given early in the course of a disorder. • Tell patient to take medication regularly; long-term therapy is required. • Do not add lactated Ringer's injection to the injectable form; will precipitate. • FDA has announced this drug may not be effective for disease states indicated.
None significant.	• Contraindicated in head trauma, cerebral hemorrhage, severe anemia. Use with caution in hypotension and glaucoma. • Monitor blood pressure, and intensity and duration of response to drug. • Medication may cause headaches, especially at first. Treat with aspirin or acetaminophen. Dosage may need to be reduced temporarily, but tolerance usually develops. • Medication should be taken regularly, even long-term, if ordered. Physiologically necessary but not habit-forming. • Additional doses may be taken before anticipated stress or at bedtime for nocturnal angina. • Not to be used for relief of acute anginal attacks. • Medication may cause orthostatic hypotension. Patient should get out of bed, go up and down stairs, or change position slowly; he should lie down at first sign of dizziness.

(continued on following page)

NAME	INDICATIONS & DOSAGE	SIDE EFFECTS
pentaerythritol tentranitrate *(continued)* Pentestan-80, Pentetra, Pentrate T.D., Pentritol, Pent-T-80, Pentylan, Peritrate♦, PETN, Petro-20 mg, P-T♦♦, P-T-T, Quintrate, Rate, Vasolate, Vasolate-80		
tolazoline hydrochloride Priscoline♦, Tazol, Toloxan, Tolzol	*Spastic peripheral vascular disorders associated with acrocyanosis, acroparesthesia, arteriosclerosis obliterans, Buerger's disease, causalgia, diabetic arteriosclerosis, gangrene, endarteritis, sequelae of frostbite, post-thrombotic conditions, Raynaud's disease, scleroderma*— **Adults:** *Oral*—25 mg 4 to 6 times daily, gradually increasing to maximum of 50 mg 6 times daily. *Parenteral*—10 to 50 mg S.C., I.V., or I.M. q.i.d. Start with low dose, increasing gradually until optimal response (as determined by appearance of flushing) is reached. *Intra-arterial*—50 to 75 mg/injection, depending on response; 1 or 2 injections may be required initially, then dose of 2 or 3 injections weekly to maintain circulation, possibly coupled with oral tolazoline between injections.	**CV:** *arrhythmias, anginal pain, hypertension, flushing,* transient postural vertigo, palpitations. **GI:** *nausea, vomiting, diarrhea, epigastric discomfort, exacerbation of peptic ulcer.* **Local:** burning at injection site. **Other:** weakness, paradoxical response in seriously damaged limbs, increased pilomotor activity, tingling, chilliness, apprehension.

INTERACTIONS	NURSING CONSIDERATIONS
	• Drug should not be discontinued abruptly—coronary vasospasm may occur. • Store medication in cool place in tightly covered, light-resistant container.
Ethyl alcohol: possible disulfiram reaction from accumulation of acetaldehyde. Use together cautiously.	• Contraindicated in coronary artery disease, active peptic ulcer, or following cerebrovascular accident. Use with caution in patients with history of peptic ulcer disease, gastritis, or known or suspected mitral stenosis. • Keep patient warm during parenteral administration to increase response. • Appearance of flushing usually indicates maximum tolerable dose. • Monitor vital signs. Watch especially for blood pressure changes, arrhythmias. • Instruct patient to avoid alcohol: chills and flushing may occur. • Due to risks, technique, and precautions, intra-arterial injection should be done only by experienced personnel, in selected cases, and only after maximum benefit has been achieved with oral and parenteral therapy. • Warn patient against exposure to cold, which can aggravate tissue damage. • Often used to distinguish between functional (vasospastic) and organic (obstructive) forms of peripheral vascular disease.

24 Antilipemics

cholestyramine
clofibrate
colestipol hydrochloride
dextrothyroxine sodium
niacin
probucol
sitosterols

Antilipemics can retard, and even arrest, atherosclerosis and its resultant complications. Atherosclerosis is associated with increased levels of certain blood lipids. Research thus far, however, has not been able to show a direct clinical relationship between lowered blood lipid levels and reduced incidence of atherosclerosis since other risk factors are reduced as well during the treatment period.

Dietary restriction and physical exercise are essential in treating all hyperlipidemias. If strict dietary therapy does not effectively lower lipid levels after 2 or 3 months, drug therapy may be started.

Hyperlipidemias may be primary or secondary to conditions such as hypothyroidism, hepatic disorders, renal failure, nephrosis, pancreatic insufficiency, malabsorption syndromes, and diabetes mellitus.

Major uses

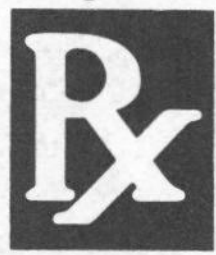

Antilipemics counteract high concentrations of lipids in the blood. They do this by lowering levels of cholesterol or triglycerides or both, to different degrees.

Mechanism of action

The drug chosen to reduce blood lipid levels depends on which fraction or fractions of the blood lipids are elevated. The table on page 339 compares the quantitative antilipemic effects of various drugs.

- Both cholestyramine and colestipol combine with bile acid to form an insoluble compound that is excreted.
- Clofibrate—used when triglycerides are high and cholesterol levels are only moderately elevated—seems to inhibit biosynthesis of cholesterol, but the exact mechanism is unknown.
- Dextrothyroxine accelerates hepatic catabolism of cholesterol and increases bile secretion to lower cholesterol levels. The drug's serious cardiovascular side effects restrict its use to young patients with no history of coronary artery disease.
- Niacin, by an unknown mechanism, decreases synthesis of low-density lipoproteins and inhibits lipolysis in adipose tissue.
- Probucol inhibits cholesterol transport from the intestine and may also decrease cholesterol synthesis. The drug appears to be more effective in patients with mild cholesterol elevations than in those with severe hypercholesterolemia.
- Sitosterols, structurally similar to cholesterol, compete with it to reduce absorption.

Absorption, distribution, metabolism, and excretion

- Cholestyramine, colestipol, and the

TYPES OF HYPERLIPOPROTEINEMIA

TYPE AND NAME	FREQUENCY	POSSIBLE TREATMENTS
I—Fat-induced hyperlipemia	Rare	• Very low-fat diet
II—Familial hyper-cholesterolemia	Common	• If severe, possibly antiplatelet therapy • Fat-controlled diet • Colestipol or cholestyramine (first choice); clofibrate or nicotinic acid (second choice)
III—Broad beta disease	Rare	• Low-calorie diet if overweight • Fat-controlled diet • Clofibrate
IV—Endogenous hypertriglycer-idemia	Common	• Low-calorie diet if overweight • Fat-controlled diet • Exercise • Clofibrate • Avoidance of oral contraceptives and estrogens
V—Mixed hyper-lipemia	Uncommon	• Diet low in cholesterol, fat, and carbohydrates • Clofibrate

sitosterols are not appreciably absorbed from the gastrointestinal (GI) tract. They are eliminated in the feces.
- Clofibrate and niacin are well absorbed from the GI tract.
- Dextrothyroxine is poorly absorbed from the GI tract.
- Probucol is very poorly absorbed from the GI tract. It is passed into the bile for elimination in the feces.

Onset and duration
Response to antilipemic therapy varies with adherence to drug and dietary regimens. Drug treatment is effective only when combined with an adequate dietary plan. (See the patient-teaching aid on the following page for selecting foods on a diet for hyperlipoproteinemia.) For maximum benefit, blood cholesterol and triglyceride levels should be tested several times during the first few months of therapy and periodically thereafter.

After administration of dietary or drug therapy, a new lipid steady-state level is reached in 4 weeks. Lipid levels should be rechecked at this time and the regimen changed, if necessary.
- Clofibrate and probucol take up to 2 months to achieve maximum effect.
- Niacin's effect is transient; therefore, free fatty acid levels rebound between meals and at night. The bedtime dose is especially important to counteract the striking rise of free fatty acid levels during the nocturnal fast.

Combination products
None.

PATIENT-TEACHING AID

SELECTING FOODS ON A DIET FOR HYPERLIPOPROTEINEMIA (TYPES II AND IV)

FOOD	FOODS INCLUDED	FOODS EXCLUDED
Meat	**II**—Lean meat, with fat trimmed off; beef (ground round or chuck, roast, pot roast, stew, steak, dried chipped beef); lamb; pork; ham; veal. Limit to 9 oz cooked/day, including fish and poultry. Limit beef, lamb, ham, and pork to 3-oz portion 3 times/week	**II**—Fried meats; fatty meats such as bacon, cold cuts, hot dogs, luncheon meats, sausage, canned meats (for example, Spam); corned beef; pork and beans; spareribs; commercially prepared ground beef or hamburger; meat canned or frozen in sauces or gravy; frozen or packaged prepared products; all organ meats (kidney, heart, brains, liver, sweetbread)
	IV—Same as for II except limit to 6 to 9 oz cooked/day	**IV**—Same as above minus all organ meats
Poultry, fish, and eggs	**II**—Skinned turkey, chicken, or Cornish hen; fish, water-packed tuna or salmon, limited amounts of shellfish (crab, clams, lobster, oysters, scallops)	**II**—Poultry skin, fish canned in oil, goose, duck, fried poultry or fish, fish roe (including caviar)
	IV—Same as for II, except 3 egg yolks/week may be substituted for 2 oz shellfish or 2 oz organ meats; shrimp allowed	**IV**—Same as above except for egg yolks and shrimp
Soups	**II, IV**—Bouillon, clear broth; any fat-free soups, cream soup made with skim milk, packaged broth-base dehydrated soups	**II, IV**—All others
Sweets	**II**—Hard candies, jams, jelly, honey, sugar	**II**—Chocolate, all other candy
	IV—Most concentrated sweets eliminated	**IV**—All candy, chocolate, jams, jelly, syrups, honey, sugar
Vegetables	**II**—2 to 4 servings/day of any vegetable (at least one dark green and one deep yellow vegetable daily) prepared with allowed fats	**II**—Buttered, creamed, or fried vegetables except when prepared with safflower or corn oil
	IV—Same as for II, except limit amounts of potatoes, corn, lima beans, dried peas, and beans	**IV**—Same as for II, except when prepared with unsaturated fats
Miscellaneous	**II, IV**—Pickles, salt, spice, herbs, vinegar, mustard, soy sauce, Worcestershire sauce, cocoa, peanut butter, olives, and nuts (except those excluded)	**II, IV**—Coconut, cashew and macadamia nuts
Beverages (nondairy)	**II**—Coffee, tea, carbonated beverages, fruit and vegetable juices	**II**—None
	IV—Same as above, but only unsweetened beverages allowed	**IV**—Sweetened beverages

FOOD	FOODS INCLUDED	FOODS EXCLUDED
Breads and cereals	**II, IV**—Enriched varieties of all breads, except egg bread, saltines, and graham crackers. Baked goods containing no whole milk or egg yolks (angel food cake). All cereals and grain products (rice, macaroni, noodles, spaghetti) **II**—Four or more servings/day **IV**—Number of servings specified for weight control	**II, IV**—Biscuits, muffins, corn bread, pancakes, waffles, French toast, hot rolls, sweet rolls, corn or potato chips, flavored crackers
Dairy products	**II**—Skim milk, nonfat buttermilk, evaporated skim milk, dried skim milk, uncreamed (no fat) cottage cheese, cheese made from skim milk plus specially prepared cheese high in polyunsaturated fat; ¼ cup creamed cottage cheese may be substituted for 1 oz meat **IV**—Same as above except that 2 oz of any cheese allowed per week	**II, IV**—Fresh, dried, evaporated, or condensed whole milk; sweet or sour cream; yogurt; ice cream or ice milk; sherbet; commercial whipped toppings; cream cheese and all other cheese, except skim milk cheese; nondairy or other cream substitutes with exceptions shown under foods included
Desserts	**II, IV**—Angel food cake, puddings or frozen desserts made with skim milk, flavored gelatin dessert, meringues, fruit ices or whips, plus desserts made with allowed fats	**II, IV**—All cake and cookie mixes, except angel food cake; any pies, cakes, cookies containing whole milk, fat, or egg yolks; allowed fats included
Fat	**II**—Safflower oil, corn oil, soft safflower margarine, commercial mayonnaise **IV**—Any unsaturated vegetable oil (safflower, corn, cottonseed, olive, and peanut), commercial mayonnaise, commercial salad dressings containing no sour cream or cheese	**II**—Butter, lard, hydrogenated shortening, and margarine; coconut oil and other oils not listed; salt pork, suet, bacon and meat drippings, gravies and sauces unless made with allowed fats and skim milk **IV**—Same as for II, except margarine made from unsaturated fat permitted
Fruits	**II**—Any fresh, frozen, canned, or dried fruit or juice of which one serving/day should be citrus fruit; avocado in small amounts two servings/day **IV**—Same as for II, except three servings/day and small amounts of avocado allowed	**II, IV**—None

NAME	INDICATIONS & DOSAGE	SIDE EFFECTS
cholestyramine Questran♦	*Primary hyperlipidemia, pruritus, and diarrhea due to excess bile acid—* **Adults:** 4 g P.O. before meals and h.s., not to exceed 32 g daily. Each scoop or packet of Questran contains 4 g cholestyramine. **Children:** 240 mg/kg/day P.O. in 3 divided doses with beverage or food. Safe dosage not established for children under 6 years.	**GI:** *constipation,* fecal impaction, hemorrhoids, *abdominal discomfort,* flatulence, *nausea,* vomiting, steatorrhea. **Skin:** *rashes,* irritation of skin, tongue, and perianal area. **Other:** *vitamin A, D, and K deficiencies from decreased absorption;* hyperchloremic acidosis with long-term use or very high dosage.
clofibrate Atromid-S♦	*Hyperlipidemia and xanthoma tuberosum—* **Adults:** 2 g P.O. daily in 4 divided doses. Some patients may respond to lower doses as assessed by serum lipid monitoring. Should not be used in children.	**Blood:** leukopenia. **CNS:** fatigue, weakness. **GI:** *nausea, diarrhea, vomiting,* stomatitis, *dyspepsia,* flatulence. **GU:** decreased libido. **Hepatic:** gallstones, *transient and reversible elevations of liver function studies.* **Skin:** rashes, urticaria, pruritus, dry skin and hair. **Other:** *myalgias and arthralgias,* resembling a flu-like syndrome; *weight gain; polyphagia;* fever.
colestipol hydrochloride Colestid	*Primary hypercholesterolemia and xanthomas—* **Adults:** 15 to 30 g P.O. daily in 2 to 4 divided doses.	**GI:** *constipation (common, may require decreasing the dosage),* fecal impaction, hemorrhoids, abdominal discomfort, flatulence, nausea, vomiting, steatorrhea. **Skin:** rashes, irritation of skin, tongue, and perianal area. **Other:** vitamin A, D, and K deficiencies from decreased absorption; hyperchloremic acidosis with long-term use or very high dosage.
dextrothyroxine sodium Choloxin♦	*Hyperlipidemia in euthyroid patients, especially when cholesterol and triglyceride levels are elevated—* **Adults:** initial dose 1 to 2 mg P.O. daily, increased by 1 to 2 mg daily at monthly intervals to a total of 4 to 8 mg daily. **Children:** initial dose 0.05 mg/kg P.O. daily, increased by 0.05 mg/kg daily at monthly intervals to a total of 4 mg daily.	**CV:** palpitations, angina pectoris, arrhythmias, ischemic myocardial changes on EKG, myocardial infarction. **EENT:** visual disturbances, ptosis. **GI:** nausea, vomiting, diarrhea, constipation, decreased appetite. **Metabolic:** *insomnia, weight loss, sweating,* flushing, hyperthermia, hair loss, menstrual irregularities.

INTERACTIONS	NURSING CONSIDERATIONS
None significant.	• To mix, sprinkle powder on surface of preferred beverage or wet food. Let stand a few minutes, then stir to obtain uniform suspension. • Mixing with carbonated beverages may result in excess foaming. To avoid, use large glass, mix slowly. • Administer all other medications at least 1 hour before or 4 to 6 hours after cholestyramine to avoid blocking their absorption. • Observe bowel habits; treat constipation as needed. Encourage a diet high in roughage and fluids. If severe constipation develops, decrease dosage, add a stool softener, or discontinue drug. • Monitor cardiotonic glycoside levels in patients receiving both medications concurrently. Should cholestyramine therapy be discontinued, cardiotonic glycoside toxicity may result unless dosage is adjusted. • Watch for signs of vitamin A, D, and K deficiencies. • May cause decreased absorption of many drugs due to binding. Check drug interaction list of individual drugs.
Oral contraceptives: may antagonize clofibrate's lipid-lowering effect. Monitor blood lipid level.	• Contraindicated in patients with severe renal or hepatic disease. • Warn patient to report flu-like symptoms to doctor immediately. • Monitor renal and hepatic function, blood counts, serum electrolyte and blood sugar levels. If liver function studies show steady rise, clofibrate should be discontinued. • Should not be used indiscriminately. May pose increased risk of gallstones and cancer. • If significant lipid lowering is not achieved within 3 months, drug should be discontinued.
Oral hypoglycemics: may antagonize response to colestipol. Monitor blood lipid level.	• Administer all other medications at least 1 hour before or 4 to 6 hours after colestipol to avoid blocking their absorption. • Monitor cardiotonic glycoside levels in patients receiving both medications concurrently. Should colestipol therapy be discontinued, cardiotonic glycoside toxicity may result unless dosage is adjusted. • Watch for signs of vitamin A, D, and K deficiencies. • Lowering dosage or adding stool softener may relieve constipation. • May cause decreased absorption of many drugs due to binding. Check drug interaction list of individual drugs.
None significant.	• Contraindicated in patients with hepatic or renal disease, or iodism. Patients with history of cardiac disease, including arrhythmias, hypertension, or angina pectoris, should receive very small doses. • May increase need for insulin, diet therapy, or oral hypoglycemics in patients with diabetes. • If the use of anticoagulants is being considered, discontinue drug 2 weeks before surgery to avoid possible potentiation of anticoagulant effect. • Observe patient for signs of hyperthyroidism, such as nervousness, insomnia, weight loss. If these occur, dosage should be decreased or drug discontinued.

NAME	INDICATIONS & DOSAGE	SIDE EFFECTS
niacin Diacin, Efacin, Niac, Niacalex, Niacels, NICL, Nicobid, Nicocap, Nico-400, Nicolar, NiCord XL, Nico-Span, Nicotinex, Ni-Span, Tega-Span, Tinic, Wampocap	*Adjunctive treatment of hyperlipidemias, especially associated with hypercholesterolemia—* **Adults:** 1.5 to 3 g daily in 3 divided doses with or after meals, increased at intervals to 6 g daily.	**CV:** *flushing* (which usually subsides in a few weeks). **GI:** *nausea,* dyspepsia, vomiting, diarrhea, anorexia, flatulence, epigastric pain. **Hepatic:** liver function study abnormalities. **Metabolic:** *glucose intolerance resulting in hyperglycemia in previously well-controlled diabetics, hyperuricemia.* **Skin:** *pruritus,* sensation of burning or stinging.
probucol Lorelco♦	*Primary hypercholesterolemia—* **Adults:** 2 tablets (500 mg total) P.O. b.i.d. with morning and evening meals. Not recommended in children.	**GI:** *diarrhea, flatulence, abdominal pain, nausea, vomiting.* **Other:** *hyperhidrosis,* fetid sweat, angioneurotic edema.
sitosterols Cytellin	*Adjunctive therapy for hypercholesterolemia or hyperbetalipoproteinemia—* **Adults:** 15 ml (3 g) P.O. before meals to a total of 45 ml (9 g) daily. May increase to 30 ml before large or high-fat meals; give fraction of usual dose before snacks.	**GI:** anorexia; *diarrhea;* abdominal cramps; *bulky, light-colored stools;* nausea.

♦ Available in U.S. and Canada. ♦♦ Available in Canada only. All other products (no symbol) available in U.S. only. Italicized side effects are common or life-threatening.

LETHAL LIPIDS

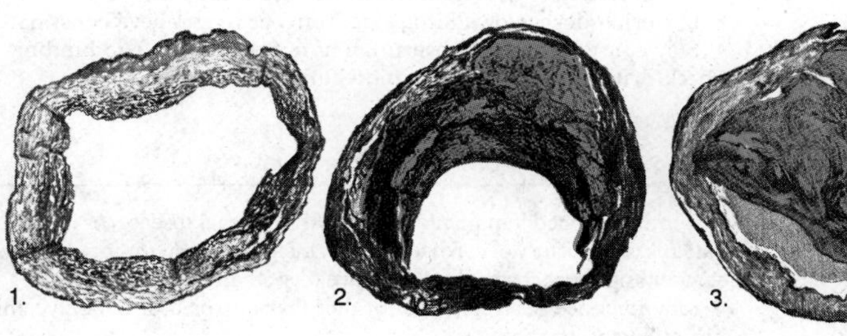

As atherosclerosis develops, a normal coronary artery (illustration 1) becomes roughened and narrowed by lipid deposits (illustration 2). This condition can be treated with antilipemic drugs and a fat-controlled diet. But if left untreated, a blood clot may develop and potentially clog the artery (illustration 3), depriving the heart of its blood supply and causing a heart attack.

INTERACTIONS	NURSING CONSIDERATIONS
None significant.	• Use cautiously in patients with gout, diabetes, gallbladder or hepatic disease, peptic ulcer. • Advise patient that pruritus and flushing noted in first few weeks of therapy usually lessen with continued use. • Begin therapy with small doses; then increase gradually. • Give with meals to minimize GI irritation. Cold water eases swallowing. • Blood glucose tests and liver function studies should be performed routinely during early therapy.
None significant.	• Contraindicated in patients with arrhythmias. Drug should be stopped in any patient whose EKG shows prolonged Q-T interval. • Drug's effect is enhanced when taken with food. • May cause cardiotoxic effects in animals. Evidence of cardiotoxicity in humans not established at this time.
None significant.	• Administer other medications 1 hour before or 4 hours after sitosterols. • Give sitosterols immediately before meals or snacks. • Mix with milk, tea, coffee, or fruit juice for palatability. • Maximum therapeutic effect occurs during 2nd and 3rd months of therapy.

ANTILIPEMICS' EFFECTS ON BLOOD LIPIDS

DRUG	EFFECT ON CHOLESTEROL	EFFECT ON TRIGLYCERIDES
cholestyramine	Marked decrease	No change or Mild increase
clofibrate	Mild decrease	Marked decrease
colestipol	Marked decrease	No change or Mild increase
dextrothyroxine	Moderate decrease	Mild decrease or Mild increase
niacin	Marked decrease	Moderate decrease
probucol	Moderate decrease	No change or Mild increase
sitosterols	Mild decrease	No change

KEY: (white down arrow) = Mild decrease; (gray down arrow) = Moderate decrease; (black down arrow) = Marked decrease; (white up arrow) = Mild increase; (O) = No change

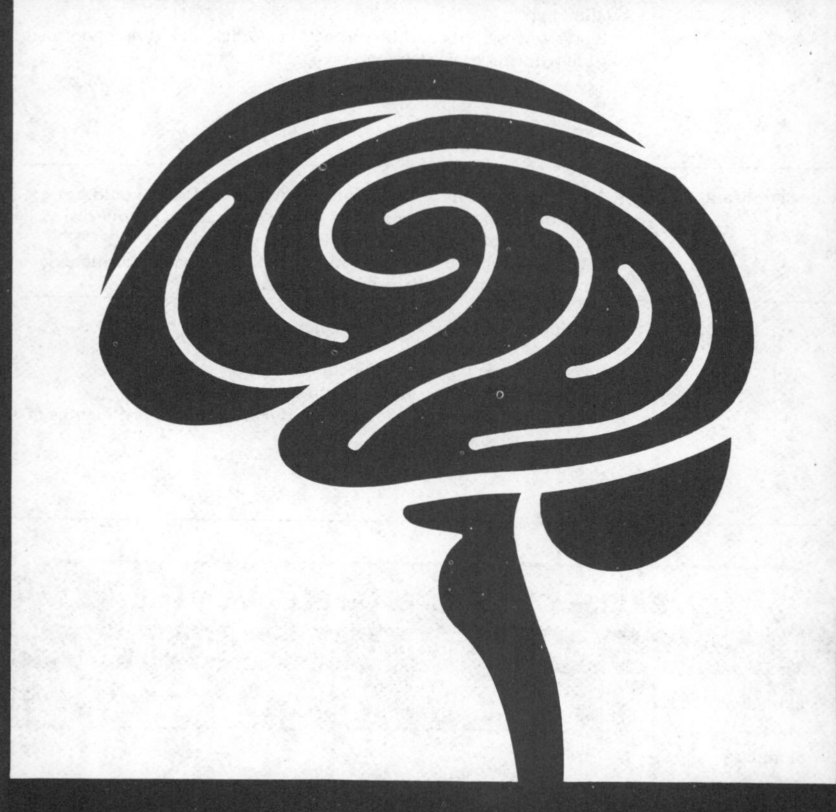

IV Central Nervous System Drugs

Nonnarcotic analgesics and antipyretics

Morphine-like analgesics
butorphanol
nalbuphine hydrochloride

Salicylates
aspirin
choline magnesium trisalicylate
choline salicylate
magnesium salicylate
salicylamide
salsalate
sodium salicylate
sodium thiosalicylate

Urinary tract analgesics
ethoxazene hydrochloride
phenazopyridine hydrochloride

Miscellaneous
acetaminophen
ethoheptazine citrate
methotrimeprazine
phenacetin
zomepirac sodium

(The nonnarcotic analgesics and antipyretics are listed in alphabetical order in the tables that follow.)

Nonnarcotic analgesics and antipyretics are probably the most common drugs in medicine. Aspirin, of course, and most salicylate derivatives are available without a doctor's prescription. Acetaminophen, and to a lesser extent phenacetin, are also widely available without prescriptions. Salicylates, acetaminophen, and phenacetin are combined with one another in varying amounts in many proprietary preparations that are widely advertised in the mass media. Both the morphine-like and urinary tract analgesics necessitate a doctor's prescription.

Major uses

Rx

• Morphine-like analgesics relieve moderate-to-severe pain.

• Salicylates relieve mild-to-moderate pain; alleviate inflammation of rheumatoid arthritis, osteoarthritis, gout, and other conditions; and reduce fever.

Aspirin also inhibits platelet aggregation, hindering coagulation.

• Urinary tract analgesics ease the pain of frequent urination (burning and urgency) associated with cystitis, prostatitis, and urethritis.

Although once thought to have antiseptic properties, urinary tract analgesics are ineffective against microorganisms responsible for urinary tract infections.

• Among the miscellaneous drugs, acetaminophen, ethotheptazine, and phenacetin relieve mild-to-moderate pain and fever. Methotrimeprazine alleviates moderate-to-severe pain; zomepirac is effective against mild-to-moderately-severe pain.

Mechanism of action

• Morphine-like analgesics bind to receptor sites in the central nervous system to alter the individual's perception of and response to pain.

• Salicylates produce analgesia by an

ill-defined effect on the hypothalamus (central action) and by blocking generation of pain impulses (peripheral action). The peripheral action may involve inhibition of prostaglandin synthesis.

Salicylates probably exert their anti-inflammatory effect by inhibiting prostaglandin synthesis; they may also inhibit the synthesis or action of other mediators of the inflammatory response.

They relieve fever by acting on the hypothalamic heat-regulating center to produce peripheral vasodilation. This increases peripheral blood supply and promotes sweating, which leads to loss of heat and cooling by evaporation.

Aspirin also appears to impede coagulation by blocking prostaglandin synthetase action, which prevents formation of platelet-aggregating substance thromboxane A_2.

• The exact mechanism of action of the urinary tract analgesics is unknown.

• Among the miscellaneous drugs, acetaminophen and phenacetin produce analgesia by blocking generation of pain impulses. This action is probably

USING NONNARCOTIC ANALGESICS EFFECTIVELY

To use aspirin and acetaminophen most effectively in relieving pain, suggest these guidelines to the doctor:

1. *Start with nonnarcotics instead of narcotics if pain is mild to moderate.* Nonnarcotics aren't addictive and generally don't produce the narcotic side effects of sedation, constipation, respiratory depression, and tolerance to analgesia.

In some patients the antipyretic effect of aspirin and acetaminophen can mask signs of infection. And patients with bleeding disorders or peptic ulcers shouldn't take aspirin. In the absence of complications, however, try nonnarcotics first.

Administer doses on a regular schedule to keep the blood salicylate level relatively stable and to maintain relief from pain and inflammation. If your patient misses one dose, he'll notice significantly less relief. (*Note:* The degree of analgesia produced by aspirin and by acetaminophen is about equal, but aspirin's anti-inflammatory effect is much greater. For pain accompanied by inflammation, as in arthritis, aspirin may provide more relief.)

2. *Continue to give nonnarcotics concurrently with narcotics, even when nonnarcotics are inadequate for pain relief.* Nonnarcotics provide a foundation of pain relief so that less narcotic is needed. The combination of these two types of drugs attacks pain simultaneously by two different mechanisms, affecting the central (narcotics) and the peripheral and central (nonnarcotics) nervous systems.

Also, narcotics and nonnarcotics have different onset, peak, and duration times. Therefore, a steady level of pain relief may be better achieved by administering tering these two drugs concurrently.

Dosage suggestions

If your patient requires narcotics only once or twice a day, suggest the doctor order 650 mg of aspirin or acetaminophen.

If the patient requires two or more doses of narcotic almost every day, ask the doctor for an order to give two nonnarcotic tablets (325 mg/tablet) on a regular schedule, for a total daily dose of 2,600 to 3,900 mg. While receiving the same total dose of nonnarcotic each day, the patient should experience a stable level of nonnarcotic pain relief. Then narcotics may be added as needed.

You can combine a narcotic analgesic and a nonnarcotic analgesic for better pain relief even when the narcotic is given by injection, provided your patient can tolerate oral aspirin or acetaminophen.

Some oral narcotics are compounded with nonnarcotics, but the dose of the latter may be inadequate. For example, Tylenol #3 and Tylenol #4 contain different amounts of codeine but the same amount of acetaminophen—325 mg—not an adult analgesic dose (see *Combination products,* p. 344). With the doctor's approval, a single tablet of Tylenol #3 or Tylenol #4 should be boosted by an additional acetaminophen dose.

If you administer narcotics and nonnarcotics several times a day, carefully calculate the total daily nonnarcotic dose so it doesn't exceed safe limits for your patient. When giving combination tablets, check the amount of each component so that you can accurately calculate the patient's total daily nonnarcotic dose.

NURSING TIPS

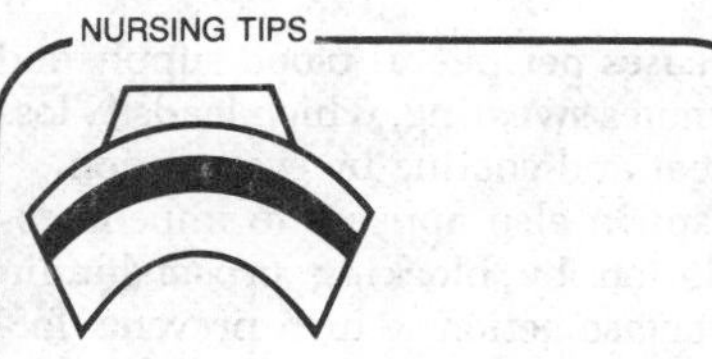

WHAT TO DO FOR ACETAMINOPHEN OVERDOSE

First, question the patient or his family to determine the exact time he took the acetaminophen overdose. If the patient ingested the drug within the past 12 hours, the doctor will usually prescribe ipecac syrup to induce vomiting, or attempt a gastric lavage.

Next, the doctor will prescribe the antidote acetylcysteine (Mucomyst). To make it palatable, mix the vial of acetylcysteine solution with a soft drink. Remember: You must administer it *orally*—not as an inhalant—to effectively counteract acetaminophen toxicity.

If the patient's comatose, you can administer the acetylcysteine solution through a nasogastric tube. Coma, however, is rare in the first phases of acetaminophen toxicity, so find out if the patient has taken another drug that could have produced the coma.

The usual initial dose of acetylcysteine is 140 mg/kg, then 70 mg/kg every 4 hours for 17 doses, to make a total dose of 1,330 mg/kg. Nausea is sometimes a side effect. If the patient vomits any dose within 1 hour after administration, tell the doctor; he'll ask you to repeat the dose.

due to inhibition of prostaglandin synthesis; it may also be due to inhibition of the synthesis or action of other substances that sensitize pain receptors to mechanical or chemical stimulation. Both drugs relieve fever by central action in the hypothalamic heat-regulating center.

Ethoheptazine's mechanism of action is unknown.

Methotrimeprazine is thought to suppress sensory impulses by acting on sites in the thalamus, hypothalamus, and reticular activating and limbic systems.

Zomepirac's mechanism of action is unknown but is probably related to inhibition of prostaglandin synthesis.

Absorption, distribution, metabolism, and excretion

All oral and I.M. forms of the analgesics and antipyretics are well absorbed. The drugs are distributed in most body tissues and fluids, largely metabolized in the liver, and eliminated as inactive metabolites in urine and—through the bile—in feces. The urinary tract analgesics are eliminated as both inactive metabolites and unchanged drug.

Onset and duration

All the nonnarcotic analgesics and antipyretics begin to act 30 to 60 minutes after oral administration and 15 to 30 minutes after I.M. injection. Peak blood levels are reached in 2 to 3 hours. Duration of action of these drugs is generally 4 to 6 hours.

Combination products

ANACIN: aspirin 400 mg and caffeine 32 mg.
A.P.C.: aspirin 227 mg, phenacetin 162 mg, and caffeine 32 mg.
A.S.A. COMPOUND: aspirin 227 mg, phenacetin 160 mg, and caffeine 32.5 mg.
BUTAZOLIDIN ALKA: phenylbutazone 100 mg, dried aluminum hydroxide gel 100 mg, and magnesium trisilicate 150 mg.
DARVOCET-N 50: acetaminophen 325 mg and propoxyphene napsylate 50 mg.
DARVON COMPOUND-65: aspirin 227 mg, phenacetin 162 mg, caffeine 32.4 mg, and propoxyphene HCl 65 mg.
DOLENE AP-65: acetaminophen 650 mg and propoxyphene HCl 65 mg.
DOLENE COMPOUND-65: aspirin 227 mg, phenacetin 162 mg, propoxyphene HCl 65 mg, and caffeine 32.4 mg.
EQUAGESIC: aspirin 250 mg, ethoheptazine citrate 75 mg, and meprobamate 150 mg.
EXCEDRIN TABLETS: aspirin 194.4 mg, acetaminophen 97.2 mg, caffeine 64.8 mg, and salicylamide 129.6 mg.
FEMCAPS: aspirin 162 mg, phenacetin

ASPIRIN'S ROLE IN TRANSIENT ISCHEMIC ATTACKS AND REYE'S SYNDROME

Aspirin, taken daily, can help prevent recurrence of transient ischemic attacks (TIAs) in men. These temporary blackouts, lasting from seconds to hours, are considered a warning sign of impending major cerebrovascular accident.

Studies show that a dose of two regular aspirin tablets twice a day, or one tablet four times a day, can reduce the risk of a TIA by 19% and the incidence of major stroke and death by 31%. Aspirin blocks production of a certain clot-promoting prostaglandin (called thromboxane A_2) in blood platelets, thus helping to prevent formation of stroke-producing clots in the brain. Since new platelets develop constantly, repeated doses of aspirin are necessary to halt synthesis of new prostaglandins. Too high a dose, however, inhibits the clot-*dissolving* prostaglandin prostacyclin, restoring danger of clotting.

Current test findings are definitive for men but not for women. Aspirin has reduced the number of minor strokes in women, but figures are insignificant. Testing is now underway to determine the efficacy of aspirin for healthy persons who have never had attacks.

Link to Reye's syndrome?

Studies done by several state health departments have shown an increased risk of Reye's syndrome in children given aspirin for fever accompanying influenza and varicella. The Center for Disease Control (C.D.C.) in Atlanta asked a panel of experts to evaluate the study data. These experts concluded that the link between Reye's syndrome and salicylates probably couldn't be attributed solely to the limitations of the studies. Therefore, they advised that the use of salicylates be avoided during influenza and varicella in children up to age 18.

The C.D.C., however, has announced that until definitive information either confirming or denying this association is available, it is advising parents and doctors of the possible increased risk of Reye's syndrome.

65 mg, caffeine 32 mg, ephedrine sulfate 8 mg, and atropine sulfate 0.0325 mg.

FIORINAL: butalbital 50 mg, aspirin 200 mg, phenacetin 130 mg, caffeine 40 mg.

SYNALGOS: promethazine HCl 6.25 mg, aspirin 194.4 mg, phenacetin 162 mg, caffeine 30 mg.

TALWIN COMPOUND CAPLETS: aspirin 325 mg and pentazocine (as HCl) 12.5 mg.

TRILISATE: choline salicylate 293 mg and magnesium salicylate 362 mg.

VANQUISH: aspirin 227 mg, acetaminophen 194 mg, caffeine 33 mg, aluminum hydroxide 25 mg, and magnesium hydroxide 50 mg.

ZACTIRIN: aspirin 325 mg and ethoheptazine citrate 75 mg.

NAME	INDICATIONS & DOSAGE	SIDE EFFECTS
acetaminophen Acephen, Atasol♦♦, Campain♦♦, Datril, Dolanex, Liquiprin, Paralgin♦♦, Phenaphen, Phendex, Robigesic♦♦, Rounox♦♦, SK-Apap, Tapar, Tempra♦, Tenlap, Tivrin♦♦, Tylenol♦, Valadol	*Mild pain or fever—* **Adults, and children over 10 years:** 325 to 650 mg P.O. or rectally q 4 hours, p.r.n. Maximum 2.6 g daily. **Children under 1 year:** 15 to 60 mg/dose. **1 year:** 60 mg/dose. **2 years:** 120 mg/dose. **3 years:** 180 mg/dose. **4 years:** 240 mg/dose. **5 to 10 years:** 325 mg/dose. May give P.O. or rectally q 4 to 6 hours. Maximum 1.2 g daily.	**Hepatic:** severe hepatotoxicity with large doses. **Skin:** rash, urticaria.
aspirin Acetal♦♦, Acetophen♦♦, Acetyl-Sal♦♦, Ancasal♦♦, A.S.A., Aspergum, Aspirjen Jr., Aspirin♦♦, Bayer Timed-Release, Buffinol, Decaprin, Ecotrin♦, Empirin, Entrophen♦♦, Measurin, Neopirine No. 25♦♦, Nova-Phase♦♦, Novasen♦♦, Rhonal♦♦, Sal-Adult♦♦, Sal-Infant♦♦, Supasa♦♦, Triaphen-10♦♦	**Adults:** *Arthritis*—2.6 to 5.2 g P.O. daily in divided doses. *Mild pain or fever*—325 to 650 mg P.O. or rectally q 4 hours, p.r.n. *Thromboembolic disorders*—325 to 650 mg P.O. daily or b.i.d. *Transient ischemic attacks*—650 mg P.O. b.i.d. or 325 mg q.i.d. **Children:** *Arthritis*—90 to 130 mg/kg P.O. daily divided q 4 to 6 hours. *Fever*—40 to 80 mg/kg P.O. or rectally daily divided q 6 hours, p.r.n. *Mild pain*—65 to 100 mg/kg P.O. or rectally daily divided q 4 to 6 hours, p.r.n.	**Blood:** *prolonged bleeding time.* **EENT:** *tinnitus and hearing loss (first signs of toxicity).* **GI:** *nausea, vomiting, GI distress, occult bleeding.* **Hepatic:** abnormal liver function studies. **Skin:** *rash.* **Other:** *hypersensitivity manifested by anaphylaxis.*
butorphanol tartrate Stadol	*Moderate-to-severe pain—* **Adults:** 1 to 4 mg I.M. q 3 to 4 hours, p.r.n.; or 0.5 to 2 mg I.V. q 3 to 4 hours, p.r.n.	**CNS:** *sedation, headache, vertigo, floating sensation,* lethargy, confusion, nervousness, unusual dreams, agitation, euphoria, hallucinations, flushing. **CV:** palpitations, fluctuation in blood pressure. **EENT:** diplopia, blurred vision. **GI:** *nausea,* vomiting, dry mouth. **Skin:** rash, hives, *clamminess, excessive sweating.* **Other:** *respiratory depression.*
choline magnesium trisalicylate Trilisate	*Arthritis, mild—* **Adults:** 1 to 2 teaspoonfuls or tablets, each tablet or teaspoonful equal to 500 mg salicylate, b.i.d.	**Blood:** *prolonged bleeding time.* **EENT:** *tinnitus and hearing loss (first signs of toxicity).* **GI:** *nausea, vomiting, GI distress, occult bleeding.*

♦ Available in U.S. and Canada. ♦♦ Available in Canada only. All other products (no symbol) available in U.S. only. Italicized side effects are common or life-threatening.

INTERACTIONS	**NURSING CONSIDERATIONS**
None significant.	• Has no anti-inflammatory effect. • Warn patient that high doses or unsupervised chronic use can cause hepatic damage. Excessive ingestion of alcoholic beverages may hasten hepatotoxicity. • Has little or no effect on prothrombin time. • For toxicity, see APPENDIX, *Drug Toxicities*.
Ammonium chloride (and other urine acidifiers): increases blood levels of aspirin products. Monitor for aspirin toxicity. *Antacids (and other urine alkalinizers):* decrease levels of aspirin products. Monitor for decreased aspirin effect. *Oral anticoagulants:* increase risk of bleeding. Avoid using together if possible.	• Contraindicated in GI ulcer, GI bleeding, aspirin hypersensitivity. Use cautiously in patients with hypoprothrombinemia, vitamin K deficiency, bleeding disorders, Hodgkin's disease (may cause profound hypothermia); in asthmatics with nasal polyps (may cause severe bronchospasm); and in children with fever due to flu or varicella. • Febrile, dehydrated children can develop toxicity rapidly. • Give with food, milk, antacid, or large glass of water to reduce GI side effects. • Warn patients to check with doctor or pharmacist before taking over-the-counter combinations containing aspirin. • Therapeutic blood salicylate level in arthritis is 20 to 30 mg/100 ml. • Alcohol may increase GI blood loss. • May cause increase in serum levels of SGOT, SGPT, alkaline phosphatase, and bilirubin. May produce false-negative test results for urine glucose by glucose oxidase methods (Clinistix, Tes-Tape) and false-positive results using Clinitest. • Keep out of reach of children—aspirin is one of the leading causes of poisoning in children. • Advise patients receiving large doses of aspirin for an extended period of time to watch for petechiae, bleeding gums, signs of GI bleeding, and to maintain adequate fluid intake. Obtain hemoglobin and prothrombin tests periodically. • For toxicity, see APPENDIX, *Drug Toxicities*.
None significant.	• Contraindicated in narcotic addiction; may precipitate narcotic abstinence syndrome. Use cautiously in head injury, increased intracranial pressure, acute MI, ventricular dysfunction, coronary insufficiency, respiratory diseases or depression, renal or hepatic dysfunction. • Unlikely to cause dependence. • Respiratory depression does not increase with increased dosage. • Subcutaneous route not recommended. • Also approved for use as a preoperative medication, as the analgesic component of balanced anesthesia, and for relief of postpartum pain.
Ammonium chloride (and other urine acidifiers): increases blood levels of salicylates. Monitor for sa-	• Contraindicated in GI ulcer, GI bleeding, aspirin hypersensitivity. Use cautiously in patients with hypoprothrombinemia, vitamin K deficiency, bleeding disorders, Hodgkin's disease (may cause profound hypothermia); and in asthmatics with nasal polyps (may cause severe bronchospasm).

(continued on following page)

NAME	INDICATIONS & DOSAGE	SIDE EFFECTS
choline magnesium trisalicylate *(continued)*	*Rheumatoid arthritis and osteoarthritis—* **Adults:** 2 to 3 teaspoonfuls or tablets b.i.d. Each tablet or teaspoonful equal in salicylate content to 650 mg aspirin.	**Hepatic:** abnormal liver function studies. **Skin:** *rash.* **Other:** *hypersensitivity manifested by anaphylaxis.*
choline salicylate Arthropan♦	*Arthritis—* **Adults:** 5 to 10 ml P.O. q.i.d. *Minor pain or fever—* **Adults:** 870 mg (5 ml) P.O. q 3 to 4 hours, p.r.n. **Children 3 to 6 years:** 105 to 210 mg P.O. q 4 hours, p.r.n. Each 870 mg (5 ml) equals 650 mg aspirin.	**Blood:** *prolonged bleeding time.* **EENT:** *tinnitus and hearing loss (first signs of toxicity).* **GI:** *nausea, vomiting, GI distress, occult bleeding.* **Hepatic:** abnormal liver function studies. **Skin:** *rash.* **Other:** *hypersensitivity manifested by anaphylaxis.*
ethoheptazine citrate Zactane	*Mild pain—* **Adults:** 75 to 150 mg P.O. t.i.d. or q.i.d.	**CNS:** dizziness, headache, syncope, nervousness. **EENT:** visual disturbances. **GI:** nausea, vomiting. **Skin:** pruritus.
ethoxazene hydrochloride Serenium	*Pain with urinary tract irritation or infection—* **Adults:** 100 mg a.c. P.O. t.i.d.	**GI:** nausea, vomiting.
magnesium salicylate Analate, Arthrin, Lorisal, Magan, Mobidin, MSG-600, Triact	**Adults:** *Arthritis*—up to 9.6 g daily in divided doses. *Mild pain or fever*—600 mg P.O. t.i.d. or q.i.d.	**Blood:** *prolonged bleeding time.* **EENT:** *tinnitus and hearing loss (first signs of toxicity).* **GI:** *nausea, vomiting, GI distress, occult bleeding.* **Hepatic:** abnormal liver function studies.

♦ Available in U.S. and Canada. ♦♦ Available in Canada only. All other products (no symbol) available in U.S. only. Italicized side effects are common or life-threatening.

INTERACTIONS	NURSING CONSIDERATIONS
licylate toxicity. *Antacids (and other urine alkalinizers):* decrease levels of salicylates. Monitor for decreased salicylate effect. *Oral anticoagulants:* increase risk of bleeding. Avoid using together if possible.	• May cause less GI distress than aspirin. If antacid is needed, give it 2 hours after meals and give choline magnesium trisalicylate before meals. • May mix drug with water, fruit juice, or carbonated drinks. • Febrile, dehydrated children can develop toxicity rapidly. • Warn patient to check with doctor before taking over-the-counter combinations containing aspirin. • Therapeutic blood salicylate level in arthritis is 20 to 30 mg/ 100 ml. • Alcohol may increase GI blood loss. • May cause an increase in serum levels of SGOT, SGPT, alkaline phosphatase, and bilirubin. May produce false-negative test results for urine glucose by glucose oxidase methods (Clinistix, Tes-Tape) and false-positive results using Clinitest. • Obtain hemoglobin and prothrombin tests periodically in patients receiving large doses over an extended period of time.
Ammonium chloride (and other urine acidifiers): increases blood levels of salicylates. Monitor for salicylate toxicity. *Antacids (and other urine alkalinizers):* decrease levels of salicylates. Monitor for decreased salicylate effect. *Oral anticoagulants:* increase risk of bleeding. Avoid using together if possible.	• Contraindicated in GI ulcer, GI bleeding, aspirin hypersensitivity. Use cautiously in patients with hypoprothrombinemia, vitamin K deficiency, bleeding disorders, Hodgkin's disease (may cause profound hypothermia); and in asthmatics with nasal polyps (may cause severe bronchospasm). • May cause less GI distress than aspirin. If antacid is needed, give it 2 hours after meals and give choline salicylate before meals. • May mix drug with water, fruit juice, or carbonated drinks. • Febrile, dehydrated children can develop toxicity rapidly. • Warn patient to check with doctor before taking over-the-counter combinations containing aspirin. • Therapeutic blood salicylate level in arthritis is 20 to 30 mg/ 100 ml. • Alcohol may increase GI blood loss. • May cause an increase in serum levels of SGOT, SGPT, alkaline phosphatase, and bilirubin. May produce false-negative test results for urine glucose by glucose oxidase methods (Clinistix, Tes-Tape) and false-positive results using Clinitest. • Obtain hemoglobin and prothrombin tests periodically in patients receiving large doses over an extended period. • For toxicity, see APPENDIX, *Drug Toxicities*.
None significant.	• May use with aspirin for arthritic pain. • Doesn't lower fever; may use alone when fever is valuable for diagnosis. • Side effects other than GI distress and pruritus usually occur only when recommended is dosage exceeded.
None significant.	• Contraindicated in hepatic and renal disease. Use cautiously in GI disorders. • Colors urine reddish-orange. May stain fabrics. • Use only as analgesic. Use with antibiotic to treat urinary tract infection.
Ammonium chloride (and other urine acidifiers): increases blood levels of aspirin products. Monitor for aspirin toxicity. *Antacids (and other	• Contraindicated in severe chronic renal insufficiency because of risk of magnesium toxicity; GI ulcer; GI bleeding; aspirin hypersensitivity. Use cautiously in hypoprothrombinemia, vitamin K deficiency, bleeding disorders, and Hodgkin's disease (may cause profound hypothermia). • Febrile, dehydrated children can develop toxicity rapidly. • Alcohol may increase GI blood loss.

(continued on following page)

NAME	INDICATIONS & DOSAGE	SIDE EFFECTS
magnesium salicylate *(continued)*		**Skin:** *rash.* **Other:** *hypersensitivity manifested by anaphylaxis.*
methotrimeprazine Levoprome, Nozinan♦♦	*Moderate-to-severe pain in nonambulatory patients—* **Adults:** 10 to 20 mg deep I.M. into large muscle mass q 4 to 6 hours p.r.n. Maximum dose 40 mg.	**Blood:** *agranulocytosis.* **CNS:** confusion, dizziness, *sedation,* weakness, amnesia, slurred speech. **CV:** *orthostatic hypotension.* **EENT:** nasal congestion. **GI:** dry mouth, nausea, vomiting. **GU:** difficulties in urination. **Local:** pain, inflammation at injection site. **Other:** chills.
nalbuphine hydrochloride Nubain	*Moderate-to-severe pain—* S.C., I.M., or I.V. **Adults:** 10 to 20 mg q 3 to 6 hours p.r.n. Maximum daily dose 160 mg.	**CNS:** *sedation,* nervousness, depression, restlessness, crying, euphoria, hostility, unusual dreams, confusion, hallucinations, delusions. **GI:** cramps, dyspepsia, bitter taste. **GU:** urinary urgency. **Skin:** itching, burning, urticaria. **Other:** *respiratory depression,* physical and psychological dependence.
phenacetin	*Mild pain or fever—* **Adults:** 300 mg P.O. q 3 to 4 hours p.r.n. Maximum 2.4 g daily.	**Blood:** methemoglobinemia in toxic doses, hemolytic anemia in G-6-PD deficiency. **GI:** nausea, vomiting. **GU:** *papillary necrosis and chronic interstitial nephritis with long-term high doses.* **Skin:** rash.
phenazopyridine hydrochloride Azodine, Azogesic, Azo-Pyridon, Azo-Standard, Azo-Sulfizin, Baridium, Di-Azo, Diridone, Phenazo♦♦, Phen-Azo, Phenazodine, Pyridiate, Pyridium♦, Urodine	*Pain with urinary tract irritation or infection—* **Adults:** 100 to 200 mg P.O. t.i.d. **Children:** 100 mg P.O. t.i.d.	**CNS:** headache. **GI:** nausea.

♦ Available in U.S. and Canada. ♦♦ Available in Canada only. All other products (no symbol) available in U.S. only. Italicized side effects are common or life-threatening.

INTERACTIONS	NURSING CONSIDERATIONS
urine alkalinizers): decrease levels of aspirin products. Monitor for decreased aspirin effect. *Oral anticoagulants:* increase risk of bleeding. Avoid using together if possible.	• Give with food, milk, antacid, or large glass of water to reduce GI side effects. • Warn patient to check with doctor before taking over-the-counter combinations containing aspirin. • Therapeutic blood salicylate level in arthritis is 20 to 30 mg/ 100 ml. • May cause an increase in serum levels of SGOT, SGPT, alkaline phosphatase, and bilirubin. May produce false-negative test results for urine glucose by glucose oxidase methods (Clinistix, Tes-Tape) and false-positive results using Clinitest. • Obtain hemoglobin and prothrombin tests periodically in patients receiving large doses over an extended period. • For toxicity, see APPENDIX, *Drug Toxicities.*
All antihypertensive agents and MAO inhibitors: increased orthostatic hypotension. Select other analgesic.	• Contraindicated in phenothiazine hypersensitivity; cardiac, renal or hepatic disease; hypotension; coma; convulsive disorders. Use with extreme caution in elderly or debilitated patients with cardiac disease or any patients who may suffer severe consequences from a sudden drop in blood pressure. • Used mainly in nonambulatory patients because of hypotension. Keep patient in bed or assist when out of bed for at least 6 hours after initial dose. Tolerance to this effect usually develops, but watch patient closely after each dose. • May mix with atropine or scopolamine but not with other drugs.
None significant.	• Contraindicated in emotional instability, drug abuse, head injury, increased intracranial pressure. Use cautiously in patients with hepatic and renal disease. These patients may overreact to customary doses. • Causes respiratory depression which at 10 mg is equal to the respiratory depression produced by 10 mg of morphine. • Psychological and physiologic dependence may occur, but it is less than that of pentazocine (Talwin). • Respiratory depression can be reversed with naloxone. • Also acts as a narcotic antagonist. • Warn patient to avoid activities that require alertness until CNS response to drug is determined.
None significant.	• Repeated use is contraindicated in anemia; cardiac, pulmonary, hepatic, or renal disease. • Contained in many analgesic combinations. Warn patient to check ingredients of combination over-the-counter products.
None significant.	• Contraindicated in renal and hepatic insufficiency. • Colors urine red or orange. May stain fabrics. • Use only as analgesic. Use with antibiotic to treat urinary tract infection. • Drug may be stopped in 3 days if pain is relieved. • May alter Clinistix or Tes-Tape results. Use Clinitest for accurate urine glucose test results. • Stop drug if skin or sclera becomes yellow-tinged. May indicate accumulation due to impaired renal excretion.

NAME	INDICATIONS & DOSAGE	SIDE EFFECTS
salicylamide Amid-Sal, Doldram, Salamide	*Mild pain or fever—* **Adults:** 650 mg P.O. q.i.d., p.r.n. **Children:** 65 mg/kg/day divided into 6 doses.	**Blood:** *prolonged bleeding time.* **EENT:** *tinnitus and hearing loss (first signs of toxicity).* **GI:** *nausea, vomiting, GI distress, occult bleeding.* **Hepatic:** abnormal liver function studies. **Skin:** *rash.* **Other:** *hypersensitivity manifested by anaphylaxis.*
salsalate Disalcid	*Minor pain or fever, arthritis—* **Adults:** 1 g P.O. b.i.d., t.i.d., or q.i.d., p.r.n.	**Blood:** *prolonged bleeding time.* **EENT:** *tinnitus and hearing loss (first signs of toxicity).* **GI:** *nausea, vomiting, GI distress, occult bleeding.* **Hepatic:** abnormal liver function studies. **Skin:** *rash.* **Other:** *hypersensitivity manifested by anaphylaxis.*
sodium salicylate Uracel	*Minor pain or fever—* **Adults:** 325 to 650 mg P.O. q 4 to 6 hours, p.r.n., or 500 mg slow I.V. infusion over 4 to 8 hours. Maximum dose 1 g daily. **Children:** 40 to 100 mg/kg P.O. q 4 to 6 hours, p.r.n.	**Blood:** *prolonged bleeding time.* **EENT:** *tinnitus and hearing loss (first signs of toxicity).* **GI:** *nausea, vomiting, GI distress, occult bleeding.* **Hepatic:** abnormal liver function studies. **Skin:** *rash.* **Other:** *hypersensitivity manifested by anaphylaxis.*

♦ Available in U.S. and Canada. ♦♦ Available in Canada only. All other products (no symbol) available in U.S. only. Italicized side effects are common or life-threatening.

INTERACTIONS	NURSING CONSIDERATIONS
Ammonium chloride (and other urine acidifiers): increases blood levels of aspirin products. Monitor for aspirin toxicity. *Antacids (and other urine alkalinizers):* decrease levels of aspirin products. Monitor for decreased aspirin effect. *Oral anticoagulants:* increase risk of bleeding. Avoid using together if possible.	• Contraindicated in GI ulcer, GI bleeding, aspirin hypersensitivity. Use cautiously in hypoprothrombinemia, vitamin K deficiency, bleeding disorders, and Hodgkin's disease (may cause profound hypothermia). • Give with food, milk, antacid, or large glass of water to reduce GI side effects. • Warn patient to check with doctor before taking over-the-counter combinations containing aspirin. • Alcohol may increase GI blood loss. • May increase serum alkaline phosphatase, bilirubin, SGOT, and SGPT levels. May produce false-negative results for urine glucose using glucose oxidase methods (Clinistix and Tes-Tape) and false-positive results using Clinitest. • Advise patients receiving large doses for an extended period to watch for petechiae, bleeding gums, and signs of GI bleeding, and to maintain adequate fluid intake. Obtain hemoglobin and prothrombin tests periodically. • For toxicity, see APPENDIX, *Drug Toxicities*.
Ammonium chloride (and other urine acidifiers): increases blood levels of aspirin products. Monitor for aspirin toxicity. *Antacids (and other urine alkalinizers):* decrease levels of aspirin products. Monitor for decreased aspirin effect. *Oral anticoagulants:* increase risk of bleeding. Avoid using together if possible.	• Contraindicated in GI ulcer, GI bleeding, aspirin hypersensitivity. Use cautiously in hypoprothrombinemia, vitamin K deficiency, bleeding disorders, and Hodgkin's disease (may cause profound hypothermia). • Give with food, milk, antacid, or large glass of water to reduce GI side effects. • Warn patient to check with doctor before taking over-the-counter combinations containing aspirin. • Therapeutic blood salicylate level in arthritis is 20 to 30 mg/100 ml. • Alcohol may increase GI blood loss. • May increase serum alkaline phosphatase, bilirubin, SGOT, and SGPT levels. May produce false-negative results for urine glucose using glucose oxidase methods (Clinistix and Tes-Tape) and false-positive results using Clinitest. • Advise patients receiving large doses for extended period to watch for petechiae, bleeding gums, and signs of GI bleeding, and to maintain adequate fluid intake. Obtain hemoglobin and prothrombin tests periodically. • For toxicity, see APPENDIX, *Drug Toxicities*.
Ammonium chloride (and other urine acidifiers): increases blood levels of aspirin products. Monitor for aspirin toxicity. *Antacids (and other urine alkalinizers):* decrease levels of aspirin products. Monitor for decreased aspirin effect. *Oral anticoagulants:* increase risk of bleeding. Avoid using together if possible.	• Contraindicated in GI ulcer, GI bleeding, aspirin hypersensitivity. Use cautiously in hypoprothrombinemia, vitamin K deficiency, bleeding disorders, asthma with nasal polyps (may cause severe bronchospasm), and Hodgkin's disease (may cause profound hypothermia). • Febrile, dehydrated children can develop toxicity rapidly. • Give with food, milk, antacid, or large glass of water to reduce GI side effects. • Enteric-coated or timed-release preparations are absorbed erratically and are ineffective for long-term therapy. • Warn patient to check with doctor before taking over-the-counter combinations containing aspirin. • Therapeutic salicylate level in arthritis is 20 to 30 mg/100 ml. • Tinnitus, headache, dizziness, confusion, fever, sweating, thirst, drowsiness, dim vision, hyperventilation, and tachycardia are signs of mild toxicity. • Alcohol may increase GI blood loss. • May increase serum alkaline phosphatase, bilirubin, SGOT, and SGPT levels. May produce false-negative results for urine glucose us-

(continued on following page)

NAME	INDICATIONS & DOSAGE	SIDE EFFECTS
sodium salicylate *(continued)*		
sodium thiosalicylate Arthrolate, Jecto Sal, Nalate, Osteolate, Thiodyne, Thiolate, Thiosal, TH Sal	*Mild pain—* **Adults:** 50 to 100 mg I.M. daily or every other day. *Arthritis—* **Adults:** 100 mg I.M. daily. *Rheumatic fever—* **Adults:** 100 to 150 mg I.M. b.i.d. until asymptomatic. *Acute gout—* **Adults:** 100 mg I.M. q 3 to 4 hours for 2 days, then 100 mg I.M. daily until asymptomatic.	**Blood:** *prolonged bleeding time.* **EENT:** *tinnitus and hearing loss (first signs of toxicity).* **GI:** *nausea, vomiting, GI distress, occult bleeding.* **Hepatic:** abnormal liver function studies. **Skin:** *rash.* **Other:** *hypersensitivity manifested by anaphylaxis.*
zomepirac sodium Zomax	*Mild-to-moderately severe pain—* **Adults:** 100 mg P.O. q 4 to 6 hours p.r.n. In mild pain, 50 mg q 4 to 6 hours may be adequate. Don't exceed 600 mg/day. Not recommended for children.	**CNS:** *drowsiness, dizziness, insomnia,* paresthesia, nervousness. **CV:** *edema, hypertension,* cardiac irregularity, palpitations. **EENT:** tinnitus. **GI:** *nausea, vomiting, diarrhea, dyspepsia,* constipation, flatulence, anorexia. **GU:** urinary frequency, urinary tract infection, elevated BUN and creatinine, vaginitis. **Skin:** rash, pruritus. **Other:** chills, alterations in sense of taste.

MORE ABOUT ZOMEPIRAC SODIUM

Zomepirac sodium (Zomax) is a nonsteroidal anti-inflammatory drug that rivals narcotics for analgesic effect but is nonaddictive. It's available only as a 100-mg, highly recognizable tablet—a yellow, scored, modified hexagon imprinted with the word ZOMAX.

The target patient

The drug is approved to treat mild to moderately severe pain, implying relief for everything from minor toothache to terminal cancer pain. But doctors may hesitate to transfer patients with narcotic-controlled chronic pain to zomepirac because its long-term effectiveness and safety haven't yet been established.

The relatively high cost of this drug (at least 30 cents per tablet) may limit its use to patients who can't get relief from aspirin. These patients will benefit most from zomepirac, especially if they can take it instead of a narcotic to relieve their pain.

Dosage: More isn't better

Your patient should begin to get relief within 30 minutes after receiving a standard dose. Explain to him that dosages above the recommended maximum (100 mg every 4 →

INTERACTIONS	NURSING CONSIDERATIONS
	ing glucose oxidase methods (Clinistix and Tes-Tape) and false-positive results using Clinitest. • Advise patients receiving large doses for extended period to watch for petechiae, bleeding gums, and signs of GI bleeding, and to maintain adequate fluid intake. Obtain hemoglobin and prothrombin tests periodically. • For toxicity, see APPENDIX, *Drug Toxicities.*
Ammonium chloride (and other urine acidifiers): increases blood levels of aspirin products. Monitor for aspirin toxicity. *Antacids (and other urine alkalinizers):* decrease levels of aspirin products. Monitor for decreased aspirin effect. *Oral anticoagulants:* increase risk of bleeding. Avoid using together if possible.	• Contraindicated in GI ulcer, GI bleeding, aspirin hypersensitivity. Use cautiously in hypoprothrombinemia, vitamin K deficiency, bleeding disorders, asthma with nasal polyps (may cause severe bronchospasm), and Hodgkin's disease (may cause profound hypothermia). • Tinnitus, headache, dizziness, confusion, fever, sweating, thirst, drowsiness, dim vision, hyperventilation, and tachycardia are signs of mild toxicity. • Alcohol may increase GI blood loss. • May increase serum alkaline phosphatase, bilirubin, SGOT, and SGPT levels. May produce false-negative results for urine glucose using glucose oxidase method (Clinistix and Tes-Tape) and false-positive results using Clinitest. • Advise patients receiving large doses for extended period to watch for petechiae, bleeding gums, and signs of GI bleeding, and to maintain adequate fluid intake. Obtain hemoglobin and prothrombin tests periodically. • For toxicity, see APPENDIX, *Drug Toxicities.*
None significant.	• Contraindicated in patients in whom aspirin and nonsteroidal anti-inflammatory drugs induce bronchospasm, rhinitis, urticaria, or other hypersensitivity reactions. Give cautiously to patients with a history of GI bleeding, fluid retention, hypertension, and heart failure. • A nonnarcotic analgesic with narcotic potency. In several studies has been shown to be as effective as morphine. • No evidence of addiction with zomepirac. • Give with food or antacids if GI symptoms occur.

to 6 hours) offer no additional pain relief and may increase side effects. Advise your patient to report side effects (drowsiness, nausea, gastrointestinal upset, diarrhea, peripheral edema, urinary tract infection, skin rash) to the doctor, and warn him against taking the drug for longer than 6 months without his doctor's knowledge.

Interaction with other drugs

Zomepirac doesn't seem to interact adversely with other drugs. Unlike aspirin, it won't increase the risk of bleeding in a patient who's also taking an oral anticoagulant, such as warfarin (Coumadin). Nor do antacids containing magnesium and aluminum (for example, Mylanta and Maalox) reduce its effectiveness. Taking zomepirac with meals, however, may alter its absorption, so advise your patient to take it 1 hour before or 2 hours after eating.

Other precautions

Patients who are hypersensitive to nonsteroidal anti-inflammatory drugs shouldn't take zomepirac. Because it impairs platelet function and may cause gastrointestinal bleeding, it could be dangerous for patients with peptic ulcers or bleeding disorders, although it's still safer than aspirin.

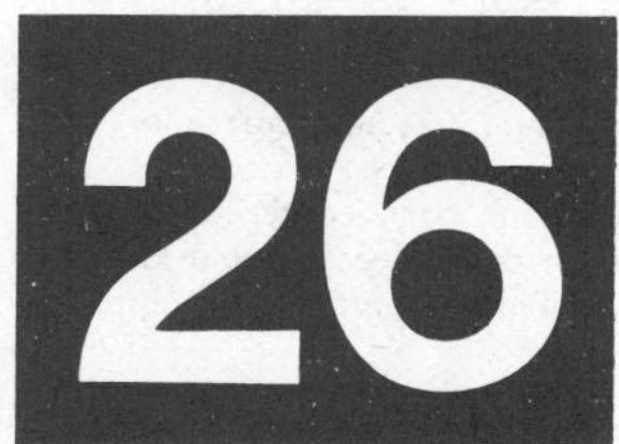

Nonsteroidal anti-inflammatory agents

fenoprofen calcium
ibuprofen
indomethacin
meclofenamate
mefenamic acid
naproxen
oxyphenbutazone
phenylbutazone
sulindac
tolmetin sodium

The nonsteroidal anti-inflammatory agents may be particularly useful when a patient cannot tolerate the gastrointestinal (GI) side effects of the salicylates. Tolmetin and the propionic-acid derivatives (fenoprofen, ibuprofen, and naproxen) are new drugs that cause fewer GI side effects than the older, established alternatives to salicylates (indomethacin, oxyphenbutazone, and phenylbutazone).

Major uses

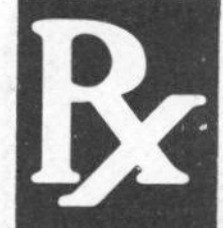

The nonsteroidal anti-inflammatory agents are used to reduce inflammation associated with osteoarthritis, rheumatoid arthritis, gout, and other conditions.

Mechanism of action

Although their exact mechanism of action is unknown, these drugs probably inhibit prostaglandin synthesis.

Absorption, distribution, metabolism, and excretion

Oral forms of the nonsteroidal anti-inflammatory agents are well absorbed from the GI tract. Distributed in most body tissues and fluids, these drugs are largely metabolized in the liver. The inactive metabolites are eliminated in urine and—through the bile—in feces.

Onset and duration

Onset after oral administration is within 30 to 60 minutes; after I.M. injection, within 15 to 30 minutes. Blood levels peak within 2 to 3 hours. Duration of action for most of the drugs is 4 to 6 hours. Optimal anti-inflammatory action develops only after 2 to 4 weeks of therapy.

- Naproxen and sulindac have a longer duration of action and are generally given twice daily.

Combination products

None.

DYSMENORRHEA: NEW INDICATION FOR PROSTAGLANDIN INHIBITORS

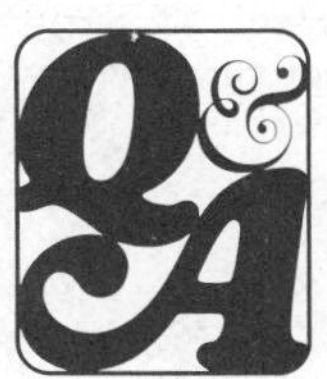

Mefenamic acid (Ponstel) and ibuprofen (Motrin) were the first prostaglandin inhibitors approved for use in dysmenorrhea, but you'll be seeing others prescribed for your patients.

Studies now show that primary dysmenorrhea (of idiopathic origin) results when the endometrium overproduces prostaglandin hormones. The cause is still unknown, but the effect is strong uterine contractions and cramping pain. Increased prostaglandin production also stimulates synthesis of vasodilators bradykinin and histamine, which may cause menstrual headaches and nausea. Thus, drugs that inhibit prostaglandins are a logical choice to relieve dysmenorrhea.

Will any prostaglandin inhibitor work?

Theoretically, all should relieve dysmenorrhea, but some, like indomethacin (Indocin), may be undesirable because of severe side effects. You'll probably see mefenamic acid and ibuprofen prescribed most often. Four daily doses of 250 mg of mefenamic acid significantly decrease the frequency and severity of symptoms and reduce the patient's need for an additional analgesic. Ibuprofen's usual dosage is 400 mg four times a day. Reduced doses of either drug may also be effective.

What side effects might patients taking mefenamic acid or ibuprofen report?

Both drugs are relatively free of side effects when dosage is below recommended levels. However, at recommended dosage, some patients may report dizziness and gastrointestinal (GI) upsets, such as nausea, heartburn, and diarrhea. If taking the drugs with food or milk doesn't relieve these symptoms, the doctor may reduce the dose. Agranulocytosis, a blood dyscrasia, rarely occurs with mefenamic acid, but periodic complete blood counts can help detect it. Encourage your patient to report all symptoms to the doctor.

When obtaining your patient's history, check for incidence of peptic ulcer or asthma. A patient with either of these conditions shouldn't take prostaglandin inhibitors since they produce GI side effects, and some patients with asthma develop allergies to them.

What other prostaglandin inhibitors might a doctor prescribe to treat dysmenorrhea?

Possible alternatives are naproxen (Naprosyn), fenoprofen (Nalfon), sulindac (Clinoril), and tolmetin (Tolectin). Aspirin and acetaminophen inhibit prostaglandins but not enough to relieve symptoms. Oral contraceptives relieve dysmenorrhea by suppressing ovulation and thus lowering prostaglandin levels, but these drugs have many side effects.

Is there any special advice I should give the patient taking a prostaglandin inhibitor?

Advise her to start the medication *after* her menstrual flow begins, unless the doctor orders otherwise. Although starting the drug a few days before her period begins may help prevent dysmenorrhea, your patient could be pregnant—and pregnant women shouldn't take a prostaglandin inhibitor.

NAME	INDICATIONS & DOSAGE	SIDE EFFECTS
fenoprofen calcium Nalfon♦	*Rheumatoid arthritis and osteoarthritis—* **Adults:** 300 to 600 mg P.O. q.i.d. Maximum 3.2 g daily.	**Blood:** prolonged bleeding time, anemia. **CNS:** headache, drowsiness, dizziness. **GI:** *epigastric distress,* nausea, *occult blood loss.* **GU:** reversible renal failure. **Skin:** pruritus, rash, urticaria.
ibuprofen Motrin♦	*Arthritis, primary dysmenorrhea, postextraction dental pain—* **Adults:** 300 to 600 mg P.O. q.i.d.	**Blood:** prolonged bleeding time. **CNS:** headache, drowsiness, dizziness. **EENT:** visual disturbances, tinnitus. **GI:** *epigastric distress,* nausea, *occult blood loss.* **GU:** reversible renal failure. **Skin:** pruritus, rash, urticaria. **Other:** aseptic meningitis, bronchospasm, edema.
indomethacin Indocid♦♦, Indocin	*Moderate to severe arthritis—* **Adults:** 25 mg P.O. b.i.d. or t.i.d. with food or antacids; may increase dose by 25 mg daily q 7 days up to 200 mg daily. *Acute gouty arthritis*—50 mg t.i.d. Reduce dose as soon as possible, then stop.	**Blood:** *hemolytic anemia, aplastic anemia, agranulocytosis,* leukopenia, *thrombocytopenic purpura,* iron deficiency anemia. **CNS:** *headache, dizziness,* depression, drowsiness, confusion, peripheral neuropathy, convulsions, psychic disturbances, syncope, *vertigo.* **CV:** hypertension, edema. **EENT:** blurred vision, corneal and retinal damage, hearing loss, tinnitus. **GI:** *nausea, vomiting,* anorexia, *diarrhea, severe GI bleeding.* **GU:** hematuria, acute renal failure. **Skin:** pruritus, urticaria. **Other:** hypersensitivity (shock-like symptoms, rash, respiratory distress, angioedema).
meclofenamate Meclomen	*Rheumatoid arthritis and osteoarthritis—* **Adults:** 200 to 400 mg/day P.O. in 3 or 4 equally divided doses.	**Blood:** leukopenia, thrombocytopenia, *agranulocytosis, aplastic anemia.* **CNS:** drowsiness, dizziness, nervousness, headache. **EENT:** blurred vision, eye irritation. **GI:** nausea, vomiting, *diarrhea,* hemorrhage. **GU:** dysuria, hematuria, nephrotoxicity.

♦ Available in U.S. and Canada. ♦♦ Available in Canada only. All other products (no symbol) available in U.S. only. Italicized side effects are common or life-threatening.

INTERACTIONS	NURSING CONSIDERATIONS
None significant.	• Contraindicated in patients with renal disease and in asthmatics with nasal polyps. Use cautiously in patients with GI disorders, cardiac disease, or allergy to other noncorticosteroid anti-inflammatory drugs. • Tell patient therapeutic effect may be delayed for 2 to 4 weeks. • Check renal, hepatic, and auditory function periodically in long-term therapy. Stop drug if abnormalities occur. • Give dose 30 minutes before or 2 hours after meals. If GI side effects occur, give with milk or meals. • Prothrombin time may be prolonged in patients receiving coumarin-type anticoagulants. Fenoprofen decreases platelet aggregation and may prolong bleeding time.
None significant.	• Contraindicated in asthmatics with nasal polyps. Use cautiously in GI disorders, allergy to other noncorticosteroid anti-inflammatory drugs, hepatic or renal disease, cardiac decompensation, or known intrinsic coagulation defects. • Tell patient therapeutic effect may be delayed for 2 to 4 weeks. • Check renal and hepatic function periodically in long-term therapy. Stop drug if abnormalities occur. • Tell patient to report to doctor immediately any GI symptoms or signs of bleeding, visual disturbances, skin rashes, weight gain, or edema. • Give with meals or milk to reduce GI side effects.
Probenecid: decreases indomethacin excretion; watch for increased incidence of indomethacin side effects. *Furosemide:* impaired response to both drugs. Avoid if possible.	• Contraindicated in aspirin allergy, GI disorders. Use cautiously in patients with epilepsy, parkinsonism, hepatic or renal disease, infection, history of mental illness, and in elderly patients. • Severe headache may occur within 1 hour. Decrease dose if headache persists. • Tell patient to notify doctor immediately if any visual or hearing changes occur. Patients taking drug long-term should have regular eye examinations and hearing tests. • Very irritating to GI tract. Give with meals. Advise patient to notify doctor of any GI side effects. • Monitor for bleeding in patients receiving anticoagulants. • Causes sodium retention; monitor for increased blood pressure in patients with hypertension. • Used investigationally as prophylaxis for gout when colchicine is not well tolerated. • Patients taking drug long-term should receive periodic testing of CBC and renal function.
None significant.	• Contraindicated in GI ulceration or inflammation. Use cautiously in patients with hepatic or renal disease, blood dyscrasias, diabetes mellitus, and in asthmatics with nasal polyps. • Warn patient against activities that require alertness until CNS response to drug is determined. • Stop drug if rash or diarrhea develops. • Should not be administered for more than 1 week at a time. • Administer with food to minimize GI side effects. • Almost identical in chemical structure to mefenamic acid. • False-positive reactions for urine bilirubin using the diazo tablet test have been reported.

(continued on following page)

NAME	INDICATIONS & DOSAGE	SIDE EFFECTS
meclofenamate *(continued)*		**Hepatic:** hepatotoxicity. **Skin:** rash, urticaria.
mefenamic acid Ponstan♦♦, Ponstel	*Mild to moderate pain, dysmenorrhea—* **Adults, and children over 14 years:** 500 mg P.O. initially, then 250 mg q 4 hours, p.r.n. Maximum therapy 1 week.	**Blood:** leukopenia, thrombocytopenia, *agranulocytosis, aplastic anemia.* **CNS:** drowsiness, dizziness, nervousness, headache. **EENT:** blurred vision, eye irritation. **GI:** nausea, vomiting, *diarrhea,* hemorrhage. **GU:** dysuria, hematuria, nephrotoxicity. **Hepatic:** hepatotoxicity. **Skin:** rash, urticaria.
naproxen Naprosyn♦	*Arthritis—* **Adults:** 250 to 500 mg P.O. b.i.d. Maximum 1,000 mg daily.	**Blood:** prolonged bleeding time. **CNS:** headache, drowsiness, dizziness. **GI:** *epigastric distress, occult blood loss,* nausea. **GU:** reversible renal failure. **Skin:** pruritus, rash, urticaria.
oxyphenbutazone Oxalid, Tandearil	*Pain, inflammation in arthritis, bursitis, superficial venous thrombosis—* **Adults:** 100 to 200 mg P.O. with food or milk t.i.d. or q.i.d. *Acute gouty arthritis—* **Adults:** 400 mg initially as single dose, then 100 mg q 4 hours for 4 days or until relief is obtained.	**Blood:** *bone marrow depression (fatal aplastic anemia, agranulocytosis, thrombocytopenia),* hemolytic anemia, leukopenia. **CNS:** restlessness, confusion, lethargy. **CV:** hypertension, *pericarditis, myocarditis, cardiac decompensation.* **EENT:** optic neuritis, blurred vision, retinal hemorrhage or detachment, hearing loss. **GI:** *nausea, vomiting, diarrhea,* ulceration, occult blood loss. **GU:** proteinuria, hematuria, glomerulonephritis, nephrotic syndrome, *renal failure.* **Hepatic:** *hepatitis.* **Metabolic:** toxic and nontoxic goiter, respiratory alkalosis, and metabolic acidosis. **Skin:** petechiae, pruritus, purpura, various dermatoses from rash to *toxic necrotizing epidermolysis.*
phenylbutazone Algoverine♦♦, Anevral♦♦, Azolid, Butagesic♦♦, Butazolidin♦, Intrabutazone♦♦, Malgesic♦♦,	*Pain, inflammation in arthritis, bursitis, acute superficial thrombophlebitis—* **Adults:** initially, 100 to 200 mg P.O. t.i.d. or q.i.d. Maximum dose 600 mg per day. When improvement is obtained, decrease	**Blood:** *bone marrow depression (fatal aplastic anemia, agranulocytosis,* thrombocytopenia), hemolytic anemia, leukopenia. **CNS:** agitation, confusion, lethargy. **CV:** hypertension, edema, *peri-*

♦ Available in U.S. and Canada. ♦♦ Available in Canada only. All other products (no symbol) available in U.S. only. Italicized side effects are common or life-threatening.

INTERACTIONS	NURSING CONSIDERATIONS
	• Patients taking drug long-term should receive periodic testing of CBC, renal and hepatic function.
None significant.	• Contraindicated in GI ulceration or inflammation. Use cautiously in patients with hepatic or renal disease, blood dyscrasias, diabetes mellitus, and in asthmatics with nasal polyps. • Warn patient against activities that require alertness until CNS response to drug is determined. • Severe hemolytic anemia may occur with prolonged use. • Stop drug if rash or diarrhea develops. • Should not be administered for more than 1 week at a time. • Administer with food to minimize GI side effects. • Can be used to treat menstrual pain. • False-positive reactions for urine bilirubin using the diazo tablet test have been reported.
None significant.	• Use cautiously in patients with renal disease, GI disorders, in those allergic to noncorticosteroid anti-inflammatory agents, and in asthmatics with nasal polyps. • Check renal and hepatic function periodically in long-term therapy. Stop drug if abnormalities occur. • If ordered, give once daily to improve patient compliance. • Monitor hemoglobin and bleeding time periodically.
Methandrostenolone: may increase oxyphenbutazone levels. Give together cautiously.	• Contraindicated in children under 14 years and in patients with senility; GI ulcer; blood dyscrasias; renal, hepatic, cardiac, and thyroid disease; polymyalgia rheumatica and temporal arteritis. Should not be used in patients receiving long-term anticoagulant therapy. • Tell patient to stop drug and notify doctor immediately if fever, sore throat, mouth ulcers, GI discomfort, black or tarry stools, bleeding, bruising, rash, or weight gain occurs. • Give with food, milk, or antacids. • Complete physical examination and laboratory evaluation are recommended before therapy. Warn patient to remain under close medical supervision and to keep all doctor and laboratory appointments. • Monitor CBC every 2 weeks or weekly in elderly patients. Report any abnormality to doctor immediately. • Record patient's weight, intake, and output daily. May cause sodium retention and edema. • Response should be seen in 2 or 3 days. Drug should be stopped if no response seen within 1 week. • Patient over age 60 should not receive drug for longer than 1 week.
Barbiturates, antidepressants: may impair phenylbutazone effect. Use together cautiously. *Cholestyramine:* may alter phenylbutazone	• Contraindicated in children under 14 years and in patients with senility; GI ulcer; blood dyscrasias; renal, hepatic, cardiac, and thyroid disease; polymyalgia rheumatica; temporal arteritis; and hypertension. Should not be used in patients receiving long-term anticoagulant therapy. • Give with food, milk, or antacids. • Patient over age 60 should not receive drug for longer than 1 week.

(continued on following page)

NAME	INDICATIONS & DOSAGE	SIDE EFFECTS
phenylbutazone *(continued)* Nadozone♦♦, Neo-Zoline♦♦, Phenbutazone♦♦, Phenylbetazone♦♦	dose to 100 mg t.i.d. or q.i.d. *Acute, gouty arthritis—* **Adults:** 400 mg initially as single dose, then 100 mg q 4 hours for 4 days or until relief is obtained.	*carditis, myocarditis, cardiac decompensation.* **EENT:** optic neuritis, blurred vision, retinal hemorrhage or detachment, hearing loss. **GI:** *nausea, vomiting, diarrhea,* ulceration, occult blood loss. **GU:** proteinuria, hematuria, glomerulonephritis, nephrotic syndrome, *renal failure.* **Hepatic:** *hepatitis.* **Metabolic:** hyperglycemia, toxic and nontoxic goiter, respiratory alkalosis, and metabolic acidosis. **Skin:** petechiae, pruritus, purpura, various dermatoses from rash to *toxic necrotizing epidermolysis.*
sulindac Clinoril	*Osteoarthritis, rheumatoid arthritis, ankylosing spondylitis—* **Adults:** 150 mg P.O. b.i.d. initially; may increase to 200 mg P.O. b.i.d. *Acute subacromial bursitis or supraspinatus tendinitis, acute gouty arthritis—* **Adults:** 200 mg P.O. b.i.d. for 7 to 14 days. Dose may be reduced as symptoms subside.	**Blood:** prolonged bleeding time, *aplastic anemia.* **CNS:** dizziness, headache, nervousness. **EENT:** tinnitus, transient visual disturbances. **GI:** *epigastric distress, occult blood loss,* nausea. **Skin:** rash, pruritus. **Other:** edema.
tolmetin sodium Tolectin♦, Tolectin DS	*Rheumatoid arthritis and osteoarthritis, juvenile rheumatoid arthritis—* **Adults:** 400 mg P.O. t.i.d. or q.i.d. Maximum 2 g daily. **Children (2 years or older):** 15 to 30 mg/kg/day in divided doses.	**Blood:** prolonged bleeding time. **CNS:** headache, dizziness, drowsiness. **GI:** *epigastric distress, occult blood loss,* nausea. **GU:** reversible renal failure. **Skin:** rash, urticaria, pruritus. **Other:** sodium retention, edema.

HOW PROSTAGLANDIN INHIBITORS WORK

Nonsteroidal anti-inflammatory agents are prostaglandin inhibitors that relieve pain and inflammation by blocking an early step in the inflammatory reaction.

Prostaglandins form when cell injury or maybe even distortion of cell membranes triggers a chain reaction: First, enzymes produced by phagocytes at the injury site split the phospholipids present within all cell membranes, freeing arachidonic acid. This normally dormant fatty acid is then activated by the enzyme cyclo-oxygenase (prostaglandin synthetase) to create the G and H series prostaglandins called endoperoxides. These highly unstable intermediate prostaglandins convert to thromboxanes and prostacyclin, which respectively promote and prevent platelet aggregation, and to series E, F, and D prostaglandins. These final prostaglandins, particularly the E series, cause inflammation and pain.

Prostaglandin inhibitors check the action of the cyclo-oxygenase enzyme complex and prevent conversion of arachidonic acid to the endoperoxides or intermediate prostaglandins. Prostaglandin inhibitors mediate but do not arrest the inflammatory response or its consequences. For example, in the patient with rheumatoid arthritis, these drugs may reduce pain, redness, and swelling, but joint destruction continues.

INTERACTIONS	NURSING CONSIDERATIONS
absorption. Give 1 hour before cholestyramine.	• Warn patient to stop drug and notify doctor immediately if fever, sore throat, mouth ulcers, GI discomfort, black or tarry stools, bleeding, bruising, rash, or weight gain occurs. • Complete physical examination and laboratory evaluation are recommended before therapy. Patient should remain under close medical supervision and keep all doctor and laboratory appointments. • Monitor CBC every 2 weeks or weekly in elderly patients. Report any abnormalities to doctor right away. • Record patient's weight, intake, and output daily. May cause sodium retention and edema. • Response should be seen in 3 to 4 days. Stop drug if no response within 1 week.
None significant.	• Contraindicated in acute asthmatics whose condition is precipitated by aspirin or other nonsteroidal anti-inflammatory agents; in patients who have active ulcers and GI bleeding. Use cautiously in patients with a history of ulcers and GI bleeding, renal dysfunction, compromised cardiac function, hypertension; or in those receiving oral anticoagulants or oral hypoglycemic agents. • To reduce GI side effects, give with food, milk, or antacids. • Patient should notify doctor and have complete visual examination if any visual disturbances occur. • Drug causes sodium retention. Patient should report edema and have blood pressure checked periodically.
None significant.	• Contraindicated in asthmatics with nasal polyps. Use cautiously in cardiac and renal disease, and GI bleeding. • Give with food, milk, or antacids to reduce GI side effects. • Tell patient therapeutic effect should begin within 1 week. • Double-strength capsule (400 mg) is available. • Extended therapy should be accompanied by periodic eye examinations and renal function studies.

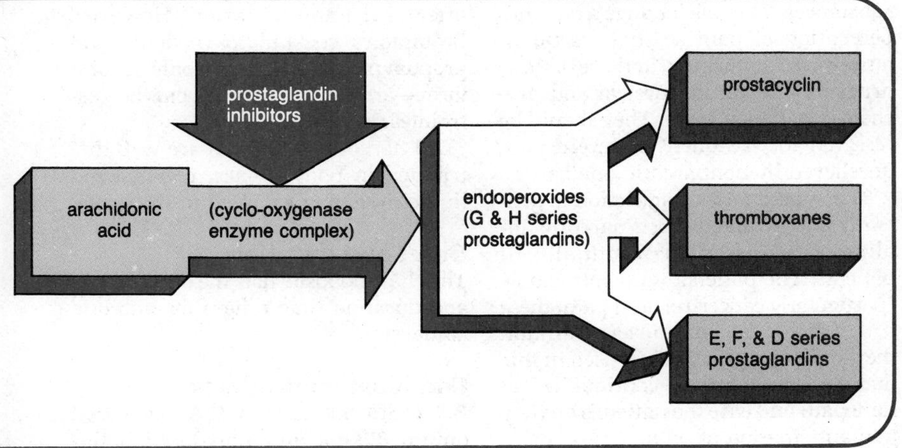

27 Narcotic analgesics

alphaprodine hydrochloride
anileridine hydrochloride
anileridine phosphate
Brompton's cocktail
codeine phosphate
codeine sulfate
fentanyl citrate
hydromorphone hydrochloride
levorphanol tartrate
meperidine hydrochloride
methadone hydrochloride
morphine sulfate
oxycodone hydrochloride
oxymorphone hydrochloride
pentazocine hydrochloride
pentazocine lactate
propoxyphene hydrochloride
propoxyphene napsylate

Narcotic analgesics are defined by the Comprehensive Drug Abuse Prevention and Control Act of 1970 as controlled substances. They can change a patient's perception of pain so that it's qualitatively less disturbing, and use of these drugs may result in physical and psychological dependence. They should be reserved for treatment of severe pain unrelieved by nonnarcotic analgesics.

The concern about addiction is generally unwarranted when narcotic analgesics are used in terminally ill patients. For patients with intractable (particularly cancer-related) pain, these drugs should be administered around the clock—not p.r.n. When used in this manner, these drugs continually relieve pain and ease the patient's anxiety and anticipation of pain.

Major uses

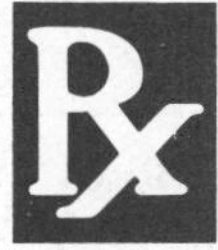

Narcotic analgesics relieve moderate to severe pain and furnish preoperative sedation, alone or in combination with tranquilizers (such as chlorpromazine, diazepam, and hydroxyzine).

Mechanism of action

Narcotic analgesics bind with opiate receptors at many sites in the central nervous system (brain, brain stem, and spinal cord), altering both perception of and emotional response to pain. The precise mechanism of action, however, is unknown.

Absorption, distribution, metabolism, and excretion

Absorption of most narcotic analgesics is more effective after parenteral than after oral administration. However, Brompton's cocktail, oxycodone, and propoxyphene—available only in oral form—are well absorbed from the gastrointestinal tract.

All narcotic analgesics are well distributed in body tissues, metabolized in the liver, and excreted in the urine.

Onset and duration

The chart opposite lists the onset, peak, and duration time ranges for narcotic analgesics.

Combination products

B & O SUPPRETTES NO. 15A: powdered opium 30 mg and powdered bella-

THERAPEUTIC ACTIVITY OF NARCOTIC ANALGESICS

DRUG	ONSET	PEAK	DURATION
alphaprodine	5 to 10 min	30 to 60 min	1 to 2 hr
anileridine	within 15 min	30 to 60 min	2 to 3 hr
Brompton's cocktail*	10 to 15 min	2 to 3 hr	3 to 8 hr
codeine	15 to 30 min	60 to 90 min	4 to 6 hr
fentanyl	5 to 15 min	within 30 min	1 to 2 hr
hydromorphone	15 to 30 min	30 to 90 min	4 to 5 hr
levorphanol	within 1 hr	60 to 90 min	4 to 5 hr
meperidine	10 to 15 min	30 to 60 min	2 to 4 hr
methadone	10 to 15 min	1 to 2 hr	4 to 6 hr†
morphine	within 20 min	30 to 90 min	4 to 7 hr
oxycodone*	10 to 15 min	60 to 90 min	4 to 5 hr
oxymorphone	5 to 10 min	30 to 90 min	4 to 5 hr
pentazocine	10 to 15 min	30 to 60 min	2 to 3 hr
propoxyphene*	15 to 60 min	2 to 3 hr	4 to 6 hr

*Oral administration. (Other values in chart are for I.M. or S.Q. administration.)
†Increases with repeated use due to cumulative effects.

donna extract 15 mg.
B & O SUPPRETTES NO. 16A: powdered opium 60 mg and powdered belladonna extract 15 mg.
EMPIRIN WITH CODEINE NO. 2: aspirin 325 mg and codeine phosphate 15 mg.
EMPIRIN WITH CODEINE NO. 3: aspirin 325 mg and codeine phosphate 30 mg.
EMPIRIN WITH CODEINE NO. 4: aspirin 325 mg and codeine phosphate 60 mg.
FIORINAL WITH CODEINE NO. 1: butalbital 50 mg, caffeine 40 mg, aspirin 200 mg, phenacetin 130 mg, and codeine phosphate 7.5 mg.
FIORINAL WITH CODEINE NO. 2♦: butalbital 50 mg, caffeine 40 mg, aspirin 200 mg, phenacetin 130 mg, and codeine phosphate 15 mg.
FIORINAL WITH CODEINE NO. 3♦: butalbital 50 mg, caffeine 40 mg, aspirin 200 mg, phenacetin 130 mg, and codeine 30 mg.
INNOVAR (INJECTION)♦: fentanyl (as the citrate) 0.05 mg and droperidol 2.5 mg per ml.
PANTOPON♦: hydrochlorides of opium

alkaloids; 20 mg is therapeutically equivalent to 15 mg morphine.
PERCOCET-5: acetaminophen 325 mg and oxycodone hydrochloride 5 mg.
PERCODAN: oxycodone hydrochloride 4.5 mg, oxycodone terephthalate 0.38 mg, and aspirin 325 mg.
PERCODAN-DEMI: oxycodone hydrochloride 2.25 mg, oxycodone terephthalate 0.19 mg, as well as aspirin 325 mg.
TYLENOL WITH CODEINE NO 1: acetaminophen 300 mg and codeine phosphate 7.5 mg.
TYLENOL WITH CODEINE NO. 2: acetaminophen 300 mg and codeine phosphate 15 mg.
TYLENOL WITH CODEINE NO. 3: acetaminophen 300 mg and codeine phosphate 30 mg.
TYLENOL WITH CODEINE NO. 4: acetaminophen 300 mg and codeine phosphate 60 mg.
TYLOX: acetaminophen 500 mg, oxycodone hydrochloride 4.5 mg, and oxycodone terephthalate 0.38 mg.

EQUIANALGESIC DOSES OF NARCOTIC ANALGESICS

DRUG	I.M.	P.O.
alphaprodine	50 mg	*
anileridine	35 mg	*
Brompton's cocktail	*	Depends on preparation
codeine	130 mg	200 mg
fentanyl	0.1 mg	*
hydromorphone	1.5 mg	8 mg
levorphanol	2 mg	4 mg
meperidine	75 mg	300 mg
methadone	10 mg	20 mg
morphine	10 mg	60 mg
oxycodone	*	30 mg
oxymorphone	1 mg	5 mg (rectal)
pentazocine	40 mg	100 mg
propoxyphene	*	About 300 mg

*Not available in this form

QUESTIONS & ANSWERS

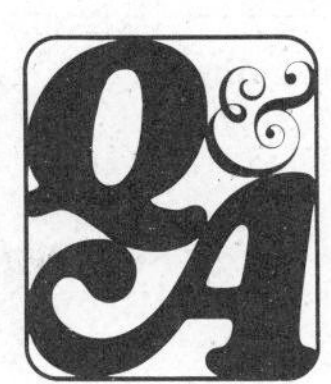

COMMON CONCERNS ABOUT NARCOTIC ANALGESICS

Will my patient become addicted?

Probably not. Most studies of hospitalized patients who received meperidine (Demerol) 100 mg I.M. every 4 hours for 10 days for acute pain relief show that less than 1% became addicted, that is, continued to take narcotics after the pain subsided. Other studies show that less than 3% of such patients became addicted.

You may withhold narcotics because they're not the best way to relieve pain or because they're causing adverse effects, such as respiratory depression, but don't withhold them simply because you fear addiction.

If your patient expresses concern about addiction, he may really mean drug tolerance or physical dependence—physiologic responses to the repeated administration of a drug. These responses subside spontaneously. Withdrawal symptoms diminish within days, and tolerance returns to normal within a month. Drug tolerance and physical dependence do not automatically lead to addiction.

Will my patient become a clockwatcher?

When a patient asks for the next dose of analgesic as soon as the prescribed interval has elapsed, he may not be receiving adequate pain relief. For instance, the doctor orders the drug to be administered every 4 hours, but pain relief lasts only 2 or 3 hours. The solution is to provide better pain relief for the patient. Usually, this means increasing the dosage or giving it more frequently, so consult the doctor.

Why do some patients need more analgesic than others?

How much drug a patient needs for pain relief depends on the intensity of his pain and the way his body uses the analgesic. Generally, the more severe the pain, the greater the amount of analgesic required to relieve it. Some adults may need twice the recommended dose.

In the past, the trend was toward undertreatment of acute pain with narcotics. One form of undertreatment is underprescribing—prescribing less than the effective dose or prescribing the dose at intervals greater than the duration of action. For most adult patients, 50 mg of meperidine I.M. every 4 hours, p.r.n. for moderate to severe pain, is undertreatment.

Some patients may require a higher dosage because their bodies use the drug differently, or because they absorb the drug poorly due to poor circulation or tissue damage, or because they metabolize or excrete the drug more rapidly than others.

Although you can't predict how a patient's body will use an analgesic, you can observe what happens and report it.

Should potentiators such as hydroxyzine (Vistaril) be added to analgesics to increase potency?

Potentiators are supposed to increase the duration of pain relief of analgesics. Most so-called potentiators simply produce a sedative effect. Increasing the analgesic dose itself will provide more effective pain relief.

NAME	INDICATIONS & DOSAGE	SIDE EFFECTS
alphaprodine hydrochloride Controlled Substance Schedule II Nisentil♦	*Moderate to severe pain*— **Adults:** 0.4 to 0.6 mg/kg I.V. or 0.4 to 1.2 mg/kg S.C. q 2 hours, p.r.n. Maximum 240 mg daily. Don't give I.M.	**CNS:** *sedation, clouded sensorium, euphoria,* convulsions with large doses. **CV:** *hypotension,* bradycardia. **GI:** *nausea, vomiting, constipation,* ileus. **GU:** *urinary retention.* **Other:** *respiratory depression,* physical dependence.
anileridine hydrochloride **anileridine phosphate** Controlled Substance Schedule II Leritine♦	*Adjunct to anesthetic*— **Adults:** 50 to 100 mg added to 500 ml 5% dextrose in water for slow I.V. infusion; initially, 5 to 10 mg followed by slow infusion of 0.6 mg/minute. Maximum dose 200 mg daily. *Moderate to severe pain*— **Adults:** 25 to 50 mg P.O., I.M., or S.C. q 4 to 6 hours, p.r.n. *Preoperatively*— **Adults:** 50 to 75 mg I.M. or S.C.	**CNS:** *sedation, clouded sensorium, euphoria,* convulsions with large doses. **CV:** *hypotension,* bradycardia. **GI:** *nausea, vomiting, constipation,* ileus. **GU:** *urinary retention.* **Local:** pain at injection site, local tissue irritation, and induration after S.C. injection; phlebitis after I.V. injection. **Other:** *respiratory depression,* physical dependence.
Brompton's cocktail (Mixture containing varying amounts of the following ingredients: morphine or methadone, cocaine or amphetamine, syrup or honey, alcohol [90% to 98%] or gin, chloroform water) Controlled Substance Schedule II	*Severe chronic pain of terminal cancer*— **Adults:** 10 to 20 ml of (standard pharmacy-prepared mixture) q 3 to 4 hours (if morphine is used) or q 6 to 8 hours (if methadone is used). Must be given around the clock. Dosage titrations can be made at 48- to 72-hour intervals. Maximum dose totally dependent on patient response.	**CNS:** *sedation, clouded sensorium, euphoria,* convulsions with large doses. **CV:** *hypotension,* bradycardia. **GI:** *nausea, vomiting, constipation,* ileus. **GU:** *urinary retention.* **Other:** *respiratory depression,* physical dependence.

♦ Available in U.S. and Canada. ♦♦ Available in Canada only. All other products (no symbol) available in U.S. only. Italicized side effects are common or life-threatening.

INTERACTIONS	NURSING CONSIDERATIONS
None significant.	• Use with extreme caution in patients with head injury, increased intracranial pressure, shock, increased cerebrospinal fluid pressure, CNS depression, asthma, COPD, respiratory depression, seizures, hepatic or renal disease, hypothyroidism, Addison's disease, alcoholism, and in elderly or debilitated patients. • Keep narcotic antagonist (naloxone) available when giving this drug I.V. • Monitor respirations of newborns exposed to drug during labor. • Rapid but short-lived effect makes drug useful in minor surgery or in urologic procedures; not useful for relief of chronic pain. • Monitor respiratory and circulatory status carefully. • Related to meperidine. • If used with other narcotic analgesics, general anesthetics, tranquilizers, sedatives, hypnotics, alcohol, tricyclic antidepressants, or MAO inhibitors, depressant effect is increased. Reduce narcotic dose. Use together with extreme caution. • For better analgesic effect, give before patient has intense pain. • When used postoperatively, encourage turning, coughing, and deep breathing to avoid atelectasis. • Warn ambulatory patients to avoid activities that require alertness. • For toxicity, see APPENDIX, *Drug Toxicities*.
None significant.	• Use with extreme caution in patients with increased intracranial pressure, increased cerebrospinal fluid pressure, CNS depression, head injury, asthma, COPD, respiratory depression, seizures, hepatic or renal disease, hypothyroidism, Addison's disease, alcoholism, shock, and in elderly or debilitated patients. • Keep narcotic antagonist (naloxone) available when giving this drug I.V. • Warn ambulatory patient to avoid activities that require alertness. • Monitor respirations of newborns exposed to drug during labor. • S.C. injection more likely to cause tissue irritation than I.M. route. • Stopping drug after long-term use may cause withdrawal symptoms. • Related to meperidine. • Carefully aspirate before S.C. or I.M. injection. Sudden I.V. injection of more than 10 mg can cause cardiac arrest. • Monitor respiratory and circulatory status carefully. • If used with other narcotic analgesics, general anesthetics, tranquilizers, sedatives, hypnotics, alcohol, tricyclic antidepressants, or MAO inhibitors, depressant effect is increased. Reduce narcotic dose. Use together with extreme caution. • For toxicity, see APPENDIX, *Drug Toxicities*.
None significant	• Use with extreme caution in patients with head injury, increased intracranial pressure, shock, increased cerebrospinal fluid pressure, CNS depression, asthma, COPD, respiratory depression, seizures, hepatic or renal disease, hypothyroidism, Addison's disease, alcoholism, and in elderly or debilitated patients. • Originated in Brompton Hospital in England to keep cancer patients in constant pain-free and euphoric state. • Not commercially prepared—must be prepared by pharmacy. • Has frequently proven to be effective when narcotic analgesics alone have failed to provide pain relief. • Around-the-clock administration reduces patient's anticipation of pain and is major reason for effectiveness. See also p. 378. • If cocaine is ingredient in mixture—advise patient to swish mixture in mouth to aid absorption, as cocaine is absorbed only through oral mucosa.

(continued on following page)

NAME	INDICATIONS & DOSAGE	SIDE EFFECTS
Brompton's cocktail *(continued)*		
codeine phosphate **codeine sulfate** Controlled Substance Schedule II	*Mild to moderate pain—* **Adults:** 15 to 60 mg P.O. or 15 to 60 mg (phosphate) S.C. or I.M. q 4 hours, p.r.n. **Children:** 3 mg/kg daily P.O. divided q 4 hours, p.r.n.	**CNS:** *sedation, clouded sensorium, euphoria,* convulsions with large doses. **CV:** *hypotension,* bradycardia. **GI:** *nausea, vomiting, constipation,* ileus. **GU:** *urinary retention.* **Other:** *respiratory depression,* physical dependence.
fentanyl citrate Controlled Substance Schedule II Sublimaze♦	*Adjunct to general anesthetic—* **Adults:** 0.05 to 0.1 mg I.V. repeated q 2 to 3 minutes, p.r.n. Dose should be reduced in elderly and poor-risk patients. *Postoperatively—* **Adults:** 0.05 to 0.1 mg I.M. q 1 to 2 hours, p.r.n. **Children 2 to 12 years:** 0.02 to 0.03 mg per 9 kg. *Preoperatively—* **Adults:** 0.05 to 0.1 mg I.M. 30 to 60 minutes before surgery.	**CNS:** *sedation, clouded sensorium, euphoria,* convulsions with large doses. **CV:** *hypotension,* bradycardia. **GI:** *nausea, vomiting, constipation,* ileus. **GU:** *urinary retention.* **Other:** *respiratory depression,* physical dependence.
hydromorphone hydrochloride Controlled Substance Schedule II Dilaudid♦	*Moderate to severe pain—* **Adults:** 2 to 4 mg P.O. q 4 to 6 hours, p.r.n.; or 2 to 4 mg I.M., S.C., or I.V. q 4 to 6 hours, p.r.n. (I.V. dose should be given over 3 to 5 minutes); or 3 mg rectal suppository at bedtime, p.r.n.	**CNS:** *sedation, clouded sensorium, euphoria,* convulsions with large doses. **CV:** *hypotension,* bradycardia. **GI:** *nausea, vomiting, constipation,* ileus. **GU:** *urinary retention.* **Local:** induration with repeated S.C. injection. **Other:** *respiratory depression,* physical dependence.

♦ Available in U.S. and Canada. ♦♦ Available in Canada only. All other products (no symbol) available in U.S. only. Italicized side effects are common or life-threatening.

INTERACTIONS	NURSING CONSIDERATIONS
	• Phenothiazines are occasionally added to increase analgesic effect and prevent nausea. • Most formulations are stable for up to 4 weeks at room temperature; storage in refrigerator may increase stability to 8 weeks.
None significant.	• Use with extreme caution in patients with head injury, increased intracranial pressure, increased cerebrospinal fluid pressure, hepatic or renal disease, hypothyroidism, Addison's disease, acute alcoholism, seizures, severe CNS depression, bronchial asthma, COPD, respiratory depression, shock, and in elderly or debilitated patients. • Warn ambulatory patient to avoid activities that require alertness. • Monitor respiratory and circulatory status and bowel function. • For full analgesic effect, give before patient has intense pain. • Codeine and aspirin have additive effect. Give together for maximum pain relief. • Do not administer discolored injection solution. • If used with general anesthetics, other narcotic analgesics, tranquilizers, sedatives, hypnotics, alcohol, tricyclic antidepressants, or MAO inhibitors, CNS depression is increased. Use together with extreme caution. Monitor patient's response. • For toxicity, see APPENDIX, *Drug Toxicities*.
None significant.	• Contraindicated in patients who have received MAO inhibitors within 14 days and who have myasthenia gravis. Use cautiously in patients with head injury, increased cerebrospinal fluid pressure, asthma, COPD, respiratory depression, seizures, hepatic or renal disease, hypothyroidism, Addison's disease, alcoholism, increased intracranial pressure, CNS depression, shock, and in elderly or debilitated patients. • Keep narcotic antagonist (naloxone) and resuscitative equipment available when giving drug I.V. • Monitor respirations of newborns exposed to drug during labor. • Use as postoperative analgesic, only in recovery room. Make sure another analgesic is ordered for later use. • Often used with droperidol (as Innovar) to produce neuroleptanalgesia. • Monitor circulatory and respiratory status carefully. • Respiratory depression, hypotension, profound sedation, and coma may result if used with other narcotic analgesics, general anesthetics, tranquilizers, alcohol, sedatives, hypnotics, tricyclic antidepressants, or MAO inhibitors. Fentanyl citrate dose should be reduced by ¼ to ⅓. Also give above drugs in reduced dosages. • For better analgesic effect, give before patient has intense pain. • When used postoperatively, encourage turning, coughing, and deep breathing to avoid atelectasis. • For toxicity, see APPENDIX, *Drug Toxicities*.
None significant.	• Contraindicated in increased intracranial pressure and status asthmaticus. Use with extreme caution in patients with increased cerebrospinal fluid pressure, respiratory depression, hepatic or renal disease, hypothyroidism, shock, Addison's disease, acute alcoholism, seizures, head injury, severe CNS depression, brain tumor, bronchial asthma, COPD, and in elderly or debilitated patients. • Warn ambulatory patient to avoid activities that require alertness. • Monitor respiratory and circulatory status and bowel function. • Keep narcotic antagonist (naloxone) available. • Respiratory depression and hypotension can occur with I.V. administration. Give very slowly and monitor constantly.

(continued on following page)

NAME	INDICATIONS & DOSAGE	SIDE EFFECTS
hydromorphone hydrochloride *(continued)*		
levorphanol tartrate Controlled Substance Schedule II Levo-Dromoran♦	*Moderate to severe pain*— **Adults:** 2 to 3 mg P.O. or S.C. q 6 to 8 hours, p.r.n.	**CNS:** *sedation, clouded sensorium, euphoria,* convulsions with large doses. **CV:** *hypotension,* bradycardia. **GI:** *nausea, vomiting, constipation,* ileus. **GU:** *urinary retention.* **Other:** *respiratory depression,* physical dependence.
meperidine hydrochloride Controlled Substance Schedule II Demer-Idine♦♦, Demerol♦, Pethidine HCl B.P.♦♦	*Moderate to severe pain*— **Adults:** 50 to 150 mg P.O., I.M., or S.C. q 3 to 4 hours, p.r.n. **Children:** 1 mg/kg P.O., I.M., or S.C. q 4 to 6 hours. Maximum—100 mg q 4 hours, p.r.n. *Preoperatively*— **Adults:** 50 to 100 mg I.M. or S.C. 30 to 90 minutes before surgery. **Children:** 1 to 2.2 mg/kg I.M. or S.C. 30 to 90 minutes before surgery.	**CNS:** *sedation, clouded sensorium, euphoria,* convulsions with large doses. **CV:** *hypotension,* bradycardia. **GI:** *nausea, vomiting, constipation,* ileus. **GU:** *urinary retention.* **Local:** pain at injection site, local tissue irritation and induration after S.C. injection; phlebitis after I.V. injection. **Other:** *respiratory depression,* physical dependence.

INTERACTIONS	NURSING CONSIDERATIONS
	• Rotate injection sites to avoid induration with subcutaneous injection. • Commonly abused narcotic. • If used with general anesthetics, other narcotic analgesics, tranquilizers, sedatives, hypnotics, alcohol, tricyclic antidepressants, or MAO inhibitors, CNS depression is increased. Hydromorphone dose should be reduced. Use together with extreme caution. Monitor patient's response. • Oral dosage form is particularly convenient for patients with chronic pain because tablets are available in 1 mg, 2 mg, 3 mg, and 4 mg. This enables these patients to titrate their own dose. • For better analgesic effect, give before patient has intense pain. • When used postoperatively, encourage turning, coughing, and deep breathing to avoid atelectasis. • For toxicity, see APPENDIX, *Drug Toxicities*.
None significant.	• Contraindicated in patients with acute alcoholism, bronchial asthma, increased intracranial pressure, respiratory depression, and anoxia. Use with extreme caution in patients with hepatic or renal disease, hypothyroidism, Addison's disease, seizures, head injury, severe CNS depression, brain tumor, COPD, shock, and in elderly or debilitated patients. • Warn ambulatory patient to avoid activities that require alertness. • Monitor circulatory and respiratory status and bowel function. • Warn patient drug has bitter taste. • Protect from light. • Keep narcotic antagonist (naloxone) available. • If used with general anesthetics, other narcotic analgesics, tranquilizers, sedatives, hypnotics, alcohol, tricyclic antidepressants, or MAO inhibitors, CNS depression is increased. Reduce levorphanol dose. Use together with extreme caution. Monitor patient's response. • For better analgesic effect, give before patient has intense pain. • When used postoperatively, encourage turning, coughing, and deep breathing to avoid atelectasis. • For toxicity, see APPENDIX, *Drug Toxicities*.
MAO inhibitors, isoniazid: increased CNS excitation or depression can be severe or fatal. Don't use together.	• Contraindicated if patient has used MAO inhibitors within 14 days. Use with extreme caution in patients with increased intracranial pressure, increased cerebrospinal fluid pressure, shock, CNS depression, head injury, asthma, COPD, respiratory depression, supraventricular tachycardias, seizures, acute abdominal conditions, hepatic or renal disease, hypothyroidism, Addison's disease, urethral stricture, prostatic hypertrophy, alcoholism, and in children under 12 years and elderly or debilitated patients. • Meperidine and active metabolite normeperidine accumulate in renal failure. Monitor for increased toxic effect in patients with poor renal function. • Meperidine may be given slow I.V., preferably as a diluted solution. S.C. injection very painful. • Keep narcotic antagonist (naloxone) available when giving this drug I.V. • Warn ambulatory patient to avoid activities that require alertness. • Monitor respirations of newborns exposed to drug during labor. Have resuscitation equipment available. • P.O. dose less than half as effective as parenteral dose. Give I.M. if possible. When changing from parenteral to P.O. route, dose should be increased. • Syrup has local anesthetic effect. Give with full glass of water. • Chemically incompatible with barbiturates. Don't mix together.

(continued on following page)

NAME	INDICATIONS & DOSAGE	SIDE EFFECTS
meperidine hydrochloride *(continued)*		
methadone hydrochloride Controlled Substance Schedule II Dolophine, Westadone	*Severe pain—* **Adults:** 2.5 to 10 mg P.O., I.M., or S.C. q 3 to 4 hours, p.r.n. *Narcotic abstinence syndrome—* **Adults:** 15 to 40 mg P.O. daily (highly individualized). **Maintenance:** 20 to 120 mg P.O. daily. Adjust dose as needed. Daily doses greater than 120 mg may require special state and federal approval.	**CNS:** *sedation, clouded sensorium, euphoria,* convulsions with large doses. **CV:** *hypotension,* bradycardia. **GI:** *nausea, vomiting, constipation,* ileus. **GU:** *urinary retention.* **Local:** pain at injection site, tissue irritation, induration following S.C. injection. **Other:** *respiratory depression,* physical dependence.
morphine sulfate♦ Controlled Substance Schedule II	*Severe pain—* **Adults:** 5 to 15 mg S.C. or I.M., or 30 to 60 mg P.O. q 4 hours, p.r.n. or around the clock. May be injected slow I.V. (over 4 to 5 minutes) diluted in 4 to 5 ml water for injection. **Children:** 0.1 to 0.2 mg/kg dose S.C. Maximum 15 mg.	**CNS:** *sedation, clouded sensorium, euphoria,* convulsions with large doses. **CV:** *hypotension,* bradycardia. **GI:** *nausea, vomiting, constipation,* ileus. **GU:** *urinary retention.* **Other:** *respiratory depression, physical dependence.*

INTERACTIONS	NURSING CONSIDERATIONS
	• Monitor respiratory and cardiovascular status carefully. Don't give if respirations are below 12/minute or if change in pupils is noted. • Watch for withdrawal symptoms if stopped abruptly after long-term use. • If used with other narcotic analgesics, general anesthetics, phenothiazines, sedatives, hypnotics, tricyclic antidepressants, or alcohol, respiratory depression, hypotension, profound sedation, or coma may occur. Reduce meperidine dose. Use together with extreme caution. • For better analgesic effect, give before patient has intense pain. • When used postoperatively, encourage turning, coughing, and deep breathing to avoid atelectasis. • For toxicity, see APPENDIX, *Drug Toxicities*.
Rifampin: withdrawal symptoms; reduced blood levels of methadone. Use together cautiously. *Ammonium chloride and other urine acidifiers, phenytoin:* may reduce methadone effect. Monitor for decreased pain control.	• Contraindicated in obstetric analgesia. Give with extreme caution in elderly or debilitated patients, or in patients with acute abdominal conditions, severe hepatic or renal impairment, hypothyroidism, Addison's disease, prostatic hypertrophy, urethral stricture, head injury, increased intracranial pressure, asthma, COPD, respiratory depression, CNS depression. • Safe use in adolescents as maintenance drug not established. • Oral dose is half as potent as injected dose. • Rotate injection sites. • Has cumulative effect; marked sedation can occur after repeated doses. • Monitor circulatory and respiratory status and bowel function. • Warn ambulatory patient to avoid activities that require alertness. • One daily dose adequate for maintenance. No advantage to divided doses. • Oral form legally required in maintenance programs. • Give maintenance doses as oral liquid. Completely dissolve tablets in 120 ml of orange juice or powdered citrus drink. • Constipation often severe with maintenance. Make sure stool softener or other laxative is ordered. • Patient treated for narcotic abstinence syndrome will usually require an additional analgesic if pain control necessary. • If used with general anesthetics, tranquilizers, sedatives, hypnotics, alcohol, tricyclic antidepressants or MAO inhibitors, respiratory depression, hypotension, profound sedation, or coma may occur. Use together with extreme caution. Monitor patient's response. • For toxicity, see APPENDIX, *Drug Toxicities*.
None significant.	• Use with extreme caution in patients with head injury, increased intracranial pressure, seizures, asthma, COPD, alcoholism, prostatic hypertrophy, severe hepatic or renal disease, acute abdominal conditions, hypothyroidism, Addison's disease, increased cerebrospinal fluid pressure, urethral stricture, cardiac arrhythmias, reduced blood volume, toxic psychosis, and in elderly or debilitated patients. • Warn ambulatory patient to avoid activities that require alertness. • Monitor circulatory and respiratory status and bowel function. Don't give if respirations are below 12/minute. • Drug of choice in relieving pain of myocardial infarction. May cause transient decrease in blood pressure. • Keep narcotic antagonist (naloxone) and resuscitative equipment available. • For better analgesic effect, give before patient has intense pain. • Respiratory depression, hypotension, profound sedation, or coma may occur if used with general anesthetics, tranquilizers, sedatives, hypnotics, alcohol, tricyclic antidepressants, or MAO inhibitors. Re-

(continued on following page)

NAME	INDICATIONS & DOSAGE	SIDE EFFECTS
morphine sulfate *(continued)*		
oxycodone hydrochloride Controlled Substance Schedule II Supeudol♦♦ Combinations: Percocet♦♦, Percocet 5, Percocet-Demi♦, Percodan♦, Percodan-Demi♦, Tylox	*Moderate pain*— **Adults:** available in U.S. only in combination with other drugs, such as aspirin, phenacetin, and caffeine (Percodan, Percodan-Demi), or acetaminophen (Percocet 5, Tylox). 1 to 2 tablets P.O. q 6 hours, p.r.n. **Adults:** (Supeudol) 1 to 3 suppositories rectally/day, p.r.n. **Children:** (Percodan-Demi) ¼ to ½ tablet P.O. q 6 hours, p.r.n.	**CNS:** *sedation, clouded sensorium, euphoria,* convulsions with large doses. **CV:** *hypotension,* bradycardia. **GI:** *nausea, vomiting, constipation,* ileus. **GU:** *urinary retention.* **Other:** *respiratory depression,* physical dependence.
oxymorphone hydrochloride Controlled Substance Schedule II Numorphan♦	*Moderate to severe pain*— **Adults:** 1 to 1.5 mg I.M. or S.C. q 4 to 6 hours, p.r.n., or 0.5 mg I.V. q 4 to 6 hours, p.r.n., or 2.5 to 5 mg rectally q 4 to 6 hours, p.r.n.	**CNS:** *sedation, clouded sensorium, euphoria,* convulsions with large doses. **CV:** *hypotension,* bradycardia. **GI:** *nausea, vomiting, constipation,* ileus. **GU:** *urinary retention.* **Other:** *respiratory depression,* physical dependence.
pentazocine hydrochloride **pentazocine lactate** Controlled Substance Schedule IV Talwin♦	*Moderate to severe pain*— **Adults:** 50 to 100 mg P.O. q 3 to 4 hours, p.r.n. Maximum 600 mg daily or 30 mg I.M., I.V., or S.C. q 3 to 4 hours, p.r.n. Maximum 360 mg daily. Doses above 30 mg I.V. or 60 mg I.M. or S.C. not recommended.	**CNS:** *sedation,* visual disturbances, hallucinations, drowsiness, dizziness, light-headedness, confusion, euphoria, headache. **GI:** nausea, vomiting, dry mouth. **GU:** urinary retention. **Local:** induration, nodules, sloughing, and sclerosis of injection site.

♦ Available in U.S. and Canada. ♦♦ Available in Canada only. All other products (no symbol) available in U.S. only. Italicized side effects are common or life-threatening.

INTERACTIONS	NURSING CONSIDERATIONS
	duce morphine dose. Use together with extreme caution. Monitor patient's response. • When used postoperatively, encourage turning, coughing, and deep breathing to avoid atelectasis. • Newly available oral solution contains 10 mg/5 ml. • For toxicity, see APPENDIX, *Drug Toxicities*.
Anticoagulants: oxycodone hydrochloride products containing aspirin may increase anticoagulant effect. Monitor clotting times. Use together cautiously.	• Use with extreme caution in patients with head injury, increased intracranial pressure, increased cerebrospinal fluid pressure, seizures, asthma, COPD, alcoholism, prostatic hypertrophy, severe hepatic or renal disease, acute abdominal conditions, urethral stricture, hypothyroidism, Addison's disease, cardiac arrhythmias, reduced blood volume, toxic psychosis, and in elderly or debilitated patients. • Don't give to children, except for Percodan-Demi and Percocet-Demi. • Warn ambulatory patient to avoid activities that require alertness. • Monitor circulatory and respiratory status and bowel function. Do not give if respirations are below 12/minute. • For full analgesic effect, give before patient has intense pain. • High level of analgesia when given P.O., but poor choice due to high risk of addiction and presence of phenacetin in some combinations. • Give after meals or with milk. • If used with general anesthetics, other narcotic analgesics, tranquilizers, sedatives, hypnotics, alcohol, tricyclic antidepressants, or MAO inhibitors, CNS depression is increased. Reduce oxycodone dose. Use together with extreme caution. Monitor patient's response. • For toxicity, see APPENDIX, *Drug Toxicities*.
None significant.	• Use with extreme caution in patients with head injury, increased intracranial pressure, seizures, asthma, COPD, alcoholism, increased cerebrospinal fluid pressure, acute abdominal conditions, prostatic hypertrophy, severe hepatic or renal disease, urethral stricture, CNS depression, respiratory depression, hypothyroidism, Addison's disease, cardiac arrhythmias, reduced blood volume, toxic psychosis, and in elderly or debilitated patients. • Warn ambulatory patient to avoid activities that require alertness. • Monitor cardiovascular and respiratory status. Don't give if respirations are below 12/minute. • Well absorbed rectally. Alternative to narcotics with more limited dosage forms. • Keep narcotic antagonist (naloxone) and resuscitative equipment available. • If used with general anesthetics, tranquilizers, sedatives, hypnotics, alcohol, tricyclic antidepressants, or MAO inhibitors, CNS depression is increased. Reduce oxymorphone dose. Use together with extreme caution. Monitor patient's response. • For better analgesic effect, give before patient has intense pain. • When used postoperatively, encourage turning, coughing, and deep breathing to avoid atelectasis. • For toxicity, see APPENDIX, *Drug Toxicities*.
None significant.	• Contraindicated in emotional instability, drug abuse, head injury, increased intracranial pressure. Use cautiously in hepatic or renal disease, myocardial infarction with nausea, respiratory depression. • Tablets not well absorbed. • Possesses narcotic antagonist properties. • Psychological and physiologic dependence may occur. • Respiratory depression can be reversed with naloxone. • Do not mix in same syringe with soluble barbiturates.

(continued on following page)

NAME	INDICATIONS & DOSAGE	SIDE EFFECTS
pentazocine *(continued)*		**Other:** *respiratory depression,* physical and psychological dependence.
propoxyphene hydrochloride Controlled Substance Schedule IV Darvon, Depronal♦♦, Dolene, Doraphen, Harmar, Myospaz, Pargesic 65, Pro-65♦♦, Pro-Pox 65, Proxagesic, Ropoxy, Scrip-Dyne, SK-65, S-Pain-65, 642♦♦ **propoxyphene napsylate** Controlled Substance Schedule IV Darvocet-N, Darvon-N♦	*Mild to moderate pain*— **Adults:** 65 mg (hydrochloride) P.O. q 4 hours, p.r.n. *Mild to moderate pain*— **Adults:** 100 mg (napsylate) P.O. q 4 hours, p.r.n.	**CNS:** dizziness, headache, sedation, euphoria, paradoxical excitement, insomnia. **GI:** nausea, vomiting, constipation. **Other:** psychological and physical dependence.

♦ Available in U.S. and Canada. ♦♦ Available in Canada only. All other products (no symbol) available in U.S. only. Italicized side effects are common or life-threatening.

WHAT YOU SHOULD KNOW ABOUT BROMPTON'S COCKTAIL

Brompton's cocktail, developed in the 1930s at Brompton Hospital, England, has these advantages over other analgesics:

- It prevents pain from starting because it's administered around the clock—usually every 4 hours. This lessens the patient's fear of the pain returning.
- It's easy to administer, since it's an oral drug. It's especially good for a patient who has a nasogastric tube in place.
- It relieves pain without clouding the patient's mind.
- Most important, many patients with cancer claim it's the only drug that relieves their pain.

Brompton's cocktail contains a narcotic analgesic, a CNS stimulant, and alcohol as a flavor enhancer. Syrup and chloroform water are added to improve the mixture's taste and texture.

Nursing considerations

- First and foremost, Brompton's cocktail must be administered regularly around the clock, not p.r.n.; administering this drug as needed negates its preventive analgesic effect.
- If a patient is to receive Brompton's cocktail at home, make sure he has a supply of medication cups, so he can accurately measure each dose. Remind him to take the preparation on a regular basis, as prescribed by the doctor, even when he's not experiencing pain. Warn him not to increase the dosage.
- Brompton's cocktail is not the best analgesic for every cancer patient. It should be used only when narcotics alone don't work, since some patients don't need the extra ingredients in this preparation. For example, a patient may not need a CNS stimulant to counteract sedation. So compare the assessment of the patient with the components in the preparation to see if the patient is receiving more medication than he requires.

For more information on Brompton's cocktail, see p. 368.

INTERACTIONS	NURSING CONSIDERATIONS
	• Warn ambulatory patient to avoid activities that require alertness. • For toxicity, see APPENDIX, *Drug Toxicities*.
None significant.	• Not to be prescribed in narcotic addiction. • Warn ambulatory patient to avoid activities that require alertness until CNS response to drug has been established. • Warn patient not to exceed recommended dosage. • Do not use caffeine or amphetamines to treat overdose: may cause fatal convulsions. Use narcotic antagonist instead. • May cause false decreases in urinary steroid excretion tests. • 65 mg propoxyphene HCl equals 100 mg propoxyphene napsylate. • Can be considered a mild narcotic analgesic. • Advise patients to limit their alcohol intake when taking this drug. • For toxicity, see APPENDIX, *Drug Toxicities*.

DRUG ERROR

COULD YOU HAVE GIVEN THIS POSTOPERATIVE OVERDOSE?

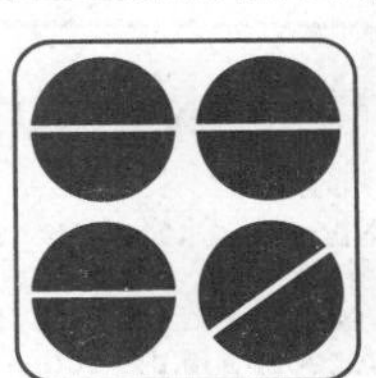

A doctor wrote an order for 25 mg of meperidine I.M. every 3 hours until 4 p.m., then 50 mg I.M., p.r.n., for pain, for a postoperative patient. Attached to the patient's chart was a warning sticker noting that he had received Innovar (fentanyl citrate with droperidol) preoperatively.

At 3 p.m. the patient complained of pain. The medication nurse checked his chart, obtained what she thought was the correct analgesic from the narcotic floor stock, and administered it.

Moments later, the charge nurse checked the meperidine control form and noticed the medication nurse hadn't signed out any doses. When questioned, the medication nurse insisted she had signed the form. When she produced the form, however, it was for morphine. She had mistakenly read *morphine* for *meperidine.*

The usual dose of morphine is 10 to 12 mg. But since this patient had received Innovar, the morphine dosage should have been reduced to 4 mg.

Having received about six times the safe dose of morphine, the patient developed respiratory depression and had to be given a narcotic antagonist to counteract the overdose.

This medication error could have been prevented if the nurse had read the order carefully. She also should have known a parenteral dose of 25 mg of morphine is too high for most surgical patients.

28 Narcotic antagonists

levallorphan tartrate
naloxone

Because of their chemical similarity to narcotics, narcotic antagonists can compete with narcotics for receptor sites. They are antidotes for overdoses of narcotics, including pentazocine and propoxyphene. Narcotic antagonists are very potent and can reverse respiratory depression caused by a narcotic dose 10 to 100 times as great, as well as the narcotic's analgesic, cardiovascular, and gastrointestinal effects.

Levallorphan is ineffective against barbiturate- or anesthetic-induced respiratory depression. Indeed, levallorphan itself can induce respiratory depression and exacerbates such depression caused by nonnarcotic drugs. Naloxone, which does not worsen nonnarcotic respiratory depression, is

NARCOTIC ANTAGONISTS: HOW THEY WORK

Narcotic antagonists can reverse the action of narcotic analgesics because they reach—and thus can affect—the same receptors in the body. This is possible because the chemical structure of these two types of drugs is similar.

The chemical structure of naloxone (a narcotic antagonist) and of oxymorphone (a narcotic analgesic) are illustrated below. As you can see, their basic structures are the same. But the groups highlighted in color are different, and these determine the drugs' effects on the patient. Naloxone has an allyl group, which makes it an antagonist; oxymorphone has a methyl group, which makes it an analgesic.

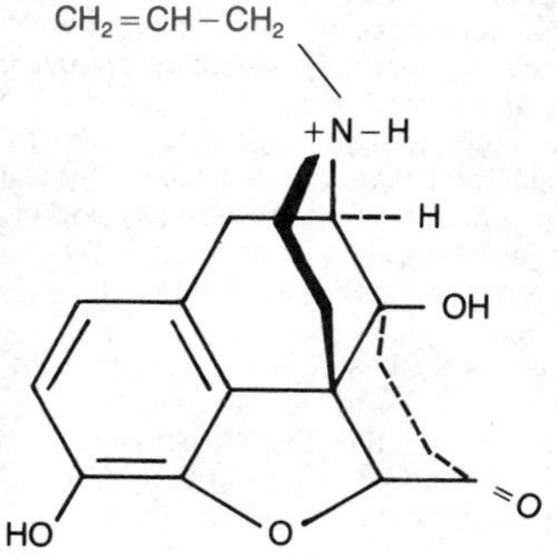

$CH_2=CH-CH_2$
+N–H
H
OH
=O
HO
O

naloxone

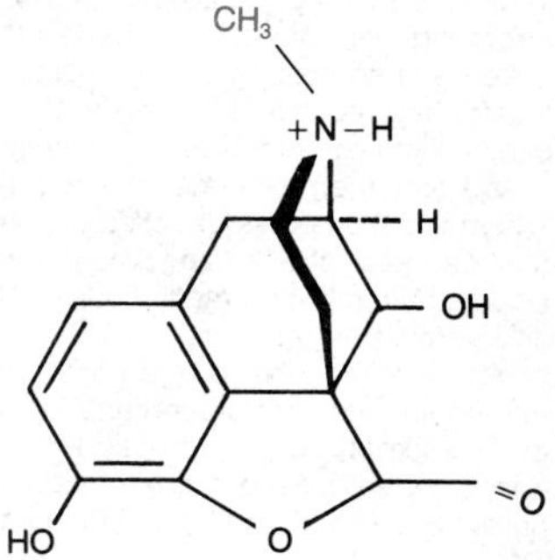

CH_3
+N–H
H
OH
=O
HO
O

oxymorphone

the antagonist of choice for respiratory depression of unknown cause.

Major uses

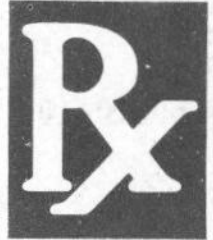

Narcotic antagonists are antidotes for narcotic-induced respiratory depression, including asphyxia neonatorum.

- Naloxone is used in diagnosis of suspected acute opiate overdosage.

Mechanism of action

Although the precise mechanism of action of narcotic antagonists is unknown, levallorphan and naloxone apparently displace previously administered narcotic analgesics from their receptors (competitive antagonism).

- Levallorphan may have some narcotic *agonist* activity (narcotic analgesic effect), especially if administered alone, not as an antidote to narcotic analgesics.
- Naloxone—administered alone—has no pharmacologic activity.

Absorption, distribution, metabolism, and excretion

Narcotic antagonists are well absorbed after parenteral administration, rapidly metabolized in the liver, and excreted in the urine.

Onset and duration

- Levallorphan's onset of action is 1 to 2 minutes when given I.V.; 2 to 5 minutes when given I.M. or subcutaneously. The drug's duration of action by all parenteral routes is 2 to 5 hours.
- Naloxone's onset of action is within 2 minutes after I.V. injection; approximately 2 to 5 minutes after I.M. or subcutaneous administration. Naloxone's duration of action when given I.V. is 45 minutes but longer when administered I.M. and subcutaneously.

Combination products

None.

QUESTIONS & ANSWERS

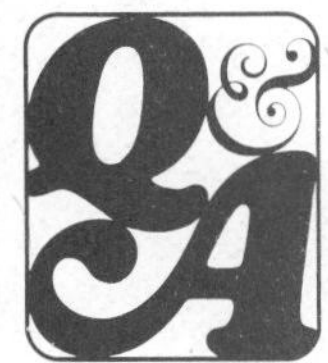

MORE BACKGROUND ON NALOXONE: AN EFFECTIVE ANTAGONIST WITH FEW SIDE EFFECTS

Why is naloxone chosen over other narcotic antagonists?

Naloxone is the most frequently used narcotic antagonist because it's the only one free of analgesic properties. And it doesn't produce unpleasant side effects, such as hallucinations, disorientation, tolerance or signs of physical dependence. It also has a high therapeutic index.

Does naloxone have any limitations?

Yes. Naloxone's duration of action is short compared with that of narcotic analgesics, so relapses are possible. When you're treating an opiate addict for an overdose, remember that large doses of naloxone may cause severe withdrawal symptoms. These symptoms are much more severe and difficult to manage than those induced by narcotic abstinence alone.

When is naloxone used?

Naloxone is used to treat coma, respiratory depression, and convulsions whenever narcotic overdose is suspected.

How is naloxone administered?

Naloxone can be given I.V., I.M., or subcutaneously. However, in patients who have abused I.V. drugs, often no I.V. sites are available. I.M. and subcutaneous injections are inappropriate when your patient requires immediate antagonist therapy. In emergencies, sublingual or intra-arterial injections may be used.

NAME	INDICATIONS & DOSAGE	SIDE EFFECTS
levallorphan tartrate Lorfan	*Severe narcotic-induced respiratory depression—* **Adults:** 1 mg I.V., then 1 to 2 doses of 0.5 mg at 10- to 15-minute intervals, p.r.n. Maximum total dose 3 mg. **Children:** 0.02 mg/kg I.V. May give 0.01 to 0.02 mg/kg in 10 to 15 minutes. **Neonates** (asphyxia neonatorum): 0.05 to 0.1 mg I.V. into umbilical vein immediately after delivery. May repeat in 5 to 10 minutes.	**CNS:** lethargy, dizziness, drowsiness, restlessness, sense of heaviness in limbs; with high doses: psychic disturbances (hallucinations, disorientation, weird dreams); in neonates: irritability, increased crying. **CV:** pallor. **EENT:** miosis, pseudoptosis. **GI:** nausea. **Other:** sweating, respiratory depression.
naloxone Narcan♦	*Narcotic-induced respiratory depression, including pentazocine and propoxyphene—* **Adults:** 0.4 mg I.V., S.C., or I.M. May repeat q 2 to 3 minutes, p.r.n., for 3 doses. *Postoperative narcotic depression—* **Adults:** 0.1 to 0.2 mg I.V. q 2 to 3 minutes, p.r.n. Adult concentration is 0.4 mg/ml. **Children:** 0.01 mg/kg dose I.M., I.V., S.C. May repeat q 2 to 3 minutes for 3 doses. *Note:* If initial dose 0.01 mg/kg does not result in clinical improvement, up to 10 times this dose (0.1 mg/kg) may be needed to be effective. **Neonates** (asphyxia neonatorum): 0.01 mg/kg I.V. into umbilical vein. May repeat q 2 to 3 minutes for 3 doses. Neonatal concentration (for children also) is 0.02 mg/ml.	*With higher-than-recommended doses:* nausea, vomiting. *In narcotic addicts:* withdrawal symptoms.

INTERACTIONS	NURSING CONSIDERATIONS
None significant.	• Contraindicated in mild respiratory depression and in narcotic addiction. (Violent withdrawal symptoms may occur.) • Monitor respiratory depth and rate. Be prepared to provide oxygen, ventilation, and other resuscitative measures. • May increase mild respiratory depression or that caused by nonnarcotic agents. Repeated doses may produce tolerance and increased respiratory depression.
None significant.	• Use cautiously in patients with cardiac irritability and narcotic addiction. • Safest drug to use when cause of respiratory depression is uncertain. • Monitor respiratory depth and rate. Be prepared to provide oxygen, ventilation, and other resuscitative measures. • Ineffective in respiratory depression caused by nonnarcotics. • May dilute adult concentration (0.4 mg) by mixing 0.5 ml with 9.5 ml sterile water or saline solution for injection to make neonatal concentration (0.02 mg/ml).

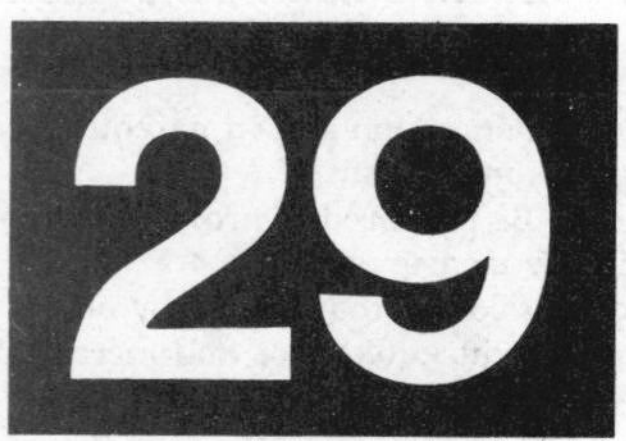

Sedatives and hypnotics

amobarbital
amobarbital sodium
aprobarbital
barbital
butabarbital
butabarbital sodium
chloral hydrate
ethchlorvynol
ethinamate
flurazepam hydrochloride
glutethimide
hexobarbital
mephobarbital
methaqualone
methaqualone hydrochloride
methotrimeprazine hydrochloride
methyprylon
paraldehyde
pentobarbital
pentobarbital sodium
phenobarbital
phenobarbital sodium
propiomazine hydrochloride
secobarbital
secobarbital sodium
talbutal
triclofos sodium

For information on temazepam, see APPENDIX, *New Drugs*.

Most of the drugs in this chapter are barbiturates (amobarbital, aprobarbital, barbital, butabarbital, hexobarbital, mephobarbital, pentobarbital, phenobarbital, secobarbital, and talbutal). Until recently, these were used extensively as nighttime sedative-hypnotics to induce sleep. However, because of the high risk of barbiturate toxicity and dependence, most doctors no longer regard them as the drugs of choice for this indication.

The benzodiazepines flurazepam and temazepam are more desirable for nighttime sedation because they have a much greater therapeutic index (margin between toxic and therapeutic dose) than the barbiturates. Also, both are generally as therapeutically effective as the barbiturates. The other drugs in this chapter (except paraldehyde) more closely resemble the barbiturates in their potential to cause toxicity and drug dependence. Methaqualone has a particularly high potential for abuse; for more details on this, see p. 406.

Major uses

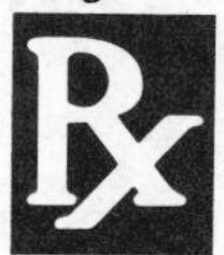

Sedatives and hypnotics are used to treat insomnia, induce sleep before operative or test procedures, and provide sedation and relief of anxiety.

- Mephobarbital and paraldehyde alleviate alcohol withdrawal syndrome.
- Phenobarbital controls acute psychotic agitation.

Mechanism of action

- Although their mechanism of action is not completely defined, barbiturates probably interfere with transmission of impulses from the thalamus to the cortex of the brain.
- Flurazepam acts on the limbic system, thalamus, and hypothalamus of the central nervous system to produce hypnotic effects.

SLEEP MEDICATIONS: ARE THEY ALWAYS NECESSARY?

Sleep problems are probably among your patients' most common complaints. Approximately 40 million Americans have trouble sleeping, but researchers say sleep medications won't necessarily help such persons. Only a small percentage of the 2 million Americans who regularly take sleep medications may actually need them. Look at these facts:

- 85% of persons who claim they have insomnia really don't. Most persons tested for insomnia in sleep laboratories fall asleep in 20 minutes.
- Relief is only temporary. After a 2-week period, effectiveness usually wanes, and patients develop a false tolerance to the drug, requiring a higher dosage to get the same effect. (*Effective* dosage increases, but the *lethal* dosage remains the same.)
- 10% of all insomniacs seen at sleep disorder treatment centers—only a small number of the people taking drugs for insomnia—are victims of *drug-induced* insomnia.

Doubling and tripling the original dosage leads to *drug dependence*. Withdrawal symptoms occur mainly at night, in the form of nightmares and restless sleep. Unfortunately, these symptoms tend to reinforce the patient's perceived need for the drug; this is especially true of anxious patients and those with chronic illnesses.

You can make a better judgment about your patient's real need for sleep medications by remembering these facts and by closely observing your patient's condition. He may be experiencing *transient* sleep difficulties, caused by psychological or environmental influences. These sleep problems can be treated successfully with hypnotics, since only short-term therapy is necessary. Insomnia may also accompany use of certain drugs (amphetamines or caffeine, for example) or withdrawal of certain substances (alcoholic beverages or nicotine, for example).

Medical conditions characterized by pain, dyspnea, physical discomfort, fear, anxiety, and depression can also affect sleep habits. Remember:

- Patients with arthritis, neurogenic pain, and various kinds of headache may experience more pain or discomfort at night than during the day. (With *decreased* external stimulation, patients are more conscious of their body sensations.)
- Patients with nocturnal leg recumbency cramps (restless leg syndrome—tingling sensations and nighttime cramps) commonly complain of sleep problems and see sleep medication as the solution.
- Besides increased pain, patients with cancer may experience fear and anxiety while trying to fall asleep, and this complicates the sleep process.
- Patients with angina pectoris and/or cardiac arrhythmias may fear attack at night and thus be afraid to sleep. This is common. Such patients who cannot readily fall asleep may become dependent on sleep medications to induce sleep.
- Some patients may actually have *sleep apnea,* a serious disorder in which they unknowingly stop breathing for as long as 2 minutes during the night, disturbing normal sleep patterns. They awake feeling tired and in need of more sleep, so may ask you for something to help them sleep. Unusually explosive, intermittent snoring may be a key to this specific diagnosis. So find out if your patient snores, and observe him while he sleeps.

Hypnotics may be useful in treating short-term sleep problems. But be alert for excessive or long-term use in your patients. And remember that insomnia is often only a symptom of other problems that need to be treated to overcome the sleeplessness.

For tips on promoting sleep without using hypnotics and sedatives, see p. 407.

Absorption, distribution, metabolism, and excretion

- The barbiturates are well absorbed from all administration routes; the sodium salts are more rapidly absorbed than the acids. They are distributed to all tissues and body fluids, with high concentrations in the brain and liver.

They are metabolized slowly in the liver. Both metabolites and unchanged drug are excreted in urine. Trace amounts are also eliminated in feces and perspiration.

- Chloral hydrate is well absorbed from the gastrointestinal (GI) tract after oral or rectal administration. It is rapidly reduced and distributed to all tissues. Both the unchanged drug and active metabolites are detected in cerebrospinal fluid (CSF), umbilical-cord blood, fetal blood, and amniotic fluid.

Chloral hydrate is metabolized in the liver and red cells. It is eliminated primarily in urine and partially in feces through the bile.

• Ethchlorvynol is rapidly absorbed from the GI tract after oral administration. Both the unchanged drug and metabolites are detected in the liver, kidneys, spleen, brain, bile, and CSF. The drug is metabolized primarily in the liver and excreted in urine.

• Ethinamate is well absorbed from the GI tract. Although it is rapidly destroyed in the tissues, its pattern of distribution is unknown. The liver is not significantly involved in the drug's metabolism. Small amounts are excreted in the urine.

• Flurazepam is well absorbed from the GI tract after oral administration. Distributed to all tissues and metabolized in the liver, it is eliminated primarily in urine and partially in feces.

• Glutethimide is absorbed irregularly from the GI tract after oral administration. The unchanged drug and active metabolites are detected in the liver, kidneys, brain, and bile. The drug is metabolized in the liver and eliminated in both urine and feces.

• Methaqualone is absorbed rapidly from the GI tract after oral administration. The unchanged drug or its metabolites or both are detected in the liver, kidneys, heart, brain, spleen, skeletal muscles, and CSF. The drug is metabolized in the liver; some of the metabolites are excreted in urine, and the remainder passes through the bile for elimination in feces.

• Methotrimeprazine is rapidly absorbed after I.M. injection. It is well distributed to body tissues, including the CSF, metabolized in the liver, and eliminated slowly in urine and feces.

• Methyprylon's absorption and distribution are not well known. The drug is metabolized in the liver. Some of its metabolites are secreted in the bile and reabsorbed; the rest are excreted in urine.

• Paraldehyde is rapidly absorbed from either the GI tract or muscles, depending on the route of administration. Although its distribution is not well known, the drug is metabolized in the liver and excreted in urine and through the lungs. Significant quantities are exhaled unchanged, emitting a characteristic odor.

• Propiomazine is well absorbed from parenteral sites; distributed throughout the body; metabolized in the liver; and eliminated in urine and, through the bile, in feces.

• Triclofos is rapidly absorbed from the GI tract. Its distribution in body tissues is unclear. It is metabolized primarily in the liver and kidneys and slowly eliminated in urine and feces.

Onset and duration

The chart on the opposite page summarizes onset and duration.

Combination products—barbiturates

BUTATRAX CAPSULES: amobarbital 20 mg and butabarbital 30 mg.

CARBRITAL KAPSEALS: pentobarbital sodium 97.5 mg and carbromal 260 mg.

ETHOBRAL CAPSULE: phenobarbital 50 mg, butabarbital sodium 30 mg, and secobarbital sodium 50 mg.

HYPTRAN TABLET: secobarbital 60 mg and phenyltoloxamine dihydrogen citrate 25 mg in outer layer (immediate release), phenyltoloxamine dihydrogen citrate 75 mg in core (delayed release).

NIDAR TABLET: phenobarbital sodium 7.5 mg, butabarbital sodium 7.5 mg, secobarbital sodium 25 mg, and pentobarbital sodium 25 mg.

TRI-BARBS CAPSULE: phenobarbital 32 mg, butabarbital sodium 32 mg, and secobarbital sodium 32 mg.

TUINAL 50 MG PULVULES: amobarbital sodium 25 mg and secobarbital sodium 25 mg.

TUINAL 100 MG PULVULES♦: amobarbital sodium 50 mg and secobarbital sodium 50 mg.

TUINAL 200 MG PULVULES♦: amobarbital sodium 100 mg and secobarbital sodium 100 mg.

THERAPEUTIC ACTIVITY OF SEDATIVES AND HYPNOTICS

ONSET AND DURATION	DRUGS P.O./I.M.	DRUGS I.V.
Ultra short-acting: few minutes' onset; short-term duration (less than 1 hour)	hexobarbital	amobarbital ethchlorvynol pentobarbital phenobarbital
Short-acting: 10 to 15 minutes' onset; 3 hours or less duration	paraldehyde pentobarbital secobarbital	
Intermediate-acting: 10 to 30 minutes' onset; 3 to 6 hours' duration	amobarbital aprobarbital butabarbital chloral hydrate ethchlorvynol ethinamate methotrimeprazine propiomazine talbutal tricloflos	
Long-acting: 30 to 60 minutes' onset; 6 or more hours' duration	barbital flurazepam glutethimide mephobarbital methaqualone methyprylon phenobarbital	

NAME	INDICATIONS & DOSAGE	SIDE EFFECTS
amobarbital Amytal♦, Isobec♦♦ **amobarbital sodium** Controlled Substance Schedule II Amytal Sodium♦	*Sedation—* **Adults:** usually 30 to 50 mg P.O. b.i.d. or t.i.d. but may range from 15 to 120 mg b.i.d. to q.i.d. **Children:** 3 to 6 mg/kg/day P.O. divided into 4 equal doses. *Insomnia—* **Adults:** 65 to 200 mg P.O. or deep I.M. at bedtime; I.M. injection not to exceed 5 ml in any one site. Maximum dose 500 mg. **Children:** 3 to 5 mg/kg deep I.M. at bedtime; I.M. injection not to exceed 5 ml in any one site. *Preanesthetic sedation—* **Adults and children:** 200 mg P.O. or I.M. 1 to 2 hours before surgery. *Manic reactions; anticonvulsant—* **Adults, and children over 6 years:** 65 to 500 mg slow I.V.; rate not to exceed 100 mg/minute. Maximum dose 1 g. **Children under 6 years:** 3 to 5 mg/kg slow I.V. or I.M.	**CNS:** *drowsiness, lethargy, hangover,* paradoxical excitement in elderly patients. **GI:** nausea, vomiting. **Skin:** rash, urticaria. **Local:** pain, irritation, sterile abscess at injection site. **Other:** *Stevens-Johnson syndrome,* angioedema.
aprobarbital Controlled Substance Schedule III Alurate	*Sedation—* **Adults:** 15 to 40 mg P.O. t.i.d. or q.i.d.; usual dose 40 mg t.i.d. *Insomnia—* **Adults:** 40 to 160 mg P.O. at bedtime.	**CNS:** *drowsiness, lethargy, hangover,* paradoxical excitement in elderly patients. **GI:** nausea, vomiting. **Skin:** rash, urticaria. **Other:** *Stevens-Johnson syndrome,* angioedema.
barbital Controlled Substance Schedule IV Barbital Sodium	*Insomnia—* **Adults:** 300 to 600 mg P.O. or I.M. 1 to 2 hours before bedtime. *Sedative—*	**CNS:** *drowsiness, lethargy, hangover,* paradoxical excitement in elderly patients. **GI:** nausea, vomiting. **Skin:** rash, urticaria.

♦ Available in U.S. and Canada. ♦♦ Available in Canada only. All other products (no symbol) available in U.S. only. Italicized side effects are common or life-threatening.

INTERACTIONS	NURSING CONSIDERATIONS
Alcohol or other CNS depressants, including other narcotic analgesics: excessive CNS and respiratory depression. Don't use together. *MAO inhibitors:* inhibit metabolism of barbiturates; may cause prolonged CNS depression. Reduce barbiturate dosage. *Rifampin:* may decrease barbiturate levels. Monitor for decreased effect.	• Contraindicated in patients with uncontrolled severe pain, respiratory disease with dyspnea or obstruction, hypersensitivity to barbiturates, previous addiction to sedatives, porphyria. Use with caution in hepatic or renal impairment. • Use injection solution within 30 minutes after opening container to minimize deterioration. Don't use cloudy or precipitated solution. Don't shake solution; mix with sterile water only. • Reserve I.V. injection for emergency treatment. Give under close supervision. Be prepared to give artificial respiration. Administer slowly I.V.; not to exceed 100 mg/minute. • Administer I.M. injection deeply. Superficial injection may cause pain, sterile abscess, and sloughing. • Because barbiturates potentiate narcotics, reduce dose when giving during labor. Excessive dose may cause respiratory depression in neonate. • Remove cigarettes of patient receiving hypnotic dose. • Supervise walking; raise bed rails, especially for elderly patients. • Long-term high dosage may cause drug dependence and severe withdrawal symptoms. Withdraw barbiturates gradually. • Prevent hoarding or self-overdosing by patients who are depressed, suicidal, or drug-dependent, or who have a history of drug abuse. Warn patient that alcohol increases effects of drug, and advise him not to perform activities requiring alertness or skill until CNS response is determined. • Watch for signs of barbiturate toxicity: coma, pupillary constriction, cyanosis, clammy skin, hypotension. Overdose can be fatal. • Monitor prothrombin times carefully when patient on amobarbital starts or ends anticoagulant therapy. Anticoagulant dose may need to be adjusted. • For toxicity, see APPENDIX, *Drug Toxicities*.
Alcohol or other CNS depressants, including narcotic analgesics: excessive CNS and respiratory depression. Don't use together. *MAO inhibitors:* inhibit metabolism of barbiturates; may cause prolonged CNS depression. Reduce barbiturate dosage. *Rifampin:* may decrease barbiturate levels. Monitor for decreased effect.	• Contraindicated in patients with uncontrolled severe pain, respiratory disease with dyspnea or obstruction, hypersensitivity to barbiturates, previous addiction to sedatives, porphyria. Use with caution in hepatic or renal impairment. • Remove cigarettes of patient receiving hypnotic dose. • Supervise walking; raise bed rails, especially for elderly patients. • Long-term high dosage may cause drug dependence and severe withdrawal symptoms. Withdraw barbiturates gradually. • Prevent hoarding or self-overdosing by patients who are depressed, suicidal, or drug-dependent, or who have a history of drug abuse. Warn patient that alcohol increases effects of drug, and advise him not to perform activities requiring alertness or skill until CNS response is determined. • Available as elixir only, with alcohol 20%. • Monitor prothrombin times carefully when patient on aprobarbital starts or ends anticoagulant therapy. Anticoagulant dose may need to be adjusted. • Watch for signs of barbiturate toxicity: coma, pupillary constriction, cyanosis, clammy skin, hypotension. Overdose can be fatal. • For toxicity, see APPENDIX, *Drug Toxicities*.
Alcohol or other CNS depressants, including narcotic analgesics: excessive CNS and respiratory	• Contraindicated in patients with uncontrolled severe pain, respiratory disease with dyspnea or obstruction, hypersensitivity to barbiturates, previous addiction to sedatives, and porphyria. Use with caution in hepatic, renal, cardiac, or respiratory impairment. • Use injection solution within 30 minutes after opening container to

(continued on following page)

NAME	INDICATIONS & DOSAGE	SIDE EFFECTS
barbital *(continued)*	**Adults:** 65 to 130 mg P.O. or I.M. b.i.d. or t.i.d.	**Local:** pain, swelling, thrombophlebitis. **Other:** *Stevens-Johnson syndrome,* angioedema.
butabarbital Buta-Barb♦♦, Butisol, Day-Barb♦♦, Medarsed, Neo-Barb♦♦ **butabarbital sodium** Controlled Substance Schedule III BBS, Butal, Butazem, Buticaps, Butisol Sodium♦, Sarisol No. 1, Soduben	*Sedation—* **Adults:** 15 to 30 mg P.O. t.i.d. or q.i.d. **Children:** 6 mg/kg P.O. divided t.i.d. Dosage range 7.5 to 30 mg P.O. t.i.d. *Preoperatively—* **Adults:** 50 to 100 mg P.O. 60 to 90 minutes before surgery. *Insomnia—* **Adults:** 50 to 100 mg P.O. at bedtime.	**CNS:** *drowsiness, lethargy, hangover,* paradoxical excitement in elderly patients. **GI:** nausea, vomiting. **Skin:** rash, urticaria. **Other:** *Stevens-Johnson syndrome,* angioedema.
chloral hydrate Controlled Substance Schedule IV Aquachloral Supprettes, Chloralvan♦♦, Cohidrate, Noctec♦, Novochlorhydrate♦♦, Oradrate, SK-Chloral Hydrate	*Sedation—* **Adults:** 250 mg P.O. or rectally t.i.d. after meals. **Children:** 8 mg/kg P.O. t.i.d. Maximum 500 mg t.i.d. *Insomnia—* **Adults:** 500 mg to 1 g P.O. or rectally 15 to 30 minutes before bedtime. **Children:** 50 mg/kg single dose.	**CNS:** *hangover, drowsiness,* nightmares, dizziness, ataxia. **GI:** *nausea,* vomiting, diarrhea, flatulence. **Skin:** hypersensitivity reactions.

INTERACTIONS	NURSING CONSIDERATIONS
depression. Don't use together. *MAO inhibitors:* inhibit metabolism of barbiturates; may cause prolonged CNS depression. Reduce barbiturate dosage. *Rifampin:* may decrease barbiturate levels. Monitor for decreased effect.	minimize deterioration. Don't use cloudy solution. • Administer I.M. injection deeply. Superficial injection may cause pain, sterile abscess, and sloughing. • Because barbiturates potentiate narcotics, reduce dose when giving during labor. Excessive dose may cause respiratory depression in neonate. • Remove cigarettes of patient receiving hypnotic dose. • Supervise walking; raise bed rails, especially for elderly patients. • Long-term high dosage may cause drug dependence and severe withdrawal symptoms. Withdraw barbiturates gradually. • Prevent hoarding or self-overdosing by patients who are depressed, suicidal, or drug-dependent, or who have a history of drug abuse. Warn patient that alcohol increases effects of drug, and advise him not to perform activities requiring alertness or skill until CNS response is determined. • No analgesic action. May cause restlessness or delirium in presence of pain. • Monitor prothrombin times carefully when patient on barbital starts or ends anticoagulant therapy. Anticoagulant dose may need to be adjusted. • Watch for signs of barbiturate toxicity: coma, pupillary constriction, cyanosis, clammy skin, hypotension. Overdose can be fatal. • For toxicity, see APPENDIX, *Drug Toxicities.*
Alcohol or other CNS depressants, including narcotic analgesics: excessive CNS and respiratory depression. Don't use together. *MAO inhibitors:* inhibit the metabolism of barbiturates; may cause prolonged CNS depression. Reduce barbiturate dosage. *Rifampin:* may decrease barbiturate levels. Monitor for decreased effect.	• Contraindicated in patients with uncontrolled severe pain, respiratory disease with dyspnea or obstruction, hypersensitivity to barbiturates, previous addiction to sedatives, porphyria. Use with caution in hepatic or renal impairment. • Remove cigarettes of patient receiving hypnotic dose. • Supervise walking; raise bed rails, especially for elderly patients. • Long-term high dosage may cause drug dependence and severe withdrawal symptoms. Withdraw barbiturates gradually. • Prevent hoarding or self-overdosing by patients who are depressed, suicidal, or drug-dependent, or who have a history of drug abuse. Warn patient that alcohol increases effects of drug, and advise him not to perform activities requiring alertness or skill until CNS response is determined. • Butisol sodium elixir is sugar-free. • Monitor prothrombin times carefully when patient on butabarbital starts or ends anticoagulant therapy. Anticoagulant dose may need to be adjusted. • Watch for signs of barbiturate toxicity: coma, pupillary constriction, cyanosis, clammy skin, hypotension. Overdose can be fatal. • Prolonged administration is not recommended: drug not shown to be effective after 14 days. A drug-free interval of at least 1 week is advised. • For toxicity, see APPENDIX, *Drug Toxicities.*
Alcohol or other CNS depressants, including narcotic analgesics: excessive CNS depression or vasodilation reaction. Use together cautiously. *Furosemide I.V.:* sweating, flushes, variable blood pres-	• Contraindicated in patients with marked hepatic or renal impairment, hypersensitivity to chloral hydrate or triclofos. Oral administration contraindicated in gastric disorders. Use with caution in severe cardiac disease, mental depression, suicidal tendencies. • Dilute or administer with liquid to minimize unpleasant taste and stomach irritation. Administer after meals. • Prevent hoarding by patients who are depressed, suicidal, or drug-dependent, or who have a history of drug abuse. Warn patient that alcohol increases effects of drug, and advise him not to perform activities requiring alertness or skill until CNS response is determined.

(continued on following page)

NAME	INDICATIONS & DOSAGE	SIDE EFFECTS
chloral hydrate *(continued)*	Maximum dose 1 g. *Premedication for EEG—* **Children:** 25 mg/kg single dose. Maximum dose 1 g.	
ethchlorvynol Controlled Substance Schedule IV Placidyl♦	*Sedation—* **Adults:** 100 to 200 mg P.O. b.i.d. or t.i.d. *Insomnia—* **Adults:** 500 mg to 1 g P.O. at bedtime. May repeat 100 to 200 mg if awakened in early a.m.	**Blood:** thrombocytopenia. **CNS:** facial numbness, drowsiness, fatigue, nightmares, dizziness, residual sedation, muscular weakness, syncope, ataxia. **CV:** hypotension. **EENT:** unpleasant aftertaste, blurred vision. **GI:** distress, nausea, vomiting. **Skin:** rashes, urticaria.
ethinamate Controlled Substance Schedule IV Valmid	*Insomnia—* **Adults:** 500 mg to 1 g P.O. 20 minutes before bedtime. Starting dose may be 250 mg for elderly or debilitated patients. *Preanesthetic—* **Adults:** 500 mg to 1 g P.O. 2½ hours preoperatively.	**Blood:** thrombocytopenia. **GI:** mild upset. **Skin:** rashes, purpura. **Other:** fever (allergic reaction).

♦ Available in U.S. and Canada. ♦♦ Available in Canada only. All other products (no symbol) available in U.S. only. Italicized side effects are common or life-threatening.

INTERACTIONS	NURSING CONSIDERATIONS
sure, uneasiness. Use together cautiously. Use a different hypnotic drug.	• Remove cigarettes of patient receiving hypnotic dose. • Supervise walking; raise bed rails, especially for elderly patients. • Large dosage may raise BUN level. • May cause false-positive results in glycosuria tests using cupric sulfate as Benedict's solution. Use Clinitest, Clinistix, or Tes-Tape. • May interfere with fluorometric tests for urine catecholamines and Reddy, Jenkins, Thorn test for urine 17-hydroxycorticosteroids. Do not administer drug for 48 hours before fluorometric test. • Aqueous solutions incompatible with alkaline substances. • Store in dark container. Store suppositories in refrigerator. • If patient is given anticoagulant, monitor for increased prothrombin times during the first several days of therapy. Anticoagulant dose may need to be adjusted.
Alcohol or other CNS depressants, including narcotic analgesics; MAO inhibitors: excessive CNS depression. Use together cautiously.	• Contraindicated in patients with uncontrolled pain and porphyria. Use cautiously in hepatic or renal impairment; in elderly or debilitated patients; in mental depression with suicidal tendencies; if patient has previously overreacted to barbiturates or alcohol. • Give with milk or food to minimize transient dizziness or ataxia caused by rapid absorption. • May cause dependence and severe withdrawal symptoms. Withdraw gradually. • Prevent hoarding or self-overdosing by patients who are depressed, suicidal, or drug-dependent, or who have a history of drug abuse. Overdosage very difficult to treat and has a high mortality. Warn patient that alcohol increases effects of drug, and advise him not to perform activities requiring alertness or skill until CNS response is determined. • Watch for signs of toxicity, such as poor muscle coordination, confusion, hypothermia, speech or vision disturbances, tremors, or weakness. • 750-mg strength contains tartrazine dye. May cause allergic reactions in susceptible patients. • Remove cigarettes of patient receiving hypnotic dose. • Supervise walking; raise bed rails, especially for elderly patients. • Slight darkening of liquid from exposure to air and light doesn't affect safety or potency, but store in tight, light-resistant container to avoid possible deterioration. • Monitor prothrombin times carefully when patient on ethchlorvynol starts or ends anticoagulant therapy. Anticoagulant dose may need to be adjusted. • Drug is effective for short-term use only; treatment period should not exceed 1 week.
None significant.	• Contraindicated for uncontrolled pain. Use cautiously in patients with mental depression, suicidal tendencies, or history of drug abuse. • Not usually given for daytime sedation because of short duration of effect. • Long-term use may cause dependence and severe withdrawal symptoms. Withdraw gradually. • Prevent hoarding or self-overdosing by patients who are depressed, suicidal, or drug-dependent, or who have a history of drug abuse. Warn patient that alcohol increases effects of drug, and advise him not to perform activities requiring alertness or skill until CNS response is determined. • Abrupt withdrawal may cause blood pressure and pulse rate changes, sweating, and hallucinations. • Remove cigarettes of patient receiving dose.

(continued on following page)

NAME	INDICATIONS & DOSAGE	SIDE EFFECTS
ethinamate *(continued)*		
flurazepam hydrochloride Controlled Substance Schedule IV Dalmane♦	*Insomnia—* **Adults:** 15 to 30 mg P.O. at bedtime.	**Blood:** leukopenia, granulocytopenia. **CNS:** *daytime sedation, dizziness, drowsiness, disturbed coordination,* lethargy, confusion, *headache.*
glutethimide Controlled Substance Schedule III Doriden♦, Rolathimide	*Insomnia—* **Adults:** 250 to 500 mg P.O. at bedtime. May be repeated, but not less than 4 hours before intended awakening. Total daily dose should not exceed 1 g. *Preoperatively—* **Adults:** 500 mg night before surgery; 500 mg to 1 g 1 hour before anesthesia. *First stage of labor—* 500 mg at onset of labor; repeat once if necessary. *Sedative—* **Adults:** 125 to 250 mg t.i.d. after meals.	**CNS:** *residual sedation,* paradoxical excitation, headache, vertigo. **EENT:** dry mouth, blurred vision. **GI:** irritation, nausea, diarrhea. **GU:** bladder atony. **Skin:** rashes, urticaria.
hexobarbital Controlled Substance Schedule III Sombulex	*Sedation—* **Adults:** 250 mg P.O., repeated as needed, q 2 to 3 hours. *Insomnia—* **Adults:** 250 to 500 mg P.O. at bedtime.	**CNS:** *drowsiness, lethargy, hangover,* paradoxical excitement in elderly patients. **GI:** nausea, vomiting. **Skin:** rash, urticaria. **Other:** *Stevens-Johnson syndrome,* angioedema.

♦ Available in U.S. and Canada. ♦♦ Available in Canada only. All other products (no symbol) available in U.S. only. Italicized side effects are common or life-threatening.

INTERACTIONS	NURSING CONSIDERATIONS
	• Supervise walking; raise bed rails, especially for elderly patients. • In overdosage, treat CNS and respiratory depression same as barbiturate intoxication; ethinamate is dialyzable. • May cause falsely elevated urine 17-ketosteroid (modified Zimmerman reaction) and 17-hydroxycorticosteroid levels (Porter-Silber test). • Prolonged therapy not recommended; drug is not effective for more than 7 days.
Cimetidine: increased sedation. Monitor carefully.	• Use cautiously in patients with impaired hepatic or renal function, mental depression, suicidal tendencies, or history of drug abuse. Use caution and low end of dosage range for elderly or debilitated patients. • Prevent hoarding or self-overdosing by patients who are depressed, suicidal, or drug-dependent, or who have a history of drug abuse. Warn patient that alcohol increases effects of drug, and advise him not to perform activities requiring alertness or skill until CNS response is determined. • Remove cigarettes of patient receiving dose. • Supervise walking; raise bed rails, especially for elderly patients.
Alcohol or other CNS depressants, including narcotic analgesics: excessive CNS depression. Use together cautiously.	• Contraindicated in uncontrolled pain, severe renal impairment, porphyria. Use cautiously in patients with mental depression, suicidal tendencies, history of drug abuse, prostatic hypertrophy, stenosing peptic ulcer, pyloroduodenal or bladder-neck obstruction, narrow-angle glaucoma, cardiac arrhythmias. • Drug is effective for short-term use only. • Remove cigarettes of patient receiving dose. • Supervise walking; raise bed rails, especially for elderly patients. • Prevent hoarding or self-overdosing by patients who are depressed, suicidal, or drug-dependent, or who have a history of drug abuse. Warn patient that alcohol increases effects of drug, and advise him not to perform activities requiring alertness or skill for 7 to 8 hours after receiving this drug. • Abrupt withdrawal may produce nausea, vomiting, nervousness, tremors, chills, fever, nightmares, insomnia, tachycardia, delirium, numbness of extremities, hallucinations, dysphagia, convulsions. Withdraw gradually. • Monitor prothrombin times carefully when patient on glutethimide starts or ends anticoagulant therapy. Anticoagulant dose may need to be adjusted.
Alcohol or other CNS depressants, including narcotic analgesics: excessive CNS and respiratory depression. Do not use together. *MAO inhibitors:* inhibit metabolism of barbiturates; may cause prolonged CNS depression. Reduce barbiturate dosage. *Rifampin:* may decrease barbiturate levels. Monitor for decreased effect.	• Contraindicated in patients with uncontrolled severe pain, respiratory disease with dyspnea or obstruction, hypersensitivity to barbiturates, previous addiction to sedatives, porphyria. Use with caution in hepatic or renal impairment. • May be used preoperatively with atropine when morphine contraindicated. • Because barbiturates potentiate narcotics, reduce dose when giving during labor. Excessive dose may cause respiratory depression in neonate. • Remove cigarettes of patient receiving hypnotic dose. • Supervise walking; raise bed rails, especially for elderly patients. • Long-term high dosage may cause drug dependence and severe withdrawal symptoms. Withdraw barbiturates gradually. • Monitor prothrombin times carefully when patient on hexobarbital starts or ends anticoagulant therapy. Anticoagulant dose may need to be adjusted. • Prevent hoarding or self-overdosing by patients who are depressed,

(continued on following page)

NAME	INDICATIONS & DOSAGE	SIDE EFFECTS
hexobarbital *(continued)*		
mephobarbital Controlled Substance Schedule IV Mebaral♦	*Sedation—* **Adults:** 32 to 100 mg P.O. t.i.d. to q.i.d. **Children:** 16 to 32 mg P.O. t.i.d. to q.i.d. *Incipient or active delirium tremens—*200 mg P.O. t.i.d.	**CNS:** drowsiness, vertigo, headache, depression, residual sedation after hypnotic dose, paradoxical excitement. **GI:** nausea, vomiting, diarrhea. **Skin:** hypersensitivity reactions, jaundice. **Other:** respiratory depression, apnea; discontinuance of hypnotic doses may induce nightmares or insomnia.
methaqualone Mequin, Quaalude, Sopor **methaqualone hydrochloride** Controlled Substance Schedule II Parest, Parest 400, Rouqualone♦♦, Sedalone♦♦, Somnafac, Somnafac Forte, Triador♦♦, Tualone♦♦, Vitalone♦♦	*Sedation (methaqualone)—* **Adults:** 75 mg P.O. t.i.d. or q.i.d. *Insomnia (methaqualone)—* **Adults:** 150 to 300 P.O. at bedtime. *Insomnia (methaqualone hydrochloride)—* **Adults:** 200 to 400 mg P.O. at bedtime.	**CNS:** headache, dizziness, fatigue, residual sedation, *transient paresthesias of extremities,* restlessness, anxiety. **EENT:** dry mouth. **GI:** anorexia, *nausea, vomiting,* epigastric discomfort.
methotrimeprazine hydrochloride Levoprome, Nozinan♦♦	*Postoperative analgesia—* **Adults, and children over 12 years:** initially, 2.5 to 7.5 mg I.M. q 4 to 6 hours, then adjust dose. *Preanesthetic medication—* **Adults, and children over 12 years:** 2 to 20 mg I.M. 45 minutes to 3 hours before surgery.	**Blood:** agranulocytosis and other dyscrasias after long-term high dosage. **CNS:** *orthostatic hypotension, fainting, weakness, dizziness,* drowsiness, excessive sedation, amnesia, disorientation, euphoria, headache, slurred speech. **CV:** *drop in blood pressure,* palpitations.

♦ Available in U.S. and Canada. ♦♦ Available in Canada only. All other products (no symbol) available in U.S. only. Italicized side effects are common or life-threatening.

INTERACTIONS	NURSING CONSIDERATIONS
	suicidal, or drug-dependent, or who have a history of drug abuse. Warn patient that alcohol increases effects of drug, and advise him not to perform activities requiring alertness or skill until CNS response is determined. • Watch for signs of toxicity: coma, pupillary constriction (pupillary dilation with severe poisoning), clammy skin, hypotension. Overdose can be fatal. • For toxicity, see APPENDIX, *Drug Toxicities*.
Alcohol or other CNS depressants, including narcotic analgesics: excessive CNS and respiratory depression. Do not use together. *MAO inhibitors:* inhibit metabolism of barbiturates; may cause prolonged CNS depression. Reduce barbiturate dosage. *Rifampin:* may decrease barbiturate levels. Monitor for decreased effect.	• Contraindicated in patients with uncontrolled severe pain, respiratory disease with dyspnea or obstruction, hypersensitivity to barbiturates, previous addiction to sedatives, porphyria. Use with caution in hepatic or renal impairment, impaired cardiac or respiratory function. • Remove cigarettes of patient receiving hypnotic dose. • Supervise walking; raise bed rails, especially for elderly patients. • Long-term high dosage may cause drug dependence and severe withdrawal symptoms. Withdraw barbiturates gradually. • Prevent hoarding or self-overdosing by patients who are depressed, suicidal, or drug-dependent, or who have a history of drug abuse. Warn patient that alcohol increases effects of drug, and advise him not to perform activities requiring alertness or skill until CNS response is determined. • Mephobarbital is metabolized to phenobarbital, the active agent. • Monitor prothrombin times carefully when patient on mephobarbital starts or ends anticoagulant therapy. Anticoagulant dose may need adjustment. • Watch for signs of toxicity. • For toxicity, see APPENDIX, *Drug Toxicities*.
Alcohol or other CNS depressants, including narcotic analgesics: excessive CNS depression. Use together cautiously.	• Contraindicated in patients with history of drug abuse. Use cautiously in patients with hepatic impairment, mental depression, suicidal tendencies. • Remove cigarettes of patient receiving hypnotic dose. • Supervise walking; raise bed rails, especially for elderly patients. • Warn patient that alcohol increases effects of drug, and advise him not to perform activities requiring alertness or skill until CNS response is determined. • After switching from another hypnotic to methaqualone, onset of satisfactory hypnotic effect requires 5 to 7 consecutive nights of therapy. • Prolonged administration of methaqualone is not recommended: drug not shown to be effective more than 14 days. • One of major drugs of abuse "on the street." Because of high abuse potential, methaqualone is rarely clinically indicated. • For toxicity, see APPENDIX, *Drug Toxicities*.
All antihypertensive agents: increased orthostatic hypotension. Don't use together.	• Contraindicated in patients receiving concurrent antihypertensive drug therapy, including MAO inhibitors; also, in patients with history of convulsive disorders; hypersensitivity to phenothiazines; severe cardiac, hepatic, or renal disease; previous overdose of CNS depressant; coma. Use with extreme caution in elderly or debilitated patient with cardiac disease or in any patient who may suffer serious consequences from a sudden drop in blood pressure. • Use low initial dose in susceptible patient; increase gradually while frequently checking pulse rate, blood pressure, and circulation. • Inject I.M. into large muscle masses. Rotate sites. Do not adminis-

(continued on following page)

NAME	INDICATIONS & DOSAGE	SIDE EFFECTS
methotrimeprazine hydrochloride *(continued)*	*Sedation, analgesia—* **Adults, and children over 12 years:** 10 to 20 mg deep I.M. q 4 to 6 hours as required. **Elderly:** 5 to 10 mg I.M. q 4 to 6 hours.	**EENT:** dry mouth, nasal congestion. **GI:** nausea, vomiting, abdominal discomfort. **GU:** difficulty urinating. **Local:** *pain, inflammation, swelling at injection site.*
methyprylon Controlled Substance Schedule III Noludar♦	*Insomnia—* **Adults:** 200 to 400 mg P.O. 15 minutes before bedtime. **Children over 3 months:** 50 mg P.O. at bedtime, increased to 200 mg, if necessary. Maximum 400 mg/day.	**CNS:** morning drowsiness, dizziness, headache, paradoxical excitation. **GI:** nausea, vomiting, diarrhea, esophagitis. **Skin:** rash.
paraldehyde Controlled Substance Schedule IV Paral	*Sedation—* **Adults:** 4 to 10 ml P.O. or rectally; or 5 ml deep I.M. in upper outer quadrant of buttock; 3 to 5 ml I.V. (in emergency only). **Children:** 0.15 ml/kg P.O., rectally, or deep I.M. *Insomnia—* **Adults:** 10 to 30 ml P.O. or rectally; 10 ml I.M. or I.V. **Children:** 0.3 ml/kg P.O., rectally, deep I.M. *Alcohol withdrawal syndrome—* **Adults:** 5 to 10 ml P.O. or rectally; or 5 ml deep I.M. q 4 to 6 hours for the first 24 hours, not to exceed a total of 60 ml P.O. or 30 ml I.M.; then q 6 hours on following days, not to exceed 40 ml P.O. or 20 ml I.M. per 24 hours. *Tetanus—* **Adults:** 4 to 5 ml I.V. (well diluted) or 12 ml (diluted 1:10)	**CV:** *I.V. administration may cause pulmonary edema or hemorrhage,* dilation of right side of heart, circulatory collapse. **GI:** irritation, *foul breath odor.* **GU:** nephrosis with prolonged use. **Skin:** *erythematous rash.* **Local:** *pain,* sterile abscesses, sloughing of skin, fat necrosis, muscular irritation, nerve damage at I.M. injection site (if injection is near nerve trunk). **Other:** *respiratory depression.*

♦ Available in U.S. and Canada. ♦♦ Available in Canada only. All other products (no symbol) available in U.S. only. Italicized side effects are common or life-threatening.

INTERACTIONS	NURSING CONSIDERATIONS
	ter subcutaneously, as local irritation results. I.V. injection not recommended. • Expect drop in blood pressure 10 to 20 minutes after I.M. injection. • Keep patient in bed or closely supervised for 6 to 12 hours after each of the first several injections because orthostatic hypotension may occur. If hypotension is severe, combat with phenylephrine, methoxamine, or levarterenol. Don't use epinephrine. • Don't use for longer than 30 days except in terminal illness or when narcotics are contraindicated. • In prolonged use, monitor liver function and blood studies periodically. • May be mixed in same syringe with reduced dose of atropine and scopolamine. Do not mix with other drugs. Protect from light.
None significant.	• Contraindicated in intermittent porphyria. Use cautiously in patients with renal or hepatic impairment. • Periodic blood counts are advisable during repeated or long-term use. • Long-term high dosage may cause drug dependence and severe life-threatening withdrawal symptoms. Withdrawal should be gradual and closely monitored. • Prevent hoarding or self-overdosing by patients who are depressed, suicidal, or drug-dependent, or who have a history of drug abuse. Warn patient that alcohol increases effect of drug, and advise him not to perform activities requiring alertness or skill until CNS response is determined. • Remove cigarettes of patient receiving hypnotic dose. • Supervise walking; raise bed rails, especially for elderly patients. • Value of this drug as a sedative has not been established. • Overdosage symptoms include somnolence, confusion, constricted pupils, respiratory depression, hypotension, coma. Hemodialysis is useful in severe intoxication. • For toxicity, see APPENDIX, *Drug Toxicities*.
Alcohol: excessive CNS depression. Use with caution. *Disulfiram (Antabuse):* increase in paraldehyde and acetaldehyde blood levels. Use together cautiously. May produce toxic disulfiram reaction.	• Contraindicated in bronchopulmonary disease or gastroenteritis with ulceration. Use cautiously in patients with hepatic impairment. • Give rectal dose in olive oil or cottonseed oil as retention enema: 1 part paraldehyde, 2 parts oil, and 200 ml 0.9% sodium chloride solution. • Dilute oral dose with iced juice or milk to mask taste and odor and to reduce GI distress. • Use fresh supply; discard bottles opened more than 24 hours. Don't use if liquid has a brownish color or vinegary odor, or if it contains a precipitate. • Drug reacts with plastic. Use glass syringe for parenteral dose, and don't put liquid in Styrofoam cup. • Give I.M. injection deeply, away from nerve trunks, and massage injection site. Do not give more than 5 ml per injection site. • Watch closely for respiratory depression, especially with repeated doses. • Long-term high dosage may cause drug dependence and severe withdrawal symptoms. Withdraw gradually, with close monitoring. • Remove cigarettes of patient receiving hypnotic dose. • Supervise walking; raise bed rails, especially for elderly patients. • Ventilate patient's room well to remove exhaled paraldehyde. • No analgesic effect. May produce excitement or delirium in presence of pain. • Oral or rectal administration of decomposed paraldehyde may

(continued on following page)

NAME	INDICATIONS & DOSAGE	SIDE EFFECTS
paraldehyde *(continued)*	via gastric tube q 4 hours, p.r.n.; 5 to 10 ml I.M., p.r.n. to control seizures.	
pentobarbital Controlled Substance Schedule II Nebralin **pentobarbital sodium** Maso-Pent, Nembutal Sodium♦, Nova-Rectal♦♦, Penital, Pentogen♦♦	*Sedation—* **Adults:** 20 to 40 mg P.O. b.i.d., t.i.d., or q.i.d. **Children:** 6 mg/kg/day P.O. in divided doses. *Insomnia—* **Adults:** 100 to 200 mg P.O. at bedtime or 150 to 200 mg deep I.M.; 100 mg initially, I.V., then additional doses up to 500 mg; 120 to 200 mg rectally. **Children:** 3 to 5 mg/kg I.M. Maximum dose: 100 mg. Rectal dosages: 2 months to 1 year, 30 mg; 1 to 4 years, 30 to 60 mg; 5 to 12 years, 60 mg; 12 to 14 years, 60 to 120 mg. *Preanesthetic medication—* **Adults:** 150 to 200 mg I.M. or P.O. in 2 divided doses.	**CNS:** *drowsiness, lethargy, hangover,* paradoxical excitement in elderly patients. **GI:** nausea, vomiting. **Skin:** rash, urticaria. **Other:** *Stevens-Johnson syndrome,* angioedema.
phenobarbital Barbipil, Barbita, Eskabarb♦, Gardenal♦, Henomint, Luminal♦, Orprine, PBR 12, Pheno-Squar, SK-Phenobarbital, Solfoton, Solu-barb, Stental **phenobarbital sodium** Controlled Substance Schedule IV Luminal Sodium♦	*Sedation—* **Adults:** 30 to 120 mg P.O. daily in 2 or 3 divided doses. **Children:** 6 mg/kg P.O. divided t.i.d. *Insomnia—* **Adults:** 100 to 320 mg P.O. or I.M. **Children:** 3 to 6 mg/kg. *Preoperative sedation—* **Adults:** 100 to 200 mg I.M. 60 to 90 minutes before surgery. **Children:** 16 to 100 mg I.M. 60 to 90 minutes before surgery. *Hyperbilirubinemia—* **Neonates:** 7 mg/kg/day P.O.	**CNS:** *drowsiness, lethargy, hangover,* paradoxical excitement in elderly patients. **GI:** nausea, vomiting. **Skin:** rash, urticaria. **Local:** pain, swelling, thrombophlebitis, necrosis, nerve injury. **Other:** *Stevens-Johnson syndrome,* angioedema.

♦ Available in U.S. and Canada. ♦♦ Available in Canada only. All other products (no symbol) available in U.S. only. Italicized side effects are common or life-threatening.

INTERACTIONS	NURSING CONSIDERATIONS
	cause severe corrosion of stomach or rectum.
Alcohol or other CNS depressants, including narcotic analgesics: excessive CNS and respiratory depression. Do not use together. *MAO inhibitors:* inhibit metabolism of barbiturates; may cause prolonged CNS depression. Reduce barbiturate dosage. *Rifampin:* may decrease barbiturate levels. Monitor for decreased effect.	• Contraindicated in patients with uncontrolled severe pain, respiratory disease with dyspnea or obstruction, hypersensitivity to barbiturates, previous addiction to sedatives, porphyria. Use with caution in hepatic or renal impairment. • Use injection solution within 30 minutes after opening container to minimize deterioration. Don't use cloudy solution. • Parenteral solution alkaline. Avoid extravasation; may cause tissue necrosis. • I.V. injection should be reserved for emergency treatment and should be given under close supervision. Be prepared to give artificial respiration. • Administer I.M. injection deeply. Superficial injection may cause pain, sterile abscess, and slough. • Do not mix with other medication. • Because barbiturates potentiate narcotics, reduce dose when giving during labor. Excessive dose may cause respiratory depression in neonate. • Remove cigarettes of patient receiving hypnotic dose. • Supervise walking; raise bed rails, especially for elderly patients. • Long-term high dosage may cause drug dependence and severe withdrawal symptoms. Withdraw barbiturates gradually. • Prevent hoarding or self-overdosing by patients who are depressed, suicidal, or drug-dependent, or who have a history of drug abuse. Warn patient that alcohol increases effects of drug, and advise him not to perform activities requiring alertness or skill until CNS response is determined. • No analgesic effect. May cause restlessness or delirium in presence of pain. • Monitor prothrombin times carefully when patient on pentobarbital starts or ends anticoagulant therapy. Anticoagulant dose may need to be adjusted. • Watch for signs of barbiturate toxicity: coma, pupillary constriction, cyanosis, clammy skin, hypotension. Overdose can be fatal. • To ensure accurate dosage, don't divide rectal suppositories. • Nembutal sodium contains tartrazine dye; may cause allergic reactions in susceptible persons. • For toxicity, see APPENDIX, *Drug Toxicities*.
Alcohol or other CNS depressants, including narcotic analgesics: excessive CNS and respiratory depression. Do not use together. *MAO inhibitors:* inhibit metabolism of barbiturates; may cause prolonged CNS depression. Reduce barbiturate dosage. *Rifampin:* may decrease barbiturate levels. Monitor for	• Contraindicated in patients with uncontrolled severe pain, respiratory disease with dyspnea or obstruction, hypersensitivity to barbiturates, previous addiction to sedatives, porphyria. Use with caution in patients with impaired hepatic, renal, cardiac, or respiratory function; hyperthyroidism; diabetes mellitus; anemia; and in elderly or debilitated patients. • Use injection solution within 30 minutes after opening container to minimize deterioration. Don't use cloudy solution. • I.V. injection should be reserved for emergency treatment and should be given under close supervision. Be prepared to give artificial respiration. • When administering I.V., do not give more than 60 mg/minute. • Give I.M. injection deeply. Superficial injection may cause pain, sterile abscess, and sloughing. • Long-term high dosage may cause drug dependence and severe withdrawal symptoms. Withdraw barbiturates gradually.

(continued on following page)

NAME	INDICATIONS & DOSAGE	SIDE EFFECTS
phenobarbital *(continued)*	from first to fifth day of life, or 5 mg/kg/day I.M. on first day, repeated P.O. on second to seventh days. *Chronic cholestasis*— **Adults:** 90 to 180 mg P.O. daily in 2 or 3 divided doses. **Children under 12 years:** 3 to 12 mg/kg/day P.O. in 2 or 3 divided doses.	
propiomazine hydrochloride Largon	*Sedation*— **Adults:** 20 to 40 mg I.M. or I.V. *Preoperatively; during surgery; in conjunction with local, nerve block, or spinal anesthetic*— **Adults:** 10 to 20 mg I.M. or I.V. *Obstetrics*— **Adults:** 20 to 40 mg I.M. or I.V. during early stages of labor, repeated q 3 hours, if necessary. *Sedation the night before surgery as a preanesthetic, or postoperatively*— **Children under 27 kg:** 0.55 to 1.1 mg/kg I.M. or I.V. **Children 6 to 12 years:** 25 mg I.M. or I.V. in a single dose. **Children 4 to 6 years:** 15 mg I.M. or I.V. in a single dose.	**CNS:** dizziness, confusion, amnesia (primarily in the elderly), restlessness. **CV:** tachycardia, rise in blood pressure, transient hypotension with rapid I.V. infusion. **EENT:** dry mouth. **GI:** distress. **Skin:** rashes. **Local:** vein irritation and thrombophlebitis after I.V. injection. **Other:** respiratory depression.
secobarbital Seconal **secobarbital sodium** Controlled Substance Schedule II Seco-8, Secogen Sodium♦♦, Seconal Sodium♦, Seral♦♦	*Sedation, preoperatively*— **Adults:** 200 to 300 mg P.O. 1 to 2 hours before surgery. **Children:** 50 to 100 mg P.O. or 4 to 5 mg/kg rectally 1 to 2 hours before surgery. *Insomnia*— **Adults:** 100 to 200 mg P.O. or I.M. **Children:** 3 to 5 mg/kg I.M., not to exceed 100 mg, with no more than 5 ml injected in any one site; 4 to 5 mg/kg rectally. *Acute tetanus convulsion*— **Adults and children:** 5.5 mg/kg I.M. or slow I.V., repeated q 3 to 4 hours, if needed; I.V. injection rate not to exceed 50 mg per 15 seconds.	**CNS:** *drowsiness, lethargy, hangover,* paradoxical excitement in elderly patients. **GI:** nausea, vomiting. **Skin:** rash, urticaria. **Other:** *Stevens-Johnson syndrome,* angioedema.

♦ Available in U.S. and Canada. ♦♦ Available in Canada only. All other products (no symbol) available in U.S. only. Italicized side effects are common or life-threatening.

INTERACTIONS	NURSING CONSIDERATIONS
decreased effect. *Primidone:* monitor for excessive phenobarbital blood levels.	• Because barbiturates potentiate narcotics, reduce dose when giving during labor. Excessive dose may cause respiratory depression in neonate. • Remove cigarettes of patient receiving hypnotic dose. • Supervise walking; raise bed rails, especially for elderly patients. • Prevent hoarding or self-overdosing by patients who are depressed, suicidal, or drug-dependent, or who have a history of drug abuse. Warn patient that alcohol increases effects of drug, and advise him not to perform activities requiring alertness or skill until CNS response is determined. • No analgesic action. May cause restlessness or delirium in presence of pain. • Monitor prothrombin times carefully when patient on phenobarbital starts or ends anticoagulant therapy. Anticoagulant dose may need to be adjusted. • Watch for signs of barbiturate toxicity: coma, pupillary constriction, cyanosis, clammy skin, hypotension. Overdose can be fatal. • For toxicity, see APPENDIX, *Drug Toxicities*.
None significant.	• Contraindicated if patients have received large doses of other CNS depressants or are comatose. Use extreme caution in patients with hypertensive crisis. • Give I.V. injection slowly to avoid transient fall in blood pressure. • Inject in large, undamaged vein to minimize irritation. Avoid extravasation. Don't inject into artery; irritation may cause severe arteriospasm, impaired circulation, and gangrene. • Do not give subcutaneously. • Do not use solution for injection if it is cloudy or contains a precipitate. • Antiemetic effect may mask signs of drug overdose or other disorders. • Warn about increased effects of alcohol, tranquilizers, antihistamines, and other CNS depressants and against performing hazardous activities requiring alertness or skill. • Supervise walking; raise bed rails, especially in elderly patients. • Propiomazine reverses vasopressor effect of epinephrine. Use norepinephrine when vasopressor effect needed.
Alcohol or other CNS depressants, including narcotic analgesics: excessive CNS and respiratory depression. Do not use together. *MAO inhibitors:* inhibit metabolism of barbiturates; may cause prolonged CNS depression. Reduce barbiturate dosage. *Rifampin:* may decrease barbiturate levels. Monitor for decreased effect.	• Contraindicated in uncontrolled severe pain, respiratory disease with dyspnea or obstruction, hypersensitivity to barbiturates, previous addiction to sedatives, porphyria. Use with caution in patients with hepatic or renal impairment; also, in pregnant women with toxemia or history of bleeding. • Use injection solution within 30 minutes after opening container to minimize deterioration. Don't use cloudy solution. • I.V. injection should be reserved for emergency treatment and should be given under close supervision. Be prepared to give artificial respiration. • Give I.M. injection deeply. Superficial injection may cause pain, sterile abscess, and slough. • Because barbiturates potentiate narcotics, reduce dose when giving during labor. Excessive dose may cause respiratory depression in neonate. • Remove cigarettes of patient receiving hypnotic dose. • Supervise walking; raise bed rails, especially for elderly patients. • Long-term high dosage may cause drug dependence and severe withdrawal symptoms. Withdraw barbiturates gradually.

(continued on following page)

NAME	INDICATIONS & DOSAGE	SIDE EFFECTS
secobarbital *(continued)*	*Acute psychotic agitation—* **Adults:** 50 mg/minute I.V. up to 250 mg I.V. initially, additional doses given cautiously after 5 minutes if desired response is not obtained. Not to exceed 500 mg total. *Status epilepticus—* **Adults and children:** 250 to 350 mg I.M. or I.V.	
talbutal Controlled Substance Schedule III Lotusate	*Sedation—* **Adults:** 30 to 60 mg P.O. b.i.d. or t.i.d. *Insomnia—* **Adults:** 120 mg P.O. at bedtime.	**CNS:** *drowsiness, lethargy, hangover,* paradoxical excitement in elderly patients. **GI:** nausea, vomiting. **Skin:** rash, urticaria. **Other:** *Stevens-Johnson syndrome,* angioedema.
triclofos sodium Triclos	*Insomnia—* **Adults:** 1.5 g P.O. 15 to 20 minutes before bedtime. *To induce sleep in EEG—* **Children under 12 years:** 22 mg/kg P.O.	**CNS:** light-headedness, dizziness, hangover, *drowsiness,* headache, ataxia. **GI:** *nausea,* vomiting, flatulence, bad taste in mouth. **Skin:** hypersensitivity reactions.

INTERACTIONS	NURSING CONSIDERATIONS
	• Prevent hoarding or self-overdosing by patients who are depressed, suicidal, or drug-dependent, or who have a history of drug abuse. Warn patient that alcohol increases effects of drug, and advise him not to perform activities requiring alertness or skill until CNS response is determined. • If patient has renal insufficiency, use sterile drug reconstituted with sterile water for injection. Avoid commercial solution containing polyethylene glycol; it may irritate kidneys. • Secobarbital in polyethylene glycol must be refrigerated. • Secobarbital sodium injection not compatible with lactated Ringer's solution. • Sterile secobarbital sodium compatible with Ringer's injection and normal saline solution. Don't mix with acidic solutions. • To reconstitute, rotate ampul. Do not shake. • Monitor prothrombin times carefully when patient on secobarbital starts or ends anticoagulant therapy. Anticoagulant dose may need to be adjusted. • Watch for signs of barbiturate toxicity: coma, pupillary constriction, cyanosis, clammy skin, hypotension. Overdose can be fatal. • For toxicity, see APPENDIX, *Drug Toxicities*.
Alcohol or other CNS depressants, including narcotic analgesics: excessive CNS and respiratory depression. Don't use together. *MAO inhibitors:* inhibit the metabolism of barbiturates; may cause prolonged CNS depression. Reduce barbiturate dosage. *Rifampin:* may decrease barbiturate levels. Monitor for decreased effect.	• Contraindicated in patients with uncontrolled severe pain, respiratory disease with dyspnea or obstruction, hypersensitivity to barbiturates, previous addiction to sedatives, porphyria. Use with caution in hepatic or renal impairment. • Remove cigarettes of patient receiving hypnotic dose. • Supervise walking; raise bed rails, especially for elderly patients. • Long-term high dosage may cause drug dependence and severe withdrawal symptoms. Withdraw barbiturates gradually. • Prevent hoarding or self-overdosing by patients who are depressed, suicidal, or drug-dependent, or who have a history of drug abuse. Warn patient that alcohol increases effects of drug, and advise him not to perform activities requiring alertness or skill until CNS response is determined. • Monitor prothrombin times carefully when patient on talbutal starts or ends anticoagulant therapy. Anticoagulant dose may need to be adjusted. • Watch for signs of barbiturate toxicity: coma, pupillary constriction, cyanosis, clammy skin, hypotension. Overdose can be fatal. • For toxicity, see APPENDIX, *Drug Toxicities*.
Alcohol or other CNS depressants, including narcotic analgesics: excessive CNS depression or vasodilation. Use together cautiously. *Furosemide I.V.:* possible sweating, flushes, variable blood pressure, uneasiness. Use together cautiously.	• Contraindicated in patients with hepatic or renal impairment, hypersensitivity to triclofos sodium or chloral hydrate; and in women in labor. Use with caution in patients with cardiac arrhythmias, severe cardiac disease, mental depression, suicidal tendencies, or drug dependency. • In prolonged use, monitor liver function and blood studies periodically. • Withdraw slowly after prolonged use to avoid delirium, tremors, hallucinations. • Prevent hoarding or self-overdosing by patients who are depressed, suicidal, or drug-dependent, or who have a history of drug abuse. Warn patient that alcohol increases effects of drug, and advise him not to perform activities requiring alertness or skill until CNS response is determined. • Supervise walking; raise bed rails, especially for elderly patients. • May cause false-positive results in glycosuria tests using cupric sulfate as Benedict's or Fehling's solution. Use Clinitest, Clinistix, or Tes-Tape.

(continued on following page)

NAME	INDICATIONS & DOSAGE	SIDE EFFECTS
triclofos sodium *(continued)*		

WHAT YOU SHOULD KNOW ABOUT METHAQUALONE ABUSE

Since its introduction in 1965, methaqualone has become one of the ten most abused drugs in the United States, according to the Federal Bureau of Narcotics and Dangerous Drugs.

Abusers find methaqualone more enjoyable and satisfying than barbiturates because it:

- produces rapid, long-lasting effects
- reduces inhibitions in social situations
- promotes a perpetual state of sedation that eases life's pressures
- substitutes for narcotics when they're not available.

Several years after its introduction, methaqualone was classified as a controlled substance. Quaalude, the most publicized brand of methaqualone, had become notorious, so many doctors stopped prescribing it and many pharmacists avoided stocking it.

Now Quaalude's manufacturer—Lemmon Company—is marketing a new brand of methaqualone: Mequin. Mequin is an alternative for doctors and pharmacists who prefer not to handle the widely abused Quaalude. (*Note:* Mequin and Quaalude are chemically and therapeutically identical.)

Meanwhile, methaqualone abuse has increased. (In 1980, methaqualone abuse was up 1.3% from 1979.) Since methaqualone overdose can result in deep coma or even death, be alert for these symptoms:

- depressed respiratory and cardiovascular activity
- increased muscle tone (ranging from hypertonia and muscle spasms to tonic-clonic convulsions)
- increased salivation
- possible increased pupil reaction to light and rapid changes in pupil size
- vomiting
- lack of response to auditory stimulus or pain. High doses can increase a person's pain threshold, so that he is unaware of injury and its resulting pain. Some users may have a sense of indestructibility.

If your patient's coming out of a coma, he may experience excitation again. Complications may include:

- oliguria
- renal failure
- toxic polyneuropathy
- myocardial damage
- cutaneous, gastrointestinal, or retinal hemorrhage
- facial or pulmonary edema.

For more information, and photographs of drugs of abuse, see special color section following p. 75.

INTERACTIONS	NURSING CONSIDERATIONS
	• May interfere with fluorometric tests for urine catecholamines and Reddy, Jenkins, Thorn test for urine 17-hydroxycorticosteroids. Don't administer drug for 48 hours before fluorometric test. • Monitor prothrombin times carefully when patient on triclofos starts or ends anticoagulant therapy. Anticoagulant dose may need to be adjusted.

PATIENT CARE

PROMOTING GOOD SLEEP WITHOUT HYPNOTICS AND SEDATIVES

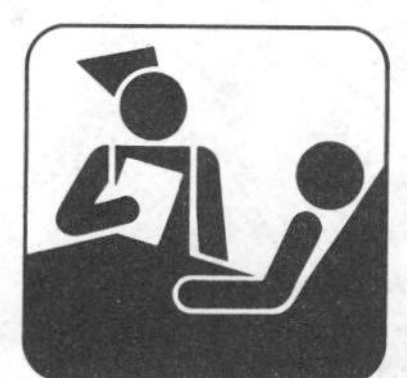

Each nursing shift can help promote good sleep without resorting to hypnotics and sedatives by following these suggestions:

Day staff

• Encourage naps in the morning rather than in the afternoon. Morning naps are mostly a continuation of REM sleep. Because it is a light sleep, it usually refreshes the patient. Also, if your patient naps in the morning, he will more likely feel tired enough by evening to fall asleep again.

• If your patient's condition permits, keep him as busy as possible during the day.

• Check your patient's history for unresolved anxiety—situations at home that may be worrying him in the hospital, such as financial problems or an invalid spouse at home. Help to relieve the anxiety by getting your patient in touch with a hospital social worker.

Evening staff

• Find out what your patient's sleep routine was at home and, whenever possible, let him follow it. Certain rituals, like a bedtime snack or sleeping with a favorite pillow, can aid sleep.

• Offer back rubs.

• Straighten bed linens.

• Pull the curtain closed to block light from the unit.

• If advisable, close the door to your patient's room.

• If your patient requires pain medication, try to give it early so he'll be relaxed by bedtime.

Night staff

• Find out who isn't sleeping and why.

• Be sure unit lights are dim and unnecessary lights are out.

• Turn off nurses' station radio or make sure the patients can't hear it.

• After establishing a successful sleep plan for a specific patient, write it down so it can be followed again.

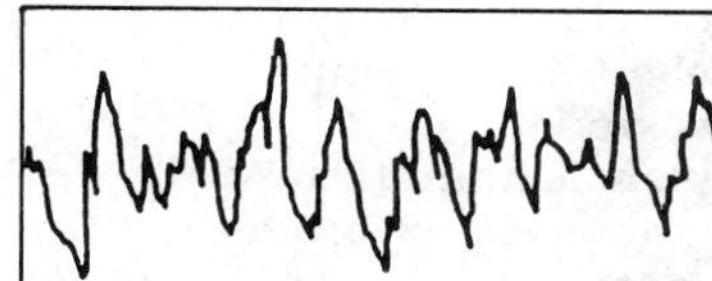

R.E.M., final sleep cycle, waves show an active EEG.

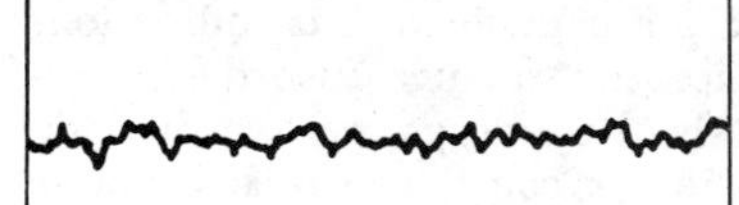

Slow, high delta waves mark the start of stage four sleep.

30 Anticonvulsants

acetazolamide
acetazolamide sodium
bromides
carbamazepine
clonazepam
diazepam
ethosuximide
ethotoin
magnesium sulfate
mephenytoin
mephobarbital
metharbital
methsuximide
paraldehyde
paramethadione
phenacemide
phenobarbital
phenobarbital sodium
phensuximide
phenytoin sodium (extended)
phenytoin sodium (prompt)
primidone
trimethadione
valproic acid
valproate sodium

Each anticonvulsant has indications for specific seizure disorders. Frequently, these drugs are used in combination for complex or mixed-seizure disorders. For indications in epileptic-type seizures, see chart on opposite page.

Seizures may be of unknown origin (idiopathic) or secondary to some organic or acquired condition.

When the etiology of seizures is known, therapy is often aimed at the underlying cause as well.

Major uses

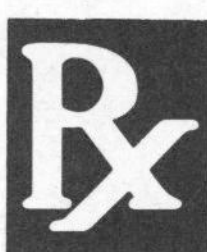

Anticonvulsants prevent or reduce the frequency or severity of seizures of idiopathic epilepsy, or seizures secondary to drugs, hypoglycemia, hypomagnesemia, meningitis, eclampsia, encephalitis, alcohol withdrawal, or accident-related brain injury.

HELPING A PATIENT DURING A GRAND MAL SEIZURE

To see your patient through the various stages of a grand mal seizure, follow these guidelines:

At onset:

- Place a stat stick or a padded tongue depressor between the patient's teeth *before* they're clenched, to keep him from biting his tongue. (After the patient has clenched his teeth, don't try to force anything between them.)
- Maintain an airway.
- Protect him from injury.
- Cushion his head, and turn it to the side.

During the *tonic phase,* the patient's teeth are clenched and his muscles are constantly tensed or contracted.

Next, the *clonic phase* appears; the patient experiences continuous and rapid spasms, with alternating relaxed and rigid states.

When the seizure is over:

- Place the patient in semiprone position or on his side, to keep his airway open.
- Watch him carefully until he's conscious again.
- Allow him to rest: many patients are lethargic and sleepy after a seizure.

USE OF ANTICONVULSANTS IN EPILEPTIC-TYPE SEIZURES

DRUG	GRAND MAL	PETIT MAL	MYOCLONIC	MIXED	PSYCHOMOTOR	STATUS EPILEPTICUS
Barbiturate derivatives						
mephobarbital	✓	✓				
metharbital	✓	✓	✓	✓		
phenobarbital	✓	✓	✓	✓	✓	
primidone	✓				✓	
Benzodiazepine derivatives						
clonazepam		✓	✓			
diazepam						✓
Hydantoin derivatives						
ethotoin	✓				✓	
mephenytoin	✓				✓	
phenacemide				✓	✓	
phenytoin	✓				✓	✓
Oxazolidone derivatives						
paramethadione		✓				
trimethadione		✓				
Succinimide derivatives						
ethosuximide		✓				
methsuximide		✓				
phensuximide		✓				
Miscellaneous						
acetazolamide		✓				
bromides*	✓	✓	✓	✓	✓	
carbamazepine	✓			✓	✓	
valproic acid		✓				

*Rarely used as drug of first or second choice

Note: Magnesium sulfate and paraldehyde are not included in this list since they are used to control nonepileptic seizures.

THERAPEUTIC ACTIVITY

THERAPEUTIC ACTIVITY OF COMMON ANTICONVULSANTS

DRUG	BLOOD LEVELS (mcg/ml)	HALF-LIFE	TIME TO REACH STEADY STATE*
carbamazepine	6 to 8	7 to 30 hr	2 to 4 days
clonazepam	0.013 to 0.072	20 to 30 hr	5 to 10 days
ethosuximide	40 to 80	2 to 3 days	5 to 8 days
methsuximide	0.1	2 to 4 hr	8 to 16 hr
phenobarbital	10 to 35	2 to 4 days	14 to 21 days
phenytoin	10 to 20	24 hr	5 to 10 days
primidone	6 to 12	3 to 12 hr	4 to 7 days
trimethadione	6 to 41	12 to 24 hr	2 to 5 days
valproic acid	50 to 100	5 to 20 hr	2 to 4 days

*Steady-state blood levels are achieved if the patient is initially given maintenance therapy rather than a loading dose.

Mechanism of action

• Acetazolamide may inhibit carbonic anhydrase in the central nervous system (CNS) and decrease abnormal paroxysmal or excessive neuronal discharge.

• Barbiturate derivatives depress monosynaptic and polysynaptic transmission in the CNS and increase the threshold for seizure activity in the motor cortex.

• Benzodiazepine derivatives appear to act on the limbic system, thalamus, and hypothalamus to produce anticonvulsant effects.

• Bromides depress all nerve tissue, but their exact mechanism of CNS depression is unknown.

• Carbamazepine and paraldehyde's mechanisms of action are unknown.

• Hydantoin derivatives stabilize neuronal membranes and limit seizure activity by either increasing efflux or decreasing influx of sodium ions across cell membranes in the motor cortex during generation of nerve impulses.

• Magnesium sulfate may decrease acetylcholine released by nerve impulse, but its anticonvulsant mechanism is unknown.

• Oxazolidone derivatives raise the threshold for cortical seizure but do not modify seizure pattern. They decrease projection of focal activity and reduce both repetitive spinal-cord transmission and spike-and-wave patterns of absence (petit mal) seizures.

• Succinimide derivatives increase

seizure threshold. They reduce the paroxysmal spike-and-wave pattern of absence seizures by depressing nerve transmisson in the motor cortex.
• Valproic acid may increase brain levels of gamma-aminobutyric acid, which transmits inhibitory nerve impulses in the CNS.

Absorption, distribution, metabolism, and excretion

Anticonvulsants are generally well absorbed from the gastrointestinal tract and widely distributed in the tissues, including the CNS. They're metabolized by the liver and excreted by the kidneys.

Because barbiturates induce microsomal enzymes in the liver, they may accelerate metabolism of other anticonvulsant drugs given concurrently.

Onset and duration

Onset and duration of action vary with each drug and from patient to patient. When parenteral preparations are used for acute episodes (status epilepticus or eclampsia, for example), onset is immediate.

Most anticonvulsants have half-lives of several hours to days, and they may require days or even weeks of therapy to achieve steady-state blood concentrations.

See chart on opposite page for details on common anticonvulsants.

Combination products

DILANTIN WITH PHENOBARBITAL♦: phenytoin sodium 100 mg and phenobarbital 16 mg.
DILANTIN WITH PHENOBARBITAL♦: phenytoin sodium 100 mg and phenobarbital 32 mg.
PHELANTIN KAPSEALS♦: phenytoin 100 mg, phenobarbital 30 mg, and methamphetamine hydrochloride 2.5 mg.

DRUG ALERT

KNOW ABOUT THE TWO FORMS OF PHENYTOIN

Oral phenytoin is often prescribed to prevent and control epileptic seizures. But phenytoin (Dilantin) is available in *two* forms; confusing one with the other may cause serious problems.

The FDA has determined that one of the phenytoins—Dilantin Kapseals—is absorbed more slowly and is longer-acting than other phenytoins. As a result, Dilantin Kapseals are designated extended-release and approved for once-a-day dosage. (All other phenytoins are designated prompt-release and labeled "not for once-a-day dosing.") Remember these points when administering phenytoins:
• Use of extended-release phenytoin may improve patient compliance. However, some patients can't be adequately controlled with a once-a-day dosage. These patients must take a prompt-release phenytoin two or three times a day.
• Prompt-release phenytoin attains higher blood levels sooner than the extended-release form. If a patient taking Dilantin Kapseals mistakenly takes a total daily dose of prompt-release phenytoin, he may experience phenytoin toxicity.

Alert your patient to the difference between the two forms of the drug. And warn him not to allow generic phenytoin to be substituted for Dilantin Kapseals after he leaves the hospital.

NAME	INDICATIONS & DOSAGE	SIDE EFFECTS
acetazolamide Acetazolam♦♦, Diamox♦, Hydrazol, Roxolamide **acetazolamide sodium** Diamox♦	*Myoclonic seizures; refractory grand mal or petit mal seizures; mixed seizures—* **Adults:** 375 mg P.O., I.M., or I.V. daily up to 250 mg q.i.d. Initial dose when used with other anticonvulsants usually 250 mg daily. **Children:** 8 to 30 mg/kg daily, divided t.i.d. or q.i.d. Maximum dose 1.5 g daily, or 300 to 900 mg/m² daily.	**Blood:** leukopenia, *aplastic anemia.* **CNS:** paresthesias, drowsiness. **EENT:** transient myopia. **GI:** anorexia, nausea, vomiting. **GU:** crystalluria, renal calculi. **Metabolic:** *hyperchloremic acidosis.* **Skin:** rash. **Local:** *pain at injection site,* sterile abscesses.
bromides Bromide, Calcium Bromide, Lanabrom, Neurosine, Peacock's Bromides, Potassium Bromide, Sodium Bromide	*Major motor and myoclonic seizures—* **Adults:** 1 to 2 g t.i.d. **Children:** 50 to 100 mg/kg daily, divided equally t.i.d. Or, 1.5 to 3 g/m² daily in divided doses t.i.d.	**CNS:** *drowsiness,* mental dullness, toxic psychosis. **Skin:** *rashes* (acneiform, morbilliform, granulomatous), Stevens-Johnson syndrome.
carbamazepine Tegretol♦	*Psychomotor, temporal lobe, and grand mal seizures; mixed seizure patterns—* **Adults, and children over 12 years:** 200 mg P.O. b.i.d. on day 1. May increase by 200 mg P.O. per day, in divided doses at 6- to 8-hour intervals. Adjust to minimum effective level when control achieved. Usual maintenance 800 to 1,200 mg daily. Don't exceed 1 g total daily dose in 12- to 15-year-olds and 1,200 mg P.O. daily in patients over 15 years. **Children under 12 years:** 10 to 20 mg/kg P.O daily in 2 to 4 divided doses.	**Blood:** *aplastic anemia, agranulocytosis,* eosinophilia, leukocytosis, *thrombocytopenia.* **CNS:** dizziness, *vertigo, drowsiness,* fatigue, *ataxia.* **CV:** congestive heart failure, hypertension, hypotension, aggravation of coronary artery disease. **EENT:** conjunctivitis, dry mouth and pharynx, blurred vision, diplopia, nystagmus. **GI:** *nausea,* vomiting, abdominal pain, diarrhea, anorexia, *stomatitis,* glossitis, *dry mouth.* **GU:** urinary frequency or retention, impotence, albuminuria, glycosuria, elevated BUN. **Hepatic:** abnormal results from

♦ Available in U.S. and Canada. ♦♦ Available in Canada only. All other products (no symbol) available in U.S. only. Italicized side effects are common or life-threatening.

INTERACTIONS	NURSING CONSIDERATIONS
Methenamine: antagonized methenamine effect. If used together, urine must be kept at pH 5.5 or lower.	• Contraindicated in sulfonamide sensitivity, chronic pulmonary disease, renal or hepatic dysfunction, Addison's disease (adrenocortical insufficiency), hyponatremia, hypokalemia, hyperchloremic acidosis, chronic noncongestive narrow-angle glaucoma. Use cautiously in hypercalciuria, diabetes mellitus, gout, and respiratory acidosis. • Obtain CBC and serum electrolytes every 3 months; serum calcium every 6 months. • Don't withdraw drug suddenly. Call doctor if side effects develop. • Warn patient to avoid activities that require alertness and good psychomotor coordination until CNS response to drug has been determined. • This drug is also a diuretic. Use diuretic precautions. • Chronic use results in tolerance to drug. • Reconstitute 500-mg vial with 5 ml sterile water for injection. Provides 100 mg/ml. Refrigerate reconstituted solution. Discard after 24 hours. • Oral liquid: soften 1 tablet in 2 teaspoonfuls of very warm water and add to 2 teaspoonfuls honey or syrup (chocolate, cherry). Don't use fruit juice. • May cause hyperglycemia in prediabetics or diabetics on insulin or oral drugs. Monitor patients carefully. • Observe and report signs of hypokalemia or metabolic acidosis.
None significant.	• Contraindicated in debilitated, dehydrated, or alcoholic patients, or in those with cerebral arteriosclerosis, organic brain damage, impaired renal function, severe depression, neurologic or psychological disorders, tuberculosis or skin disorders (acne, dermatitis herpetiformis). Especially in adults, use may lead to chronic toxicity (mental, psychic, GI, and neurologic disturbances; skin eruptions). May be mistaken for acute alcohol intoxication, tabes dorsalis, cerebral tumor, uremia, or multiple sclerosis. • Watch closely for toxicity. In adults, blood levels above 5 mEq/liter may cause toxicity. • Bromides are better tolerated in children than in adults. Therapeutic blood level in children usually 20 to 25 mEq/liter (200 mg/100 ml), but range is 10 to 35 mEq/liter. • Effect may not be seen for 2 to 3 weeks. • Notify doctor if side effects develop.
Troleandomycin, erythromycin: may increase carbamazepine blood levels. Use cautiously. *Propoxyphene:* may raise carbamazepine levels. Use another analgesic.	• Contraindicated in patients with bone marrow depression, hypersensitivity to carbamazepine or tricyclic antidepressants. Use cautiously in cardiac, renal, or hepatic damage, or increased intraocular pressure. • Warn patient to avoid activities that require alertness and good psychomotor coordination until CNS response to drug has been determined. • Never stop the drug suddenly when treating seizures or status epilepticus. Notify doctor immediately if side effects occur. • Obtain CBC, platelet and reticulocyte counts, and serum iron levels weekly for first 3 months, then monthly. If bone marrow depression develops, stop drug. Obtain urinalysis, BUN, and liver function studies every 3 months. Periodic eye examinations are recommended. • Tell patient to notify doctor immediately if fever, sore throat, mouth ulcers, or easy bruising occurs. • Therapeutic anticonvulsant blood level is 3 to 9 mcg/ml. • When used for trigeminal neuralgia, an attempt should be made every 3 months to decrease dose or stop drug.

(continued on following page)

NAME	INDICATIONS & DOSAGE	SIDE EFFECTS
carbamazepine *(continued)*	*Trigeminal neuralgia*— **Adults:** 100 mg P.O. b.i.d. with meals on day 1. Increase by 100 mg q 12 hours until pain relieved. Don't exceed 1.2 g daily. Maintenance dose 200 to 400 mg P.O. b.i.d.	liver-function studies. **Metabolic:** water intoxication. **Skin:** rash, urticaria. **Other:** diaphoresis, fever, chills.
clonazepam Controlled Substance Schedule IV Clonopin, Rivotril♦	*Petit mal and petit mal variant (Lennox syndrome); akinetic and myoclonic seizures*— **Adults:** initial dose should not exceed 1.5 mg P.O. per day, divided into 3 doses. May be increased by 0.5 to 1 mg q 3 days until seizures controlled. Maximum recommended daily dose is 20 mg. **Children up to 10 years or 30 kg:** 0.01 to 0.03 mg/kg P.O. daily (not to exceed 0.05 mg/kg daily), divided q 8 hours. Increase dosage by 0.25 to 0.5 mg q third day to a maximum maintenance dose of 0.1 mg to 0.2 mg/kg daily.	**Blood:** leukopenia, thrombocytopenia, eosinophilia. **CNS:** *drowsiness, ataxia, behavioral disturbances (especially in children),* slurred speech, tremor, confusion. **EENT:** *increased salivation,* diplopia, nystagmus, abnormal eye movements. **GI:** constipation, gastritis, change in appetite, nausea, abnormal thirst, sore gums. **GU:** dysuria, enuresis, nocturia, urinary retention. **Skin:** rash. **Other:** respiratory depression.
diazepam Controlled Substance Schedule IV Valium♦	*Status epilepticus*— **Adults:** 5 to 10 mg slow I.V. push 5 mg/minute; may repeat q 10 minutes up to maximum total dose of 30 mg. Use 2 to 5 mg in elderly or debilitated patients. May repeat therapy in 2 to 4 hours with caution if seizures recur. **Children:** 0.1 to 0.3 mg/kg slow I.V. push (1 mg/minute over 3 minutes). May repeat q 15 minutes for 2 doses. Maximum single dose: children under 5 years—5 mg; children over 5 years—10 mg. *Adjunctive use in convulsive disorders*— **Adults and children:** 2 to 10 mg P.O. b.i.d., t.i.d., or q.i.d.	**Blood:** neutropenia. **CNS:** fatigue, *drowsiness, ataxia,* dizziness, headache, dysarthria, slurred speech, tremor. **CV:** hypotension, bradycardia, *cardiovascular collapse.* **EENT:** diplopia, blurred vision, nystagmus. **GI:** nausea, constipation, change in salivation. **GU:** incontinence, urinary retention. **Local:** *pain, phlebitis at injection site.* **Skin:** rash, urticaria.
ethosuximide Zarontin♦	*Petit mal seizures*— **Adults, and children over 6 years:** initially, 250 mg P.O. b.i.d. May increase by 250 mg q 4 to 7 days up to 1.5 g daily. **Children 3 to 6 years:** 250 mg P.O. daily or 125 mg P.O. b.i.d. May increase by 250 mg q 4 to 7 days up to 1.5 g daily.	**Blood:** leukopenia, eosinophilia, *agranulocytosis,* pancytopenia, *aplastic anemia.* **CNS:** *drowsiness,* headache, *fatigue, dizziness,* ataxia, irritability, hiccups, *euphoria, lethargy.* **EENT:** myopia. **GI:** *nausea, vomiting,* diarrhea, gum hypertrophy, weight loss, cramps, tongue swelling, *an-*

INTERACTIONS	NURSING CONSIDERATIONS
None significant.	• Contraindicated in hepatic disease; chlordiazepoxide, diazepam, or other benzodiazepine sensitivity; acute narrow-angle glaucoma. Use with caution in chronic respiratory disease, impaired renal function, open-angle glaucoma. • Warn patient to avoid activities that require alertness and good psychomotor coordination until CNS response to drug has been determined. • Never withdraw drug suddenly. Call doctor at once if side effects develop. • Obtain periodic CBC and liver function tests. • Monitor patient for oversedation. • Withdrawal symptoms similar to barbiturates.
None significant.	• Contraindicated in shock, psychosis, coma, acute alcohol intoxication with depression of vital signs, acute narrow-angle glaucoma. Use cautiously in elderly or debilitated patients; those with limited pulmonary reserve; those in whom blood pressure drop might cause cardiovascular complications; and also those with history of anxiety states with suicidal tendencies, blood dyscrasias, hepatic or renal damage, open-angle glaucoma, or alcoholism. • Monitor respirations every 5 to 15 minutes and before each I.V. repeated dose. Have emergency resuscitative equipment and oxygen at bedside. • Do not mix with other drugs or I.V. fluids. • Do not use small veins such as those on dorsum of hand or wrist. • Avoid extravasation. • Give slowly I.V. at rate not exceeding 5 mg/minute. Watch for phlebitis at injection site. • Do not infuse drug through plastic tubing. Do not store in plastic syringe. • Drug should not be withdrawn abruptly. • Tell patient to avoid heavy use of alcohol or other CNS depressants. • For toxicity, see APPENDIX, *Drug Toxicities*.
None significant.	• Contraindicated in hypersensitivity to succinimide derivatives. Use cautiously in hepatic or renal disease. • Never withdraw drug suddenly. Abrupt withdrawal may precipitate petit mal seizures. Call doctor immediately if side effects develop. • Warn patient to avoid activities that require alertness and good psychomotor coordination until CNS response to drug has been determined. • Obtain CBC every 3 months. • Therapeutic blood levels 40 to 80 mcg/ml. • May increase frequency of grand mal seizures when used alone in

(continued on following page)

NAME	INDICATIONS & DOSAGE	SIDE EFFECTS
ethosuximide *(continued)*		*orexia, epigastric and abdominal pain.* **GU:** vaginal bleeding. **Skin:** urticaria, pruritic and erythematous rashes, hirsutism.
ethotoin Peganone	*Grand mal or psychomotor seizures—* **Adults:** initially, 250 mg P.O. q.i.d. after meals. May increase slowly over several days to 3 g daily divided q.i.d. **Children:** initially, 250 mg P.O. b.i.d. May increase up to 250 mg P.O. q.i.d.	**Blood:** thrombocytopenia, leukopenia, *agranulocytosis,* pancytopenia, megaloblastic anemia. **CNS:** fatigue, insomnia, dizziness, headache, numbness. **CV:** chest pain. **EENT:** diplopia, nystagmus. **GI:** nausea, vomiting, diarrhea, gingival hyperplasia (rare). **Skin:** rash. **Other:** fever, lymphadenopathy.
magnesium sulfate	*Hypomagnesemic seizures—* **Adults:** 1 to 2 g (as 10% solution) I.V. over 15 minutes, then 1 g I.M. q 4 to 6 hours, based on patient's response and magnesium blood levels. **Children:** seizures secondary to hypomagnesemia in acute nephritis—0.2 ml/kg of 50% solution I.M. q 4 to 6 hours, p.r.n. or 100 mg/kg of 10% solution I.V. very slowly. Titrate dosage according to magnesium blood levels and seizure response. *Prevention or control of seizures in preeclampsia or eclampsia—* **Women:** initially, 4 g I.V. in 250 ml 5% dextrose in water and 4 g deep I.M. each buttock; then 4 g deep I.M. into alternate buttock q 4 hours, p.r.n. Subsequent doses based on magnesium blood levels and urinary magnesium excretion. Do not exceed 40 g daily.	**CNS:** sweating, drowsiness, depressed reflexes, flaccid paralysis, hypothermia. **CV:** hypotension, flushing, *circulatory collapse,* depressed cardiac function, heart block. **Other:** *respiratory paralysis,* hypocalcemia.
mephenytoin Mesantoin♦	*Refractory grand mal, focal, or psychomotor seizures—* **Adults:** 50 to 100 mg P.O. daily. May increase by 50 to 100 mg at weekly intervals up to 200 mg P.O. t.i.d. **Children:** initial dose 50 to 100 mg P.O. daily or 100 to 450 mg/m² P.O. daily in 3 di-	**Blood:** *leukopenia,* neutropenia, *agranulocytosis,* thrombocytopenia, pancytopenia, eosinophilia. **CNS:** ataxia, *drowsiness,* fatigue, irritability, choreiform movements, depression, tremor, sleeplessness, dizziness (usually transient). **EENT:** photophobia, conjunctivi-

♦ Available in U.S. and Canada. ♦♦ Available in Canada only. All other products (no symbol) available in U.S. only. Italicized side effects are common or life-threatening.

INTERACTIONS	NURSING CONSIDERATIONS
	patients who have mixed types of seizures. • May cause positive direct Coombs' test.
Alcohol, folic acid, loxapine succinate: monitor for decreased ethotoin activity. *Oral anticoagulants, antihistamines, chloramphenicol, diazepam, diazoxide, disulfiram, isoniazid, phenylbutazone, phenyramidol, salicylates, sulfamethizole, valproate:* monitor for increased ethotoin activity and toxicity.	• Contraindicated in patients with hydantoin hypersensitivity and in hepatic or hematologic disorders. Use cautiously in patients receiving other hydantoin derivatives. • Never withdraw drug suddenly. Call doctor at once if side effects develop. • Warn patient to avoid activities that require alertness and good psychomotor coordination until CNS response to drug has been determined. • Obtain CBC and urinalysis when therapy starts and monthly thereafter. • Give after meals. Schedule doses as evenly as possible over 24 hours. • Stop at once if lymphadenopathy or lupus-like syndrome develops. • Heavy use of alcohol may diminish benefits of drug. • Hydantoin derivative of choice in young adults who are prone to gingival hyperplasia caused by phenytoin.
Neuromuscular blocking agents: may cause increased neuromuscular blockade. Use cautiously.	• Use cautiously in patients with impaired renal function, myocardial damage, heart block, and in women in labor. • Keep I.V. calcium gluconate available to reverse magnesium intoxication; however, don't use in digitalized patient due to danger of arrhythmias. • Monitor vital signs every 15 minutes when giving drug I.V. • Watch for respiratory depression and signs of heart block. Respirations should be approximately 16 per minute before each dose given. • Monitor intake and output. Urinary output should be 100 ml or more in 4-hour period before each dose. • Check magnesium blood levels after repeated doses. Disappearance of knee jerk and patellar reflexes is a sign of pending magnesium toxicity. • Maximum infusion rate is 150 mg per minute. Rapid drip will induce uncomfortable feeling of heat. • Call doctor if side effects develop. • Especially when given I.V. to toxemic mothers within 24 hours before delivery, observe newborn for signs of magnesium toxicity, including neuromuscular or respiratory depression. • Signs of hypermagnesemia begin to appear at blood levels of 4 mEq/liter. • I.V. infusion should not be faster than 150 mg/minute.
Alcohol, folic acid, loxapine succinate: monitor for decreased mephenytoin activity. *Oral anticoagulants, antihistamines, chloramphenicol, diazepam, diazoxide, disulfiram, isoniazid,*	• Contraindicated in hydantoin hypersensitivity. Use cautiously in patients receiving other hydantoin derivatives. • Tell patient to notify doctor if fever, sore throat, bleeding, or rash occurs. • Check CBC and platelet count initially and every 2 weeks thereafter, up to 2 weeks after full dose attained; then monthly for first year and every 3 months thereafter. Stop drug if neutrophil count becomes less than 1,600/mm³. • Never withdraw drug suddenly. Call doctor if side effects develop.

(continued on following page)

NAME	INDICATIONS & DOSAGE	SIDE EFFECTS
mephenytoin *(continued)*	vided doses. May increase slowly by 50 to 100 mg at weekly intervals up to 200 mg P.O. t.i.d., divided q 8 hours. Dosage must be adjusted individually.	tis, diplopia, nystagmus. **GI:** gingival hyperplasia, nausea and vomiting (with prolonged use). **Skin:** *rashes, exfoliative dermatitis.* **Other:** hypertrichosis, edema, dysarthria, lymphadenopathy, polyarthropathy, pulmonary fibrosis.
mephobarbital Controlled Substance Schedule IV Mebaral♦, Mentabal, Mephoral	*Grand or petit mal seizures—* **Adults:** 400 to 600 mg P.O. daily or in divided doses. **Children:** 6 to 12 mg/kg P.O. daily, divided q 6 to 8 hours (smaller doses are given initially and increased over 4 to 5 days as needed).	**Blood:** megaloblastic anemia, agranulocytosis, thrombocytopenia. **CNS:** dizziness, headache, hangover, confusion, paradoxical excitation, exacerbation of existing pain, drowsiness. **CV:** hypotension. **GI:** nausea, vomiting, epigastric pain. **Skin:** urticaria, morbilliform rash, blisters, purpura, erythema multiforme. **Other:** allergic reactions (facial edema).
metharbital Controlled Substance Schedule III Gemonil	*Grand or petit mal seizures; myoclonic or mixed seizures—* **Adults:** initially, 100 mg P.O. daily to t.i.d. May increase to 800 mg daily in divided doses. **Children:** 5 to 15 mg/kg P.O. daily, divided t.i.d. May increase to 50 to 100 mg P.O. daily, b.i.d., or t.i.d.	**Blood:** megaloblastic anemia, *agranulocytosis,* thrombocytopenia. **CNS:** dizziness, irritability, drowsiness, headache, confusion, excitation. **CV:** hypotension. **GI:** nausea, vomiting, discomfort. **Skin:** rash, urticaria, purpura, erythema multiforme.
methsuximide Celontin♦	*Refractory petit mal seizures—* **Adults and children:** initially, 300 mg P.O. daily. May increase by 300 mg weekly. Maximum daily dosage of 1.2 g in divided doses.	**Blood:** eosinophilia, leukopenia, monocytosis, pancytopenia. **CNS:** *drowsiness, ataxia, dizziness,* irritability, nervousness, headache, insomnia, confusion, depression, aggressiveness. **EENT:** blurred vision, photophobia, periorbital edema. **GI:** *nausea, vomiting, anorexia,* diarrhea, weight loss, abdominal or epigastric pain. **Skin:** urticaria, pruritic and erythematous rashes.

♦ Available in U.S. and Canada. ♦♦ Available in Canada only. All other products (no symbol) available in U.S. only. Italicized side effects are common or life-threatening.

INTERACTIONS	NURSING CONSIDERATIONS
phenylbutazone, phenyramidol, salicylates, sulfamethizole, valproate: monitor for increased mephenytoin activity and toxicity.	• Warn patient to avoid activities that require alertness and good psychomotor coordination until CNS response to drug has been determined. • Therapeutic blood level is 5 to 20 mcg/ml. • Heavy use of alcohol may diminish benefit of drug.
Alcohol and other CNS depressants, including narcotic analgesics: excessive CNS depression. Use cautiously. *MAO inhibitors:* potentiated barbiturate effect. Monitor patient for increased CNS and respiratory depression. *Rifampin:* may decrease barbiturate levels. Monitor for decreased effect.	• Contraindicated in barbiturate hypersensitivity, porphyria, and respiratory disease with dyspnea or obstruction. Use cautiously in hepatic, renal, cardiac, or respiratory function impairment, and in myasthenia gravis and myxedema. • Never withdraw drug suddenly. Call doctor at once if side effects develop. • Warn patient to avoid activities that require alertness and good psychomotor coordination until CNS response to drug has been determined. • Store in light-resistant container. • In adults, give total or largest dose at night if seizures occur then. • Three quarters of drug metabolized to phenobarbital; therapeutic blood levels as phenobarbital are 15 to 40 mcg/ml. • Monitor prothrombin times carefully when patient on mephobarbital starts or ends anticoagulant therapy. Anticoagulant dose may need to be adjusted. • For toxicity, see APPENDIX, *Drug Toxicities.*
Alcohol and other CNS depressants, including narcotic analgesics: excessive CNS depression. Use cautiously. *MAO inhibitors:* potentiated barbiturate effect. Monitor patient for increased CNS and respiratory depression. *Rifampin:* may decrease barbiturate levels. Monitor for decreased effect.	• Contraindicated in barbiturate hypersensitivity, in manifest or latent porphyria, and in respiratory disease with dyspnea or obstruction. Use cautiously in hepatic, cardiac, or renal impairment. • Don't stop drug abruptly. Call doctor at once if side effects develop. • Warn patient to avoid activities that require alertness and good psychomotor coordination until response to drug is determined. • Monitor prothrombin times carefully when patient on metharbital starts or ends anticoagulant therapy. Anticoagulant dose may need to be adjusted. • For toxicity, see APPENDIX, *Drug Toxicities.*
None significant.	• Contraindicated in hypersensitivity to succinimide derivatives. Use cautiously in hepatic or renal dysfunction. • Never change or withdraw drug suddenly. Abrupt withdrawal may precipitate petit mal seizures. Call doctor immediately if side effects develop. • Warn patient to avoid activities that require alertness and good psychomotor coordination until CNS response to drug has been determined. • Obtain CBC every 3 months; urinalysis and liver function tests every 6 months. • May color urine pink or brown. • Therapeutic blood levels 40 to 100 mcg/ml.

NAME	INDICATIONS & DOSAGE	SIDE EFFECTS
paraldehyde Controlled Substance Schedule IV Paral	*Refractory grand mal seizures, status epilepticus—* **Adults:** 5 to 10 ml I.M. (divide 10 ml dose into 2 injections); 0.2 to 0.4 ml/kg in 0.9% saline injection I.V. **Children:** 0.15 ml/kg dose deep I.M. q 4 to 6 hours, p.r.n.; or 0.3 ml/kg rectally in olive oil q 4 to 6 hours; or 1 ml per year of age not to exceed 5 ml, repeated in 1 hour, p.r.n.; or dilute 5 ml in 95 ml 0.9% saline injection for I.V. infusion and titrate dose beginning at 5 ml/hour.	**CV:** *I.V. administration may cause pulmonary edema or hemorrhage,* dilatation of right side of heart, *circulatory collapse.* **GI:** irritation, *foul breath odor.* **GU:** nephrosis with prolonged use. **Skin:** *erythematous rash.* **Local:** *pain,* sterile abscesses, sloughing of skin, fat necrosis, muscular irritation, nerve damage (if injection is near nerve trunk) at I.M. injection site. **Other:** respiratory depression.
paramethadione Paradione♦	*Refractory petit mal seizures—* **Adults:** initially, 300 mg P.O. t.i.d. May increase by 300 mg weekly, up to 600 mg q.i.d., if needed. **Children over 6 years:** 0.9 g P.O. daily in divided doses t.i.d. or q.i.d. **Children 2 to 6 years:** 0.6 g P.O. daily in divided doses t.i.d. or q.i.d. **Children under 2 years:** 0.3 g P.O. daily in divided doses b.i.d.	**Blood:** neutropenia, leukopenia, eosinophilia, thrombocytopenia, pancytopenia, *agranulocytosis, hypoplastic and aplastic anemia.* **CNS:** *drowsiness,* fatigue, vertigo, headache, paresthesias, irritability. **CV:** hypertension, hypotension. **EENT:** hemeralopia, photophobia, diplopia, epistaxis, retinal hemorrhage. **GI:** nausea, vomiting, abdominal pain, weight loss, bleeding gums. **GU:** albuminuria, vaginal bleeding. **Hepatic:** abnormal liver function tests. **Skin:** acneiform or morbilliform rash, *exfoliative dermatitis,* erythema multiforme, petechiae, alopecia. **Other:** lymphadenopathy, lupus erythematosus.
phenacemide Phenurone	*Refractory, mixed psychomotor, grand mal, petit mal, and petit mal variant seizures—* **Adults:** 500 mg P.O. t.i.d. May increase by 500 mg weekly up to 5 g daily, p.r.n. **Children 5 to 10 years:** 250 mg P.O. t.i.d. May increase by 250 mg weekly, up to 1.5 g daily, p.r.n.	**Blood:** *aplastic anemia, agranulocytosis,* leukopenia. **CNS:** drowsiness, dizziness, insomnia, headaches, paresthesias, *depression, suicidal tendencies,* aggressiveness. **GI:** anorexia, weight loss. **GU:** nephritis with marked albuminuria. **Hepatic:** hepatitis, jaundice. **Skin:** rashes.

♦ Available in U.S. and Canada. ♦♦ Available in Canada only. All other products (no symbol) available in U.S. only. Italicized side effects are common or life-threatening.

INTERACTIONS	NURSING CONSIDERATIONS
Alcohol: increased CNS depression. Use with caution. *Disulfiram:* increased paraldehyde and acetaldehyde blood levels; possible toxic disulfiram reaction. Use together cautiously.	• Contraindicated in gastroenteritis with ulceration. Use cautiously in impaired hepatic function or in asthma or other pulmonary disease. • Use fresh supply. Don't expose to air. Don't use if liquid is brown, has a vinegary odor, or if container has been open longer than 24 hours. • Watch closely for respiratory depression, especially in repeated doses. • Drug reacts with plastic. Use glass syringe and bottle for parenteral dose. Prepare fresh I.V. solution every 4 hours. I.V. administration very hazardous. • Give I.M. dose deeply, away from nerve trunks; massage injection site. • Dilute paraldehyde in olive oil or cottonseed oil 1:2 for rectal administration. Give as retention enema. May also use 200 ml normal saline solution to prepare enema. • Keep patient's room well ventilated to remove exhaled paraldehyde. • Long-term high dosage may cause drug dependence and severe withdrawal symptoms. • Oral or rectal administration of decomposed paraldehyde may cause severe corrosion of stomach or rectum.
None significant.	• Contraindicated in renal and hepatic dysfunction, severe blood dyscrasias. Use cautiously in retinal or optic nerve diseases. • Never withdraw drug suddenly. Call doctor at once if side effects develop. • Therapeutic blood levels 6 to 71 mcg/ml. • Stop drug if scotomata or signs of hepatitis, systemic lupus erythematosus, lymphadenopathy, skin rash, nephrosis, hair loss, or grand mal seizures appear. • Tell patient to report sore throat, fever, malaise, bruises, petechiae, or epistaxis to doctor immediately. Advise patient to wear dark glasses if photophobia occurs. Warn him not to drive car or operate machinery until CNS response to drug has been determined. • Obtain liver function studies and urinalysis before therapy; then monthly. • Dilute oral solution with water before giving. • Monitor CBC. Discontinue drug if neutrophil count falls below 2,500/mm^3. • 300-mg capsule contains tartrazine. May cause allergy in susceptible patients.
None significant.	• Contraindicated in patients with preexisting personality disturbances. Use with caution in patients with hepatic dysfunction, history of allergy, and when a hydantoin is used concomitantly. • Obtain liver function tests, CBCs, and urinalyses before and at monthly intervals during therapy. • Tell patient to report sore throat or fever to doctor immediately. • Warn patient to avoid activities that require alertness or good psychomotor coordination until CNS response to drug has been determined. • Never withdraw drug suddenly. Call doctor at once if side effects develop. • Tell patient's family to watch for personality or psychological changes and report them to doctor at once.

(continued on following page)

NAME	INDICATIONS & DOSAGE	SIDE EFFECTS
phenacemide *(continued)*		
phenobarbital Bar, Barbipil, Barbita, Eskabarb♦, Floramine, Gardenal♦♦, Henomint, Luminal♦, Nova-Pheno♦♦, Orprine, PB, PBR, Pheno-Squar, Solfoton, Solu-Barb, Stental **phenobarbital sodium** Controlled Substance Schedule IV Luminal Sodium♦	*All forms of epilepsy, febrile seizures in children—* **Adults:** 100 to 200 mg P.O. daily, divided t.i.d. or given as single dose at bedtime. **Children:** 4 to 6 mg/kg P.O. daily, divided q 12 hours. *Status epilepticus—* **Adults:** 90 to 120 mg I.V., followed by 30 to 60 mg q 10 to 15 minutes, as needed, up to 500 mg total. **Children:** 5 to 10 mg/kg I.V. May repeat q 10 to 15 minutes up to total of 20 mg/kg. I.V. injection rate should not exceed 60 mg/minute.	**CNS:** *drowsiness, lethargy, hangover,* paradoxical excitement in elderly patients. **GI:** nausea, vomiting. **Skin:** rash, Stevens-Johnson syndrome, urticaria. **Other:** angioedema.
phensuximide Milontin♦	*Petit mal seizures—* **Adults and children:** 500 mg to 1 g P.O. b.i.d. to t.i.d.	**Blood:** transient leukopenia, pancytopenia, *agranulocytosis.* **CNS:** muscular weakness, *drowsiness,* dizziness, ataxia, headache. **GI:** nausea, vomiting, anorexia. **GU:** urinary frequency, renal damage, hematuria. **Skin:** pruritus, eruptions, erythema.
phenytoin sodium (extended) Dilantin♦ **phenytoin sodium (prompt)** Di-Phen, Diphenylan, Ditan	*Grand mal and psychomotor seizures, nonepileptic seizures (post-head trauma, Reye's syndrome)—* **Adults:** loading dose 900 mg to 1.5 g I.V. at 50 mg/minute or P.O. divided t.i.d., then start maintenance dose of 300 mg P.O. daily (extended only) or divided t.i.d. (extended or prompt). **Children:** loading dose 15 mg/kg I.V. at 50 mg/minute or P.O. divided q 8 to 12 hours, then start maintenance dose of 5 to 7 mg/kg P.O. or I.V. daily, divided q 12 hours.	**Blood:** thrombocytopenia, leukopenia, *agranulocytosis,* pancytopenia, macrocytosis, megaloblastic anemia. **CNS:** *ataxia,* slurred speech, confusion, dizziness, insomnia, nervousness, twitching, headache. **CV:** hypotension, *ventricular fibrillation.* **EENT:** *nystagmus, diplopia,* blurred vision. **GI:** *nausea, vomiting, gingival hyperplasia (especially children).* **Hepatic:** *toxic hepatitis.* **Skin:** scarlatiniform or morbilliform rash; bullous, *exfoliative,* or purpuric *dermatitis;* Stevens-

♦ Available in U.S. and Canada. ♦♦ Available in Canada only. All other products (no symbol) available in U.S. only. Italicized side effects are common or life-threatening.

INTERACTIONS	NURSING CONSIDERATIONS
	• Extremely toxic. Use drug only when other anticonvulsants are ineffective. • Notify doctor if patient develops jaundice or other signs of hepatitis, abnormal urinary findings, or WBC below 4,000/mm³.
Alcohol and other CNS depressants, including narcotic analgesics: excessive CNS depression. Use cautiously. *MAO inhibitors:* potentiated barbiturate effect. Monitor for increased CNS and respiratory depression. *Rifampin:* may decrease barbiturate levels. Monitor for decreased effect. *Primidone:* monitor for excessive phenobarbital blood levels. *Valproic acid:* increased phenobarbital levels. Monitor for toxicity.	• Contraindicated in patients with barbiturate hypersensitivity, porphyria, hepatic dysfunction, respiratory disease with dyspnea or obstruction, nephritis, and in lactating women. Use cautiously in patients with hyperthyroidism, diabetes mellitus, anemia, and in elderly or debilitated patients. • I.V. injection should be reserved for emergency treatment and should be given slowly under close supervision. Monitor respirations closely. • Watch for barbiturate toxicity signs, such as coma, asthmatic breathing, cyanosis, clammy skin, hypotension. Overdose can be fatal. • Warn patient to avoid activities that require alertness and good psychomotor coordination until CNS response to drug is determined. • Don't stop drug abruptly. Call doctor immediately if side effects develop. • Full therapeutic effects not seen for 2 to 3 weeks, except when loading dose is used. • Do not use injection solution if it contains a precipitate. • Therapeutic blood levels are 15 to 40 mg/ml. • Monitor prothrombin times carefully when patient on phenobarbital starts or ends anticoagulant therapy. Anticoagulant dose may need to be adjusted. • Do not mix parenteral form with acidic solutions: precipitation may result. • For toxicity, see APPENDIX, *Drug Toxicities.*
None significant.	• Contraindicated in hypersensitivity to succinimide derivatives. Use cautiously in patients with hepatic or renal disease. • Never withdraw drug suddenly. Abrupt withdrawal may precipitate petit mal seizures. Call doctor immediately if side effects develop. • Obtain CBCs every 3 months; urinalyses and liver function tests every 6 months. • May color urine pink or red to reddish brown. • Therapeutic blood level 40 to 80 mcg/ml. • May increase incidence of grand mal seizures if used alone to treat patients with mixed seizure types.
Alcohol, folic acid, loxapine: monitor for decreased phenytoin activity. *Oral anticoagulants, antihistamines, chloramphenicol, diazepam, diazoxide, disulfiram, isoniazid, phenylbutazone, phenyramidol, salicylates, sulfamethizole, valproate:* monitor for increased phenytoin activity and toxicity.	• Contraindicated in phenacemide or hydantoin hypersensitivity, bradycardia, SA and AV block, Stokes-Adams syndrome. Use cautiously in patients with hepatic or renal dysfunction, hypotension, myocardial insuffienciency, respiratory depression, and in elderly or debilitated patients, or patients receiving other hydantoin derivatives. • Don't withdraw drug suddenly. Call doctor at once if side effects develop. • Warn patient to avoid activities that require alertness and good psychomotor coordination until CNS response to drug is determined. • Don't mix drug with 5% dextrose in water because it will precipitate. Clear I.V. tubing first with normal saline solution. Never use cloudy solution. May mix with normal saline solution at a concentration of 100 mg/50 ml if necessary. • Do not give I.M. unless dosage adjustments are made. Drug may precipitate at injection site, cause pain, and give erratic blood levels. • Obtain CBC and serum calcium every 6 months. Doctor may order folic acid and vitamin B_{12} if megaloblastic anemia is evident.

(continued on following page)

NAME	INDICATIONS & DOSAGE	SIDE EFFECTS
phenytoin sodium *(continued)*	*A loading dose is given if patient has not taken phenytoin in the past. If patient has not received phenytoin previously or has no detectable blood level, use loading dose—* **Adults:** 900 mg to 1.5 g I.V. divided into t.i.d. at 50 mg/minute. Do not exceed 500 mg each dose. **Children:** 15 mg/kg I.V. at 50 mg/minute. *If patient has been receiving phenytoin but has missed one or more doses and has subtherapeutic levels—* **Adults:** 100 to 300 mg I.V. at 50 mg/minute. **Children:** 5 to 7 mg/kg I.V. at 50 mg/minute. May repeat lower dose in 30 minutes if needed. *Neuritic pain (migraine, trigeminal neuralgia, Bell's palsy)—* **Adults:** 200 to 400 mg P.O. daily.	Johnson syndrome; lupus erythematosus; hirsutism; toxic epidermal necrolysis. **Local:** pain, necrosis, and inflammation at injection site. **Other:** periarteritis nodosa, lymphadenopathy, hyperglycemia, osteomalacia, hypertrichosis.
primidone Mysoline♦, Sertan♦♦	*Grand mal, psychomotor, and focal seizures—* **Adults, and children over 8 years:** 250 mg P.O. daily. Increase by 250 mg weekly, up to maximum 2 g daily, divided q.i.d. **Children under 8 years:** 125 mg P.O. daily. Increase by 125 mg weekly, up to maximum 1 g daily, divided q.i.d.	**Blood:** leukopenia, eosinophilia. **CNS:** *drowsiness, ataxia,* emotional disturbances, vertigo, hyperirritability, fatigue. **EENT:** *diplopia,* nystagmus, edema of the eyelids. **GI:** anorexia, *nausea, vomiting.* **GU:** impotence, polyuria. **Skin:** morbilliform rash, alopecia. **Other:** edema, thirst.
trimethadione Tridione, Trimedone♦♦	*Refractory petit mal seizures—* **Adults:** initially, 300 mg P.O. t.i.d. May increase by 300 mg weekly up to 600 mg P.O. q.i.d. **Children:** 20 to 50 mg/kg P.O. daily, divided q 6 to 8 hours. May increase by 150 to 300 mg. Usual maintenance 40 mg/kg or 1 g/m² P.O. daily in divided doses t.i.d. or q.i.d.	**Blood:** neutropenia, leukopenia, eosinophilia, thrombocytopenia, pancytopenia, *agranulocytosis, hypoplastic and aplastic anemia.* **CNS:** *drowsiness,* fatigue, *malaise,* insomnia, dizziness, headache, paresthesias, irritability. **CV:** hypertension, hypotension. **EENT:** *hemeralopia,* diplopia, photophobia, epistaxis, retinal hemorrhage. **GI:** nausea, vomiting, anorexia, abdominal pain, bleeding gums. **GU:** nephrosis, albuminuria, vaginal bleeding.

♦ Available in U.S. and Canada. ♦♦ Available in Canada only. All other products (no symbol) available in U.S. only. Italicized side effects are common or life-threatening.

INTERACTIONS	NURSING CONSIDERATIONS
	• Drug may color urine pink or red to reddish brown. • Tell patient to carry identification stating that he's taking phenytoin. • Stress importance of good oral hygiene and regular dental examinations. Gingivectomy may be necessary periodically. • Drug should be stopped if rash appears. If rash is scarlet or measles-like, drug may be resumed after rash clears. If rash reappears, therapy should be stopped. If rash is exfoliative, purpuric, or bullous, don't resume drug. • Use only clear solution for injection. Slight yellow color acceptable. Don't refrigerate. • Divided doses given with or after meals may decrease GI side effects. • Available as suspension. Shake well before each dose. Use solid form (chewable tablets or capsules) if possible. • Therapeutic blood level is 10 to 20 mcg/ml. • Heavy use of alcohol may diminish benefits of drug. • Phenytoin levels may be decreased in mononucleosis. Monitor for increased seizure activity. • Dilantin brand is the only oral form that can be given on a once-daily basis. Toxic levels may result if any other brand is given once daily. • Advise patient not to change brands once stabilized on therapy. • The drug was formerly known as diphenylhydantoin. • For more information on phenytoin, see pages 411 and 427.
Phenytoin: stimulated conversion of primidone to phenobarbital. Observe for increased phenobarbital effect.	• Contraindicated in phenobarbital hypersensitivity, porphyria. • Don't withdraw drug suddenly. Call doctor at once if side effects develop. • Warn patient to avoid activities that require alertness and good psychomotor coordination until CNS response to drug has been determined. • Therapeutic blood levels of primidone 7 to 15 mcg/ml. Therapeutic blood levels of phenobarbital 15 to 40 mcg/ml. • CBC and routine blood chemistry should be done every 6 months. • Partially converted to phenobarbital; use cautiously with phenobarbital. • Shake liquid suspension well. • For toxicity, see APPENDIX, *Drug Toxicities.*
None significant.	• Contraindicated in paramethadione and trimethadione hypersensitivity, severe blood dyscrasias, severe hepatic dysfunction. Use with extreme caution in retinal and optic nerve diseases. • Don't withdraw drug suddenly. Abrupt withdrawal may precipitate petit mal seizures. Call doctor immediately if side effects develop. • Check CBC, hepatic function, and urinalysis before starting therapy and monthly thereafter. Drug should be stopped if neutrophil count falls below 2,500/mm^3. • Watch for impending toxicity; may precipitate grand mal seizure. • Warn patient to report skin rash, alopecia, sore throat, fever, bruises, or epistaxis to doctor immediately. • Warn patient to avoid activities requiring alertness and good psychomotor coordination until CNS response to drug has been determined. • Suggest sunglasses if vision blurs in bright light. Notify doctor. • If scotomata or rash occurs, drug should be stopped. • Therapeutic blood levels 20 to 40 mcg/ml.

(continued on following page)

NAME	INDICATIONS & DOSAGE	SIDE EFFECTS
trimethadione *(continued)*		**Skin:** acneiform and morbilliform rash, *exfoliative dermatitis,* erythema multiforme, petechiae, alopecia. **Other:** lymphadenopathy.
valproic acid Depakene **valproate sodium** Depakene Syrup	*Simple and complex absence seizures (including petit mal), mixed seizure types (including absence seizures), investigationally in major motor (grand mal, tonic clonic) seizures—* **Adults and children:** initially, 15 mg/kg P.O. daily divided b.i.d. or t.i.d.; then may increase by 5 to 10 mg/kg daily at weekly intervals up to maximum of 30 mg/kg daily, divided b.i.d. or t.i.d.	Because drug usually used in combination with other anticonvulsants, side effects reported may not be caused by valproic acid alone. **Blood:** inhibited platelet aggregation, thrombocytopenia, increased bleeding time. **CNS:** *sedation,* emotional upset, depression, psychosis, aggression, hyperactivity, behavioral deterioration, muscle weakness, tremors. **GI:** *nausea, vomiting,* indigestion, diarrhea, abdominal cramps, constipation, increased appetite and weight gain, *anorexia,* pancreatitis. **Hepatic:** *enzyme elevations, toxic hepatitis.* **Other:** alopecia.

◆ Available in U.S. and Canada. ◆◆ Available in Canada only. All other products (no symbol) available in U.S. only. Italicized side effects are common or life-threatening.

INTERACTIONS	NURSING CONSIDERATIONS
	• May increase incidence of grand mal seizures if used alone to treat patients who have mixed types of seizures.
None significant.	• Use cautiously in hepatic dysfunction. • Don't withdraw suddenly. Call doctor at once if side effects develop. • Obtain liver function studies, platelet counts, and prothrombin time before starting drug and every 2 months thereafter. • Warn patient to avoid activities that require alertness and good psychomotor coordination until response to drug is determined. • May give drug with food or milk to reduce GI side effects. Advise against chewing capsules; causes irritation of mouth and throat. • Tremors may indicate the need for dosage reduction. • Advise patients to take with meals; will produce more uniform blood levels. • May produce false-positive test for ketones in urine. • Available as tasty red syrup. Keep out of reach of children. • Syrup is more rapidly absorbed. Peak effect within 15 minutes. • Syrup shouldn't be mixed with carbonated beverages; may be irritating to mouth and throat.

QUESTIONS & ANSWERS

DRUG OR DISEASE: WHICH BRINGS ON ATAXIA?

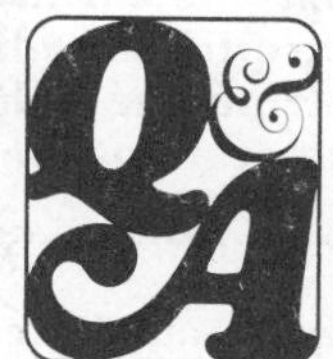

Is ataxia caused by the grand mal convulsion or too much phenytoin?

Grand mal epileptic seizures can cause cerebellar dysfunction—staggered gait, ataxia, slurred speech, and tensed muscles. Unfortunately, too much phenytoin—a drug that's commonly used to *treat* grand mal seizures—can also produce ataxia. In fact, this is one of the major warning signs of phenytoin toxicity.

To help determine whether the ataxia is caused by the drug or the disease, observe the patient closely. Clinical signs can be the first indication that phenytoin blood levels are too high.

If your patient becomes ataxic, *notify the doctor immediately.* Ask if phenytoin dosage should be reduced or stopped until drug levels have been determined.

If ataxia persists even though phenytoin blood levels are normal (10 to 20 mcg/ml), your patient's ataxia is probably due to epilepsy, not drug therapy.

31 Antidepressants

Monoamine oxidase inhibitors
isocarboxazid
phenelzine sulfate
tranylcypromine

Tetracyclic antidepressants
maprotiline hydrochloride

Tricyclic antidepressants
amitriptyline hydrochloride
amoxapine
desipramine hydrochloride
doxepin hydrochloride
imipramine hydrochloride
nortriptyline hydrochloride
protriptyline hydrochloride
trimipramine maleate

(All drugs are listed in alphabetical order in the tables that follow.)

Tricyclic antidepressants (TCAs) are the drugs of choice for most types of depression. Since their introduction in the late 1950s, they have totally supplanted amphetamines and other psychomotor stimulants for this indication. This change has occurred because of the TCAs' effectiveness and relative lack of side effects.

Monoamine oxidase inhibitors (MAO inhibitors, or MAOIs) are another class of antidepressants. These can cause more serious side effects than the TCAs; thus they are generally reserved until two TCAs have been tried unsuccessfully. Despite the official warning against the combined use of a TCA and an MAO inhibitor, reports have documented the success of combination therapy.

Tetracyclic antidepressants are the most recent class of drugs to come on the market.

With all classes of antidepressants, the biggest problem in the past has been underdosage, that is, reluctance or failure to prescribe maximum recommended dose. The latest trend in psychotropic drug therapy is higher dosage for greater therapeutic effectiveness.

Major uses

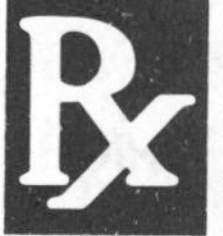

All antidepressants are used to treat psychotic and neurotic endogenous depression and to prevent recurrent depression.

- Imipramine is used to treat enuresis in children and adolescents.
- MAO inhibitors may be effective in closely supervised patients who are unresponsive to other antidepressant therapy for severe reactive or endogenous depression.

Mechanism of action

- Tricyclic and tetracyclic antidepressants are thought to increase the amount of norepinephrine or serotonin, or both, in the central nervous system by blocking their reuptake by the presynaptic neurons. This action allows these neurotransmitters to accumulate.
- MAO inhibitors block MAO (which helps metabolize neurotransmitters at synapse), causing buildup of certain neurotransmitters and probably resulting in antidepressant action.

HELPING THE DEPRESSED PATIENT

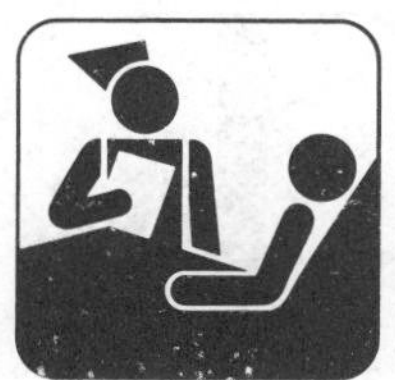

In most cases, a patient becomes depressed because he's suffered some real or imagined loss, for example, a loved one, his job or his self-esteem. Expect temporary depression in a patient who's grieving; it's a normal part of the grieving process. And expect it with certain physical disorders, such as Parkinson's disease or a fluid and electrolyte imbalance.

Certain medications can also cause depression in some patients. If drug-induced depression is severe, you may ask the doctor to consider switching the patient to another drug.

Try to discover the cause of a patient's depression, in case it's something physical you can correct. But don't waste precious time trying to analyze his problem. Do what you can to offer emotional support while assessing his physical condition. If his depression seems severe or prolonged, refer him immediately. Don't risk a possible suicide attempt.

Recognizing depression

Learn to recognize the physical and emotional signs of depression. Watch for:

- erratic sleep patterns, especially early-morning insomnia
- apathy, including lack of interest in appearance
- appetite loss
- complaints of headache, fatigue, or reduced sex drive
- profound sadness, with crying spells
- hostility toward self and others
- irritability, particularly toward those who are energetic or lively
- morbid preoccupation with self
- anxiety or despair, with strongly expressed fears of death.

If your patient shows any of these signs, document what you observe in your notes. Then report his depression to the doctor for further evaluation.

How to help

While you're waiting for a more extensive assessment of your patient's condition, do your best to relieve his stress. Use the following guidelines to plan his care.

- First, accept the patient as he is. Don't reject him by saying things like, "What's the matter with you?" or, "Things aren't really that bad." Such remarks imply he has no right to feel depressed. Be friendly but matter of fact. Don't act too sympathetic, or you'll encourage clinging behavior.
- Reinforce your patient's positive behavior by praising him when he does something well.
- Your patient's depression may prevent him from making decisions. Guide his decision-making by offering positive suggestions. Don't increase his stress by asking, "Mr. Carson, when are you going to get up and exercise?" Instead, say, "I'll be back in 5 minutes, so we can walk down the hall."
- Promote good nutrition and adequate fluid intake. Encourage your patient to eat by providing small meals, snacks, and appetizing finger foods. Ask his family to bring his favorite foods from home. Make sure he gets enough fluids and bulk to prevent elimination problems.
- Provide an environment that your patient can cope with easily. Do your best to minimize noise and confusion.
- Encourage your patient to talk about his feelings. Since you can't be with him every minute, ask him to write down his feelings throughout the day so you can discuss them later.
- Promote natural sleep with back rubs, soothing conversation, or a warm bath. Avoid using medications to induce sleep.

The road back

By maintaining a calm, positive manner, you may ease the depressed patient's stress and lift his spirits. But remember, the risk of suicide increases when the patient's depression first begins to lift.

However, don't consider yourself a failure if you can't help him. His depression may be so severe that he'll require psychiatric help. Never feel you have to succeed with every depressed patient; just do the best you can. By relieving even a little stress you may help more than you realize.

PATIENT-TEACHING AID

FOODS TO AVOID WHEN TAKING MAO INHIBITORS

Dear Patient:

When your doctor prescribes an antidepressant, ask him if it's an MAO inhibitor. If it is, avoid foods with high-tyramine content. These include:

- most cheeses, but especially blue, Boursault, brick, Brie, Camembert, cheddar, Emmentaler, Gruyère, mozzarella, Parmesan, Romano, Roquefort, and Stilton
- caviar
- herring
- sausage meats, especially bologna, pepperoni, salami, and summer sausage
- yeast extracts, that is, those foods containing live yeast, such as compressed yeast cakes. (Cooking kills yeast cells, so baked goods won't cause adverse reactions.)
- chocolate
- Chianti wine and imported beers. (Feel free to drink white wines because they're made without the grape pulp and seeds, the possible source of the amino acid tyramine present in red wines.)

Absorption, distribution, metabolism, and excretion

- Tricyclic and tetracyclic antidepressants have rapid and uniformly good absorption after oral administration.
- All antidepressants are widely distributed to body tissues.
- Tricyclic and tetracyclic antidepressants are metabolized in the liver and excreted by the kidneys as inactive metabolites. Most of the drugs and metabolites are excreted within 72 hours.
- MAO inhibitors are rapidly and uniformly absorbed after oral administration, metabolized by the liver, and excreted by the kidneys, usually within 24 hours. Although their half-lives are short, the pharmacologic effects of these drugs are long-lasting because they permanently inactivate enzymes.

Onset and duration

- Tricyclic and tetracyclic antidepressants produce sedative effects within a few hours after oral administration. Also, anticholinergic side effects occur soon after therapy begins. Antidepressant effects occur 7 to 14 days after onset of therapy due to slow effect on the brain's neurotransmitter metabolism.

  The claim that some of the newer TCAs (amoxapine and trimipramine) supply a more rapid onset of action is not well substantiated.
- Of the MAO inhibitors, isocarboxazid and phenelzine have a very slow onset that may not occur for several weeks or months. Effects may persist for up to 3 weeks after therapy is stopped.

  Tranylcypromine has a more rapid onset of action (usually several days), and MAO activity is restored 3 to 5 days after the drug's discontinued.

Combination products

ETRAFON 2-10♦: perphenazine 2 mg and amitriptyline HCl 10 mg.
ETRAFON: perphenazine 2 mg and amitriptyline HCl 25 mg.
ETRAFON-A: perphenazine 4 mg and amitriptyline 10 mg.
ETRAFON-FORTE: perphenazine 4 mg and amitriptyline 25 mg.
LIMBITROL 10-25: chlordiazepoxide 10 mg and amitriptyline (as HCl) 25 mg.
TRIAVIL-2-10, TRIAVIL-4-10, TRIAVIL-2-25, TRIAVIL-4-25 are products identical to the Etrafon products listed above. Triavil is also available as TRIAVIL-4-50 (perphenazine 4 mg and amitriptyline HCl 50 mg).

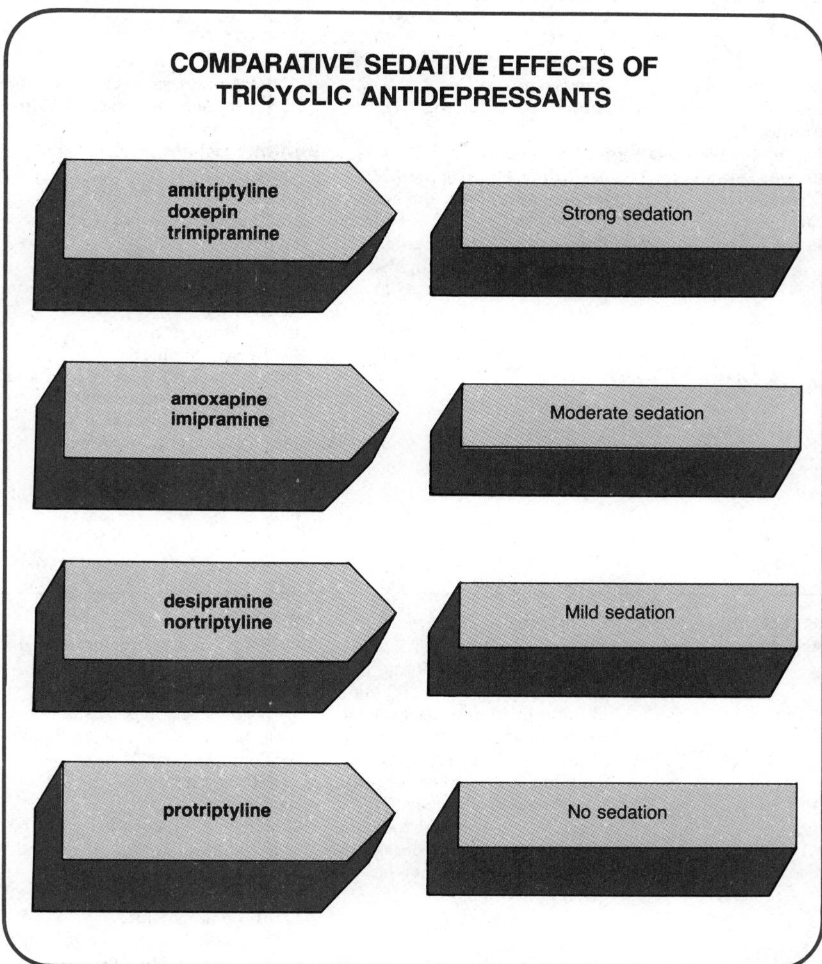
COMPARATIVE SEDATIVE EFFECTS OF TRICYCLIC ANTIDEPRESSANTS
amitriptyline
doxepin
trimipramine
Strong sedation
amoxapine
imipramine
Moderate sedation
desipramine
nortriptyline
Mild sedation
protriptyline
No sedation

NAME	INDICATIONS & DOSAGE	SIDE EFFECTS
amitriptyline hydrochloride Amavil, Amiline♦♦, Amitid, Amitril, Deprex♦♦, Elavil♦, Endep, Levate♦♦, Meravil♦♦, Novotriptyn♦♦, Rolavil	*Endogenous and other depression—* **Adults:** 50 to 100 mg P.O. h.s., increasing to 200 mg daily; maximum 300 mg daily if needed; or 20 to 30 mg I.M. q.i.d. Alternatively, the entire dosage can be given at bedtime. **Elderly and adolescents:** 30 mg P.O. daily in divided doses. May be increased to 150 mg.	**Blood:** *agranulocytosis.* **CNS:** *drowsiness,* excitation, seizures, tremors, weakness, confusion, headache. **CV:** *orthostatic hypotension, tachycardia, EKG changes,* hypertension. **EENT:** *blurred vision,* tinnitus, mydriasis. **GI:** *dry mouth, constipation,* nausea, vomiting, anorexia, paralytic ileus. **GU:** *urinary retention.* **Skin:** rash, urticaria. **Other:** *sweating, weight gain and craving for sweets,* allergy. **Abrupt cessation after long-term therapy:** nausea, headache, malaise. (Does not indicate addiction.)
amoxapine Asendin	*Endogenous and other depression—* **Adults:** initial dose 50 mg P.O. t.i.d. May increase to 100 mg t.i.d. on third day of treatment. Increases above 300 mg daily should be made only if 300 mg daily has been ineffective during a trial period of at least 2 weeks. When effective dosage is established, entire dosage (not exceeding 300 mg) may be given at bedtime.	**Blood:** *agranulocytosis.* **CNS:** *drowsiness,* excitation, seizures, tremors, weakness, confusion, headache. **CV:** *orthostatic hypotension, tachycardia, EKG changes,* hypertension. **EENT:** *blurred vision,* tinnitus, mydriasis. **GI:** *dry mouth, constipation,* nausea, vomiting, anorexia, paralytic ileus. **GU:** *urinary retention.* **Skin:** rash, urticaria. **Other:** *sweating, weight gain and craving for sweets,* allergy. **Abrupt cessation after long-term therapy:** nausea, headache, malaise. (Does not indicate addiction.)
desipramine hydrochloride Norpramin♦, Pertofrane♦	*Endogenous and other depression—* **Adults:** 75 to 150 mg P.O. daily in divided doses, increasing to maximum 200 mg daily. Alternatively, the entire dosage can be given at bedtime. **Elderly and adolescents:** 25 to 50 mg P.O. daily, increasing gradually to maximum 100 mg daily.	**Blood:** *agranulocytosis.* **CNS:** *drowsiness,* excitation, seizures, tremors, weakness, confusion, headache. **CV:** *orthostatic hypotension, tachycardia, EKG changes,* hypertension. **EENT:** *blurred vision,* tinnitus, mydriasis. **GI:** *dry mouth, constipation,* nausea, vomiting, anorexia, paralytic ileus.

♦ Available in U.S. and Canada. ♦♦ Available in Canada only. All other products (no symbol) available in U.S. only. Italicized side effects are common or life-threatening.

INTERACTIONS	NURSING CONSIDERATIONS
MAO inhibitors: may cause severe excitation, hyperpyrexia, convulsions, usually with high dose. Use together cautiously. *Epinephrine, levarterenol:* increase hypertensive effect. Use with caution. *Barbiturates:* decrease TCA blood levels. Monitor for decreased antidepressant effect. *Methylphenidate:* increases TCA blood levels. Monitor for enhanced antidepressant effect.	• Contraindicated during acute recovery phase of myocardial infarction, and in patients with prostatic hypertrophy. Use with caution in patients who are suicide risks or who have a history of seizures; in patients with urinary retention, narrow-angle glaucoma, increased intraocular pressure, cardiovascular disease, impaired hepatic function, hyperthyroidism; and in patients receiving thyroid medications, electroshock therapy, or elective surgery. • Reduce dose in elderly or debilitated persons and adolescents. • Do not withdraw abruptly. • If psychotic signs increase, dose should be reduced. Chart mood changes. Watch for suicidal tendencies. Allow minimum supply of tablets to lessen suicide risk. • Check for urinary retention and constipation. Increase fluids to lessen constipation. Suggest stool softener, if needed. • Warn patient to avoid activities that require alertness and good psychomotor coordination until CNS response to drug is determined. Drowsiness and dizziness usually subside after first few weeks. • Has strong anticholinergic effects; one of the most sedating tricyclic antidepressants. Avoid combining with alcohol or other depressants. • Expect time lag of up to 10 to 14 days before noticeable effect. Full effect usually appears in 30 days. • Dry mouth may be relieved with sugarless hard candy or gum. • Advise the patient not to take any other drugs (prescription or over-the-counter) without first consulting the doctor.
MAO inhibitors: may cause severe excitation, hyperpyrexia, convulsions, usually with high dose. Use together cautiously. *Epinephrine, levarterenol:* increase hypertensive effect. Use with caution. *Barbiturates:* decrease TCA blood levels. Monitor for decreased antidepressant effect. *Methylphenidate:* increases TCA blood levels. Monitor for enhanced antidepressant effect.	• Contraindicated in acute recovery phase of myocardial infarction, and in prostatic hypertrophy. Use with caution in patients who are suicide risks or who have a history of seizures; in patients with urinary retention, narrow-angle glaucoma, increased intraocular pressure, cardiovascular disease, impaired hepatic function, hyperthyroidism; and in patients receiving thyroid medications, electroshock therapy, or elective surgery. • Reduce dose in elderly or debilitated persons and adolescents. • Do not withdraw abruptly. • If psychotic signs increase, reduce dose. Chart mood changes. Watch for suicidal tendencies. Allow minimum supply of tablets to lessen suicide risk. • Check for urinary retention and constipation. Increase fluids to lessen constipation. Suggest stool softener, if needed. • Warn patient to avoid activities that require alertness and good psychomotor coordination until CNS response to drug is determined. Drowsiness and dizziness usually subside after first few weeks. • Dry mouth may be relieved with sugarless hard candy or gum. • Beneficial response may occur within 4 to 7 days. • Whenever possible, patient should take full dose at bedtime.
MAO inhibitors: may cause severe excitation, hyperpyrexia, convulsions, usually with high dose. Use together cautiously. *Epinephrine, levarterenol:* increase hypertensive effect. Use with caution. *Barbiturates:* decrease TCA blood	• Contraindicated during acute recovery phase of myocardial infarction, in patients with prostatic hypertrophy. Use with caution in patients with cardiovascular disease, urinary retention, narrow-angle glaucoma, thyroid disease, seizure disorders, blood dyscrasias, impaired hepatic function; in patients who are suicide risks; and in those receiving electroshock therapy, thyroid medication, or elective surgery. • Reduce dose in elderly or debilitated persons, and adolescents. • Do not withdraw abruptly. • Orthostatic hypotension not as severe with this drug compared to that with other tricyclics. • If psychotic signs increase, dose should be decreased. Chart mood

(continued on following page)

NAME	INDICATIONS & DOSAGE	SIDE EFFECTS
desipramine hydrochloride *(continued)*		**GU:** *urinary retention.* **Skin:** rash, urticaria. **Other:** *sweating, weight gain and craving for sweets,* allergy. **Abrupt cessation after long-term therapy:** nausea, headache, malaise. (Does not indicate addiction.)
doxepin hydrochloride Adapin, Sinequan♦	*Endogenous and other depression—* **Adults:** initially, 50 to 75 mg P.O. daily in divided doses, to maximum 300 mg daily. Alternatively, entire dosage may be given at bedtime.	**Blood:** *agranulocytosis.* **CNS:** *drowsiness,* excitation, seizures, tremors, weakness, confusion, headache. **CV:** *orthostatic hypotension, tachycardia, EKG changes,* hypertension. **EENT:** *blurred vision,* tinnitus, mydriasis. **GI:** *dry mouth, constipation,* nausea, vomiting, anorexia, paralytic ileus. **GU:** *urinary retention.* **Skin:** rash, urticaria. **Other:** *sweating, weight gain and craving for sweets,* allergy. **Abrupt cessation after long-term therapy:** nausea, headache, malaise. (Does not indicate addiction.)
imipramine hydrochloride Antipress, Imavate, Impril♦♦, Janimine, Novopramine♦♦, Praminil♦♦, Presamine, Ropramine, SK-Pramine, Tofranil♦, W.D.D.	*Endogenous and other depression—* **Adults:** 75 to 100 mg P.O. or I.M. daily in divided doses, with 25- to 50-mg increments up to 200 mg. Maximum 300 mg daily. Alternatively, the entire dosage may be given at bedtime. (I.M. route rarely used.) *Childhood enuresis—* 25 to 75 mg P.O. daily.	**Blood:** *agranulocytosis.* **CNS:** *drowsiness,* excitation, seizures, tremors, weakness, confusion, headache. **CV:** *orthostatic hypotension, tachycardia, EKG changes,* hypertension. **EENT:** *blurred vision,* tinnitus, mydriasis. **GI:** *dry mouth, constipation,* nausea, vomiting, anorexia, paralytic ileus. **GU:** *urinary retention.* **Skin:** rash, urticaria. **Other:** *sweating, weight gain and craving for sweets,* allergy.

INTERACTIONS	NURSING CONSIDERATIONS
levels. Monitor for decreased antidepressant effect. *Methylphenidate:* increases TCA blood levels. Monitor for enhanced antidepressant effect.	changes. Watch for suicidal tendencies. To lessen suicide risk, allow minimum supply of tablets. • Check for urinary retention and constipation. Increase fluids to lessen constipation. Suggest stool softener, if needed. • Warn patient to avoid activities that require alertness and good psychomotor coordination until response to drug is determined. Drowsiness and dizziness usually subside after a few weeks. • Dry mouth may be relieved with sugarless hard candy or gum. • Drug has anticholinergic effect, is a metabolite of imipramine, and produces less sedation than amitriptyline or doxepin. Alcohol may antagonize effects of desipramine. • Because it produces less tachycardia and other anticholinergic effects compared with other tricyclics, desipramine is often prescribed for cardiac patients. • Expect time lag of 10 to 14 days before noticeable effects. Full effect usually appears in 30 days. • Advise patient not to take any other drugs (prescription or over-the-counter) without first consulting the doctor.
MAO inhibitors: may cause severe excitation, hyperpyrexia, convulsions, usually with high dose. Use together cautiously. *Barbiturates:* decrease TCA blood levels. Monitor for decreased antidepressant effect. *Methylphenidate:* increases TCA blood levels. Monitor for enhanced antidepressant effect.	• Contraindicated in patients with urinary retention, narrow-angle glaucoma, or prostatic hypertrophy. Use with caution in suicide risks. • Reduce dose in elderly or debilitated persons, adolescents, and those receiving other medications (especially anticholinergics). • Dilute oral concentrate with 120 ml water, milk, or juice (orange, grapefruit, tomato, prune, or pineapple). Avoid carbonated beverages. • Have patient take most of daily dose at bedtime. • If psychotic symptoms increase, dose should be decreased. Chart mood changes. Watch for suicidal tendencies. • Check for urinary retention and constipation. Increase fluids to lessen constipation. Suggest stool softener, if needed. • Warn patient to avoid activities that require alertness and good psychomotor coordination until CNS response to drug is determined. Drowsiness and dizziness usually subside after a few weeks. • Expect time lag of 10 to 14 days before effect is noticeable. Full effect usually appears within 30 days. • Dry mouth may be relieved with sugarless hard candy or gum. • Has strong anticholinergic effects; one of the most sedating tricyclic antidepressants. Avoid combining with alcohol or other depressants. • Advise patient not to take any other drugs (over-the-counter or prescription) without first consulting the doctor.
MAO inhibitors: may cause severe excitation, hyperpyrexia, convulsions, usually with high dose. Use together cautiously. *Epinephrine, levarterenol:* increase hypertensive effect. Use with caution. *Barbiturates:* decrease TCA blood levels. Monitor for decreased antidepressant effect. *Methylphenidate:* in-	• Contraindicated during acute recovery phase of myocardial infarction; in patients with prostatic hypertrophy. Use with extreme caution in patients with cardiovascular disease, urinary retention, narrow-angle glaucoma or increased intraocular pressure, thyroid disease, seizure disorders, blood dyscrasias, impaired hepatic function; in patients who are suicide risks; and in those receiving electroshock therapy, thyroid medication, or elective surgery. • Reduce dose in elderly or debilitated persons, adolescents, and patients with aggravated psychotic symptoms. • Do not withdraw abruptly. • If psychotic signs increase, dose should be reduced. Chart mood changes. Watch for suicidal tendencies. To lessen suicide risk, allow minimum tablet supply. • Check for urinary retention and constipation. Increase fluids to lessen constipation. Suggest stool softener, if needed. • Warn patient to avoid activities that require alertness and good

(continued on following page)

NAME	INDICATIONS & DOSAGE	SIDE EFFECTS
imipramine hydrochloride *(continued)*		**Abrupt cessation after long-term therapy:** nausea, headache, malaise. (Does not indicate addiction.)
isocarboxazid Marplan♦	*Depression—* **Adults:** 30 mg P.O. daily in divided doses. Reduce to 10 to 20 mg daily when condition improves. Not recommended for children under 16 years.	**CNS:** dizziness, vertigo, weakness, headache, overactivity, hyperreflexia, tremors, muscle twitching, mania, *insomnia,* confusion, memory impairment, fatigue. **CV:** *orthostatic hypotension,* arrhythmias, paradoxical hypertension. **EENT:** blurred vision. **GI:** dry mouth, *anorexia,* nausea, diarrhea, constipation. **GU:** altered libido. **Skin:** rash. **Other:** peripheral edema, sweating, weight changes.
maprotiline hydrochloride Ludiomil	*Treatment of depression associated with depressive neurosis and manic-depressive illness—* **Adults:** initial dose of 75 mg daily for patients with mild-to-moderate depression. The dosage may be increased as required to a dose of 150 mg daily. Maximum dose is 225 mg in patients who are not hospitalized. More severely depressed, hospitalized patients may receive up to 300 mg daily.	**Blood:** *agranulocytosis.* **CNS:** *drowsiness,* excitation, seizures, tremors, weakness, confusion, headache. **CV:** *orthostatic hypotension, tachycardia, EKG changes,* hypertension. **EENT:** *blurred vision,* tinnitus, mydriasis. **GI:** *dry mouth, constipation,* nausea, vomiting, anorexia, paralytic ileus. **GU:** *urinary retention.*

♦ Available in U.S. and Canada. ♦♦ Available in Canada only. All other products (no symbol) available in U.S. only. Italicized side effects are common or life-threatening.

INTERACTIONS	NURSING CONSIDERATIONS
creases TCA blood levels. Monitor for enhanced antidepressant effect.	psychomotor coordination until CNS response to drug is determined. Drowsiness and dizziness usually subside after a few weeks. • Expect time lag of 10 to 14 days before noticeable effect. Full effect usually appears in 30 days. • Dry mouth may be relieved with sugarless hard candy or gum. • Avoid combining with alcohol or other depressants. • Advise patient not to take any other drugs (prescription or over-the-counter) without first consulting the doctor.
Amphetamines, ephedrine, levodopa, meperidine, metaraminol, methotrimeprazine, methylphenidate, phenylephrine, phenylpropanolamine: pressor effects of these drugs are enhanced by isocarboxazid. Use together very cautiously. *Alcohol, barbiturates, and other sedatives; tranquilizers; narcotics; dextromethorphan; tricyclic antidepressants:* unpredictable interaction. Use with caution and in reduced dosage.	• Contraindicated in elderly or debilitated patients, and in patients with severe hepatic or renal impairment; congestive heart failure; pheochromocytoma; hypertensive, cardiovascular, or cerebrovascular disease; severe or frequent headaches. Also contraindicated with foods containing tryptophan or tyramine and excess caffeine. Also during therapy with other MAO inhibitor (including pargyline HCl, phenelzine sulfate, tranylcypromine sulfate) or within 10 days of such therapy; within 10 days of elective surgery requiring general anesthetic, cocaine, or local anesthetic containing sympathomimetic vasoconstrictors. Use cautiously with other psychotropic drugs or with spinal anesthetic; in hyperactive, agitated, or schizophrenic patients; in suicide risks; and in patients with diabetes or epilepsy. • Recommended only when TCA or electroshock therapy is ineffective or contraindicated. • If patient develops symptoms of overdosage (palpitations or frequent headaches, or severe orthostatic hypotension), hold dose and notify doctor. • Watch for suicidal tendencies. • Dose is usually reduced to maintenance level as soon as possible. • Do not withdraw drug abruptly. • Weigh patient biweekly; check for edema and urinary retention. • Warn patient to avoid foods high in tyramine or tryptophan; large amounts of caffeine; and self-medication with over-the-counter cold, hay fever, or diet preparations. • Incidence of orthostatic hypotension is high. Supervise walking. Tell patient to get out of bed slowly, sitting up first for 1 minute. Wearing elastic stockings may help minimize orthostatic hypotension. • Have phentolamine available to counteract severe hypertension. • Continue precautions 10 days after stopping drug. • Expect time lag of 1 to 4 weeks before noticeable effect. • Drug is MAO inhibitor and is generally less effective than tricyclic antidepressant. Avoid combining with alcohol or other depressant. • Obtain baseline blood pressure readings, CBC, and liver function studies before beginning therapy, and continue to monitor throughout treatment.
MAO inhibitors: may cause severe excitation, hyperpyrexia, convulsions, usually with high dose. Use together cautiously. *Epinephrine, levarterenol:* increase hypertensive effect. Use with caution. *Barbiturates:* decrease maprotiline blood levels. Monitor	• Contraindicated during acute recovery phase of myocardial infarction, in patients with prostatic hypertrophy. Use with caution in cardiovascular disease, urinary retention, narrow-angle glaucoma, thyroid disease or medication, seizure disorders, blood dyscrasias, impaired hepatic functon; in patients who are suicide risks; and in those receiving electroshock therapy or elective surgery. • Reduce dose in elderly or debilitated persons, and adolescents. • Do not withdraw abruptly. • If psychotic signs increase, reduce dose. Chart mood changes. Watch for suicidal tendencies. To lessen suicide risk, allow minimum supply of tablets. • Check for urinary retention and constipation. Increase fluids to lessen constipation. Suggest stool softener, if needed.

(continued on following page)

NAME	INDICATIONS & DOSAGE	SIDE EFFECTS
maprotiline hydrochloride *(continued)*		**Skin:** rash, urticaria. **Other:** *sweating, weight gain and craving for sweets,* allergy. **Abrupt cessation after long-term therapy:** nausea, headache, malaise. (Does not indicate addiction.)
nortriptyline hydrochloride Aventyl♦, Pamelor	*Endogenous and other depression*— **Adults:** 25 mg P.O. t.i.d. or q.i.d., gradually increasing to maximum 100 mg daily. Alternatively, entire dose may be given at bedtime.	**Blood:** *agranulocytosis.* **CNS:** *drowsiness,* excitation, seizures, tremors, weakness, confusion, headache. **CV:** *orthostatic hypotension, tachycardia, EKG changes,* hypertension. **EENT:** *blurred vision,* tinnitus, mydriasis. **GI:** *dry mouth, constipation,* nausea, vomiting, anorexia, paralytic ileus. **GU:** *urinary retention.* **Skin:** rash, urticaria. **Other:** *sweating, weight gain and craving for sweets,* allergy. **Abrupt cessation after long-term therapy:** nausea, headache, malaise. (Does not indicate addiction.)
phenelzine sulfate Nardil♦	*Endogenous and other depression*— **Adults:** 45 mg P.O. daily in divided doses, increasing rapidly to 60 mg daily. Maximum 90 mg daily. Not recommended for children under 16 years.	**CNS:** dizziness, vertigo, headache, overactivity, hyperreflexia, tremors, muscle twitching, mania, jitters, *insomnia,* confusion, memory impairment, drowsiness, weakness, fatigue. **CV:** paradoxical hypertension, *orthostatic hypotension,* arrhythmias. **GI:** dry mouth, *anorexia,* nausea, constipation. **Other:** peripheral edema, sweating, weight changes.

♦ Available in U.S. and Canada. ♦♦ Available in Canada only. All other products (no symbol) available in U.S. only. Italicized side effects are common or life-threatening.

INTERACTIONS	NURSING CONSIDERATIONS
for decreased antidepressant effect. *Methylphenidate:* increases maprotiline blood levels. Monitor for enhanced antidepressant effect.	• Warn patient to avoid activities that require alertness and good psychomotor coordination until CNS response to drug is determined. Drowsiness and dizziness usually subside after a few weeks. • Dry mouth may be relieved with sugarless hard candy or gum. • Beneficial response may occur within 4 to 7 days. • Whenever possible, patient should take full dose at bedtime. • The first tetracyclic antidepressant.
MAO inhibitors: may cause severe excitation, hyperpyrexia, convulsions, usually with high dose. Use together cautiously. *Epinephrine, levarterenol:* increase hypertensive effect. Use with caution. *Barbiturates:* decrease TCA blood levels. Monitor for decreased antidepressant effect. *Methylphenidate:* increases TCA blood levels. Monitor for enhanced antidepressant effect.	• Contraindicated during acute recovery phase of myocardial infarction and in patients with prostatic hypertrophy. Use with caution in patients with cardiovascular disease, urinary retention, glaucoma, thyroid disease, seizure disorders, impaired hepatic function, blood dyscrasias; in patients who are suicide risks; or in those receiving electroshock therapy, thyroid medicaton, or elective surgery. • Reduce dose in elderly or debilitated persons, and adolescents. • Do not withdraw abruptly. • If psychotic signs increase, dose should be reduced. Chart mood changes. Watch for suicidal tendencies. To lessen suicide risk, allow minimum tablet supply. • Check for urinary retention and constipation. Increase fluids to lessen constipation. Suggest stool softener, if needed. • Warn patient to avoid activities that require alertness and good psychomotor coordination until CNS response to drug is determined. Drowsiness and dizziness usually subside after a few weeks. • Expect time lag of 10 to 14 days before noticeable effects. Full effect usually appears in 30 days. • Dry mouth may be relieved with sugarless hard candy or gum. • Drug is tricyclic antidepressant, similar in anticholinergic effects to other tricyclics. Avoid combining with alcohol or other depressants. • Advise patient not to use other drugs (prescription or over-the-counter) without first consulting the doctor.
Amphetamines, ephedrine, levodopa, meperidine, metaraminol, methotrimeprazine, methylphenidate, phenylephrine, phenylpropanolamine: enhance pressor effects. Use together cautiously. *Alcohol, barbiturates, and other sedatives; tranquilizers; narcotics; dextromethorphan; tricyclic antidepressants:* unpredictable interaction. Use with caution and in reduced dosage.	• Contraindicated in elderly or debilitated patients, and in patients with hepatic impairment, congestive heart failure, pheochromocytoma, hypertension, cardiovascular or cerebrovascular disease, severe or frequent headaches; also contraindicated with foods containing tryptophan (broad beans) or tyramine and excess caffeine or chocolate. Also contraindicated during therapy with other MAO inhibitor, including pargyline HCl, isocarboxazid, tranylcypromine sulfate, or within 10 days of such therapy; within 10 days of elective surgery requiring general anesthetic, cocaine, or local anesthetic containing sympathomimetic vasoconstrictors; in hyperactive, agitated, or schizophrenic patients. Use cautiously with antihypertensive drugs containing thiazide diuretics or with spinal anesthetic; in suicide risk, diabetes, epilepsy. • Use only when TCA or electroshock therapy is ineffective or contraindicated. • If patient develops symptoms of overdose (severe hypotension, palpitations, or frequent headaches), hold dose and notify doctor. • Watch for suicidal tendencies. • Expect time lag of 1 to 4 weeks before noticeable effect. • Dose is usually reduced to maintenance level as soon as possible. • Store drug in tight container, away from heat and light. • Have phentolamine (Regitine) available to counteract severe hypertension. • Warn patient to avoid foods high in tyramine or tryptophan; large amounts of caffeine; and self-medication with over-the-counter cold, hay fever, or diet preparations.

(continued on following page)

NAME	INDICATIONS & DOSAGE	SIDE EFFECTS
phenelzine sulfate *(continued)*		
protriptyline hydrochloride Triptil♦♦, Vivactil	*Endogenous and other depression—* **Adults:** 15 to 40 mg P.O. daily in divided doses, increasing gradually to maximum 60 mg daily.	**Blood:** *agranulocytosis.* **CNS:** excitation, seizures, tremors, weakness, confusion, headache. **CV:** *orthostatic hypotension, tachycardia, EKG changes,* hypertension. **EENT:** *blurred vision,* tinnitus, mydriasis. **GI:** *dry mouth, constipation,* nausea, vomiting, anorexia, paralytic ileus. **GU:** *urinary retention.* **Skin:** rash, urticaria. **Other:** *sweating, weight gain and craving for sweets,* allergy. **Abrupt cessation after long-term therapy:** nausea, headache, malaise. (Does not indicate addiction.)
tranylcypromine sulfate Parnate♦	*Endogenous or other depression—* **Adults:** 10 mg P.O. b.i.d. Increase to maximum 30 mg daily, if necessary, after 2 weeks. Not recommended for children under 16 years.	**CNS:** dizziness, vertigo, headache, overactivity, hyperreflexia, tremors, muscle twitching, mania, jitters, confusion, memory impairment, fatigue. **CV:** *orthostatic hypotension,* arrhythmias, paradoxical hypertension. **EENT:** blurred vision. **GI:** dry mouth, *anorexia,* nausea, diarrhea, constipation, abdominal pain. **GU:** changed libido, impotence. **Skin:** rash. **Other:** peripheral edema, sweating, weight changes, chills.

♦ Available in U.S. and Canada. ♦♦ Available in Canada only. All other products (no symbol) available in U.S. only. Italicized side effects are common or life-threatening.

INTERACTIONS	NURSING CONSIDERATIONS
	• Incidence of orthostatic hypotension is high. Supervise walking. Tell patient to get out of bed slowly, sitting up first for 1 minute. • Continue precautions 10 days after stopping drug; long-lasting effects. Wearing elastic stockings may help minimize orthostatic hypotension. • Drug is MAO inhibitor and is generally less effective than tricyclic antidepressant. Avoid combining with alcohol or other depressants. • Obtain baseline blood pressure readings, CBC, and liver function studies before beginning therapy, and continue to monitor throughout treatment.
MAO inhibitors: may cause severe excitation, hyperpyrexia, convulsions, and death, usually with high dose. Use together cautiously. *Epinephrine, levarterenol:* increase hypertensive effect. Use with caution. *Barbiturates:* decrease TCA blood levels. Monitor for decreased antidepressant effect. *Methylphenidate:* increases TCA blood levels. Monitor for enhanced antidepressant effect.	• Contraindicated during acute recovery phase of myocardial infarction and in patients with prostatic hypertrophy. Use with caution in the elderly and in patients with cardiovascular disease, urinary retention, increased intraocular tension, thyroid disease, seizure disorders, blood dyscrasias; in suicide risks; and in those receiving electroshock therapy, thyroid medication, or elective surgery. • Reduce dose in elderly or debilitated persons, and adolescents. • Do not withdraw abruptly. • Watch for increased psychotic signs, anxiety, agitation, or cardiovascular reactions; dose should be reduced if they occur. Chart mood changes. Watch for suicidal tendencies. To lessen suicide risk, allow minimum supply of tablets. • Check for urinary retention and constipation. Increase fluids to lessen constipation. Suggest stool softener, if needed. • Warn patient to avoid activities that require alertness and good psychomotor coordination until CNS response to drug is determined. Drowsiness and dizziness usually subside after a few weeks. • Dry mouth may be relieved with sugarless hard candy or gum. • Expect time lag of 7 to 14 days before effect is noticeable. • Drug is possibly the most rapid-acting but least-sedating tricyclic antidepressant. May even have an amphetamine-like effect. • Do not give entire dose at bedtime as patient may develop insomnia. • Advise patient not to use other drugs (prescription or over-the-counter) without first consulting the doctor.
Amphetamines, ephedrine, levodopa, meperidine, metaraminol, methotrimeprazine, methylphenidate, phenylephrine, phenylpropanolamine: pressor effects of these drugs are enhanced by tranylcypromine. Use together cautiously. *Alcohol, barbiturates, and other sedatives; tranquilizers; narcotics; dextromethorphan; tricyclic antidepressants:* use with caution and in reduced dosage.	• Contraindicated in patients with severe hepatic or renal impairment; congestive heart failure; pheochromocytoma, hypertension, or cardiovascular or cerebrovascular disease; severe or frequent headaches; in patients taking antihypertensive drugs or diuretics; in elderly or debilitated patients; in patients for whom close supervision is not possible; and in hyperactive, agitated, or schizophrenic patients. Also contraindicated with foods containing tryptophan or tyramine and with excess caffeine. Also contraindicated during therapy with other MAO inhibitor (including pargyline HCl, phenelzine sulfate, isocarboxazid) or within 7 days of such therapy; within 7 days of elective surgery requiring general anesthetic, cocaine, or local anesthetic containing sympathomimetic vasoconstrictors. Use cautiously with anti-Parkinson drugs, spinal anesthetic; in renal disease, diabetes, epilepsy, hyperthyroidism; and in suicide risks. • Use only when TCA or electroshock therapy is ineffective or contraindicated. • If patient develops symptoms of overdose (palpitations, severe orthostatic hypotension), hold dose and notify doctor. • Watch for suicidal tendencies. • Dose is usually reduced to maintenance level as soon as possible. • Do not withdraw drug abruptly.

(continued on following page)

NAME	INDICATIONS & DOSAGE	SIDE EFFECTS
tranylcypromine sulfate *(continued)*		
trimipramine maleate Surmontil	*Endogenous and other depression—* **Adults:** 75 mg daily in divided doses, increased to 200 mg per day. Dosages over 300 mg per day not recommended. *Enuresis—* **Children over 6 years:** initial dose 25 mg P.O. 1 hour before bedtime; if no response, increase dose to 50 mg in children under 12 years, and to 75 mg in children over 12 years.	**Blood:** *agranulocytosis.* **CNS:** *drowsiness,* excitation, seizures, tremors, weakness, confusion, headache. **CV:** *orthostatic hypotension, tachycardia, EKG changes,* hypertension. **EENT:** *blurred vision,* tinnitus, mydriasis. **GI:** *dry mouth, constipation,* nausea, vomiting, anorexia, paralytic ileus. **GU:** *urinary retention.* **Skin:** rash, urticaria. **Other:** *sweating, weight gain and craving for sweets,* allergy. **Abrupt cessation after long-term therapy:** nausea, headache, malaise. (Does not indicate addiction.)

INTERACTIONS	NURSING CONSIDERATIONS
	• Have phentolamine (Regitine) available to counteract severe hypertension. • Warn patient to avoid foods high in tyramine or trytophan; large amounts of caffeine; and self-medication with over-the-counter cold, hay fever, or reducing preparations. • Tell patient to get out of bed slowly, sitting up for 1 minute. Wearing elastic stockings may help minimize orthostatic hypotension. • Continue precautions for 7 days after stopping drug; effects last that long. • Expect time lag of 1 to 3 weeks before effect is noticeable. • More rapid onset of action than isocarboxazid or phenelzine sulfate. • MAO inhibitor most likely to cause hypertensive crisis in presence of high-tyramine ingestion. Generally less effective than a tricyclic antidepressant. Avoid combining with alcohol or other depressants. • Obtain baseline blood pressure readings, CBC, and liver function tests before beginning therapy, and continue to monitor throughout treatment.
MAO inhibitors: may cause severe excitation, hyperpyrexia, convulsions, usually with high dose. Use together cautiously. *Epinephrine, levarterenol:* increase hypertensive effect. Use with caution. *Barbiturates:* decrease TCA blood levels. Monitor for decreased antidepressant effect. *Methylphenidate:* increases TCA blood levels. Monitor for enhanced antidepressant effects.	• Contraindicated during acute recovery phase of myocardial infarction; in patients with prostatic hypertrophy. Use with extreme caution in patients with cardiovascular disease, urinary retention, narrow-angle glaucoma or increased intraocular pressure, thyroid disease, seizure disorders, blood dyscrasias, impaired hepatic function. Also contraindicated in patients who are suicide risks and in those receiving electroshock therapy, thyroid medication, or elective surgery. • Reduce dose in elderly or debilitated persons, and adolescents. • Do not withdraw abruptly. • Watch for increased psychotic signs; dose should be reduced if they occur. Chart mood changes. Watch for suicidal tendencies. Allow only minimum supply of tablets to lessen suicide risk. • Check for urinary retention and constipation. Increase fluids to lessen constipation. Suggest stool softener, if necessary. • Warn patient to avoid activities that require alertness and good psychomotor coordination until CNS response to drug has been determined. Drowsiness and dizziness usually subside after a few weeks. • Don't combine with alcohol or other depressants. • Expect time lag of 10 to 14 days before noticeable effect. Full effect usually appears in 30 days. • Dry mouth may be relieved with sugarless hard candy or gum. • Most common tricyclic used for enuresis, but effectiveness may decrease over time. Similar in anticholinergic effects to other tricyclics. • Advise patient not to use other drugs (prescription or over-the-counter) without first consulting the doctor.

32 Tranquilizers

chlordiazepoxide hydrochloride
chlormezanone
clorazepate dipotassium
diazepam
hydroxyzine hydrochloride
hydroxyzine pamoate
lorazepam
meprobamate
oxazepam
prazepam
tybamate

For information on alprazolam and halazepam, see APPENDIX, *New Drugs*.

Tranquilizers reduce anxiety without inducing sleep; they're indicated for patients suffering from various neuroses or mild depression. Most tranquilizers have muscle-relaxant and anticonvulsant properties. They produce a dose-dependent, nonspecific depression of the central nervous system (CNS) and closely resemble sedative-hypnotic drugs (barbiturates) in pharmacologic properties.

Major uses

Rx Tranquilizers are used to:
- treat anxiety
- relax skeletal muscle
- prevent and treat alcohol withdrawal symptoms (especially chlordiazepoxide, diazepam, and lorazepam) and convulsions
- treat status epilepticus (especially I.V. diazepam)
- supply premedication for I.V. general anesthetic for short procedures (especially diazepam and lorazepam).

Mechanism of action

- Benzodiazepines (chlordiazepoxide, clorazepate, diazepam, lorazepam, oxazepam, and prazepam) appear to depress the CNS at the limbic and subcortical levels of the brain, with sedative, skeletal-muscle relaxant, and anticonvulsant effects. They can produce dependence.
- The mechanisms of the other tranquilizers are still unclear.

Absorption, distribution, metabolism, and excretion

- Benzodiazepines are very well absorbed when given orally. Well distributed to body tissues and fluids, they're all metabolized in the gastrointestinal tract and the liver to either active or inactive metabolites. These metabolites are then excreted by the kidneys.

Chlordiazepoxide and diazepam absorption, after I.M. injection, is variable, painful, and unpredictable.

Lorazepam absorption, after I.M. injection, is much more dependable and less painful than that of diazepam and chlordiazepoxide.

- Chlormezanone, hydroxyzine, meprobamate, and tybamate are well absorbed orally, distributed to most body tissues, metabolized in the liver, and eliminated in both the urine and feces.

Onset and duration

- All benzodiazepines have a fairly prompt onset of action (1 to 2 hours); diazepam has the fastest (about 1 hour). Generally, those agents that are changed into active (long-acting) metabolites have longer duration of action (up to 24 hours) than those that are not changed. The long therapeutic half-lives of the active metabolites permit once-daily dosing when steady-state levels are reached.

Lorazepam and oxazepam, with shorter half-lives, must be given two to four times daily (see chart below).

- Chlormezanone acts within 15 to 30 minutes, and its effect lasts 6 hours.
- Hydroxyzine acts within 15 to 20 minutes, and its effect lasts 4 to 6 hours.
- Meprobamate begins its therapeutic action in 1 hour, peaks in 2 to 3 hours, and has a half-life of about 10 hours.
- Tybamate has an onset and peak similar to meprobamate but a shorter half-life (3 hours).

Combination products

DEPROL: meprobamate 400 mg and benactyzine HCl 1 mg.

EQUAGESIC: meprobamate 150 mg, ethoheptazine citrate 75 mg, and aspirin 250 mg.

LIBRAX CAPSULES: chlordiazepoxide hydrochloride 5 mg and clidinium bromide 2.5 mg.

LIMBITROL 5-12.5: chlordiazepoxide 5 mg and amitriptyline (as HCl) 12.5 mg.

LIMBITROL 10-25: chlordiazepoxide 10 mg and amitriptyline (as HCl) 25 mg.

MENRIUM 5-2: chlordiazepoxide 5 mg and esterified estrogens 0.2 mg.

MENRIUM 5-4: chlordiazepoxide 5 mg and esterified estrogens 0.4 mg.

MENRIUM 10-4: chlordiazepoxide 10 mg and esterified estrogens 0.4 mg.

MILPATH-400: meprobamate 400 mg and tridihexethyl chloride 25 mg.

MILPREM-400: meprobamate 400 mg and conjugated estrogens 0.45 mg.

MILTRATE-10: meprobamate 200 mg and pentaerythritol tetranitrate 10 mg.

PMB 400: meprobamate 400 mg and conjugated estrogens 0.45 mg.

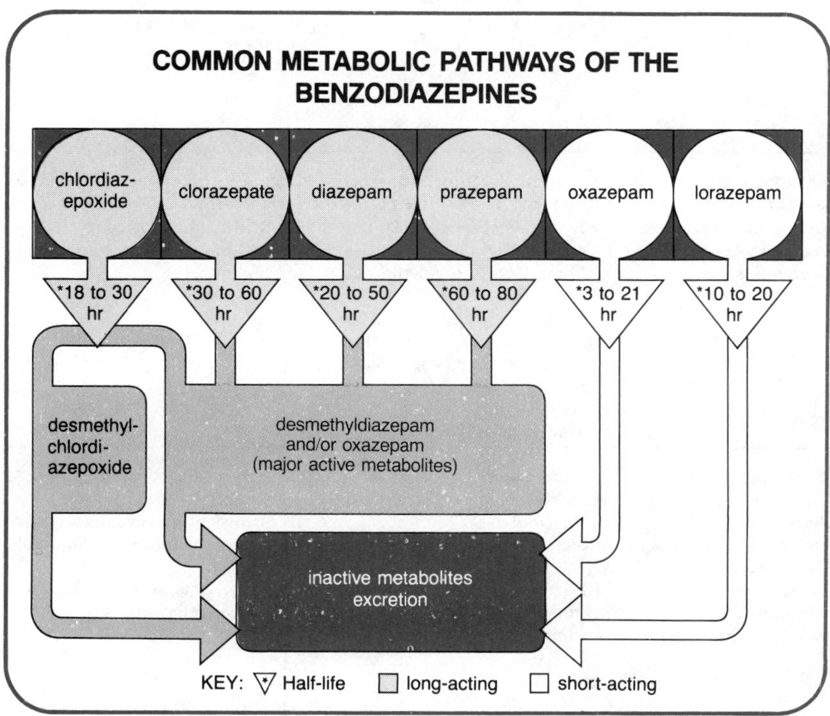

NAME	INDICATIONS & DOSAGE	SIDE EFFECTS
chlordiazepoxide hydrochloride Controlled Substance Schedule IV A-poxide, Chlordiazachel, Corax♦♦, C-Tran♦♦, J-Liberty, Libritabs, Librium♦, Medilium♦♦, Nack♦♦, Novopoxide♦♦, Protensin♦♦, Relaxil♦♦, Sereen, SK-Lygen, Solium♦♦, Tenax, Trilium♦♦, Zetran	*Mild-to-moderate anxiety and tension—* **Adults:** 5 to 10 mg t.i.d. or q.i.d. **Children over 6 years:** 5 mg P.O. b.i.d. to q.i.d. Maximum 10 mg P.O. b.i.d. to t.i.d. *Severe anxiety and tension—* **Adults:** 20 to 25 mg t.i.d. or q.i.d. *Withdrawal symptoms of acute alcoholism—* **Adults:** 50 to 100 mg P.O., I.M., or I.V. Maximum 300 mg daily. *Preoperative apprehension and anxiety—* **Adults:** 5 to 10 mg P.O. t.i.d. or q.i.d. on day preceding surgery; or 50 to 100 mg I.M. 1 hour before surgery. **Note:** parenteral form not recommended for children under 12 years.	**CNS:** *drowsiness, lethargy, hangover,* fainting. **CV:** transient hypotension. **GI:** nausea, vomiting, abdominal discomfort. **Local:** *pain at injection site.*
chlormezanone Fenarol, Trancopal♦	*Mild anxiety and tension, muscle relaxation—* **Adults:** 100 to 200 mg P.O. t.i.d. or q.i.d. **Children 5 to 12 years:** 50 to 100 mg P.O. t.i.d. or q.i.d.	**CNS:** *drowsiness,* mental depression, headache, dizziness, ataxia, lethargy, muscular weakness. **CV:** edema. **GI:** nausea, anorexia, dry mouth. **GU:** urinary retention. **Skin:** rash.
clorazepate dipotassium Controlled Substance Schedule IV Tranxene♦	*Acute alcohol withdrawal—* **Adults:** day 1—30 mg P.O. initially, followed by 30 to 60 mg P.O. in divided doses; day 2—45 to 90 mg P.O. in divided doses; day 3—22.5 to 45 mg P.O. in divided doses; day 4—15 to 30 mg P.O. in divided doses; gradually reduce daily dose to 7.5 to 15 mg. *Anxiety—* **Adults:** 15 to 60 mg P.O. daily.	**CNS:** *drowsiness, lethargy, hangover,* fainting. **CV:** transient hypotension. **GI:** nausea, vomiting, abdominal discomfort.
diazepam Controlled Substance Schedule IV D-Tran♦♦, E-Pam♦♦, Erital♦♦, Meval♦♦, NeoCalme♦♦, Novodipam♦♦, Paxel♦♦, Serenack♦♦,	*Tension, anxiety, adjunct in convulsive disorders or skeletal-muscle spasm—* **Adults:** 2 to 10 mg P.O. t.i.d. or q.i.d. **Children over 6 months:** 1 to 2.5 mg P.O. t.i.d. or q.i.d. *Tension, anxiety, muscle*	**CNS:** *drowsiness, lethargy, hangover,* fainting. **CV:** transient hypotension. **GI:** nausea, vomiting, abdominal discomfort. **Local:** desquamation, pain, phlebitis at injection site.

♦ Available in U.S. and Canada. ♦♦ Available in Canada only. All other products (no symbol) available in U.S. only. Italicized side effects are common or life-threatening.

INTERACTIONS	**NURSING CONSIDERATIONS**
Cimetidine: increased sedation. Monitor carefully.	• Use with caution in patients with mental depression, blood dyscrasias, hepatic or renal disease, or in those undergoing anticoagulant therapy. • Dosage should be reduced in elderly or debilitated patients. • Possibility of abuse, addiction. Do not withdraw drug abruptly; withdrawal symptoms may occur. • Warn patient to avoid activities that require alertness and good psychomotor coordination until CNS response to drug is determined. • Warn patient not to combine drug with alcohol or other depressants. • Although package recommends I.M. use only, this drug may be given I.V. • Injectable form (as hydrochloride) comes as two ampuls—diluent and powdered drug. Read directions carefully. For I.M., add 2 ml of diluent to powder and agitate gently until clear. Use immediately. I.M. form may be erratically absorbed. • For I.V., use 5 ml of saline injection or sterile water for injection as diluent; do not give packaged diluent I.V. Give slowly over 1 minute. • Keep powder away from light; mix just before use; discard remainder. • Do not mix injectable form with any other parenteral drug. • Caution patient against giving medication to others. • Drug should not be prescribed regularly for everyday stress. • For toxicity, see APPENDIX, *Drug Toxicities*.
None significant.	• Use with caution in hepatic or renal disease. • Dosage should be reduced in elderly or debilitated patients. • Possibility of abuse, addiction exists. Do not withdraw drug abruptly; withdrawal symptoms may occur. • Warn patient to avoid activities that require alertness and good psychomotor coordination until CNS response to drug is determined. • Warn patient not to combine drug with alcohol or other depressants. • Rapid onset of action (15 to 30 minutes), with effects lasting 4 to 6 hours. • Chemically unrelated to other antianxiety agents. • Suggest sugarless chewing gum or hard candy to relieve dry mouth.
Cimetidine: increased sedation. Monitor carefully.	• Contraindicated in patients with acute narrow-angle glaucoma, depressive neuroses, psychotic reactions, and in children under 18 years. Use with caution when hepatic or renal damage is present. • Dosage should be reduced in elderly or debilitated patients. • Possibility of abuse, addiction exists. Do not withdraw drug abruptly; withdrawal symptoms may occur. • Warn patient to avoid activities requiring alertness and good psychomotor coordination until CNS response to drug is determined. • Warn patient not to combine drug with alcohol or other depressants. • Suggest sugarless chewing gum or hard candy to relieve dry mouth. • Caution patient against giving medication to others. • Drug should not be prescribed regularly for everyday stress.
Cimetidine: increased sedation. Monitor carefully.	• Contraindicated in shock, coma, acute alcohol intoxication, acute narrow-angle glaucoma, psychosis; in oral form for children under 6 months. Use with caution in patients with blood dyscrasias, hepatic or renal damage, depression, open-angle glaucoma; in elderly and debilitated patients; and in those with limited pulmonary reserve. • Dosage should be reduced in elderly or debilitated patients. • Possibility of abuse, addiction exists. Do not withdraw drug abruptly; withdrawal symptoms may occur.

(continued on following page)

NAME	INDICATIONS & DOSAGE	SIDE EFFECTS
diazepam *(continued)* Stress-Pam♦♦, Valium♦, Vivol♦♦	*spasm, endoscopic procedures, seizures—* **Adults:** 5 to 10 mg I.V. initially, up to 30 mg in 1 hour or possibly more for cardioversion or status epilepticus, depending on response. **Children 5 years and over:** 1 mg I.V. or I.M. slowly q 2 to 5 minutes to maximum 10 mg. Repeat q 2 to 4 hours. **Children 30 days to 5 years:** 0.2 to 0.5 mg I.V. or I.M. slowly q 2 to 5 minutes to maximum 5 mg. Repeat q 2 to 4 hours. *Tetanic muscle spasms—* **Children over 5 years:** 5 to 10 mg I.M. or I.V. q 3 to 4 hours, p.r.n. **Infants over 30 days:** 1 to 2 mg I.M. or I.V. q 3 to 4 hours, p.r.n.	
hydroxyzine hydrochloride Atarax♦, Hyzine-50, Quiess, Vistaril (parenteral) **hydroxyzine pamoate** Vistaril (oral)	*Anxiety and tension—* **Adults:** 25 to 100 mg P.O. t.i.d. or q.i.d. *Anxiety, tension, hyperkinesia—* **Children over 6 years:** 50 to 100 mg P.O. daily in divided doses. **Children under 6 years:** 50 mg P.O. daily in divided doses. *Preoperative and postoperative adjunctive therapy—* **Adults:** 25 to 100 mg I.M. q 4 to 6 hours. **Children:** 1.1 mg/kg I.M. q 4 to 6 hours.	**CNS:** *drowsiness*, involuntary motor activity. **GI:** *dry mouth.* **Local:** marked discomfort at site of I.M. injection.
lorazepam Controlled Substance Schedule IV Ativan♦	*Anxiety, tension, agitation, irritability, especially in anxiety neuroses or organic (especially GI or CV) disorders—* **Adults:** 2 to 6 mg P.O. daily in divided doses. Maximum 10 mg daily. *Insomnia—* **Adults:** 2 to 4 mg P.O. h.s. *Sedation, anxiety, and as a premedication before operative procedure—* **Adults:** 2 to 4 mg I.M. or I.V.	**CNS:** *drowsiness, lethargy, hangover*, fainting. **CV:** transient hypotension. **GI:** abdominal discomfort.
meprobamate Controlled Substance Schedule IV	*Anxiety and tension—* **Adults:** 1.2 to 1.6 g P.O. in 3 or 4 equally divided doses. Maxi-	**Blood:** *thrombocytopenia, leukopenia*, eosinophilia. **CNS:** *drowsiness*, ataxia, dizzi-

♦ Available in U.S. and Canada. ♦♦ Available in Canada only. All other products (no symbol) available in U.S. only. Italicized side effects are common or life-threatening.

INTERACTIONS	NURSING CONSIDERATIONS
	• Warn patient to avoid activities that require alertness and good psychomotor coordination until CNS response to drug is determined. • Warn patient not to combine drug with alcohol or other depressants. • Do not dilute with solutions or mix with other drugs. See Chapter 6, UNDERSTANDING INTRAVENOUS SOLUTION COMPATIBILITY. • Avoid extravasation. Do not inject into small veins. • Watch daily for phlebitis at injection site. • Give I.V. slowly, at rate not exceeding 5 mg per minute. • I.V. route is more reliable; I.M. absorption is variable, to be discouraged. • Drug of choice (I.V. form) for status epilepticus. • Do not store diazepam in plastic syringes. • Caution patient against giving medication to others. • Drug should not be prescribed regularly for everyday stress. • For toxicity, see APPENDIX, *Drug Toxicities.*
None significant.	• Contraindicated in patients in shock or comatose states. • Dosage should be reduced in elderly or debilitated patients. • Possibility of abuse, addiction exists. Do not withdraw drug abruptly; withdrawal symptoms may occur. • Warn patient to avoid activities that require alertness and good psychomotor coordination until CNS response to drug is determined. • Warn patient not to combine drug with alcohol or other depressants. • Observe for excessive sedation due to potentiation with other CNS drugs. • Used as an antiemetic and antianxiety drug. • Used in psychogenically induced allergic conditions, such as chronic urticaria and pruritus. • Parenteral form (hydroxyzine HCl) for I.M. use only, never I.V. • Aspirate injection carefully to prevent inadvertent intravascular injection. Inject deep into a large muscle. • Suggest sugarless hard candy or gum to relieve dry mouth.
Cimetidine: increased sedation. Monitor carefully.	• Contraindicated in myasthenia gravis, acute narrow-angle glaucoma, psychosis, mental depression. Use with caution in organic brain syndrome, renal or hepatic impairment. • Dosage should be reduced in elderly or debilitated patients. • Possibility of abuse, addiction exists. Do not withdraw drug abruptly; withdrawal symptoms may occur. • When administering I.M., inject deep into muscle mass. Don't dilute. • When administering I.V., dilute with an equal volume of sterile water for injection, sodium chloride injection, or 5% dextrose injection. • Warn patient to avoid activities that require alertness or good psychomotor coordination until CNS response to drug is determined. • Warn patient not to combine drug with alcohol or other depressants. • Caution patient against giving medication to others. • Drug should not be prescribed regularly for everyday stress. • For toxicity, see APPENDIX, *Drug Toxicities.*
None significant.	• Contraindicated in patients with hypersensitivity to meprobamate, carisoprodol, mebutamate, tybamate, carbromal; and in those with renal insufficiency or porphyria. Use with caution in patients with

(continued on following page)

NAME	INDICATIONS & DOSAGE	SIDE EFFECTS
meprobamate *(continued)* Arcoban, Bamate, Bamo-400, Equanil, Kalmm, Lan-Dol♦♦, Maso-Bamate, Meditran, Mep-E, Mepriam, Meprocon, Meprotabs, Meribam, Miltown♦, Neo-Tran♦♦, Novomepro♦♦, Pax-400, Quietal♦♦, Saronil, Sedabamate, SK-Bamate, Tranmep	mum 2.4 g daily. **Children 6 to 12 years:** 100 to 200 mg P.O. b.i.d. or t.i.d. Not recommended for children under 6 years.	ness, slurred speech, headache, vertigo. **CV:** palpitation, tachycardia, hypotension. **GI:** anorexia, nausea, vomiting, diarrhea, stomatitis. **Skin:** pruritus, urticaria, erythematous maculopapular rash.
oxazepam Controlled Substance Schedule IV Serax♦	*Alcohol withdrawal—* **Adults:** 15 to 30 mg P.O. t.i.d. or q.i.d. *Severe anxiety—* **Adults:** 15 to 30 mg P.O. t.i.d. or q.i.d. *Tension, mild-to-moderate anxiety—* **Adults:** 10 to 15 mg P.O. t.i.d. or q.i.d.	**CNS:** *drowsiness, lethargy, hangover,* fainting. **CV:** transient hypotension. **GI:** nausea, vomiting, abdominal discomfort.
prazepam Controlled Substance Schedule IV Centrax, Verstran	*Anxiety—* **Adults:** 30 mg P.O. in divided doses. Range 20 to 60 mg daily. May be administered as single daily dose at bedtime. Start with 20 mg.	**CNS:** *drowsiness, lethargy, hangover,* fainting. **CV:** transient hypotension. **GI:** nausea, vomiting, discomfort.
tybamate Controlled Substance Schedule IV Tybatran	*Anxiety and tension—* **Adults:** 750 mg to 2 g P.O. daily in divided doses; maximum 3 g daily. **Children 6 to 12 years:** 20 to 25 mg/kg daily, divided into 3 or 4 doses.	**Blood:** dyscrasias. **CNS:** *drowsiness,* dizziness, fatigue, weakness, ataxia, depressive or panic reactions, paradoxical irritability, excitement, confusion, euphoria, insomnia, headache, paresthesias. **CV:** flushing, light-headedness, hypotension, palpitation, tachycardia, fainting. **GI:** nausea, anorexia, dry mouth, glossitis. **Skin:** urticaria, pruritus, pruritus ani, rash.

♦ Available in U.S. and Canada. ♦♦ Available in Canada only. All other products (no symbol) available in U.S. only. Italicized side effects are common or life-threatening.

INTERACTIONS	NURSING CONSIDERATIONS
	impaired hepatic or renal function, in lactating women, and in patients with suicidal tendencies. • Dosage should be reduced in elderly or debilitated patients. • Possibility of abuse, addiction exists. Withdraw drug gradually (over 2 weeks) or withdrawal symptoms may occur. • Warn patient to avoid activities that require alertness or good psychomotor coordination until CNS response to drug is determined. • Warn patient not to combine drug with alcohol or other depressants. • Give I.M. deep into muscle. • Give P.O. with meals to reduce gastric distress. • Therapeutic blood levels 0.5 to 2 mg/100 ml; levels above 20 mg/100 ml may cause coma and death. • Periodic evaluation of CBC and liver function studies are indicated in patients receiving high doses.
Cimetidine: increased sedation. Monitor carefully.	• Contraindicated in psychoses. Use cautiously in patients with history of convulsive disorders, drug allergies, blood dyscrasias, renal disease, depression. • Dose should be reduced in elderly or debilitated patients. • Possibility of abuse, addiction exists. Do not withdraw drug abruptly; withdrawal symptoms may occur. • Warn patient to avoid activities that require alertness or good psychomotor coordination until CNS response to drug is determined. • Warn patient not to combine drug with alcohol or other depressants. • Fewer cumulative effects than most other benzodiazepines due to short half-life. • Caution patient against giving medication to others. • Drug should not be prescribed for everyday stress. • For toxicity, see APPENDIX, *Drug Toxicities*.
Cimetidine: increased sedation. Monitor carefully.	• Contraindicated in patients with acute narrow-angle glaucoma, psychosis, and psychiatric disorders not showing anxiety. Use with caution in renal or hepatic impairment. • Dosage should be reduced in elderly or debilitated patients. • Possibility of abuse, addiction exists. Do not withdraw drug abruptly; withdrawal symptoms may occur. • Warn patient to avoid activities that require alertness and good psychomotor coordination until CNS response to drug is determined. • Warn patient not to combine drug with alcohol or other depressants. • Caution patient against giving medication to others. • Drug should not be prescribed for everyday stress. • For toxicity, see APPENDIX, *Drug Toxicities*.
None significant.	• Contraindicated in patients with history of hypersensitivity to tybamate or related compounds, such as meprobamate, carisoprodol, or mebutamate; in patients with convulsive disorders, drug allergies, blood dyscrasias, or porphyria; and in lactating women. Use with caution in hepatic or renal dysfunction. • Dosage should be reduced in elderly or debilitated patients. • Possibility of abuse, addiction exists. Do not withdraw drug abruptly; withdrawal symptoms may occur. • Warn patient to avoid activities that require alertness and good psychomotor coordination until CNS response to drug is determined. • Warn patient not to combine drug with alcohol or other depressants. • Shorter-acting than meprobamate. • Periodic evaluation of CBC, liver and kidney function studies are advised in patients receiving high doses or prolonged therapy. • Suggest sugarless hard candy or gum to relieve dry mouth.

33 Antipsychotics

acetophenazine maleate
butaperazine maleate
carphenazine maleate
chlorpromazine hydrochloride
chlorprothixene
droperidol
fluphenazine decanoate
fluphenazine enanthate
fluphenazine hydrochloride
haloperidol
loxapine succinate
mesoridazine besylate
molindone hydrochloride
perphenazine
piperacetazine
prochlorperazine edisylate
prochlorperazine maleate
promazine hydrochloride
thioridazine hydrochloride
thiothixene
thiothixene hydrochloride
trifluoperazine hydrochloride
triflupromazine hydrochloride

Antipsychotic (neuroleptic) drugs may help control the symptoms but not the causes of organic psychoses. These agents modify thought disorders, blunted affect (deadened emotions and apathy), and behaviors associated with psychomotor and mental retardation. They lessen symptoms of paranoia, as well as agitation, hallucinations, delusions, and autistic behavior. Some of them are also used as antiemetics, antihistamines, or antipruritics.

The antipyschotics may help patients become more receptive to psychotherapy. Since their introduction in the early 1950s, they have greatly reduced the number of persons requiring institutionalization for psychotic disorders.

Antipsychotics can be classified on the basis of chemical structure into five groups, as shown in the chart on the opposite page. Many clinicians believe that one of these groups, the phenothiazines, should be treated as three distinct drug classes because of their differences in side effects (sedative properties, cardiovascular effects, and potential for inducing neuromuscular or extrapyramidal reactions). The three classes include aliphatics (which may cause sedation and anticholinergic effects), piperidines (which may cause sedation), and piperazines (which may cause extrapyramidal reactions).

Because antipsychotics cause many side effects, they should be reserved for severe mental illnesses. For lesser disturbances, antianxiety drugs (benzodiazepines) are safer and probably more efficient. Patients undergoing antipsychotic drug therapy, however, should take their medications exactly as ordered. Symptoms of psychoses may return if these patients stop taking the medications.

Major uses

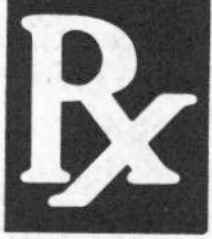

Antipsychotics may be used to treat symptoms of acute and chronic psychoses, especially those attended by increased psychomotor activity (including manic phase of manic-depressive illness, or bipolar

RELATIVE EFFECTS OF ANTIPSYCHOTICS

CHEMICAL CLASSIFICATION AND DRUG	THERAPEUTICALLY EQUIVALENT ORAL DOSE (mg)	SEDATION	EXTRAPYRAMIDAL REACTIONS
Butyrophenones			
haloperidol	2	○	●
Dibenzoxazepine			
loxapine*	10	◍	●
Dihydroindole			
molindone	10	◍	◍ to ●
Phenothiazines			
Aliphatic			
chlorpromazine†	100	●	◍
triflupromazine	25	●	◍
Piperidine			
mesoridazine	50	●	○
piperacetazine	10	◍	◍
thioridazine	100	●	○
Piperazine			
acetophenazine	20	◍	●
butaperazine	10	◍	●
carphenazine	25	◍	●
fluphenazine	2	○ to ◍	●
perphenazine	8	○ to ◍	●
prochlorperazine	15	◍	●
trifluoperazine	5	◍	●
Thioxanthines			
chlorprothixene	100	●	○ to ◍
thiothixene	4	○	●

KEY: ○ = mild ◍ = moderate ● = heavy or severe

* Only drug in this group that is commercially available

† Chlorpromazine (100 mg), the first drug to be used as an antipsychotic, is the reference compound for all other drugs in this category

EXTRAPYRAMIDAL SYMPTOMS (EPS) CAUSED BY ANTIPSYCHOTIC DRUGS

Extrapyramidal (parkinsonian) symptoms are common, dramatic side effects of antipsychotic drugs. These symptoms, defined below, result from a relative increase in cholinergic effects in the extrapyramidal system that has been brought on by dopamine blockade. Low-dose phenothiazines (such as prochlorperazine, trifluoperazine, or fluphenazine) and haloperidol are probably the most frequent causes of such effects.

Many doctors don't prescribe anti-EPS drugs until EPS symptoms develop, because about 70% of patients on antipsychotics do *not* develop significant EPS. Also, excessive doses of anti-EPS drugs may produce a toxic psychosis or delirium. This is sometimes mistaken for a relapse of the patient's pretreatment psychosis. Stopping the anti-EPS drug helps determine the cause of such a condition.

Although antipsychotic drugs are not believed to cause birth defects, these drugs may cause fetal EPS if given to the mother in the last month of pregnancy.

SYMPTOMS	DEFINITIONS
Akathisia	Discomforting feeling of insomnia, restlessness, and compulsion to walk about, with marked inability to sit still. Symptoms are first seen in 2 to 4 weeks, with a peak in 6 to 10 weeks. They decline in 12 to 16 weeks.
Akinesia	Diminished muscular movements, weakness, unusual numbness or tingling sensations. Symptoms are first seen during the first 2 weeks, with a peak in 1 week. They decline in 3 to 4 weeks.
Dystonia	Uncoordinated jerking or spastic movements of neck, face, eyes, tongue, torso, arm or leg muscles; backward rolling of the eyes in their sockets (oculogyric crisis); sideways twisting of the neck (torticollis); protrusion of the tongue ("thick" tongue); drooling; spasms of back muscles (opisthotonos). Symptoms are seen in the first few days, with a peak in 1 week. They decline in 2 weeks.
Rigidity	Abnormally high muscle tone or tension, "cogwheel" resistance to movement, unchanging blank facial expression (masked facies), stiff mechanical gait. Symptoms are first seen in ½ to 2 weeks, with a peak in 2 to 4 weeks. They decline in 5 to 10 weeks.
Tremor	Fine quivering motions due to alternating rapid contractions, especially of the arm muscles. Symptoms are first seen in ½ to 2 weeks, with a peak in 2 to 6 weeks. They decline in 8 to 16 weeks.

disorders, and schizophrenia).

- Chlorpromazine and prochlorperazine may control nausea and vomiting.
- Haloperidol and thioridazine are more commonly used than other antipsychotics to control agitation in organic brain syndrome.

Mechanism of action

- As antipsychotics, these drugs block postsynaptic dopamine receptors in the brain. They also produce alpha-adrenergic blocking and depress release of hypothalamic and some pituitary hormones.
- As antiemetics, the drugs inhibit the medullary chemoreceptor trigger zone.
- As antiagitative drugs, they cause indirect reduction of stimuli to the brain stem reticular system.

Absorption, distribution, metabolism, and excretion

Although absorption after oral administration of these agents is efficient (faster with liquid concentrate than with tablets), it varies markedly from patient to patient. Absorption after I.M.

administration is generally more complete (about one half the oral dose produces equal effect).

The agents are well distributed to body tissues, and highest concentrations of unchanged drug occur in the brain. Metabolites predominate in the lungs, liver, kidneys, and spleen.

All antipsychotics are metabolized in the liver; the metabolites are eliminated in the urine and—through the bile—in feces.

Onset and duration

- Onset of action is 2 to 6 hours for most drugs given orally and I.M., although haloperidol's onset (administered I.M.) is much shorter (20 to 30 minutes).
- Although symptoms may diminish with the first few doses, maximal effects may require weeks to months to develop.
- Long half-lives generally permit once-daily dosing (usually at bedtime).
- Divided doses are sometimes necessary for drugs causing significant hypotension (thioridazine and chlorpromazine, for example).

Administering large doses of the prescribed antipsychotic at the beginning of drug therapy (rapid neuroleptization) is becoming more popular. Drugs such as haloperidol and thiothixene are given hourly until symptoms abate.

Combination products

COMBID: prochlorperazine maleate 10 mg and isopropamide iodide 5 mg.
ESKATROL: prochlorperazine maleate 7.5 mg and dextroamphetamine sulfate 15 mg.
ETRAFON 2-10: perphenazine 2 mg and amitriptyline HCl 10 mg.
ETRAFON A: perphenazine 2 mg and amitriptyline HCl 25 mg.
ETRAFON-FORTE: perphenazine 4 mg and amitriptyline HCl 25 mg.
LIMBITROL 10-25: chlordiazepoxide 10 mg and amitriptyline (as HCl) 25 mg.
LIMBITROL 5-12.5: chlordiazepoxide 5 mg and amitriptyline (as HCl) 12.5 mg.
TRIAVIL 2-10, TRIAVIL 4-10, TRIAVIL 2-25 are identical to Etrafon products listed above; TRIAVIL 4-50: perphenazine 4 mg and amitriptyline HCl 50 mg.

NAME	INDICATIONS & DOSAGE	SIDE EFFECTS
acetophenazine maleate Tindal	*Psychotic disorders—* **Adults:** initially, 20 mg P.O. t.i.d. or q.i.d. Daily dosage ranges from 40 to 80 mg in outpatients, or 80 to 120 mg in hospitalized patients, but in severe psychotic states up to 600 mg daily has been safely administered. Smallest effective dose should be used at all times.	**Blood:** *transient leukopenia, agranulocytosis.* **CNS:** *extrapyramidal reactions (high incidence),* sedation (low incidence), pseudoparkinsonism, EEG changes, dizziness. **CV:** *orthostatic hypotension,* tachycardia, EKG changes. **EENT:** *ocular changes, blurred vision.* **GI:** *dry mouth, constipation.* **GU:** *urinary retention,* dark urine, menstrual irregularities, gynecomastia, inhibited ejaculation. **Hepatic:** *cholestatic jaundice, abnormal liver function tests.* **Metabolic:** hyperprolactinemia. **Skin:** *mild photosensitivity,* dermal allergic reactions, *exfoliative dermatitis.* **Other:** weight gain, increased appetite. **After abrupt withdrawal:** gastritis, nausea, vomiting, dizziness, tremors, feeling of warmth or cold, sweating, tachycardia, headache, insomnia.
butaperazine maleate Repoise	*Psychotic disorders—* **Adults:** initially, 5 to 10 mg P.O. t.i.d. Increase gradually to maximum 100 mg daily. Use lowest effective dose.	**Blood:** *transient leukopenia, agranulocytosis.* **CNS:** *extrapyramidal reactions (high incidence),* sedation (low incidence), pseudoparkinsonism, EEG changes, dizziness. **CV:** *orthostatic hypotension,* tachycardia, EKG changes. **EENT:** *ocular changes, blurred vision.* **GI:** *dry mouth, constipation.* **GU:** *urinary retention,* dark urine, menstrual irregularities, gynecomastia, inhibited ejaculation. **Hepatic:** *cholestatic jaundice, abnormal liver function tests.* **Metabolic:** hyperprolactinemia. **Skin:** *mild photosensitivity,* dermal allergic reactions, *exfoliative dermatitis.* **Other:** weight gain, increased appetite.

INTERACTIONS	NURSING CONSIDERATIONS
Antacids: inhibit absorption of oral phenothiazines. Separate antacid and phenothiazine doses by at least 2 hours. *Barbiturates:* may decrease phenothiazine effect. Observe patient.	• Contraindicated in CNS depression, bone marrow depression, subcortical damage, and coma; also with use of spinal or epidural anesthetic, or adrenergic blocking agents. Use cautiously with other CNS depressants, anticholinergics; in elderly or debilitated patients; and in patients with hepatic disease, arteriosclerosis or cardiovascular disease (may cause sudden drop in blood pressure), exposure to extreme heat or cold (including antipyretic therapy), respiratory disorders, hypocalcemia, convulsive disorders (may lower seizure threshold), severe reactions to insulin or electroshock therapy, suspected brain tumor or intestinal obstruction, glaucoma, or prostatic hypertrophy. • Hold dose and notify doctor if patient develops symptoms of blood dyscrasias (fever, sore throat, infection, cellulitis, weakness), persistent (longer than a few hours) extrapyramidal reactions, or any such reaction during pregnancy. • Dose of 20 mg is therapeutic equivalent of 100 mg chlorpromazine. • Monitor therapy by weekly bilirubin tests during first month, periodic blood tests (CBC, liver function), and ophthalmic tests (long-term use). • Check intake/output for urinary retention or constipation. • Tell patient to use sunscreening agents and protective clothing to avoid photosensitivity reactions. • Warn against activities requiring alertness or good psychomotor coordination until CNS response to drug is determined. • Obtain baseline measures of blood pressure before starting therapy and monitor routinely. Watch for orthostatic hypotension. Advise patient to get up slowly. • Dry mouth may be relieved with sugarless gum, sour hard candy, or rinsing with mouthwash. • Avoid combining with alcohol or other depressants. • Do not withdraw drug abruptly unless required by severe side effects. • Patient on maintenance may take medication at bedtime to facilitate sleep and decrease sedation during daytime. • For toxicity, see APPENDIX, *Drug Toxicities*.
Antacids: inhibit absorption of oral phenothiazines. Separate antacid and phenothiazine doses by at least 2 hours. *Barbiturates:* may decrease phenothiazine effect. Observe patient.	• Contraindicated in CNS depression, bone marrow depression, subcortical damage, and coma; also contraindicated with use of spinal or epidural anesthetic, or adrenergic blocking agents. Use cautiously with other CNS depressants, anticholinergics; in elderly or debilitated patients; in patients with hepatic disease, arteriosclerosis or cardiovascular disease (may cause sudden drop in blood pressure), exposure to extreme heat or cold (including antipyretic therapy), respiratory disorders, hypocalcemia, convulsive disorders (may lower seizure threshold), severe reactions to insulin or electroshock therapy, suspected brain tumor or intestinal obstruction, glaucoma, or prostatic hypertrophy; and in acutely ill or dehydrated children. • Hold dose and notify doctor if patient develops symptoms of jaundice, blood dyscrasias (fever, sore throat, infection, cellulitis, weakness), persistent (longer than a few hours) extrapyramidal reactions, or any such reaction in children. • Patients on maintenance may take medication at bedtime to facilitate sleep and decrease sedation during the daytime. • Monitor therapy by weekly bilirubin tests during first month, periodic blood tests (CBC, liver function), and ophthalmic tests (long-term use). • Check intake/output for urinary retention or constipation. • Watch patient for possible addiction.

(continued on following page)

NAME	INDICATIONS & DOSAGE	SIDE EFFECTS
butaperazine maleate *(continued)*		**After abrupt withdrawal:** gastritis, nausea, vomiting, dizziness, tremors, feeling of warmth or cold, sweating, tachycardia, headache, insomnia.
carphenazine maleate Proketazine	*Psychotic disorders—* **Adults:** initially, 12.5 to 50 mg P.O., b.i.d. or t.i.d. Increase gradually to maximum 100 mg daily.	**Blood:** *transient leukopenia, agranulocytosis.* **CNS:** *extrapyramidal reactions (high incidence),* sedation (low incidence), pseudoparkinsonism, EEG changes, dizziness. **CV:** *orthostatic hypotension,* tachycardia, EKG changes. **EENT:** *ocular changes, blurred vision.* **GI:** *dry mouth, constipation.* **GU:** *urinary retention,* dark urine, menstrual irregularities, gynecomastia, inhibited ejaculation. **Hepatic:** *cholestatic jaundice, abnormal liver function tests.* **Metabolic:** hyperprolactinemia. **Skin:** *mild photosensitivity,* dermal allergic reactions, *exfoliative dermatitis.* **Other:** weight gain, increased appetite. **After abrupt withdrawal:** gastritis, nausea, vomiting, dizziness, tremors, feeling of warmth or cold, sweating, tachycardia, headache, insomnia.
chlorpromazine hydrochloride Chlorprom♦♦, Chlor-Promanyl♦♦, Chlorzine, Klomazine,	*Intractable hiccups—* **Adults:** 25 to 50 mg P.O. or I.M. t.i.d. or q.i.d. *Mild alcohol withdrawal, acute intermittent porphyria, and tetanus—*	**Blood:** *transient leukopenia, agranulocytosis.* **CNS:** *extrapyramidal reactions (moderate incidence), sedation (high incidence),* pseudoparkinsonism, EEG changes, dizziness.

♦ Available in U.S. and Canada. ♦♦ Available in Canada only. All other products (no symbol) available in U.S. only. Italicized side effects are common or life-threatening.

INTERACTIONS	NURSING CONSIDERATIONS
	• Tell patient to use sunscreening agents and protective clothing to avoid photosensitivity reactions. • Warn against activities that require alertness or good psychomotor coordination until CNS response to drug is determined. Drowsiness and dizziness usually subside after first few weeks. • Obtain baseline measures of blood pressure before starting therapy and monitor regularly. Watch for orthostatic hypotension. Advise patient to get up slowly. • If dry mouth or nasal congestion occurs, explain that symptoms may diminish in a week or two. Dry mouth may be relieved with sugarless gum, sour hard candy, or rinsing with mouthwash. • Do not withdraw drug abruptly unless required by severe side effects. • Avoid combining with alcohol or other depressants. • Dose of 10 mg is therapeutic equivalent of 100 mg chlorpromazine. • For toxicity, see APPENDIX, *Drug Toxicities*.
Antacids: inhibit absorption of oral phenothiazines. Separate antacid and phenothiazine doses by at least 2 hours. *Barbiturates:* may decrease phenothiazine effect. Observe patient.	• Contraindicated in CNS depression, bone marrow depression, subcortical damage, and coma; also contraindicated with use of spinal or epidural anesthetic, or adrenergic blocking agents. Use cautiously with other CNS depressants, anticholinergics; in elderly or debilitated patients; in patients with hepatic disease, arteriosclerosis or cardiovascular disease (may cause sudden drop in blood pressure), exposure to extreme heat or cold (including antipyretic therapy), respiratory disorders, hypocalcemia, convulsive disorders (may lower seizure threshold), severe reactions to insulin or electroshock therapy, suspected brain tumor or intestinal obstruction, glaucoma, or prostatic hypertrophy; and in acutely ill or dehydrated children. • Hold dose and notify doctor if patient develops symptoms of jaundice, blood dyscrasias (fever, sore throat, infection, cellulitis, weakness) or persistent (longer than a few hours) extrapyramidal reactions. • Monitor therapy by weekly bilirubin tests during first month, periodic blood tests (CBC, liver function), and ophthalmic tests (long-term use). • Check intake/output for urinary retention or constipation. • Tell patient to use sunscreening agents and protective clothing to avoid photosensitivity reactions. • Warn against activities that require alertness or good psychomotor coordination until CNS response to drug is determined. Drowsiness and dizziness usually subside after a few weeks. • Obtain baseline measures of blood pressure before starting therapy and monitor regularly. Watch for orthostatic hypotension. Advise patient to get up slowly. • Avoid combining with alcohol or other depressants. • Do not withdraw drug abruptly unless required by severe side effects. • Dry mouth may be relieved by sugarless gum, sour hard candy, or rinsing with mouthwash. • Dose of 25 mg is therapeutic equivalent of 100 mg chlorpromazine. • For toxicity, see APPENDIX, *Drug Toxicities*.
Antacids: inhibit absorption of oral phenothiazines. Separate antacid and phenothiazine doses by at least 2 hours.	• Contraindicated in CNS depression, bone marrow depression, subcortical damage, Reye's syndrome, and coma; also contraindicated with use of spinal or epidural anesthetic, or adrenergic blocking agents. Use cautiously with other CNS depressants, anticholinergics; in elderly or debilitated patients; in patients with hepatic disease, arteriosclerosis or cardiovascular disease (may cause sudden drop in

(continued on following page)

NAME	INDICATIONS & DOSAGE	SIDE EFFECTS
chlorpromazine hydrochloride *(continued)* Klorazine, Largactil♦♦, Ormazine, Promachel, Promachlor, Promapar, Promaz, Sonazine, Terpium, Thoradex, Thorazine	**Adults:** 25 to 50 mg I.M. t.i.d. or q.i.d. *Nausea and vomiting—* **Adults:** 10 to 25 mg P.O. or I.M. q 4 to 6 hours, p.r.n.; or 50 to 100 mg rectally q 6 to 8 hours, p.r.n. **Children:** 0.25 mg/kg P.O. q 4 to 6 hours; or 0.25 mg/kg I.M. q 6 to 8 hours; or 0.5 mg/kg rectally q 6 to 8 hours. *Psychosis—* **Adults:** 500 mg P.O. daily in divided doses, increasing gradually to 2 g; or 25 to 50 mg I.M. q 1 to 4 hours, p.r.n. **Children:** 0.25 mg/kg P.O. q 4 to 6 hours; or 0.25 mg/kg I.M. q 6 to 8 hours; or 0.5 mg/kg rectally q 6 to 8 hours. Maximum dose is 40 mg in children under 5 years, and 75 mg in children 5 to 12 years.	**CV:** *orthostatic hypotension,* tachycardia, EKG changes. **EENT:** *ocular changes, blurred vision.* **GI:** *dry mouth, constipation.* **GU:** *urinary retention,* dark urine, menstrual irregularities, gynecomastia, inhibited ejaculation. **Hepatic:** *cholestatic jaundice, abnormal liver function tests.* **Metabolic:** hyperprolactinemia. **Skin:** *mild photosensitivity,* dermal allergic reactions, *exfoliative dermatitis.* **Local:** pain on I.M. injection, sterile abscess. **Other:** weight gain, increased appetite. **After abrupt withdrawal:** gastritis, nausea, vomiting, dizziness, tremors, feeling of warmth or cold, sweating, tachycardia, headache, insomnia.
chlorprothixene Taractan, Tarasan♦♦	*Psychotic disorders—* **Adults:** initially, 10 mg P.O. t.i.d. or q.i.d. Increase gradually to maximum 600 mg daily. **Children over 6 years:** 10 to 25 mg P.O. t.i.d. or q.i.d. *Agitation of severe neurosis, depression, schizophrenia—* **Adults:** 25 to 50 mg P.O. or I.M. t.i.d. or q.i.d. Increase as needed up to maximum 600 mg.	**Blood:** *transient leukopenia, agranulocytosis.* **CNS:** *extrapyramidal reactions (high incidence),* sedation (low incidence), pseudoparkinsonism, EEG changes, dizziness. **CV:** *orthostatic hypotension,* tachycardia, EKG changes. **EENT:** *ocular changes, blurred vision.* **GI:** *dry mouth, constipation.* **GU:** *urinary retention,* dark urine, menstrual irregularities, gynecomastia, inhibited ejaculation. **Hepatic:** *cholestatic jaundice, abnormal liver function tests.*

INTERACTIONS	NURSING CONSIDERATIONS
Anticholinergics (including antidepressant and antiparkinson agents): increased anticholinergic activity, aggravated parkinson-like symptoms. Use with caution. *Barbiturates:* may decrease phenothiazine effect. Observe patient. *Lithium:* possible decreased response to chlorpromazine. Observe patient.	blood pressure), exposure to extreme heat or cold (including antipyretic therapy), respiratory disorders, hypocalcemia, convulsive disorders (may lower seizure threshold), severe reactions to insulin or electroshock therapy, suspected brain tumor or intestinal obstruction, glaucoma, or prostatic hypertrophy; and in acutely ill or dehydrated children. • Hold dose and notify doctor if patient develops jaundice, symptoms of blood dyscrasias (fever, sore throat, infection, cellulitis, weakness), persistent (longer than a few hours) extrapyramidal reactions, or any such reaction in pregnancy or in children. • Monitor therapy by weekly bilirubin tests during first month, periodic blood tests (CBC, liver function), and ophthalmic tests (long-term use). • Check intake/output for urinary retention or constipation. • Tell patient to use sunscreening agents and protective clothing to avoid photosensitivity reactions. • Warn against activities that require alertness or good psychomotor coordination until CNS response to drug is determined. Drowsiness and dizziness usually subside after first few weeks. • Obtain baseline measures of blood pressure before starting therapy and monitor regularly. Watch for orthostatic hypotension, especially with parenteral administration. Monitor blood pressure before and after I.M. administration. Keep patient supine for 1 hour afterward. Advise patient to get up slowly. • Avoid combining with alcohol or other depressants. • Give deep I.M. only in upper outer quadrant of buttocks. Massage slowly afterward to prevent sterile abscess. Injection may sting. • Prevent contact dermatitis by keeping drug off patient's skin and clothes. • Protect liquid concentrate from light. Dilute with fruit juice, milk, or semisolid food just before administration. • Slight yellowing of injection or concentrate is common; does not affect potency. Discard markedly discolored solutions. • Do not withdraw drug abruptly unless required by severe side effects. • Dry mouth may be relieved by sugarless gum, sour hard candy, or rinsing with mouthwash. • An aliphatic; has greater tendency to cause anticholinergic side effects than other phenothiazines. • For toxicity, see APPENDIX, *Drug Toxicities.*
None significant.	• Contraindicated in coma, CNS depression, bone marrow depression, circulatory collapse, congestive heart failure, cardiac decompensation, coronary artery or cerebrovascular disorders, subcortical damage; with use of spinal or epidural anesthetic, or adrenergic blocking agents. Use cautiously with other CNS depressants, anticholinergics; in elderly or debilitated patients; in patients with hepatic or renal disease, arteriosclerosis or cardiovascular disease (may cause sudden drop in blood pressure), exposure to extreme heat or cold (including antipyretic therapy), respiratory disorders, hypocalcemia, convulsive disorders (may lower seizure threshold), severe reactions to insulin or electroshock therapy, suspected brain tumor or intestinal obstruction, glaucoma, or prostatic hypertrophy; and in acutely ill or dehydrated children. • Hold dose and notify doctor if patient develops symptoms of blood dyscrasias (fever, sore throat, infection, cellulitis, weakness), jaundice, persistent (longer than a few hours) extrapyramidal reactions, or any such reactions in children.

(continued on following page)

NAME	INDICATIONS & DOSAGE	SIDE EFFECTS
chlorprothixene *(continued)*		**Metabolic:** hyperprolactinemia. **Skin:** *mild photosensitivity,* dermal allergic reactions, *exfoliative dermatitis.* **Local:** pain on I.M. injection, sterile abscess. **Other:** weight gain, increased appetite. **After abrupt withdrawal:** gastritis, nausea, vomiting, dizziness, tremors, feeling of warmth or cold, sweating, tachycardia, headache, insomnia.
droperidol Inapsine♦	*Premedication—* **Adults:** 2.5 to 10 mg (1 to 4 ml) I.M. 30 to 60 minutes preoperatively. **Children 2 to 12 years:** 1 to 1.5 mg (0.4 to 0.6 ml) I.M. per 20 to 25 lbs of body weight. *As induction agent—* **Adults:** 2.5 mg (1 ml) I.V. per 20 to 25 lbs with analgesic and/or general anesthetic. **Children 2 to 12 years:** 1 to 1.5 mg (0.4 to 0.6 ml) I.V. per 20 to 25 lbs. Dose should be titrated. **Elderly, debilitated patients:** initial dose should be decreased. *Maintenance dose with general anesthetic—*1.25 to 2.5 mg (0.5 to 1 ml) I.V.	**CNS:** extrapyramidal reactions (dystonia, akathisia), upward rotation of eyes and oculogyric crises, extended neck, flexed arms, fine tremor of limbs, dizziness, chills or shivering, facial sweating, restlessness. **CV:** hypotension, tachycardia.
fluphenazine decanoate Modecate,	*Psychotic disorders—* **Adults:** initially, 0.5 to 10 mg fluphenazine HCl P.O. daily in	**Blood:** *transient leukopenia, agranulocytosis.* **CNS:** *extrapyramidal reactions*

♦ Available in U.S. and Canada. ♦♦ Available in Canada only. All other products (no symbol) available in U.S. only. Italicized side effects are common or life-threatening.

INTERACTIONS	NURSING CONSIDERATIONS
	• Monitor therapy by weekly bilirubin tests during first month, periodic blood tests (CBC, liver function) before and during therapy, and ophthalmic tests (long-term therapy). • Check intake/output for urinary retention or constipation. • Tell patient to use sunscreening agents and protective clothing to avoid photosensitivity reactions. • Warn against activities that require alertness or good psychomotor coordination until CNS response to drug is determined. Drowsiness and dizziness usually subside after first few weeks. • Obtain baseline measures of blood pressure before starting therapy and monitor regularly. Watch for orthostatic hypotension, especially with parenteral administration, since adrenergic blockage is high. Keep patient supine for 1 hour afterward. Advise patient to change positions slowly. • Avoid combining with alcohol or other depressants. • Give deep I.M. only in upper outer quadrant of buttocks or midlateral thigh. Massage slowly afterward to prevent sterile abscess. Injection may sting. • Dilute liquid concentrate with fruit juice, milk, or semisolid food just before administration. • Protect medication from light. Slight yellowing of injection or concentrate is common; does not affect potency. Discard markedly discolored solutions. • Do not withdraw drug abruptly unless required by severe side effects. • Prevent contact dermatitis by keeping drug off patient's skin and clothes. • Dry mouth may be relieved by sugarless gum, sour hard candy, or rinsing with mouthwash. • Dose of 100 mg is the therapeutic equivalent of 100 mg chlorpromazine.
None significant.	• Use cautiously in elderly or debilitated patients; and in patients with hypotension or other cardiovascular disease, impaired hepatic or renal function, Parkinson's disease. • Watch for extrapyramidal reactions. Call doctor at once if any occur. • Approved by FDA *only* for use preoperatively and during induction and maintenance of anesthesia. • A butyrophenone compound, related to haloperidol; has greater tendency to cause extrapyramidal reactions than other antipsychotics. • Keep intravenous fluids and vasopressors handy for hypotension. • If used with a narcotic analgesic such as fentanyl (Sublimaze), be familiar with the special properties of each drug, particularly the widely differing durations of action. Watch for respiratory depression, apnea, and muscular rigidity, which could lead to respiratory arrest if untreated. Have narcotic antagonist and CPR equipment on hand. • Monitor vital signs frequently; notify doctor of any changes immediately. • Give intravenous injections slowly. • Do not place patient in Trendelenburg position (that is, shock position); severe hypotension and deeper anesthesia may result, causing respiratory arrest. • Has been used to prevent cisplatin-associated nausea and vomiting.
Antacids: inhibit absorption of oral phenothiazines. Separate	• Contraindicated in coma, CNS depression, bone marrow depression or other blood dyscrasia, subcortical damage, hepatic damage, renal insufficiency; and with use of spinal or epidural anesthetic, or

(continued on following page)

NAME	INDICATIONS & DOSAGE	SIDE EFFECTS
fluphenazine *(continued)* Decanoate♦♦, Prolixin Decanoate **fluphenazine enanthate** Moditen♦, Prolixin Enanthate **fluphenazine hydrochloride** Moditen Hydrochloride♦♦, Permitil Hydrochloride, Prolixin Hydrochloride	divided doses q 6 to 8 hours; may increase cautiously to 20 mg. Higher doses (50 to 100 mg) have been given. Maintenance: 1 to 5 mg P.O. daily. I.M. doses are ⅓ to ½ oral doses. Lower doses for geriatric patients (1 to 2.5 mg daily). **Children:** 0.25 to 3.5 mg fluphenazine HCl P.O. daily in divided doses q 4 to 6 hours; or ⅓ to ½ of oral dose I.M.; maximum 10 mg daily. **Adults, and children over 12 years:** 12.5 to 25 mg of long-acting esters (fluphenazine decanoate and enanthate) I.M. or S.C. q 1 to 6 weeks. Maintenance: 25 to 100 mg, p.r.n.	*(high incidence),* sedation (low incidence), pseudoparkinsonism, EEG changes, dizziness. **CV:** *orthostatic hypotension,* tachycardia, EKG changes. **EENT:** *ocular changes, blurred vision.* **GI:** *dry mouth, constipation.* **GU:** *urinary retention,* dark urine, menstrual irregularities, gynecomastia, inhibited ejaculation. **Hepatic:** *cholestatic jaundice, abnormal liver function tests.* **Metabolic:** hyperprolactinemia. **Skin:** *mild photosensitivity,* dermal allergic reactions, *exfoliative dermatitis.* **Other:** weight gain, increased appetite. **After abrupt withdrawal:** gastritis, nausea, vomiting, dizziness, tremors, feeling of warmth or cold, sweating, tachycardia, headache, insomnia.
haloperidol Haldol♦	*Psychotic disorders—* **Adults:** dosage varies for each patient. Initial range is 0.5 to 5 mg P.O. b.i.d. or t.i.d.; or 2 to 5 mg I.M. q 4 to 8 hours, increasing rapidly if necessary for prompt control. Maximum 100 mg P.O. daily. Doses over 100 mg have been used for patients with severely resistant	**Blood:** transient leukopenia and leukocytosis. **CNS:** *high incidence of severe extrapyramidal reactions,* low incidence of sedation. **CV:** low incidence of cardiovascular effects with therapeutic dosages. **EENT:** blurred vision, dry mouth. **GU:** urinary retention, menstrual irregularities, gynecomastia.

♦ Available in U.S. and Canada. ♦♦ Available in Canada only. All other products (no symbol) available in U.S. only. Italicized side effects are common or life-threatening.

INTERACTIONS	NURSING CONSIDERATIONS
antacid and phenothiazine doses by at least 2 hours. *Barbiturates:* may decrease phenothiazine effect. Observe patient.	adrenergic blocking agents. Use cautiously with other CNS depressants, anticholinergics; in elderly or debilitated patients; in acutely ill or dehydrated children; and in patients with hepatic disease, pheochromocytoma, arteriosclerotic, cerebrovascular, or cardiovascular disease (may cause sudden drop in blood pressure), peptic ulcer, exposure to extreme heat or cold (including antipyretic therapy), respiratory disorders, hypocalcemia, convulsive disorders (may lower seizure threshold), severe reactions to insulin or electroshock therapy, suspected brain tumor or intestinal obstruction, glaucoma, or prostatic hypertrophy. • Hold dose and notify doctor if patient develops symptoms of blood dyscrasias (fever, sore throat, infection, cellulitis, weakness), persistent (longer than a few hours) extrapyramidal reactions, or any such reactions in pregnancy or in children. • Monitor therapy by weekly bilirubin tests during first month, periodic blood tests (CBC, liver function), periodic renal function and ophthalmic tests (long-term use). • Check intake/output for urinary retention or constipation. • Tell patient to use sunscreening agents and protective clothing to avoid photosensitivity reactions. • Warn against activities that require alertness and good psychomotor coordination until CNS response to drug is determined. Drowsiness and dizziness usually subside after first few weeks. • Avoid combining with alcohol or other depressants. • Obtain baseline measures of blood pressure before starting therapy and monitor regularly. Watch for orthostatic hypotension, especially with parenteral administration. Monitor blood pressure before and after I.M. administration. Keep patient supine for 1 hour afterward. Advise him to change positions slowly. • Decanoate and enanthate may be given subcutaneously. • For long-acting forms (decanoate and enanthate), which are oil preparations, use a dry needle of at least 21G. Allow 24 to 96 hours for onset of action. Important: Note and report adverse side effects in patients taking the long-acting drug forms. • Prevent contact dermatitis by keeping drug off patient's skin and clothes. • Dilute liquid concentrate with water, fruit juice, milk, or semisolid food just before administration. • Protect medication from light. Slight yellowing of injection or concentrate is common; does not affect potency. Discard markedly discolored solutions. • Dry mouth may be relieved by sugarless gum, sour hard candy, or rinsing with mouthwash. • Do not withdraw drug abruptly unless required by severe side effects. • Dose of 2 mg is therapeutic equivalent of 100 mg chlorpromazine. • For toxicity, see APPENDIX, *Drug Toxicities.*
Lithium: lethargy and confusion with high doses. Observe patient. *Methyldopa:* possible symptoms of dementia. Observe patient.	• Contraindicated in parkinsonism, coma, or CNS depression. Use with caution in elderly and debilitated patients; in severe cardiovascular disorders, allergies, glaucoma, urinary retention; and in conjunction with anticonvulsant, anticoagulant, antiparkinson, or lithium medications. • Warn patient against activities that require alertness and good psychomotor coordination until CNS response to drug is determined. Drowsiness and dizziness usually subside after a few weeks. • Avoid combining with alcohol or other depressants. • Protect medication from light. Slight yellowing of injection or con-

(continued on following page)

NAME	INDICATIONS & DOSAGE	SIDE EFFECTS
haloperidol *(continued)*	conditions. *Control of tics, vocal utterances in Gilles de la Tourette's syndrome—* **Adults:** 0.5 to 5 mg P.O. b.i.d. or t.i.d., increasing p.r.n.	**Skin:** rash.
loxapine succinate Daxolin, Loxapac♦♦, Loxitane, Loxitane-C	*Psychotic disorders—* **Adults:** 10 mg P.O. or I.M. b.i.d. to q.i.d., rapidly increasing to 60 to 100 mg P.O. daily for most patients; dose varies from patient to patient.	**Blood:** *transient leukopenia.* **CNS:** *extrapyramidal reactions (moderate incidence), sedation (moderate incidence),* pseudoparkinsonism, EEG changes, dizziness. **CV:** *orthostatic hypotension,* tachycardia, EKG changes. **EENT:** *blurred vision.* **GI:** *dry mouth, constipation.* **GU:** *urinary retention,* dark urine, menstrual irregularities, gynecomastia. **Skin:** *mild photosensitivity,* dermal allergic reactions, *exfoliative dermatitis.* **Other:** weight gain, increased appetite.
mesoridazine besylate Serentil♦	*Alcoholism—* **Adults, and children over 12 years:** 25 mg P.O. b.i.d. up to maximum 200 mg daily. *Behavioral problems associated with chronic brain syndrome—* **Adults, and children over 12 years:** 25 mg P.O. t.i.d. up to maximum of 300 mg daily. *Psychoneurotic manifestations (anxiety)—* **Adults, and children over 12 years:** 10 mg P.O. t.i.d. up to maximum 150 mg daily. *Schizophrenia—* **Adults, and children over 12 years:** initially, 50 mg P.O. t.i.d. or 25 mg I.M. repeated in 30 to 60 minutes, p.r.n.	**Blood:** *transient leukopenia, agranulocytosis.* **CNS:** extrapyramidal reactions (low incidence), *sedation (high incidence),* EEG changes, dizziness. **CV:** *orthostatic hypotension,* tachycardia, EKG changes. **EENT:** *ocular changes, blurred vision,* pigmentary retinopathy. **GI:** *dry mouth, constipation.* **GU:** *urinary retention,* dark urine, menstrual irregularities, gynecomastia, inhibited ejaculation. **Hepatic:** *cholestatic jaundice, abnormal liver function tests.* **Metabolic:** hyperprolactinemia. **Skin:** *mild photosensitivity,* dermal allergic reactions, *exfoliative dermatitis.* **Local:** pain at I.M. injection site, sterile abscess. **Other:** weight gain, increased appetite. **After abrupt withdrawal:** gastritis, nausea, vomiting, dizziness, tremors, feeling of warmth or cold, sweating, tachycardia, headache, insomnia.

INTERACTIONS	NURSING CONSIDERATIONS
	centrate is common; does not affect potency. Discard markedly discolored solutions. • Do not withdraw drug abruptly unless required by severe side effects. • Dry mouth may be relieved by sugarless gum, sour hard candy, and rinsing with mouthwash. • Dose of 2 mg is therapeutic equivalent of 100 mg chlorpromazine. • Only butyrophenone compound used as an antipsychotic in the United States.
None significant.	• Contraindicated in coma, severe CNS depression, drug-induced depressed states. Use with caution in epilepsy, cardiovascular disorders, glaucoma, urinary retention, suspected intestinal obstruction or brain tumor, renal damage. • Warn against activities that require alertness and good psychomotor coordination until CNS response to drug is determined. Drowsiness and dizziness usually subside after first few weeks. • Avoid combining with alcohol or other depressants. • Obtain baseline measures of blood pressure before starting therapy and monitor regularly. Advise patient to get up slowly to avoid orthostatic hypotension. • Dilute liquid concentrate with orange or grapefruit juice just before giving. • Dry mouth may be relieved by sugarless gum, sour hard candy, or rinsing with mouthwash. • Periodic ophthalmic tests recommended. • Tricyclic dibenzoxazepine; the only dibenzoxazepine derivative. • Dose of 10 mg is therapeutic equivalent of 100 mg chlorpromazine.
Antacids: inhibit absorption of oral phenothiazines. Separate antacid and phenothiazine doses by at least 2 hours. *Barbiturates:* may decrease phenothiazine effect. Observe patient.	• Contraindicated in coma, CNS depression, bone marrow depression, subcortical damage, and with use of spinal or epidural anesthetic or adrenergic blocking agents. Use cautiously with other CNS depressants, anticholinergics; in elderly or debilitated patients; in acutely ill or dehydrated children; and in patients with hepatic disease, arteriosclerosis or cardiovascular disease (may cause sudden drop in blood pressure), exposure to extreme heat or cold (including antipyretic therapy), respiratory disorders, hypocalcemia, convulsive disorders, severe reactions to insulin or electroshock therapy, suspected brain tumor or intestinal obstruction, glaucoma, or prostatic hypertrophy. • Hold dose and notify doctor if patient develops jaundice, symptoms of blood dyscrasias (fever, sore throat, infection, cellulitis, weakness), persistent (longer than a few hours) extrapyramidal reactions, or any such reactions in pregnancy or in children over 12 years. • Monitor therapy by weekly bilirubin tests during first month, periodic blood tests (CBC, liver function), and ophthalmic tests (long-term use). • Check intake/output for urinary retention or constipation. • Tell patient to use sunscreening agents and protective clothing to avoid photosensitivity reactions. • Warn against activities that require alertness and good psychomotor coordination until CNS response to drug is determined. Drowsiness and dizziness usually subside after a few weeks. • Avoid combining with alcohol or other depressants. • Obtain baseline measures of blood pressure before starting therapy and monitor regularly. Watch for orthostatic hypotension, especially with parenteral administration. Advise patient to change positions slowly.

(continued on following page)

NAME	INDICATIONS & DOSAGE	SIDE EFFECTS
mesoridazine besylate *(continued)*		
molindone hydrochloride Lidone, Moban	*Psychotic disorders—* **Adults:** 50 to 75 mg P.O. daily, increasing to maximum 225 mg daily. Doses up to 400 mg may be required.	**Blood:** *transient leukopenia.* **CNS:** *extrapyramidal reactions (moderate incidence), sedation (moderate incidence),* pseudoparkinsonism, EEG changes, dizziness. **CV:** *orthostatic hypotension,* tachycardia, EKG changes. **EENT:** *blurred vision.* **GI:** *dry mouth, constipation.* **GU:** *urinary retention,* dark urine, menstrual irregularities, gynecomastia, inhibited ejaculation. **Hepatic:** *cholestatic jaundice, abnormal liver function tests.* **Metabolic:** hyperprolactinemia. **Skin:** *mild photosensitivity,* dermal allergic reactions, *exfoliative dermatitis.* **Other:** weight gain, increased appetite.
perphenazine Phenazine♦♦, Trilafon♦	*Hospitalized psychiatric patients—* **Adults:** initially, 8 to 16 mg P.O. b.i.d., t.i.d., or q.i.d., increasing to 64 mg daily. **Children over 12 years:** 6 to 12 mg P.O. daily in divided doses. *Mental disturbances, acute alcoholism, nausea, vomiting, hiccups—* **Adults, and children over 12 years:** 5 to 10 mg I.M., p.r.n. Maximum 15 mg daily in ambulatory, 30 mg daily in hospitalized patients.	**Blood:** *transient leukopenia, agranulocytosis.* **CNS:** *extrapyramidal reactions (high incidence),* sedation (low incidence), pseudoparkinsonism, EEG changes, dizziness. **CV:** *orthostatic hypotension,* tachycardia, EKG changes. **EENT:** *ocular changes, blurred vision.* **GI:** *dry mouth, constipation.* **GU:** *urinary retention,* dark urine, menstrual irregularities, gynecomastia, inhibited ejaculation. **Hepatic:** *cholestatic jaundice, abnormal liver function tests.* **Metabolic:** hyperprolactinemia. **Skin:** *mild photosensitivity,* dermal allergic reactions, *exfoliative dermatitis.*

♦ Available in U.S. and Canada. ♦♦ Available in Canada only. All other products (no symbol) available in U.S. only. Italicized side effects are common or life-threatening.

INTERACTIONS	NURSING CONSIDERATIONS
	• Give deep I.M. only in upper outer quadrant of buttocks. Massage slowly afterward to prevent sterile abscess. Injection may sting. • Protect medication from light. Slight yellowing of injection or concentrate is common; does not affect potency. Discard markedly discolored solutions. • Prevent contact dermatitis by keeping drug off patient's skin and clothes. • Dry mouth may be relieved with sugarless gum, sour hard candy, or rinsing with mouthwash. • Do not withdraw drug abruptly unless required by severe side effects. • Drug is a piperidine phenothiazine (a metabolite of thioridazine). • Dose of 50 mg is therapeutic equivalent of 100 mg chlorpromazine. • For toxicity, see APPENDIX, *Drug Toxicities*.
None significant.	• Contraindicated in coma or severe CNS depression. Use with caution when increased physical activity would be harmful, as this agent increases activity; in seizures (may lower seizure threshold), suicide risk, suspected brain tumor, or intestinal obstruction. • Warn against activities that require alertness or good psychomotor coordination until CNS response to drug is determined. Drowsiness and dizziness usually subside after first few weeks. • Avoid combining with alcohol or other depressants. • Dry mouth may be relieved with sugarless gum, sour hard candy, or rinsing with mouthwash. • Drug is the only dihydroindolone derivative. • Dose of 20 mg is therapeutic equivalent of 100 mg chlorpromazine. • No injection available. • Liquid oral concentrate is available. • Lidone capsules contain tartrazine dye. May cause allergy in susceptible patients. • May be administered in a single daily dose.
Antacids: inhibit absorption of oral phenothiazines. Separate antacid and phenothiazine doses by at least 2 hours. *Barbiturates:* may decrease phenothiazine effect. Observe patient.	• Contraindicated in coma, CNS depression, bone marrow depression, subcortical damage, use of spinal or epidural anesthetic or adrenergic blocking agents. Use cautiously with other CNS depressants, anticholinergics; in elderly or debilitated patients; in acutely ill or dehydrated children; and in patients with hepatic disease, arteriosclerosis or cardiovascular disease (may cause sudden drop in blood pressure), exposure to extreme heat or cold (including antipyretic therapy), respiratory disorders, hypocalcemia, convulsive disorders (may lower seizure threshold), severe reactions to insulin or electroshock therapy, suspected brain tumor or intestinal obstruction, glaucoma, prostatic hypertrophy. • Hold dose and notify doctor if patient develops jaundice, symptoms of blood dyscrasias (fever, sore throat, infection, cellulitis, weakness), persistent (longer than a few hours) extrapyramidal reactions, or any such reactions in pregnancy or in children. • Monitor therapy by weekly bilirubin tests during first month, periodic blood tests (CBC, liver function), and ophthalmic tests (long-term use). • Check intake/output for urinary retention or constipation. • Avoid combining with alcohol or other depressants.

(continued on following page)

NAME	INDICATIONS & DOSAGE	SIDE EFFECTS
perphenazine *(continued)*		**Local:** pain at I.M. injection site, sterile abscess. **Other:** weight gain, increased appetite. **After abrupt withdrawal:** gastritis, nausea, vomiting, dizziness, tremors, feeling of warmth or cold, sweating, tachycardia, headache, insomnia.
piperacetazine Quide♦	*Psychotic disorders—* **Adults:** initially, 10 mg P.O. b.i.d. to q.i.d. Dosage may be gradually increased to 160 mg daily if necessary.	**Blood:** *transient leukopenia, agranulocytosis.* **CNS:** extrapyramidal reactions (low incidence), *sedation (high incidence),* EEG changes, dizziness. **CV:** *orthostatic hypotension,* tachycardia, EKG changes. **EENT:** *ocular changes, blurred vision,* pigmentary retinopathy. **GI:** *dry mouth, constipation.* **GU:** *urinary retention,* dark urine, menstrual irregularities, gynecomastia, inhibited ejaculation. **Hepatic:** *cholestatic jaundice, abnormal liver function tests.* **Metabolic:** hyperprolactinemia. **Skin:** *mild photosensitivity,* dermal allergic reactions, *exfoliative dermatitis.* **Other:** weight gain, increased appetite. **After abrupt withdrawal:** gastritis, nausea, vomiting, dizziness, tremors, feeling of warmth or cold, sweating, tachycardia, headache, insomnia.

INTERACTIONS | **NURSING CONSIDERATIONS**

- Tell patient to use sunscreening agents and protective clothing to avoid photosensitivity reactions.
- Warn against activities that require alertness or good psychomotor coordination until CNS response to drug is determined. Drowsiness and dizziness usually subside after a few weeks.
- Obtain baseline measures of blood pressure before starting therapy and monitor regularly. Watch for orthostatic hypotension, especially with parenteral administration. Keep patient supine for 1 hour afterward. Advise patient to change positions slowly.
- Give deep I.M. only in upper outer quadrant of buttocks. Massage slowly afterward to prevent sterile abscess. Injection may sting.
- Do not withdraw drug abruptly unless required by severe side effects.
- Protect drug from light. Slight yellowing of injection or concentrate is common; does not affect potency. Discard markedly discolored solutions.
- Prevent contact dermatitis by keeping drug off patient's skin and clothes.
- Dilute liquid concentrate with fruit juice, milk, carbonated beverage, or semisolid food just before giving. Exceptions: oral concentrate causes turbidity or precipitation in colas, black coffee, grape or apple juice, or tea. Do not mix with these liquids.
- Dry mouth may be relieved with sugarless gum, sour hard candy, or rinsing with mouthwash.
- Dose of 8 mg is therapeutic equivalent of 100 mg chlorpromazine.
- For toxicity, see APPENDIX, *Drug Toxicities.*

Antacids: inhibit absorption of oral phenothiazines. Separate antacid and phenothiazine doses by at least 2 hours.
Barbiturates: may decrease phenothiazine effect. Observe patient.

- Contraindicated in coma, CNS depression, bone marrow depression, thrombocytopenia and other blood dyscrasias, subcortical damage, and with use of spinal or epidural anesthetic or adrenergic blocking agents. Use cautiously with other CNS depressants, anticholinergics; in elderly or debilitated patients; in patients with hepatic disease, arteriosclerosis or cardiovascular disease (may cause sudden drop in blood pressure), exposure to extreme heat or cold (including antipyretic therapy), respiratory disorders, hypocalcemia, convulsive disorders (may lower seizure threshold), severe reactions to insulin or electroshock therapy, suspected brain tumor or intestinal obstruction, glaucoma, or prostatic hypertrophy.
- Hold dose and notify doctor if patient develops jaundice, symptoms of blood dyscrasias (fever, sore throat, infection, cellulitis, weakness), persistent (longer than a few hours) extrapyramidal reactions, or any such reactions during pregnancy.
- Monitor therapy by weekly bilirubin tests during first month, periodic blood tests (CBC, liver function), and ophthalmic tests (long-term use).
- Check intake/output for urinary retention or constipation.
- Tell patient to use sunscreening agents and protective clothing to avoid photosensitivity reactions.
- Monitor blood pressure. Obtain baseline measures of blood pressure before starting therapy. Watch for orthostatic hypotension.
- Warn against activities that require alertness or good psychomotor coordination until CNS response to drug is determined. Drowsiness and dizziness usually subside after a few weeks.
- Avoid combining with alcohol or other depressants.
- Do not withdraw drug abruptly unless required by severe side effects.
- Dry mouth may be relieved with sugarless gum, sour hard candy, or rinsing with mouthwash.

(continued on following page)

NAME	INDICATIONS & DOSAGE	SIDE EFFECTS
piperacetazine *(continued)*		
prochlorperazine edisylate **prochlorperazine maleate** Compazine, Stemetil♦♦	*Mild-to-moderate emotional disturbances—* **Adults:** 5 to 10 mg P.O. t.i.d. or q.i.d.; extended-release 15 mg P.O. in a.m. or 10 mg q 12 hours; 25 mg rectally b.i.d.; 5 to 10 mg I.M. q 3 to 4 hours. **Children weighing 18 to 38.5 kg:** 5 mg P.O. or rectally b.i.d., to maximum of 15 mg daily. **Children weighing 13.5 to 17.5 kg:** 2.5 mg P.O. or rectally b.i.d. or t.i.d., up to maximum 10 mg daily. **Children weighing 9 to 13 kg:** 2.5 mg P.O. or rectally daily or b.i.d. to maximum 7.5 mg daily. I.M. dose 0.13 mg/kg; repeat if necessary. Not recommended in children under 9 kg. *Psychomotor agitation in schizophrenia; manic phase of manic-depressive psychosis; involutional toxic and senile psychoses—* **Adults:** initially, 10 mg P.O. t.i.d. to q.i.d., increasing up to 50 to 150 mg daily; or 10 to 20 mg I.M. q 1 to 4 hours, p.r.n., up to 100 mg daily, until symptoms are controlled. Prolonged I.M. dosage 10 to 20 mg q 4 to 6 hours.	**Blood:** *transient leukopenia, agranulocytosis.* **CNS:** *extrapyramidal reactions (high incidence),* sedation (low incidence), pseudoparkinsonism, EEG changes, dizziness. **CV:** *orthostatic hypotension,* tachycardia, EKG changes. **EENT:** *ocular changes, blurred vision.* **GI:** *dry mouth, constipation.* **GU:** *urinary retention,* dark urine, menstrual irregularities, gynecomastia, inhibited ejaculation. **Hepatic:** *cholestatic jaundice, abnormal liver function tests.* **Metabolic:** hyperprolactinemia. **Skin:** *mild photosensitivity,* dermal allergic reactions, *exfoliative dermatitis.* **Local:** pain at I.M. injection site, sterile abscess. **Other:** weight gain, increased appetite. **After abrupt withdrawal:** gastritis, nausea, vomiting, dizziness, tremors, feeling of warmth or cold, sweating, tachycardia, headache, insomnia.

♦ Available in U.S. and Canada. ♦♦ Available in Canada only. All other products (no symbol) available in U.S. only. Italicized side effects are common or life-threatening.

INTERACTIONS	NURSING CONSIDERATIONS
	• Protect tablets from light. • Drug is a piperidine phenothiazine. • Dose of 10 mg is therapeutic equivalent of 100 mg chlorpromazine. • For toxicity, see APPENDIX, *Drug Toxicities*.
Antacids: inhibit absorption of oral phenothiazines. Separate antacid and phenothiazine doses by at least 2 hours. *Barbiturates:* may decrease phenothiazine effect. Observe patient.	• Contraindicated in coma, depression, CNS depression, bone marrow depression, subcortical damage, pediatric surgery, and with use of spinal or epidural anesthetic, adrenergic blocking agents, or alcohol. Use cautiously with other CNS depressants, anticholinergics; in elderly or debilitated patients; in patients with hepatic disease, arteriosclerosis or cardiovascular disease (may cause sudden drop in blood pressure), exposure to extreme heat or cold (including antipyretic therapy), respiratory disorders, hypocalcemia, vomiting in children, convulsive disorders (may lower seizure threshold) or severe reactions to insulin or electroshock therapy, suspected brain tumor or intestinal obstruction, glaucoma, or prostatic hypertrophy; and in acutely ill or dehydrated children. • Hold dose and notify doctor if patient develops jaundice, symptoms of blood dyscrasias (fever, sore throat, infection, cellulitis, weakness), persistent (longer than a few hours) extrapyramidal reactions, or any such reactions during pregnancy or in children. • Monitor therapy by weekly bilirubin tests during first month, periodic blood tests (CBC, liver function), and ophthalmic tests (long-term use). • Check intake/output for urinary retention or constipation. • Tell patient to use sunscreening agents and protective clothing to avoid photosensitivity reactions. • Warn against activities that require alertness or good psychomotor coordination until CNS response to drug is determined. Drowsiness and dizziness usually subside after a few weeks. • Avoid combining with alcohol or other depressants. • Obtain baseline measures of blood pressure. Monitor blood pressure and heart rate regularly. Watch for orthostatic hypotension, especially with parenteral administration. Advise patient to change positions slowly. • Give deep I.M. only in upper outer quadrant of buttocks. Massage slowly afterward to prevent sterile abscess. Injection may sting. • Do not mix in same syringe with another drug. • Do not give subcutaneously. • Protect from light. Slight yellowing of injection or concentrate is common; does not affect potency. Discard markedly discolored solutions. • Prevent contact dermatitis by keeping drug off patient's skin and clothes. • Dilute liquid concentrate with at least 60 ml fruit juice, milk, coffee, tea, carbonated beverages, or semisolid food just before giving. • Do not withdraw drug abruptly unless required by severe side effects. • Dry mouth may be relieved with sugarless gum, sour hard candy, or rinsing with mouthwash. • Piperazine phenothiazine; most commonly used as an antiemetic. • If more than 4 doses are needed in 24-hour period, notify doctor. • Injectable form may be mixed with solutions of 5% dextrose, 10% dextrose, 10% fructose, 5% invert sugar, 10% invert sugar, normal saline, Ringer's injection, lactated Ringer's I.V. infusion, and dextrose-saline combinations. • For toxicity, see APPENDIX, *Drug Toxicities*.

NAME	INDICATIONS & DOSAGE	SIDE EFFECTS
promazine hydrochloride Promabec◆◆, Promanyl◆◆, Promazettes◆◆, Sparine◆	*Psychosis—* **Adults:** 25 to 200 mg P.O. or I.M. q 4 to 6 hours, up to 1 g daily. I.V. dose in concentrations no greater than 25 mg/ml for acutely agitated patients. Initial dose 50 to 150 mg; repeat within 5 to 10 minutes if necessary. **Children over 12 years:** 10 to 25 mg P.O. or I.M. q 4 to 6 hours.	**Blood:** *transient leukopenia, agranulocytosis.* **CNS:** *extrapyramidal reactions (moderate incidence), sedation (high incidence),* pseudoparkinsonism, EEG changes, dizziness. **CV:** *orthostatic hypotension,* tachycardia, EKG changes. **EENT:** *ocular changes, blurred vision.* **GI:** *dry mouth, constipation.* **GU:** *urinary retention,* dark urine, menstrual irregularities, gynecomastia, inhibited ejaculation. **Hepatic:** *cholestatic jaundice, abnormal liver function tests.* **Metabolic:** hyperprolactinemia. **Skin:** *mild photosensitivity,* dermal allergic reactions, *exfoliative dermatitis.* **Local:** pain at I.M. injection site, sterile abscess. **Other:** weight gain, increased appetite. **After abrupt withdrawal:** gastritis, nausea, vomiting, dizziness, tremors, feeling of warmth or cold, sweating, tachycardia, headache, insomnia.
thioridazine hydrochloride Mellaril◆, Novoridazine◆◆	*Psychosis—* **Adults:** initially, 50 to 100 mg P.O. t.i.d., with gradual increments up to 800 mg daily in divided doses, if needed. Dosage varies. Dose above 800 mg may be associated with ocular toxicity (pigmentary retinopathy). *Depressive neurosis, alcohol withdrawal, dementia in geriatric patients, behavioral prob-*	**Blood:** *transient leukopenias, agranulocytosis.* **CNS:** extrapyramidal reactions (low incidence), *sedation (high incidence),* EEG changes, dizziness. **CV:** *orthostatic hypotension,* tachycardia, EKG changes. **EENT:** *ocular changes, blurred vision,* pigmentary retinopathy. **GI:** *dry mouth, constipation.*

◆ Available in U.S. and Canada. ◆◆ Available in Canada only. All other products (no symbol) available in U.S. only. Italicized side effects are common or life-threatening.

INTERACTIONS	NURSING CONSIDERATIONS
Antacids: inhibit absorption of oral phenotniazines. Separate antacid and phenothiazine doses by at least 2 hours. *Anticholinergics (including antidepressant and antiparkinson agents):* increased anticholinergic activity, aggravated parkinson-like symptoms. Use with caution. *Barbiturates:* may decrease phenothiazine effect. Observe patient.	• Contraindicated in coma, CNS depression, bone marrow depression, subcortical damage, and with use of spinal or epidural anesthetic or adrenergic blocking agents. Use cautiously with other CNS depressants, anticholinergics; in elderly or debilitated patients; in patients with hepatic disease, arteriosclerosis or cardiovascular disease (may cause sudden drop in blood pressure), exposure to extreme heat or cold (including antipyretic therapy), respiratory disorders, hypocalcemia, convulsive disorders (may lower seizure threshold), severe reactions to insulin or electroshock therapy, suspected brain tumor or intestinal obstruction, glaucoma, prostatic hypertrophy; and in acutely ill or dehydrated children. • Hold dose and notify doctor if patient develops jaundice, symptoms of blood dyscrasias (fever, sore throat, infection, cellulitis, weakness), persistent (longer than a few hours) extrapyramidal reactions, or such reactions during pregnancy or in children. • Monitor therapy by weekly bilirubin tests during first month, periodic blood tests (CBC, liver function), and ophthalmic tests (long-term use). • Check intake/output for urinary retention or constipation. • Tell patient to use sunscreening agents and protective clothing to avoid photosensitivity reactions. • Warn against activities that require alertness or good psychomotor coordination until CNS response to drug is determined. Drowsiness and dizziness usually subside after a few weeks. • Avoid combining with alcohol or other depressants. • Monitor blood pressure with patient lying and standing before starting therapy, and routinely throughout course of treatment. • Watch for orthostatic hypotension, especially with parenteral administration. Keep patient supine for 1 hour afterward. Advise patient to change positions slowly. • Give deep I.M. only in upper outer quadrant of buttocks. Massage slowly afterward to prevent sterile abscess. Injection may sting. • Protect drug from light. Slight yellowing of injection or concentrate is common; does not affect potency. Discard markedly discolored solutions. • Prevent contact dermatitis by keeping drug off patient's skin and clothes. • Dilute liquid concentrate with fruit juice, milk, semisolid food, or chocolate-flavored drinks just before giving. For best taste, use at least 10 ml of diluent per 25 mg drug. • Do not withdraw drug abruptly unless required by severe side effects. • Dry mouth may be relieved with sugarless gum, sour hard candy, or rinsing with mouthwash. • Drug is an aliphatic phenothiazine; it's seldom prescribed for psychiatric treatment.
Antacids: inhibit absorption of oral phenothiazines. Separate antacid and phenothiazine doses by at least 2 hours. *Barbiturates:* may decrease phenothiazine effect. Observe patient.	• Contraindicated in coma, CNS depression, bone marrow depression, hypertensive or hypotensive cardiac disease, subcortical damage, and with use of spinal or epidural anesthetic or adrenergic blocking agents. Use cautiously with other CNS depressants, anticholinergics; in elderly or debilitated patients; in patients with hepatic disease, arteriosclerosis or cardiovascular disease (may cause sudden drop in blood pressure), exposure to extreme heat or cold (including antipyretic therapy), respiratory disorders, hypocalcemia, convulsive disorders, severe reactions to insulin or electroshock therapy, suspected brain tumor or intestinal obstruction, glaucoma, or prostatic hypertrophy; and in acutely ill or dehydrated children.

(continued on following page)

NAME	INDICATIONS & DOSAGE	SIDE EFFECTS
thioridazine hydrochloride *(continued)*	*lems in children—* **Adults:** initially, 25 mg P.O. t.i.d. Maintenance dose is 20 to 200 mg daily. **Children over 2 years:** 0.5 to 3 mg/kg daily in divided doses.	**GU:** *urinary retention,* dark urine, menstrual irregularities, gynecomastia, inhibited ejaculation. **Hepatic:** *cholestatic jaundice.* **Metabolic:** hyperprolactinemia. **Skin:** *mild photosensitivity,* dermal allergic reactions, *exfoliative dermatitis.* **Other:** weight gain, increased appetite. **After abrupt withdrawal:** gastritis, nausea, vomiting, dizziness, tremors, feeling of warmth or cold, sweating, tachycardia, headache, insomnia.
thiothixene **thiothixene hydrochloride** Navane♦	*Acute agitation—* **Adults:** 4 mg I.M. b.i.d. to q.i.d. Maximum 30 mg daily I.M. Change to P.O. as soon as possible. *Mild-to-moderate psychosis—* **Adults:** initially, 2 mg P.O. t.i.d. May increase gradually to 15 mg daily. *Severe psychosis—* **Adults:** initially, 5 mg P.O. b.i.d. May increase gradually to 15 to 30 mg daily. Maximum recommended daily dose 60 mg. Not recommended in children under 12 years.	**Blood:** *transient leukopenia, agranulocytosis.* **CNS:** *extrapyramidal reactions (high incidence),* sedation (low incidence), pseudoparkinsonism, EEG changes, dizziness. **CV:** *orthostatic hypotension,* tachycardia, EKG changes. **EENT:** *ocular changes, blurred vision.* **GI:** *dry mouth, constipation.* **GU:** *urinary retention,* dark urine, menstrual irregularities, gynecomastia, inhibited ejaculation. **Hepatic:** *cholestatic jaundice.* **Metabolic:** hyperprolactinemia. **Skin:** *mild photosensitivity,* dermal allergic reactions, *exfoliative dermatitis.* **Local:** pain at I.M. injection site, sterile abscess. **Other:** weight gain, increased appetite. **After abrupt withdrawal:** gastritis, nausea, vomiting, dizziness,

♦ Available in U.S. and Canada. ♦♦ Available in Canada only. All other products (no symbol) available in U.S. only. Italicized side effects are common or life-threatening.

INTERACTIONS	NURSING CONSIDERATIONS
	• Hold dose and notify doctor if patient develops jaundice, symptoms of blood dyscrasias (fever, sore throat, infection, cellulitis, weakness), persistent (longer than a few hours) extrapyramidal reactions, or such reactions during pregnancy or in children. • Monitor therapy by weekly bilirubin tests during first month, periodic blood tests (CBC, liver function), and ophthalmic tests (long-term therapy). • Check intake/output for urinary retention or constipation. • Watch for blurred vision, dry mouth; high incidence of anticholinergic effects. • Tell patient to use sunscreening agents and protective clothing to avoid photosensitivity reactions. • Monitor blood pressure. • Warn against activities that require alertness or good psychomotor coordination until response to drug is determined. Drowsiness and dizziness usually subside after a few weeks. • Avoid combining with alcohol or other depressants. • Watch for orthostatic hypotension, especially with parenteral administration. Advise patient to change positions slowly. • Prevent contact dermatitis by keeping drug off patient's skin and clothes. • Dilute liquid concentrate with water or fruit juice just before giving. • Do not withdraw abruptly unless required by severe side effects. • Dry mouth may be relieved with sugarless gum, sour hard candy, or rinsing with mouthwash. • Piperidine phenothiazine; used to continue antipsychotic therapy when parkinsonian effects require withdrawal of other phenothiazines. • Dose of 100 mg is the therapeutic equivalent of 100 mg chlorpromazine. • For toxicity, see APPENDIX, *Drug Toxicities*.
None significant.	• Contraindicated in convulsive seizures, circulatory collapse, coma, CNS depression, blood dyscrasias, bone marrow depression, alcohol withdrawal, akathisia or restlessness, subcortical damage, and with use of spinal or epidural anesthetic or adrenergic blocking agents. Use cautiously with other CNS depressants, anticholinergics; in elderly or debilitated patients; and in patients with hepatic disease, arteriosclerosis or cardiovascular disease (may cause sudden drop in blood pressure), exposure to extreme heat or cold (including antipyretic therapy) or undue sunlight, respiratory disorders, hypocalcemia, severe reactions to insulin or electroshock therapy, suspected brain tumor or intestinal obstruction, glaucoma, or prostatic hypertrophy. • Hold dose and notify doctor if patient develops jaundice, symptoms of blood dyscrasias (fever, sore throat, infection, cellulitis, weakness), persistent (longer than a few hours) extrapyramidal reactions, or any such reactions during pregnancy. • Monitor therapy by weekly bilirubin tests during first month, periodic blood tests (CBC, liver function), and ophthalmic tests (long-term therapy). • Check intake/output for urinary retention or constipation. • Tell patient to use sunscreening agents and protective clothing to avoid photosensitivity reactions. • Warn against activities that require alertness or good psychomotor coordination until CNS response to drug is determined. Drowsiness and dizziness usually subside after a few weeks. • Avoid combining with alcohol or other depressants. • Watch for orthostatic hypotension, especially with parenteral

(continued on following page)

NAME	INDICATIONS & DOSAGE	SIDE EFFECTS
thiothixene *(continued)*		tremors, feeling of warmth or cold, sweating, tachycardia, headache, insomnia.
trifluoperazine hydrochloride Clinazine♦♦, Novoflurazine♦♦, Pentazine♦♦, Solazine♦♦, Stelazine♦, Terfluzine♦♦, Triflurin♦♦, Tripazine♦♦	*Anxiety states—* **Adults:** 1 to 2 mg P.O. b.i.d. *Schizophrenia and other psychotic disorders—* **Adults:** outpatients—1 to 2 mg P.O. b.i.d., up to 4 mg daily; hospitalized—2 to 5 mg P.O. b.i.d.; may gradually increase to 40 mg daily. 1 to 2 mg I.M. q 4 to 6 hours, p.r.n. More than 6 mg daily is rarely needed. **Children 6 to 12 years (hospitalized or under close supervision):** 1 mg P.O. daily or b.i.d.; may increase gradually to 15 mg daily.	**Blood:** *transient leukopenia, agranulocytosis.* **CNS:** *extrapyramidal reactions (high incidence),* sedation (low incidence), pseudoparkinsonism, EEG changes, dizziness. **CV:** *orthostatic hypotension,* tachycardia, EKG changes. **EENT:** *ocular changes, blurred vision.* **GI:** *dry mouth, constipation.* **GU:** *urinary retention,* dark urine, menstrual irregularities, gynecomastia, inhibited ejaculation. **Hepatic:** *cholestatic jaundice.* **Metabolic:** hyperprolactinemia. **Skin:** *mild photosensitivity,* dermal allergic reactions, *exfoliative dermatitis.* **Local:** pain at I.M. injection site, sterile abscess. **Other:** weight gain, increased appetite. **After abrupt withdrawal:** gastritis, nausea, vomiting, dizziness, tremors, feeling of warmth or cold, sweating, tachycardia, headache, insomnia.

♦ Available in U.S. and Canada. ♦♦ Available in Canada only. All other products (no symbol) available in U.S. only. Italicized side effects are common or life-threatening.

INTERACTIONS	NURSING CONSIDERATIONS
	administration. Keep patient supine for 1 hour afterward. Advise patient to change positions slowly. • Give I.M. only in upper outer quadrant of buttocks or midlateral thigh. Massage slowly afterward to prevent sterile abscess. Injection may sting. • I.M. form must be stored in refrigerator. • Slight yellowing of injection or concentrate is common; does not affect potency. Discard markedly discolored solutions. • Prevent contact dermatitis by keeping drug off patient's skin and clothes. • Dilute liquid concentrate with fruit juice, milk, or semisolid food just before giving. • Do not withdraw abruptly unless required by severe side effects. • Dry mouth may be relieved with sugarless gum, sour hard candy, or rinsing with mouthwash. • Drug is a thioxanthene derivative but produces responses similar to phenothiazines and butyrophenones. • Dose of 4 mg is therapeutic equivalent of 100 mg chlorpromazine.
Antacids: inhibit absorption of oral phenothiazines. Separate antacid and phenothiazine doses by at least 2 hours. *Barbiturates:* may decrease phenothiazine effect. Observe patient.	• Contraindicated in coma, CNS depression, bone marrow depression, subcortical damage, and with use of spinal or epidural anesthetic or adrenergic blocking agents. Use cautiously with other CNS depressants, anticholinergics; in elderly or debilitated patients; in patients with hepatic disease, arteriosclerosis or cardiovascular disease (may cause drop in blood pressure), exposure to extreme heat or cold (including antipyretic therapy), respiratory disorders, hypocalcemia, convulsive disorders, severe reactions to insulin or electroshock therapy, suspected brain tumor or intestinal obstruction, glaucoma, or prostatic hypertrophy; and in acutely ill or dehydrated children. • Hold dose and notify doctor if patient develops jaundice, symptoms of blood dyscrasias (fever, sore throat, infection, cellulitis, weakness), persistent (longer than a few hours) extrapyramidal reactions, or any such reactions during pregnancy or in children. • Monitor therapy by weekly bilirubin tests during first month, periodic blood tests (CBC, liver function), and ophthalmic tests (long-term therapy). • Check intake/output for urinary retention or constipation. • Tell patient to use sunscreening agents and protective clothing to avoid photosensitivity reactions. • Warn against activities that require alertness or good psychomotor coordination until CNS response to drug is determined. Drowsiness and dizziness usually subside after a few weeks. • Avoid combining with alcohol or other depressants. • Watch for orthostatic hypotension, especially with parenteral administration. Keep patient supine for 1 hour afterward. Advise patient to change positions slowly. • Give deep I.M. only in upper outer quadrant of buttocks. Massage slowly afterward to prevent sterile abscess. Injection may sting. • Protect drug from light. Slight yellowing of injection or concentrate is common; does not affect potency. Discard markedly discolored solutions. • Prevent contact dermatitis by keeping drug off patient's skin and clothes. • Dilute liquid concentrate with 60 ml of tomato or fruit juice, carbonated beverages, coffee, tea, milk, water, or semisolid food just before giving. • Do not withdraw abruptly unless required by severe side effects. • Dry mouth may be relieved with sugarless gum, sour hard candy, or rinsing with mouthwash.

(continued on following page)

NAME	INDICATIONS & DOSAGE	SIDE EFFECTS
trifluoperazine hydrochloride *(continued)*		
triflupromazine hydrochloride Vesprin	*Acute, severe agitation—* **Adults:** 60 to 150 mg I.M. in 2 or 3 divided doses. **Children over 2½ years:** 0.2 to 0.25 mg/kg in divided doses. Maximum dose 10 mg daily. *Nausea and vomiting—* **Adults:** 20 to 30 mg P.O. daily; or 1 to 3 mg I.V. daily; or 5 to 15 mg I.M. daily up to maximum 60 mg daily. **Children:** 0.2 mg/kg P.O. or I.M. up to maximum 10 mg daily. *Psychotic disorders (mild-to-moderate symptoms)—* **Adults:** 10 to 25 mg P.O. b.i.d. **Children over 2½ years:** 10 mg P.O. t.i.d. **Elderly or debilitated patients:** 10 mg P.O. b.i.d. or t.i.d.; increase gradually to desired effect. *Severe symptoms—* **Adults:** 50 mg P.O. b.i.d. or t.i.d. **Children over 2½ years:** 2 mg/kg P.O. in 3 divided doses; may increase gradually to 150 mg daily.	**Blood:** *transient leukopenia, agranulocytosis.* **CNS:** *extrapyramidal reactions (moderate incidence), sedation (high incidence),* pseudoparkinsonism, EEG changes, dizziness. **CV:** *orthostatic hypotension,* tachycardia, EKG changes. **EENT:** *ocular changes, blurred vision.* **GI:** *dry mouth, constipation.* **GU:** *urinary retention,* dark urine, menstrual irregularities, gynecomastia, inhibited ejaculation. **Hepatic:** *cholestatic jaundice.* **Metabolic:** hyperprolactinemia. **Skin:** *mild photosensitivity,* dermal allergic reactions, *exfoliative dermatitis.* **Local:** pain at I.M. injection site, sterile abscess. **Other:** weight gain, increased appetite. **After abrupt withdrawal:** gastritis, nausea, vomiting, dizziness, tremors, feeling of warmth or cold, sweating, tachycardia, headache, insomnia.

♦ Available in U.S. and Canada. ♦♦ Available in Canada only. All other products (no symbol) available in U.S. only. Italicized side effects are common or life-threatening.

INTERACTIONS	NURSING CONSIDERATIONS
	• Drug is a prototype piperazine phenothiazine. • Dose of 5 mg is therapeutic equivalent of 100 mg chlorpromazine. • For toxicity, see APPENDIX, *Drug Toxicities.*
Antacids: inhibit absorption of oral phenothiazines. Separate antacid and phenothiazine doses by at least 2 hours. *Anticholinergics (including antidepressant and antiparkinson agents):* increased anticholinergic activity, aggravated parkinson-like symptoms. Use with caution. *Barbiturates:* may decrease phenothiazine effect. Observe patient.	• Contraindicated in coma, CNS depression, blood dyscrasias, bone marrow depression, subcortical brain damage, and with use of spinal or epidural anesthetic or adrenergic blocking agents. Use cautiously with other CNS depressants, anticholinergics; in elderly or debilitated patients; in patients with hepatic disease, arteriosclerosis or cardiovascular disease (may cause sudden drop in blood pressure), exposure to extreme heat or cold (including antipyretic therapy), respiratory disorders, pheochromocytoma, hypocalcemia, convulsive disorders, severe reactions to insulin or electroshock therapy, suspected brain tumor or intestinal obstruction, glaucoma, prostatic hypertrophy; and in acutely ill or dehydrated children. • Hold dose and notify doctor if patient develops jaundice, symptoms of blood dyscrasias (fever, sore throat, infection, cellulitis, weakness), persistent (longer than a few hours) extrapyramidal reactions, or any such reactions during pregnancy or in children. • Monitor therapy by weekly bilirubin tests during first month, periodic blood tests (CBC, liver function), and ophthalmic tests in long-term therapy. • Check intake/output for urinary retention or constipation. • Watch for hypothermia reactions. • Tell patient to use sunscreening agents and protective clothing to avoid photosensitivity reactions. • Warn against activities that require alertness or good psychomotor coordination until response to drug is determined. Drowsiness and dizziness usually subside after a few weeks. • Avoid combining with alcohol or other depressants. • Watch for orthostatic hypotension, especially with parenteral administration. Keep patient supine for 1 hour afterward. Advise patient to change positions slowly. • Give I.M. only in upper outer quadrant of buttocks. Massage slowly afterward to prevent sterile abscess. Injection may sting. • Protect drug from light. Slight yellowing of injection or concentrate is common; does not affect potency. Discard markedly discolored solutions. • Keep liquid suspension tightly closed. • Prevent contact dermatitis by keeping drug off patient's skin and clothes. • Do not withdraw abruptly unless required by severe side effects. • Dry mouth may be relieved with sugarless gum, sour hard candy, or rinsing with mouthwash. • Drug is an aliphatic phenothiazine. • Dose of 25 mg is therapeutic equivalent of 10 mg chlorpromazine.

34 Miscellaneous psychotherapeutics

lithium carbonate
lithium citrate

Lithium salts have been used throughout the world for more than 20 years to combat manic-depressive illness (bipolar disorders). In the United States, however, lithium has been used only since 1970. (Many deaths had occurred during the 1940s when lithium was improperly used as a salt substitute.)

Under proper supervision, lithium may prevent up to 80% of manic and depressive episodes. Episodes that occur during lithium therapy are usually less severe and shorter than those that might occur without such therapy. Close monitoring to maintain therapeutic lithium blood levels allows safe use of this drug. However, lithium's toxic level is very close to its therapeutic level.

Consistent dietary sodium and fluid intake are necessary every day to help prevent toxicity. Conditions that may

PATIENT-TEACHING AID

WHAT YOU SHOULD KNOW ABOUT LITHIUM

Dear Patient:

To get the most from your drug therapy, follow these instructions carefully:

- If you experience diarrhea, vomiting, drowsiness, muscle weakness and coordination failure, tremors, restlessness, or confusion, call the doctor immediately. But don't abruptly stop taking your drug.
- Expect transient nausea, frequent urination, and thirst during the first few days of therapy.
- Expect a time lag of 1 to 3 weeks before you notice the drug's beneficial effects.
- Avoid activities that require complete mental alertness, such as operating machinery or driving, until your response to the drug is determined.
- Don't switch brands of lithium without asking the doctor first.
- Drink a full glass of water when you take your medication. Also, taking your medication after meals helps minimize nausea.
- Carry an identification card that gives instructions and toxicity and emergency information (available from your pharmacy).

HOW TO DETERMINE DAILY LITHIUM DOSAGE

Oral administration of lithium can effectively control recurrent and chronic mania. Lithium does not impair intellectual activity, consciousness, or range or quality of emotional life. It does help patients to fully experience joy, grief, tenderness, sexual desire, and other normal effects.

When determining daily dosage, the blood lithium concentration should be maintained between 1 and 1.5 mEq/liter, which may be measured with a flame photometer. For long-term control, the blood levels should be adjusted to remain between 0.6 and 1.5 mEq/liter, which usually requires 300 mg P.O. three times daily.

To determine the appropriate daily lithium dosage:

- Give a 600-mg priming dose.
- Measure lithium level in a blood sample collected 24 hours later. Next, refer to the chart below to match the 24-hour blood level to the dosage required. (This chart minimizes blood fluctuation between 0.6 and 1.2 mEq/liter.)

If patient's 24-hour blood level after single loading dose is:	Lithium dosage required is:
less than 0.05	1,200 mg three times a day
0.05 to 0.09	900 mg three times a day
0.10 to 0.14	600 mg three times a day
0.15 to 0.19	300 mg four times a day
0.20 to 0.23	300 mg three times a day
0.24 to 0.3	300 mg twice a day
more than 0.3	300 mg twice a day*

Toxicity may occur if blood levels are more than 1.5 mEq/liter. Signs to watch for include nausea, abdominal cramps, vomiting, diarrhea, thirst, and polyuria. Reverse the toxic symptoms by promptly discontinuing the drug.

*Use extreme caution.

cause excess sodium and water loss (such as sweating or diarrhea) may require supplemental fluid or salt administration.

Major uses

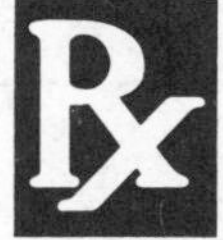

Lithium salts are used to treat acute manic or hypomanic episodes of manic-depressive disorders and to prevent their recurrence.

They're also used investigationally to stimulate white cell production in patients receiving antineoplastic drugs.

Mechanism of action

Lithium alters chemical transmitters in the central nervous system, possibly by interfering with ionic pump mechanisms in brain cells.

Its exact mechanism of action in mania, however, is unknown.

Absorption, distribution, metabolism, and excretion

Lithium is readily absorbed orally. It is distributed to body tissues, with highest concentrations in the kidneys and lowest concentrations in brain tissue. The drug is almost entirely excreted through the kidneys as unchanged lithium ions.

Onset and duration

Blood levels of lithium peak within 2 to 4 hours. The antimanic action is delayed for 5 to 10 days.

Combination products

None.

NAME	INDICATIONS & DOSAGE	SIDE EFFECTS
lithium carbonate Carbolith♦♦, Eskalith, Lithane♦, Lithizine♦♦, Lithobid, Lithonate, Lithotabs **lithium citrate** Lithonate-S	*Prevention or control of mania*— **Adults:** 300 to 600 mg P.O. up to 4 times daily, increasing on the basis of blood levels to achieve optimal dosage. Recommended therapeutic lithium blood levels: 1 to 1.5 mEq/liter for acute mania; 0.6 to 1.2 mEq/liter for maintenance therapy; and 2 mEq/liter as maximum. **Adults:** 5 ml lithium citrate (liquid) contains 8 mEq lithium equal to 300 mg lithium carbonate.	**Blood:** *leukocytosis of 14,000 to 18,000 (reversible).* **CNS:** tremors, drowsiness, headache, confusion, restlessness, dizziness, psychomotor retardation, stupor, lethargy, coma, blackouts, epileptiform seizures, EEG changes, worsened organic brain syndrome, impaired speech, ataxia, muscle weakness, incoordination, hyperexcitability. **CV:** *reversible EKG changes,* arrhythmia, hypotension, peripheral circulatory collapse, allergic vasculitis, ankle and wrist edema. **EENT:** tinnitus, impaired vision. **GI:** nausea, vomiting, anorexia, diarrhea, fecal incontinence, dry mouth, thirst, metallic taste. **GU:** *polyuria,* glycosuria, incontinence, renal toxicity. **Metabolic:** transient hyperglycemia, goiter, hypothyroidism (lowered T_3, T_4, and PBI, but elevated ^{131}I uptake), hyponatremia. **Skin:** pruritus, rash, diminished or lost sensation, drying and thinning of hair.

♦ Available in U.S. and Canada. ♦♦ Available in Canada only. All other products (no symbol) available in U.S. only. Italicized side effects are common or life-threatening.

LITHIUM MAY REDUCE INFECTION RISK DURING CANCER CHEMOTHERAPY

Studies indicate that lithium carbonate may prevent infectious complications in patients undergoing cancer chemotherapy.

In a landmark study reported in the *New England Journal of Medicine* (January 31, 1980), 20 patients were given 300 mg of lithium three times daily, from 24 hours before chemotherapy until 48 hours before the next chemotherapy cycle. Here's how their reactions to chemotherapy differed from 25 patients who hadn't received lithium. →

INTERACTIONS	NURSING CONSIDERATIONS
Diuretics: increased reabsorption of lithium by kidneys, with possible toxic effect. Use with extreme caution, and monitor lithium and electrolyte levels (especially sodium). *Haloperidol:* encephalopathic syndrome (lethargy, tremors, extrapyramidal symptoms). Watch for syndrome, and stop drug if it occurs. *Aminophylline, sodium bicarbonate, and sodium chloride:* ingestion of these salts increases lithium excretion. Avoid salt loads and monitor lithium levels. *Probenecid, methyldopa:* increased effect of lithium. Monitor for lithium toxicity.	• Contraindicated if therapy cannot be closely monitored. Use with caution with haloperidol, other antipsychotics, neuromuscular blocking agents, and diuretics; in elderly or debilitated persons; and in thyroid disease, epilepsy, renal or cardiovascular disease, brain damage, severe debilitation or dehydration, and sodium depletion. • Monitor baseline EKG, thyroid and renal studies, and electrolyte levels. Monitor lithium blood levels 8 to 12 hours after first dose, usually before a.m. dose, two or three times weekly first month, then weekly to monthly on maintenance. • When blood levels of lithium are below 1.5 mEq/liter, side effects generally remain mild. • Check fluid intake and output, especially when surgery is scheduled. • Warn patient and family to watch for signs of toxicity (diarrhea, vomiting, drowsiness, muscle weakness, ataxia) and to expect transient nausea, polyuria, thirst, and discomfort during first few days. Call doctor if toxic symptoms appear, but do not stop drug abruptly. • Expect time lag of 1 to 3 weeks before drug's beneficial effects are noticed. • Weigh patient daily; check for signs of edema or sudden weight gain. • Adjust fluid and salt ingestion to compensate if excessive loss occurs through protracted sweating. Under normal conditions, patients should have fluid intake of 2,500 to 3,000 ml/day and a balanced diet with adequate salt intake. • Have outpatient follow-up of thyroid and renal functions every 6 to 12 months. Palpate thyroid to check for enlargement. • Patient should carry identification/instruction card (available from pharmacy) with toxicity and emergency information. • Warn ambulatory patient to avoid activities that require alertness and good psychomotor coordination until CNS response to drug is determined. • Administer with plenty of water, and after meals to minimize GI upset. • Check urine for specific gravity and report level below 1.015, which may indicate diabetes insipidus syndrome. • Has been used to treat syndrome of inappropriate ADH. • Tell patient not to switch brands of lithium or to take other drugs (prescription or over-the-counter) without doctor's guidance. • Investigationally used to increase white cells in patients undergoing cancer chemotherapy. • Also used investigationally for treatment of cluster headaches, aggression, organic brain syndrome, and tardive dyskinesia. • For toxicity, see APPENDIX, *Drug Toxicities.*

They experienced:
- fewer days with severe neutropenia
- fewer days hospitalized with neutropenia and fever
- no neutropenic febrile episodes, in contrast with six cases in the control group
- no infection-related deaths, in contrast with five in the control group
- significantly longer infection-free survival
- fewer antineoplastic dose reductions
- shorter and less frequent delays in treatment.

Patients given lithium had higher leukocyte and neutrophil counts throughout their chemotherapy treatment than those who were not given lithium.

Thus, this study concludes that administration of lithium between chemotherapy cycles reduces the risk of infection-related mortality, which is due to the leukocyte and neutrophil depression that commonly develops between treatment cycles. However, further study is needed to check the safety and efficacy of this regimen.

35 Cerebral stimulants

amphetamine hydrochloride
amphetamine phosphate
amphetamine sulfate
benzphetamine hydrochloride
caffeine
caffeine, citrated
caffeine sodium benzoate
chlorphentermine hydrochloride
clortermine hydrochloride
deanol acetamidobenzoate
dextroamphetamine phosphate
dextroamphetamine sulfate
diethylpropion hydrochloride
fenfluramine hydrochloride
mazindol
methamphetamine hydrochloride
methylphenidate hydrochloride
pemoline
phendimetrazine tartrate
phenmetrazine hydrochloride
phentermine hydrochloride

Amphetamines are the prototypes for central nervous system (CNS) stimulants. They're the first agents to have been used as appetite suppressants (anorexigenics). Recently, however, the Food and Drug Administration proposed that weight reduction in obesity be deleted as an approved indication for these drugs. Their use as anorexigenics should be limited to short-term weight control only as prescribed by a doctor.

Amphetamines, or "uppers" in street language, are common drugs of abuse (many are pictured in the special color section following p. 75).

Also included in this class are isomers of amphetamines (amphetamine-like drugs). These have less potential for abuse because their euphoric effects aren't as great.

All the agents discussed in this chapter, except caffeine and deanol, are officially listed by the Drug Enforcement Agency as controlled substances.

Major uses

Rx

• The amphetamines and amphetamine-like drugs may suppress appetite, promote weight reduction in exogenous obesity, and supply short-term adjunctive therapy for weight control and dieting.
• Deanol, dextroamphetamine, methamphetamine, methylphenidate, and pemoline are used as therapeutic adjuncts in minimal brain dysfunction in children, such as hyperkinesia.
• Dextroamphetamine and methylphenidate are used to treat narcolepsy.

Mechanism of action

• Amphetamines and amphetamine-like drugs, caffeine, methylphenidate, and pemoline are sympathomimetics whose main sites of activity appear to be the cerebral cortex and the reticular activating system. They probably promote nerve impulse transmission by releasing stored noreinephrine from nerve terminals in the brain.
• In children with hyperkinesia, amphetamines have a paradoxical calming effect that is probably related to the actions of the drug on CNS neurotrans-

mitters. The mechanism by which amphetamines produce mental and behavioral effects in children, however, has not been established.

• Deanol probably elicits a CNS-stimulating effect by increasing brain levels of choline—a precursor of acetylcholine.

Absorption, distribution, metabolism, and excretion

Cerebral stimulants are readily absorbed from the gastrointestinal tract. They are well distributed to most body tissues, with high concentrations in the brain and cerebrospinal fluid.

• Amphetamines and amphetamine-like drugs are excreted by the kidneys, largely unchanged, in about 3 hours. They and fenfluramine hydrochloride are excreted more readily in acidic urine than they are in alkaline urine.

• Caffeine, deanol, and methylphenidate are partially metabolized by the liver and excreted by the kidneys.

• Pemoline probably undergoes the greatest metabolic change of these drugs, with more than 50% being metabolized to pemoline dione, an active metabolite, before being excreted by the kidneys.

Onset and duration

Onset is usually within 1 to 2 hours. Duration is from 4 to 10 hours, with most drugs requiring multiple doses for continued anorexigenic effect. Some are longer-acting (6 to 12 hours).

Combination products

AMPHAPLEX-10/OBETROL-10: dextroamphetamine saccharate 2.5 mg, amphetamine aspartate 2.5 mg, amphetamine sulfate 2.5 mg, and dextroamphetamine sulfate 2.5 mg.

AMPHAPLEX-20/OBETROL-20: dextroamphetamine saccharate 5 mg, amphetamine aspartate 5 mg, amphetamine sulfate 5 mg, and dextroamphetamine sulfate 5 mg.

BIPHETAMINE 12½: dextroamphetamine 6.25 mg and amphetamine 6.25 mg.

BIPHETAMINE 20: dextroamphetamine 10 mg and amphetamine 10 mg.

ESKATROL: dextroamphetamine sulfate 15 mg and prochlorperazine maleate 7.5 mg.

NURSING TIPS

DEALING WITH AMPHETAMINE ADDICTION

Prevention

• Educate the patient concerning the misuse of caffeine and amphetamines.

• Prevent medically induced amphetamine addiction by:

—teaching the obese patient who is taking amphetamines to report such symptoms as nervousness, insomnia, and cardiac palpitations.

—observing the depressed patient who is being treated with amphetamines for insomnia, loss of appetite, restlessness, and agitation.

—watching the patient on powerful central nervous system stimulants such as dextroamphetamine, which is twice as potent as amphetamine. Dextroamphetamine, in large doses, is more likely to cause fatigue, mental depression, increased blood pressure, cyanosis, respiratory failure, disorientation, hallucinations, convulsions, and coma.

• Alert the doctor to drug-induced symptoms you've observed. He may want to stop medication.

Patient care

• Be aware of your own attitude toward drug addiction and abuse. Respect the amphetamine addict as a human being; his motivation will be increased. Be straightforward with him. Be firm in setting limits, but do not irritate or humiliate him unnecessarily when enforcing them.

• Make a special effort to establish a supportive relationship with the addicted patient during his withdrawal from amphetamines. This critical stage of rehabilitation can have a favorable effect on the patient's final recovery.

For more information as well as photographs of drugs of abuse, see special color section following page 75.

NAME	INDICATIONS & DOSAGE	SIDE EFFECTS
amphetamine hydrochloride **amphetamine phosphate** **amphetamine sulfate** Controlled Substance Schedule II Benzedrine♦	*Minimal brain dysfunction—* **Children 6 years and older:** 5 mg P.O. daily, with 5-mg increments weekly, p.r.n. **Children 3 to 5 years:** 2.5 mg P.O. daily, with 2.5-mg increments weekly, p.r.n. *Narcolepsy—* **Adults:** 5 to 60 mg P.O. daily in divided doses. **Children over 12 years:** 10 mg P.O. daily, with 10-mg increments weekly, p.r.n. **Children 6 to 12 years:** 5 mg P.O. daily, with 5-mg increments weekly, p.r.n. *Short-term adjunct in exogenous obesity—* **Adults:** single 10- or 15-mg long-acting capsule daily, or 2 if needed, up to 30 mg daily; or 5 to 30 mg daily in divided doses 30 to 60 minutes before meals. Not recommended for children under 12 years old.	**CNS:** *restlessness,* tremor, *hyperactivity, talkativeness, insomnia,* irritability, dizziness, headache, chills, overstimulation, dysphoria. **CV:** *tachycardia, palpitations,* hypertension, hypotension. **GI:** nausea, vomiting, cramps, dry mouth, diarrhea, constipation, metallic taste, anorexia, weight loss. **Other:** urticaria, impotence, changes in libido.
benzphetamine hydrochloride Controlled Substance Schedule III Didrex	*Short-term adjunct in exogenous obesity—* **Adults:** 25 to 50 mg P.O. daily, b.i.d., or t.i.d.	**CNS:** *restlessness,* tremor, *hyperactivity, talkativeness, insomnia,* irritability, dizziness, headache, chills, overstimulation, dysphoria. **CV:** *tachycardia, palpitations,* hypertension, hypotension. **GI:** nausea, vomiting, cramps, dry mouth, diarrhea, constipation, metallic taste, anorexia, weight loss. **Skin:** urticaria. **Other:** impotence, changes in libido.

♦ Available in U.S. and Canada. ♦♦ Available in Canada only. All other products (no symbol) available in U.S. only. Italicized side effects are common or life-threatening.

INTERACTIONS	NURSING CONSIDERATIONS
MAO inhibitors: severe hypertension; possible hypertensive crisis. Don't use together. *Sodium bicarbonate, acetazolamide:* increased renal reabsorption. Monitor for enhanced effect. *Ammonium chloride, ascorbic acid:* observe for decreased amphetamine effect. *Phenothiazines, haloperidol:* observe for decreased amphetamine effect.	• Contraindicated in symptomatic cardiovascular diseases, hyperthyroidism, nephritis, angina pectoris, moderate to severe hypertension, parkinsonism due to arteriosclerosis, certain types of glaucoma, advanced arteriosclerosis, agitated states, or patients with history of drug abuse. Use with caution in patients with diabetes mellitus and in elderly, debilitated, or hyperexcitable patients. • Psychic dependence or habituation may occur, especially in patients with history of drug addiction. Avoid prolonged administration. When used long-term, lower dosage gradually to prevent acute rebound depression. • When used for obesity, make sure patient is also on a weight-reduction program. Give drug 30 to 60 minutes before meals. • Fatigue may result as drug effects wear off. Patient will need more rest. • Tell patient to avoid caffeine, which increases the effects of amphetamines and related amines. • Check vital signs regularly for signs of excessive stimulation. • Urinary acidification enhances renal excretion; urinary alkalinization enhances renal reabsorption and recycling. • When tolerance to anorexigenic effect develops, dosage should not be increased, but drug discontinued. • Discourage use to combat fatigue. • Warn patient to avoid activities that require alertness or good psychomotor coordination until CNS response to drug is determined. • May alter daily insulin needs in patients with diabetes. Monitor blood and urine sugars. • Use as analeptic is usually discouraged, since CNS stimulation superimposed on CNS depression can lead to neuronal instability and seizures. • May reverse beneficial effect of antihypertensives. Monitor blood pressure.
MAO inhibitors: severe hypertension; possible hypertensive crisis. Don't use together. *Sodium bicarbonate, acetazolamide:* increased renal reabsorption. Monitor for enhanced effects. *Ammonium chloride, ascorbic acid:* observe for decreased benzphetamine effects. *Phenothiazines, haloperidol:* observe for decreased benzphetamine effects.	• Contraindicated in symptomatic cardiovascular diseases, hyperthyroidism, nephritis, angina pectoris, moderate to severe hypertension, parkinsonism due to arteriosclerosis, certain types of glaucoma, advanced arteriosclerosis, agitated states, or patients with history of drug abuse. Use with caution in patients with diabetes mellitus and in elderly, debilitated, or hyperexcitable patients. • Psychic dependence or habituation may occur, especially in patients with history of drug addiction. Avoid prolonged administration. When used long-term, lower dosage gradually to prevent acute rebound depression. • Use in conjunction with weight-reduction program. Give 30 to 60 minutes before meals. • Fatigue may result as drug effects wear off. Patient will need more rest. • Tell patient to avoid caffeine, which increases the effects of amphetamines and related amines. • Check vital signs regularly for signs of excessive stimulation. • Urinary acidification enhances renal excretion; urinary alkalinization enhances renal reabsorption and recycling. • When tolerance to anorexigenic effect develops, dosage should not be increased, but drug discontinued. • Warn patient to avoid activities that require alertness or good psychomotor coordination until CNS response to drug is determined. • May alter daily insulin needs in patients with diabetes. Monitor blood and urine sugars.

NAME	INDICATIONS & DOSAGE	SIDE EFFECTS
caffeine Ban-Drowz, Kirkaffeine, Nodoz, Stim 250, Stim-Tabs, Tirend, Vivarin **caffeine, citrated** **caffeine sodium benzoate injection**	*Respiratory and central nervous system stimulant—* **Adults:** 100 to 200 mg anhydrous caffeine P.O.; 500 mg to 1 g caffeine sodium benzoate I.M. or I.V. in emergency only.	**CNS:** *stimulation, insomnia,* restlessness, nervousness, mild delirium, headache, excitement, agitation, muscle tremors, twitches. **CV:** *tachycardia.* **GI:** nausea, vomiting. **GU:** *diuresis.* **Skin:** hyperesthesia.
chlorphentermine hydrochloride Controlled Substance Schedule III Chlorophen, Pre-Sate♦	*Short-term adjunct in exogenous obesity—* **Adults:** 65 mg P.O. taken after breakfast.	**CNS:** *insomnia,* overstimulation, nervousness, dizziness, paradoxical sedation, headache. **CV:** *tachycardia, palpitations,* increased blood pressure. **GI:** nausea, dry mouth, constipation. **Skin:** urticaria.
clortermine hydrochloride Controlled Substance Schedule III Voranil	*Short-term adjunct in exogenous obesity—* **Adults:** 50 mg P.O. taken at midmorning.	**CNS:** *restlessness,* dizziness, *insomnia,* euphoria, tremor, headache. **CV:** *tachycardia, palpitations,* arrhythmias, increased blood pressure. **GI:** dry mouth, diarrhea, constipation. **Skin:** urticaria. **Other:** impotence, libido changes.
deanol acetamidobenzoate Deaner, Deaner-100♦♦, Deaner-250	*Minimal brain dysfunction—* **Children over 6 years:** initially, 500 mg P.O. daily after breakfast; may reduce to maintenance 250 to 500 mg daily. Dose adjusted to patient's needs and response. *Dyskinesia, blepharospasm—* **Adults:** 600 mg to 1.6 g P.O. daily.	**CNS:** insomnia, mild overstimulation, irritability, headache, muscle twitching, tenseness. **CV:** postural hypotension. **EENT:** increased nasal and oral secretions. **GI:** constipation. **Skin:** transient rash. **Other:** dyspnea.
dextroamphetamine phosphate	*Narcolepsy—* **Adults:** 5 to 60 mg P.O. daily in divided doses.	**CNS:** *restlessness,* tremor, *hyperactivity, talkativeness, insomnia,* irritability, dizziness, headache,

♦ Available in U.S. and Canada. ♦♦ Available in Canada only. All other products (no symbol) available in U.S. only. Italicized side effects are common or life-threatening.

INTERACTIONS	NURSING CONSIDERATIONS
None significant.	• Contraindicated in patients with gastric or duodenal ulcer. • Tolerance or psychological dependence may develop. • Be alert for signs of overdose: GI pain, mild delirium, insomnia, diuresis, dehydration, and fever. Treat with short-acting barbiturates, gastric emesis, or lavage. • Single dose should not exceed 1 g. • Caffeine does not reverse alcohol intoxication or depressant effects of alcohol. Overvigorous therapy with caffeine may aggravate depression in an already depressed patient. • Use as analeptic is discouraged.
MAO inhibitors: severe hypertension; possible hypertensive crisis. Don't use together. *Sodium bicarbonate, acetazolamide:* increased renal reabsorption. Monitor for enhanced effects. *Ammonium chloride, ascorbic acid:* observe for decreased chlorphentermine effects.	• Contraindicated in hyperexcitability states, hyperthyroidism, hypertension, angina pectoris, severe cardiovascular disease, glaucoma, or patients with history of drug abuse. • Psychic dependence and habituation may occur. When tolerance to anorexigenic effect develops, dose should not be increased, but drug discontinued. • May alter daily insulin needs in patients with diabetes. Monitor blood and urine sugars. • Teach patient a good dietary plan and exercise program. • Withdraw drug gradually. • Fatigue may result as drug effects wear off. Patient will need more rest. • Tell patient to avoid caffeine, which increases the effects of amphetamines and related amines. • Check vital signs regularly. Observe for signs of excessive stimulation. • Urinary acidification enhances renal excretion; urinary alkalinization enhances renal reabsorption and recycling.
MAO inhibitors: severe hypertension; possible hypertensive crisis. Don't use together. *Sodium bicarbonate, acetazolamide:* increased renal reabsorption. Monitor for enhanced effects. *Ammonium chloride, ascorbic acid:* observe for decreased clortermine effects.	• Contraindicated in hyperthyroidism, glaucoma, severe hypertension, cardiovascular diseases, agitated states, and patients with history of drug abuse. Use with caution in diabetes mellitus. Insulin requirements may be altered. Monitor blood and urine sugars. • Warn patient to avoid activities that require alertness or good psychomotor coordination until CNS response to drug is determined. • Be sure patient is following a sensible dietary regimen. • Drug should be discontinued when tolerance develops. • Fatigue may result as drug effects wear off. Patient will need more rest. • Tell patient to avoid caffeine, which increases the effects of amphetamines and related amines. • Check vital signs regularly. Observe for signs of excessive stimulation. • Urinary acidification enhances renal excretion; urinary alkalinization enhances renal reabsorption and recycling.
None significant.	• Contraindicated in patients with grand mal epilepsy. • In long-term use, monitor child closely for signs of growth suppression. • Beneficial effects may not appear until after several weeks of therapy. • Used with some success in treatment of tardive dyskinesia.
MAO inhibitors: severe hypertension; possible hypertensive	• Contraindicated in patients with hyperthyroidism, nephritis, severe hypertension, angina pectoris or other severe cardiovascular disease, some types of glaucoma, or history of drug abuse. Use with caution

(continued on following page)

NAME	INDICATIONS & DOSAGE	SIDE EFFECTS
dextroamphetamine *(continued)* **dextroamphetamine sulfate** Controlled Substance Schedule II Dexampex, Dexedrine♦, Ferndex, Robese, Spancap #1 and #4, Tidex	**Children over 12 years:** 10 mg P.O. daily, with 10-mg increments weekly, p.r.n. **Children 6 to 12 years:** 5 mg P.O. daily, with 5-mg increments weekly, p.r.n. *Short-term adjunct in exogenous obesity—* **Adults:** single 10- to 15-mg long-acting capsule, up to 30 mg daily; or in divided doses, 5 to 10 mg ½ hour before meals. *Minimal brain dysfunction—* **Children 6 years and over:** 5 mg once daily or b.i.d., with 5-mg increments weekly, p.r.n. **Children 3 to 5 years:** 2.5 mg P.O. daily, with 2.5-mg increments weekly, p.r.n.	chills, overstimulation, dysphoria. **CV:** *tachycardia, palpitations,* hypertension, hypotension. **GI:** nausea, vomiting, cramps, dry mouth, diarrhea, constipation, metallic taste, anorexia, weight loss. **Skin:** urticaria. **Other:** impotence, changes in libido.
diethylpropion hydrochloride Controlled Substance Schedule IV Dietec♦♦, D.I.P.♦♦, Nobesine♦♦, NuDispoz, Regibon♦♦, Ro-Diet, Tenuate♦, Tepanil	*Short-term adjunct in exogenous obesity—* **Adults:** 25 mg P.O. before meals, t.i.d.; or 75 mg controlled-release tablet P.O. in midmorning.	**CNS:** headache, *nervousness,* dizziness. **CV:** *tachycardia, palpitations,* rise in blood pressure. **EENT:** blurred vision. **GI:** nausea, abdominal cramps, dry mouth, diarrhea, constipation. **Skin:** urticaria. **Other:** impotence, libido changes, menstrual upset.
fenfluramine hydrochloride Controlled Substance Schedule IV Pondimin♦	*Short-term adjunct in exogenous obesity—* **Adults:** initially, 20 mg P.O. t.i.d. before meals. Maximum 40 mg t.i.d. Adjust dosage according to patient's response.	**CNS:** dizziness, incoordination, headache, euphoria or depression, anxiety, *insomnia,* weakness or fatigue, agitation. **CV:** *palpitations,* hypotension, hypertension, chest pain. **EENT:** eye irritation, and blurring of vision. **GI:** diarrhea, dry mouth, nausea, vomiting, abdominal pain,

♦ Available in U.S. and Canada. ♦♦ Available in Canada only. All other products (no symbol) available in U.S. only. Italicized side effects are common or life-threatening.

INTERACTIONS	NURSING CONSIDERATIONS
crisis. Don't use together. *Sodium bicarbonate, acetazolamide:* increased renal reabsorption. Monitor for enhanced amphetamine effects. *Ammonium chloride, ascorbic acid:* observe for decreased amphetamine effects. *Phenothiazines, haloperidol:* observe for decreased amphetamine effects.	in patients with diabetes mellitus and in elderly, debilitated, or hyperexcitable patients. • Psychic dependence or habituation may occur, especially in patients with history of drug addiction. Avoid prolonged administration. When used long-term, lower dosage gradually to prevent acute rebound depression. • When used for obesity, be sure patient is also on a weight-reduction program. Give 30 to 60 minutes before meals. Avoid giving within 6 hours of bedtime. • Fatigue may result as drug effects wear off. Patient will need more rest. • Tell patient to avoid caffeine, which increases the effects of amphetamines and related amines. • Check vital signs regularly. Observe for signs of excessive stimulation. • Urinary acidification enhances renal excretion; urinary alkalinization enhances renal reabsorption and recycling. • When tolerance to anorexigenic effect develops, dosage should not be increased, but drug discontinued. • Discourage use to combat fatigue. • Warn patient to avoid activities that require alertness or good psychomotor coordination until CNS response to drug is determined. • May alter daily insulin needs in patients with diabetes. • Use as analeptic is usually discouraged, since CNS stimulation superimposed on CNS depression can lead to neuronal instability and seizures.
MAO inhibitors: hypertension; possible hypertensive crisis. Don't use together.	• Contraindicated in patients with hyperthyroidism, hypertension, angina pectoris, severe cardiovascular disease, glaucoma, or history of drug abuse. Use with caution in epilepsy, diabetes mellitus, or hyperexcitability states. May alter insulin requirements. Monitor blood and urine sugars. • When tolerance to anorexigenic effect develops, dosage should not be increased, but drug discontinued. • Habituation or psychic dependence may occur. • Be sure patient is also on a weight-reduction program. • Can be used to stop nighttime eating. Rarely causes insomnia. • Fatigue may result as drug effects wear off. Patient will need more rest. • Tell patient to avoid caffeine, which increases the effects of amphetamines and related amines. • Check vital signs regularly. Observe for signs of excessive stimulation. • Urinary acidification enhances renal excretion; urinary alkalinization enhances renal reabsorption and recycling. • Use as analeptic is usually discouraged, since CNS stimulation superimposed on CNS depression can lead to neuronal instability and seizures.
MAO inhibitors: severe hypertension; possible hypertensive crisis. Don't use together.	• Contraindicated in patients with glaucoma, hypersensitivity to sympathomimetic amines, symptomatic cardiovascular disease, alcoholism, or history of drug abuse. Use with caution in patients with hypertension, history of mental depression, diabetes mellitus. • Because of possible hypoglycemia, patients with diabetes may have altered insulin or sulfonylurea requirements. Monitor blood and urine sugars. • Check vital signs regularly. Observe patient for signs of excessive sedation, depression, or excessive stimulation. Closely monitor blood pressure.

(continued on following page)

NAME	INDICATIONS & DOSAGE	SIDE EFFECTS
fenfluramine hydrochloride *(continued)*		constipation. **GU:** dysuria, increased urinary frequency, impotence, increased libido. **Skin:** rashes, urticaria, burning sensation. **Other:** sweating, chills, fever.
mazindol Controlled Substance Schedule IV Sanorex♦	*Short-term adjunct in exogenous obesity—* **Adults:** 1 mg t.i.d. 1 hour before meals, or 2 mg daily 1 hour before lunch. Use lowest effective dose.	**CNS:** *nervousness,* restlessness, dizziness, *insomnia,* dysphoria, headache, depression, drowsiness, weakness, tremors. **CV:** *palpitations, tachycardia.* **GI:** dry mouth, nausea, constipation, diarrhea, unpleasant taste. **GU:** difficulty initiating micturition, impotence, libido changes. **Skin:** rash, clamminess, pallor. **Other:** shivering, excessive sweating.
methamphetamine hydrochloride Controlled Substance Schedule II Desoxyn, Methampex, Obedrin-LA	*Minimal brain dysfunction—* **Children 6 years and over:** 2.5 to 5 mg P.O. once daily or b.i.d., with 5-mg increments weekly, p.r.n. Usual effective dosage is 20 to 25 mg daily. *Short-term adjunct in exogenous obesity—* **Adults:** 2.5 to 5 mg P.O. once to t.i.d. 30 minutes before meals; or 1 long-acting 5- to 15-mg tablet daily before breakfast.	**CNS:** *nervousness, insomnia,* irritability, *talkativeness,* dizziness, headache, hyperexcitability, tremor. **CV:** hypertension or hypotension, *tachycardia, palpitations,* cardiac arrhythmias. **EENT:** blurred vision, mydriasis. **GI:** nausea, vomiting, abdominal cramps, diarrhea or constipation, dry mouth, anorexia, metallic taste. **Skin:** urticaria. **Other:** impotence, libido changes.
methylphenidate hydrochloride Controlled Substance Schedule II Methidate♦♦, Ritalin♦	*Minimal brain dysfunction (hyperkinetic behavior disorders)—* **Children 6 years and over:** initial dose 5 to 10 mg P.O. daily before breakfast and lunch, with 5- to 10-mg increments weekly as needed, up to 60 mg daily. *Narcolepsy—* **Adults:** 10 mg P.O. b.i.d. or t.i.d. ½ hour before meals. Dos-	**CNS:** *nervousness, insomnia,* dizziness, headache, akathisia, dyskinesia. **CV:** *palpitations,* angina, *tachycardia,* changes in blood pressure and pulse rate. **EENT:** difficulty with accommodation and blurring of vision. **GI:** nausea, dry throat, abdominal pain, anorexia, weight loss. **Skin:** rash, urticaria, *exfoliative dermatitis,* erythema multiforme.

♦ Available in U.S. and Canada. ♦♦ Available in Canada only. All other products (no symbol) available in U.S. only. Italicized side effects are common or life-threatening.

INTERACTIONS	NURSING CONSIDERATIONS
	• Be sure patient is on a weight-reduction program. • Tolerance or dependence may occur. Avoid prolonged administration. • Fatigue may result as drug effects wear off. Patient will need more rest. • Tell patient to avoid caffeine, which increases the effects of amphetamines and related amines.
MAO inhibitors: severe hypertension; possible hypertensive crisis. Don't use together.	• Contraindicated in patients with glaucoma, cardiovascular disease including arrhythmias, agitated states, and history of drug abuse. Use with caution in diabetes mellitus, hypertension, hyperexcitability states. • Warn patient to avoid activities that require alertness or good psychomotor coordination until CNS response to drug has been determined. • Fatigue may result as drug effects wear off. Patient will need more rest. • Tell patient to avoid caffeine, which increases the effects of amphetamines and related amines. • Check vital signs regularly. Observe for signs of excessive stimulation. • Tolerance or dependence may develop. Avoid prolonged use. • Be sure patient is also on a weight-reduction program. • May alter insulin needs in patients with diabetes. Monitor blood and urine sugars.
MAO inhibitors: severe hypertension; possible hypertensive crisis. Don't use together. *Sodium bicarbonate, acetazolamide:* increased renal reabsorption. Monitor for enhanced effects. *Ammonium chloride, ascorbic acid:* observe for decreased amphetamine effects. *Phenothiazines, haloperidol:* observe for decreased amphetamine effects.	• Contraindicated in patients with hypertension, hyperthyroidism, nephritis, angina pectoris or other severe cardiovascular disease, glaucoma, parkinsonism due to arteriosclerosis, agitated states, or history of drug abuse. Use with caution in patients with diabetes mellitus; and in patients who are elderly, debilitated, asthenic, psychopathic, or who have a history of suicidal or homicidal tendencies. • Warn that potential for abuse is high. Discourage use to combat fatigue. • May alter insulin needs in patients with diabetes. Monitor blood and urine sugars. • When used for obesity, be sure patient is on a weight-reduction program. • Tell patient to avoid caffeine, which increases the effects of amphetamines and related amines. • Check vital signs regularly. Observe for signs of excessive stimulation. • Urinary acidification enhances renal excretion; urinary alkalinization enhances renal reabsorption and recycling. • When tolerance to anorexigenic effect develops, dosage should not be increased, but drug discontinued. • Warn patient to avoid activities that require alertness or good psychomotor coordination until CNS response to drug is determined.
MAO inhibitors: severe hypertension; possible hypertensive crisis. Don't use together.	• Contraindicated in patients with symptomatic cardiac disease, hyperthyroidism, moderate to severe hypertension, angina pectoris, advanced arteriosclerosis, severe depression of either endogenous or exogenous form, glaucoma, parkinsonism; history of drug abuse or dependency; history of marked anxiety, tension, or agitation. Use with caution in elderly, debilitated, or hyperexcitable patients and those with history of cardiovascular disease, diabetes, or seizures. • Closely monitor blood pressure. Observe for signs of excessive stimulation. • Discourage use to combat fatigue. • Used in treatment for nocturnal enuresis in children. • Observe for interactions, as treatment of other disease states may

(continued on following page)

NAME	INDICATIONS & DOSAGE	SIDE EFFECTS
methylphenidate hydrochloride *(continued)*	age varies with patient needs. Dosage range is 5 to 50 mg daily.	
pemoline Controlled Substance Schedule IV Cylert	*Minimal brain dysfunction*— **Children 6 years and over:** initially, 37.5 mg P.O. given in the morning. Daily dose can be raised by 18.75 mg weekly. Effective dosage range 56.25 to 75 mg daily; maximum is 112.5 mg daily.	**CNS:** *insomnia,* malaise, irritability, fatigue, mild depression, dizziness, headache, drowsiness, hallucinations, nervousness (large doses), seizures. **CV:** tachycardia (large doses). **GI:** anorexia, abdominal pain, nausea, diarrhea. **Hepatic:** liver enzyme elevations. **Skin:** rash.
phendimetrazine tartrate Controlled Substance Schedule IV Adphen, Anorex, Bacarate, Banobese, Bontril PDM, Delcozine, Di-Ap-Trol, Ex-Obese, Limit, Melfiat, Metra, Minus, Obalan, Obepar, Obeval, Obezine, Phenazine♦, Phenzine, Plegine, Ropledge, Sprx 1,2,3, Sprx-105, Statobex, Trimstat, Trimtabs, Weightrol	*Short-term adjunct in exogenous obesity*— **Adults:** 35 mg P.O. 2 to 3 times daily 1 hour before meals. Maximum dosage is 70 mg t.i.d. Use lowest effective dosage. Adjust dose to individual response.	**CNS:** *nervousness,* dizziness, *insomnia,* tremor, headache. **CV:** *tachycardia, palpitations,* rise in blood pressure. **EENT:** blurred vision. **GI:** dry mouth, nausea, abdominal cramps, diarrhea or constipation. **GU:** dysuria.
phenmetrazine hydrochloride Controlled Substance Schedule II Preludin	*Short-term adjunct in exogenous obesity*— **Adults:** 25 mg P.O. b.i.d. or t.i.d. 1 hour before meals, up to 75 mg daily; or single 50- to 75-mg extended-release tablet daily in midmorning.	**CNS:** *nervousness,* dizziness, *insomnia,* headache. **CV:** *tachycardia, palpitations,* increased blood pressure. **EENT:** blurred vision. **GI:** dry mouth, nausea, abdominal cramps, constipation. **Skin:** urticaria. **Other:** libido changes, impotence.

♦ Available in U.S. and Canada. ♦♦ Available in Canada only. All other products (no symbol) available in U.S. only. Italicized side effects are common or life-threatening.

INTERACTIONS	NURSING CONSIDERATIONS
	be affected. May alter daily insulin needs in patients with diabetes. Monitor blood and urine sugars. May decrease seizure threshold in patients with seizure disorders. • Drug of choice for minimal brain dysfunction. Usually stopped postpuberty. • Periodic CBC, differential, and platelet counts advised with long-term use. • Tolerance, psychic dependence, or habituation may develop, especially in patients with history of drug addiction. High abuse potential. Avoid prolonged administration. When used long-term, lower dosage gradually to prevent acute rebound depression. • Fatigue may result as drug effects wear off. • Tell patient to avoid caffeine, which increases the effects of amphetamines and related amines. • Warn patient to avoid activities that require alertness or good psychomotor coordination until CNS response to drug is determined. • Monitor height and weight in children on prolonged therapy.
None significant.	• Use with caution in patients with impaired renal function. Drug may accumulate. • Safety and efficacy for more than 2 years of administration has not been established. Closely monitor patients on long-term therapy for possible hepatic function abnormalities and for growth suppression. • Structurally dissimilar to amphetamines or methylphenidate. • Therapeutic effects may not be evident for 2 to 3 weeks.
MAO inhibitors: severe hypertension; possible hypertensive crisis. Don't use together. *Sodium bicarbonate, acetazolamide:* increased renal reabsorption. Monitor for enhanced effects. *Ammonium chloride, ascorbic acid:* observe for decreased phendimetrazine effects. *Phenothiazines, haloperidol:* observe for decreased effect.	• Contraindicated in hyperthyroidism, hypertension, angina pectoris or other severe cardiovascular disease, glaucoma. Use with caution in hyperexcitability states or patients with history of addiction. • Warn patient to avoid activities that require alertness or good psychomotor coordination until CNS response to drug has been determined. • Be sure patient is following weight-reduction program. • Tolerance or dependence can develop. Not advised for prolonged use. • Fatigue may result as drug effects wear off. Patient will need more rest. • Tell patient to avoid caffeine, which increases the effects of amphetamines and related amines. • Check vital signs regularly. Observe for signs of excessive stimulation. • Urinary acidification enhances renal excretion; urinary alkalinization enhances renal reabsorption and recycling. • May alter daily insulin needs in patients with diabetes. Monitor blood and urine sugars.
MAO inhibitors: severe hypertension; possible hypertensive crisis. Don't use together. *Sodium bicarbonate, acetazolamide:* increased renal reabsorption. Monitor for	• Contraindicated in patients with hyperthyroidism, hypertension, angina pectoris or other cardiovascular disease, glaucoma, or history of drug abuse. Use with caution in hyperexcitability states. • Tolerance or dependence may develop. High abuse potential. Not advised for prolonged use. • Be sure patient is also following weight-reduction program. • Fatigue may result as drug effects wear off. Patient will need more rest. • Tell patient to avoid caffeine drinks, which increase the effects of

(continued on following page)

NAME	INDICATIONS & DOSAGE	SIDE EFFECTS
phenmetrazine hydrochloride *(continued)*		
phentermine hydrochloride Controlled Substance Schedule IV Adipex, Anoxine, Fastin, Ionamin♦, Parmine, Phentrol, Rolaphent, Wilpowr	*Short-term adjunct in exogenous obesity*— **Adults:** 8 mg P.O. t.i.d. ½ hour before meals; or 15 to 30 mg daily before breakfast (resin complex).	**CNS:** *nervousness,* dizziness, *insomnia.* **CV:** *palpitations, tachycardia,* increased blood pressure. **GI:** dry mouth, unpleasant taste, nausea, constipation, diarrhea. **Skin:** urticaria. **Other:** libido changes, impotence.

♦ Available in U.S. and Canada. ♦♦ Available in Canada only. All other products (no symbol) available in U.S. only. Italicized side effects are common or life-threatening.

CAFFEINE CONTENT OF SOME COMMON FOODS, BEVERAGES, AND NONPRESCRIPTION DRUGS (IN MG)

Coffee, 5 oz (150 ml)	
Drip	146
Percolated	110
Instant	53
Decaffeinated	2
Tea, 5 oz (150 ml)	
brewed 1 minute	9 to 33
brewed 3 minutes	20 to 46
brewed 5 minutes	20 to 50
Canned ice tea, 12 oz (360 ml)	22 to 36
Cocoa beverage	
Water mix, 6 oz (180 ml)	10
Milk chocolate, 1 oz (30 ml)	35
Baking chocolate, 1 oz (30 ml)	35
Soft drinks, 12 oz (360 ml)	
Mountain Dew	52
Tab	44
Sunkist Orange	42
Shasta Cola	42
Dr. Pepper	38
Sugar-free Dr. Pepper	37
Pepsi	37
RC Cola	36
Diet-Rite Cola	34
Diet Pepsi	34
Coca-cola	34
7-Up	0
Sprite	0
Diet 7-Up	0

INTERACTIONS	NURSING CONSIDERATIONS
enhanced effects. *Ammonium chloride, ascorbic acid:* observe for decreased phenmetrazine effects. *Phenothiazines, haloperidol:* observe for decreased effect.	amphetamines and related amines. • Check vital signs regularly. Observe for signs of excessive stimulation. • Urinary acidification enhances renal excretion; urinary alkalinization enhances renal reabsorption and recycling.
MAO inhibitors: severe hypertension; possible hypertensive crisis. Don't use together. *Sodium bicarbonate, acetazolamide:* increased renal reabsorption. Monitor for enhanced effects. *Ammonium chloride, ascorbic acid:* observe for decreased phentermine effects. *Phenothiazines, haloperidol:* observe for decreased effect.	• Contraindicated in hyperthyroidism, hypertension, angina pectoris or other severe cardiovascular disease, glaucoma. Use with caution in hyperexcitability states or patients with history of drug addiction. • Tolerance or dependence may develop. Avoid prolonged administration. • Use with weight-reduction program. Give 30 minutes before meals. • Fatigue may result as drug effects wear off. Patient will need more rest. • Tell patient to avoid caffeine, which increases the effects of amphetamines and related amines. • Check vital signs regularly. Observe for signs of excessive stimulation. • Urinary acidification enhances renal excretion; urinary alkalinization enhances renal reabsorption and recycling.

RC-100	0
Diet Sunkist Orange	0
Fanta Orange	0
Fresca	0
Hires Root Beer	0
Stimulants (standard dose)	
Caffedrine Capsules	200
NoDoz Tablets	200
Vivarin Tablets	200
Pain relievers (standard dose)	
Anacin	64
Excedrin	134
Midol	65
Plain aspirin, any brand	0
Diuretics (standard dose)	
Aqua-Ban	200
Permathene H_2Off	200
Pre-Mens Forte	100
Cold remedies (standard dose)	
Coryban-D	30
Dristan	32
Triaminicin	30
Weight-control aids (daily dose)	
Dexatrim	200
Dietac	200
Prolamine	280

36 Respiratory stimulants

ammonia, aromatic spirits
doxapram hydrochloride
nikethamide
pentylenetetrazol

Respiratory stimulants, or analeptics, have limited usefulness in treating respiratory depression in patients with postanesthetic apnea caused by drugs other than muscle relaxants.

Doxapram is the most common respiratory stimulant. Aromatic spirits of ammonia are essentially smelling salts and are still commonly used. Pentylenetetrazol and nikethamide are seldom used today.

All these drugs except ammonia are dangerous because they're epileptogenic, or able to precipitate seizures.

Major uses

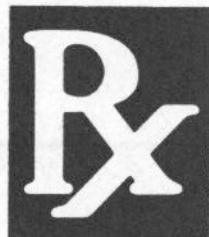

The respiratory stimulants combat effects of central nervous system depressants.

• Ammonia stimulates res-

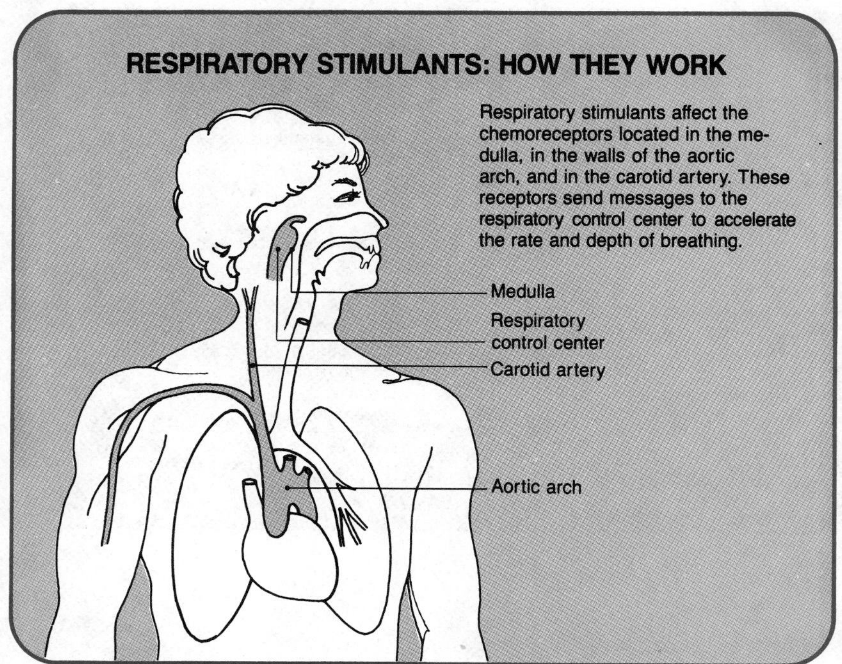
RESPIRATORY STIMULANTS: HOW THEY WORK
Respiratory stimulants affect the chemoreceptors located in the medulla, in the walls of the aortic arch, and in the carotid artery. These receptors send messages to the respiratory control center to accelerate the rate and depth of breathing.
Medulla
Respiratory control center
Carotid artery
Aortic arch

piration through peripheral irritation. It is also sometimes used as an antacid and a carminative.

- Pentylenetetrazol enhances physical and mental activity in elderly patients.

Mechanism of action

Respiratory stimulants act either directly on the central respiratory centers in the medulla or indirectly on the chemoreceptors.

- Ammonia causes irritation of the sensory receptors in the nasal membranes, producing reflex stimulation of the respiratory centers.

Absorption, distribution, metabolism, and excretion

Generally, respiratory stimulants are quickly absorbed after oral (pentylenetetrazol) or I.V. administration and well distributed to the body tissues.

- Doxapram is rapidly metabolized in the liver and eliminated in both urine and feces.
- Nikethamide is partly metabolized in the liver to niacinamide, which is excreted in the urine as N-methylniacinamide.
- Pentylenetetrazol is metabolized in the liver to at least five inactive metabolites, which are largely excreted in the urine.

Onset and duration

Onset of respiratory stimulants is quick, usually within 1 to 2 minutes; duration varies (usually 2 to 15 minutes).

- Pentylenetetrazol (the only orally administered drug in this group) has an onset of 1 to 2 hours and a duration of 4 to 6 hours.

Combination products

NICO-METRAZOL: pentylenetetrazol 100 mg and niacin 50 mg.

CLEARING A PATIENT'S AIRWAY

When an unconscious patient lies in supine position, his relaxed muscles allow his lower jaw to drop backward and permit the back of his tongue to block his airway (illustration 1). To relieve this obstruction easily and quickly, use the head-tilt maneuver (illustration 2). This raises the tongue from the back of the throat and, in some cases, may be enough to start the patient breathing.

If tilting the patient's head doesn't open his airway, try the jaw thrust. Place your fingers behind the angles of the patient's jaw and push forward. Exert enough pressure to maintain the head tilt.

Caution: If you suspect a neck injury, don't use the head-tilt maneuver. Try opening the airway with a modified jaw thrust. Push the jaw forward, but don't hyperextend the neck or move the head to either side.

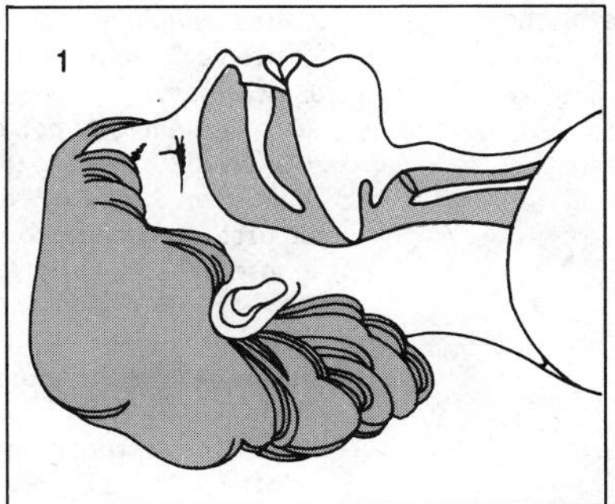

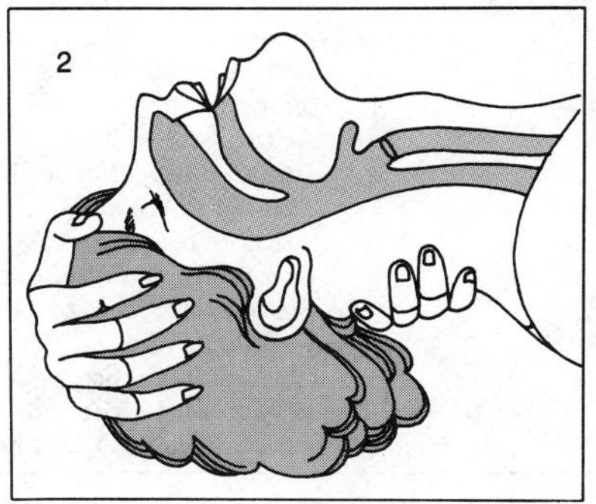

NAME	INDICATIONS & DOSAGE	SIDE EFFECTS
ammonia, aromatic spirits	*Fainting—* **Adults and children:** inhale as needed.	None reported.
doxapram hydrochloride Dopram♦	*Postanesthesia respiratory stimulant, drug-induced central nervous system depression, and chronic pulmonary disease associated with acute hypercapnia—* **Adults:** 0.5 to 1 mg/kg of body weight (up to 2 mg/kg in CNS depression), I.V. injection or infusion. Maximum 4 mg/kg, up to 3 g in 1 day. Infusion rate 1 to 3 mg/minute (initial: 5 mg/minute for postanesthesia). *Chronic obstructive pulmonary disease—* **Adults:** infusion, 1 to 2 mg/minute. Maximum 3 mg/minute for a maximum duration of 2 hours.	**CNS:** seizures, headache, dizziness, apprehension, disorientation, pupillary dilation, bilateral Babinski signs, flushing, sweating, paresthesias. **CV:** chest pain and tightness, variations in heart rate, hypertension, lowered T waves. **GI:** nausea, vomiting, diarrhea. **GU:** urinary retention, or stimulation of the bladder with incontinence. **Other:** sneezing, coughing, laryngospasm, bronchospasm, hiccups, rebound hypoventilation, pruritus.
nikethamide Coramine♦, Kardonyl♦♦	*Acute alcoholism—* **Adults:** 1.25 to 5 g I.V.; repeat as necessary. *Carbon monoxide poisoning—* **Adults:** 1.25 to 2.5 g I.V. initially, then 1.25 g q 5 minutes for first hour, depending on response. *Cardiac arrest associated with anesthetic overdose—* **Adults:** 125 to 250 mg intracardially. *Combat respiratory paralysis—* **Adults:** 3.75 g I.V.; repeat as required. *Overcome respiratory depression—* **Adults:** 1.25 to 2.5 g I.V. *Shock—* **Adults:** 2.5 to 3.75 g I.V. or I.M. initially; repeat as indicated. *Shorten narcosis—* **Adults:** 1 g I.V. or I.M. *Adjunct in neonatal asphyxia—* **Neonates:** 375 mg injected into umbilical vein. Oral maintenance: **Adults and children:** 3 to 5 ml oral solution q 4 to 6 hours.	**CNS:** seizure, restlessness, muscle twitching or fasciculations, fear. **CV:** increased heart rate and blood pressure. **EENT:** unpleasant burning or itching at back of nose, sneezing, coughing. **GI:** nausea, vomiting. **Other:** increased respiratory rate, flushing, feeling of warmth, sweating.

♦ Available in U.S. and Canada. ♦♦ Available in Canada only. All other products (no symbol) available in U.S. only. Italicized side effects are common or life-threatening.

INTERACTIONS	NURSING CONSIDERATIONS
None significant.	• Stimulates mucous membranes of upper respiratory tract.
MAO inhibitors: potentiate adverse cardiovascular effects. Use together cautiously.	• Contraindicated in convulsive disorders; head injury; cardiovascular disorders; frank uncompensated heart failure; severe hypertension; cerebrovascular accidents; respiratory failure or incompetence secondary to neuromuscular disorders, muscle paresis, flail chest, obstructed airway, pulmonary embolism, pneumothorax, restrictive respiratory disease, acute bronchial asthma, extreme dyspnea; hypoxia not associated with hypercapnia. Use with caution in bronchial asthma, severe tachycardia or cardiac arrhythmias, cerebral edema or increased cerebrospinal fluid pressure, hyperthyroidism, pheochromocytoma, or profound metabolic disorders. • Establish adequate airway before administering drug. Prevent patient from aspirating vomitus by placing him on his side. • Monitor blood pressure, heart rate, deep tendon reflexes, and arterial blood gases before giving drug and every 30 minutes afterward to avoid overdosage. • Be alert for signs of overdosage: hypertension, tachycardia, arrhythmias, skeletal muscle hyperactivity, dyspnea. Discontinue if patient shows signs of increased arterial carbon dioxide or oxygen tension, or if mechanical ventilation is started. May give I.V. injection of anticonvulsant for convulsions. • Use only in surgical or emergency room situations. • Do not combine with alkaline solutions such as thiopental sodium; doxapram is acidic.
None significant.	• Monitor patient's respiratory rate and volume frequently during therapy. • Mechanical support of breathing is often preferred over nikethamide. • Don't inject intra-arterially; arterial spasm and thrombosis may result. • Watch for signs of overdosage: muscle tremors or spasm, retching, tachycardia, arrhythmias, hyperpyrexia, hyperpnea, convulsions, psychotic reactions, postictal depression. May give I.V. injection of diazepam or barbiturate such as thiopental sodium for convulsions. Induced emesis and gastric lavage aren't effective.

NAME	INDICATIONS & DOSAGE	SIDE EFFECTS
pentylenetetrazol Metrazol, Nelex-100, Nioric, Petrazole	*Overdose of CNS depressants*— **Adults:** 100 to 500 mg I.V. Repeat, if necessary, followed by 100 to 200 mg I.M., p.r.n. *In depression from barbiturates*— 5 ml of 10% solution I.V. within 3 to 5 seconds. If necessary, may be repeated until patient awakens. *To improve mental and physical activity in elderly patients*— **Adults:** 100 to 200 mg P.O. t.i.d.	Few side effects with oral administration; narrow margin of safety with parenteral administration. *Signs of overdose:* **CNS:** fasciculations, clonic convulsions. **CV:** slight increases in blood pressure, bradycardia. **GI:** nausea, vomiting. **Other:** hypersalivation, coughing, hyperthermia.

INTERACTIONS	NURSING CONSIDERATIONS
None significant.	• Use with caution in patients with a history of seizures or focal brain lesion. If dosage is high, use with caution in patients with cardiac disease. • Analeptic use is not recommended. • May cause false-positive response to human chorionic gonadotropin pregnancy test.

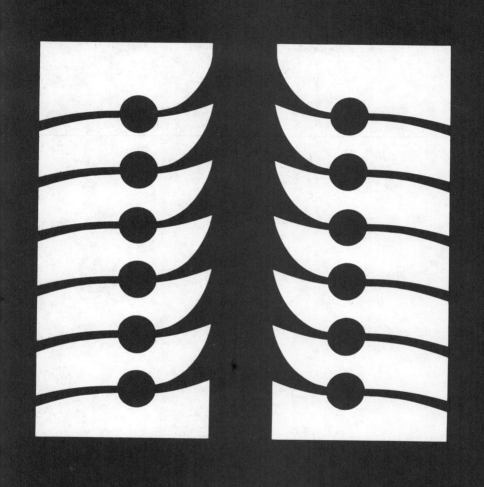

V Autonomic Nervous System Drugs

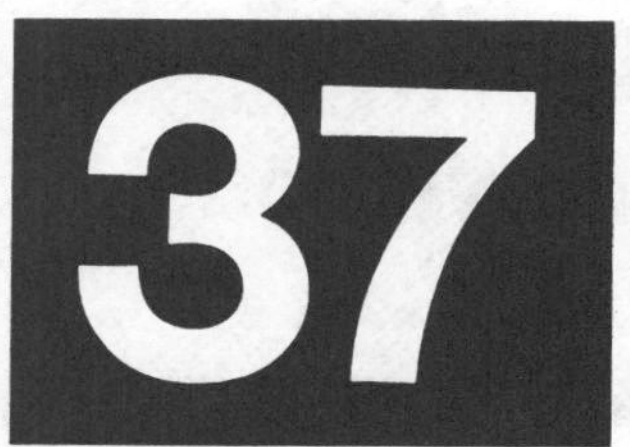

Cholinergics (parasympathomimetics)

ambenonium chloride
bethanechol chloride
edrophonium chloride
neostigmine bromide
neostigmine methylsulfate
physostigmine salicylate
pyridostigmine bromide

Cholinergics mimic the action of acetylcholine in that they produce parasympathetic responses. They are not organ-specific. When bethanechol, for example, is administered to treat postoperative urinary retention, it is distributed through the body, and other organs innervated by the parasympathetic system are activated. Thus, these drugs can produce a therapeutic effect at one location (such as preventing urinary retention in the bladder) and annoying side effects at another (such as causing excess production of saliva by the salivary glands).

The parasympathetic division of the autonomic nervous system innervates various body organs and systems and acts on the heart, gastrointestinal (GI) tract, urinary bladder, and respiratory tract. The parasympathetic division works in concert with its sympathetic counterpart to provide continuous control of those functions which occur without conscious thought (for example, digestion, respiration, and maintenance of blood pressure).

When stimulated, parasympathetic nerves release acetylcholine from their nerve endings. This chemical binds to specific sites (muscarinic receptors) in the tissue innervated by the parasympathetic nerve. This interaction starts the mechanisms that result in a typical parasympathetic response. Some of the organs innervated by the parasympathetic system, and their response to parasympathetic stimulation, are shown in the chart on the opposite page.

Nerves that innervate skeletal muscle also release acetylcholine when stimulated. The released acetylcholine binds to specific sites in skeletal muscle, triggering contraction. Disordered release of acetylcholine from these nerves or impaired binding with skeletal muscle leads to profound muscle weakness (myasthenia gravis). Drugs that promote the accumulation of acetylcholine at skeletal muscle sites (for example, neostigmine) improve muscular performance in patients with this disease.

Major uses

- Ambenonium, neostigmine, and pyridostigmine are used to treat symptoms of myasthenia gravis.
- Bethanechol is used to prevent and treat postoperative urinary retention, postoperative gastric atony and retention, abdominal distention, and megacolon.
- Edrophonium aids differential diagnosis of myasthenia gravis.
- Neostigmine is used to prevent and treat postoperative urinary retention.
- Neostigmine and pyridostigmine reverse the effect of neuromuscular blocking agents used in surgery.

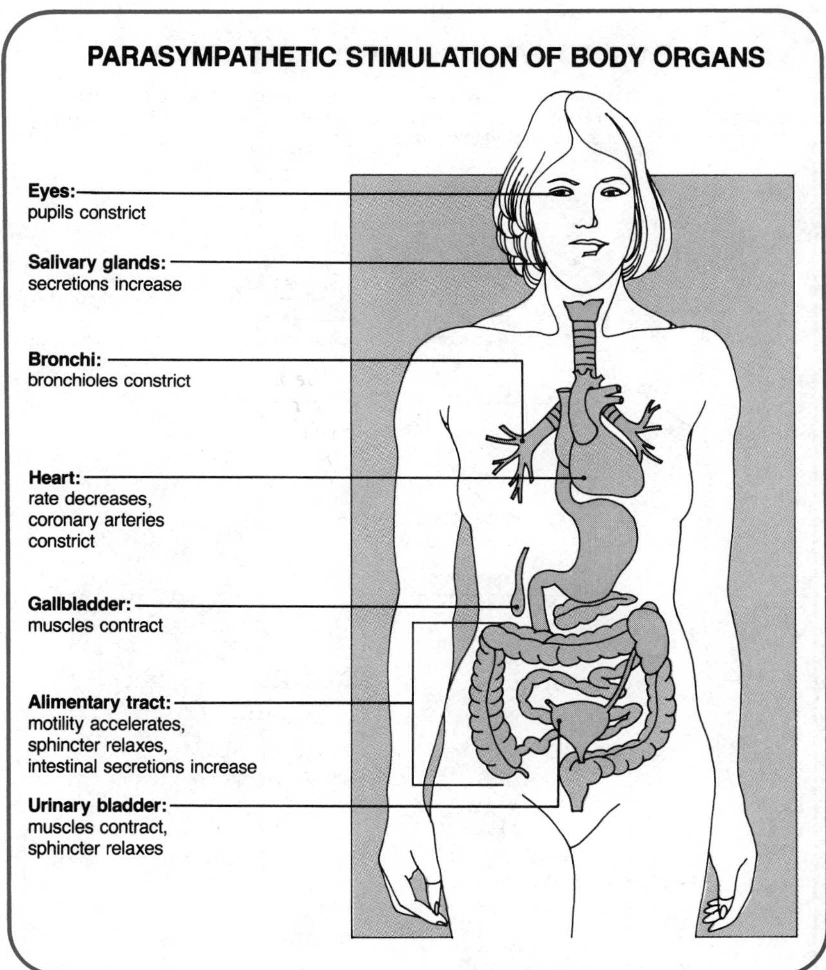

• Physostigmine is an antidote in anticholinergic poisoning, particularly poisoning caused by tricyclic antidepressants.

Mechanism of action

• Ambenonium, edrophonium, neostigmine, physostigmine, and pyridostigmine inhibit the destruction of acetylcholine released from the parasympathetic nerves. Acetylcholine accumulates, promoting increased stimulation of the receptor.

• Bethanechol and neostigmine directly bind to muscarinic receptors, mimicking the action of acetylcholine.

Absorption, distribution, metabolism, and excretion

All cholinergics except physostigmine are poorly absorbed orally. They are widely distributed to organs innervated by the parasympathetic nervous system, metabolized by the liver, and excreted by the kidneys as water-soluble metabolites.

• Physostigmine is the only cholinergic drug that effectively crosses the blood-brain barrier, making it useful for tricyclic antidepressant and anti-

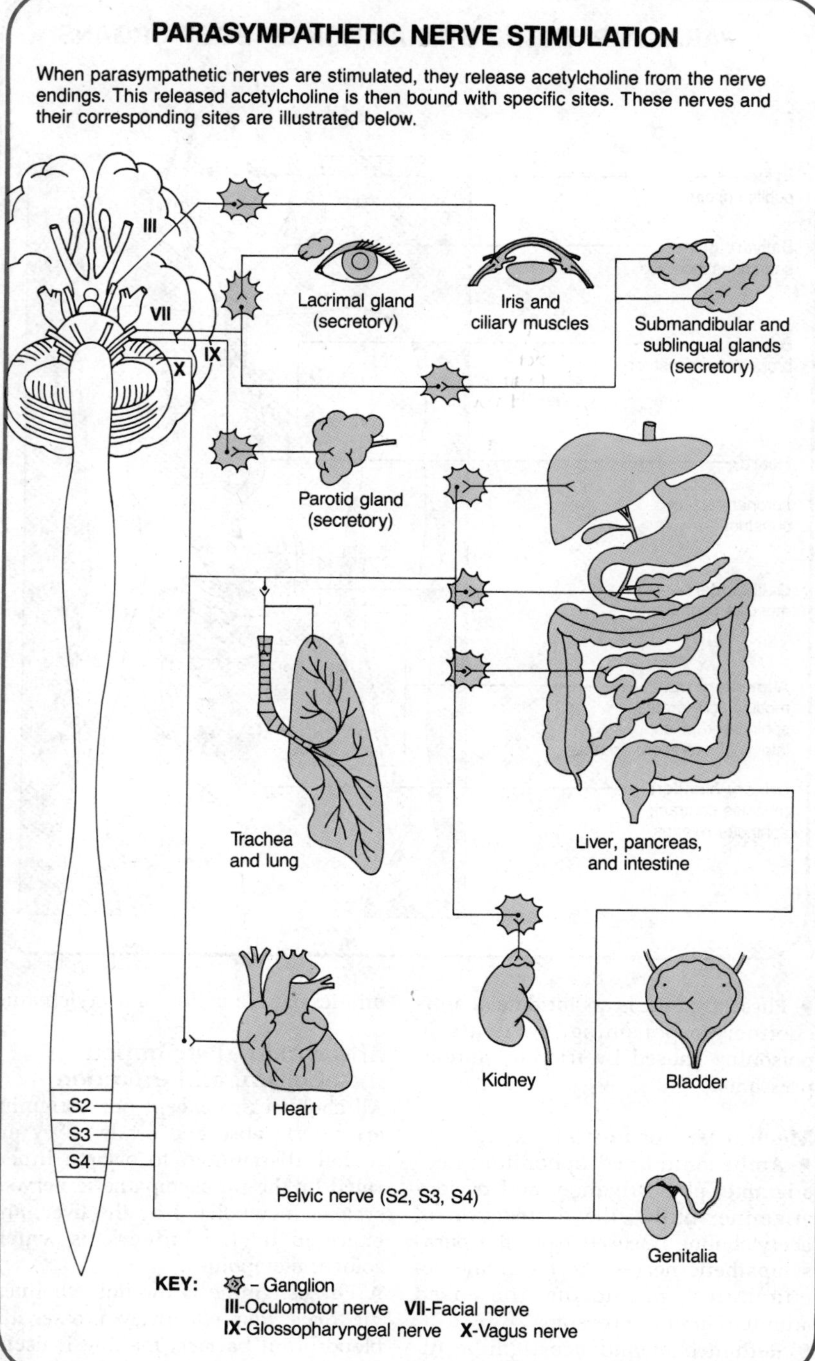
PARASYMPATHETIC NERVE STIMULATION
When parasympathetic nerves are stimulated, they release acetylcholine from the nerve endings. This released acetylcholine is then bound with specific sites. These nerves and their corresponding sites are illustrated below.
III
VII
IX
X
Lacrimal gland (secretory)
Iris and ciliary muscles
Submandibular and sublingual glands (secretory)
Parotid gland (secretory)
Trachea and lung
Liver, pancreas, and intestine
Heart
Kidney
Bladder
S2
S3
S4
Pelvic nerve (S2, S3, S4)
Genitalia
KEY: – Ganglion
III-Oculomotor nerve VII-Facial nerve
IX-Glossopharyngeal nerve X-Vagus nerve

PATIENT-TEACHING AID

WHAT YOU SHOULD KNOW ABOUT CHOLINERGICS

Dear Patient:

Since your bladder isn't contracting effectively, it's retaining urine. Bacteria grows in accumulated urine, resulting in frequent infections. Therefore, your doctor has prescribed a cholinergic drug to strengthen the contraction of your bladder and reduce urine retention.

To get the most from your drug therapy, follow these instructions carefully:

- If you have a history of low blood pressure, heart trouble, allergies, or hyperthyroidism, or have stomach or intestinal problems, tell the doctor.
- Be sure not to take any prescription or nonprescription drug while you're being treated with a cholinergic drug without first checking with the doctor.
- Take your medication on an empty stomach, about an hour before meals if possible. If you take it after meals, you may feel nauseated or start vomiting.
- If you experience diarrhea—the most common side effect of cholinergics—take a mixture of kaolin-pectin (Kaopectate).
- Call the doctor immediately if you begin to feel light-headed, particularly when you get up in the morning.

Note: When you begin drug therapy, you may notice a temporary worsening of bladder symptoms. After your doctor assesses your response to this drug, he may change your medication dosage.

cholinergic poisoning.

Onset and duration

- Ambenonium's onset and duration are variable. The drug's effects on skeletal muscle usually lasts 4 to 8 hours.
- Bethanechol has an onset between 60 and 90 minutes (occasionally as soon as 30 minutes) after oral administration. Therapeutic effects persist for about 1 hour. After subcutaneous injection, onset occurs within 5 to 15 minutes, and action peaks in 15 to 30 minutes. Therapeutic effects wane thereafter and disappear after 2 hours.
- Edrophonium's onset, after I.V. infusion, occurs within 30 to 60 seconds; therapeutic activity lasts 5 to 10 minutes. When the drug is given I.M., onset occurs in 2 to 10 minutes, and its duration of action is 5 to 30 minutes.
- Neostigmine has an onset of action on the GI tract 2 to 4 hours after oral administration, 10 to 30 minutes after I.M. injection. Duration of action on skeletal muscle, after I.M. injection, is 2½ to 4 hours.
- Physostigmine's onset occurs in 3 to 8 minutes after parenteral administration; its duration of action is 30 minutes to 5 hours.
- Pyridostigmine's action on skeletal muscle begins within 30 to 45 minutes when the drug is given orally. Its action persists 3 to 6 hours. After I.M. injection, onset occurs within 15 minutes. After I.V. infusion, onset occurs in 2 to 5 minutes; its duration of action is 2 to 3 hours.

Combination products

None.

NAME	INDICATIONS & DOSAGE	SIDE EFFECTS
ambenonium chloride Mytelase♦	*Symptomatic treatment of myasthenia gravis in patients who cannot take neostigmine bromide and pyridostigmine bromide—* **Adults:** dose must be individualized for each patient, but usually ranges from 5 to 25 mg P.O. q 3 to 4 hours while awake. Starting dose usually 5 mg P.O. q 3 to 4 hours. Increase gradually and adjust at 1- to 2-day intervals to avoid drug accumulation and overdosage. May range from 5 mg to as much as 75 mg per dose.	**CNS:** headache, dizziness, muscle weakness, convulsions, mental confusion, jitters, sweating, respiratory depression. **CV:** bradycardia, hypotension. **EENT:** miosis. **GI:** *nausea, vomiting, diarrhea, abdominal cramps,* increased salivation. **GU:** urinary frequency, incontinence. **Other:** bronchospasm, *muscle cramps,* bronchoconstriction.
bethanechol chloride Duvoid, Mictrol-10, Mictrol-25, Myotonachol, Urecholine♦, Urolax, Vesicholine	*Acute postoperative and postpartum nonobstructive (functional) urinary retention, neurogenic atony of urinary bladder with retention, abdominal distention, megacolon—* **Adults:** 10 to 30 mg P.O. t.i.d. to q.i.d. Never give I.M. or I.V. When used for urinary retention, some patients may require 50 to 100 mg P.O. per dose. Use such doses with extreme caution. Test dose: 2.5 mg S.C. repeated at 15- to 30-minute intervals to total of 4 doses to determine the minimal effective dose; then use	*Dose-related:* **CNS:** headache, malaise. **CV:** bradycardia, hypotension, *cardiac arrest,* tachycardia. **EENT:** lacrimation, miosis. **GI:** *abdominal cramps, diarrhea,* salivation, nausea, vomiting, belching, borborygmus. **GU:** urinary urgency. **Skin:** flushing, sweating. **Other:** bronchoconstriction.

♦ Available in U.S. and Canada. ♦♦ Available in Canada only. All other products (no symbol) available in U.S. only. Italicized side effects are common or life-threatening.

INTERACTIONS	NURSING CONSIDERATIONS
Procainamide, quinidine: may reverse cholinergic effect on muscle. Observe for lack of drug effect.	• Contraindicated in patients with mechanical obstruction of intestine or urinary tract, bradycardia, hypotension. • Use with extreme caution in patients with bronchial asthma. • Use cautiously in patients with epilepsy, recent coronary occlusion, vagotonia, hyperthyroidism, cardiac arrhythmias, peptic ulcer. • Avoid large dose in patients with decreased gastrointestinal motility or megacolon. • Discontinue all other cholinergics before administering this drug. • Watch patient very closely for side effects, particularly if total dose is greater than 200 mg daily. Side effects may indicate drug toxicity. Notify doctor immediately if they develop. • Monitor and document vital signs frequently, being especially careful to check respirations. Always have atropine injection readily available and be prepared to give atropine 0.5 mg subcutaneously or slow I.V. push as ordered, and provide respiratory support as needed. • Administer each dose exactly as ordered, on time. Amount and frequency of dosage should vary with patient's activity level. The doctor will probably order larger doses to be given when patient is fatigued, for example, in the afternoon and at mealtime. • If muscle weakness is severe, doctor must determine if this is caused by drug toxicity or exacerbation of myasthenia gravis. A test dose of edrophonium I.V. will aggravate drug-induced weakness but will temporarily relieve weakness that results from the disease. • Observe and record the patient's variations in muscle strength. Show him how to do it himself. • When given for myasthenia gravis, explain to patient that this drug will relieve symptoms of lid ptosis, double vision, difficulty in chewing and swallowing, trunk and limb weakness. Stress the importance of taking this drug exactly as ordered. Explain to patient and his family that he must take this drug for the rest of his life. Teach them about the disease and the drug's effect on symptoms. • Monitor intake and output. • Patient may develop resistance to drug. • Seek approval when indicated for hospitalized patient to have bedside supply of tablets to take himself. Patients with long-standing disease often insist on this. • Give with milk or food to produce fewer muscarinic side effects. • Advise patient to carry an identification card indicating that he has myasthenia gravis. • For toxicity, see APPENDIX, *Drug Toxicities.*
Procainamide, quinidine: may reverse cholinergic effects on muscle. Observe for lack of drug effect.	• Contraindicated in patients with uncertain strength or integrity of bladder wall; when increased muscular activity of GI or urinary tract is harmful; in mechanical obstructions of GI or urinary tract; in hyperthyroidism, peptic ulcer, latent or active bronchial asthma, cardiac or coronary artery disease, vagotonia, epilepsy, Parkinson's disease, bradycardia, chronic obstructive pulmonary disease, hypotension. Use cautiously in hypertension, vasomotor instability, peritonitis, or other acute inflammatory conditions of GI tract. • *Never* give I.M. or I.V.; could cause circulatory collapse, hypotension, severe abdominal cramping, bloody diarrhea, shock, cardiac arrest. • Should stop all other cholinergics before giving this drug. • Watch closely for side effects that may indicate drug toxicity, especially with subcutaneous administration. • Monitor vital signs frequently, being especially careful to check respirations. Always have atropine injection readily available and be prepared to give atropine 0.5 mg subcutaneously or slow I.V. push as ordered, and provide respiratory support if needed.

(continued on following page)

NAME	INDICATIONS & DOSAGE	SIDE EFFECTS
bethanechol chloride *(continued)*	minimal effective dose q 6 to 8 hours. All doses must be adjusted individually.	
edrophonium chloride Tensilon♦	*As a curare antagonist (to reverse neuromuscular blocking action)—* **Adults:** 10 mg I.V. given over 30 to 45 seconds. Dose may be repeated as necessary to 40 mg maximum dose. Larger doses may potentiate rather than antagonize effect of curare. *Diagnostic aid in myasthenia gravis (the Tensilon test)—* **Adults:** 1 to 2 mg I.V. within 15 to 30 seconds, then 8 mg if no response (increase in muscular strength). **Children over 34 kg:** 2 mg I.V. If no response within 45 seconds, give 1 mg q 45 seconds to maximum of 10 mg. **Children up to 34 kg:** 1 mg I.V. If no response within 45 seconds, give 1 mg q 45 seconds to maximum of 5 mg. **Infants:** 0.5 mg I.V. *To differentiate myasthenic crisis from cholinergic crisis—* **Adults:** 1 mg I.V. If no response in 1 minute, repeat dose once. Increased muscular strength confirms myasthenic crisis; no increase or exaggerated weakness confirms cholinergic crisis. *Paroxysmal supraventricular tachycardia—* **Adults:** 10 mg I.V. given over 1 minute or less.	**CNS:** weakness, respiratory paralysis, sweating. **CV:** hypotension, bradycardia. **EENT:** miosis. **GI:** nausea, vomiting, *diarrhea, abdominal cramps,* excessive salivation. **Other:** increased bronchial secretions, bronchospasm, muscle cramps, muscle fasciculation.
neostigmine bromide Prostigmin Bromide♦ **neostigmine methylsulfate** Prostigmin♦	*Antidote for tubocurarine—* **Adults:** 0.5 to 2 mg I.V. slowly. Repeat p.r.n. Give 0.6 to 1.2 mg atropine sulfate I.V. before antidote dose. *Functional amenorrhea*—1 mg I.M. or S.C. daily for 3 days. *Postoperative abdominal distention and bladder atony—*	**CNS:** dizziness, muscle weakness, mental confusion, jitters, sweating, respiratory depression. **CV:** bradycardia, hypotension. **EENT:** miosis. **GI:** *nausea, vomiting, diarrhea, abdominal cramps,* excessive salivation. **Skin:** rash (bromide).

♦ Available in U.S. and Canada. ♦♦ Available in Canada only. All other products (no symbol) available in U.S. only. Italicized side effects are common or life-threatening.

INTERACTIONS	NURSING CONSIDERATIONS
	• If used to treat urinary retention, make sure bedpan is handy. Monitor intake and output. • When used to prevent abdominal distention and GI distress, the doctor may also order a rectal tube inserted to help passage of gas. • Poor and variable oral absorption requires larger oral doses. Oral and subcutaneous doses are *not* interchangeable. • Drug usually effective 5 to 15 minutes after injection and 30 to 90 minutes after oral use. • Give on empty stomach; if taken after meals, may cause nausea and vomiting. • For toxicity, see APPENDIX, *Drug Toxicities*.
Procainamide, quinidine: may reverse cholinergic effects on muscle. Observe for lack of drug effect.	• Contraindicated in mechanical obstruction of intestine or urinary tract, bradycardia, hypotension. Use cautiously in hyperthyroidism, cardiac disease, peptic ulcer, bronchial asthma. • Should stop all other cholinergics before giving this drug. • Watch closely for side effects; may indicate toxicity. • Monitor vital signs frequently, being especially careful to check respirations. Always have atropine injection readily available and be prepared to give atropine 0.5 mg subcutaneously or slow I.V. push as ordered, and provide respiratory support as needed. • When giving drug to differentiate myasthenic crisis from cholinergic crisis, observe patient's muscle strength closely. • Edrophonium not effective against muscle relaxation induced by decamethonium bromide and succinylcholine chloride. • This cholinergic has the most rapid onset but shortest duration; therefore not used for treatment of myasthenia gravis. • For easier parenteral administration, use a tuberculin syringe with an I.V. needle. • I.M. route may be used in children due to difficulty with I.V. route: for children under 34 kg, inject 2 mg I.M.; children over 34 kg, 5 mg I.M. Expect same reactions as with I.V. test, but these appear after 2- to 10-minute delay. • For toxicity, see APPENDIX, *Drug Toxicities*.
Procainamide, quinidine: may reverse cholinergic effect on muscle. Observe for lack of drug effect.	• Contraindicated in hypersensitivity to cholinergics or to bromide, mechanical obstruction of the intestine or urinary tract, bradycardia, hypotension. Use with extreme caution in bronchial asthma. Use cautiously in epilepsy, recent coronary occlusion, peritonitis, vagotonia, hyperthyroidism, cardiac arrhythmias, or peptic ulcer. • Should stop all other cholinergics before giving this drug. • Watch closely for side effects; may indicate toxicity. • Monitor vital signs frequently, being especially careful to check respirations. Always have atropine injection readily available and be

(continued on following page)

NAME	INDICATIONS & DOSAGE	SIDE EFFECTS
neostigmine *(continued)*	**Adults:** 0.5 to 1 mg I.M. or S.C. q 4 to 6 hours. *Postoperative ileus—* **Adults:** 0.25 to 1 mg I.M. or S.C. q 4 to 6 hours. *Treatment of myasthenia gravis—* **Adults:** 15 to 30 mg t.i.d. (range 15 to 375 mg/day); or 0.5 to 2 mg I.M. or I.V. q 1 to 3 hours. Dose must be individualized, depending on response and tolerance of side effects. Therapy may be required day and night. **Children:** 7.5 to 15 mg P.O. t.i.d. to q.i.d. *Note:* 1:1,000 solution of injectable solution contains 1 mg/1 ml; 1:2,000 solution contains 0.5 mg/ml.	**Other:** bronchospasm, *muscle cramps,* bronchoconstriction.
physostigmine salicylate Antilirium♦	*Anticholinergic poisoning—* **Adults:** 0.5 to 4 mg I.M. or I.V. q 2 hours. *Tricyclic antidepressant poisoning—* **Adults:** 0.5 to 3 mg I.M. or I.V. (1 mg per minute I.V.) repeated as necessary if life-threatening signs recur (coma, convulsions, arrhythmias).	**CNS:** hallucinations, muscular twitching, muscle weakness, ataxia, *restlessness, excitability, sweating.* **CV:** irregular pulse, palpitations. **EENT:** miosis. **GI:** nausea, vomiting, epigastric pain, *diarrhea, excessive salivation.* **Other:** bronchospasm, bronchial constriction, dyspnea.
pyridostigmine bromide Mestinon♦, Regonol♦	*Curariform antagonist—* **Adults:** 10 to 30 mg I.V. preceded by atropine sulfate 0.6 to 1.2 mg I.V. *Myasthenia gravis—*	**CNS:** headache (with high doses), weakness, sweating, convulsions. **CV:** bradycardia, hypotension. **EENT:** miosis. **GI:** abdominal cramps, nausea,

INTERACTIONS	NURSING CONSIDERATIONS
	prepared to give atropine 0.5 mg subcutaneously or slow I.V. push as ordered, and provide respiratory support as needed. • Difficult to judge optimum dose. Help doctor by documenting patient's response after each dose. Show patient how to observe and record variations in muscle strength. • When using for myasthenia gravis, explain that this drug will relieve lid ptosis, double vision, difficulty in chewing and swallowing, trunk and limb weakness. Stress importance of taking drug exactly as ordered. Explain that drug may have to be taken for life. Explain drug's effect on myasthenic symptoms. • If patient has dysphagia, schedule dose 30 minutes before each meal. • When used to prevent abdominal distention and GI distress, the doctor may order a rectal tube inserted to help passage of gas. • Patients sometimes develop a resistance to neostigmine. • When used for functional amenorrhea, check for vaginal bleeding and instruct patient to report any vaginal bleeding. If no bleeding in 72 hours after third injection, patient has nonfunctional amenorrhea. • If muscle weakness is severe, doctor determines if it is caused by drug-induced toxicity or exacerbation of myasthenia gravis. Test dose of edrophonium I.V. will aggravate drug-induced weakness but will temporarily relieve weakness caused by disease. • Hospitalized patients with long-standing myasthenia may request bedside supply of tablets. This will enable patient to take each dose precisely as ordered. Seek approval for self-medication program according to hospital policy, but continue to oversee medication regimen. • GI side effects may be reduced by taking drug with milk or food. • Advise patient to carry an identification card indicating that he has myasthenia gravis. • For toxicity, see APPENDIX, *Drug Toxicities.*
Procainamide, quinidine: may reverse cholinergic effects on muscle. Observe for lack of drug effect.	• Use cautiously in preexisting conditions: mechanical obstruction of intestine or urinary tract, bronchial asthma, gangrene, diabetes, cardiovascular disease, vagotonia, bradycardia, hypotension, epilepsy, Parkinson's disease, hyperthyroidism, peptic ulcer. • Watch closely for side effects, particularly CNS disturbances. Use side rails if patient becomes restless or hallucinates. Side effects may indicate drug toxicity. • Monitor vital signs frequently, being especially careful to check respirations. Position patient to make breathing easier. Always have atropine injection readily available and be prepared to give atropine 0.5 mg subcutaneously or slow I.V. push as ordered, and provide respiratory support as needed. Best administered in presence of doctor. • Use only clear solution. Darkening may indicate loss of potency. • Give I.V. at controlled rate; use slow, direct injection at no more than 1 mg/minute. • Only cholinergic that crosses blood/brain barrier; therefore the only one useful for treating CNS effects of anticholinergic or tricyclic antidepressant toxicity. • Effectiveness often immediate and dramatic but may be transient and may require repeat dose. • For toxicity, see APPENDIX, *Drug Toxicities.*
Procainamide, quinidine: may reverse cholinergic effects on muscle. Observe for lack of drug effect.	• Contraindicated in mechanical obstruction of intestine or urinary tract, bradycardia, hypotension. Use with extreme caution in bronchial asthma. Use cautiously in epilepsy, recent coronary occlusion, vagotonia, hyperthyroidism, cardiac arrhythmias, peptic ulcer. Avoid large doses in decreased gastrointestinal motility or megacolon.

(continued on following page)

NAME	INDICATIONS & DOSAGE	SIDE EFFECTS
pyridostigmine bromide *(continued)*	**Adults:** 60 to 180 mg P.O. b.i.d. or q.i.d. Usual dose 600 mg daily but higher doses may be needed (up to 1,500 mg per day). Give 1/30 of oral dose I.M. or I.V. Dose must be adjusted for each patient, depending on response and tolerance of side effects.	vomiting, diarrhea, excessive salivation. **Skin:** rash. **Local:** thrombophlebitis. **Other:** bronchospasm, bronchoconstriction, increased bronchial secretions, muscle cramps.

◆ Available in U.S. and Canada. ◆◆ Available in Canada only. All other products (no symbol) available in U.S. only. Italicized side effects are common or life-threatening.

INTERACTIONS	NURSING CONSIDERATIONS
	• Difficult to judge optimum dosage. Help doctor by recording patient's response after each dose. • Should stop all other cholinergics before giving this drug. • Watch closely for side effects; may indicate toxicity. • Monitor vital signs frequently, being especially careful to check respirations. Position patient to make breathing easier. Always have atropine injection readily available and be prepared to give atropine 0.5 mg subcutaneously or slow I.V. push as ordered, and provide respiratory support as needed. • If muscle weakness is severe, doctor determines if it is caused by drug-induced toxicity or exacerbation of myasthenia gravis. Test dose of edrophonium I.V. will aggravate drug-induced weakness but will temporarily relieve weakness caused by disease. • When using for myasthenia gravis, stress importance of taking drug exactly as ordered, on time, in evenly spaced doses. If doctor has ordered extended-release tablets, explain how these work. Patient must take them at the same time each day, at least 6 hours apart. Explain that he may have to take this drug for life. Tell about drug's effect on myasthenic symptoms. • Has longest duration of the cholinergics used for myasthenia gravis. • Available in 60-mg tablets, sustained-release (180-mg) tablets, injection, and syrup. • For toxicity, see APPENDIX, *Drug Toxicities*.

Cholinergic blockers (parasympatholytics)

atropine sulfate
benztropine mesylate
biperiden hydrochloride
biperiden lactate
chlorphenoxamine hydrochloride
cycrimine hydrochloride
glycopyrrolate
procyclidine hydrochloride
scopolamine hydrobromide
trihexyphenidyl hydrochloride

Cholinergic blockers inhibit the action of acetylcholine released by parasympathetic and some sympathetic nerves. Because parasympathetic nerves innervate many organs, parasympatholytic action can be widespread. The effects of parasympatholytics are typically opposite those of parasympathetic stimulation. For example, parasympathetic (vagal) stimulation of the heart decreases heart rate, whereas atropine, a parasympatholytic drug, increases heart rate.

Several of these drugs (for example, benztropine and trihexyphenidyl) can enter the brain, where they antagonize the actions of cerebral acetylcholine. The cholinergic blockers help to control the clinical effects of parkinsonism (a disease partly attributable to overactivity of certain cholinergic pathways in the brain) and dyskinesias associated with the use of major tranquilizers.

Parasympatholytic drugs are not organ-specific. The administration of atropine to reverse severe bradycardia, for example, can dry oral and respiratory secretions. Likewise, the use of benztropine for parkinsonism can produce urinary retention, especially in men with prostatic hypertrophy. (For cholinergic blockers used specifically for gastrointestinal disorders, see Chapter 50, GASTROINTESTINAL ANTICHOLINERGICS.)

Major uses

Rx

- Atropine may be used for poisoning due to organic phosphate insecticides and certain mushrooms.
- Atropine and scopolamine, as preanesthetic medications, are used to reduce salivary and respiratory secretions.
- Benztropine, biperiden, cycrimine, procyclidine, and trihexyphenidyl are used to treat parkinsonism and extrapyramidal reactions associated with the use of neuroleptics.

Mechanism of action

Cholinergic blockers inhibit the effect of acetylcholine—as the neurotransmitter for impulses in the parasympathetic nervous system—at the junction between postganglionic nerve endings and effector organs.

Absorption, distribution, metabolism, and excretion

Cholinergic blockers generally are well absorbed from the gastrointestinal (GI) tract. They are widely distributed to body organs innervated by the parasympathetic nervous system and ex-

WHAT CHOLINERGIC BLOCKERS DO

INNERVATED ORGAN	When body naturally releases neurohormone acetylcholine:	When cholinergic blockers are given:
Heart	▼	▲
Bronchioles	▲	▼
GI tract	▲	▼
Bladder	▲	▼
Bladder sphincter	▼	▲
Blood vessels	▼	▲
Sweat and salivary glands	▲	▼

KEY: ▼ = relaxes or dilates ▲ = constricts or stimulates

creted unchanged in the urine.

- Atropine, benztropine, biperiden, scopolamine, and trihexyphenidyl are more likely to penetrate the central nervous system than the other cholinergic blockers.

Onset and duration

All cholinergic blockers take effect within 30 minutes when injected I.M. or subcutaneously, and within 30 to 60 minutes when given orally.

The duration of these agents (except benztropine) is from 2 to 6 hours when given I.M. or subcutaneously, and from 4 to 6 hours when given orally. Effects of large doses can last as long as 24 hours.

- Benztropine's duration of action is 24 hours after I.M., subcutaneous, or oral administration.

Combination products

Cholinergic blocking agents are available in tablets and capsules, combined with varying amounts of sedatives.

NAME	INDICATIONS & DOSAGE	SIDE EFFECTS
atropine sulfate	*Antidote for anticholinesterase insecticide poisoning—* **Adults and children:** 2 mg I.M. or I.V. repeated at hourly intervals until muscarinic symptoms disappear. Severe cases may require up to 6 mg I.M. or I.V. q 1 hour. *Preoperatively for diminishing secretions and blocking cardiac vagal reflexes—* **Adults:** 0.4 to 0.6 mg I.M. 45 to 60 minutes before anesthetic. **Children:** 0.01 mg/kg I.M. up to a maximum dose of 0.4 mg 45 to 60 minutes before anesthetic.	With usual doses of 0.4 to 0.6 mg, there are few side effects other than dry mouth. However, individual tolerance varies greatly. **CNS:** disorientation, restlessness, irritability, incoherence, hallucinations, headache. **CV:** palpitations, tachycardia, paradoxical bradycardia with doses less than 0.4 mg. **EENT:** *dilated pupils, blurred vision,* photophobia, increased intraocular pressure, eye pain, dysphagia. **GI:** *constipation, mouth dryness,* nausea, vomiting. **GU:** *urinary hesitancy or retention.* **Skin:** flushing, dryness. **Other:** bronchial plugging, fever. Side effects above may be due to pending atropine toxicity and are dose-related.
benztropine mesylate Cogentin♦	*Acute dystonic reaction—* **Adults:** 2 mg I.V. or I.M. followed by 1 to 2 mg P.O. b.i.d. to prevent recurrence. *Parkinsonism—* **Adults:** 0.5 to 6 mg P.O. daily. Initial dose 0.5 mg to 1 mg. Increase 0.5 mg every 5 to 6 days. Adjust dosage to meet individual requirements.	**CNS:** disorientation, restlessness, irritability, incoherence, hallucinations, headache, sedation, depression, muscular weakness. **CV:** palpitations, tachycardia, paradoxical bradycardia. **EENT:** dilated pupils, blurred vision, photophobia, difficulty swallowing. **GI:** *constipation, mouth dryness,* nausea, vomiting, epigastric distress. **GU:** urinary hesitancy or retention. Some side effects may be due to pending atropine-like toxicity and are dose-related.
biperiden hydrochloride Akineton♦ **biperiden lactate** Akineton Lactate♦	*Extrapyramidal disorders—* **Adults:** 2 to 6 mg P.O. daily, b.i.d., or t.i.d., depending on severity. Usual dose is 2 mg daily, or 2 mg I.M. or I.V. q ½ hour, not to exceed 4 doses or 8 mg total daily. *Parkinsonism—* **Adults:** 2 mg P.O. t.i.d. to q.i.d.	**CNS:** disorientation, euphoria, restlessness, irritability, incoherence, dizziness, increased tremor. **CV:** transient postural hypotension. **EENT:** blurred vision. **GI:** *constipation, mouth dryness,* nausea, vomiting, epigastric distress. **GU:** urinary hesitancy or retention. Side effects are dose-related and may resemble atropine toxicity.

♦ Available in U.S. and Canada. ♦♦ Available in Canada only. All other products (no symbol) available in U.S. only. Italicized side effects are common or life-threatening.

INTERACTIONS	**NURSING CONSIDERATIONS**
None significant.	• Contraindicated in narrow-angle glaucoma, obstructive uropathy, obstructive disease of GI tract, myasthenia gravis, paralytic ileus, intestinal atony, unstable cardiovascular status in acute hemorrhage, and toxic megacolon. Use with caution in autonomic neuropathy, hyperthyroidism, coronary artery disease, cardiac arrhythmias, congestive heart failure, hypertension, hiatal hernia associated with reflux esophagitis, hepatic or renal disease, ulcerative colitis; in patients over 40 years because of the increased incidence of glaucoma; and in children under 6 years. Use with caution in hot or humid environments. Drug-induced heatstroke possible. • Check all dosages carefully. Even slight overdose could lead to toxicity. • Monitor vital signs carefully. Watch closely for side effects, especially in elderly or debilitated patients. Call doctor promptly. • When given I.V., may cause paradoxical initial bradycardia. Usually disappears within 2 minutes. • Monitor intake/output. Drug causes urinary retention and hesitancy; have patient void before receiving the drug. • Many of the side effects (such as dry mouth and constipation) are an extension of the drug's pharmacologic activity and may be expected. • For toxicity, see APPENDIX, *Drug Toxicities*.
Amantadine: anticholinergic side effects, such as confusion and hallucinations. Reduce dosage before administering amantadine.	• Contraindicated in narrow-angle glaucoma. Use cautiously in patients with prostatic hypertrophy, tendency to tachycardia, and in elderly or debilitated patients; produces atropine-like side effects. • Monitor vital signs carefully. Watch closely for side effects, especially in elderly or debilitated patients. Call doctor promptly. • Never discontinue this drug abruptly. Dosage must be reduced gradually. • Warn patient to avoid activities that require alertness until CNS response to drug is determined. If patient is to receive single daily dose, give at bedtime. • Explain that drug may take 2 to 3 days to exert full effect. • Monitor intake/output; urinary hesitancy and retention may develop. • Watch for intermittent constipation, distention, abdominal pain; may be onset of paralytic ileus. • Relieve dry mouth with fluids, ice chips, gum, or hard candy. • To help prevent gastric irritation, administer after meals. • For toxicity, see APPENDIX, *Drug Toxicities*.
None significant.	• Use with caution in prostatism, cardiac arrhythmias, narrow-angle glaucoma. • Monitor vital signs carefully. Watch closely for side effects, especially in elderly or debilitated patients. Call doctor promptly. • Give oral doses with or after meals to decrease GI side effects. • When giving parenterally, keep patient supine. Parenteral administration may cause transient postural hypotension and coordination disturbances. • I.V. injections should be made very slowly. • Because of possible dizziness, help patient when he gets out of bed. • Tolerance may develop, requiring increased dosage. • In severe parkinsonism, tremors may increase as spasticity is relieved. • Warn patient to avoid activities that require alertness until CNS response to drug is determined.

(continued on following page)

NAME	INDICATIONS & DOSAGE	SIDE EFFECTS
biperiden *(continued)*		
chlorphenoxamine hydrochloride Phenoxene♦	*Parkinsonism—* **Adults:** 50 mg P.O. t.i.d.; in severe cases, 300 to 400 mg daily, 100 mg t.i.d. to q.i.d.	**CNS:** drowsiness, sedation, increased tremors. **EENT:** blurred vision. **GI:** *constipation, dry mouth,* nausea, vomiting, epigastric distress.
cycrimine hydrochloride Pagitane Hydrochloride	*Idiopathic and arteriosclerotic parkinsonism—* **Adults:** initially, 1.25 to 2.5 mg P.O. t.i.d.; gradually increase dosage to 5 mg q.i.d. *Postencephalitic parkinsonism—* **Adults:** 5 mg t.i.d. or up to 5 mg q 2 hours while awake.	**CNS:** disorientation, incoherence, weakness, drowsiness, dizziness. **EENT:** blurred vision. **GI:** epigastric distress, sore mouth and tongue, *constipation, mouth dryness.* Also transient nausea and anorexia 30 minutes to 1 hour after administration. **Skin:** flushing, dryness, rash. **Other:** fever.
glycopyrrolate Robinul	*To reverse neuromuscular blockade—* **Adults:** 0.2 mg I.V. for each 1 mg neostigmine or equivalent dose of pyridostigmine. May be given intravenously without dilution or may be added to dextrose injection and given by infusion. *Preoperatively to diminish secretions and block cardiac vagal reflexes—* **Adults:** 0.002 mg/lb of body weight I.M. 30 to 60 minutes before anesthetic.	**CNS:** disorientation, irritability, incoherence, weakness, nervousness, drowsiness, dizziness, headache. **CV:** palpitations, tachycardia, paradoxical bradycardia. **EENT:** *dilated pupils, blurred vision,* photophobia, increased intraocular pressure, difficulty swallowing. **GI:** *constipation, mouth dryness,* nausea, vomiting, epigastric distress. **GU:** urinary hesitancy or retention. **Skin:** flushing, dryness, rash. **Local:** burning at injection site. **Other:** bronchial plugging, fever.
procyclidine hydrochloride	*Parkinsonism, muscle rigidity—* **Adults:** initially, 2 to 2.5 mg	**CNS:** light-headedness, giddiness. **EENT:** blurred vision, mydriasis.

♦ Available in U.S. and Canada. ♦♦ Available in Canada only. All other products (no symbol) available in U.S. only. Italicized side effects are common or life-threatening.

INTERACTIONS	NURSING CONSIDERATIONS
	• Monitor intake/output; urinary hesitancy and retention may develop. • Relieve dry mouth with fluids, ice chips, gum, or hard candy. • For toxicity, see APPENDIX, *Drug Toxicities*.
None significant.	• Use cautiously in narrow-angle glaucoma, tachycardia, or prostatic hypertrophy. • Monitor vital signs carefully. Watch closely for side effects, especially in elderly or debilitated patients. Call doctor promptly. • Warn patient to avoid activities that require alertness until CNS response to drug is determined. • Administer doses with milk after meals to decrease GI side effects. • In severe parkinsonism, tremors may increase as spasticity is relieved. • Tolerance may develop, requiring increased dosage. • Relieve dry mouth with fluids, ice chips, gum, or hard candy. • For toxicity, see APPENDIX, *Drug Toxicities*.
None significant.	• Use with caution in narrow-angle glaucoma; in the elderly with arteriosclerotic changes; in tachycardia or tendency toward urinary retention. • Monitor vital signs carefully. • Watch closely for side effects, especially vertigo, disorientation, and weakness. Call doctor promptly if these develop; he may want to stop drug or reduce dosage. • Explain that mild side effects, such as dry mouth, blurred vision, epigastric distress, disappear with continued administration. • Administer doses with milk or after meals to decrease GI side effects. • Relieve dry mouth with fluids, ice chips, gum, or hard candy. • For toxicity, see APPENDIX, *Drug Toxicities*.
None significant.	• Contraindicated in narrow-angle glaucoma, obstructive uropathy, obstructive disease of the GI tract, myasthenia gravis, paralytic ileus, intestinal atony, unstable cardiovascular status in acute hemorrhage, toxic megacolon. Use with caution in patients with autonomic neuropathy, hyperthyroidism, coronary artery disease, cardiac arrhythmias, congestive heart failure, hypertension, hiatal hernia associated with reflux esophagitis, hepatic or renal disease, ulcerative colitis, and in patients over 40 years because of increased incidence of glaucoma. Use with caution in hot or humid environments. Drug-induced heatstroke possible. • Check all dosages carefully. Even slight overdose could lead to toxicity. • Don't mix with I.V. solution containing sodium chloride or bicarbonate. • Monitor vital signs carefully. Watch closely for side effects, especially in elderly or debilitated patients. Call doctor promptly. • Monitor intake/output. Causes urinary retention or hesitancy. • Warn patient to avoid activities that require alertness until CNS response to drug is determined. • Side effects less likely than with other parasympatholytics, unless dosages are excessive. • For toxicity, see APPENDIX, *Drug Toxicities*.
None significant.	• Contraindicated in narrow-angle glaucoma. Use cautiously in tachycardia, hypotension, urinary retention, or prostatic hypertrophy.

(continued on following page)

NAME	INDICATIONS & DOSAGE	SIDE EFFECTS
procyclidine hydrochloride *(continued)* Kemadrin♦, Procyclid♦♦	P.O. t.i.d., after meals. Increase as needed to maximum 60 mg daily. Also used to relieve extrapyramidal dysfunction that accompanies treatment with phenothiazines and rauwolfia derivatives. Also controls sialorrhea from neuroleptic medications.	**GI:** *constipation, mouth dryness,* nausea, vomiting, epigastric distress. **Skin:** rash.
scopolamine hydrobromide	*Postencephalitic parkinsonism and other spastic states*— **Adults:** 0.5 to 1 mg P.O. t.i.d. to q.i.d.; 0.3 to 0.6 mg S.C., I.M., or I.V. (with suitable dilution) t.i.d. to q.i.d. **Children:** 0.006 mg/kg P.O. or S.C. t.i.d. to q.i.d.; or 0.2 mg/m².	**CNS:** disorientation, restlessness, irritability, incoherence, headache. **CV:** palpitations, tachycardia, paradoxical bradycardia. **EENT:** dilated pupils, blurred vision, photophobia, increased intraocular pressure, difficulty swallowing. **GI:** *constipation, mouth dryness,* nausea, vomiting, epigastric distress. **GU:** urinary hesitancy or retention. **Skin:** flushing, dryness. **Other:** bronchial plugging, fever, depressed respirations. Side effects may be due to pending atropine-like toxicity and are dose-related. Individual tolerance varies greatly.
trihexyphenidyl hydrochloride Aparkane♦♦, Artane♦, Hexaphen, Novohexidyl♦♦, T.H.P., Tremin, Trihexane, Trihexidyl, Trihexy♦♦, Trixyl♦♦	*Drug-induced parkinsonism*— **Adults:** 1 mg P.O. 1st day, 2 mg 2nd day, then increase 2 mg every 3 to 5 days until total of 6 to 10 mg given daily. Usually given t.i.d. with meals and, if needed, q.i.d. (last dose should be before bedtime). Postencephalitic parkinsonism may require 12 to 15 mg total daily dose.	**CNS:** nervousness, dizziness, headache, restlessness, agitation, hallucinations, euphoria, delusion, amnesia. **CV:** tachycardia. **EENT:** blurred vision, mydriasis, increased intraocular pressure. **GI:** constipation, *dry mouth, nausea.* **GU:** urinary hesitancy or retention. Side effects are dose-related.

♦ Available in U.S. and Canada. ♦♦ Available in Canada only. All other products (no symbol) available in U.S. only. Italicized side effects are common or life-threatening.

INTERACTIONS	NURSING CONSIDERATIONS
	• Watch closely for mental confusion, disorientation, agitation, hallucinations, and psychotic symptoms, especially in elderly. Call doctor promptly if these occur. • In severe parkinsonism, tremors may increase as spasticity is relieved. • Give after meals to minimize GI distress. • Warn patient to avoid activities that require alertness until CNS response to drug is determined. • Relieve dry mouth with fluids, ice chips, gum, or hard candy. • For toxicity, see APPENDIX, *Drug Toxicities*.
None significant.	• Contraindicated in narrow-angle glaucoma, obstructive uropathy, obstructive disease of the GI tract, asthma, chronic pulmonary disease, myasthenia gravis, paralytic ileus, intestinal atony, unstable cardiovascular status in acute hemorrhage, or toxic megacolon. Use with caution in patients with autonomic neuropathy, hyperthyroidism, coronary artery disease, cardiac arrhythmias, congestive heart failure, hypertension, hiatal hernia associated with reflux esophagitis, hepatic or renal disease, ulcerative colitis; in patients over 40 years because of the increased incidence of glaucoma; and in children under 6 years. Use with caution in hot or humid environments. Drug-induced heatstroke possible. • Some patients become temporarily excited or disoriented. This disappears when sedative effect is complete. Use safety precautions. • Warn patients to avoid activities requiring alertness until CNS response to drug is determined. • Monitor intake/output; urinary hesitancy or retention may develop. • Tolerance may develop when given over a long period of time. • Many of the side effects (such as dry mouth, constipation) are an extension of the drug's pharmacologic activity and may be expected. • For toxicity, see APPENDIX, *Drug Toxicities*.
Amantadine: anticholinergic side effects, such as confusion and hallucinations. Reduce dosage before administering amantadine.	• Use cautiously in patients with narrow-angle glaucoma; cardiac, hepatic, or renal disorders; hypertension; obstructive disease of the gastrointestinal and the genitourinary tracts; possible prostatic hypertrophy; patients over 60 years; and those with arteriosclerosis or history of drug hypersensitivities. • Warn patient to avoid activities that require alertness until CNS response to drug is determined. • Causes nausea if given before meals. • Relieve dry mouth with fluids, ice chips, gum, or hard candy. • Patient may develop a tolerance to this drug. • Monitor intake/output; urinary hesitancy or retention may develop. • Gonioscopic evaluation and close monitoring of intraocular pressures advised, especially in patients over 40 years. • For toxicity, see APPENDIX, *Drug Toxicities*.

NEW TREATMENT FOR DRY MOUTH

Moi-stir is a new nonprescription mouth moistener produced by Kingswood Laboratories. It relieves dry mouth (depressed salivary function), a common side effect of anticholinergic drugs.

Moi-stir contains sorbitol, sodium carboxymethylcellulose, potassium chloride, dibasic sodium phosphate, calcium chloride, sodium chloride, and magnesium chloride. Use Moi-stir cautiously in patients on sodium- or potassium-restricted diets. It's supplied in 120-ml bottles; a manual spray pump delivers about 0.5 ml of the moistener per stroke. Advise patients to spray Moi-stir one or two times into the mouth, as needed.

Adrenergics (sympathomimetics)

dobutamine hydrochloride
dopamine hydrochloride
ephedrine sulfate
epinephrine
epinephrine bitartrate
epinephrine hydrochloride
ethylnorepinephrine hydrochloride
isoetharine hydrochloride 1%
isoetharine mesylate
isoproterenol hydrochloride
isoproterenol sulfate
mephentermine sulfate
metaproterenol sulfate
metaraminol bitartrate
methoxamine hydrochloride
methoxyphenamine hydrochloride
norepinephrine injection (formerly levarterenol bitartrate)
pseudoephedrine hydrochloride
terbutaline sulfate

For information on albuterol, see APPENDIX, *New Drugs*.

Adrenergics produce their effect by either mimicking the actions of epinephrine or norepinephrine at receptor sites in the sympathetic nervous system, or displacing natural norepinephrine from neural storage sites. Because these drugs do not simulate all classes of adrenergic receptors equally, their effects and indications for use differ.

As with most drugs, the actions of adrenergics are not organ- or site-specific: they may occur at other than the desired sites.

The sympathetic nervous system innervates numerous organs (for example, the heart, blood vessels, respiratory tract, liver, urinary bladder, and intestines) and significantly affects the regulation of many body functions. When stimulated, sympathetic nerves release norepinephrine (except for sympathetic nerves that innervate sweat glands, which release acetylcholine). Norepinephrine combines with receptor sites on the innervated organ to elicit a response.

The three major types of receptors within the sympathetic system are alpha, beta, and dopaminergic. Stimulation of alpha receptors causes vasoconstriction and uterine and sphincter contraction. Beta receptors are divided into two subgroups, $beta_1$ and $beta_2$. $Beta_1$ receptors are largely in the heart; when stimulated, they increase the rate and force of myocardial contraction and the rate of atrioventricular node conduction. $Beta_2$ receptors are primarily in the bronchi, blood vessels, and uterus; stimulation produces bronchodilation, vasodilation, and uterine relaxation, respectively. Dopaminergic receptors are primarily in splanchnic blood vessels; stimulation dilates these vessels.

The adrenal medulla is a major part of the sympathetic nervous system. During times of danger or acute stress, it releases large amounts of epinephrine into the systemic circulation. Epinephrine activates alpha and beta receptors, ultimately producing physiologic and metabolic effects that prepare the person to cope with the stress (as in the fight-or-flight response).

Major uses

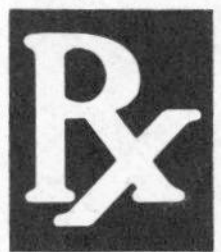

• Dobutamine, dopamine, mephentermine, metaraminol, methoxamine, and norepinephrine raise blood pressure and cardiac output in severely decompensated states, such as cardiogenic shock and heart failure.
• Ephedrine, ethylnorepinephrine, isoetharine, isoproterenol, metaproterenol, and terbutaline relieve bronchoconstriction.
• Epinephrine and isoproterenol are used to treat heart block, certain arrhythmias such as paroxysmal atrial tachycardia, and cardiac arrest.
• Epinephrine, methoxyphenamine, and pseudoephedrine are used to treat anaphylaxis and other allergic reactions (common in asthmatic attacks) and to relieve congestion.

Mechanism of action

Adrenergics simulate or increase the effect of epinephrine and norepinephrine on alpha- and beta-adrenergic receptors within the sympathetic nervous system. Effects vary and include bronchodilation, release of glucose from the liver, increase in heart rate and ventricular contractility, central nervous system excitation, dilation (beta effect) of blood vessels in skeletal muscles, and constriction (alpha effect) of blood vessels in cutaneous areas.

Absorption, distribution, metabolism, and excretion

• Dobutamine and dopamine are not absorbed from the GI tract and must be given parenterally. They're metabolized by the liver to inactive compounds and excreted in urine.
• Ephedrine is rapidly absorbed after oral, I.M., or subcutaneous administration. Some of the drug is metabolized by the liver; both unchanged compound and metabolites are excreted in the urine.
• Epinephrine and ethylnorepinephrine are not well absorbed from the GI tract after oral administration. Absorption is efficient, however, after I.M. or subcutaneous injection. The drugs are extensively metabolized in the liver and excreted in the urine.
• Isoetharine is rapidly absorbed from the respiratory tract after inhalation. It is partly metabolized by enzymes in the lungs and other tissues. Both the parent compound and metabolite are excreted in the urine.
• Isoproterenol is irregularly absorbed after oral or sublingual administration, but is well absorbed following parenteral administration or oral inhalation. It is metabolized in the liver and other tissues and excreted in the urine.
• Mephentermine is not absorbed from the GI tract and must be given parenterally. It is metabolized in the liver and excreted in the urine; excretion is increased in an acidic urine.
• Metaproterenol, well absorbed after oral administration, is subject to the first-pass effect. Conjugates of the parent compound are excreted in the urine.
• Metaraminol is erratically absorbed from the GI tract after being given orally, so must be given parenterally. Distribution, metabolism, and route of excretion are not completely known. Its pharmacologic effects are stopped by its uptake into body tissues.
• Methoxamine is not absorbed from the GI tract, so must be given parenterally. Its metabolism and excretion patterns are unclear.
• Methoxyphenamine is active when given orally and widely distributed to body tissues. It is excreted in urine.
• Norepinephrine is not absorbed after oral administration and is poorly absorbed after subcutaneous injection. The drug is taken up by nerve endings where it is metabolized; it is also metabolized by the liver and other tissues. Metabolites are excreted in urine.
• Pseudoephedrine, effective when administered orally, is metabolized by the liver. The metabolites are excreted in the urine. Excretion increases in an acidic urine.

THERAPEUTIC ACTIVITY

THERAPEUTIC ACTIVITY OF ADRENERGICS

DRUG	ROUTE	ONSET	DURATION
dobutamine	I.V.	within 2 min	until shortly after infusion is stopped
dopamine	I.V.	within 5 min	less than 10 min, or as long as infusion is continued
ephedrine	P.O.	less than 1 hr	4 to 12 hr, depending on form of P.O. dosage
epinephrine	I.M. S.C.	3 to 5 min	20 to 30 min
ethylnor-epinephrine	I.M. S.C.	3 to 5 min	20 to 30 min
isoetharine	inhalation	rapid; peaks in 5 to 15 min	1 to 4 hr
isoproterenol	I.V. P.O.	immediate 20 min	as long as infusion is continued 1 hr
mephentermine	I.M. I.V.	5 to 15 min immediate	1 to 4 hr 15 to 30 min after injection
metaproterenol	inhalation P.O.	1 min; peaks in 1 hr 15 min; peaks in 1 hr	up to 4 hr up to 4 hr
metaraminol	I.M. I.V. S.C.	within 10 min 1 to 2 min 5 to 20 min	1 hr 5 to 15 min 1 hr
methoxamine	I.M. I.V.	15 to 20 min immediate	60 to 90 min 5 to 15 min
methoxy-phenamine	P.O.	30 to 60 min	3 to 4 hr
norepinephrine	I.V.	immediate	until shortly after infusion is stopped
pseudo-ephedrine	P.O.	30 min	4 to 6 hr
terbutaline	P.O. S.C.	20 to 30 min 10 to 20 min	6 hr 4 to 6 hr

• Terbutaline is partially absorbed after oral administration but is well absorbed subcutaneously. It is eliminated in the urine and feces in both metabolized and unchanged form.

Onset and duration

The chart on the opposite page summarizes the onset and duration of the adrenergics.

Combination products

Only a few of the many combinations are included here as examples of this group.

Inhalants

DUO-MEDIHALER: isoproterenol hydrochloride 0.16 mg and phenylephrine bitartrate 0.24 mg per dose.

Oral bronchodilators

AMESEC♦: aminophylline 130 mg, ephedrine HCl 25 mg, and amobarbital 25 mg.

BRONCHOBID DURACAPS: theophylline 260 mg and ephedrine HCl 35 mg.

MARAX♦: theophylline 130 mg, ephedrine sulfate 25 mg, and hydroxyzine HCl 10 mg.

QUADRINAL♦: theophylline calcium salicylate 65 mg, ephedrine hydrochloride 24 mg, potassium iodide 320 mg, and phenobarbital 24 mg.

QUIBRON PLUS: theophylline 150 mg, ephedrine hydrochloride 25 mg, guaifenesin 100 mg, and butabarbital 20 mg.

TEDRAL SA♦: theophylline 180 mg, ephedrine hydrochloride 48 mg, and phenobarbital 25 mg.

(OTC) ASMA-LIEF: theophylline 130 mg, ephedrine hydrochloride 24 mg, and phenobarbital 8 mg.

(OTC) TEDRAL: theophylline 130 mg, ephedrine hydrochloride 24 mg, and phenobarbital 8 mg.

(OTC) THALFED: theophylline 120 mg, ephedrine hydrochloride 25 mg, and phenobarbital 8 mg.

Decongestants

ACTIFED: pseudoephedrine hydrochloride 60 mg and triprolidine hydrochloride 2.5 mg.

CONGESPRIN: phenylephrine hydrochloride 1.25 mg and aspirin 81 mg.

DRISTAN: phenylephrine hydrochloride 5 mg, chlorpheniramine maleate 2 mg, aspirin 325 mg, and caffeine 16.2 mg.

HISTASPAN-PLUS: phenylephrine hydrochloride 20 mg and chlorpheniramine maleate 8 mg.

NALDECON: phenylpropanolamine hydrochloride 40 mg, phenylephrine hydrochloride 10 mg, chlorpheniramine maleate 5 mg, and phenyltoloxamine citrate 15 mg.

ORNEX: phenylpropanolamine hydrochloride 18 mg and acetaminophen 325 mg.

PHENERGAN-D: pseudoephedrine hydrochloride 60 mg and promethazine hydrochloride 6.25 mg.

SINUTAB-II: phenylpropanolamine hydrochloride 25 mg and acetaminophen 325 mg.

TRIAMINIC: phenylpropanolamine hydrochloride 50 mg, pyrilamine maleate 25 mg, and pheniramine maleate 25 mg.

NAME	INDICATIONS & DOSAGE	SIDE EFFECTS
dobutamine hydrochloride Dobutrex	*Refractory heart failure and as adjunct in cardiac surgery—* **Adults:** 2.5 to 10 mcg/kg/minute as an I.V. infusion. Rarely, infusion rates up to 40 mcg/kg/minute have been required. May be reconstituted with 5% dextrose in water, normal saline solution, or lactated Ringer's solution.	**CNS:** headache. **CV:** *increased heart rate, hypertension, premature ventricular beats,* angina, nonspecific chest pain. **GI:** nausea, vomiting. **Other:** shortness of breath.
dopamine hydrochloride Intropin♦	*To treat shock and correct hemodynamic imbalances; to improve perfusion to vital organs, increase cardiac output; to correct hypotension—* **Adults:** 2 to 5 mcg/kg/minute I.V. infusion, up to 50 mcg/kg/minute. Titrate the dosage to the desired hemodynamic and/or renal response.	**CNS:** headache. **CV:** ectopic beats, tachycardia, anginal pain, palpitations, *hypotension.* Less frequently, bradycardia, widening of QRS complex, conduction disturbances, vasoconstriction. **GI:** nausea, vomiting. **Local:** necrosis and tissue sloughing with extravasation. **Other:** piloerection, dyspnea.
ephedrine sulfate Ectasule Minus III	*To correct hypotensive states; to support ventricular rate in Adams-Stokes syndrome—* **Adults:** 25 to 50 mg I.M. or S.C., or 10 to 25 mg I.V. p.r.n. to maximum 150 mg/24 hours. **Children:** 3 mg/kg S.C. or I.V.	**CNS:** *insomnia, nervousness,* dizziness, headache, muscle weakness, sweating, euphoria, confusion, delirium. **CV:** *palpitations,* tachycardia, hypertension. **EENT:** nose and throat dryness.

INTERACTIONS	NURSING CONSIDERATIONS
Propranolol, metoprolol: These beta blockers may make dobutamine ineffective. Do not use together.	• Contraindicated in idiopathic hypertrophic subaortic stenosis. • A unique agent. Increases contractility of failing heart without inducing marked tachycardia, except at high doses. • Dobutamine is chemical modification of isoproterenol. • Often used with nitroprusside for additive effects. • EKG, blood pressure, pulmonary wedge pressure, and cardiac output should be monitored continuously. Also monitor urinary output. • Incompatible with alkaline solutions. Do not mix with sodium bicarbonate injection. • Infusions of up to 72 hours produce no more adverse effects than shorter infusions. • Oxidation of drug may slightly discolor admixtures containing dobutamine. This does not indicate a significant loss of potency. • Intravenous solutions remain stable for 24 hours.
Ergot alkaloids: extreme elevations in blood pressure. Don't use together. *Phenytoin:* may lower blood pressure of dopamine-stabilized patients. Monitor carefully.	• Contraindicated in uncorrected tachyarrhythmias, pheochromocytoma, ventricular fibrillation. Use cautiously in patients with occlusive vascular disease, cold injuries, diabetic endarteritis, arterial embolism; also, in pregnant patients and those taking MAO inhibitors. • Not a substitute for blood or fluid volume deficit. If volume deficit exists, it should be replaced before vasopressors are administered. • Use large vein, as in antecubital fossa, to minimize risk of extravasation. Watch site carefully for signs of extravasation. If it occurs, stop infusion immediately and call doctor. He may want to counteract effect by infiltrating the area with 5 to 10 mg phentolamine and 10 to 15 ml normal saline solution. • Check blood pressure, pulse rate, urinary output, and extremity color and temperature often during infusion. Titrate infusion rate according to findings, using doctor's guidelines. Use a microdrip or infusion pump to regulate flow rate. • Observe patient closely for side effects. If adverse effects develop, dosage may need to be adjusted or discontinued. • If a disproportionate rise in the diastolic pressure (a marked decrease in pulse pressure) is observed in patients receiving dopamine, decrease infusion rate and observe carefully for further evidence of predominant vasoconstrictor activity, unless such an effect is desired. • Most patients satisfactorily maintained on less than 20 mcg/kg/minute. • If doses exceed 50 mcg/kg/minute, check urinary output often. If urine flow decreases without hypotension, consider reducing dose. • If drug is stopped, watch closely for sudden drop in blood pressure. • Don't mix with alkaline solutions. Use 5% dextrose in water, normal saline solution, or combination of 5% dextrose in water and saline solution. Mix just before use. See Chapter 6, UNDERSTANDING INTRAVENOUS SOLUTION COMPATIBILITY. • Dopamine solutions deteriorate after 24 hours. Discard at that time or earlier if solution is discolored. • Do not mix other drugs in bottle containing dopamine. • Do not give alkaline drugs (sodium bicarbonate, phenytoin sodium) through I.V. line containing dopamine.
MAO inhibitors and tricyclic antidepressants: when given with sympathomimetics, may cause severe hypertension (hypertensive crisis). Don't	• Contraindicated in patients with porphyria, severe coronary artery disease, cardiac arrhythmias, narrow-angle glaucoma, psychoneurosis, and in patients on MAO-inhibitor therapy. Use with caution in elderly patients and those with hypertension, hyperthyroidism, nervous or excitable states, cardiovascular disease, prostatic hypertrophy. • Not a substitute for blood or fluid volume deficit. Volume deficit should be replaced before vasopressors are administered.

(continued on following page)

NAME	INDICATIONS & DOSAGE	SIDE EFFECTS
ephedrine sulfate *(continued)*	daily, divided into 4 to 6 doses. *Bronchodilator or nasal decongestant—* **Adults:** 12.5 to 50 mg P.O. b.i.d., t.i.d., or q.i.d. Maximum 400 mg/day in 6 to 8 divided doses. **Children:** 2 to 3 mg/kg P.O. daily in 4 to 6 divided doses.	**GI:** nausea, vomiting, anorexia. **GU:** urinary retention, painful urination due to visceral sphincter spasm.
epinephrine Inhalants: Bronkaid Mist♦, Primatene Mist **epinephrine bitartrate** Inhalants: AsthmaHaler, Medihaler-Epi♦ **epinephrine hydrochloride** Adrenalin Chloride, Asmolin, Sus-Phrine♦	*Bronchospasm, hypersensitivity reactions, and anaphylaxis—* **Adults:** 0.1 to 0.5 ml of 1:1,000 S.C. or I.M. Repeat q 10 to 15 minutes, p.r.n. Or 0.1 to 0.25 ml 1:1,000 I.V. **Children:** 0.01 ml (10 mcg) of 1:1,000/kg S.C. Repeat q 20 minutes to 4 hours, p.r.n.; 0.005 ml/kg of 1:200 (Sus-Phrine). Repeat q 8 to 12 hours, p.r.n. *Hemostatic—* **Adults:** 1:50,000 to 1:1,000, applied topically. *Acute asthmatic attacks (inhalation)—* **Adults and children:** 1 or 2 inhalations of 1:100 or 2.25% racemic, p.r.n.; 0.2 mg/dose usual content. *To prolong local anesthetic effect—* **Adults and children:** 0.2 to 0.4 ml of 1:1,000 intraspinal; 1:500,000 to 1:50,000 local mixed with local anesthetic. *To restore cardiac rhythm in cardiac arrest—* **Adults:** 0.5 to 1 mg I.V. or into endotracheal tube. May be given intracardiac if no I.V. route or intratracheal route available. **Children:** 10 mcg/kg I.V. or 5 to 10 mcg (0.05 to 0.1 ml of 1:10,000)/kg intracardiac. *Note:* 1 mg = 1 ml of 1:1,000 or 10 ml of 1:10,000.	**CNS:** *nervousness,* tremor, euphoria, anxiety, coldness of extremities, vertigo, *headache,* sweating, cerebral hemorrhage, disorientation, agitation. In patients with Parkinson's disease, the drug increases rigidity and tremor. **CV:** *palpitations;* widened pulse pressure; hypertension; *tachycardia; ventricular fibrillation; cerebrovascular accident;* anginal pain; EKG changes, including a decrease in the T-wave amplitude. **Metabolic:** *hyperglycemia,* glycosuria. **Other:** pulmonary edema, dyspnea, *pallor.*
ethylnorepinephrine hydrochloride Bronkephrine	*To relieve bronchospasm due to asthma—* **Adults:** 0.5 to 1 ml S.C. or I.M. **Children:** 0.1 to 0.5 ml S.C. or I.M.	**CNS:** *headache,* dizziness. **CV:** changes in blood pressure, *elevation in pulse rate,* palpitations. **GI:** nausea.

♦ Available in U.S. and Canada. ♦♦ Available in Canada only. All other products (no symbol) available in U.S. only. Italicized side effects are common or life-threatening.

INTERACTIONS	**NURSING CONSIDERATIONS**
use together. *Methyldopa:* may inhibit effect of ephedrine. Give together cautiously.	• Give I.V. injection slowly. • Hypoxia, hypercapnia, and acidosis, which may reduce effectiveness or increase the incidence of adverse effects, must be identified and corrected before or during ephedrine administration. • Effectiveness decreases after 2 to 3 weeks. Then increased dosage may be needed. Tolerance develops, but drug is not known to cause addiction. • To prevent insomnia, avoid giving within 2 hours before bedtime. • Warn patient not to take over-the-counter drugs that contain ephedrine without informing doctor.
Tricyclic antidepressants: when given with sympathomimetics, may cause severe hypertension (hypertensive crisis). Don't give together. *Propranolol:* vasoconstriction and reflex bradycardia. Monitor patient carefully.	• Contraindicated in narrow-angle glaucoma, shock (other than anaphylactic shock), organic brain damage, cardiac dilatation, and coronary insufficiency. Also during general anesthesia with halogenated hydrocarbons or cyclopropane and in labor (may delay second stage). Use with extreme caution in patients with long-standing bronchial asthma and emphysema who have developed degenerative heart disease. Use with caution in elderly patients, and those with hyperthyroidism, angina, hypertension, psychoneurosis, diabetes. • Don't mix with alkaline solutions. Use 5% dextrose in water, normal saline solution, or a combination of 5% dextrose in water and saline solution. Mix just before use. See Chapter 6, UNDERSTANDING INTRAVENOUS SOLUTION COMPATIBILITY. • Epinephrine is rapidly destroyed by oxidizing agents, such as iodine, chromates, nitrates, nitrites, oxygen, and salts of easily reducible metals such as iron. • Epinephrine solutions deteriorate after 24 hours. Discard after that time or before if solution is discolored or contains precipitate. Keep solution in light-resistant container, and don't remove before use. • Massage site after injection to counteract possible vasoconstriction. Repeated local injection can cause necrosis at site due to vasoconstriction. • Avoid intramuscular administration of oil injection into buttocks. Gas gangrene may occur because epinephrine reduces oxygen tension of the tissues, encouraging the growth of contaminating organisms. • This drug may widen patient's pulse pressure. • In the event of a sharp blood pressure rise, rapid-acting vasodilators, such as the nitrites or alpha-adrenergic blocking agents, can be given to counteract the marked pressor effect of large doses of epinephrine. • Observe patient closely for side effects. If adverse effects develop, dosage may need to be adjusted or discontinued. • If patient has acute hypersensitivity reactions, it may be necessary to instruct him to self-inject epinephrine at home. • Drug of choice in emergency treatment of acute anaphylactic reactions, including anaphylactic shock.
None significant.	• Use with caution in patients with cardiovascular disease or history of stroke. • Safer than epinephrine for use in hypertensive or severely ill patients in whom significant pressor effects are undesirable. • Valuable when used in children due to low incidence of adverse effects; may be useful in diabetic asthmatics due to low glycogenolytic activity. • Choose anatomic injection site carefully to avoid inadvertent intraneural or intravascular injection.

NAME	INDICATIONS & DOSAGE	SIDE EFFECTS
isoetharine hydrochloride 1% Bronkosol **isoetharine mesylate** Bronkometer	*Bronchial asthma and reversible bronchospasm that may occur with bronchitis and emphysema—* **Adults:** (hydrochloride): administered by hand nebulizer (3 to 7 inhalations, undiluted), oxygen aerosolization (0.5 ml, 1:3 dilution with saline), or IPPB (0.5 ml, 1:3 dilution with saline). **Adults:** (mesylate): 1 to 2 inhalations. Occasionally, more may be required.	**CNS:** *tremor, headache,* dizziness, excitement. **CV:** *palpitations,* increased heart rate. **GI:** nausea, vomiting.
isoproterenol hydrochloride Isuprel♦, Proternol (tabs) Inhalants: Norisodrine, Vapo-Iso **isoproterenol sulfate** Iso-Autohaler, Luf-Iso Inhalation, Medihaler-Iso♦, Norisodrine	*Bronchial asthma and reversible bronchospasm (hydrochloride)—* **Adults:** 10 to 20 mg S.L. q 6 to 8 hours. **Children:** 5 to 10 mg S.L. q 6 to 8 hours. Not recommended for children under 6 years. *Bronchospasm (sulfate)—* **Adults and children:** acute dyspneic episodes: 1 inhalation initially. May repeat if needed after 2 to 5 minutes. Maintenance: 1 to 2 inhalations q.i.d. to 6 times daily. May repeat once more 10 minutes after second dose. Not more than 3 doses should be administered for each attack. *Heart block and ventricular arrhythmias (sulfate)—* **Adults:** initially, 0.02 to 0.06 mg I.V. Subsequent doses 0.01 to 0.2 mg I.V. or 5 mcg/ minute I.V.; or 0.2 mg I.M. initially, then 0.02 to 1 mg, p.r.n. **Children:** may give ½ of initial adult dose. *Maintenance for Stokes-Adams disease or AV block (sulfate)—* **Adults:** 30 to 180 mg timed-release tablets P.O. daily swallowed whole. *Shock (sulfate)—* **Adults and children:** 0.5 to 5 mcg/ minute by continuous I.V. infusion. Usual concentration: 1 mg (5 ml) in 500 ml 5% dextrose in water. Adjust rate according to heart rate, central venous pressure, blood pressure, and urine flow.	**CNS:** *headache,* mild tremor, weakness, dizziness, nervousness, insomnia. **CV:** *palpitations,* tachycardia, anginal pain; blood pressure may be elevated and then fall. **GI:** nausea, vomiting. **Metabolic:** hyperglycemia. **Other:** sweating, flushing of face, bronchial edema and inflammation.

♦ Available in U.S. and Canada. ♦♦ Available in Canada only. All other products (no symbol) available in U.S. only. Italicized side effects are common or life-threatening.

INTERACTIONS	NURSING CONSIDERATIONS
None significant.	• Use cautiously in patients with hyperthyroidism, hypertension, coronary disease, or those with sensitivity to sympathomimetics. • Excessive use can lead to decreased effectiveness. • Monitor for severe paradoxical bronchoconstriction after excessive use. Discontinue immediately if bronchoconstriction occurs. • Although isoetharine has minimal effects on the heart, use cautiously in patients receiving general anesthetics that sensitize the myocardium to sympathomimetic drugs. • Instruct patient in the use of aerosol and mouthpiece.
Propranolol and other beta blockers: blocked effect of isoproterenol and vice versa. Monitor patient carefully if used together.	• Contraindicated in tachycardia caused by digitalis intoxication and in patients with preexisting arrhythmias, especially tachycardia, because chronotropic effect on the heart may aggravate such disorders. Contraindicated in recent myocardial infarction. Use cautiously in coronary insufficiency, diabetes, hyperthyroidism. • Not a substitute for blood or fluid volume deficit. If deficit exists, it should be replaced before vasopressors are administered. • If heart rate exceeds 110 beats/minute, it may be advisable to decrease infusion rate or temporarily stop infusion. Doses sufficient to increase the heart rate to more than 130 beats/minute may induce ventricular arrhythmias. • If precordial distress or anginal pain occurs, stop drug immediately. • When administering I.V. isoproterenol for shock, closely monitor blood pressure, CVP, EKG, arterial blood gas measurements, and urinary output. Carefully adjust infusion rate according to these measurements. • Oral and sublingual tablets are poorly and erratically absorbed. • Teach patient how to take sublingual tablet properly. Tell him to hold tablet under tongue until it dissolves and is absorbed and not to swallow saliva until that time. Prolonged use of sublingual tablets can cause tooth decay. Instruct patient to rinse mouth with water between doses. Will also help prevent dryness of oropharynx. • If possible, don't give at bedtime because it interrupts sleep patterns. • Oral tablets not for sublingual use; must be swallowed whole, not broken. Store in cool, dry place in airtight, light-resistant container. Keep bottle tightly capped after opening. • This drug may cause slight rise in systolic blood pressure and slight to marked drop in diastolic blood pressure. • Use a microdrip or infusion pump to regulate infusion flow rate. • Observe patient closely for side effects. Dosage may need to be adjusted or discontinued. • Teach patient to perform oral inhalation correctly. See patient-teaching aid on p. 545 for instructions on using a metered-dose nebulizer. • Instructions for metered-powder nebulizer are the same, except that deep inhalation is not necessary. • Patient may develop a tolerance to this drug. Warn against overuse. • Warn patient using oral inhalant that drug may turn sputum and saliva pink. • May aggravate ventilation perfusion abnormalities; even while ease of breathing is improved, arterial oxygen tension may fall paradoxically. • Discard inhalation solution if it is discolored or contains precipitate.

NAME	INDICATIONS & DOSAGE	SIDE EFFECTS
mephentermine sulfate Wyamine♦	*Hypotension following spinal anesthesia—* **Adults:** 30 to 45 mg I.V. in a single injection, then 30 mg I.V. repeated p.r.n. Maintenance of blood pressure: continuous I.V. infusion of 0.1% solution of mephentermine in 5% dextrose in water. *Hypotension following spinal anesthesia during obstetric procedures—* **Adults:** initially, 15 mg I.V., p.r.n. *Prevention of hypotension during spinal anesthesia—* **Adults:** 30 to 40 mg I.M. 10 to 20 minutes prior to anesthesia. *Treatment of shock and hypotension—* **Adults:** 0.5 mg/kg I.V. **Children:** 0.4 mg/kg I.V.	**CNS:** euphoria, nervousness, anxiety, tremor, incoherence, drowsiness, convulsions. **CV:** arrhythmias, marked elevation of blood pressure (with large doses).
metaproterenol sulfate Alupent♦, Metaprel	*Acute episodes of bronchial asthma—* **Adults and children:** 2 to 3 inhalations. Should not repeat inhalations more often than q 3 to 4 hours. Should not exceed 12 inhalations daily. *Bronchial asthma and reversible bronchospasm—* **Adults:** 20 mg P.O. q 6 to 8 hours. **Children over 9 years or over 27 kg:** 20 mg P.O. q 6 to 8 hours. (0.4 mg to 0.9 mg/kg/dose t.i.d.) **Children 6 to 9 years or less than 27 kg:** 10 mg P.O. q 6 to 8 hours. (0.4 mg to 0.9 mg/kg/dose t.i.d.) Not recommended for children under 6 years.	**CNS:** nervousness, weakness, drowsiness, tremor. **CV:** tachycardia, hypertension, palpitations; *with excessive use, cardiac arrest.* **GI:** vomiting, nausea, bad taste in mouth. **Other:** paradoxical bronchiolar constriction with excessive use.
metaraminol bitartrate Aramine♦	*Prevention of hypotension—* **Adults:** 2 to 10 mg I.M. or S.C. *Severe shock—* **Adults:** 0.5 to 5 mg direct I.V. followed by I.V. infusion. *Treatment of hypotension due to shock—* **Adults:** 15 to 100 mg in 500 ml normal saline solution or 5% dextrose in water I.V. infusion. Adjust rate to maintain blood pressure. *All indications—*	**CNS:** apprehension, restlessness, dizziness, headache, tremor, weakness; with excessive use, convulsions. **CV:** hypertension; hypotension; precordial pain; palpitations; arrhythmias, including sinus or ventricular tachycardia; bradycardia; premature supraventricular beats; atrioventricular dissociation. **GI:** nausea, vomiting. **GU:** decreased urinary output. **Metabolic:** hyperglycemia.

♦ Available in U.S. and Canada. ♦♦ Available in Canada only. All other products (no symbol) available in U.S. only. Italicized side effects are common or life-threatening.

INTERACTIONS	NURSING CONSIDERATIONS
None significant.	• Contraindicated in concealed hemorrhage or hypotension from hemorrhage, except in emergencies; also in patients receiving phenothiazines, or who have received MAO inhibitors within 2 weeks. Use cautiously in arteriosclerosis, cardiovascular disease, hyperthyroidism, hypertension, chronic illness. • Not a substitute for blood or fluid volume deficit. If deficit exists, it should be replaced before vasopressors are administered. • During infusion, check blood pressure every 5 minutes until stabilized; then every 15 minutes. • Observe patient closely for side effects. If adverse effects develop, dosage may need to be adjusted or discontinued. • Monitor blood pressure even after stopping drug. • I.M. route may be used since drug is not irritating to tissue. • I.V. drug is not irritating to tissue, and extravasation is not dangerous. To prepare 0.1% I.V. solution: add 16.6 ml mephentermine (30 mg/ml) to 500 ml 5% dextrose in water. • Can be given I.V. undiluted. • May increase uterine contractions during third trimester of pregnancy. • Hypercapnia, hypoxia, and acidosis may reduce effectiveness or increase adverse effects. Identify and correct before and during administration.
None significant.	• Contraindicated in tachycardia, and in arrhythmias associated with tachycardia. Use with caution in hypertension, coronary artery disease, hyperthyroidism, diabetes. • Safe use of inhalant in children under 12 years not established. • Teach patient how to administer metered dose correctly. Instructions: shake container; exhale through nose; administer aerosol while inhaling deeply on mouthpiece of inhaler; hold breath for a few seconds, then exhale slowly. Allow 2 minutes between inhalations. Store drug in light-resistant container. • Tell patient to notify doctor if no response is derived from dosage. Warn against changing dose without calling doctor.
MAO inhibitors: may cause severe hypertension (hypertensive crisis). Don't use together.	• Contraindicated in peripheral or mesenteric thrombosis, pulmonary edema, hypercarbia, and acidosis; also during anesthesia with cyclopropane and halogenated hydrocarbon anesthetics. Use cautiously in patients with hypertension, thyroid disease, diabetes, cirrhosis, or malaria, and those receiving digitalis. • Not a substitute for blood or fluid volume deficit. Fluid deficit should be replaced before vasopressors are administered. • Keep solution in light-resistant container, away from heat. • Use large veins, as in antecubital fossa, to minimize risk of extravasation. Watch infusion site carefully for signs of extravasation. If it occurs, stop infusion immediately and call doctor. • During infusion, check blood pressure every 5 minutes until stabilized; then every 15 minutes. Check pulse rates, urinary output, and

(continued on following page)

NAME	INDICATIONS & DOSAGE	SIDE EFFECTS
metaraminol bitartrate *(continued)*	**Children:** 0.01 mg/kg as single I.V. injection; 1 mg/25 ml 5% dextrose in water as I.V. infusion. Adjust rate to maintain blood pressure in normal range. 0.1 mg/kg I.M. as single dose, p.r.n. Allow at least 10 minutes to elapse before increasing dose because maximum effect is not immediately apparent.	**Skin:** flushing, pallor, sweating. **Local:** irritation upon extravasation. **Other:** *metabolic acidosis in hypovolemia, increased body temperature, respiratory distress.*
methoxamine hydrochloride Vasoxyl♦	*Moderate fall in blood pressure—* **Adults:** 5 to 10 mg I.M. *Paroxysmal supraventricular tachycardia—* **Adults:** 5 to 15 mg I.V. injected slowly. 10 to 20 mg I.M. Allow 15 minutes before additional increased doses to evaluate effects of initial dose and prevent a cumulative effect. *Prevention of hypotension during spinal anesthesia—* **Adults:** 10 to 15 mg I.M. before or with spinal anesthesia. *Support and restoration of blood pressure during anesthesia (including cyclopropane); termination of paroxysmal supraventricular tachycardia; emergency situations; systolic falls below 60 mm Hg—* **Adults:** initially, 3 to 5 mg slow I.V. injection, followed by 10 to 15 mg I.M. to prolong effect. **Children:** direct I.V. dose is 80 mcg/kg of body weight or 2.5 mg/m² of body-surface area, injected slowly.	**CNS:** paresthesias, chills, severe headache, restlessness, tremors, dizziness, anxiety, nervousness. **CV:** hypertension, bradycardia, cardiac depression, precordial pain, heart failure in diseased myocardium. **GI:** projectile vomiting. **GU:** urinary urgency, decreased urinary output. **Skin:** gooseflesh, pallor. **Other:** respiratory distress, *metabolic acidosis.*

♦ Available in U.S. and Canada. ♦♦ Available in Canada only. All other products (no symbol) available in U.S. only. Italicized side effects are common or life-threatening.

INTERACTIONS	NURSING CONSIDERATIONS
	color and temperature of extremities. Titrate infusion rate according to findings, using doctor's guidelines. • Use a microdrip or infusion pump to regulate infusion flow rate. • Observe patient closely for side effects. If adverse effects develop, dosage may need to be adjusted or discontinued. • For I.V. therapy, use 2-bottle setup so I.V. can continue if this drug is stopped. • Blood pressure should be raised to slightly less than the patient's normal level. Be careful to avoid excessive blood pressure response. Rapidly induced hypertensive response can cause acute pulmonary edema, arrhythmias, and cardiac arrest. • Because of prolonged action, a cumulative effect is possible. With an excessive vasopressor response, elevated blood pressure may persist after the drug is stopped. • Urinary output may decrease initially, then increase as blood pressure reaches normal level. Report persistent decreased urinary output. • When discontinuing therapy with this drug, slow infusion rate gradually. Continue monitoring vital signs, watching for possible severe drop in blood pressure. Keep equipment nearby to start drug again, if necessary. Pressor therapy should not be reinstated until the systolic blood pressure falls below 70 to 80 mm Hg. • Keep emergency drugs on hand to reverse effects of metaraminol: atropine for reflex bradycardia; phentolamine to decrease vasopressor effects; propranolol for arrhythmias. • Closely monitor patients with diabetes. Adjustment in insulin dose may be needed. • Metaraminol should not be mixed with other drugs. See Chapter 6, UNDERSTANDING INTRAVENOUS SOLUTION COMPATIBILITY.
None significant.	• Contraindicated in patients with severe heart disease or in those taking MAO inhibitors; in shock due to myocardial infarction, or peripheral or mesenteric vascular thrombosis; and in elderly or pregnant patients. Use cautiously in hyperthyroidism or hypertension, and after use of ergot alkaloids. • Should not be used with local anesthetics to prolong their effect. • Not a substitute for blood volume or fluid volume deficit. If deficit exists, replace before vasopressors are given. Hypoxia and acidosis should also be corrected before or during therapy. • Methoxamine solutions deteriorate after 24 hours. Discard after that time or before if discolored or contains precipitate. • Has potent, prolonged pressor action. Does not increase cardiac rate or irritability of cyclopropane-sensitized heart. • Does not stimulate CNS. • Monitor response by checking blood pressure. Adjust dose accordingly. Blood pressure should be raised to slightly less than normal level. In previously normotensive patients, systolic blood pressure should be maintained at 80 to 100 mm Hg; in previously hypertensive patients, systolic blood pressure should be maintained at 30 to 40 mm Hg below usual level. • Observe patient closely for side effects. Dosage may need to be adjusted or discontinued. • Keep these emergency drugs on hand to reverse effects of methoxamine: atropine for reflex bradycardia and phentolamine for increased vasopressor effects. • Monitor blood pressure and pulse rate even after stopping drug. Report sudden changes.

NAME	INDICATIONS & DOSAGE	SIDE EFFECTS
methoxyphenamine hydrochloride Orthoxine Hydrochloride	*To treat allergies and bronchial asthma—* **Adults:** 100 mg P.O. q 4 to 6 hours. Maximum dose, 600 mg/day. **Children:** 25 to 50 mg P.O. q 4 to 6 hours.	**CNS:** insomnia, nervousness, dizziness, headache, anxiety. **CV:** palpitations, tachycardia, hypertension. **GI:** nausea, vomiting, dry mouth. **Other:** sweating, flushing.
norepinephrine injection (formerly levarterenol bitartrate) Levophed♦	*To restore blood pressure in acute hypotensive states—* **Adults:** initially, 8 to 12 mcg/minute I.V. infusion, then adjust to maintain normal blood pressure. Average maintenance dose 2 to 4 mcg/minute.	**CNS:** *headache,* anxiety, weakness, dizziness, tremor, restlessness, insomnia. **CV:** bradycardia, severe hypertension, marked increase in peripheral resistance, decreased cardiac output, arrhythmias, *ventricular tachycardia, fibrillation,* bigeminal rhythm, atrioventricular dissociation, precordial pain. **GU:** *decreased urinary output.* **Metabolic:** *metabolic acidosis,* hyperglycemia, increased glycogenolysis. **Local:** irritation with extravasation. **Other:** fever, respiratory difficulty.
pseudoephedrine hydrochloride Besan, Cenafed, D-Feda, Eltor♦♦, First Sign, Gyrocaps, Novafed, Robidrine♦♦, Ro-Fedrin, Sudabid,	*Nasal and eustachian tube decongestant—* **Adults:** 60 mg P.O. q 4 hours. **Children 6 to 12 years:** 30 mg P.O. q 4 hours. Maximum 120 mg/day. **Children 2 to 6 years:** 15 mg P.O. q 4 hours. Maximum	**CNS:** *anxiety,* transient stimulation, tremors, dizziness, headache, insomnia, *nervousness.* **CV:** arrhythmias, *palpitations,* tachycardia. **GI:** anorexia, nausea, vomiting, dry mouth. **GU:** difficulty in urination.

♦ Available in U.S. and Canada. ♦♦ Available in Canada only. All other products (no symbol) available in U.S. only. Italicized side effects are common or life-threatening.

INTERACTIONS	NURSING CONSIDERATIONS
None significant.	• Contraindicated in those who have used MAO inhibitors within past 2 weeks. Use cautiously in hypertension, hyperthyroidism, acute coronary disease, cardiac decompensation, diabetes mellitus. • Only "possibly effective" in treating bronchial asthma, acute urticaria, allergic rhinitis, gastrointestinal allergy, and allergic headaches. • Effectiveness decreases after 2 to 3 weeks. Then increased dose may be needed. • Avoid giving this drug within 2 hours of bedtime; insomnia may result. • Warn against using over-the-counter drugs containing sympathomimetics without informing doctor.
Tricyclic antidepressants: when given with sympathomimetics, may cause severe hypertension (hypertensive crisis). Don't give together.	• Contraindicated in mesenteric or peripheral vascular thrombosis, pregnancy, profound hypoxia, hypercarbia, hypotension from blood volume deficits, or during cyclopropane and halothane anesthesia. Use cautiously in hypertension, hyperthyroidism, severe cardiac disease. Use with extreme caution in patients receiving MAO inhibitors or tricyclic antidepressants. • Not a substitute for blood or fluid volume deficit. If deficit exists, it should be replaced before vasopressors are administered. • Norepinephrine solutions deteriorate after 24 hours. Discard after that time. • Use large vein, as in antecubital fossa, to minimize risk of extravasation. Check site frequently for signs of extravasation. If it occurs, stop infusion immediately and call doctor. He may counteract effect by infiltrating area with 5 to 10 mg phentolamine and 10 to 15 ml normal saline solution. Also check for blanching along course of infused vein; may progress to superficial slough. During infusion, check blood pressure every 2 minutes until stabilized; then every 5 minutes. Also check pulse rates, urinary output, and color and temperature of extremities. Titrate infusion rate according to findings, using doctor's guidelines. In previously hypertensive patients, blood pressure should be raised no more than 40 mm Hg below preexisting systolic pressure. • Never leave patient unattended during infusion. • Use a microdrip or infusion pump to regulate infusion flow rate. • For I.V. therapy, use two-bottle setup with Y-port so I.V. can continue if norepinephrine is stopped. • Report decreased urinary output to doctor immediately. • If prolonged I.V. therapy is necessary, change injection site frequently. • When stopping drug, slow infusion rate gradually. Monitor vital signs, even after drug is stopped. Watch for possible severe drop in blood pressure. • Keep emergency drugs on hand to reverse effects of norepinephrine: atropine for reflex bradycardia; propranolol for arrhythmias; phentolamine for increased vasopressor effects. • Administer in dextrose and saline solution; saline solution alone is not recommended.
MAO inhibitors: may cause severe hypertension (hypertensive crisis). Don't use together.	• Contraindicated in patients with severe hypertension or severe coronary artery disease; in those receiving MAO inhibitors; and in breast-feeding mothers. Use cautiously in hypertension, cardiac disease, glaucoma, hyperthyroidism, or prostatic hypertrophy. • Tell patient to stop drug if he becomes unusually restless and to notify doctor promptly. • Warn against using over-the-counter products containing ephedrine or other sympathomimetic amines.

(continued on following page)

NAME	INDICATIONS & DOSAGE	SIDE EFFECTS
pseudoephedrine hydrochloride *(continued)* Sudafed♦, Sudafed SA	60 mg/day. Extended-relief tablets: **Adults, and children over 12 years:** 60 to 120 mg P.O. q 12 hours. This form contraindicated for children under 12 years.	**Skin:** pallor.
terbutaline sulfate Brethine, Bricanyl ♦	*Bronchodilator—* **Adults:** 2.5 to 5 mg P.O. q 8 hours; or 0.25 mg S.C. If no improvement in 15 to 30 minutes, repeat dose. Do not exceed 0.5 mg in 4 hours. **Children 12 to 15 years:** 2.5 mg P.O. t.i.d. Not recommended for children under 12 years.	**CNS:** *nervousness, tremors, headache,* drowsiness, sweating. **CV:** palpitations, increased heart rate. **GI:** vomiting, nausea.

♦ Available in U.S. and Canada. ♦♦ Available in Canada only. All other products (no symbol) available in U.S. only. Italicized side effects are common or life-threatening.

PATIENT-TEACHING AID

WHAT YOU SHOULD KNOW ABOUT OVER-THE-COUNTER BRONCHODILATORS

Dear Patient:

Epinephrine is the principal drug in over-the-counter (OTC) bronchodilators. Even if you have no underlying health problems, you may experience some unpleasant side effects with this drug. So consider these points before taking any OTC bronchodilators.

- Tolerance develops suddenly.
- Since epinephrine is a short-duration drug, rebound bronchospasms may occur, tempting you to overdose.
- If you don't keep the inhaler's mouthpiece perfectly clean, you risk spraying harmful bacteria into your bronchial tubes.
- If you swallow the drug, epigastric distress (severe pains in your upper abdomen) may occur.
- Epinephrine can severely compromise the effectiveness of other drugs. For example, its hyperglycemic effect can create a need for increased insulin or increased oral hypoglycemic dosages.
- Both normal and excessive doses of epinephrine can produce headaches, anxiety, dizziness, tachycardia (rapid heartbeat), tremor, nausea, bronchial irritation, dried secretions, and mucous plug obstructions in otherwise healthy patients. Acute epinephrine toxicity can cause severe hypertension, pulmonary edema, and cardiac arrhythmias.

Underlying conditions that magnify the potential dangers of epinephrine use include hypertension, hyperthyroidism, diabetes, cardiovascular disease, and pregnancy. If you suffer from narrow-angle glaucoma, benign prostatic hypertrophy, or Parkinson's disease, using epinephrine can worsen your condition.

In any case, make sure you have your doctor's permission before you use any OTC bronchodilator.

INTERACTIONS	NURSING CONSIDERATIONS
	• Tell patient not to take drug within 2 hours of bedtime because it can cause insomnia. • Tell patient he can relieve dry mouth with sugarless gum or sour hard candy.
MAO inhibitors: when given with sympathomimetics, may cause severe hypertension (hypertensive crisis). Don't use together. *Propranolol and other beta blockers:* blocked effects. Monitor patient carefully if used together.	• Use cautiously in patients with diabetes, hypertension, hyperthyroidism, severe cardiac disease, or cardiac arrhythmias. • Protect injection from light. Do not use if discolored. • Make sure patient and his family understand why drug is necessary. • Give subcutaneous injections in lateral deltoid area. • Tolerance may develop with prolonged use.

PATIENT-TEACHING AID

HOW TO USE A METERED-DOSE NEBULIZER

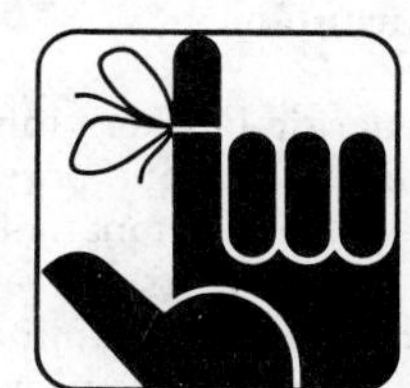

Dear Patient:

You will be taking the drug your doctor has prescribed as an aerosol. To get the most from your therapy, follow these instructions carefully:

• Insert the drug container into the short end of the plastic mouthpiece so that the container nozzle engages in the small hole (illustration 1).

• Then, holding the apparatus so that the drug container is upside down, place the mouthpiece well into your mouth, closing your lips tightly over it (illustration 2).

• Exhale through your nose as completely as possible.

• Then, inhale deeply through your mouth, while pressing the container firmly into the mouthpiece to release the medication.

• After you've released the medication, before you exhale, hold your breath for several seconds.

1

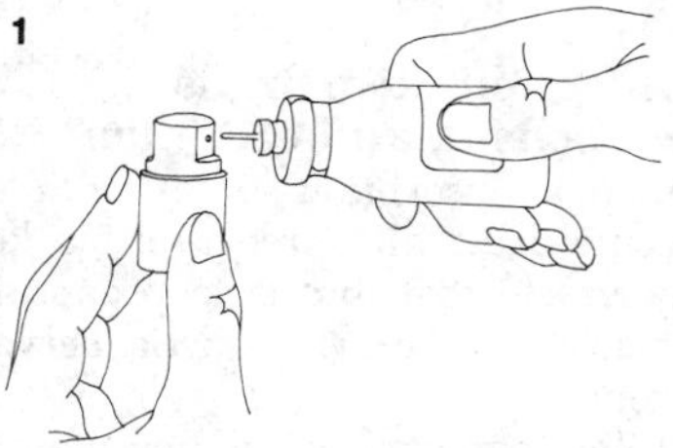

2

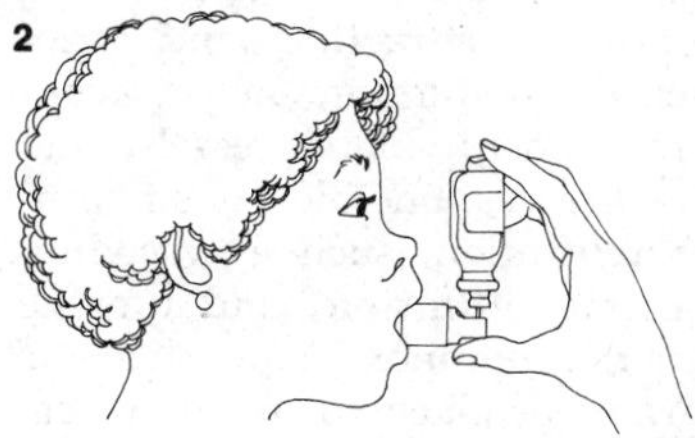

This patient-teaching aid may be reproduced by office copier for distribution to patients.

40 Adrenergic blockers (sympatholytics)

dihydroergotamine mesylate
ergotamine tartrate
methysergide maleate
phenoxybenzamine hydrochloride
phentolamine hydrochloride
phentolamine mesylate
propranolol

Adrenergic blockers inhibit the effects of epinephrine and norepinephrine released from sympathetic nerve endings, as well as the effects of other sympathomimetic amines.

The sympathetic nervous system has two types of receptors: alpha and beta. Stimulation of alpha receptors—located in smooth muscle—causes smooth-muscle contraction, such as vasoconstriction and sphincteric and uterine contraction. The alpha blockers are dihydroergotamine, ergotamine, methysergide, phenoxybenzamine, and phentolamine.

Beta receptors are classified as $beta_1$ and $beta_2$. $Beta_1$ receptors—located mainly in the heart—increase heart rate, cardiac contraction, and atrioventricular conduction. $Beta_2$ receptors—in bronchi, blood vessels, and uterus—are responsible for smooth-muscle relaxation, such as vasodilation, bronchodilation, and uterine relaxation. Propranolol, a prophylactic in migraine headache, is the only beta blocker discussed in this chapter. For more information on propranolol and the other beta blockers, see Chapter 21, ANTIARRHYTHMICS, and Chapter 22, ANTIHYPERTENSIVES.

Major uses

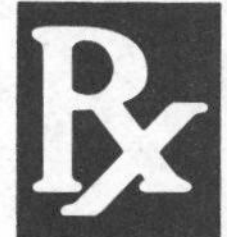

- Dihydroergotamine, ergotamine, methysergide, and propranolol are effective in prophylaxis and treatment of vascular headaches.
- Phenoxybenzamine is used to treat symptoms of spastic peripheral vascular disease. Both phentolamine and phenoxybenzamine furnish temporary relief of hypertension caused by pheochromocytoma.

Mechanism of action

- Alpha blockers inhibit the effects of epinephrine, norepinephrine, and other sympathomimetic amines on both smooth muscle and exocrine glands, preventing sympathetic stimulation.
- Methysergide specifically blocks serotonin (a neurotransmitter); other alpha blockers may also have some antiserotonin effects.
- Propranolol's beta-blocking action prevents vasodilation of the cerebral arteries.

Absorption, distribution, metabolism, and excretion

Although absorption varies with the specific drug, all adrenergic blockers are widely distributed to organs innervated by the sympathetic nervous system.

- Dihydroergotamine and ergotamine are well absorbed after parenteral administration. Ergotamine is also well absorbed orally, and rapidly and well absorbed sublingually. The distribution, metabolism, and excretion of the ergot alkaloids are still not completely defined.

- Methysergide and propranolol are well absorbed orally, metabolized in the liver, and excreted in the urine.
- Phenoxybenzamine is variably absorbed when given orally; it is excreted by the kidneys as both the parent compound and inactive metabolites.
- Little is known about phentolamine absorption, distribution, metabolism, and excretion.

Onset and duration

- Onset of the adrenergic blockers after oral administration varies from 30 minutes for ergot alkaloids to several hours for phenoxybenzamine. Duration of action varies from 3 to 4 hours for the ergot alkaloids, methysergide, and propranolol to 3 to 4 days for phenoxybenzamine and phentolamine.
- Onset after I.M. or subcutaneous injection of ergot alkaloids is 15 to 30 minutes. Onset after I.V. administration (recommended for acute symptomatic episodes) is immediate.

DRUG ADVANCES

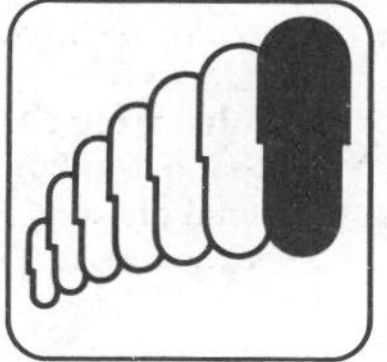

ANOTHER USE FOR PROPRANOLOL

The Food and Drug Administration has approved a new use for propranolol: prevention of migraine headaches.

The benefits of propranolol in migraine therapy were discovered by chance. Migraine sufferers taking propranolol for angina pectoris mentioned to their doctors that they weren't having as many migraine headaches. So doctors theorized that the propranolol lessened migraine attacks.

Subsequent studies showed that two-thirds of all patients with chronic migraine headaches reported good-to-excellent responses when treated with propranolol for some, the number of headaches was cut in half.

How does propranolol prevent migraine headaches? The most likely cause of migraine headaches is the dilation of cerebral blood vessels. Propranolol's beta-blocking action prevents this vasodilation.

Combination products

ALLYGESIC W/ERGOTAMINE: ergotamine tartrate 1 mg, allobarbital 15 mg, aspirin 150 mg, acetaminophen 100 mg, and aluminum aspirin 100 mg.
CAFERGOT: ergotamine tartrate 1 mg and caffeine 100 mg.
CAFERGOT SUPPOSITORIES: ergotamine tartrate 2 mg and caffeine 100 mg.
CAFERGOT P-B (SUPPOSITORIES): ergotamine tartrate 2 mg, caffeine 100 mg, pentobarbital 30 mg, and levorotatory belladonna alkaloids 0.125 mg.
ERGOCAF: ergotamine tartrate 1 mg and caffeine 100 mg.
MIGRAL: ergotamine tartrate 1 mg, caffeine 50 mg, and cyclizine HCl 25 mg.
WIGRAINE♦: ergotamine tartrate 1 mg, caffeine 100 mg, levorotatory belladonna alkaloids 0.1 mg, and phenacetin 130 mg.
WIGRAINE SUPPOSITORIES: ergotamine tartrate 1 mg, caffeine 100 mg, levorotatory belladonna alkaloids 0.1 mg, and phenacetin 130 mg.

NAME	INDICATIONS & DOSAGE	SIDE EFFECTS
dihydroergotamine mesylate D.H.E. 45	*Vascular or migraine headache—* **Adults:** 1 mg I.M. or I.V. May repeat q 1 to 2 hours, p.r.n., up to total of 3 mg. Maximum weekly dose is 6 mg.	**CV:** numbness and tingling in fingers and toes, transient tachycardia or bradycardia, precordial distress and pain, increased arterial pressure. **GI:** nausea, vomiting. **Skin:** itching. **Other:** weakness in legs, muscle pains in extremities, localized edema.
ergotamine tartrate Ergomar♦, Ergostat, Gynergen♦, Medihaler-Ergotamine♦	*Vascular or migraine headache—* **Adults:** initially, 2 mg P.O. S.L., then 1 to 2 mg P.O. q hour or S.L. q ½ hour, to maximum 6 mg daily and 10 mg weekly; or initially, 0.25 mg I.M. or S.C.; repeat in 40 minutes if needed. Maximum dose 0.5 mg/24 hours and 1 mg/week; or 1 inhalation initially, if not relieved in 5 minutes, use another inhalation. May repeat inhalations at least 5 minutes apart up to maximum of 6 per 24 hours.	**CV:** numbness and tingling in fingers and toes, transient tachycardia or bradycardia, precordial distress and pain, increased arterial pressure, angina pectoris. **GI:** nausea, vomiting, diarrhea, abdominal cramps. **Skin:** itching. **Other:** weakness in legs, muscle pains in extremities, localized edema.
methysergide maleate Sansert♦	*Prevention of frequent, severe, uncontrollable, or disabling migraine or vascular headache—* **Adults:** 2 to 4 mg P.O. b.i.d. with meals.	**Blood:** neutropenia, eosinophilia. **CNS:** insomnia, drowsiness, *euphoria, vertigo,* ataxia, *lightheadedness,* hyperesthesia, weakness, *hallucinations or feelings of dissociation.* **CV:** *fibrotic thickening of cardiac valves and aorta, inferior vena cava, and common iliac branches;* vasoconstriction, causing chest pain, abdominal pain, vascular insufficiency of lower limbs; cold, numb, painful extremities with or without paresthesias and diminished or absent pulses; postural hypotension; tachycardia; peripheral edema; murmurs; bruits. **EENT:** nasal stuffiness. **GI:** nausea, vomiting, diarrhea, constipation, epigastric pain. **Skin:** hair loss, dermatitis, sweating, flushing, rash.

♦ Available in U.S. and Canada. ♦♦ Available in Canada only. All other products (no symbol) available in U.S. only. Italicized side effects are common or life-threatening.

INTERACTIONS	NURSING CONSIDERATIONS
Propranolol and other beta blockers: blocked natural pathway for vasodilation in patients receiving ergot alkaloids and thus could result in excessive vasoconstriction. Watch closely if drugs are used together.	• Contraindicated in patients with peripheral and occlusive vascular disease, coronary artery disease, hypertension, hepatic or renal dysfunction, sepsis. • Avoid prolonged administration; don't exceed recommended dosage. • Tell patient to report any feeling of coldness in extremities or tingling of fingers and toes due to vasoconstriction. Severe vasoconstriction may result in tissue damage. • Most effective when used to prevent migraine or soon after onset. Provide a quiet, low-light environment to help patient relax. • Help patient evaluate underlying causes of stress. • Protect ampuls from heat and light. Discard if solution is discolored. • Best results are obtained by adjusting the dose in order to determine the most effective minimal dose.
Propranolol and other beta blockers: blocked natural pathway for vasodilation in patients receiving ergot alkaloids and thus could result in excessive vasoconstriction. Watch closely if drugs are used together.	• Contraindicated in patients with peripheral and occlusive vascular diseases, coronary artery disease, hypertension, hepatic or renal dysfunction, sepsis. • Avoid prolonged administration; don't exceed recommended dosage. • Most effective when used during prodromal stage or as soon after onset as possible. • Provide a quiet, low-light environment to help patient relax. • Help patient evaluate underlying causes of physical or emotional stress, which may precipitate attacks. • Instruct patient on long-term therapy to check for and report feeling of coldness in extremities or tingling of fingers and toes due to vasoconstriction. Severe vasoconstriction may result in tissue damage. • Store drug in light-resistant container. • Sublingual tablet is preferred during early stage of attack because of its rapid absorption. • Warn patient not to increase dosage without first consulting the doctor. • Obtain an accurate dietary history from patient to determine if a relationship exists between certain foods and onset of headache.
None significant.	• Contraindicated in patients with severe hypertension, arteriosclerosis, peripheral vascular insufficiency, renal or hepatic disease, severe coronary artery diseases, thromboembolic disorders, phlebitis or cellulitis of lower limbs, fibrotic processes, valvular heart disease; and in debilitated patients. Use cautiously in patients with peptic ulcers or suspected coronary artery disease. EKG and cardiac status evaluation advisable before giving to patients over 40 years. • GI effects may be prevented by gradual introduction of medication and by administering with meals. • Obtain laboratory studies of cardiac and renal function, blood count, and sedimentation rate before and during therapy. • Stop drug every 6 months; then restart after at least 3 or 4 weeks. • Tell patient not to stop drug abruptly; may cause rebound headaches. Stop gradually over 2 to 3 weeks. • Patient should keep daily weight record and report unusually rapid weight gain. Teach him to check for peripheral edema. Explain and suggest low-salt diet if necessary. • Give drug for 3 weeks before evaluating effectiveness. • Tell patient to report to doctor promptly if he experiences cold, numb, or painful hands and feet; leg cramps when walking; pelvic, chest, or flank pain. • Not for treatment of migraine or vascular headache in progress, or

(continued on following page)

NAME	INDICATIONS & DOSAGE	SIDE EFFECTS
methysergide maleate *(continued)*		**Other:** *retroperitoneal fibrosis,* causing general malaise, fatigue, weight gain, backache, low-grade fever, urinary obstruction; *pulmonary fibrosis,* causing dyspnea, tightness and pain in chest, pleural friction rubs and effusion, arthralgia, myalgia.
phenoxybenzamine hydrochloride Dibenzyline	*To control or prevent hypertension and sweating associated with pheochromocytoma; Raynaud's syndrome; frostbite; acrocyanosis—* **Adults:** initially, 10 mg P.O., then increase by 10 mg q 4 days to a maximum of 60 mg daily.	**CNS:** sedation, fatigue, lassitude. **CV:** tachycardia, *postural hypotension with dizziness.* **EENT:** miosis, nasal congestion. **GI:** irritation. **GU:** inhibition of ejaculation.
phentolamine hydrochloride Regitine, Rogitine♦♦ **phentolamine mesylate**	*To control or prevent hypertension before or during pheochromocytomectomy—* **Adults:** 50 to 100 mg P.O. 4 to 6 times daily; or 5 mg I.M. or I.V. 1 to 2 hours preoperatively. May repeat if needed. During surgery, 5 mg I.V. may be given as needed. **Children:** 25 mg P.O. daily, divided q 4 to 6 hours; or 1 mg I.M. or I.V. 1 to 2 hours preoperatively. May repeat if needed. During surgery, 1 mg I.V. may be given as needed. *To treat extravasation*—infiltrate area with 5 to 10 mg phentolamine in 10 ml normal saline solution. Must be done within 12 hours.	**CV:** acute and prolonged hypotension, tachycardia, cardiac arrhythmia, angina, orthostatic hypotension, flushing. **EENT:** nasal congestion. **GI:** nausea, vomiting, diarrhea, exacerbation of peptic ulcer.
propranolol Inderal♦	*Prevention of frequent, severe, uncontrollable, or disabling migraine or vascular headache—* **Adults:** initially, 80 mg daily in divided doses. Usual maintenance dose: 160 to 240 mg daily, divided t.i.d. or q.i.d.	**CNS:** *fatigue, lethargy,* vivid dreams, hallucinations. **CV:** *bradycardia, hypotension, congestive heart failure,* peripheral vascular disease. **GI:** nausea, vomiting, diarrhea. **Metabolic:** hypoglycemia without symptoms. **Skin:** rash. **Other:** *increased airway resistance,* fever.

♦ Available in U.S. and Canada. ♦♦ Available in Canada only. All other products (no symbol) available in U.S. only. Italicized side effects are common or life-threatening.

INTERACTIONS	NURSING CONSIDERATIONS
	for treatment of tension (muscle contraction) headaches. • Indicated only for patients who are unresponsive to other drugs and who can be kept under close medical supervision.
None significant.	• Contraindicated whenever a fall in blood pressure is undesirable. Use cautiously in cerebral or coronary arteriosclerosis, renal damage, or respiratory disease. • May aggravate symptoms of respiratory infections. • Safe use in pregnancy has not been established, but drug has been used during the third trimester to treat hypertension caused by pheochromocytoma without apparent harm to mother or fetus. • Reduce gastric irritation by giving with milk or in divided doses. • Instruct patient to change position slowly to prevent possible hypotension. Advise him to dangle his legs for a few minutes before standing if he has been lying down. • Place overdosed patient in Trendelenburg position. Treat hypotension with I.V. infusion of norepinephrine. • Full therapeutic effect may not be seen for several weeks. • Store drug in airtight containers, protected from light.
None significant.	• Contraindicated in angina, coronary artery disease, or in history of myocardial infarction. Use with caution in gastritis or peptic ulcer. • If cardiac arrhythmias occur, don't give cardiotonic glycosides until cardiac rhythm returns to normal. • Place overdosed patient in Trendelenburg position. Treat hypotension with I.V. infusion of norepinephrine. • Monitor blood pressure closely, especially after parenteral administration. Patient should be in supine position when receiving drug parenterally. • To reconstitute injection, add 1 ml sterile water for injection to 5-mg vial of drug. Use immediately after reconstitution.
Insulin, hypoglycemic drugs (oral): can alter requirements for these drugs in previously stabilized diabetics. Monitor for hypoglycemia. *Cardiotonic glycosides:* excessive bradycardia and increased depressant effect on myocar-	• Contraindicated in diabetes mellitus, asthma, or allergic rhinitis; during ethyl ether anesthesia; in sinus bradycardia and in heart block greater than first degree; in cardiogenic shock; in right ventricular failure secondary to pulmonary hypertension. Use with caution in congestive heart failure or respiratory disease. • Withdraw drug slowly in patients with coronary artery disease. Abrupt withdrawal might precipitate myocardial infarction or aggravate angina or pheochromocytoma. Abrupt withdrawal in thyrotoxicosis may exacerbate hyperthyroidism or precipitate thyroid storm. In thyrotoxicosis, propranolol may mask clinical signs of hyperthyroidism. • Don't stop before surgery for pheochromocytoma. Before any surgi-

(continued on following page)

NAME	INDICATIONS & DOSAGE	SIDE EFFECTS
propranolol *(continued)*		

♦ Available in U.S. and Canada. ♦♦ Available in Canada only. All other products (no symbol) available in U.S. only. Italicized side effects are common or life-threatening.

THE ROLE OF HORMONES IN MIGRAINE ATTACKS

Four times more women than men experience migraine headaches after they've reached puberty. Researchers associate the hormonal changes that occur during puberty and that remain throughout adulthood in women with the onset and frequency of migraine attacks. Here's what studies have shown on these hormone-related factors:

• *Menstrual cycle.* In one study, 60% of the women sufferers related their attacks to their menstrual cycle, though individual differences existed: 28% reported migraines premenstrually; 20% during menstruation; 25% postmenstrually; and 8% at midcycle. A related study showed migraine attacks occurred when women experienced a rapid drop in their blood estrogen level after it had been elevated for several days.

• *Oral contraceptives.* These appeared to affect the frequency of migraine attacks. One study revealed that some women with no previous migraine history suffered from migraines while on the pill; 70% of these women said their headaches disappeared once they stopped using the pill. Migraine headaches also appeared for the first time in women on estrogen replacement therapy after a hysterectomy or menopause. When these women reduced or discontinued their use of estrogen, the number of headaches decreased by 58%.

Most doctors agree that women migraine sufferers should not take oral contraceptives or other female hormone preparations. This is particularly important when the migraine is of the classical or complicated type because of the risk of stroke.

• *Pregnancy.* In one study of women migraine sufferers, about 77% said their attacks either disappear completely, occur less frequently, or are milder during pregnancy.

Although hormones may affect the onset and frequency of migraine attacks, several other factors, including emotional stress, fatigue, and environmental stimuli (noise, crowds, bright lights), may contribute to the migraine syndrome. The cause of migraine headaches, however, has not been clearly established.

Adapted with permission from "Hormones and Migraine," *National Migraine Foundation Newsletter,* No. 33, Summer 1980.

INTERACTIONS	NURSING CONSIDERATIONS
dium. Monitor pulse rate. *Aminophylline:* antagonized beta-blocking effects of propranolol. Use together cautiously. *Isoproterenol, glucagon:* antagonized propranolol effect. May be used therapeutically and in emergencies.	cal procedure, notify anesthesiologist that patient is receiving propranolol. • Monitor blood pressure frequently. If patient develops excessive hypotension, notify doctor. Tell patient that orthostatic hypotension can be minimized by rising slowly and avoiding sudden position changes. • Drug masks common signs of shock and hypoglycemia.

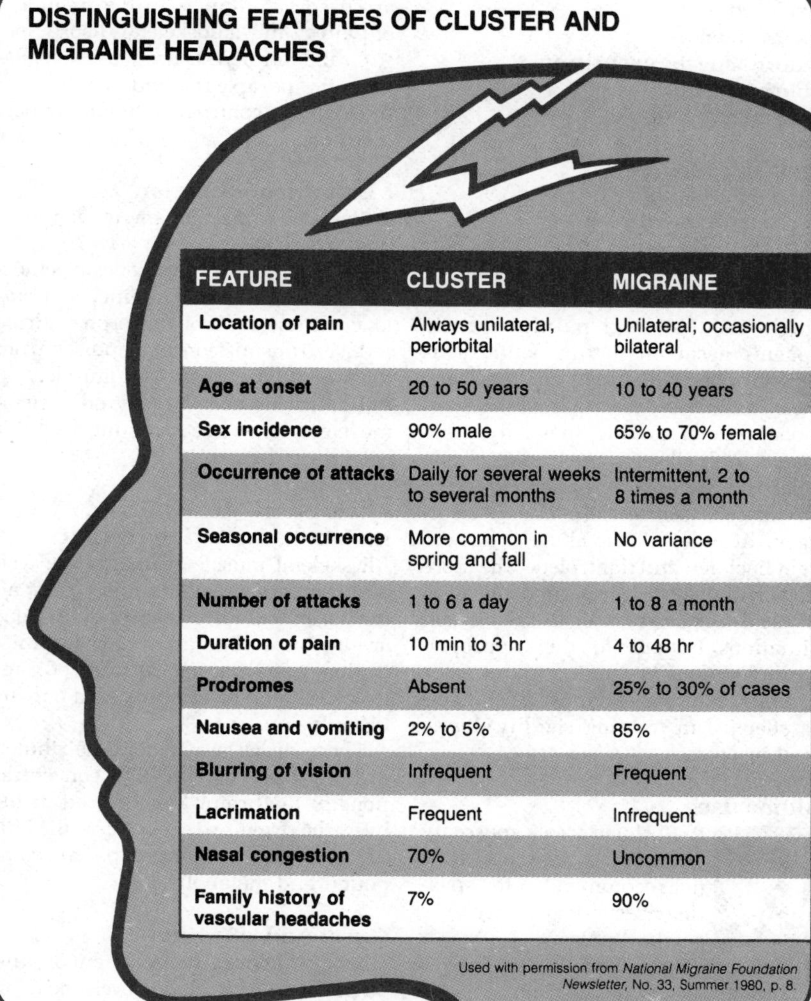

DISTINGUISHING FEATURES OF CLUSTER AND MIGRAINE HEADACHES

FEATURE	CLUSTER	MIGRAINE
Location of pain	Always unilateral, periorbital	Unilateral; occasionally bilateral
Age at onset	20 to 50 years	10 to 40 years
Sex incidence	90% male	65% to 70% female
Occurrence of attacks	Daily for several weeks to several months	Intermittent, 2 to 8 times a month
Seasonal occurrence	More common in spring and fall	No variance
Number of attacks	1 to 6 a day	1 to 8 a month
Duration of pain	10 min to 3 hr	4 to 48 hr
Prodromes	Absent	25% to 30% of cases
Nausea and vomiting	2% to 5%	85%
Blurring of vision	Infrequent	Frequent
Lacrimation	Frequent	Infrequent
Nasal congestion	70%	Uncommon
Family history of vascular headaches	7%	90%

Used with permission from *National Migraine Foundation Newsletter*, No. 33, Summer 1980, p. 8.

Skeletal muscle relaxants

baclofen
carisoprodol
chlorphenesin carbamate
chlorzoxazone
cyclobenzaprine
dantrolene sodium
metaxalone
methocarbamol
orphenadrine citrate

Skeletal muscle relaxants can be divided into two categories: those routinely used to treat painful muscle spasms associated with acute, self-limiting conditions, such as lower back pain, and those used to treat more serious skeletal muscle spasticity associated with disease, such as multiple sclerosis, or spasticity secondary to spinal cord transection. The first category includes all the above drugs except baclofen and dantrolene, the more powerful drugs of the second category. These drugs must not be used in trivial situations, but only for their appropriate indications.

None of the skeletal muscle relaxants is effective in treating rigidity due to parkinsonism.

Major uses

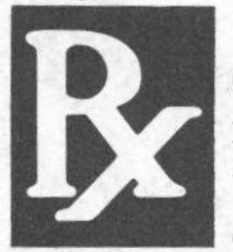

- Baclofen treats spasticity of multiple sclerosis. It is not recommended for spasticity secondary to stroke or cerebral palsy.
- Carisoprodol, chlorphenesin, chlorzoxazone, cyclobenzaprine, metaxalone, methocarbamol, and orphenadrine are used as adjuncts in the treatment of painful musculoskeletal disorders.
- Oral dantrolene is used to treat spasticity in paraplegia and hemiplegia; the I.V. form controls malignant hyperthermia.

Mechanism of action

- Baclofen's mechanism of action is unclear.
- Carisoprodol, chlorphenesin, chlorzoxazone, cyclobenzaprine, metaxalone, methocarbamol, and orphenadrine reduce transmission of impulses from the spinal cord to skeletal muscle.
- Dantrolene acts directly on skeletal muscle to interfere with intracellular calcium movement.

Absorption, distribution, metabolism, and excretion

All skeletal muscle relaxants are well absorbed after oral administration; all the parenteral forms except dantrolene are well absorbed after I.M. administration. (The parenteral form of dantrolene should be administered only by I.V. infusion.)

These drugs are widely distributed in body tissues, with high concentrations in the brain. Metabolized in the liver, the drugs are excreted by the kidneys as both unchanged parent compound and metabolites.

Onset and duration

Onset is generally between 30 and 60 minutes, and blood levels peak in 2 to 3 hours. Duration is 4 to 6 hours.

DANTROLENE CONTROLS MALIGNANT HYPERTHERMIA

Malignant hyperthermia—also known as malignant hyperpyrexia—occurs when a genetically susceptible patient is exposed to inhalation anesthetics. Standard presurgery screening (taking the patient's history, for example) may not detect patients predisposed to this condition. Since 1962, when malignant hyperthermia was first recognized, researchers have concentrated on finding the treatment for this rare but deadly condition. Both procainamide and dantrolene sodium have been studied for their usefulness in controlling malignant hyperthermia, but only dantrolene (I.V.) has proved successful enough to be approved for this use.

How does dantrolene work during a malignant hyperthermia crisis? The crisis begins when an inhalation anesthetic, such as halothane, is administered to a susceptible patient. This patient apparently has a defect in his muscle cell membranes that allows the anesthetic to trigger a sudden rise of calcium within muscle cells.

The increased amount of calcium sets off a series of biochemical reactions that increase the metabolic rate, eventually liberating heat. Muscle contractions also increase, liberating more heat.

The most consistent early symptom of malignant hyperthermia is sudden, unexplained tachycardia. The patient's temperature rises, ranging from 39° to 42° C. (102.2° to 107.6° F.). Rapid breathing, cyanotic mottling of the skin, hypotension, acidosis, muscle rigidity, and cardiac arrhythmias usually follow, causing even more calcium to flow into the muscle cells. If this cycle continually repeats itself, the patient dies.

Dantrolene presumably breaks the cycle by interfering with the release of calcium ions within the muscle fiber. If this drug is administered before bradycardia or cardiac arrest develops, the patient will probably recover.

During and after a malignant hyperthermia crisis, focus your patient care plan on three major nursing problems: elevated temperature, anoxia, and tachycardia. Here's a summary of such a plan:

For elevated temperature:
- Monitor temperature.
- Initiate cooling measures with a light cover, sponging, or hypothermia blanket, depending on your orders.
- Keep the patient clean and dry. Provide good mouth care.
- Increase fluids.
- Observe seizure precautions.
- Assess neurologic function.

For anoxia:
- Monitor respirations.
- Administer oxygen.
- Limit the patient's activity.

For tachycardia:
- Monitor apical pulse rate.
- Assess the patient's cardiovascular system.
- Limit the patient's activity.

When you prepare the patient for discharge, explain what happened, and suggest he wear a medical identification bracelet or necklace that will inform others of his susceptibility to malignant hyperthermia in case of an emergency.

Combination products

NORGESIC: orphenadrine citrate 25 mg, aspirin 225 mg, phenacetin 160 mg, and caffeine 30 mg.

NORGESIC FORTE: orphenadrine citrate 50 mg, aspirin 450 mg, phenacetin 320 mg, and caffeine 60 mg.

PARAFON FORTE♦: chlorzoxazone 250 mg and acetaminophen 300 mg.

ROBAXISAL♦: methocarbamol 400 mg and aspirin 325 mg.

SOMA COMPOUND♦: carisoprodol 200 mg, phenacetin 160 mg, and caffeine 32 mg.

SOMA COMPOUND WITH CODEINE: carisoprodol 200 mg, phenacetin 160 mg, caffeine 32 mg, and codeine phosphate 16 mg.

NAME	INDICATIONS & DOSAGE	SIDE EFFECTS
baclofen Lioresal	*Spasticity in multiple sclerosis, spinal cord injury*— **Adults:** initially, 5 mg t.i.d. for 3 days, 10 mg t.i.d. for 3 days, 15 mg t.i.d. for 3 days, 20 mg t.i.d. for 3 days. Increase according to response up to maximum 80 mg daily.	**CNS:** *drowsiness, dizziness,* headache, *weakness, fatigue,* confusion, insomnia. **CV:** hypotension. **EENT:** nasal congestion. **GI:** *nausea,* constipation. **GU:** urinary frequency. **Hepatic:** increased SGOT, alkaline phosphatase. **Metabolic:** hyperglycemia. **Skin:** rash, pruritus. **Other:** ankle edema, excessive perspiration, weight gain.
carisoprodol Rela♦, Soma♦	*As an adjunct in acute, painful musculoskeletal conditions*— **Adults, and children over 12 years:** 350 mg P.O. t.i.d. and at bedtime. Not recommended for children under 12 years.	**CNS:** *drowsiness, dizziness,* vertigo, ataxia, tremor, agitation, irritability, headache, depressive reactions, insomnia. **CV:** orthostatic hypotension, tachycardia, facial flushing. **GI:** nausea, vomiting, hiccups, increased bowel activity, epigastric distress. **Skin:** rash, *erythema multiforme,* pruritus. **Other:** asthmatic episodes, fever, angioneurotic edema, *anaphylaxis.*
chlorphenesin carbamate Maolate	*As an adjunct in short-term, acute, painful musculoskeletal conditions*— **Adults:** initial dose 800 mg P.O. t.i.d. Maintenance 400 mg P.O. q.i.d. for maximum of 8 weeks.	**Blood:** blood dyscrasia. **CNS:** *drowsiness, dizziness,* confusion, headache, weakness. Dose-related side effects include paradoxical stimulation, agitation, insomnia, nervousness, headache. **GI:** *nausea, epigastric distress.* **Other:** *anaphylaxis.*
chlorzoxazone Paraflex	*As an adjunct in acute, painful musculoskeletal conditions*— **Adults:** 250 to 750 mg P.O. t.i.d. or q.i.d. **Children:** 20 mg/kg P.O. daily divided t.i.d. or q.i.d.	**CNS:** *drowsiness, dizziness, lightheadedness,* malaise, headache, overstimulation. **GI:** anorexia, nausea, vomiting, heartburn, abdominal distress, constipation, diarrhea. **GU:** urine discoloration (orange or purple-red).

♦ Available in U.S. and Canada. ♦♦ Available in Canada only. All other products (no symbol) available in U.S. only. Italicized side effects are common or life-threatening.

INTERACTIONS	NURSING CONSIDERATIONS
None significant.	• Use cautiously in patients with impaired renal function, stroke (minimal benefit, poor tolerance), epilepsy, and when spasticity is used to maintain motor function. • Give with meals or milk to prevent gastric distress. • Amount of relief determines if dosage (and drowsiness) can be reduced. • Tell patient to avoid activities that require alertness until CNS response to drug is determined. Drowsiness is usually transient. • Watch for increased incidence of seizures in epileptics. • Watch for sensitivity reactions such as fever, skin eruptions, respiratory distress. • Advise patient to follow doctor's orders regarding rest, physical therapy. • Do not withdraw abruptly unless required by severe side effects; may precipitate hallucinations or rebound spasticity. • Overdosage treatment is supportive only; do not induce emesis or use a respiratory stimulant in obtunded patients. • Used investigationally for treatment of unstable bladder.
None significant.	• Contraindicated in hypersensitivity to related compounds (including meprobamate, tybamate); or intermittent porphyria. Use with caution in impaired hepatic or renal function. • Watch for idiosyncratic reactions after first to fourth dose (weakness, ataxia, visual and speech difficulties, fever, skin eruptions, mental changes) or severe reactions, including bronchospasm, hypotension, anaphylactic shock. Hold dose and notify doctor immediately of any unusual reactions. • Record amount of relief to determine whether dosage can be reduced. • Warn patient to avoid activities that require alertness until CNS response to drug is determined. Drowsiness is transient. • Avoid combining with alcohol or other depressants. • Advise patient to follow doctor's orders regarding rest and physical therapy. • Do not stop drug abruptly; mild withdrawal effects, such as insomnia, headache, nausea, abdominal cramps, may result. • For treatment of anaphylaxis, see inside front cover.
None significant.	• Use cautiously in hepatic disease or impaired renal function. • Safe use for periods over 8 weeks not established. • Take with meals or milk to prevent gastric distress. • Amount of relief determines if dosage (and drowsiness) can be reduced. • Watch for sensitivity reactions such as fever, skin eruptions, and respiratory distress. Hold dose and notify doctor of unusual reactions. • Monitor blood studies. • Watch for unusual bleeding and infections that may indicate blood dyscrasia. • For treatment of anaphylaxis, see inside front cover.
None significant.	• Contraindicated in impaired hepatic function. Use cautiously in patients with a history of drug allergies. • Record amount of relief to determine whether dosage can be reduced. • Watch for signs of hepatic dysfunction. Hold dose and notify doctor. • Warn patient to avoid activities that require alertness until CNS response to drug is determined. Drowsiness is transient.

(continued on following page)

NAME	INDICATIONS & DOSAGE	SIDE EFFECTS
chlorzoxazone *(continued)*		**Hepatic:** hepatic dysfunction. **Skin:** urticaria, redness, itching, petechiae, bruising.
cyclobenzaprine Flexeril♦	*Short-term treatment of muscle spasm—* **Adults:** 10 mg P.O. t.i.d. for 7 days. Maximum: 60 mg/day for 2 to 3 weeks.	**CNS:** *drowsiness,* euphoria, weakness, headache, insomnia, nightmares, paresthesias, dizziness. **CV:** tachycardia. **EENT:** blurred vision. **GI:** abdominal pain, dyspepsia, peculiar taste, constipation, dry mouth. **GU:** urinary retention. **Skin:** rash, urticaria, pruritus. **Other:** in high doses, watch for side effects like those of other tricyclic drugs (amitriptyline, imipramine).
dantrolene sodium Dantrium♦, Dantrium I.V.	*Spasticity and sequelae secondary to severe chronic disorders (multiple sclerosis, cerebral palsy, spinal cord injury, stroke)—* **Adults:** 25 mg P.O. daily. Increase gradually in increments of 25 mg, up to 100 mg b.i.d. to q.i.d. to maximum of 400 mg/day. Each dosage level should be maintained for 4 to 7 days in order to determine effectiveness. **Children:** 1 mg/kg/day P.O. b.i.d. to q.i.d. Increase gradually as needed by1 mg/kg/day to maximum of 100 mg q.i.d. *Management of malignant hyperthermia—* **Adults and children:** 1 mg/kg I.V. initially; may repeat dose up to cumulative dose of 10 mg/kg.	**Blood:** eosinophilia. **CNS:** *muscle weakness, drowsiness,* dizziness, light-headedness, malaise, headache, confusion, nervousness, insomnia. **CV:** tachycardia, blood pressure changes. **EENT:** excessive tearing, visual disturbances. **GI:** anorexia, constipation, cramping, dysphagia, *severe diarrhea.* **GU:** urinary frequency, incontinence, nocturia, dysuria, crystalluria, difficulty achieving erection. **Hepatic:** *hepatitis.* **Skin:** eczematoid eruption, pruritus, urticaria, photosensitivity. **Other:** abnormal hair growth, drooling, sweating, pleural effusion, myalgia, chills, fever.

INTERACTIONS	NURSING CONSIDERATIONS
	• Avoid combining with alcohol or other depressants. • Expect urine color to change. • Advise patient to follow doctor's orders regarding rest and physical therapy. • Give with meals or milk to prevent gastric distress.
None significant.	• Contraindicated in patients who have received MAO inhibitors within 14 days; during acute recovery phase of myocardial infarction; in heart block, arrhythmias, conduction disturbances, or congestive heart failure. Use cautiously in patients with urinary retention, narrow-angle glaucoma, increased intraocular pressure, cardiovascular disease, impaired hepatic function, seizures; and in elderly or debilitated patients. • Withdrawal symptoms (nausea, headache, malaise) may occur if drug is stopped abruptly after long-term use. • Watch for symptoms of overdose, including possible cardiotoxicity. Notify doctor immediately and have physostigmine available. • Check intake and output. Be alert for urinary retention. If constipation is a problem, increase fluid intake and get an order for a stool softener. • Warn patient to avoid activities that require alertness until CNS response to drug is determined. Drowsiness and dizziness usually subside after 2 weeks. • Avoid combining alcohol or other depressants with cyclobenzaprine. • Dry mouth may be relieved with sugarless candy or gum.
None significant.	***The following are considerations for the P.O. form only:*** • Contraindicated when spasticity is used to maintain motor function; in spasms in rheumatic disorders; lactation. Use with caution in patients with severely impaired cardiac or pulmonary function or preexisting hepatic disease; in females; and in patients over 35 years. • Safety and efficacy in long-term use not established; value may be determined by therapeutic trial. Do not give more than 45 days if no benefits obtained. • Give with meals or milk to prevent gastric distress. • Prepare oral suspension for single dose by dissolving capsule contents in juice or other suitable liquid. For multiple dose, use acid vehicle, such as citric acid in USP Syrup; refrigerate. Use in several days. • Record amount of relief to determine whether dosage can be reduced. • Watch for hepatitis (fever, jaundice), severe diarrhea or weakness, or sensitivity reactions (fever, skin eruptions). Hold dose and notify doctor. • Warn patient to avoid driving and other hazardous activities until CNS response to drug is determined. Side effects should subside after 4 days. • Tell patient to avoid combining with alcohol or other depressants; to avoid photosensitivity reactions by using sunscreening agents and protective clothing; to report abdominal discomfort or GI problems immediately; and to follow doctor's orders regarding rest and physical therapy. ***The following are considerations for the I.V. form only:*** • Administer as soon as malignant hyperthermia reaction is recognized. • Reconstitute each vial by adding 60 ml of sterile water for injection and shaking vial until clear. • Protect contents from light and use within 6 hours.

NAME	INDICATIONS & DOSAGE	SIDE EFFECTS
metaxalone Skelaxin♦	*As an adjunct in acute, painful musculoskeletal conditions—* **Adults, and children over 12 years:** 800 mg P.O. t.i.d. or q.i.d.	**Blood:** leukopenia, hemolytic anemia. **CNS:** *drowsiness,* dizziness, headache, nervousness, irritability, exacerbation of grand mal epilepsy. **GI:** *nausea, vomiting.* **Hepatic:** jaundice. **Skin:** light rash with or without pruritus.
methocarbamol Delaxin, Forbaxin, Metho-500, Robamol, Robaxin♦, Romethocarb, Spenaxin	*As an adjunct in acute, painful musculoskeletal conditions—* **Adults:** 1.5 g P.O. for 2 to 3 days, then 1 g P.O. q.i.d., or not more than 500 mg (5 ml) I.M. into each gluteal region. May repeat q 8 hours. Or 1 to 3 g/day (10 to 30 ml) I.V. directly into vein at 3 ml/minute, or 10 ml may be added to no more than 250 ml of 5% dextrose in water or normal saline solution. Maximum dose 3 g/day. *Supportive therapy in tetanus management—* **Adults:** 1 to 2 g into tubing of running I.V. or 1 to 3 g in infusion bottle q 6 hours. **Children:** 15 mg/kg I.V. q 6 hours.	**Blood:** hemolysis, increased hemoglobin (I.V. only). **CNS:** drowsiness, dizziness, lightheadedness, headache, vertigo, mild muscular incoordination (I.M. or I.V. only), convulsions (I.V. only). **CV:** hypotension, bradycardia (I.M. or I.V. only). **GI:** *nausea, anorexia, GI upset.* **GU:** red blood cells in urine (I.V. only), discoloration of urine. **Skin:** urticaria, pruritus, rash. **Local:** thrombophlebitis, extravasation (I.V. only). **Other:** fever, metallic taste, flushing, *anaphylactic reactions (I.M. or I.V. only).*
orphenadrine citrate Flexon, Myolin, Norflex♦, Ro-Orphena, Tega-Flex, X-Otag	*Adjunctive treatment in painful, acute musculoskeletal conditions—* **Adults:** 100 mg P.O. b.i.d., or 60 mg I.V. or I.M. q 12 hours, p.r.n.	**CNS:** disorientation, restlessness, irritability, weakness, *drowsiness,* headache. **CV:** palpitations, tachycardia. **EENT:** dilated pupils, blurred vision, difficulty swallowing. **GI:** constipation, *dry mouth,* nausea, vomiting, paralytic ileus, epigastric distress. **GU:** urinary hesitancy or retention.

INTERACTIONS	NURSING CONSIDERATIONS
None significant.	• Contraindicated in patients with impaired hepatic or renal function, and in those with a history of drug-induced hemolytic or other anemias. • Test hepatic function periodically. May cause abnormalities in liver function studies; repeat tests after drug is discontinued. • Record amount of relief to determine if dosage can be reduced. • Watch for sensitivity reactions such as rash with pruritus. • Warn patient to avoid combining with alcohol or other depressants. • Advise patient to follow orders regarding rest, physical therapy. • Give with meals or milk to prevent gastric distress. • False-positive results in glucose tests if cupric sulfate is used. Use glucose oxidase instead.
None significant.	• Contraindicated in patients with impaired renal function (injectable form), myasthenia gravis, epilepsy (injectable form); in children under 12 years (except in tetanus); and in patients receiving anticholinesterase agents. • I.V. irritates veins, may cause phlebitis, aggravates seizures, may cause fainting if injected rapidly. • In tetanus management, use methocarbamol with tetanus antitoxin, penicillin, tracheotomy, and aggressive supportive care. Long course of I.V. methocarbamol required. • Watch for sensitivity reactions such as fever, skin eruptions. • Warn patient to avoid activities that require alertness until CNS response to drug is determined. Drowsiness subsides. • Avoid combining with alcohol or other depressants. • Advise patient to follow doctor's orders regarding rest and physical therapy. • Tell patient urine may turn green, black, or brown. • Give with meals or milk to prevent gastric distress. • Watch for orthostatic hypotension, especially with parenteral administration. Keep patient supine for 15 minutes afterward, and supervise ambulation. Advise patient to get up slowly. • Give I.V. slowly. Maximum rate 300 mg (3 ml)/minute. Give I.M. deeply, only in upper outer quadrant of buttocks, with maximum of 5 ml in each buttock, and inject slowly. Do not give subcutaneously. • Have epinephrine, antihistamines, corticosteroids available. • Prepare liquid by crushing tablets into water or saline solution. Give through nasogastric tube. • Obtain WBC count periodically during prolonged therapy. • For treatment of anaphylaxis, see inside front cover.
None significant.	• Contraindicated in patients with narrow-angle glaucoma; prostatic hypertrophy; pyloric, duodenal, or bladder-neck obstruction; myasthenia gravis; tachycardia; severe hepatic or renal disease; ulcerative colitis. Use cautiously in elderly or debilitated patients with cardiac disease, arrhythmias; and in those exposed to high temperatures. • Check all dosages carefully. Even a slight overdose can lead to toxicity. Early signs are excessive dry mouth, dilated pupils, blurred vision, skin flushing, fever. • Monitor vital signs carefully. • When given I.V., may cause paradoxical initial bradycardia. Usually disappears in 2 minutes. • Monitor intake and output. Causes urinary retention and hesitancy; have patient void before taking the drug. • Relieve dry mouth with fluids, ice chips, gum, or hard candy. • Patient may develop a tolerance to this drug.

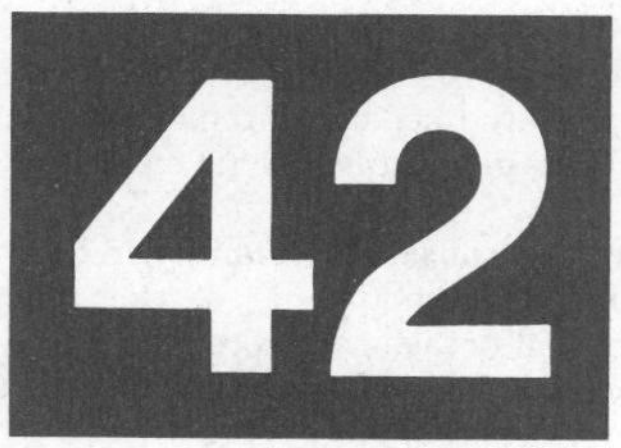

Neuromuscular blockers

decamethonium bromide
gallamine triethiodide
hexafluorenium bromide
metocurine iodide
pancuronium bromide
succinylcholine chloride
tubocurarine chloride

Neuromuscular blockers are sometimes called peripherally acting skeletal muscle relaxants. They must be used parenterally (unlike the centrally acting skeletal muscle relaxants in Chapter 41 that are commonly given orally).

Potentially dangerous drugs, neuromuscular blockers should be administered either by a doctor or under his direct supervision. They effectively paralyze skeletal muscle, thereby reducing anesthetic requirements and facilitating manipulation during surgery. However, because they also paralyze muscles essential for respiration (diaphragm and intercostals), mechanical ventilatory support must be available whenever they're administered.

Major uses

Rx Neuromuscular blockers potentiate surgical anesthetics, allowing use of a lighter level of anesthesia. They facilitate intubation, abdominal surgical procedures, correction of dislocations, and setting of fractures.

They're also used to control respirations of patients on mechanical ventilators, muscle contraction in electroconvulsive therapy, and muscle spasms in convulsive states (tetanus, status epilepticus, drug intoxication, and black widow spider bites).

- Hexafluorenium enhances the action of succinylcholine.
- Tubocurarine aids differential diagnosis of myasthenia gravis.

Mechanism of action

These agents block transmission of nerve impulses at the skeletal neuromuscular junction by one of two mechanisms:

- Decamethonium and succinylcholine (depolarizing agents) prolong depolarization of the muscle end-plate. (Hexafluorenium inhibits the enzymatic breakdown of succinylcholine, prolonging its duration.)
- Gallamine, metocurine, pancuronium, and tubocurarine (nondepolarizing agents) prevent acetylcholine from binding to the receptors on the muscle end-plate, thus blocking depolarization.

Absorption, distribution, metabolism, and excretion

Neuromuscular blockers are ineffective orally because they're poorly absorbed from the gastrointestinal tract; they're slowly and unpredictably absorbed from I.M. injection sites. Rapidly distributed from I.V. sites, these drugs (except succinylcholine) are poorly metabolized and remain effective in the body until they're eliminated in urine and—through the bile—in feces as unchanged drug.

- Succinylcholine is hydrolyzed by pseudocholinesterase in the blood and liver.

Onset and duration

- Decamethonium has an onset of 1 to 3 minutes after I.V. administration and a duration of 4 to 8 minutes. Recovery occurs 15 to 20 minutes after injection.
- Gallamine begins to work within 1 to 3 minutes after I.V. administration; its peak effect occurs in about 3 minutes. Duration of action depends on total dosage and number of doses administered.
- Hexafluorenium takes effect rapidly after I.V. administration; its action lasts 15 to 30 minutes.
- Metocurine and tubocurarine take effect within 1 to 3 minutes after I.V. administration; duration is 25 to 90 minutes. The drugs accumulate after repeated doses.
- Pancuronium's onset occurs within a few minutes after I.V. administration. Its duration is 25 to 60 minutes, or more prolonged when large doses are given.
- Succinylcholine, administered I.V., takes effect in 1 to 3 minutes; its duration is only 5 minutes but can be prolonged when used with hexafluorenium.

Combination products

None.

WHERE NEUROMUSCULAR BLOCKING AGENTS ACT

Neuromuscular blocking agents block acetylcholine at the neuromuscular synapse. Here's how they work:

The basic unit of the nervous system is the nerve cell or neuron. It consists of a central cell body and threadlike projections of cytoplasm known as nerve fibers. These are of two types: the axon, which conducts impulses away from the cell body, and the dendrite, which conducts impulses to the cell body. Most neurons have multiple dendrites and a single axon.

Axons are surrounded by a white fatty substance called myelin, which insulates and protects the delicate inner fiber.

Neurons receive and transmit impulses at junctions called synapses, where one structure almost touches another. When information flows, one of the structures releases acetylcholine, a transmitting chemical that crosses the narrow cleft between them and activates the receiving cell. This is where the synapse is blocked (colored area in diagram).

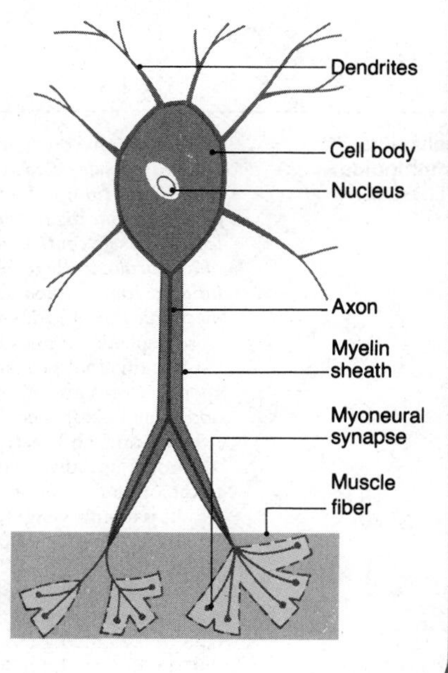

NAME	INDICATIONS & DOSAGE	SIDE EFFECTS
decamethonium bromide Syncurine♦	*Adjunct to anesthetic to induce skeletal muscle relaxation; facilitate intubation, lessen muscle contractions in pharmacologically or electrically induced convulsions; assist with mechanical ventilation—* Dose depends on anesthetic used, individual needs, and response. Doses are representative and must be adjusted. **Adults:** initially, 0.5 to 3 mg I.V., at a rate of 0.5 mg to 1 mg/minute, then 0.5 to 1 mg q 10 to 30 minutes for sustained relaxation. **Children and infants:** initially, 0.05 to 0.08 mg/kg I.V., then 0.02 to 0.03 mg/kg at 10- to 30-minute intervals.	**CV:** bradycardia, tachycardia, hypotension and hypertension. **Other:** *dose-related prolonged apnea,* residual muscle weakness, increased oropharyngeal secretions, allergic or idiosyncratic hypersensitivity reactions, *postoperative muscle pain.*
gallamine triethiodide Flaxedil♦	*Adjunct to anesthetic to induce skeletal muscle relaxation; facilitate intubation; reduction of fractures and dislocations; lessen muscle contractions in pharmacologically or electrically induced convulsions; assist with mechanical ventilation—* Dose depends on anesthetic used, individual needs, and response. Doses are representative and must be adjusted. **Adults, and children over 1 month:** initially, 1 mg/kg I.V. to maximum of 100 mg, regardless of patient's weight; then 0.5 mg to 1 mg/kg q 30 to 40 minutes. **Children under 1 month but over 5 kg (11 lb):** initially, 0.25 to 0.75 mg/kg I.V., then 0.01 to 0.05 mg/kg q 30 to 40 minutes.	**CV:** tachycardia. **Other:** *respiratory paralysis, dose-related prolonged apnea,* residual muscle weakness, increased oropharyngeal secretions, allergic or idiosyncratic hypersensitivity reactions.

INTERACTIONS	NURSING CONSIDERATIONS
Aminoglycoside antibiotics (including amikacin, gentamicin, kanamycin, neomycin, streptomycin); polymyxin antibiotics (polymyxin B sulfate, colistin); clindamycin, quinidine: potentiated neuromuscular blockade, leading to increased skeletal muscle relaxation and possible respiratory paralysis. Use cautiously during surgical and postoperative periods. *Narcotic analgesics:* potentiated neuromuscular blockade, leading to increased skeletal muscle relaxation and possible respiratory paralysis. Use with extreme caution.	• Contraindicated in hypersensitivity to bromides, impaired renal function, shock, myasthenia gravis, surgical procedures lasting longer than 20 minutes. Use cautiously in patients undergoing surgery in Trendelenburg or lithotomy positions; in patients recently digitalized; in elderly or debilitated patients; and in hepatic or pulmonary impairment, respiratory depression, myasthenic syndrome of lung cancer, dehydration, thyroid disorders, collagen disease, porphyria, electrolyte disturbances, fractures, muscle spasms, and (in large doses) cesarean section. • Seldom used due to uncertain effects and lack of suitable antidote. • Multiple doses not often recommended; may cause reduced response, prolonged apnea. • Monitor baseline electrolyte determinations (electrolyte imbalance, especially potassium, calcium, and magnesium, can potentiate neuromuscular effects) and vital signs, especially respiration. • Check intake/output (renal dysfunction prolongs duration of action, since drug is unchanged before excretion). • Maintain clear airway. Have emergency respiratory support (endotracheal equipment, ventilator, oxygen, atropine, neostigmine, or edrophonium) on hand. • Reassure patient that postoperative stiffness is normal and will soon subside. • Use only fresh solutions. • Give I.V. slowly (not more than 1 mg/minute). • Do not give without direct supervision of doctor or experienced clinician.
Aminoglycoside antibiotics (amikacin, gentamicin, kanamycin, neomycin, streptomycin); polymyxin antibiotics (polymyxin B sulfate, colistin); clindamycin; quinidine: potentiated neuromuscular blockade, leading to increased skeletal muscle relaxation and possible respiratory paralysis. Use cautiously during surgical and postoperative periods. *Narcotic analgesics:* potentiated neuromuscular blockade, leading to increased skeletal muscle relaxation and possible respiratory paralysis. Use with extreme caution, and reduce dose of gallamine.	• Contraindicated in patients with hypersensitivity to iodides, impaired renal function, myasthenia gravis; patients in shock; and patients in whom tachycardia may be hazardous. Use cautiously in elderly or debilitated patients; those with hepatic or pulmonary impairment, respiratory depression, myasthenic syndrome of lung cancer, dehydration, thyroid disorders, collagen diseases, porphyria, electrolyte disturbances, fractures, muscle spasms; and patients undergoing cesarean section. • Monitor baseline electrolyte determinations (electrolyte imbalance can potentiate neuromuscular effects). • Watch respirations for early symptoms of paralysis, inability to keep eyelids open and eyes focused, difficulty in swallowing and speaking. Notify doctor immediately. • Take vital signs every 15 minutes, especially for developing tachycardia. Notify doctor immediately of changes. • Measure intake/output (renal dysfunction prolongs duration of action, since drug is unchanged before excretion). • Keep airway clear. Have emergency respiratory support (endotracheal equipment, ventilator, oxygen, atropine, neostigmine) on hand. • Reassure patient that postoperative stiffness is normal and will soon subside. • Determine whether patient has iodide allergy. • Protect drug from light or excessive heat; use only fresh solutions. • Do not mix solution with meperidine HCl or barbiturate solutions. • Give I.V. slowly (over 30 to 90 seconds). • Do not give without direct supervision of doctor.

NAME	INDICATIONS & DOSAGE	SIDE EFFECTS
hexafluorenium bromide Mylaxen	*Adjunct for use with succinylcholine to prolong neuromuscular blockade and reduce muscular fasciculations—* Dose depends on individual needs and response. Doses are representative and must be adjusted. **Adults and children:** use in ratio of 2 mg/1 mg succinylcholine. Maximum hexafluorenium bromide 10 to 36 mg; should not be administered more frequently than q 15 to 30 minutes.	**CNS:** *prolonged neuromuscular blockade.* **CV:** hypotension, hypertension, tachycardia, bradycardia. **EENT:** increased intraocular pressure. **Other:** increased bronchial tone, *bronchospasm.*
metocurine iodide Metubine	*Adjunct to anesthetic to induce skeletal muscle relaxation; facilitate intubation, reduction of fractures and dislocations—* Dose depends on anesthetic used, individual needs, and response. Doses are representative and must be adjusted. Administer as sustained injection over 30 to 60 seconds. **Adults:** given cyclopropane: 2 to 4 mg I.V. (2.68 mg average). Given ether: 1.5 to 3 mg I.V. (2.1 mg average). Given nitrous oxide: 4 to 7 mg I.V. (4.79 mg average). Supplemental injections of 0.5 to 1 mg in 25 to 90 minutes, repeated p.r.n. *Lessen muscle contractions in pharmacologically or electrically induced convulsions—* **Adults:** 1.75 to 5.5 mg I.V.	**CV:** hypotension secondary to histamine release, ganglionic blockade in rapid dose or overdose. **Other:** *dose-related prolonged apnea,* residual muscle weakness, increased oropharyngeal secretions, allergic or idiosyncratic hypersensitivity reactions, *bronchospasm.*
pancuronium bromide Pavulon♦	*Adjunct to anesthetic to induce skeletal muscle relaxation; facilitate intubation, lessen muscle contractions in pharmacologically or electrically induced convulsions; assist with mechanical ventilation—* Dose depends on anesthetic used, individual needs, and re-	**CV:** tachycardia, increased blood pressure. **Local:** burning sensation. **Skin:** transient rashes. **Other:** excessive sweating and salivation, *prolonged dose-related apnea,* residual muscle weakness, allergic or idiosyncratic hypersensitivity reactions.

♦ Available in U.S. and Canada. ♦♦ Available in Canada only. All other products (no symbol) available in U.S. only. Italicized side effects are common or life-threatening.

INTERACTIONS	NURSING CONSIDERATIONS
None reported for this drug alone; always used with succinylcholine. See succinylcholine.	• Contraindicated in hypersensitivity to bromides and in bronchial asthma. Use cautiously in elderly or debilitated patients; in renal, hepatic, or pulmonary impairment, respiratory depression, myasthenia gravis, myasthenic syndrome of lung cancer, dehydration, thyroid disorders, collagen diseases, porphyria, electrolyte disturbances, and glaucoma; and during ocular surgery and (in large doses) cesarean section. • Not used extensively in clinical practice. • Monitor baseline electrolyte determinations (electrolyte imbalance potentiates neuromuscular effects) and vital signs (watch respirations closely). • Keep airway clear. Have emergency respiratory support (endotracheal equipment, ventilator, oxygen, atropine, neostigmine) on hand. • Reassure patient that postoperative stiffness is normal and will soon subside. • Determine whether patient has bromide allergy. • Use only fresh solutions; do not give without direct supervision of doctor.
Aminoglycoside antibiotics (including amikacin, gentamicin, kanamycin, neomycin, streptomycin); polymyxin antibiotics (polymyxin B sulfate, colistin); clindamycin; quinidine: potentiated neuromuscular blockade, leading to increased skeletal muscle relaxation and possible respiratory paralysis. Use cautiously during surgical and postoperative periods. *Narcotic analgesics:* potentiated neuromuscular blockade, leading to increased skeletal muscle relaxation and possible respiratory paralysis. Use with extreme caution, and reduce dose of metocurine iodide.	• Contraindicated in patients with hypersensitivity to iodides and those in whom histamine release is a hazard (asthmatic or atopic patients). Use cautiously in elderly or debilitated patients; and in renal, hepatic, or pulmonary impairment, respiratory depression, myasthenia gravis, myasthenic syndrome of lung cancer, dehydration, thyroid disorders, collagen diseases, porphyria, electrolyte disturbances, hyperthermia, and (in large doses) cesarean section. • Neostigmine, edrophonium, and epinephrine may be used to reverse effects of metocurine because of their anticurare effects. • Dose of 1 mg is the therapeutic equivalent of 3 mg *d*-tubocurarine chloride. • Monitor baseline electrolyte determinations (electrolyte imbalance, especially potassium, calcium, and magnesium, can potentiate neuromuscular effects) and vital signs, especially respiration. • Measure intake and output (renal dysfunction prolongs duration of action, since drug is mainly unchanged before excretion). • Keep airway clear. Have emergency respiratory support (endotracheal equipment, ventilator, oxygen, atropine, edrophonium, epinephrine, and neostigmine) on hand. • Reassure patient that postoperative stiffness is normal and will soon subside. • Determine whether patient has iodide allergy. • Store solution away from heat and sunlight; do not mix with barbiturates, methohexital, or thiopental (precipitate will form). Use fresh solutions only. • Do not give without direct supervision of doctor.
Aminoglycoside antibiotics (including amikacin, gentamicin, kanamycin, neomycin, streptomycin); polymyxin antibiotics (polymyxin B sulfate, colistin); clindamycin; quinidine: potentiated	• Contraindicated in hypersensitivity to bromides; preexisting tachycardia; and in patients for whom even a minor increase in heart rate is undesirable. Use cautiously in elderly or debilitated patients; renal, hepatic, or pulmonary impairment, respiratory depression, myasthenia gravis, myasthenic syndrome of lung cancer, dehydration, thyroid disorders, collagen diseases, porphyria, electrolyte disturbances, hyperthermia, toxemic states, and (in large doses) cesarean section. • Dose of 1 mg is the approximate therapeutic equivalent of 5 mg *d*-tubocurarine chloride.

(continued on following page)

NAME	INDICATIONS & DOSAGE	SIDE EFFECTS
pancuronium bromide *(continued)*	sponse. Doses are representative and must be adjusted. **Adults:** initially, 0.04 to 0.1 mg/kg I.V.; then 0.01 mg/kg q 30 to 60 minutes. **Children over 10 years:** initially, 0.04 to 0.1 mg/kg I.V., then $^1/_5$ initial dose q 30 to 60 minutes.	
succinylcholine chloride Anectine♦, Anectine Flo-Pack Powder, Sucostrin, Sux-Cert	*Adjunct to anesthetic to induce skeletal muscle relaxation; facilitate intubation and assist with mechanical ventilation or orthopedic manipulations (drug of choice); lessen muscle contractions in pharmacologically or electrically induced convulsions—* Dose depends on anesthetic used, individual needs, and response. Doses are representative and must be adjusted. **Adults:** 25 to 75 mg I.V., then 2.5 mg/minute, p.r.n., or 2.5 mg/kg I.M. up to maximum 150 mg I.M. in deltoid muscle. **Children:** 1 to 2 mg/kg I.M. or I.V. Maximum I.M. dose 150 mg. (Children may be less sensitive to succinylcholine than adults.)	**CV:** bradycardia, tachycardia, hypertension, hypotension, arrhythmias. **EENT:** increased intraocular pressure. **Other:** *prolonged respiratory depression, apnea, malignant hyperthermia,* muscle fasciculation, *postoperative muscle pain,* myoglobinemia, excessive salivation, allergic or idiosyncratic hypersensitivity reactions.

♦ Available in U.S. and Canada. ♦♦ Available in Canada only. All other products (no symbol) available in U.S. only. Italicized side effects are common or life-threatening.

INTERACTIONS	NURSING CONSIDERATIONS
neuromuscular blockade, leading to increased skeletal muscle relaxation and possible respiratory paralysis. Use cautiously during surgical and postoperative periods. *Lithium, narcotic analgesics:* potentiated neuromuscular blockade, leading to increased skeletal muscle relaxation and possible respiratory paralysis. Use with extreme caution, and reduce dose of pancuronium.	• Causes no histamine release or hypotension. • Monitor baseline electrolyte determinations (electrolyte imbalance can potentiate neuromuscular effects) and vital signs (watch respiration and heart rate closely). • Measure intake and output (renal dysfunction may prolong duration of action, since 25% of the drug is unchanged before excretion). • Have emergency respiratory support (endotracheal equipment, ventilator, oxygen, atropine, neostigmine) on hand. • Allow succinylcholine effects to subside before giving pancuronium. • Store in refrigerator. Do not store in plastic containers or syringes, although plastic syringes may be used for administration. • Do not mix with barbiturate solutions; use only fresh solutions. • Do not give without direct supervision of doctor.
Aminoglycoside antibiotics (including amikacin, gentamicin, kanamycin, neomycin, paromomycin, streptomycin); polymyxin antibiotics (polymyxin B sulfate, colistin); echothiophate: potentiated neuromuscular blockade, leading to increased skeletal muscle relaxation and possible respiratory paralysis. Use cautiously during surgical and postoperative periods. *Narcotic analgesics, lidocaine, procaine, methotrimeprazine:* potentiated neuromuscular blockade, leading to increased skeletal muscle relaxation and possible respiratory paralysis. Use with extreme caution. *MAO inhibitors, lithium, cyclophosphamide:* prolonged apnea. Use with caution. *Magnesium sulfate (parenterally):* poten-	• Contraindicated in abnormally low plasma pseudocholinesterase levels. Use with caution in patients with personal or family history of malignant hypertension or hyperthermia; elderly or debilitated patients; and in hepatic, renal, or pulmonary impairment, respiratory depression, severe burns or trauma, electrolyte imbalances, quinidine or digitalis therapy, hyperkalemia, paraplegia, spinal neuraxis injury, degenerative or dystrophic neuromuscular disease, myasthenia gravis, myasthenic syndrome of lung cancer, dehydration, thyroid disorders, collagen diseases, porphyria, fractures, muscle spasms, glaucoma, eye surgery or penetrating eye wounds, pheochromocytoma, and (in large doses) cesarean section. • Drug of choice for short procedures (less than 3 minutes) and for orthopedic manipulations; use caution in fractures or dislocations. • Duration of action prolonged to 20 minutes by continuous I.V. infusion or single-dose administration, along with hexafluorenium bromide. • Repeated or continuous infusions of succinylcholine alone not advised; may cause reduced response or prolonged apnea. • Monitor baseline electrolyte determinations and vital signs (check respiration every 5 to 10 minutes during infusion). • Keep airway clear. Have emergency respiratory support (endotracheal equipment, ventilator, oxygen, atropine, neostigmine) on hand. • Reassure patient that postoperative stiffness is normal and will soon subside. • Store injectable form in refrigerator. Store powder form at room temperature, tightly closed. Use immediately after reconstitution. Do not mix with alkaline solutions (thiopental, sodium bicarbonate, barbiturates). • Give test dose (10 mg I.M. or I.V.) after patient has been anesthetized. Normal response (no respiratory depression or transient depression lasting less than 5 minutes) indicates drug may be given. Do not give if patient develops respiratory paralysis sufficient to permit endotracheal intubation. (Recovery within 30 to 60 minutes.) • Do not give without direct supervision of doctor. • Give deep I.M., preferably high into the deltoid muscle.

(continued on following page)

NAME	INDICATIONS & DOSAGE	SIDE EFFECTS
succinylcholine chloride *(continued)*		
tubocurarine chloride Tubarine♦♦	*Adjunct to anesthetic to induce skeletal muscle relaxation; facilitate intubation, orthopedic manipulations—* Dose depends on anesthetic used, individual needs, and response. Doses listed are representative and must be adjusted. **Adults:** 1 unit/kg or 0.15 mg/kg I.V. slowly over 60 to 90 seconds. Average, initially, 40 to 60 units I.V. May give 20 to 30 units in 3 to 5 minutes. For longer procedures, give 20 units, p.r.n. **Children:** 1 unit/kg or 0.15 mg/kg. *Assist with mechanical ventilation—* **Adults and children:** initially, 0.0165 mg/kg I.V. (average 1 mg or 7 units), then adjust subsequent doses to patient's response. *Diagnose myasthenia gravis—* **Adults and children:** 0.0041 to 0.033 mg/kg I.V. or $^1/_{15}$ to $^1/_5$ normal adult dose for electroshock. Positive result: profound exaggeration of myasthenic symptoms. Dose may also be given I.M. when necessary. *Lessen muscle contractions in pharmacologically or electrically induced convulsions—* **Adults and children:** 1 unit/kg or 0.15 mg/kg slowly over 60 to 90 seconds. Initial dose 20 units (3 mg) less than calculated dose.	**CV:** hypotension, circulatory depression. **Other:** profound and prolonged muscle relaxation, *respiratory depression to the point of apnea,* hypersensitivity, idiosyncrasy, residual muscle weakness, *bronchospasm.*

♦ Available in U.S. and Canada. ♦♦ Available in Canada only. All other products (no symbol) available in U.S. only. Italicized side effects are common or life-threatening.

INTERACTIONS	NURSING CONSIDERATIONS
tiated neuromuscular blockade, increased skeletal muscle relaxation, and possible respiratory paralysis. Use with caution, preferably with reduced doses. *Cardiotonic glycosides:* possible cardiac arrhythmias. Use together cautiously.	
Aminoglycoside antibiotics (including amikacin, gentamicin, kanamycin, neomycin, paromomycin, streptomycin); polymyxin antibiotics (polymyxin B sulfate, colistin): potentiated neuromuscular blockade, leading to increased skeletal muscle relaxation and possible respiratory paralysis. Use cautiously during surgical and postoperative periods. *Quinidine:* prolonged neuromuscular blockade. Use together with caution. Monitor closely. *Thiazide diuretics, furosemide, ethacrynic acid, amphotericin B, propranolol, methotrimeprazine, narcotic analgesics:* potentiated neuromuscular blockade, leading to increased respiratory paralysis. Use with extreme caution during surgical and postoperative periods.	• Contraindicated in patients for whom histamine release is a hazard (asthmatics). Use cautiously in elderly or debilitated patients; in hepatic or pulmonary impairment, respiratory depression, myasthenia gravis, myasthenic syndrome of lung cancer, dehydration, thyroid disorders, collagen diseases, porphyria, electrolyte disturbances, fractures, muscle spasms, and (in large doses) cesarean section. • Small margin of safety between therapeutic dose and dose causing respiratory paralysis. • Used to diagnose myasthenia gravis, but procedure is hazardous. • Allow succinylcholine effects to subside before giving tubocurarine. • Monitor baseline electrolyte determinations (electrolyte imbalance can potentiate neuromuscular effects). • Watch respirations closely for early symptoms of paralysis—inability to keep eyelids open and eyes focused or difficulty in swallowing and speaking; notify doctor immediately. • Check vital signs every 15 minutes. Notify doctor at once of changes. • Measure intake and output (renal dysfunction prolongs duration of action, since much of drug is unchanged before excretion). • Keep airway clear. Have emergency respiratory support (endotracheal equipment, ventilator, oxygen, atropine, edrophonium, epinephrine, and neostigmine) on hand. • Reassure patient that postoperative stiffness is normal and will soon subside. • Decrease dose if inhalation anesthetics are used. • Do not mix with barbiturates. Use only fresh solutions and discard if discolored. • Give I.V. slowly (60 to 90 seconds); give deep I.M. in deltoid muscle. • Do not give without direct supervision of doctor.

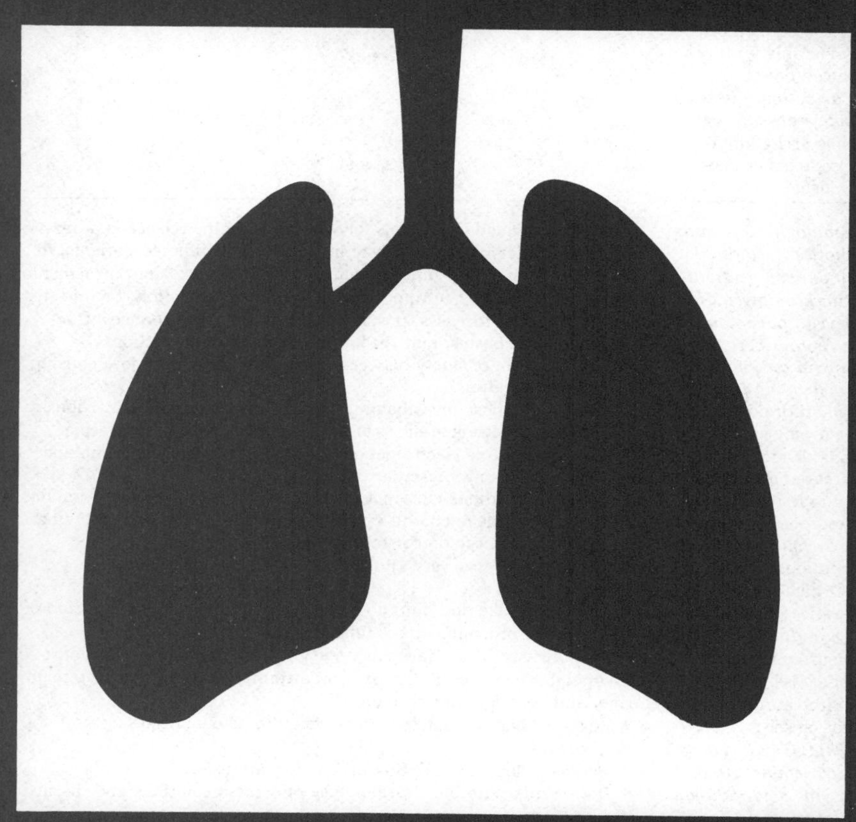

VI Respiratory Tract Drugs

43 Antihistamines

azatadine maleate
brompheniramine maleate
carbinoxamine maleate
chlorpheniramine maleate
clemastine fumarate
cyproheptadine hydrochloride
dexchlorpheniramine maleate
dimethindene maleate
diphenhydramine hydrochloride
diphenylpyraline hydrochloride
doxylamine succinate
methdilazine hydrochloride
promethazine hydrochloride
trimeprazine tartrate
tripelennamine hydrochloride
triprolidine hydrochloride

Antihistamines are thought to block the physiologic action of histamine, the humoral compound that causes symptoms associated with allergic reactions. They compete with histamine for receptor sites (by the process of competitive inhibition: see Chapter 1, PHARMACOLOGY FOR NURSES, for a detailed discussion of this concept).

Many compounds from different chemical classes are called antihistamines. The chart on the opposite page identifies the drugs in each class and their basic chemical structures. All antihistamines have *qualitatively* similar pharmacologic effects. *Quantitatively,* however, they may differ in potency and range of effect. Drowsiness, a side effect common to all antihistamines, may vary in intensity from drug to drug—and sometimes from patient to patient.

Major uses

Rx

• Antihistamines (except cyproheptadine, methdilazine, and trimeprazine) are used to relieve symptoms of allergy-related rhinitis and conjunctivitis. Antihistamines are also included in combination drug prepa-

NURSING TIPS

A NOTE ABOUT ANTIHISTAMINE INTERACTIONS

Although most antihistamine drug interactions are *not* serious, be aware of these and caution your patients accordingly:

• **Alcohol.** When a patient taking antihistamines drinks alcoholic beverages, he may become very drowsy. His alertness, motor coordination, and judgment may also be impaired.

• **Anticonvulsants.** If your patient has epilepsy and is undergoing phenytoin treatment, he may experience double vision, abnormal eye movements, a staggering gait, and slurred speech. If he is also taking phenobarbital, he may become very drowsy and less alert.

• **CNS depressants.** If your patient is taking barbiturates or other sleep medications, phenothiazines or other antipsychotics, or benzodiazepines or other tranquilizers, antihistamines may make him excessively drowsy.

COMMON ANTIHISTAMINES

CLASS	DERIVATIVES	CHEMICAL STRUCTURE*
ethanolamine	carbinoxamine, clemastine, diphenhydramine, diphenylpyraline, doxylamine	$R_1-O-C-C-N(R_2)(R_3)$
ethylenediamine	tripelennamine	$R_1-N-C-C-N(R_2)(R_3)$
alkylamine (propylamine)	brompheniramine, chlorpheniramine, dexchlorpheniramine, dimethindene, triprolidine	$R_1-C-C-C-N(R_2)(R_3)$
phenothiazine	methdilazine, promethazine, trimeprazine	$R_1-N-C-C-N(R_2)(R_3)$ (phenothiazine ring system with S)
miscellaneous	azatadine, cyproheptadine	Atypical structures; these drugs don't belong to a major antihistamine class.

*R_1, R_2, and R_3 represent chemical modifications that can be made to the basic antihistamine structure which either increase or decrease its activity.

Note: Piperidine derivatives (buclizine, cyclizine, and meclizine) are discussed in Chapter 49, EMETICS AND ANTIEMETICS.

rations because of the benefits they produce in the treatment of common cold symptoms.

• Cyproheptadine, methdilazine, and trimeprazine are used to treat mild, uncomplicated urticaria or pruritus resulting from allergic dermatoses.

• Diphenhydramine is used as a nighttime sedative.

• Diphenhydramine is a therapeutic adjunct for anaphylaxis or less severe allergic reactions caused by drugs, blood, or plasma. It is also used as a local anesthetic in dental procedures.

• Promethazine is used to prevent motion sickness.

Mechanism of action

• Antihistamines compete with histamine for H_1-receptor sites on effector cells. They can prevent but they can't reverse histamine-mediated responses, particularly histamine's effects on the smooth muscle of the bronchial tubes, gastrointestinal tract, uterus, and blood vessels.

• Anticholinergic actions of antihistamines dry the nasal mucosa and also relieve vertigo and motion sickness.

• Diphenhydramine, structurally re-

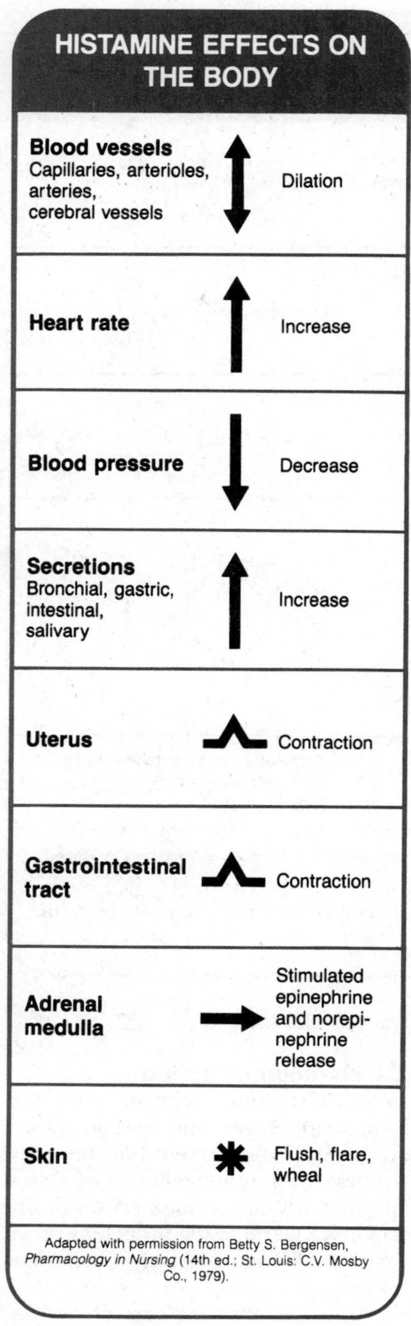

HISTAMINE EFFECTS ON THE BODY
Blood vessels
Capillaries, arterioles, arteries, cerebral vessels
Dilation
Heart rate
Increase
Blood pressure
Decrease
Secretions
Bronchial, gastric, intestinal, salivary
Increase
Uterus
Contraction
Gastrointestinal tract
Contraction
Adrenal medulla
Stimulated epinephrine and norepinephrine release
Skin
Flush, flare, wheal

Adapted with permission from Betty S. Bergensen, *Pharmacology in Nursing* (14th ed.; St. Louis: C.V. Mosby Co., 1979).

lated to local anesthetics, provides anesthesia by preventing initiation and transmission of nerve impulses.

Absorption, distribution, metabolism, and excretion

Antihistamines are well absorbed after oral or parenteral administration. They are distributed to most body tissues, extensively metabolized in the liver, and excreted in the urine as inactive metabolites within 24 hours.

Onset and duration

Antihistamines begin to act within 15 to 30 minutes; blood levels peak in about 1 hour. Duration of action varies, but symptoms are usually relieved for 4 to 6 hours. Action of the sustained-release forms may last 8 to 12 hours.

Combination products

ACTIFED: pseudoephedrine hydrochloride 60 mg and triprolidine hydrochloride 2.5 mg.
ALLEREST: phenylpropanolamine hydrochloride 18.7 mg and chlorpheniramine maleate 2 mg.
ALLERGY RELIEF MEDICINE: phenylpropanolamine hydrochloride 37.5 mg and chlorpheniramine maleate 4 mg.
ANAFED: pseudoephedrine hydrochloride 120 mg and chlorpheniramine maleate 8 mg.
BENDECTIN: doxylamine succinate 10 mg; pyridoxine hydrochloride 10 mg.
CHLOR-TRIMETON DECONGESTANT: chlorpheniramine maleate 4 mg and pseudoephedrine sulfate 60 mg.
CODIMAL DH: hydrocodone bitartrate 1.66 mg, phenylephrine hydrochloride 5 mg, pyrilamine maleate 8.33 mg, potassium guaiacolsulfonate 83.3 mg, sodium citrate 216 mg, and citric acid 50 mg.
COLREX DECONGESTANT: phenylpropanolamine hydrochloride 25 mg, phenylephrine hydrochloride 10 mg, chlorpheniramine maleate 4 mg, and tripelennamine hydrochloride 50 mg.
CONEX D.A.: phenylpropanolamine hydrochloride 50 mg and phenyltoloxamine citrate 50 mg.
CO-PYRONIL PULVULES: cyclopentamine hydrochloride 12.5 mg and pyr-

robutamine phosphate 15 mg.
COVANAMINE LIQUID: phenylpropanolamine hydrochloride 6.25 mg, phenylephrine hydrochloride 3.75 mg, chlorpheniramine maleate 1 mg, and pyrilamine maleate 6.25 mg.
DEMAZIN SYRUP: phenylephrine hydrochloride 2.5 mg, chlorpheniramine maleate 1 mg, and alcohol 7.5%.
DIMETANE DECONGESTANT: phenylephrine hydrochloride 10 mg and brompheniramine maleate 4 mg.
DIMETAPP EXTENTABS: brompheniramine maleate 12 mg, phenylephrine hydrochloride 15 mg, and phenylpropanolamine hydrochloride 15 mg.
DISOPHROL CHRONOTAB: dexbrompheniramine maleate 6 mg and pseudoephedrine sulfate 120 mg.
DRIXORAL♦: dexbrompheniramine maleate 6 mg and pseudoephedrine sulfate 120 mg.
DUO-HIST: pseudoephedrine hydrochloride 120 mg and brompheniramine maleate 12 mg.
DUPHRENE: phenylephrine hydrochloride 5 mg, chlorpheniramine maleate 1 mg, and pyrilamine maleate 12.5 mg.
FERNHIST: phenylpropanolamine hydrochloride 25 mg, chlorpheniramine maleate 2 mg, and pyrilamine maleate 12.5 mg.
HISA-CLOPANE PULVULES: cyclopentamine hydrochloride 12.5 mg and chlorpheniramine maleate 4 mg.
HISTALET FORTE: phenylpropanolamine hydrochloride 50 mg, phenylephrine hydrochloride 10 mg, chlorpheniramine maleate 4 mg, and pyrilamine maleate 25 mg.
HISTALET SYRUP: pseudoephedrine hydrochloride 45 mg, chlorpheniramine maleate 3 mg, and alcohol 0.45%.
HISTASPAN-D: chlorpheniramine maleate 8 mg, phenylephrine hydrochloride 20 mg, and methscopolamine nitrate 2.5 mg.
HISTA-VADRIN: phenylpropanolamine hydrochloride 40 mg, phenylephrine hydrochloride 5 mg, and chlorpheniramine maleate 6 mg.
NALDECON: phenylephrine hydrochloride 10 mg, phenylpropanolamine hydrochloride 40 mg, phenyltoloxamine citrate 15 mg, and chlorpheniramine maleate 5 mg.
NALDECON SYRUP: phenylpropanolamine hydrochloride 20 mg, phenylephrine hydrochloride 5 mg, chlorpheniramine maleate 2.5 mg, and phenyltoloxamine citrate 7.5 mg.
NEOTEP: chlorpheniramine maleate 9 mg and phenylephrine hydrochloride 21 mg.
NOLAMINE: chlorpheniramine maleate 4 mg, phenindamine tartrate 24 mg, and phenylpropanolamine hydrochloride 50 mg.
NOVAFED A: pseudoephedrine hydrochloride 120 mg and chlorpheniramine maleate 8 mg.
NOVAHISTINE ELIXIR: phenylpropanolamine hydrochloride 18.7 mg, chlorpheniramine maleate 2 mg, and alcohol 5%/5 ml.
ORNADE: isopropamide iodide 2.5 mg, phenylpropanolamine hydrochloride 50 mg, and chlorpheniramine maleate 8 mg.
PHENERGAN-D: pseudoephedrine hydrochloride 60 mg, promethazine hydrochloride 6.25 mg.
POLY-HISTINE-D: phenylpropanolamine hydrochloride 50 mg, phenyltoloxamine dihydrogen citrate 16 mg, pheniramine maleate 16 mg, and phenindamine tartrate 16 mg.
RELEMINE: phenylpropanolamine hydrochloride 25 mg, phenylephrine hydrochloride 15 mg, chlorpheniramine maleate 4 mg, and pyrilamine maleate 25 mg.
RHINEX D-LAY: acetaminophen 300 mg, salicylamide 300 mg, phenylpropanolamine hydrochloride 60 mg, and chlorpheniramine maleate 4 mg.
RONDEC: carbinoxamine maleate 4 mg and pseudoephedrine hydrochloride 60 mg.
RONDEC TABLETS: pseudoephedrine hydrochloride 60 mg and carbinoxamine maleate 4 mg.
TRIAMINIC TABLETS: phenylpropanolamine hydrochloride 50 mg, pheniramine maleate 25 mg, and pyrilamine maleate 25 mg.

NAME	INDICATIONS & DOSAGE	SIDE EFFECTS
azatadine maleate Optimine♦	*Rhinitis, allergy symptoms, chronic urticaria*— **Adults:** 1 to 2 mg P.O. b.i.d. Maximum 4 mg daily.	**Blood:** thrombocytopenia. **CNS (especially in the elderly):** *drowsiness, dizziness,* vertigo, disturbed coordination. **CV:** hypotension, palpitations. **GI:** anorexia, *nausea,* vomiting, *dry mouth and throat.* **GU:** urinary retention. **Skin:** urticaria, rash. **Other:** thickening of bronchial secretions.
brompheniramine maleate Dimetane♦, Dimetane-Ten, Rolabromophen, Spentane, Veltane	*Rhinitis, allergy symptoms*— **Adults:** 4 to 8 mg P.O. t.i.d. or q.i.d.; or (timed-release) 8 to 12 mg P.O. b.i.d. or t.i.d.; or 5 to 20 mg q 6 to 12 hours I.M., I.V., or S.C. Maximum 40 mg daily. **Children over 6 years:** 2 to 4 mg t.i.d. or q.i.d.; or (timed-release) 8 to 12 mg q 12 hours; or 0.5 mg/kg daily I.M., I.V., or S.C. divided t.i.d. or q.i.d. **Children under 6 years:** 0.5 mg/kg daily P.O., I.M., I.V., or S.C. divided t.i.d. or q.i.d.	**Blood:** thrombocytopenia, *agranulocytosis.* **CNS (especially in the elderly):** dizziness, tremors, irritability, insomnia, *drowsiness.* **CV:** hypotension, palpitations. **GI:** anorexia, nausea, vomiting, *dry mouth and throat.* **GU:** urinary retention. **Skin:** urticaria, rash. **After parenteral administration:** local reaction, sweating, syncope.
carbinoxamine maleate Clistin, Clistin RA	*Rhinitis, allergy symptoms*— **Adults:** 4 to 8 mg P.O. t.i.d. to q.i.d., or (timed-release) 8 to 12 mg q 8 to 12 hours. **Children over 6 years:** 4 mg P.O. t.i.d. to q.i.d. **Children 3 to 6 years:** 2 to 4 mg P.O. t.i.d. to q.i.d. **Children 1 to 3 years:** 2 mg P.O. t.i.d. to q.i.d.	**CNS (especially in the elderly):** *drowsiness, dizziness.* **GI:** anorexia, nausea, vomiting, *dry mouth.*
chlorpheniramine maleate Allerid-O.D., AL-R,	*Rhinitis, allergy symptoms*— **Adults:** 2 to 4 mg P.O. t.i.d. or q.i.d.; or (timed-release) 8 to	**CNS (especially in the elderly):** sedation, *drowsiness.* **CV:** hypotension, palpitations.

INTERACTIONS	NURSING CONSIDERATIONS
None significant.	• Contraindicated in acute asthmatic attack. Use cautiously in elderly patients, and in patients with increased intraocular pressure, hyperthyroidism, cardiovascular or renal disease, hypertension, bronchial asthma, narrow-angle glaucoma, urinary retention, prostatic hypertrophy, bladder-neck obstruction. • Warn patient against drinking alcoholic beverages during therapy and against activities that require alertness until CNS response to drug is determined. • Reduce GI distress by giving with food or milk. • Coffee or tea may reduce drowsiness. Sugarless gum, sour hard candy, or ice chips may relieve dry mouth. • Titrate each patient's dose; response to drug varies. • If tolerance develops, another antihistamine may be substituted. • Warn patient to stop taking drug 4 days before allergy skin tests; otherwise, accuracy of tests may be affected. • Monitor blood counts during long-term therapy; watch for signs of blood dyscrasias.
None significant.	• Contraindicated in acute asthmatic attack. Use cautiously in elderly patients, and in patients with increased intraocular pressure, hyperthyroidism, cardiovascular or renal disease, hypertension, bronchial asthma, narrow-angle glaucoma, urinary retention, prostatic hypertrophy, bladder-neck obstruction. • Warn patient against drinking alcoholic beverages during therapy and against activities that require alertness until CNS response to drug is determined. • Reduce GI distress by giving with food or milk. • Coffee or tea may reduce drowsiness. Sugarless gum, sour hard candy, or ice chips may relieve dry mouth. • Titrate each patient's dose; response to drug varies. • If tolerance develops, another antihistamine may be substituted. • Warn patient to stop taking drug 4 days before allergy skin tests; otherwise, accuracy of tests may be affected. • Injectable form containing 10 mg/ml can be given diluted or undiluted very slowly I.V. The 100 mg/ml injection should not be given I.V. • Monitor blood count during long-term therapy; observe for signs of blood dyscrasias.
None significant.	• Contraindicated in acute asthmatic attack. Use cautiously in elderly patients, and in patients with increased intraocular pressure, hyperthyroidism, cardiovascular or renal disease, hypertension, bronchial asthma, narrow-angle glaucoma, urinary retention, prostatic hypertrophy, bladder-neck obstruction. • Warn patient against drinking alcoholic beverages during therapy and against driving or other activities that require alertness until CNS response to drug is determined. • Reduce GI distress by giving with food or milk. • Coffee or tea may reduce drowsiness. Sugarless gum, sour hard candy, or ice chips may relieve dry mouth. • Titrate each patient's dose; response to drug varies. • If tolerance develops, another antihistamine may be substituted. • Warn patient to stop taking drug 4 days before allergy skin tests; otherwise, accuracy of tests may be affected.
None significant.	• Contraindicated in acute asthmatic attack. Use cautiously in elderly patients, and in patients with increased intraocular pressure, hyperthyroidism, cardiovascular or renal disease, hypertension, bronchial

(continued on following page)

NAME	INDICATIONS & DOSAGE	SIDE EFFECTS
chlorpheniramine maleate *(continued)* Chloramate, Chlormene, Chlortab, Chlor-Trimeton, Chlor-Tripolon♦♦, Ciramine, Histalon♦♦, Histaspan, Histex, Histrey, Novopheniram♦♦, Pyranistan, Teldrin	12 mg P.O. b.i.d. or t.i.d.; or 5 to 40 mg I.M., I.V., or S.C. Give I.V. injection over 1 minute. **Children 6 to 12 years:** 2 mg P.O. t.i.d. or q.i.d.; or (timed-release) 8 mg P.O. daily or b.i.d. **Children 2 to 6 years:** 1 mg P.O. t.i.d. or q.i.d.	**GI:** epigastric distress, *dry mouth.* **GU:** urinary retention. **Other:** thickening of bronchial secretions. **After parenteral administration:** local stinging, burning sensation, pallor, weak pulse, transient hypotension.
clemastine fumarate Tavist, Tavist-1	*Rhinitis, allergy symptoms—* **Adults:** 1.34 to 2.68 mg once daily. Maximum recommended daily dosage is 8.04 mg; or (timed-release) 1.34 mg (long-acting tablet) b.i.d., not to exceed 8.04 mg (6 long-acting tablets) per day. *Allergic skin manifestation of urticaria and angioedema—* **Adults:** 2.68 mg up to t.i.d. maximum.	**Blood:** hemolytic anemia, thrombocytopenia, *agranulocytosis.* **CNS (especially in the elderly):** *sedation, drowsiness.* **CV:** hypotension, palpitations, tachycardia. **GI:** epigastric distress, anorexia, nausea, vomiting, constipation, *dry mouth.* **GU:** urinary retention. **Skin:** rash, urticaria. **Other:** thickening of bronchial secretions.
cyproheptadine hydrochloride Periactin♦, Vimicon♦♦	*Allergy symptoms, pruritus—* **Adults:** 4 mg P.O. t.i.d. or q.i.d. Maximum 0.5 mg/kg daily. **Children 7 to 14 years:** 4 mg P.O. b.i.d. or t.i.d. **Children 2 to 6 years:** 2 mg P.O. b.i.d. or t.i.d.	**CNS (especially in the elderly):** *drowsiness,* dizziness, headache, fatigue. **GI:** anorexia, nausea, vomiting, *dry mouth.* **Skin:** rash. **Other:** weight gain.
dexchlorpheniramine maleate Polaramine♦	*Rhinitis, allergy symptoms, contact dermatitis, pruritus—* **Adults:** 1 to 2 mg P.O. t.i.d. or q.i.d.; or (timed-release) 4 to 6 mg b.i.d. or t.i.d. **Children under 12 years:** 0.15 mg/kg P.O. daily divided	**CNS (especially in the elderly):** *drowsiness,* dizziness. **GI:** nausea, *dry mouth.* **GU:** polyuria, dysuria.

♦ Available in U.S. and Canada. ♦♦ Available in Canada only. All other products (no symbol) available in U.S. only. Italicized side effects are common or life-threatening.

INTERACTIONS	NURSING CONSIDERATIONS
	asthma, narrow-angle glaucoma, urinary retention, prostatic hypertrophy, bladder-neck obstruction. • Warn patient against drinking alcoholic beverages and using other CNS depressants during therapy and against driving or other activities that require alertness until CNS response to drug is determined. • Coffee or tea may reduce drowsiness. • Titrate each patient's dose; response to drug varies. • If tolerance develops, another antihistamine may be substituted. • Warn patient to stop taking drug 4 days before allergy skin tests; otherwise, accuracy of tests may be affected. • Only injectable forms *without* preservatives can be given I.V. Give *slowly*. • If symptoms occur after parenteral dose, stop drug. Notify doctor.
None significant.	• Contraindicated in acute asthmatic attack. Use cautiously in elderly patients, and in patients with increased intraocular pressure, hyperthyroidism, cardiovascular or renal disease, hypertension, bronchial asthma, narrow-angle glaucoma, urinary retention, prostatic hypertrophy, bladder-neck obstruction. • Warn patient against drinking alcoholic beverages during therapy and against driving or other activities that require alertness until CNS response to drug is determined. • Coffee or tea may reduce drowsiness. Sugarless gum, sour hard candy, or ice chips may relieve dry mouth. • Titrate each patient's dose; response to drug varies. • If tolerance develops, another antihistamine may be substituted. • Warn patient to stop taking drug 4 days before allergy skin tests; otherwise, accuracy of tests may be affected. • Tablets are available as 1.34 and 2.68 mg. Long-acting tablets are 1.34 mg. • Monitor blood counts during long-term therapy; observe for signs of blood dyscrasias.
None significant.	• Contraindicated in acute asthmatic attack. Use cautiously in elderly patients, and in patients with increased intraocular pressure, hyperthyroidism, cardiovascular or renal disease, hypertension, bronchial asthma, narrow-angle glaucoma, urinary retention, prostatic hypertrophy, bladder-neck obstruction. • Warn patient against drinking alcoholic beverages during therapy and against driving or other activities that require alertness until CNS response to drug is determined. • Reduce GI distress by giving with food or milk. • Coffee or tea may reduce drowsiness. Sugarless gum, sour hard candy, or ice chips may relieve dry mouth. • Titrate each patient's dose; response to drug varies. • If tolerance develops, another antihistamine may be substituted. • Warn patient to stop taking drug 4 days before allergy skin tests; otherwise, accuracy of tests may be affected. • Used experimentally to stimulate appetite and increase weight gain in children.
None significant.	• Contraindicated in acute asthmatic attack. Use cautiously in elderly patients, and in patients with increased intraocular pressure, hyperthyroidism, cardiovascular or renal disease, hypertension, bronchial asthma, narrow-angle glaucoma, urinary retention, prostatic hypertrophy, bladder-neck obstruction. • Warn patient against drinking alcoholic beverages during therapy and against driving or other activities that require alertness until CNS

(continued on following page)

NAME	INDICATIONS & DOSAGE	SIDE EFFECTS
dexchlor-pheniramine maleate *(continued)*	into 4 doses. Do not use timed-release tablets for children younger than 6 years.	
dimethindene maleate Forhistal, Triten	*Allergy symptoms*— **Adults, and children over 6 years:** (timed-release) 2.5 mg P.O. daily b.i.d.	**CNS (especially in the elderly):** *drowsiness,* dizziness, insomnia, irritability, headache. **GI:** anorexia, nausea, vomiting, *dry mouth,* diarrhea. **GU:** urinary frequency.
diphenhydramine hydrochloride Allerdryl, Baramine, Bax, Benachlor, Benadryl♦, Benahist, Ben-Allergin, Bendylate, Bentrac, Bonyl, Eldadryl, Fenylhist, Hyrexin, Nordryl, Notose, Phen-Amin 50, Phenamine, Rodryl, Rohydra, SK-Diphenhydramine, Span-Lanin, Valdrene, Wehdryl	*Rhinitis, allergy symptoms, motion sickness, antiparkinsonism*— **Adults:** 25 to 50 mg P.O. t.i.d. to q.i.d.; or 10 to 50 mg deep I.M. or I.V. Maximum 400 mg daily. **Children under 12 years:** 5 mg/kg daily P.O., deep I.M., or I.V. divided q.i.d. Maximum 300 mg daily. *Sedation*— **Adults:** 25 to 50 mg P.O., deep I.M., p.r.n.	**CNS (especially in the elderly):** *drowsiness,* confusion, insomnia, headache, vertigo. **CV:** palpitations. **EENT:** photosensitivity, diplopia, nasal stuffiness. **GI:** *nausea,* vomiting, diarrhea, *dry mouth,* constipation. **GU:** dysuria. **Skin:** urticaria.
diphenylpyraline hydrochloride Diafen, Hispril	*Rhinitis, allergy symptoms*— **Adults:** 2 mg P.O. q 4 hours, p.r.n.; or (timed-release) 5 mg P.O. q 12 hours. **Children over 6 years:** 2 mg P.O. q 6 hours, p.r.n.; or (timed-release) 5 mg P.O. daily. **Children 2 to 6 years:** 1 to 2 mg P.O. q 8 hours, p.r.n.	**CNS (especially in the elderly):** *drowsiness,* dizziness, headache. **EENT:** nasal congestion. **GI:** *dry mouth and throat,* epigastric distress. **Skin:** flushing.

♦ Available in U.S. and Canada. ♦♦ Available in Canada only. All other products (no symbol) available in U.S. only. Italicized side effects are common or life-threatening.

INTERACTIONS	NURSING CONSIDERATIONS
	response to drug is determined. • Coffee or tea may reduce drowsiness. • Titrate each patient's dose; response to drug varies. • If tolerance develops, another antihistamine may be substituted. • Warn patient to stop taking drug 4 days before allergy skin tests; otherwise, accuracy of tests may be affected.
None significant.	• Contraindicated in acute asthmatic attack. Use cautiously in elderly patients, and in patients with increased intraocular pressure, hyperthyroidism, cardiovascular or renal disease, hypertension, bronchial asthma, narrow-angle glaucoma, urinary retention, prostatic hypertrophy, bladder-neck obstruction. • Warn patient against drinking alcoholic beverages during therapy and against driving or other activities that require alertness until CNS response to drug is determined. • Reduce GI distress by giving with food or milk. • Coffee or tea may reduce drowsiness. Sugarless gum, sour hard candy, or ice chips may relieve dry mouth. • Titrate each patient's dose; response to drug varies. • If tolerance develops, another antihistamine may be substituted. • Warn patient to stop taking drug 4 days before allergy skin tests; otherwise, accuracy of tests may be affected.
None significant.	• Contraindicated in acute asthmatic attack. Use cautiously in narrow-angle glaucoma, prostatic hypertrophy, peptic ulcer, pyloroduodenal and bladder-neck obstruction; in newborns, and in asthmatic, hypertensive, or cardiac patients. • Alternate injection sites to prevent irritation. Administer deep I.M. into large muscle. • Warn patient against drinking alcoholic beverages during therapy and against driving or other hazardous activities until CNS response to drug is determined. • Reduce GI distress by giving with food or milk. • Coffee or tea may reduce drowsiness. Sugarless gum, sour hard candy, or ice chips may relieve dry mouth. • Titrate each patient's dose; response to drug varies. • If tolerance develops, another antihistamine may be substituted. • Warn patient to stop taking drug 4 days before allergy skin tests; otherwise, accuracy of tests may be affected. • Used with epinephrine in anaphylaxis. • One of most sedating antihistamines; often used as a nighttime sedative.
None significant.	• Contraindicated in acute asthmatic attack. Use cautiously in elderly patients, and in patients with increased intraocular pressure, hyperthyroidism, cardiovascular or renal disease, hypertension, diabetes mellitus, bronchial asthma, narrow-angle glaucoma, urinary retention, prostatic hypertrophy, bladder-neck obstruction. • Warn patient against drinking alcoholic beverages during therapy and against driving or other activities that require alertness until CNS response to drug is determined. • Reduce GI distress by giving with food or milk. • Coffee or tea may reduce drowsiness. Sugarless gum, sour hard candy, or ice chips may relieve dry mouth. • Titrate each patient's dose; response to drug varies. • If tolerance develops, another antihistamine may be substituted. • Warn patient to stop taking drug 4 days before allergy skin tests; otherwise, accuracy of tests may be affected.

NAME	INDICATIONS & DOSAGE	SIDE EFFECTS
doxylamine succinate Bendectin, Decapryn, Unisom	*Rhinitis, allergy symptoms—* **Adults:** 12.5 to 25 mg P.O. q 4 to 6 hours, p.r.n. **Children 6 to 12 years:** 6.25 to 12.5 mg P.O. q 4 to 6 hours, p.r.n. *Nausea and vomiting of pregnancy—* **Adults:** 2 Bendectin tablets at bedtime. Maximum 4 tablets daily.	**CNS (especially in the elderly):** *drowsiness,* dizziness, insomnia, disorientation, confusion, tremor, irritability, vertigo. **CV:** palpitations. **GI:** *dry mouth and throat.*
methdilazine hydrochloride Dilosyn♦♦, Tacaryl	*Pruritus—* **Adults:** 8 mg P.O. b.i.d. to q.i.d. or (chewable tablets) 7.2 mg P.O. b.i.d. to q.i.d. **Children over 3 years:** 4 mg P.O. b.i.d. to q.i.d. or (chewable tablets) 3.6 mg P.O. b.i.d. to q.i.d.	**CNS (especially in the elderly):** *drowsiness,* dizziness, headache. **GI:** nausea, *dry mouth and throat.* **Hepatic:** cholestatic jaundice. **Skin:** rash.
promethazine hydrochloride Ganphen, Histantil♦♦, K-Phen, Methazine, Pentazine♦, Phencen-50, Phenergan♦, Promethamead, Promethazine, Prorex, Provigan, Remsed, Rolamethazine, Sigazine	*Motion sickness—* **Adults:** 25 mg P.O. b.i.d. **Children:** 12.5 to 25 mg P.O., I.M., or rectally b.i.d. *Nausea—* **Adults:** 12.5 to 25 mg P.O., I.M., or rectally q 4 to 6 hours, p.r.n. **Children:** 0.25 to 0.5 mg/kg I.M. or rectally q 4 to 6 hours, p.r.n. *Rhinitis, allergy symptoms—* **Adults:** 12.5 mg P.O. q.i.d.; or 25 mg P.O. at bedtime. **Children:** 6.25 to 12.5 mg P.O. t.i.d. or 25 mg P.O. at bedtime. *Sedation—* **Adults:** 25 to 50 mg P.O., I.M. at bedtime or p.r.n. **Children:** 12.5 to 25 mg P.O., I.M., or rectally at bedtime.	**CNS (especially in the elderly):** *sedation,* confusion, restlessness, tremors, *drowsiness.* **CV:** hypotension. **EENT:** transient myopia, nasal congestion. **GI:** anorexia, nausea, vomiting, constipation, *dry mouth.* **Other:** *photosensitivity.*

♦ Available in U.S. and Canada. ♦♦ Available in Canada only. All other products (no symbol) available in U.S. only. Italicized side effects are common or life-threatening.

INTERACTIONS	NURSING CONSIDERATIONS
None significant.	• Contraindicated in acute asthmatic attack. Use cautiously in elderly patients, and in patients with increased intraocular pressure, hyperthyroidism, cardiovascular or renal disease, hypertension, bronchial asthma, narrow-angle glaucoma, urinary retention, prostatic hypertrophy, bladder-neck obstruction. • Warn patient against drinking alcoholic beverages during therapy and against driving or other activities that require alertness until CNS response to drug is determined. • Coffee or tea may reduce drowsiness. Sugarless gum, sour hard candy, or ice chips may relieve dry mouth. • Titrate each patient's dose; response to drug varies. • If tolerance develops, another antihistamine may be substituted. • Warn patient to stop taking drug 4 days before allergy skin tests; otherwise, accuracy of tests may be affected.
Phenothiazines: increased effects. Don't use together.	• Contraindicated in acute asthmatic attack. Use cautiously in elderly or debilitated patients; acutely ill or dehydrated children; and in patients with pulmonary, hepatic, or cardiovascular disease, asthma, hypertension, narrow-angle glaucoma, peptic ulcer, prostatic hypertrophy, bladder-neck obstruction, CNS depression. • Warn patient against drinking alcoholic beverages during therapy and against driving or other activities that require alertness until CNS response to drug is determined. • Reduce GI distress by giving with food or milk. • Coffee or tea may reduce drowsiness. Sugarless gum, sour hard candy, or ice chips may relieve dry mouth. • Titrate each patient's dose; response to drug varies. • If tolerance develops, another antihistamine may be substituted. • Available as chewable tablet for children. Instruct child to chew completely and swallow promptly; may cause local anesthetic effect in mouth. • Warn patient to stop taking drug 4 days before allergy skin tests; otherwise, accuracy of tests may be affected.
Phenothiazines: increased effects. Don't give together.	• Contraindicated in narrow-angle glaucoma, peptic ulcer, intestinal obstruction, prostatic hypertrophy, bladder-neck obstruction, epilepsy, bone-marrow depression, coma, CNS depression, pregnancy (except during labor), lactation; in newborns and acutely ill or dehydrated children. Use cautiously in pulmonary, hepatic, or cardiovascular disease; asthma; hypertension; and in elderly or debilitated patients. • Warn patient against drinking alcoholic beverages during therapy and against driving or other activities that require alertness until CNS response to drug is determined. • Reduce GI distress by giving with food or milk. • Coffee or tea may reduce drowsiness. Sugarless gum, sour hard candy, or ice chips may relieve dry mouth. • Titrate each patient's dose; response to drug varies. • If tolerance develops, another antihistamine may be substituted. • Warn patient to stop taking drug 4 days before allergy skin tests; otherwise, accuracy of tests may be affected. • Pronounced sedative effect limits use in many ambulatory patients. • May cause false-positive immunologic urine pregnancy test (Gravindex). Also may interfere with blood grouping in ABO system. • When treating motion sickness, tell patient to take first dose 30 to 60 minutes before travel. On succeeding days of travel, he should take dose upon arising and with evening meal. • Inject deep I.M. into large muscle mass. • Warn patient about possible photosensitivity reaction and precautions he should take to avoid it.

NAME	INDICATIONS & DOSAGE	SIDE EFFECTS
trimeprazine tartrate Panectyl♦♦, Temaril	*Pruritus*— **Adults:** 2.5 mg P.O. q.i.d.; or (timed-release) 5 mg P.O. b.i.d. **Children 3 to 12 years:** 2.5 mg P.O. h.s. or t.i.d., p.r.n. **Children 6 months to 3 years:** 1.25 mg P.O. h.s. or t.i.d., p.r.n.	**Blood:** *agranulocytosis,* leukopenia. **CNS (especially in the elderly):** *drowsiness,* dizziness, confusion, headache, restlessness, tremors, irritability, insomnia. **CV:** hypotension, palpitations, tachycardia. **GI:** anorexia, nausea, vomiting, *dry mouth and throat.* **GU:** urinary frequency or retention. **Skin:** urticaria, rash.
tripelennamine hydrochloride PBZ-SR, Pyribenzamine♦, Ro-Hist	*Rhinitis, allergy symptoms*— **Adults:** 25 to 50 mg P.O. q 4 to 6 hours; or (timed-release) 100 mg b.i.d. to t.i.d. Maximum 600 mg daily. **Children over 5 years:** 50 mg P.O. q 8 to 12 hours (timed-release). **Children under 5 years:** 5 mg/kg daily P.O. in 4 to 6 divided doses. Maximum 300 mg daily.	**CNS (especially in the elderly):** *drowsiness,* dizziness, confusion, restlessness, tremors, irritability, insomnia. **CV:** palpitations. **GI:** anorexia, diarrhea or constipation, *nausea, vomiting, dry mouth.* **GU:** urinary frequency or retention. **Skin:** urticaria, rash. **Other:** thickening of bronchial secretions.
triprolidine hydrochloride Actidil♦	*Colds and allergy symptoms*— **Adults:** 2.5 mg P.O. t.i.d. or q.i.d. **Children over 6 years:** 1.25 mg t.i.d. or q.i.d. **Children under 6 years:** 0.3 to 0.6 mg t.i.d. or q.i.d.	**CNS (especially in the elderly):** *drowsiness,* dizziness, confusion, restlessness, insomnia. **GI:** anorexia, diarrhea or constipation, nausea, vomiting, *dry mouth.* **GU:** urinary frequency or retention. **Skin:** urticaria, rash.

♦ Available in U.S. and Canada. ♦♦ Available in Canada only. All other products (no symbol) available in U.S. only. Italicized side effects are common or life-threatening.

INTERACTIONS	NURSING CONSIDERATIONS
Phenothiazines: increased effects. Don't use together.	• Contraindicated in acute asthmatic attack. Use cautiously in pulmonary, hepatic, or cardiovascular disease; asthma; hypertension; narrow-angle glaucoma; peptic ulcer; intestinal obstruction; prostatic hypertrophy; bladder-neck obstruction; epilepsy, bone-marrow depression; coma; CNS depression; in elderly or debilitated patients, and acutely ill or dehydrated children. • Warn patient against drinking alcoholic beverages during therapy and against driving or other activities that require alertness until CNS response to drug is determined. • Reduce GI distress by giving with food or milk. • Coffee or tea may reduce drowsiness. Sugarless gum, sour hard candy, or ice chips may relieve dry mouth. • Titrate each patient's dose; response to drug varies. • If tolerance develops, another antihistamine may be substituted. • Warn patient to stop taking drug 4 days before allergy skin tests; otherwise, accuracy of tests may be affected. • Monitor blood counts during long-term therapy.
None significant.	• Contraindicated in acute asthmatic attack. Use cautiously in elderly patients, and in patients with increased intraocular pressure, hyperthyroidism, cardiovascular or renal disease, hypertension, or bronchial asthma, narrow-angle glaucoma, urinary retention, prostatic hypertrophy, bladder-neck obstruction. • Warn patient against drinking alcoholic beverages during therapy and against driving or other activities that require alertness until CNS response to drug is determined. • Reduce GI distress by giving with food or milk. • Coffee or tea may reduce drowsiness. Sugarless gum, sour hard candy, or ice chips may relieve dry mouth. • Titrate each patient's dose; response to drug varies. • If tolerance develops, another antihistamine may be substituted. • Warn patient to stop taking drug 4 days before allergy skin tests; otherwise, accuracy of tests may be affected.
None significant.	• Contraindicated in acute asthma. Use cautiously in elderly patients, and in patients with increased intraocular pressure, hyperthyroidism, cardiovascular or renal disease, hypertension, diabetes mellitus, bronchial asthma, narrow-angle glaucoma, urinary retention, prostatic hypertrophy, bladder-neck obstruction. • Warn patient against drinking alcoholic beverages during therapy and against driving or other activities that require alertness until CNS response to drug is determined. • Reduce GI distress by giving with food or milk. • Coffee or tea may reduce drowsiness. Sugarless gum, sour hard candy, or ice chips may relieve dry mouth. • Titrate each patient's dose; response to drug varies. • Warn patient to stop taking drug 4 days before allergy skin tests; otherwise, accuracy of tests may be affected.

Expectorants and antitussives

Expectorants
acetylcysteine
ammonium chloride
guaifenesin (formerly glyceryl guaiacolate)
hydriodic acid
iodinated glycerol
potassium iodide (SSKI)
terpin hydrate
tyloxapol

Antitussives
benzonatate
chlophedianol hydrochloride
codeine
codeine phosphate
codeine sulfate
dextromethorphan hydrobromide
diphenhydramine hydrochloride
hydrocodone bitartrate
hydromorphone hydrochloride
levopropoxyphene napsylate
noscapine hydrochloride

(All drugs are listed in alphabetical order in the tables that follow.)

Expectorants may decrease sputum viscosity and ease expectoration. Although they are used to loosen secretions (provide mucolytic action) in chronic pulmonary disorders and the common cold, their therapeutic efficacy is doubtful. Nevertheless, these agents are included in many prescription and over-the-counter cough and cold preparations. These agents should probably be used only in conjunction with a total-care plan that includes adequate fluid intake and a cool mist or steam vaporizer.

Antitussives, or cough suppressants, reduce the frequency of a cough, especially when it is dry and nonproductive. Cough suppression is desirable

DO EXPECTORANTS REALLY HELP?

You're probably familiar with traditional expectorants, such as guaifenesin, potassium iodide and other iodides, terpin hydrate, and syrup of ipecac. But did you know that all these drugs have been the subjects of studies to determine the actual effectiveness of expectorants?

Guaifenesin (Robitussin), the most popular expectorant, has come under especially close scrutiny. It's been found:

- no better then the placebo in controlled studies.
- ineffective as an expectorant in patients with chronic bronchitis.
- effective in some studies but only when extremely high doses are administered.

Fortunately, new and effective trends have developed in expectorant therapy. These include the use of:

- *mucolytic agents,* which lower sputum viscosity and aid expectoration
- *corticosteroids,* which reduce mucus volume and lower sputum viscosity, and are effective in severe conditions such as bronchial asthma
- *oral, parenteral, mist, or steam hydration,* which helps to loosen thick secretions. (Administer hydration only under a doctor's order. Since water increases mucus volume, further airway obstruction can result. Use hydration with a bronchodilator, a heated ultrasonic nebulizer, or a similar device if ordered. If not ordered, consult the doctor about their use.)

when a chronic cough produces extreme fatigue (as in lung cancer). Most patients with a common cold don't need antitussives; cough drops will do.

Major uses

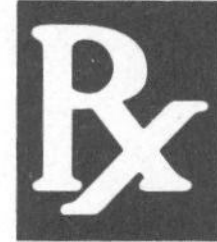

• Expectorants may facilitate expectoration in pneumonia, bronchitis, cystic fibrosis, tuberculosis, emphysema, atelectasis, and bronchial asthma.
• Antitussives suppress nonproductive coughs.

Mechanism of action

• Expectorants may increase production of respiratory tract fluids to help liquefy and reduce the viscosity of thick, tenacious secretions. Tyloxapol also lowers surface tension of sputum to facilitate expectoration.
• Antitussives suppress the cough reflex by direct action on the cough center in the medulla (brain) or by peripheral action on sensory nerve endings. Benzonatate, chlophedianol, and diphenhydramine also act as local anesthetics.

Absorption, distribution, metabolism, and excretion

All expectorants and antitussives are well absorbed after oral administration, metabolized in the liver, and excreted in the urine.
• Acetylcysteine and tyloxapol are also well absorbed after inhalation.
• Potassium iodide is also excreted through the respiratory tract.

Onset and duration

Expectorants and antitussives begin to act within 30 minutes. Their effects generally last 4 to 6 hours; benzonatate, however, may act as long as 8 hours.

Combination products

Preparations are available in the following combinations: expectorants with decongestants or antihistamines, or both; antitussives with decongestants or antihistamines, or both; expectorants and antitussives; expectorants and antitussives with decongestants or antihistamines, or both.

PATIENT CARE

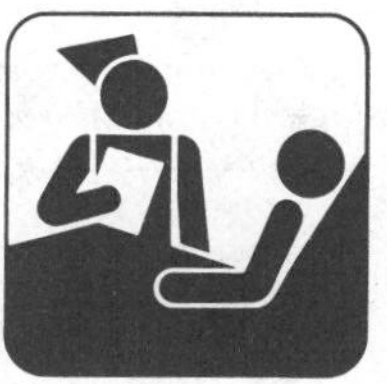

HOW TO FOSTER PRODUCTIVE COUGHING

Effective coughing usually helps a patient dislodge pulmonary secretions. (A productive cough raises sputum; a nonproductive cough results in a dry, hacking sound.)

Teach your patient productive coughing
• First, have him sit in a chair or on the edge of the bed. Make sure his feet are supported with a stool if they don't reach the floor.
• Then, have him hunch his body forward slightly. Tell him to take several slow and deep breaths, to bend his head forward, and to cough two or three times in rapid succession.
• Urge him to breathe deeply again and to repeat the entire exercise several times.
• A patient who has just had surgery should splint his incision before he coughs. Include instructions for splinting in your preoperative teaching. Show him how to position his hands above and below the incision. Explain why splinting is important so he'll remember to do it.
• If your patient has such severe pain after surgery that he can't splint his own incision effectively, help him. Hold a drawsheet or towel against his incision. Then encourage him to deep breathe and cough, as explained above.

Monitor and control the patient's cough
• Record the type of cough and its frequency, and the amount, color, odor, and consistency of the sputum.
• Instruct the patient to cough into several layers of tissues and to dispose of them properly.
• Ask the patient to report any side effects of prescribed expectorants or antitussives.

You should limit or ban the patient's smoking and visitors' smoking in the patient's room. And make sure the patient's fluid intake is adequate.

NAME	INDICATIONS & DOSAGE	SIDE EFFECTS
acetylcysteine Airbron♦♦, Mucomyst♦, NAC♦♦	*Pneumonia, bronchitis, tuberculosis, cystic fibrosis, emphysema, atelectasis (adjunct), complications of thoracic or cardiovascular surgery—* **Adults and children:** 1 to 2 ml of 10% to 20% solution by direct instillation into trachea as often as every hour; or 3 to 5 ml of 20% solution, or 6 to 10 ml of 10% solution, by mouthpiece t.i.d. or q.i.d. *Acetaminophen toxicity—* 140 mg/kg initially P.O., followed by 70 mg/kg q 4 hours for 17 doses (a total of 1,330 mg/kg).	**EENT:** *rhinorrhea, hemoptysis.* **GI:** *stomatitis, nausea.* **Other:** *bronchospasm (especially in asthmatics).*
ammonium chloride	*As expectorant—* **Adults:** 250 to 500 mg P.O. q 2 to 4 hours.	**CNS:** headache, drowsiness, confusion, excitation alternating with coma, twitching, hyperreflexia, EEG abnormalities. **CV:** bradycardia. **GI:** *anorexia, nausea, vomiting.* **GU:** renal impairment, glycosuria. **Metabolic:** acidosis, decreased potassium, hypocalcemic tetany, hyperglycemia. **Skin:** rash. **Other:** thirst.
benzonatate Tessalon♦	*Nonproductive cough—* **Adults, and children over 10 years:** 100 mg P.O. t.i.d.; up to 600 mg daily. **Children under 10 years:** 8 mg/kg P.O. in 3 to 6 divided doses.	**CNS:** dizziness, drowsiness. **EENT:** nasal congestion, sensation of burning in eyes. **GI:** nausea, constipation. **Skin:** rash.
chlophedianol hydrochloride Ulo, Ulone♦♦	*Nonproductive cough—* **Adults, and children over 12 years:** 25 mg P.O. t.i.d. or q.i.d. **Children 6 to 12 years:** 12.5 to 25 mg P.O. t.i.d. or q.i.d. **Children 2 to 6 years:** 12.5 mg P.O. t.i.d. or q.i.d.	**CNS:** *drowsiness,* dizziness, excitation, irritability, nightmares, hallucinations. **GI:** *nausea,* vomiting.
codeine **codeine phosphate** **codeine sulfate** Controlled Substance Schedule II	*Nonproductive cough—* **Adults:** 8 to 20 mg P.O. q 4 to 6 hours. Maximum 120 mg/24 hours. **Children:** 1 to 1.5 mg/kg P.O. daily in 4 divided doses. Maximum 60 mg/24 hours.	**CNS:** *dizziness, sedation.* **CV:** palpitations. **GI:** *nausea,* vomiting; with repeated doses, *constipation.* **Skin:** pruritus. **Other:** tolerance and physical dependence.

♦ Available in U.S. and Canada. ♦♦ Available in Canada only. All other products (no symbol) available in U.S. only. Italicized side effects are common or life-threatening.

INTERACTIONS	NURSING CONSIDERATIONS
None significant.	• Use cautiously in patients with asthma or severe respiratory insufficiency; in elderly or debilitated patients. • Classified as a mucolytic. • Use plastic, glass, stainless steel, or another nonreactive metal when administering by nebulization. Handbulb nebulizers not recommended because output too small and particle size too large. • After opening, store in refrigerator; use within 96 hours. • Incompatible with oxytetracycline, tetracycline, and erythromycin lactobionate. • Monitor cough type and frequency. For maximum effect, instruct patient to clear his airway by coughing before aerosol administration. • Available in combination with isoproterenol in a 4-ml vial. • Large doses are used P.O. to treat acetaminophen overdose. For dose in acetaminophen toxicity, see APPENDIX, *Drug Toxicities*.
Spironolactone: systemic acidosis. Use cautiously.	• Contraindicated in hepatic or renal impairment. Use cautiously in pulmonary insufficiency, congestive heart failure. • Give with full glass of water. • Monitor cough type and frequency. • Encourage deep-breathing exercises. • Watch for potentiated diuresis when used with diuretics. • Also used to acidify urine.
None significant.	• Patient should not chew perles or leave in mouth to dissolve; local anesthesia will result. • A cough suppressant; don't use when cough is valuable as diagnostic sign or is beneficial (as after thoracic surgery). • Monitor cough type and frequency. • Use with percussion and chest vibration. • Maintain fluid intake to help liquefy sputum.
None significant.	• An antitussive; don't use when cough is valuable diagnostic sign or beneficial (as after thoracic surgery). • Monitor cough type and frequency. • Use with percussion and chest vibration. • CNS side effects disappear when drug is stopped.
None significant.	• Contraindicated in increased intracranial or CSF pressure. Use cautiously in debilitated patients, in dehydrated postoperative patients; in those with asthma, emphysema, head injury, history of drug abuse, hepatic or renal disease, hypothyroidism, Addison's disease, acute alcoholism, seizures, severe CNS depression, chronic obstructive pulmonary disease, psychosis; after thoracotomies or laparotomies; and when other CNS depressants are given. Monitor patient carefully. • Use with percussion and chest vibration. • Warn patient against driving or other activities that require alert-

(continued on following page)

NAME	INDICATIONS & DOSAGE	SIDE EFFECTS
codeine *(continued)*		
dextromethorphan hydrobromide Balminil DM♦♦, Broncho-Grippol-DM♦♦, Contratuss♦♦, Pertussin 8-hour, Romilar Chewable Tablets for Children, St. Joseph Cough Syrup for Children, Sedatuss♦♦, Silence Is Golden. More commonly available in combination products such as Benylin-DM, Coryban-D Cough Syrup, Dimacol, Naldetuss, Novahistine DMX, Ornacol, Phenergan Expectorant with Dextromethorphan, Robitussin DM, Romilar CF, Rondec-DM, Triaminicol, Trind-DM, Tussi-Organidin-DM, 2G-DM	*Nonproductive cough*— **Adults:** 10 to 20 mg q 4 hours, or 30 mg q 6 to 8 hours. Maximum 120 mg/day. **Children 6 to 12 years:** 5 to 10 mg q 4 hours, or 15 mg q 6 to 8 hours. Maximum 60 mg/day. **Children 2 to 6 years:** 2.5 mg q 4 hours, or 7.5 mg q 6 to 8 hours. Maximum 30 mg/day.	**CNS:** drowsiness. **GI:** nausea.
diphenhydramine hydrochloride Allerdryl, Baramine, Bax, Benachlor, Benadryl♦, Benahist, Ben-Allergin, Bendylate, Bentrac, Benylin Cough Syrup♦♦, Eldadryl, Fenylhist, Hyrexin, Nordryl, Notose, Phen-Amin 50, Phenamine, Rodryl, Rohydra, Valdrene, Wehdryl	*Nonproductive cough*— **Adults:** 25 mg P.O. q 4 hours (not to exceed 100 mg/day). **Children 6 to 12 years:** 12.5 mg P.O. q 4 hours (not to exceed 50 mg/day). **Children 2 to 6 years:** 6.25 mg P.O. q 4 hours (not to exceed 25 mg/day).	**CNS:** *sedation,* confusion, restlessness, insomnia, headache. **CV:** palpitations. **EENT:** diplopia, blurred vision, nasal congestion. **GI:** *dry mouth and throat,* nausea, vomiting, diarrhea, constipation. **GU:** dysuria. **Skin:** urticaria.
guaifenesin (formerly glyceryl guaiacolate) Anti-Tuss, Balminil♦♦, Bowtussin, Colrex,	*Productive and nonproductive cough*— **Adults:** 100 to 200 mg P.O. q 2 to 4 hours. Maximum 800 mg/day. **Children:** 12 mg/kg P.O. daily	**CNS:** drowsiness. **GI:** vomiting and nausea occur with large doses.

♦ Available in U.S. and Canada. ♦♦ Available in Canada only. All other products (no symbol) available in U.S. only. Italicized side effects are common or life-threatening.

INTERACTIONS	NURSING CONSIDERATIONS
	ness until CNS response to drug is determined. • An antitussive; don't use when cough is a valuable diagnostic sign or beneficial (as after thoracic surgery). • Monitor cough type and frequency.
MAO inhibitors: hypotension, coma, hyperpyrexia, and death have occurred. Do not use together.	• Contraindicated in patients currently taking or within 2 weeks of stopping MAO inhibitors. • Produces no analgesia or addiction and little or no CNS depression. • An antitussive; don't use when cough is valuable diagnostic sign or beneficial (as after thoracic surgery). • Instruct patient not to take fluids immediately after taking drug. • Use with percussion and chest vibration. • Do not mix dextromethorphan syrups together with penicillins, tetracyclines, salicylates, phenobarbital, hydriodic acid, or high concentrations of sodium or potassium iodide. • Monitor cough type and frequency. • Available in most over-the-counter cough medicines.
None significant.	• Contraindicated in acute asthma, narrow-angle glaucoma, prostatic hypertrophy, peptic ulcer, pyloroduodenal and bladder-neck obstruction. Use cautiously in asthmatic, hypertensive, or cardiac patients. • Warn patient against drinking alcoholic beverages during therapy and against driving or other activities that require alertness until CNS response to drug is determined. • Liquid preparations are recommended for antitussive effect. • Instruct patient not to take fluids immediately after taking drug. • Coffee and tea may reduce drowsiness. Sugarless gum, sour hard candy, or ice chips may relieve dry mouth. • If tolerance develops, another antihistamine may be substituted. • Warn patient to stop taking drug 4 days before allergy skin tests; otherwise, accuracy of tests may be affected.
None significant.	• May interfere with certain laboratory tests for 5-hydroxyindoleacetic acid and vanillylmandelic acid. • Watch for bleeding gums, hematuria, and bruising if given to patients on heparin. Should such symptoms appear, guaifenesin should be discontinued. • Liquefies thick, tenacious sputum; maintain fluid intake. Advise

(continued on following page)

NAME	INDICATIONS & DOSAGE	SIDE EFFECTS
guaifenesin *(continued)* Cosin-GG, Demo-Cineol♦♦, Dilyn, 2/G, G-100, G-200, GG-CEN, Glycotuss, Gly-O-Tussin, Glytuss, G-Tussin, Guaiatussin, Hytuss, Malotuss, Motussin♦♦, Nortussin, Proco, Recsei-Tuss, Resyl♦♦, Robitussin♦, Sedatuss♦♦, Tursen, Tussanca♦♦, Wal-Tussin DM	in 6 divided doses.	
hydriodic acid	*Chronic bronchitis, bronchial asthma*— **Adults:** 1.25 to 5 ml syrup well diluted in water P.O. b.i.d. or t.i.d.	**EENT:** tooth damage.
hydrocodone bitartrate Controlled Substance Schedule II Coditrate, Codone, Corutol DH♦♦, Dicodethal, Dicodid, Hycodan♦, Robidone♦♦	*Nonproductive cough*— **Adults:** 5 to 10 mg P.O. t.i.d. or q.i.d., p.r.n. Maximum single dose 15 mg. **Children:** 0.6 mg/kg P.O. daily in 3 or 4 divided doses.	**CNS:** *drowsiness, dizziness.* **EENT:** dryness of throat. **GI:** *nausea, constipation.* **Other:** tolerance and physical dependence after long-term use.
hydromorphone hydrochloride Controlled Substance Schedule II Dilaudid Cough Syrup♦	*Cough*— **Adults:** 1 mg P.O. q 3 to 4 hours, p.r.n. **Children 6 to 12 years:** 0.5 mg P.O. q 3 to 4 hours, p.r.n.	**CNS:** *dizziness, somnolence,* respiratory depression. **CV:** hypotension. **GI:** *nausea,* vomiting, anorexia, constipation.
iodinated glycerol Organidin♦	*Bronchial asthma, bronchitis, emphysema (adjunct)*— **Adults:** 60 mg P.O. q.i.d. (tablets), or 20 drops (solution) P.O. q.i.d. with fluids, or 1 teaspoonful (elixir) P.O. q.i.d. **Children:** up to ½ adult dose based on child's weight.	*After long-term use:* **GI:** *nausea,* gastrointestinal distress. **Skin:** *eruptions.* **Other:** acute parotitis, thyroid enlargement.

♦ Available in U.S. and Canada. ♦♦ Available in Canada only. All other products (no symbol) available in U.S. only. Italicized side effects are common or life-threatening.

INTERACTIONS	NURSING CONSIDERATIONS
	patient to take with a glass of water whenever possible. • Monitor cough type and frequency. • An expectorant. • Encourage deep-breathing exercises. • Although very popular expectorant, many medical authorities doubt its efficacy.
None significant.	• Dilute well. Use straw to avoid injuring teeth; syrup is very acidic. • Liquefies thick, tenacious sputum; maintain fluid intake. Advise patient to take with a glass of water whenever possible. • Don't use if syrup is deep brown color. • Monitor cough type and frequency. • Encourage deep-breathing exercises. • An expectorant.
CNS depressants: increased sedation. Use together cautiously.	• Contraindicated in glaucoma. Use cautiously in asthma, emphysema, drug dependence; after thoracotomy or laparotomy; in debilitated or dehydrated patients. • Warn patient against driving or other activities that require alertness until CNS response to drug is determined. • Evaluate patient's need for drug, which is addictive. • An antitussive; don't use when cough is valuable diagnostic sign or beneficial (as after thoracic surgery). • Use with percussion and chest vibration. • Monitor cough type and frequency.
CNS depressants: increased sedation. Use together cautiously.	• Contraindicated in increased intracranial pressure, status asthmaticus. Use cautiously in hepatic or renal disease, hypothyroidism, Addison's disease, acute alcoholism, seizures, head injury, severe CNS depression, brain tumor, bronchial asthma, chronic obstructive pulmonary disease, or psychosis. • Warn patient against driving and other activities that require alertness until CNS response to drug is determined. • Monitor respirations, pupil size, bowel function during therapy. • An antitussive; don't use when cough is valuable diagnostic sign or beneficial (as after thoracic surgery). • Use with percussion or chest vibration. • Monitor cough type and frequency. • Addictive.
None significant.	• Contraindicated in hypothyroidism, iodine sensitivity. • Skin rash or other hypersensitivity reaction may require stopping drug. • May liquefy thick, tenacious sputum; maintain fluid intake. • Monitor cough type and frequency. • Encourage deep-breathing exercises. • An expectorant.

NAME	INDICATIONS & DOSAGE	SIDE EFFECTS
levopropoxyphene napsylate Novrad	*Nonproductive cough—* **Adults:** 50 to 100 mg q 4 hours. **Children 23 to 45 kg:** 50 mg q 4 hours. **Children up to 23 kg:** 25 mg q 4 hours.	**CNS:** *drowsiness,* jitters, *dizziness,* headache. **EENT:** visual disturbances, dry mouth. **GI:** *nausea,* vomiting, diarrhea, *epigastric burning.* **GU:** urinary frequency or urgency. **Skin:** rash, urticaria.
noscapine hydrochloride Noscatuss♦♦, Tusscapine	*Nonproductive cough—* **Adults:** 15 to 30 mg P.O. q 4 to 6 hours as chewable tablet. **Children 6 to 12 years:** 7.5 to 15 mg P.O. t.i.d. or q.i.d. as syrup. **Children 2 to 6 years:** 5 to 10 mg P.O. t.i.d. or q.i.d. as syrup.	**CNS:** slight drowsiness. **EENT:** acute vasomotor rhinitis, conjunctivitis. **GI:** nausea.
potassium iodide (SSKI)	*Chronic bronchitis, bronchial asthma—* **Adults:** 300 to 600 mg P.O. q 2 hours until desired response obtained. **Children:** 0.25 to 1 ml of saturated solution (1 g/ml) b.i.d., t.i.d., or q.i.d. *Nuclear radiation protection—* **Adults and children:** 0.13 ml P.O. of SSKI immediately before or after initial exposure will block 90% of radioactive iodine. Same dose given 3 to 4 hours after exposure will provide 50% block. Should be administered for up to 10 days under medical supervision. **Infants under 1 year:** ½ adult dose.	**GI:** nonspecific small bowel lesions, *nausea,* vomiting, *epigastric pain,* metallic taste. **Metabolic:** goiter, hyperthyroid adenoma, hypothyroidism (with excessive use), collagen disease-like syndrome. **Skin:** rash. **Prolonged use:** chronic iodine poisoning, soreness of mouth, coryza, sneezing, swelling of eyelids.
terpin hydrate Creoterp, Terp	*Excessive bronchial secretions—* **Adults:** 5 to 10 ml P.O. of elixir.	None.
tyloxapol Alevaire	*Bronchitis, emphysema, pulmonary abscess, bronchiectasis, atelectasis (by inhalation only)—* **Adults:** up to 500 ml 0.125% solution q 12 to 24 hours by continuous aerosol inhalation, adjusting rate of flow, p.r.n.; or 10 to 20 ml 0.125% solution by intermittent inhalation for 30 to 90 minutes t.i.d. or q.i.d.	**GI:** *nausea.* **Local:** irritation.

INTERACTIONS	NURSING CONSIDERATIONS
None significant.	• Contraindicated in first trimester of pregnancy. • An antitussive; don't use when cough is valuable diagnostic sign or beneficial (as after thoracic surgery). • Tell patient not to take fluids just after liquid preparation. • Use with percussion or chest vibration. • Monitor cough type and frequency. • Warn patient against driving or other activities that require mental alertness until CNS response to drug is determined.
None significant.	• An antitussive; don't use when cough is valuable diagnostic sign or is beneficial (as after thoracic surgery). Use cautiously in sedated or debilitated patients. • Tell patient not to take fluids just after liquid preparation. • Use with percussion and chest vibration. • Monitor cough type and frequency.
Lithium carbonate: may cause hypothyroidism. Don't use together.	• Contraindicated in iodine hypersensitivity, tuberculosis, hyperkalemia, acute bronchitis, hyperthyroidism. • Maintain fluid intake to help liquefy sputum. • Has strong, salty, metallic taste. Dilute with milk or fruit juice to reduce GI distress and disguise taste. • If given over long period, sudden withdrawal may precipitate thyroid storm. • Monitor cough type and frequency. • Encourage deep-breathing exercises. • If skin rash appears, discontinue use. Contact doctor. • An expectorant. • Warn patient not to use any over-the-counter drugs without first consulting doctor.
None significant.	• Contraindicated on empty stomach, in peptic ulcer or severe diabetes mellitus. Use cautiously in patients with history of alcohol or drug abuse. • Don't give in large doses; high alcoholic content of elixir (86 proof). • Monitor cough type and frequency.
None significant.	• Aerosols may induce bronchial spasm in some patients with asthma. • A surfactant with detergent properties. • Lowers surface tension and reduces viscosity of thick, tenacious sputum to facilitate expectoration; maintain fluid intake. Most benefit results from humidification of inspired air. • Monitor cough type and frequency. • Encourage deep-breathing exercises. • If used as a vehicle, add phenylephrine or isoproterenol just before use.

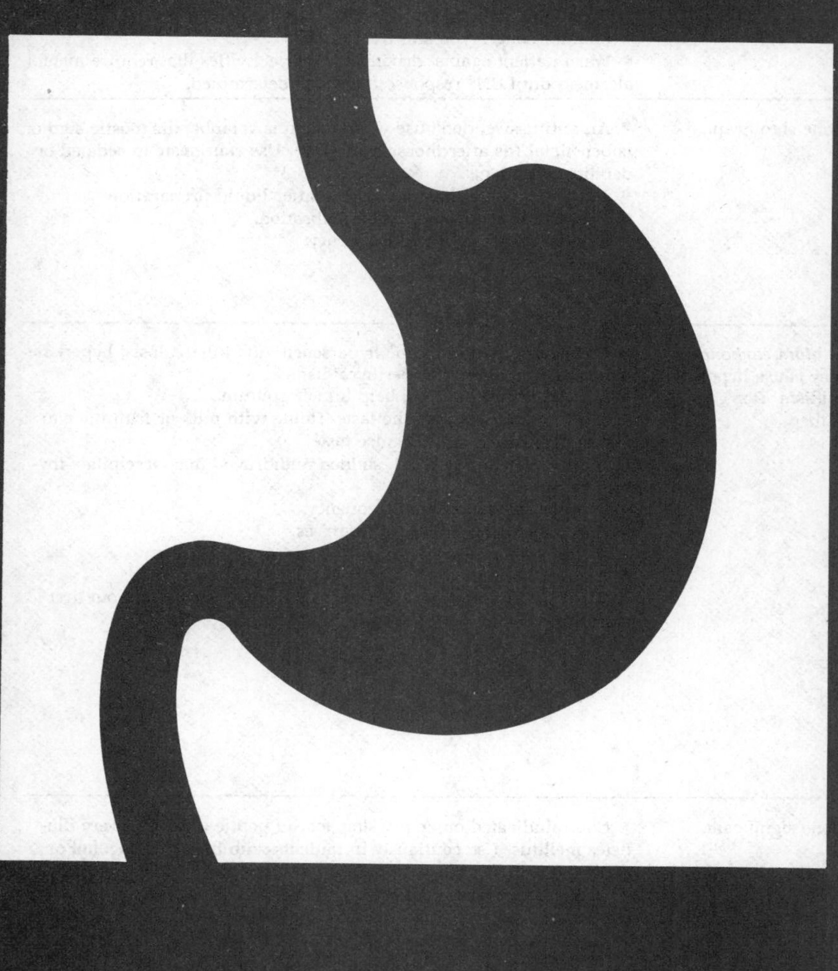

VII Gastrointestinal Tract Drugs

Antacids, adsorbents, and antiflatulents

activated charcoal
aluminum carbonate
aluminum hydroxide
aluminum phosphate
calcium carbonate
dihydroxyaluminum aminoacetate
dihydroxyaluminum sodium carbonate
magaldrate
magnesia magma (MOM)
magnesium carbonate
magnesium oxide
magnesium trisilicate
oxethazaine
simethicone
sodium bicarbonate

Antacids are used to treat peptic ulcers (localized lesions of the gastric and duodenal mucosa). They may consist of various combinations of aluminum, calcium, and magnesium salts; magaldrate; and oxethazaine. But most of them are combinations of aluminum and magnesium salts. Although the antacidic properties of the inorganic salts cited have been known for more than 2,000 years, until the modern era their use was mainly empirical and subjective. Today, however, the use and action of the antacids are well known and medically respected.

The products vary in their ability to neutralize acid. Adequate doses and proper timing of administration promote healing of duodenal ulcers.

Many patients on salt-restricted diets may not realize that the antacids they're taking contain sodium in the form of the salt sodium chloride. Sometimes the salt content is high enough to aggravate conditions such as congestive heart failure and hypertension. The chart on the opposite page offers a guide to the sodium content of 20 popular antacid preparations.

Adsorbents (specifically, activated charcoal) effectively inhibit gastroin-

NURSE'S GUIDE TO PEPTIC ULCER DISEASE

Signs and symptoms
- Gnawing or burning epigastric pain an hour after meals
- Pain relieved by food or antacid
- Pain that wakens patient at night
- Feeling of fullness
- Hematemesis or melena

Possible causes
- Stress (contributing factor)
- Hypersecretion of gastric acid (determined through gastric analysis) combined with a decrease in mucosal protective factors, such as mucus production
- History of prolonged use of aspirin, alcohol, corticosteroids, or caffeine

Nursing considerations
- Administer medications, as ordered.
- Frequently give the patient antacids and small meals, to help relieve GI distress.
- Encourage the patient not to smoke.
- Provide a diet that is free of substances that increase acid secretion, such as caffeine, alcohol, and fatty foods.
- Be alert for gastric perforation: sudden, intense, epigastric pain; possible referred pain to one or both shoulders; tender abdomen with muscle guarding; and diminished or absent bowel sounds.

testinal (GI) absorption of various drugs, chemicals, and toxins. However, activated charcoal doesn't adsorb cyanide, ethanol, methanol, iron, sodium chloride, alkalis, mineral acids, or organic solvents.

Antiflatulents, such as simethicone, have a defoaming action. They're usually combined with antacids to relieve hyperacidity and gas.

Major uses

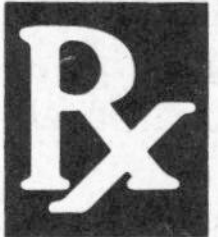

• Antacids neutralize gastric acidity and help control ulcer pain. They're also used to treat the retrosternal burning sensation (heartburn) due to reflux esophagitis.
• Adsorbents are general-purpose antidotes in acute episodes of certain oral poisonings (phenol ingestion and acetaminophen overdose, for example).
• Antiflatulents relieve painful symptoms of excess gas in the digestive tract.

Mechanism of action

• Antacids reduce total acid load in the GI tract and elevate gastric pH to reduce pepsin activity. They also strengthen the gastric mucosal barrier and increase esophageal sphincter tone. They don't seem to have a coating effect on ulcers.

Oxethazaine is a potent local anesthetic that may adhere to receptor sites, producing a prolonged topical anesthetic effect on the gastric mucosa.
• Adsorbents adhere to many drugs and chemicals, inhibiting their absorption from the GI tract.
• Antiflatulents, by the defoaming action of simethicone, disperse or prevent formation of mucus-surrounded gas pockets in the GI tract. These preparations form a film in the GI tract that causes gas bubbles to collapse.

Absorption, distribution, metabolism, and excretion

• Absorption of antacids varies. Prolonged use of antacids that contain magnesium or calcium may cause systemic absorption of magnesium or calcium ions in toxic quantities. Excessive aluminum antacid therapy can lead to hypophosphatemia. Antacids are distributed throughout the GI tract and are eliminated primarily in feces.
• Adsorbents are neither absorbed in the GI tract nor metabolized. They are eliminated unchanged in the feces.

COMPARATIVE POTENCY AND SODIUM CONTENT OF SOME ANTACIDS

PRODUCT	NEUTRALIZING CAPACITY (mEq/5 ml)	SODIUM CONTENT (mg/5 ml)
AlternaGEL	12	2
Aludrox	14	1.16
Amphojel	6.5	6.93
Camalox	18	2.5
Delcid	42	15
Di-Gel	12.5	8.5
Gelusil	12	0.7
Gelusil-II	24	1.3
Gelusil-M	15	1.2
Kolantyl	10.5	2.2
Maalox	13.5	1.35
Maalox Plus	13.5	1.3
Maalox TC	28.3	0.8
Mylanta	12.7	0.68
Mylanta II	25.4	1.14
Riopan	13.5	0.3
Riopan Plus	13.5	0.3
Simeco	22	6.93 to 13.86
Titralac	19	11
Trisogel	17	9.3

• Because antiflatulents are physiologically inactive, they're not absorbed in the GI tract and don't interfere with gastric secretion or nutrient absorption. They're eliminated unchanged in the feces.

Onset and duration

• Antacids' onset of action is generally immediate. Duration of action is usually only 1 hour when taken on an empty stomach but as long as 3 hours if taken after meals.
• Adsorbents' onset of action is immediate. Duration varies, depending on amount of poison swallowed and absorbed, as well as amount of activated charcoal given.
• Antiflatulents' onset of action is immediate; duration of effect is as long as 3 hours.

Combination products

ALMA-MAG # 4: aluminum hydroxide 260 mg and magnesium trisilicate 488 mg.
ALUDROX TABLETS: aluminum hydroxide 233 mg, magnesium hydroxide 83 mg, and sodium 1.6 mg.
ALUDROX SUSPENSION: aluminum hydroxide 307 mg, magnesium hydroxide 103 mg, and sodium 1.1 mg/5 ml.
ALUSCOP: magnesium hydroxide 180 mg and dihydroxyaluminum aminoacetate.
A-M-T: aluminum hydroxide 162 mg and magnesium trisilicate 250 mg.
BISODOL: magnesium hydroxide 178 mg, calcium carbonate 194 mg, and sodium 0.036 mg.
CAMALOX♦: aluminum hydroxide 225 mg, magnesium hydroxide 200 mg, and calcium carbonate 250 mg.
CREAMALIN: aluminum hydroxide 248 mg, magnesium hydroxide 75 mg, and sodium < 41 mg.
DELCID SUSPENSION: aluminum hydroxide 600 mg, magnesium hydroxide 665 mg, and sodium < 15 mg/5 ml.
DI-GEL: aluminum hydroxide and magnesium carbonate 282 mg, magnesium hydroxide 85 mg, simethicone 25 mg, and sodium 10.6 mg.
ESTOMUL-M: aluminum hydroxide and magnesium carbonate 500 mg, magnesium oxide 45 mg, and sodium 16 mg.
EUGEL: aluminum hydroxide and magnesium hydroxide 175 mg, calcium carbonate 325 mg, and glycine 100 mg.
FLACID: aluminum hydroxide and magnesium carbonate 282 mg, magnesium hydroxide 85 mg, and simethicone 25 mg.
GAVISCON♦: aluminum hydroxide 80 mg, magnesium trisilicate 20 mg, sodium bicarbonate 70 mg, alginic acid 200 mg, and approximately 0.8 mEq sodium.
GELUSIL♦: aluminum hydroxide 200 mg, magnesium hydroxide 200 mg, simethicone 25 mg, and sodium 1.4 mg.
GELUSIL-II: aluminum hydroxide 400 mg, magnesium hydroxide 400 mg, simethicone 30 mg, and sodium 2.7 mg.
GELUSIL-M: aluminum hydroxide 300 mg, magnesium hydroxide 200 mg, simethicone 25 mg, and sodium 3 mg.
KAMADROX: aluminum hydroxide 194 mg, calcium carbonate 146 mg, and magnesium trisilicate 259 mg.
KOLANTYL TABLETS: aluminum hydroxide 300 mg, magnesium oxide 185 mg, and sodium < 15 mg.
KOLANTYL WAFERS♦: aluminum hydroxide 180 mg and magnesium hydroxide 170 mg.
KUDROX: aluminum hydroxide and magnesium carbonate 400 mg and sodium 17 mg.
MAALOX NO. 1: aluminum hydroxide 200 mg and magnesium hydroxide 200 mg.
MAALOX NO. 2: aluminum hydroxide 400 mg and magnesium hydroxide 400 mg.
MAALOX PLUS♦: aluminum hydroxide 200 mg, magnesium hydroxide 200 mg, simethicone 25 mg, and sodium 1.6 mg.
MAALOX THERAPEUTIC CONCENTRATE: aluminum hydroxide 600 mg, magnesium hydroxide 300 mg, and sodium 1.25 mg.
MAGNAGEL: aluminum hydroxide and magnesium carbonate 325 mg.
MAGNALUM: aluminum hydroxide 260

mg and magnesium trisilicate 488 mg.
MAGNATRIL: aluminum hydroxide 260 mg, magnesium hydroxide 130 mg, and magnesium trisilicate 455 mg.
MYLANTA♦: aluminum hydroxide 200 mg, magnesium hydroxide 200 mg, simethicone 20 mg, and sodium 0.5 mg.
MYLANTA-II♦: aluminum hydroxide 400 mg, magnesium hydroxide 400 mg, simethicone 30 mg, and sodium 1 mg.
NEUTRACOMP: aluminum hydroxide 128 mg and magnesium trisilicate 400 mg.
NEUTRALOX: aluminum hydroxide 300 mg and magnesium hydroxide 150 mg.
PAMA: aluminum hydroxide 260 mg and magnesium trisilicate 260 mg.
RATIO: calcium carbonate 400 mg and magnesium carbonate 50 mg.
RIOPAN PLUS CHEW TABLETS: magaldrate 480 mg, simethicone 20 mg, and sodium < 0.65 mg.
RIOPAN PLUS SUSPENSION; magaldrate 400 mg, simethicone 20 mg, and sodium < 0.65 mg/5 ml.
RULOX #1: aluminum hydroxide 200 mg, magnesium hydroxide 200 mg, and sodium 0.84 mg.
RULOX #2: aluminum hydroxide 400 mg, magnesium hydroxide 400 mg, and sodium 1.8 mg.
SILAIN-GEL: aluminum hydroxide 282 mg, magnesium hydroxide 285 mg, simethicone 25 mg, and sodium 4.8 mg.
SIMECO SUSPENSION: aluminum hydroxide 365 mg, magnesium hydroxide 300 mg, simethicone 30 mg, and sodium 0.3 to 0.6 mEq/5 ml.
SPASTOSED: calcium carbonate 226 mg and magnesium carbonate 162 mg.
SPENOX #2: aluminum hydroxide 400 mg, magnesium hydroxide 400 mg, and sodium 1.8 mg.
SYNTROGEL: aluminum hydroxide and magnesium carbonate 220 mg, magnesium hydroxide 120 mg, and sodium 7.6 mg.
TITRALAC LIQUID: calcium carbonate 1,000 mg, glycine 300 mg, and sodium 11 mg/5 ml.
TITRALAC TABLETS: calcium carbonate 420 mg, glycine 180 mg, and sodium 0.3 mg.
TRIMAGEL: aluminum hydroxide 250 mg and magnesium trisilicate 500 mg.
TRISOGEL: aluminum hydroxide 98 mg and magnesium trisilicate 293 mg.
UNIVOL♦♦: aluminum hydroxide and magnesium carbonate co-dried gel 300 mg and magnesium hydroxide 100 mg.
WINGEL: aluminum hydroxide 180 mg, magnesium hydroxide 160 mg, and sodium < 2.5 mg.

NAME	INDICATIONS & DOSAGE	SIDE EFFECTS
activated charcoal Charcocaps, Charcodote, Charcotabs, Digestalin	*Flatulence or dyspepsia—* **Adults:** 600 mg to 5 g P.O. *Poisoning—* **Adults and children:** 5 to 10 times estimated weight of drug or chemical ingested. Minimum dose 30 g in 250 ml water to make a slurry. Give orally, preferably within 30 minutes of poisoning. Larger doses are necessary if food is in the stomach. For treatment of poisoning or overdosage with acetaminophen, amphetamines, aspirin, antimony, atropine, arsenic, barbiturates, camphor, cocaine, cardiotonic glycosides, glutethimide, ipecac, malathion, morphine, poisonous mushrooms, opium, oxalic acid, parathion, phenol, phenothiazines, potassium permanganate, propoxyphene, quinine, strychnine, sulfonamides, tricyclic antidepressants.	**GI:** black stools.
aluminum carbonate Basaljel♦	*As antacid—* **Adults:** suspension: 5 to 10 ml, P.O. p.r.n. Extra-strength suspension: 2.5 to 5 ml, p.r.n. Tablets: 1 to 2, p.r.n. Capsules: 1 to 2, p.r.n. *To prevent formation of urinary phosphate stones (with low-phosphate diet)—* **Adults:** suspension: 15 to 30 ml suspension P.O. in water or juice 1 hour after meals and h.s.; 5 to 15 ml P.O. extra-strength in water or juice 1 hour after meals and h.s.; 2 to 6 tablets or capsules 1 hour after meals and h.s.	**GI:** anorexia, *constipation,* intestinal obstruction. **Metabolic:** hypophosphatemia.
aluminum hydroxide ALternaGel, Alu-Cap, Al-U-Creme,	*Antacid—* **Adults:** 600 mg P.O. (5 to 10 ml of most products) 1 hour after meals and h.s.; 300- or 600-mg	**GI:** anorexia, *constipation,* intestinal obstruction. **Metabolic:** hypophosphatemia.

INTERACTIONS	NURSING CONSIDERATIONS
None significant.	• Because activated charcoal absorbs and inactivates syrup of ipecac, give after emesis. • Don't give in ice cream. Ice cream decreases absorptive capacity. • Powder form most effective. Mix with tap water to form consistency of thick syrup. May add small amount of fruit juice or flavoring to make more palatable. • Space doses at least 1 hour apart from other drugs if activated charcoal is being used for any indication other than poisoning. • Warn patient that feces will be black.
None significant.	• Use cautiously in elderly patients, especially those with decreased bowel motility (those receiving antidiarrheals, antispasmodics, or anticholinergics), dehydration, fluid restriction, chronic renal disease, and suspected intestinal obstruction. • Record amount and consistency of stools. Manage constipation with laxatives or stool softeners; alternate with magnesium-containing antacids (contraindicated in renal disease). • Shake suspension well; give with small amount of water or fruit juice to assure passage to stomach. When administering through nasogastric tube, be sure tube is placed correctly and is patent; follow antacid with water to clear tube. • Watch long-term, high-dose use in patient on restricted sodium intake. • Warn patient not to take aluminum carbonate indiscriminately and not to switch antacids without doctor's advice. • Because it contains aluminum, it is used in patients with renal failure to help control hyperphosphatemia. Binds phosphate in GI tract. • Monitor serum phosphate levels. • Watch for symptoms of hypophosphatemia with prolonged use (anorexia, malaise, muscle weakness); can also lead to resorption of calcium and bone demineralization. • Make patient responsible for taking his own antacid while hospitalized if he is able. • May cause enteric-coated drugs to be released prematurely in stomach. Separate doses by 1 hour.
None significant.	• Use cautiously in elderly patients, especially those with decreased bowel motility (those receiving antidiarrheals, antispasmodics, or anticholinergics), dehydration, fluid restriction, chronic renal disease, and suspected intestinal obstruction.

(continued on following page)

NAME	INDICATIONS & DOSAGE	SIDE EFFECTS
aluminum hydroxide *(continued)*	tablet, chewed before swallowing, taken with milk or water 5 to 6 times daily after meals and h.s.	
Aluminett, Amphojel♦, Basaljel♦♦, Dialume, Hydroxal, No-Co-Gel, Nutrajel	*Hyperphosphatemia in renal failure—* **Adults:** 500 mg to 2 g b.i.d. to q.i.d.	
aluminum phosphate Phosphaljel	*Antacid—* **Adults:** 15 to 30 ml P.O. undiluted q 2 hours between meals and h.s.	**GI:** *constipation,* intestinal obstruction.
calcium carbonate Alka-2, Amitone, Calcilac, Calglycine, Dicarbosil, El-Da-Mint, Equilet, Gustalac, Mallamint, P.H. Tablets, Spentacid, Titracid, Titralac, Trialea, Tums	*Antacid—* **Adults:** 1-g tablet, 4 to 6 times daily, chewed well and taken with water; or 1 g of suspension (5 ml of most products) 1 hour after meals and h.s.	**GI:** *constipation,* gastric distention, flatulence, acid-rebound, *nausea.* **Metabolic:** *hypercalcemia;* if taken with milk—milk-alkali syndrome.

♦ Available in U.S. and Canada. ♦♦ Available in Canada only. All other products (no symbol) available in U.S. only. Italicized side effects are common or life-threatening.

INTERACTIONS	NURSING CONSIDERATIONS
	• Record amount and consistency of stools. Manage constipation with laxatives or stool softeners; alternate with magnesium-containing antacids (contraindicated in renal disease.) • Shake suspension well; give with small amount of milk or water to assure passage to stomach. When administering through nasogastric tube, be sure tube is placed correctly and is patent. After instilling antacid, flush tube with water. • Watch long-term, high-dose use in patient on restricted sodium intake. • Warn patient not to take aluminum hydroxide indiscriminately and not to switch antacids without doctor's advice. • Because it contains aluminum, it is used in patients with renal failure to help control hyperphosphatemia. Binds phosphate in the GI tract. • Monitor serum phosphate levels. • Watch for symptoms of hypophosphatemia with prolonged use (anorexia, malaise, muscle weakness); can also lead to resorption of calcium and bone demineralization. • Make patient responsible for taking his own antacid while hospitalized if he is able. • May cause enteric-coated drugs to be released prematurely in stomach. Separate doses by 1 hour.
None significant.	• Use cautiously in elderly patients, especially those with decreased bowel motility (those receiving antidiarrheals, antispasmodics, or anticholinergics), dehydration, fluid restriction, chronic renal disease, and suspected intestinal obstruction. • Record amount and consistency of stools. Manage constipation with laxatives or stool softeners; alternate with magnesium-containing antacids (contraindicated in renal disease). • Shake well; give alone or with small amount of milk or water. When administering through nasogastric tube, be sure tube is placed correctly and is patent; after instilling, flush tube with water to facilitate passage to stomach and maintain tube patency. • Watch long-term, high-dose use in patient on restricted sodium intake. • Warn patient not to take aluminum phosphate indiscriminately and not to switch antacids without doctor's advice. • This drug is a very weak antacid. • Can reverse hypophosphatemia induced by aluminum hydroxide. • Make patient responsible for taking his own antacid while hospitalized if he is able. • May cause enteric-coated drugs to be released prematurely in stomach. Separate doses by 1 hour.
None significant.	• Contraindicated in severe renal disease. Use cautiously in elderly patients, especially those with decreased bowel motility (those receiving antidiarrheals, antispasmodics, anticholinergics), dehydration, fluid restriction, chronic renal disease, and suspected intestinal obstruction. • Do not administer with milk or other foods high in vitamin D. Can cause milk-alkali syndrome (headache, confusion, distaste for food, nausea, vomiting, hypercalcemia, hypercalciuria, calcinosis, hyperphosphatemia). • Record amount and consistency of stools. Manage constipation with laxatives or stool softeners. • Watch for symptoms of hypercalcemia (nausea, vomiting, headache, mental confusion, anorexia).

(continued on following page)

NAME	INDICATIONS & DOSAGE	SIDE EFFECTS
calcium carbonate *(continued)*		
dihydroxyaluminum aminoacetate Alkam, Hyperacid, Robalate♦	*Antacid*— **Adults:** 0.5 to 1 g (1 to 2 tablets) after meals and h.s., chewed before swallowing and taken with milk or water.	**GI:** anorexia, *constipation,* intestinal obstruction. **Metabolic:** hypophosphatemia.
dihydroxyaluminum sodium carbonate Rolaids	*Antacid*— **Adults:** chew 1 to 2 tablets (334 to 668 mg), p.r.n.	**GI:** anorexia, *constipation,* intestinal obstruction.
magaldrate (aluminum-magnesium complex) Riopan♦	*Antacid*— **Adults:** suspension: 400 to 800 mg (5 to 10 ml) P.O. between meals and h.s. with water. Tablet: 400 to 800 mg (1 to 2 tablets) P.O. with water between meals and h.s. Chewable tablet: 400 to 800 mg (1 to 2	**GI:** mild constipation or diarrhea.

♦ Available in U.S. and Canada. ♦♦ Available in Canada only. All other products (no symbol) available in U.S. only. Italicized side effects are common or life-threatening.

INTERACTIONS	NURSING CONSIDERATIONS
	• Monitor serum calcium levels, especially in mild renal impairment. • Warn patient not to take calcium carbonate indiscriminately and not to switch antacids without doctor's advice. • Make patient responsible for taking his own antacid while hospitalized if he is able. • Has been known to cause rebound hyperacidity. • Emphasize that it is *not* candy. • May cause enteric-coated tablets to be released prematurely in stomach. Separate doses by 1 hour.
None significant.	• Use cautiously in elderly patients, especially those with decreased bowel motility (those receiving antidiarrheals, antispasmodics, or anticholinergics), dehydration, fluid restriction, chronic renal disease, and suspected intestinal obstruction. • Record amount and consistency of stools. Less constipating than aluminum hydroxide. Manage constipation with laxatives or stool softeners; alternate with magnesium-containing antacids (contraindicated in renal disease). • Watch for symptoms of hypophosphatemia with prolonged use (anorexia, malaise, muscle weakness); can also lead to resorption of calcium and bone demineralization. • Monitor serum phosphate levels. • Watch long-term, high-dose use in patient on restricted sodium intake. • Warn patient not to take dihydroxyaluminum aminoacetate indiscriminately and not to switch antacids without doctor's advice. • Make patient responsible for taking his own antacid while hospitalized if he is able. • May cause enteric-coated drugs to be released prematurely in stomach. Separate doses by 1 hour.
None significant.	• Use cautiously in elderly patients, especially those with decreased bowel motility (those receiving antidiarrheals, antispasmodics, or anticholinergics), dehydration, fluid restriction, chronic renal disease, and suspected intestinal obstruction. • Has high sodium content and may increase sodium and water retention. • Record amount and consistency of stools. Manage constipation with laxatives or stool softeners; alternate with magnesium-containing antacids (contraindicated in renal disease). • Watch long-term, high-dose use in patient on restricted sodium intake. • Warn patient not to take dihydroxyaluminum sodium carbonate indiscriminately. • Make patient responsible for taking his own antacid while hospitalized if he is able. • Emphasize that it is *not* candy. • May cause enteric-coated drugs to be released prematurely in stomach. Separate doses by 1 hour.
None significant.	• Contraindicated in severe renal disease. Use cautiously in elderly patients, especially those with decreased bowel motility (those receiving antidiarrheals, antispasmodics, or anticholinergics), dehydration, fluid restriction, and mild renal impairment. • Record amount and consistency of stools. • Monitor serum magnesium in patients with mild renal impairment. Symptomatic hypermagnesemia usually occurs only in severe renal failure.

(continued on following page)

NAME	INDICATIONS & DOSAGE	SIDE EFFECTS
magaldrate *(continued)*	tablets) chewed before swallowing, between meals and h.s.	
magnesia magma (MOM) (magnesium hydroxide) Milk of Magnesia, Mint-O-Mag	*Antacid*— **Adults:** 5 to 10 ml P.O. or 1 to 2 tablets chewed before swallowing q.i.d., usually after meals and h.s. *Oral replacement therapy in mild hypomagnesemia*— **Adults:** 5 to 10 ml P.O. q.i.d., usually after meals and h.s. Monitor serum magnesium response.	**GI:** *diarrhea,* abdominal pain, nausea. **Metabolic:** hypermagnesemia.
magnesium carbonate	*Antacid*— **Adults:** 0.5 to 2 g of powder product P.O. or chewable tablets between meals with ½ glass of water. *Laxative*— **Adults:** 8 g of powder product P.O. or chewable tablets with water h.s.	**GI:** *diarrhea,* gastric distention, flatulence, abdominal pain, nausea. **Metabolic:** hypermagnesemia.

INTERACTIONS	NURSING CONSIDERATIONS
	• Shake suspension well; give with small amount of water to assure passage to stomach. When administering through nasogastric tube, be sure tube is placed properly and is patent. After instilling, flush tube with water to assure passage to stomach and maintain tube patency. • Not usually used in patients with renal failure (although it contains aluminum) to help control hypophosphatemia, since it contains magnesium, which may accumulate in renal failure. • Good for patient on restricted sodium intake; very low sodium content. • Warn patient not to take magaldrate indiscriminately and not to switch antacids without doctor's advice. • Make patient responsible for taking his own antacid while hospitalized if he is able. • May cause enteric-coated drugs to be released prematurely in stomach. Separate doses by 1 hour.
None significant.	• Contraindicated in severe renal disease. Use cautiously in elderly patients and in patients with mild renal impairment. • Usually not used as antacid, even though it is very effective and potent, due to increased frequency of stools. Usually used as laxative. • Record amount and consistency of stools. • Shake suspension well; give with small amount of water when used as antacid. When administering through nasogastric tube, be sure tube is placed properly and is patent. After instilling, flush tube with water to assure passage to stomach and maintain tube patency. • With prolonged use and some degree of renal impairment, watch for symptoms of hypermagnesemia (hypotension, nausea, vomiting, depressed reflexes, respiratory depression, coma). Monitor serum magnesium levels. • May cause enteric-coated drugs to be released prematurely in stomach. Separate doses by 1 hour. • If diarrhea occurs with antacid doses, suggest alternative preparation. • Subcathartic doses also used as oral magnesium replacement therapy in hypomagnesemia. • Warn patient not to take magnesia magma indiscriminately and not to switch antacids without doctor's advice. • Make patient responsible for taking his own antacid while hospitalized if he is able.
None significant.	• Contraindicated in severe renal disease. Use cautiously in elderly patients and in patients with mild renal impairment. • With prolonged use and some degree of renal impairment, watch for symptoms of hypermagnesemia (hypotension, nausea, vomiting, depressed reflexes, respiratory depression, coma). Monitor serum magnesium levels. • When used as laxative, do not give other oral drugs 1 to 2 hours before or after. • Record amount and consistency of stools. • Warn patient not to take magnesium carbonate indiscriminately and not to switch antacids without doctor's advice. • Make patient responsible for taking his own antacid while hospitalized if he is able. • May cause enteric-coated drugs to be released prematurely in stomach. Separate doses by 1 hour.

NAME	INDICATIONS & DOSAGE	SIDE EFFECTS
magnesium oxide Mag-Ox, Maox, Niko-Mag, Oxabid, Par-Mag, Uro-Mag	*Antacid—* **Adults:** 250 mg to 1 g P.O. with water or milk after meals and h.s. *Laxative—* **Adults:** 4 g P.O. with water or milk, usually h.s. *Oral replacement therapy in mild hypomagnesemia—* **Adults:** 650-mg to 1.3-g tablet or capsule daily. Monitor serum magnesium response.	**GI:** *diarrhea,* nausea, abdominal pain. **Metabolic:** hypermagnesemia.
magnesium trisilicate Trisomin	*Antacid—* **Adults:** 1- to 4-g tablet t.i.d. chewed well and taken with ½ glass of water.	**GI:** *diarrhea,* gastric distention, flatulence, nausea, abdominal pain. **GU:** possible formation of silica renal calculi with prolonged use. **Metabolic:** hypermagnesemia.
oxethazaine Oxaine (oxethazaine in aluminum hydroxide gel)	*Adjunctive therapy for hyperacidity—* **Adults:** 10 to 20 mg P.O. suspended in 5 to 10 ml aluminum hydroxide gel (equivalent to 5 to 10 ml of commercial product) q.i.d. 15 minutes before meals and h.s.	**CNS:** with high doses (120 mg oxethazaine daily): dizziness, faintness, drowsiness. **GI:** anorexia, *constipation,* intestinal obstruction.
simethicone Mylicon, Silain	*Flatulence, functional gastric bloating—* **Adults, and children over 12 years:** 40 to 100 mg P.O. after each meal and h.s.	**GI:** expulsion of excessive liberated gas as belching, rectal flatus.

♦ Available in U.S. and Canada. ♦♦ Available in Canada only. All other products (no symbol) available in U.S. only. Italicized side effects are common or life-threatening.

INTERACTIONS	NURSING CONSIDERATIONS
None significant.	• Contraindicated in severe renal disease. Use cautiously in elderly patients and in patients with mild renal impairment. • With prolonged use and some degree of renal impairment, watch for symptoms of hypermagnesemia (hypotension, nausea, vomiting, depressed reflexes, respiratory depression, coma). Monitor serum magnesium levels. • When used as laxative, do not give other oral drugs 1 to 2 hours before or after. • If diarrhea occurs on antacid doses, suggest alternate preparation. • Warn patient not to take magnesium oxide indiscriminately and not to switch antacids without doctor's advice. • Make patient responsible for taking his own antacid while hospitalized if he is able. • May cause enteric-coated drugs to be released prematurely in stomach. Separate doses by 1 hour.
None significant.	• Contraindicated in severe renal disease. Use cautiously in elderly patients and in patients with mild renal impairment. • With prolonged use and some degree of renal impairment, watch for symptoms of hypermagnesemia (hypotension, nausea, vomiting, depressed reflexes, respiratory depression, coma). Monitor serum magnesium levels. • If diarrhea occurs on antacid doses, suggest alternate preparation. • Warn patient not to take magnesium trisilicate indiscriminately and not to switch antacids without doctor's advice. • Make patient responsible for taking his own antacid while hospitalized if he is able. • May cause enteric-coated drugs to be released prematurely in stomach. Separate doses by 1 hour.
None significant.	• Use cautiously in elderly patients, especially those with decreased bowel motility (those receiving antidiarrheals, antispasmodics, or anticholinergics), dehydration, fluid restriction, chronic renal disease, suspected intestinal obstruction. • Record amount and consistency of stools. Manage constipation with laxatives or stool softeners. • Shake suspension well; give with small amount of water to assure passage to stomach. When administering antacids through nasogastric tube, be sure tube is placed correctly and is patent; after instilling, flush tube with water to assure passage to stomach and maintain tube patency. • Caution: Local anesthetic can affect gastric mucosa for up to 6 hours. Prolonged use may mask extension of ulcerative disease and may lead to perforation. Also may mask symptoms of gastric neoplasm. • Warn patient not to take oxethazaine indiscriminately and not to switch antacids without doctor's advice. • Make patient responsible for taking his own antacid while hospitalized if he is able. • May cause enteric-coated drugs to be released prematurely in stomach. Separate doses by 1 hour.
None significant.	• Observe patient for drug effectiveness. • Warn patient not to take simethicone indiscriminately. • Tablets should be chewed, not swallowed whole.

NAME	INDICATIONS & DOSAGE	SIDE EFFECTS
sodium bicarbonate Bell-ans, Soda Mint	*Antacid—* **Adults:** 300 mg P.O. to 2-g tablets chewed well and taken with full glass of water, p.r.n.	**GI:** *gastric distention, belching, flatulence.* **GU:** renal calculi or crystals. **Metabolic:** systemic alkalosis (prolonged use), sodium and water retention; if taken with milk—milk-alkali syndrome.

♦ Available in U.S. and Canada. ♦♦ Available in Canada only. All other products (no symbol) available in U.S. only. Italicized side effects are common or life-threatening.

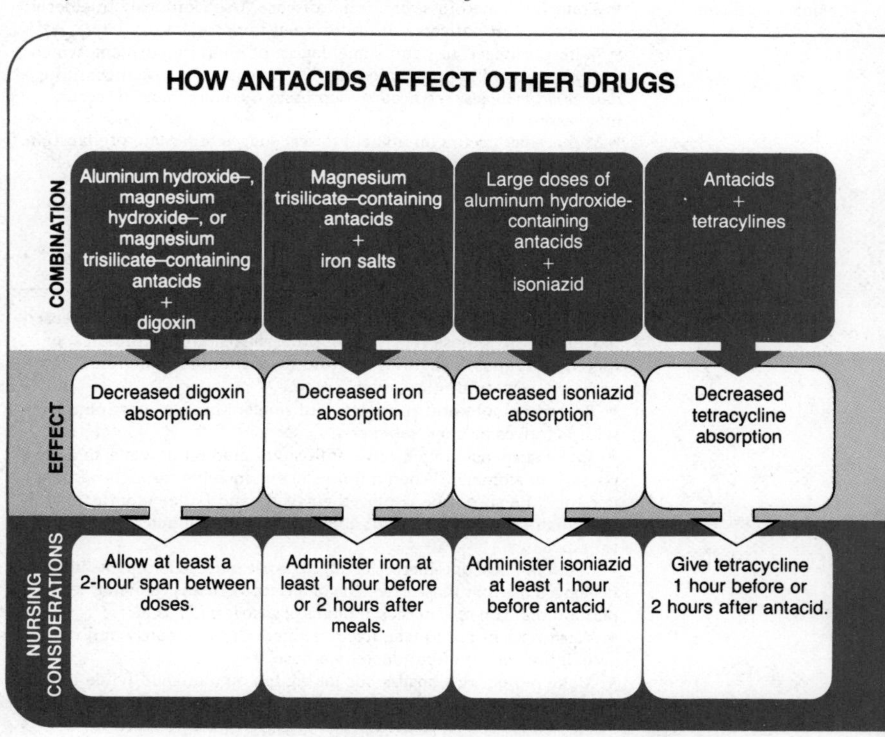

HOW ANTACIDS AFFECT OTHER DRUGS
COMBINATION
Aluminum hydroxide–, magnesium hydroxide–, or magnesium trisilicate–containing antacids + digoxin
Magnesium trisilicate–containing antacids + iron salts
Large doses of aluminum hydroxide-containing antacids + isoniazid
Antacids + tetracylines
EFFECT
Decreased digoxin absorption
Decreased iron absorption
Decreased isoniazid absorption
Decreased tetracycline absorption
NURSING CONSIDERATIONS
Allow at least a 2-hour span between doses.
Administer iron at least 1 hour before or 2 hours after meals.
Administer isoniazid at least 1 hour before antacid.
Give tetracycline 1 hour before or 2 hours after antacid.

INTERACTIONS	NURSING CONSIDERATIONS
None significant.	• Contraindicated in congestive heart failure, hypertension, advanced renal disease, sodium restrictions, tendency toward edema; in patients losing chloride from continuous GI suction; and in patients receiving diuretics that cause hypochloremic alkalosis. Also contraindicated for long-term use. Use cautiously in elderly patients and in patients with mild renal impairment. • Discourage use as antacid. Offer nonabsorbable alternative antacid if it is to be used repeatedly. • Make patient responsible for taking his own antacid while hospitalized if he is able. • Do not administer with milk; can cause milk-alkali syndrome (headache, confusion, distaste for food, nausea, vomiting, hypercalcemia, hypercalciuria, calcinosis, hyperphosphatemia). • May be used with caution to treat chronic metabolic acidosis.

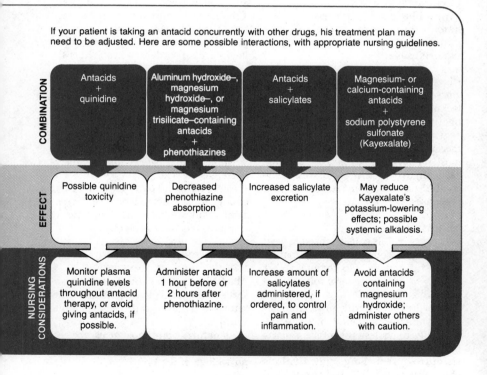

If your patient is taking an antacid concurrently with other drugs, his treatment plan may need to be adjusted. Here are some possible interactions, with appropriate nursing guidelines.

COMBINATION	Antacids + quinidine	Aluminum hydroxide–, magnesium hydroxide–, or magnesium trisilicate–containing antacids + phenothiazines	Antacids + salicylates	Magnesium- or calcium-containing antacids + sodium polystyrene sulfonate (Kayexalate)
EFFECT	Possible quinidine toxicity	Decreased phenothiazine absorption	Increased salicylate excretion	May reduce Kayexalate's potassium-lowering effects; possible systemic alkalosis.
NURSING CONSIDERATIONS	Monitor plasma quinidine levels throughout antacid therapy, or avoid giving antacids, if possible.	Administer antacid 1 hour before or 2 hours after phenothiazine.	Increase amount of salicylates administered, if ordered, to control pain and inflammation.	Avoid antacids containing magnesium hydroxide; administer others with caution.

46 Digestants

bile salts
dehydrocholic acid
glutamic acid hydrochloride
hydrochloric acid, diluted
ketocholanic acids
pancreatin
pancrelipase

Digestants promote digestion in the gastrointestinal tract. Used in patients lacking such digestive substances as bile salts, gastric acid, or pancreatic enzymes, they can provide replacement therapy in specific deficiencies. The most widely used digestants are bile salts, hydrochloric acid, and pancreatic enzymes (pancreatin and pancrelipase).

Major uses

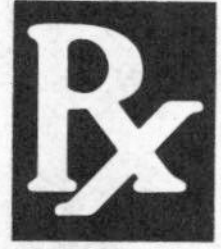

- Bile salts are used to treat uncomplicated constipation and to help maintain normal cholesterol solubility in the bile.
- Dehydrocholic and ketocholanic acids (synthetic bile salts) increase the solubility of cholesterol, preventing its buildup in recurring biliary calculi or strictures, recurring noncalculous cholangitis, biliary dyskinesia and chronic partial obstruction of the common bile duct, prolonged drainage from biliary fistulas or drainage of infected bile duct through a T tube, and sclerosing choledochitis. They may also prevent bacterial accumulation after biliary tract surgery.
- Glutamic acid hydrochloride and dilute hydrochloric acid (gastric acidifiers) are used to treat hypochlorhydria and achlorhydria.
- Pancreatin and pancrelipase (enzymes) supplement or replace exocrine pancreatic secretions, which are lacking in such disorders as cystic fibrosis.

Mechanism of action

- Bile salts, dehydrocholic acid, and ketocholanic acid stimulate bile flow from the liver, promoting normal digestion and absorption of fats, fat-soluble vitamins, and cholesterol.
- Glutamic and hydrochloric acids replace gastric acid.
- Pancreatin and pancrelipase replace endogenous exocrine pancreatic enzymes and aid intestinal digestion of starches, fats, and proteins.

Absorption, distribution, metabolism, and excretion

About 80% to 90% of bile salts are reabsorbed primarily in the ileum. They return to the liver and reenter the bile acid pool.

As natural body substances, the rest of these digestants assume the normal physiology of the body.

Onset and duration

Onset and duration of digestants are unknown.

Combination products

ACCELERASE-PB CAPSULES: lipase 4,000 units, amylase 15,000 units, protease 15,000 units, cellulase 2 mg, mixed

conjugated bile salts 65 mg, calcium carbonate 20 mg, l-alkaloids of belladonna 0.2 mg, and phenobarbital 16 mg.
BILOGEN TABLETS: pancreatin 250 mg, ox bile extract 120 mg, oxidized mixed ox bile acids 75 mg, and desoxycholic acid 30 mg.
BILRON♦: bile salts and iron.
BUTIBEL-ZYME TABLETS: proteolytic enzyme 10 mg, amylolytic enzyme 20 mg, lipolytic enzyme 100 mg, cellulolytic enzyme 5 mg, iron ox bile 30 mg, belladonna extract 15 mg, and sodium butabarbital 15 mg.
CHOLAN-HMB TABLETS: dehydrocholic acid 250 mg, homatropine methylbromide 2.5 mg, and phenobarbital 8 mg.
COTAZYM-B TABLETS: lipase 4,000 units, amylase 15,000 units, protease 15,000 units, cellulase 2 mg, and mixed conjugated bile salts 65 mg.
DONNAZYME TABLETS: pancreatin 300 mg, pepsin 150 mg, bile salts 150 mg, hyoscyamine sulfate 0.0518 mg, atropine sulfate 0.0097 mg, hyoscine hydrobromide 0.0033 mg, and phenobarbital 8.1 mg.
ENTOZYME TABLETS♦: pancreatin 300 mg, pepsin 250 mg, and bile salts 150 mg.
ENZYPAN TABLETS: pancreatin (in sufficient quantity to digest 19 g protein, 43 g starch, 10 g fat), pepsin 9 mg, and desiccated ox bile 56 mg.
FESTAL ENTERIC-COATED TABLETS: protease 17 units, amylase 10 units, lipase 10 units, bile constituents 25 mg, and hemicellulase 50 mg.
FESTALAN TABLETS: protease 17 units, amylase 10 units, lipase 10 units, lipase 10 units, bile constituents 25 mg, hemicellulase 50 mg, and atropine methylnitrate 1 mg.
KANULASE TABLETS: pancreatin 500 mg, pepsin 150 mg, ox bile extract 100 mg, cellulase 9 mg, and glutamic acid hydrochloride 200 mg.
MURIPSIN TABLETS: glutamic acid hydrochloride 500 mg and pepsin 35 mg.
PHAZYME TABLETS (enteric-coated): pancreatin 240 mg and simethicone 60 mg.
PHAZYME-95 TABLETS (enteric-coated): pancreatin 240 mg and simethicone 95 mg.
PHAZYME PB TABLETS (enteric-coated): pancreatin 240 mg, phenobarbital 15 mg, and simethicone 60 mg.
PROBILAGOL LIQUID: d-sorbitol 4.5 g and homatropine methylbromide 1 mg per 5 ml.
RO-BILE TABLETS (enteric-coated): enzyme concentrate 75 mg (lipase equivalent to 750 mg pancreatin, amylase and protease equivalent to 300 mg pancreatin), ox bile extract 100 mg, dehydrocholic acid 30 mg, belladonna extract 8 mg, and pepsin 260 mg.

SOME BACKGROUND ON ENZYMES

Enzymes are complex protein catalysts that increase chemical reaction rates without being changed in the process. They consist of a pure protein portion (apoenzyme) and a nonprotein portion (coenzyme), which, when combined, form the activated enzyme.

Enzymes are selective. Each enzyme works on only one compound or type of substance, which is called its substrate.

Enzymes are efficient. One key enzyme in the nervous system may produce a reaction up to a million times faster than any inorganic catalyst could. A relatively small amount of an enzyme can transform large quantities of its substrate; invertase, for example, can convert one million times its weight of sucrose into invert sugar.

The earliest names for enzymes ended in *-in* to indicate protein composition, such as pepsin and trypsin. Some enzymes were named for their source or method of separation.

Today, an enzyme is usually named by adding *-ase* to the root of its substrate (urease breaks down urea) or to the process it catalyzes (peptidases break peptide bonds).

NAME	INDICATIONS & DOSAGE	SIDE EFFECTS
bile salts Biso, Chobile, Ox-Bile Extract Enseals	*Uncomplicated constipation—* **Adults and children:** 300 to 500 mg enteric-coated tablets b.i.d. or t.i.d. after meals; or 150 to 450 mg capsules with or after meals.	**GI:** loose stools and mild cramping (with large doses).
dehydrocholic acid Bio-Cholin♦♦, Cholan-DH, Cholyphyl♦♦, Decholin♦, Dycholium♦♦, Hepahydrin, Idrocrine♦♦, Neocholan	*Constipation, biliary tract conditions—* **Adults:** 250 to 500 mg P.O. b.i.d. to t.i.d. after meals for 4 to 6 weeks.	None reported.
glutamic acid hydrochloride Acidulin♦	*Hypoacidity—* **Adults:** 1 to 3 capsules P.O. t.i.d. before meals.	**Metabolic:** systemic acidosis in massive overdose.
hydrochloric acid, diluted	*Hypoacidity—* **Adults:** 2 to 8 ml P.O. well diluted in 25 to 50 ml water.	**Metabolic:** systemic acidosis in massive overdose. **Other:** *tooth enamel damage.*
ketocholanic acids Ketochol	*Constipation, biliary tract conditions—* **Adults:** 250 mg to 500 mg P.O. t.i.d. with meals.	None reported.
pancreatin Beef Viokase, Elzyme, Panteric Double Strength, Viokase	*Exocrine pancreatic secretion insufficiency, digestive aid in cystic fibrosis—* **Adults and children:** 325 mg to 1 g P.O. with meals.	**GI:** *nausea,* diarrhea with high doses.

♦ Available in U.S. and Canada. ♦♦ Available in Canada only. All other products (no symbol) available in U.S. only. Italicized side effects are common or life-threatening.

INTERACTIONS	NURSING CONSIDERATIONS
None significant.	• Contraindicated in marked hepatic dysfunction, except in malnutrition with steatorrhea and vitamin K deficiency with hypoprothrombinemia. • Use Ox-Bile Extract cautiously in obstructive jaundice. • Don't use Ox-Bile Extract if other preparations are available, since it doesn't provide an adequate amount of conjugated bile salts.
None significant.	• Contraindicated in complete mechanical biliary obstruction. Use cautiously in prostatic hypertrophy, acute hepatitis, asthmatic bronchitis, elderly patients, partial GI or GU tract obstruction. • Do not use when patient is nauseated or vomiting, or has abdominal pain. • Simultaneous administration of bile salts may be needed in biliary fistula. • Used to prevent bacterial accumulation after biliary tract surgery. • Probably much less effective than natural bile salts in lowering surface tension and promoting absorption. • Don't use dehydrocholic acid to accelerate rate of healing in patients with jaundice. • Frequent use may result in dependence on laxatives.
None significant.	• Contraindicated in gastric hyperacidity or peptic ulcer. • Use instead of hydrochloric acid so tooth enamel won't be damaged; however, glutamic acid HCl is not as effective in increasing gastric pH. • Gastric acidifier.
None significant.	• Contraindicated in gastric hyperacidity or peptic ulcer. • Sip, during meal, through glass straw to protect tooth enamel. • Alleviates primary functional hypoacidity or hypoacidity caused by organic disease such as pernicious anemia, certain allergies, chronic gastritis, other chronic debilitating diseases, or gastric resection. • Gastric acidifier; usual dose not sufficient to release free acid in stomach; no evidence that even larger doses are beneficial for this.
None significant.	• Use cautiously in elderly patients and in those with prostatic hypertrophy, acute hepatitis, asthmatic bronchitis, partial GI or GU tract obstruction. • Bile salt; derived from beef bile. • Approximately equivalent to 250 mg dehydrocholic acid. • Do not use when patient is nauseated or vomiting, or has abdominal pain. • Frequent use may result in dependence on laxatives.
None significant.	• Use cautiously in patients who are hypersensitive to pork. Bovine preparations are available for these patients, but are less effective. • Balance fat, protein, and starch intake properly to avoid indigestion. Dosage varies according to degree of maldigestion and malabsorption, amount of fat in diet, and enzyme activity of individual preparations. • Pancreatin therapy shouldn't delay or replace treatment of primary disorder. • Use only after confirmed diagnosis of exocrine pancreatic insufficiency. Not effective in GI disorders unrelated to pancreatic enzyme deficiency. • For infants, mix powder with applesauce and give with meals. Avoid inhalation of powder. Older children may swallow capsules with food.

(continued on following page)

NAME	INDICATIONS & DOSAGE	SIDE EFFECTS
pancreatin *(continued)*		
pancrelipase Cotazym♦, Ilozyme, Ku-Zyme HP, Pancrease	*Dose must be titrated to patient's response. Exocrine pancreatic secretion insufficiency, cystic fibrosis in adults and children, steatorrhea and other disorders of fat metabolism secondary to insufficient pancreatic enzymes—* **Adults and children:** dosage range 1 to 3 capsules or tablets P.O. before or with meals and 1 capsule or tablet with snack; or 1 to 2 powder packets before meals or snacks.	**GI:** *nausea,* diarrhea with high doses.

♦ Available in U.S. and Canada. ♦♦ Available in Canada only. All other products (no symbol) available in U.S. only. Italicized side effects are common or life-threatening.

COMPARISON OF SOME POPULAR PANCREATIC ENZYME PRODUCTS

DIGESTANT	TRADE NAME	ENZYME CONTENT (UNITS)			FAT DIGESTION INDEX*
		Lipase	Amylase	Protease	
pancreatin	Beef Viokase				
	Tablet (1)	1,950	4,000	16,250	0.5
	Powder (1 tsp)	13,500	28,125	112,500	3.2
	Viokase				
	Tablet (1)	6,500	48,000	32,000	1.4
	Powder (1 tsp)	45,000	337,500	225,000	9.2
pancrelipase	Cotazym				
	Capsule (1)	8,000	30,000	30,000	1
	Packet (1)	16,000	60,000	60,000	2
	Cherry-flavored packet (1)	40,000	150,000	150,000	5
	Ilozyme				
	Tablet (1)	9,600	40,000	40,000	1.6

*Relative fat digestion activity. For example, the activity of a Beef Viokase tablet is half that of a Cotazyme capsule (0.5 vs. 1).

Adapted with permission from W.W. Waring, "Current Management of Cystic Fibrosis," in L.A. Barness et al., eds., *Advances in Pediatrics,* Vol. 23 (Chicago: Yearbook Medical Publishers, 1976).

INTERACTIONS	NURSING CONSIDERATIONS
	• Adequate replacement decreases number of bowel movements and improves stool consistency. • Enteric coating on some products may reduce availability of enzyme in upper portion of jejunum where it is primarily required. • Store in tight containers at room temperature.
None significant.	• Contraindicated in patients with severe pork hypersensitivity. • Therapy shouldn't delay or replace treatment of primary disorder. • Use only after confirmed diagnosis of exocrine pancreatic insufficiency. Not effective in GI disorders unrelated to enzyme deficiency. • Lipase activity greater than with other pancreatic enzymes. • For infants, mix powder from capsules with applesauce and give at mealtime. Avoid inhalation of powder. Older children may swallow capsules with food. • Dosage varies with degree of maldigestion and malabsorption, amount of fat in diet, and enzyme activity of individual preparations. • Adequate replacement decreases number of bowel movements and improves stool consistency. • Enteric coating on some products may reduce availability of enzyme in upper portion of jejunum where it is primarily required. • Crushing or chewing of capsule interferes with the enteric coating.

PARENT-TEACHING AID

WHAT YOU SHOULD KNOW ABOUT YOUR CHILD'S PANCREATIC ENZYME REPLACEMENT THERAPY

Dear Parent:

Your doctor has prescribed pancreatic enzyme replacement therapy to improve your child's digestion and absorption of fat and protein. To help your child benefit from his therapy, follow these instructions:

- Give your child pancreatic enzymes with snacks as well as with regular meals. After he starts pancreatic enzyme replacement therapy, his appetite will be dramatically decreased.
- If your child can't tolerate or is allergic to pork, be sure to tell the doctor. (Many enzyme preparations are made with pork.)
- If the pancreatic enzyme is in powder form, mix it with applesauce or other fruit to make it more palatable.
- Don't mix enzymes with foods containing protein. The enzymes would immediately break down the proteins and turn the food into a watery substance.
- To facilitate the absorption of fats and proteins, give enzymes at the beginning of a meal.
- Don't let the enzymes remain on your child's lips and skin; his skin may begin to break down.
- If you know your child will be eating a greasy meal, call the doctor; he'll probably increase the amount of enzymes your child should take with this meal.
- If your child has diarrhea, call the doctor; he'll probably decrease the amount of enzymes your child is taking.

Symptoms of inadequate pancreatic replacement and excessive intake of fat include abdominal cramps and distention, light-colored mushy stools, foul-smelling gas, rectal seepage of oil, rectal prolapse, and failure to thrive despite a voracious appetite. Call the doctor if any of these occur so he can adjust your child's replacement regimen accordingly.

47 Antidiarrheals

bismuth subcarbonate
bismuth subgallate
bismuth subsalicylate
diphenoxylate hydrochloride (with atropine sulfate)
kaolin and pectin mixtures
lactobacillus
loperamide
opium tincture
opium tincture, camphorated

For information on calcium polycarbophil, see APPENDIX, *New Drugs*.

Antidiarrheals reduce the fluidity of the stool and the frequency of defecation.

Diarrhea is the abnormally frequent passage of watery stools with an average daily weight above 300 g. (Healthy adults have an average daily fecal weight of 100 to 150 g.)

In the absence of other symptoms, diarrhea usually reflects a minor and transient gastrointestinal (GI) disorder. In more serious conditions, however, it is usually one of several symptoms. Diarrhea may be caused by foods or drugs, laxative abuse, allergies, endocrine dysfunction, malabsorption, neurologic or inflammatory diseases, mechanical obstruction, parasitic infection, gastric resection, or radiation poisoning.

Major uses

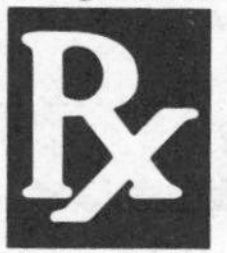

- All antidiarrheals are used to treat acute, mild, or chronic stages of nonspecific diarrhea.
- Bismuth subgallate also neutralizes or absorbs fecal odors in patients with a colostomy or ileostomy.
- Loperamide also reduces the volume of ileostomy discharge and decreases daily fecal volume and fluid and electrolyte loss.

Mechanism of action

- Bismuth subcarbonate, subgallate, and subsalicylate have a mild water-binding capacity; they also may adsorb toxins and provide protective coating for intestinal mucosa.
- Diphenoxylate hydrochloride and opium tinctures increase smooth-muscle tone in the GI tract, inhibit motility and propulsion, and diminish digestive secretions.
- Kaolin and pectin decrease the stool's fluid content, although *total* water loss seems to remain the same.
- Lactobacillus cultures may suppress the growth of pathogenic microorganisms to help reestablish normal intestinal flora.
- Loperamide inhibits peristaltic activity, prolonging transit of intestinal contents.

Absorption, distribution, metabolism, and excretion

Adsorbent antidiarrheals (bismuth salts, kaolin, pectin, and lactobacillus) are not systemically absorbed.

- Diphenoxylate hydrochloride is well absorbed from the GI tract, metabolized in the liver, and eliminated in both urine and feces.
- Loperamide is poorly absorbed orally,

TREATING DIARRHEA

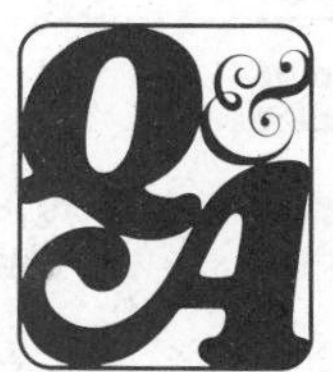

What's best for diarrhea? Lomotil, Imodium ... or codeine?

Since the actions of Lomotil and Imodium are practically identical, both drugs are fine choices. The doctor will probably order either 5 mg (2 tablets) of Lomotil or 2 to 4 mg (1 to 2 capsules) of Imodium until your patient's diarrhea subsides.

Although the doctor may prefer codeine phosphate over Lomotil and Imodium—especially in the treatment of chronic diarrhea—codeine is not specific for diarrhea treatment. And remember, compared with Lomotil and Imodium, codeine is more habit-forming; it's a more controlled substance. Codeine is classified as a Schedule II substance whereas Lomotil and Imodium are classified as Schedule V drugs. (For more information on controlled substance schedule numbers, see special color section following p. 75.)

metabolized in the liver, and eliminated primarily in feces.

- Opium tinctures are absorbed moderately from the GI tract as morphine, metabolized in the liver, and excreted in urine.

Onset and duration

- Bismuth salts, kaolin, pectin, and lactobacillus begin to act within 30 minutes; their therapeutic effects can last 4 to 6 hours.
- Diphenoxylate hydrochloride begins to act within 45 to 60 minutes. Its effect lasts as long as 4 hours.
- Loperamide's peak levels occur in 4 hours; half-life is about 40 hours.
- Opium tinctures begin to act rapidly. Duration of action varies.

Combination products

CORRECTIVE MIXTURE: zinc sulfocarbolate 10 mg, phenyl salicylate 22 mg, bismuth subsalicylate 85 mg, pepsin 45 mg, and alcohol 1.5% in 5-ml suspension.

CORRECTIVE MIXTURE WITH PAREGORIC: paregoric 0.6 ml, zinc sulfocarbolate 10 mg, phenyl salicylate 22 mg, bismuth subsalicylate 85 mg, pepsin 45 mg, and alcohol 2% in 5-ml suspension.

DONNAGEL SUSPENSION♦: kaolin 6 g, pectin 142.8 mg, hyoscyamine sulfate 0.1037 mg, atropine sulfate 0.0194 mg, hyoscine hydrobromide 0.0065 mg, and alcohol 3.8% in 30-ml suspension.

DONNAGEL-MB♦♦: kaolin 6 g, pectin 142.8 mg, and alcohol 3.8% in 30-ml suspension.

DONNAGEL-PG: powdered opium 24 mg, kaolin 6 g, pectin 142.8 mg, hyoscyamine sulfate 0.1037 mg, atropine sulfate 0.0194 mg, hyoscine hydrobromide 0.0065 mg, and alcohol 5% in 30-ml suspension.

KENPECTIN-P: opium 16.27 mg (equivalent to 3.7 ml paregoric), kaolin 5.85 g, pectin 195 mg, alcohol 6%, and aluminum hydroxide 650 mg in 30-ml suspension.

PAREPECTOLIN: opium 15 mg (equivalent to paregoric 3.7 ml), kaolin 5.85 g, pectin 162 mg, and alcohol 0.69% in 30-ml suspension.

PECTOCEL: kaolin 5.85 g, pectin 292.5 mg, and zinc phenolsulfonate 73.13 mg in 30-ml suspension.

PEKTAMALT: kaolin 6.5 g, pectin 600 mg, potassium gluconate 1.1 g, and sodium citrate 318 mg in 30-ml suspension.

POLYMAGMA PLAIN: activated attapulgite 500 mg, pectin 45 mg, and hydrated alumina powder 50 mg.

NAME	INDICATIONS & DOSAGE	SIDE EFFECTS
bismuth subcarbonate **bismuth subgallate** Devrom	*Deodorize fecal odors in colostomy and ileostomy (subcarbonate)—* **Adults:** 600 mg P.O. t.i.d. after each meal. *Mild, nonspecific diarrhea (subgallate)—* **Adults:** 1 to 2 tablets chewed or swallowed whole t.i.d.	**CNS:** personality changes. Prolonged use (especially in colostomy and ileostomy patients) may lead to reversible deterioration of mental ability, confusion, tremors, and impaired coordination. **GI:** *transient darkened tongue and stool* (both with subgallate); fecal impaction or ulceration (in infants, elderly, or debilitated patients) after chronic use; *constipation.*
bismuth subsalicylate Pepto-Bismol	*Mild, nonspecific diarrhea—* **Adults:** 30 ml or 2 tablets P.O. q ½ to 1 hour up to a maximum of 8 doses and for no longer than 2 days. **Children 10 to 14 years:** 20 ml. **Children 6 to 10 years:** 10 ml. **Children 3 to 6 years:** 5 ml.	**GI:** temporary darkening of tongue and stools. **Other:** salicylism (high doses).
diphenoxylate hydrochloride (with atropine sulfate) Controlled Substance Schedule V Colonaid, Diaction, Lofene, Loflo, Lomo-Plus, Lomotil♦, Lonox, Lotrol, Ro-Diphen-Atro, SK-Diphenoxylate	*Acute, nonspecific diarrhea—* **Adults:** initially, 5 mg P.O. q.i.d., then adjust dose to individual response. **Children 2 to 12 years:** 0.3 to 0.4 mg/kg P.O. daily in divided doses, using liquid form only. Don't use in children under 2 years.	**CNS:** *sedation, dizziness,* headache, drowsiness, lethargy, restlessness, depression, euphoria. **CV:** tachycardia. **EENT:** mydriasis. **GI:** *dry mouth,* nausea, vomiting, abdominal discomfort or distention, *paralytic ileus,* anorexia, fluid retention in bowel (may mask depletion of extracellular fluid and electrolytes, especially in young children treated for acute gastroenteritis). **GU:** urinary retention. **Skin:** pruritus, urticaria, rash. **Other:** possibly physical dependence in long-term use, angioedema, respiratory depression.
kaolin and pectin mixtures Baropectin, Kaoparin, Kaopectate♦, Kapectin, Keotin, Pargel, Pecto-Kalin, Pectokay	*Mild, nonspecific diarrhea—* **Adults:** 60 to 120 ml P.O. after each bowel movement. **Children over 12 years:** 60 ml P.O. after each bowel movement. **Children 6 to 12 years:** 30 to 60 ml P.O. after each bowel movement. **Children 3 to 6 years:** 15 to 30 ml P.O. after each bowel movement.	**GI:** drug absorbs nutrients and enzymes; fecal impaction or ulceration in infants, elderly, debilitated patients after chronic use; constipation.
lactobacillus Bacid♦, DoFUS, Lactinex♦	*Diarrhea, especially that caused by antibiotics—* **Adults:** 2 capsules (Bacid) P.O.	**GI:** (with Bacid and DoFUS) increased intestinal flatus at beginning of therapy; subsides with

♦ Available in U.S. and Canada. ♦♦ Available in Canada only. All other products (no symbol) available in U.S. only. Italicized side effects are common or life-threatening.

INTERACTIONS	NURSING CONSIDERATIONS
None significant.	• GI adsorbent. • Don't use in place of specific therapy for underlying cause. • May reduce absorption of other P.O. drugs, requiring dosage adjustment. • Store in tight, light-resistant containers.
None significant.	• Has been used successfully to treat *turista* (traveler's diarrhea). • Warn patient that this drug contains a large amount of salicylate. Should be used cautiously in patients already taking aspirin products.
None significant.	• Contraindicated in acute diarrhea resulting from poison until toxic material is eliminated from GI tract; in acute diarrhea caused by organisms that penetrate intestinal mucosa; in diarrhea resulting from antibiotic-induced pseudomembranous enterocolitis; in jaundiced patients. Use cautiously in children, and in hepatic disease, narcotic dependence, pregnancy. Use cautiously in acute ulcerative colitis. Stop therapy immediately if abdominal distention or other signs of toxic megacolon develop. • Risk of physical dependence increases with high dosage and long-term use. Discourage long-term or unsupervised use. Atropine sulfate is included to discourage abuse. • Warn patient not to exceed recommended dosage. • Dehydration, especially in young children, may increase risk of delayed toxicity. Correct fluid and electrolyte disturbances before starting drug. • Dose of 2.5 mg as effective as 5-ml camphorated tincture of opium. • Not indicated in treatment of antibiotic-induced diarrhea.
None significant.	• Contraindicated in suspected obstructive bowel lesions. • Don't use for more than 2 days. • Don't use in place of specific therapy for underlying cause. • May reduce absorption of other P.O. drugs, requiring dosage adjustments. • GI absorbent.
None significant.	• Bacid and DoFUS contraindicated in fever. • Don't use Bacid for more than 2 days. • Store in refrigerator.

(continued on following page)

NAME	INDICATIONS & DOSAGE	SIDE EFFECTS
lactobacillus *(continued)*	b.i.d., t.i.d., or q.i.d., preferably with milk; or 4 tablets or 1 packet (Lactinex) P.O. t.i.d. or q.i.d., preferably with food, milk, or juice; or 1 tablet (DoFUS) P.O. daily before meals.	continued therapy.
loperamide Controlled Substance Schedule V Imodium♦	*Acute, nonspecific diarrhea—* **Adults:** initially, 4 mg P.O., then 2 mg after each unformed stool. Maximum 16 mg daily. *Chronic diarrhea—* **Adults:** initially, 4 mg P.O., then 2 mg after each unformed stool until diarrhea subsides. Adjust dose to individual response.	**CNS:** drowsiness, fatigue, dizziness. **GI:** dry mouth; abdominal pain, distention, or discomfort; *constipation;* nausea; vomiting. **Skin:** rash.
opium tincture **opium tincture, camphorated** Controlled Substance Schedule III Paregoric♦	*Acute, nonspecific diarrhea—* **Adults:** 0.6 ml opium tincture (range 0.3 to 1 ml) P.O. q.i.d. Maximum dose 6 ml daily; or 5 to 10 ml camphorated opium tincture daily b.i.d., t.i.d., or q.i.d. until diarrhea subsides. **Children:** 0.25 to 0.5 ml/kg camphorated opium tincture daily, b.i.d., t.i.d., or q.i.d. until diarrhea subsides.	**GI:** nausea, vomiting. **Other:** physical dependence after long-term use.

NURSING TIPS

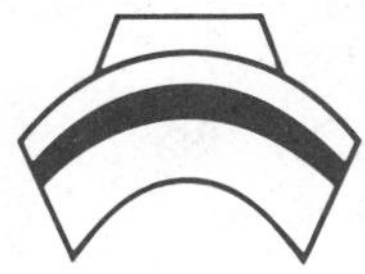

ADVISING PATIENTS ABOUT TRAVELER'S DIARRHEA

Traveler's diarrhea, or *turista,* is a self-limiting but acute form of diarrhea caused by ingesting food or water contaminated with bacteria (usually enterotoxigenic *Escherichia coli*). When on vacation, your patient can prevent it by:

- drinking only boiled or carbonated water.
- not eating ice, salads, or unpeeled fruit.

Prophylactic drug therapy may be the best way to prevent traveler's diarrhea, and may include:

- doxycycline—an extremely effective →

INTERACTIONS	NURSING CONSIDERATIONS
	• Controversial form of diarrhea treatment. • Diet containing large amounts of carbohydrate (up to 400 g), such as lactose, lactulose, and dextrin, may be more effective than lactobacillus in reestablishing normal flora after antibiotic therapy. • May be used prophylactically in patients with history of antibiotic-induced diarrhea.
None significant.	• Contraindicated in acute diarrhea resulting from poison until toxic material is removed from GI tract, when constipation must be avoided, and in acute diarrhea caused by organisms that penetrate intestinal mucosa. Use cautiously in patients with severe prostatic hypertrophy, hepatic disease, and history of narcotic dependence. • Stop drug immediately if abdominal distention or other symptoms develop in patients with acute ulcerative colitis. • In acute diarrhea, stop drug if no improvement within 48 hours; in chronic diarrhea, stop drug if no improvement after giving 16 mg daily for at least 10 days. • Appears to have low potential for abuse. • Warn patient not to exceed recommended dosage. • Produces antidiarrheal action similar to diphenoxylate HCl but without as many CNS side effects; three times more potent than diphenoxylate HCl.
None significant.	• Contraindicated in acute diarrhea resulting from poisons until toxic material is removed from GI tract, and in acute diarrhea caused by organisms that penetrate intestinal mucosa. Use cautiously in asthma, severe prostatic hypertrophy, hepatic disease, narcotic dependence. • Risk of physical dependence increases with long-term use. Discourage long-term or unsupervised use. • An effective and prompt-acting antidiarrheal. • Opium content of opium tincture 25 times greater than camphorated tincture of opium. Camphorated opium tincture is more dilute, and teaspoonful doses easier to measure than dropper quantities of opium tincture. • Not used as widely today as in past, but unique because dose can be adjusted precisely to patient's needs. • Milky fluid forms when camphorated opium tincture is added to water. • Camphorated opium tincture 0.06 to 0.5 ml daily has been used to treat infants with mild narcotic physical dependence.

agent against enterotoxigenic *E. coli* and thus far the most effective preventive treatment. However, it's ineffective against *Salmonella* or *Shigella* organisms. Since doxycycline is a tetracycline, watch its adverse effects, such as photosensitivity and increased skin pigmentation.

• neomycin, iodochlorhydroxyquin (Entero-vioform*), or a variety of sulfonamides.

• a bismuth subsalicylate suspension such as Pepto-Bismol. This may be effective only when large doses are taken.

If your patient loses a lot of fluid, he'll need to replenish the loss with an oral hydration formula containing glucose and salts. A pharmacist can mix and pack these ingredients before your patient leaves.

Antimotility agents (such as Paregoric or tincture of opium) can relieve the abdominal cramps associated with traveler's diarrhea. But don't be fooled by kaolin-pectin preparations; they may alter stool consistency, but they don't relieve any other symptoms of the disease.

*Not available in the United States

48 Laxatives

barley-malt extract
bisacodyl
cascara sagrada
castor oil
danthron
docusate calcium (formerly dioctyl calcium sulfosuccinate)
docusate potassium (formerly dioctyl potassium sulfosuccinate)
docusate sodium (formerly dioctyl sodium sulfosuccinate)
glycerin
lactulose
magnesium salts
methylcellulose
mineral oil
phenolphthalein
psyllium
senna
sodium biphosphate
sodium phosphate

Laxatives (also historically known as cathartics, drastics, and purgatives) ease the passage of feces from the colon and rectum. The accumulation of feces in the lower bowel results from constipation, which is defined as a decrease in the frequency of fecal elimination, characterized by the passage of hard, dry stools. In an effort to alleviate constipation, many people overuse laxatives.

Laxatives can be classified according to the way they work: Hyperosmolar, bulk-forming, lubricant, emollient or stool softener, or stimulant.

Major uses

Rx Laxatives may relieve or prevent constipation. They are used to evacuate the bowel before rectal or bowel examination, exposure of abdominal X-ray films, barium enema, or various surgical procedures.

- The docusate salts are commonly used to soften stools and prevent straining during defecation.
- Lactulose is also used to treat hepatic encephalopathy.

Mechanism of action

- Bulk-forming laxatives absorb water and expand to increase bulk and moisture content of the stool. The increased bulk encourages peristalsis and bowel movement.
- Emollient laxatives, or stool softeners, reduce surface tension of interfacing liquid contents of the bowel. This mechanism, or detergent activity, promotes incorporation of additional liquid into the stool, forming a softer mass.
- Among the hyperosmolar laxatives, glycerin draws water from the tissues into the feces and thus stimulates reflex evacuation.

Lactulose produces an osmotic effect in the colon and is biodegraded by the intestinal flora into lactic, formic, and acetic acids. Distention of the bowel from fluid accumulation promotes peristalsis and bowel movement.

The saline agents (magnesium salts, sodium diphosphate, and sodium

HOW LAXATIVES WORK

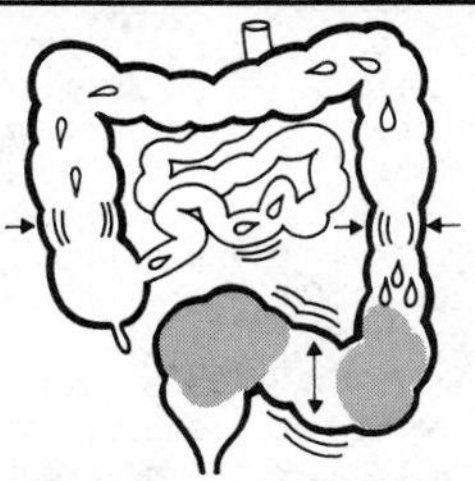

HYPEROSMOLAR LAXATIVES

Lactulose and *glycerin* produce an osmotic effect in the colon, leading to fluid accumulation, bowel distention, and peristalsis. This is also the major effect of saline laxatives; with these, however, water is drawn into the small intestine as well as the colon.

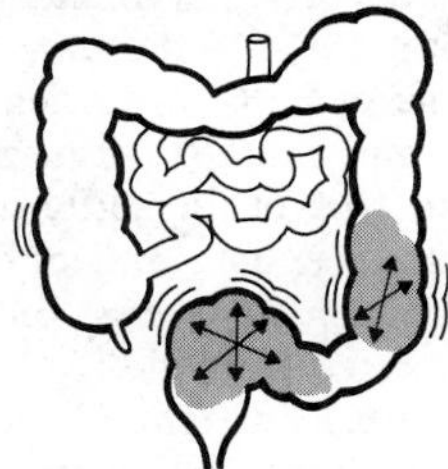

BULK-FORMING LAXATIVES

Barley-malt extract, methylcellulose, and *psyllium* absorb water and expand to increase bulk. They encourage peristalsis of the colon and small intestine by distention.

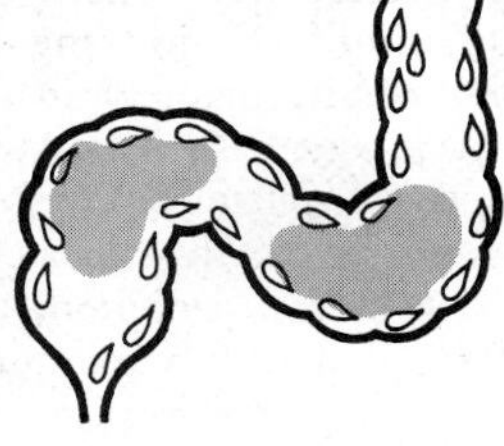

LUBRICANT LAXATIVES

Mineral oil increases water retention by creating a barrier between the colon wall and feces that prevents colonic reabsorption of fecal water.

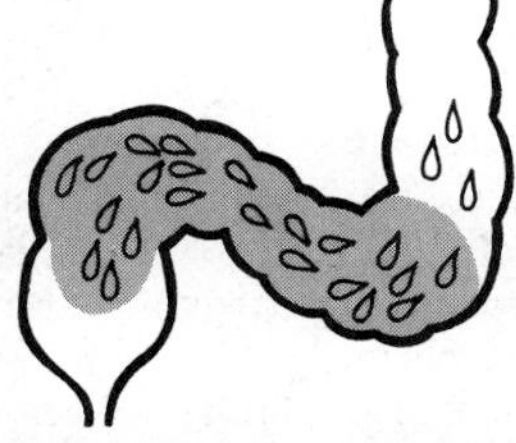

EMOLLIENT LAXATIVES OR STOOL SOFTENERS

Docusate salts reduce surface tension of interfacing liquid bowel contents. This detergent activity promotes fluid accumulation and a softer stool in the small intestine and the colon.

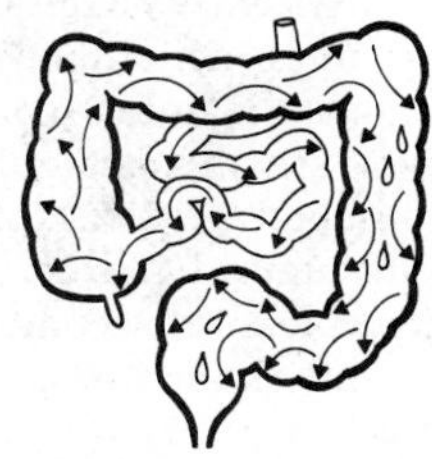

STIMULANT LAXATIVES

Bisacodyl, cascara sagrada, castor oil, danthron, phenolphthalein, and *senna* may irritate the intestine's smooth muscle or stimulate the colonic intramural plexus. They also promote fluid accumulation in the colon and small intestine.

PREVENTING LAXATIVE ABUSE

Your patient may be taking a laxative needlessly, too frequently, or too long.

He may think he's constipated because of his childhood conditioning or because of myths about the need for daily bowel movements. So tell your patient he's not necessarily constipated if he fails to have a bowel movement every day.

Occasionally, constipation is due to a disorder of the colon, but most cases may be attributed to life-style (diet, stress, medications, travel). If symptoms of simple constipation—mild anorexia, distention, and abdominal discomfort—aren't relieved by laxative therapy within 1 week, tell your patient to stop taking the laxative and consult a doctor.

Excessive laxative use can cause diarrhea and vomiting, resulting in fluid and electrolyte losses, particularly hypokalemia. Laxative abuse can produce a loss of tone in both smooth and striated muscle.

Prolonged laxative use can cause the following anatomic changes in the colon: loss of innervation, atrophy of smooth muscle, and pigmentation. These changes may lead to tissue damage and a condition known as cathartic colon.

Help your patient break the laxative habit. Inform him of natural methods of treating constipation: proper diet, exercise, and adequate fluid intake. (Also, give a copy of the patient-teaching aid "How to Prevent or Relieve Constipation," p. 643.)

phosphate) produce an osmotic effect in the small intestine by drawing water into the intestinal lumen. Fluid accumulation produces distention, which then encourages peristalsis and bowel movement. Saline laxatives also promote cholecystokinin secretion, stimulating intestinal motility and inhibiting fluid and electrolyte absorption from the jejunum and ileum.

• Lubricant laxatives increase water retention in the stool by creating a barrier between colon wall and feces that prevents colonic reabsorption of fecal water.

• Stimulant laxatives may increase peristalsis by direct effect on the smooth muscle of the intestine. Although the precise mechanism is unknown, stimulant laxatives are thought either to irritate the musculature or to stimulate the colonic intramural plexus. These drugs also promote fluid accumulation in the colon and small intestine, increasing the laxative effect.

Absorption, distribution, metabolism, and excretion

• Bulk-forming laxatives are not absorbed systemically.

• Emollient laxatives are systemically absorbed and eliminated in the bile.

• Among the hyperosmolar laxatives, glycerin suppositories and lactulose are not absorbed systemically.

About 20% of the magnesium in magnesium salts is systemically absorbed and excreted in urine.

Up to 10% of the sodium content of sodium phosphate and of sodium biphosphate enemas may be absorbed and excreted in urine.

• The lubricant laxative mineral oil, in its nonemulsified form, is not significantly absorbed; as much as one half of emulsified mineral oil may be absorbed.

• Stimulant laxatives are slightly absorbed and are metabolized in the liver. The metabolites are eliminated either in urine or—through the bile—in feces.

Combination products

AGORAL: mineral oil 28% and white phenolphthalein 1.3% in emulsion, with tragacanth, agar, egg albumin, acacia, and glycerin.

CASYLLIUM: psyllium husk powder 4.1 g, debittered fluidextract cascara 3 ml, and prune powder 1.2 g/6 g.

COMFOLAX-PLUS: docusate sodium 100 mg and casanthranol 30 mg.

CORRECTOL: yellow phenolphthalein 64.8 mg and docusate sodium 100 mg.

DIALOSE: docusate sodium 100 mg and sodium carboxymethylcellulose 400 mg.

DIALOSE-PLUS: docusate sodium 100 mg

LAXATIVE ACTION AT A GLANCE

CLASS AND DRUG	SITE OF ACTION	TIME BEFORE BOWEL MOVEMENT
Bulk-forming laxatives		
barley-malt extract methylcellulose psyllium	Small intestine and colon	12 to 72 hr
Emollient laxatives		
docusate salts	Small intestine and colon	12 to 72 hr
Hyperosmolar laxatives		
glycerin	Colon	15 to 30 min
lactulose	Colon	24 to 48 hr
saline laxatives (magnesium and sodium salts)	Small intestine and colon	30 min to 3 hr
Lubricant laxatives		
mineral oil	Colon	6 to 8 hr
Stimulant laxatives		
bisacodyl	Colon	6 to 10 hr
cascara sagrada	Colon	6 to 8 hr
castor oil	Small intestine	2 to 6 hr
danthron	Colon	8 hr
phenolphthalein	Colon	6 to 8 hr
senna	Colon	6 to 10 hr

and casanthranol 30 mg.

DORBANTYL: docusate sodium 50 mg and danthron 25 mg.

DORBANTYL FORTE: docusate sodium 100 mg and danthron 50 mg.

DOXAN-TABLETS: docusate sodium 60 mg and danthron 50 mg.

DOXIDAN♦: docusate calcium 60 mg and danthron 50 mg.

D-S-S PLUS: docusate sodium 100 mg and casanthranol 30 mg.

GENTLAX S: docusate sodium 50 mg and standardized senna concentrate 187 mg.

HALEY'S M-O: mineral oil (25%) and magnesium hydroxide.

HYDROCIL, FORTIFIED: blond psyllium coating 50% and casanthranol (with dextrose) 30 mg/6 g.

KONDREMUL WITH CASCARA♦: heavy mineral oil 55%, cascara sagrada extract 660 mg/15 ml, and Irish moss as emulsifier.

KONDREMUL WITH PHENOLPHTHALEIN♦: heavy mineral oil 55%, white phenolphthalein 147 mg/15 ml, and Irish moss as emulsifier.

OXIPHEN: phenolphthalein 32.4 mg, cascara sagrada extract 32.4 mg, aloin 8.1 mg, sodium glycocholate 16.2 mg, and sodium taurocholate 16.2 mg.

PERI-COLACE♦ (capsules): docusate sodium 100 mg and casanthranol 30 mg.

PERI-COLACE (syrup): docusate sodium 60 mg and casanthranol 30 mg per 15 ml.

PETROGALAR WITH PHENOLPHTHALEIN: mineral oil 65% and phenolphthalein 0.3%.

SENOKOT-S♦: docusate sodium 50 mg and standardized senna concentrate 187 mg.

SENOKOT WITH PSYLLIUM: psyllium 1 g and standardized senna concentrate 326 mg/tsp.

STIMULAX: docusate sodium 250 mg and casanthranol 30 mg.

SYLLAMALT: malt soup extract 3.5 g and powdered psyllium seed husks 3.5 g per rounded tsp.

SYLLAMALT EFFERVESCENT: malt-soup extract 1.75 g, powdered psyllium seed husks 1.75 g, sodium bicarbonate, and citric acid per rounded tsp.

NAME	INDICATIONS & DOSAGE	SIDE EFFECTS
barley-malt extract Maltsupex	*Constipation—* **Adults:** 4 tablets P.O. with meals and at bedtime for 4 days, then 2 to 4 tablets at bedtime; or 2 tablespoonfuls powder or liquid b.i.d. for 3 to 4 days, until stools become soft, then 1 to 2 tablespoonfuls at bedtime. **Children over 2 months:** ½ to 2 tablespoonfuls in milk or on cereal daily or b.i.d. **Infants 1 or 2 months:** ½ tablespoonful daily with milk or cereal. To prevent constipation, may add 1 to 2 teaspoonfuls to each day's feeding.	**GI:** loose stools. **Other:** laxative dependence with frequent or long-term use.
bisacodyl Biscolax♦, Codylax, Dulcolax♦, Dulcolax Micro-enema♦♦, Fleet Bisacodyl, Rolax, Theralax	*Chronic constipation; preparation for delivery, surgery, or rectal or bowel examination—* **Adults:** 10 to 15 mg P.O. in evening or before breakfast. Up to 30 mg may be used for thorough evacuation needed for examinations or surgery. **Children:** 5 to 10 mg P.O. Rectal: **Adults, and children over 2 years:** 10 mg. **Under 2 years:** 5 mg. Enema: **Adults:** 1.25 oz. **Children under 6 years:** approximately ½ contents of micro enema.	**CNS:** muscle weakness in excessive use. **GI:** *nausea, abdominal cramps,* diarrhea in high doses, *burning sensation in rectum with suppositories.* **Metabolic:** alkalosis, hypokalemia, tetany, protein-losing enteropathy in excessive use. **Other:** laxative dependence in long-term or excessive use.
cascara sagrada Cas-Evac **cascara sagrada aromatic fluidextract** **cascara sagrada fluidextract**	*Acute constipation; preparation for bowel or rectal examination—* **Adults:** 325 mg cascara sagrada tablets P.O. h.s.; or 1 ml fluidextract daily; or 5 ml aromatic fluidextract daily; or 1.25 to 2.5 ml Cas-Evac liquid b.i.d.; or 2.5 to 5 ml Cas-Evac liquid h.s. **Children 2 to 12 years:** ½ adult dose. **Children under 2 years:** ¼ adult dose.	**GI:** *nausea;* vomiting; diarrhea; loss of normal bowel function with excessive use; *abdominal cramps,* especially in severe constipation; malabsorption of nutrients; cathartic colon (syndrome resembling ulcerative colitis both radiologically and pathologically) after chronic misuse; discoloration of rectal mucosa after long-term use. **Metabolic:** hypokalemia, protein enteropathy, electrolyte imbalance in excessive use. **Other:** laxative dependence in long-term or excessive use.

♦ Available in U.S. and Canada. ♦♦ Available in Canada only. All other products (no symbol) available in U.S. only. Italicized side effects are common or life-threatening.

INTERACTIONS	NURSING CONSIDERATIONS
None significant.	• Contraindicated in abdominal pain, nausea, vomiting, or other symptoms of appendicitis or acute surgical abdomen, and in intestinal obstruction or ulceration, disabling adhesion, or difficulty swallowing. • In patients with diabetes, allow for carbohydrate content of approximately 14 g/tablespoon of liquid, 13 g/tablespoon of powder, and 0.6 g/tablet. • Tell patient to take with at least 8 oz (240 ml) liquid. • For short-term use. Before giving, determine if patient has adequate fluid intake, exercise, and diet. Tell him that dietary sources of bulk include bran and other cereals, fresh fruit, and vegetables. • Infants usually need diet change to increase bulk in addition to laxative. • Laxative effect usually takes 12 to 24 hours; may be delayed 3 days. • Bulk laxative; increases bulk and water content of stool. • Not absorbed systemically; nontoxic. • Reduces fecal pH. Especially useful in constipated postpartum mothers, debilitated patients, infants, patients with chronic laxative abuse, irritable bowel syndrome, diverticular disease, and to clear the colon before barium enema examination.
None significant.	• Contraindicated in patients with abdominal pain, nausea, vomiting, or other symptoms of appendicitis or acute surgical abdomen, or in rectal fissures or ulcerated hemorrhoids. • Tell patient to swallow enteric-coated tablet whole to avoid GI irritation. Don't give with milk or antacids. Begins to act 6 to 12 hours after oral administration. • Soft, formed stool usually produced 15 to 60 minutes after rectal administration. Time administration of drug so as not to interfere with scheduled activities or sleep. • Tablets and suppositories may be used together to cleanse colon before and after surgery and before barium enema. • Use for short-term treatment. Stimulant laxative, class of laxative most abused. Discourage excessive use. • Before giving for constipation, determine if patient has adequate fluid intake, exercise, and diet. Tell him that dietary sources of bulk include bran and other cereals, fresh fruit, and vegetables. • Store tablets and suppositories at temperature below 86° F. (30° C.). • Tell patient to report adverse side effects to the doctor.
None significant.	• Contraindicated in abdominal pain, nausea, vomiting, or other symptoms of appendicitis or acute surgical abdomen; in acute surgical delirium, fecal impaction, intestinal obstruction or perforation. Use cautiously when rectal bleeding is present. • Aromatic cascara fluidextract is less active and less bitter than nonaromatic fluidextract. • Liquid preparations more reliable than solid dosage forms. • Drug of choice among stimulant laxatives. Use for short-term treatment. • Before giving for constipation, determine if patient has adequate fluid intake, exercise, and diet. Tell him that dietary sources of bulk include bran and other cereals, fresh fruit, and vegetables. • May turn alkaline urine red-pink and acidic urine yellow-brown. • Monitor serum electrolytes during prolonged use.

NAME	INDICATIONS & DOSAGE	SIDE EFFECTS
castor oil Alphamul, Neoloid♦	*Preparation for rectal or bowel examination, or surgery; acute constipation (rarely)—* **Adults:** 15 to 60 ml P.O. as liquid or 1.25 to 3.7 mg P.O. as tablet. **Children over 2 years:** 5 to 15 ml P.O. **Children under 2 years:** 1.25 to 7.5 ml P.O. **Infants:** up to 4 ml P.O. Increased dose produces no greater effect.	**GI:** *nausea;* vomiting; diarrhea; loss of normal bowel function with excessive use; *abdominal cramps,* especially in severe constipation; malabsorption of nutrients; cathartic colon (syndrome resembling ulcerative colitis both radiologically and pathologically) in chronic misuse. May cause constipation after catharsis. **GU:** pelvic congestion in menstruating women. **Metabolic:** hypokalemia, protein enteropathy, other electrolyte imbalance in excessive use. **Other:** laxative dependence in long-term or excessive use.
danthron Dorbane♦, Duolax, Modane♦, Modane Mild♦, Weslax	*Acute constipation, preparation for rectal or bowel examination, postsurgical and postpartum constipation—* **Adults and children:** 37.5 to 150 mg P.O. after or with evening meal.	**GI:** *nausea;* vomiting; diarrhea; loss of normal bowel function in excessive use; *abdominal cramps,* especially in severe constipation; malabsorption of nutrients; cathartic colon (syndrome resembling ulcerative colitis radiologically and pathologically) in chronic misuse; discoloration of rectal mucosa in long-term use. **Metabolic:** hypokalemia, protein enteropathy, electrolyte imbalance in excessive use. **Other:** laxative dependence in long-term or excessive use.
docusate calcium (formerly dioctyl calcium sulfosuccinate) Surfak♦	*Stool softener—* **Adults and older children:** 50 to 300 mg (docusate sodium) P.O. daily or 240 mg (docusate calcium and docusate potassium) P.O. daily until bowel movements are normal; or 5 ml (250 mg) (docusate potassium) enema.	**EENT:** throat irritation. **GI:** bitter taste, mild abdominal cramping, diarrhea. **Other:** laxative dependence in long-term or excessive use.

♦ Available in U.S. and Canada. ♦♦ Available in Canada only. All other products (no symbol) available in U.S. only. Italicized side effects are common or life-threatening.

INTERACTIONS	NURSING CONSIDERATIONS
None significant.	• Contraindicated in ulcerative bowel lesions; during menstruation; in abdominal pain, nausea, vomiting, or other symptoms of appendicitis or acute surgical abdomen; in anal or rectal fissures; fecal impaction; intestinal obstruction or perforation. Use cautiously in rectal bleeding. • Failure to respond may indicate acute condition requiring surgery. • Give with juice or carbonated beverage to mask oily taste. Ice held in mouth before taking drug will help prevent tasting it. • Shake emulsion well. Store below 4.4° C. (40° F.). Don't freeze. • Give on empty stomach for best results. • Produces complete evacuation after 3 hours. Tell patient that after castor oil has emptied bowel, he will not have bowel movement for 1 to 2 days. • Time drug administration so that it doesn't interfere with scheduled activities or sleep. • Monitor serum electrolytes during prolonged use. • Generally used before diagnostic testing or therapy requiring thorough evacuation of GI tract. • Use for short-term treatment. Not recommended for routine use; useful for acute constipation not responsive to milder laxatives. • Before giving for constipation, determine if patient has adequate fluid intake, exercise, and diet. Tell him that dietary sources of bulk include bran and other cereals, fresh fruit, and vegetables. • Stimulant laxative. • Increased intestinal motility lessens absorption of concomitantly administered P.O. drugs. Reschedule dose.
None significant.	• Contraindicated in abdominal pain, nausea, vomiting, or other symptoms of appendicitis or acute surgical abdomen; in intestinal obstruction or perforation; and in hepatic dysfunction. Use cautiously in rectal bleeding or fecal impaction. • Give with fruit juice or carbonated beverage to mask oily taste. • Give on empty stomach for best results. • Produces complete evacuation of bowel in 6 to 24 hours. Tell patient that he will not have another bowel movement for 1 to 2 days. Time drug administration so that it doesn't interfere with scheduled activities or sleep. • Generally used before diagnostic testing or therapy requiring thorough evacuation of GI tract. • Agent of choice for cardiac patients; reduces strain of evacuation. • Use for short-term treatment. Not recommended for routine use; useful for acute constipation not responsive to milder laxatives. • Before giving for constipation, determine if patient has adequate fluid intake, exercise, and diet. Tell him that dietary sources of bulk include bran and other cereals, fresh fruit, and vegetables. • May discolor alkaline urine red-pink and acidic urine yellow-brown. • Monitor serum electrolytes during prolonged use.
None significant.	• Sodium salts: use cautiously in patients on sodium-restricted diets, or with edema, congestive heart failure, renal dysfunction. • Potassium salts: contraindicated in renal dysfunction. • Give liquid in milk, fruit juice, or infant formula to mask bitter taste. • Not for use in treating existing constipation, but prevents constipation from developing. • Laxative of choice in patients who should not strain during defecation, such as those recovering from myocardial infarction or rectal

(continued on following page)

NAME	INDICATIONS & DOSAGE	SIDE EFFECTS
docusate *(continued)* **docusate potassium (formerly dioctyl potassium sulfosuccinate)** Kasof, Rectalad Enema **docusate sodium (formerly dioctyl sodium sulfosuccinate)** Bu-Lax, Colace, Comfolax, Disonate, Doctate, Doxinate, D.S.S., Dynoctol, Laxinate, Regutol, Roctate	**Children over 12 years:** 2 ml (100 mg) (docusate potassium) enema. **Children 6 to 12 years:** 40 to 120 mg (docusate sodium) P.O. daily. **Children 3 to 6 years:** 20 to 60 mg (docusate sodium) P.O. daily. **Children under 3 years:** 10 to 40 mg (docusate sodium) P.O. daily. Higher doses are for initial therapy. Adjust dose to individual response. Usual dose in children and adults with minimal needs: 50 to 150 mg (docusate calcium) P.O. daily.	
glycerin	*Constipation—* **Adults, and children over 6 years:** 3 g as a suppository; or 5 to 15 ml as an enema. **Children under 6 years:** 1 to 1.5 g as a suppository; or 2 to 5 ml as an enema.	**GI:** *cramping pain,* rectal discomfort, hyperemia of rectal mucosa.
lactulose Cephulac♦, Chronulac♦	*Treatment of constipation—* **Adults:** 15 to 30 ml P.O. daily. *To prevent and treat portal-systemic encephalopathy, including hepatic precoma and coma in patients with severe hepatic disease—* **Adults:** initially, 20 to 30 g P.O. (30 to 45 ml) t.i.d. or q.i.d., until 2 or 3 soft stools are produced daily. Usual dose is 60 to 100 g daily in divided doses. Can also be given by retention enema in at least 100 ml of fluid.	**GI:** abdominal cramps, belching, diarrhea, gaseous distention, flatulence.
magnesium salts Concentrated Milk of Magnesia, Magnesium Citrate, Magnesium Sulfate, Milk of Magnesia	*Constipation, to evacuate bowel before surgery—* **Adults, and children over 6 years:** 15 g magnesium sulfate P.O. in glass of water; 10 to 20 ml concentrated milk of magnesia P.O.; or 15 to 30 ml milk of magnesia P.O.; or 5 to 10 oz magnesium citrate at bedtime. *Laxative—* **Adults:** 30 to 60 ml, usually h.s., Milk of Magnesia P.O.	**GI:** *abdominal cramping, nausea.* **Metabolic:** fluid and electrolyte disturbances if used daily. **Other:** laxative dependence in long-term or excessive use.

♦ Available in U.S. and Canada. ♦♦ Available in Canada only. All other products (no symbol) available in U.S. only. Italicized side effects are common or life-threatening.

INTERACTIONS	NURSING CONSIDERATIONS
	surgery; in disease of rectum and anus that makes passage of firm stool difficult; or postpartum constipation. • Acts within 24 to 48 hours to produce firm, semisolid stool. • Instruct patient that dietary sources of bulk include bran and other cereals, fresh fruit, and vegetables. • Emollient laxative or stool softener; doesn't stimulate intestinal peristaltic movements. • Store at 15° to 30° C. (59° to 86° F.). Protect liquid from light.
None significant.	• A hyperosmolar laxative used mainly to reestablish proper toilet habits in laxative-dependent patients.
None significant.	• Contraindicated in patients who need low-galactose diet. Use cautiously in diabetes mellitus. • Reduce dosage if diarrhea occurs. Replace fluid loss. • If desired, minimize drug's sweet taste by diluting with water or fruit juice or giving with food. • Store at room temperature, preferably below 30° C. (86° F.). Don't freeze.
None significant.	• Contraindicated in abdominal pain, nausea, vomiting, or other symptoms of appendicitis or acute surgical abdomen; in myocardial damage, heart block, imminent delivery, fecal impaction, rectal fissures, intestinal obstruction or perforation, renal disease. Use cautiously in rectal bleeding. • Shake suspension well; give with large amount of water when used as laxative. When administering through nasogastric tube, be sure tube is placed properly and is patent. After instilling, flush tube with water to assure passage to stomach and maintain tube patency. • For short-term therapy; don't use longer than 1 week. • When used as laxative, don't give oral drugs 1 to 2 hours before or after. • Saline laxative; produces watery stool in 3 to 6 hours. Time drug

(continued on following page)

NAME	INDICATIONS & DOSAGE	SIDE EFFECTS
magnesium salts *(continued)*	**Children:** 7.5 to 30 ml h.s. Milk of Magnesia P.O.	
methylcellulose Cellothyl, Cologel, Hydrolose, Syncelose	*Chronic constipation—* **Adults:** 5 to 20 ml liquid P.O. t.i.d. with a glass of water; or 15 ml syrup P.O. morning and evening. **Children:** 5 to 10 ml P.O. daily or b.i.d.	**GI:** *nausea,* vomiting, diarrhea (all after excessive use); esophageal, gastric, small intestinal, or colonic strictures when drug is chewed or taken in dry form; *abdominal cramps,* especially in severe constipation. **Other:** laxative dependence in long-term or excessive use.
mineral oil Agoral Plain, Fleet Mineral Oil Enema, Kondremul Plain♦, Neo-Cultol, Petrogalar Plain, Saf-Tip Oil Retention Enema	*Constipation; preparation for bowel studies or surgery—* **Adults:** 15 to 30 ml P.O., usually h.s.; or 4 oz enema. **Children:** 5 to 15 ml P.O. h.s.; or 1 to 2 oz enema.	**GI:** *nausea;* vomiting; diarrhea in excessive use; *abdominal cramps,* especially in severe constipation; decreased absorption of nutrients and fat-soluble vitamins, resulting in deficiency; slowed healing after hemorrhoidectomy; and increased risk of rectal infections due to seepage from rectum. **Other:** laxative dependence in long-term or excessive use.
phenolphthalein Alophen, Espotabs, Evac-U-Gen, Evac-U-Lac, Ex-Lax, Feen-A-Mint, Phenolax	*Constipation—* **Adults:** 60 to 200 mg P.O., preferably h.s.	**GI:** diarrhea; *colic in large doses;* factitious nausea; vomiting; loss of normal bowel function in excessive use; *abdominal cramps,* especially in severe constipation; malabsorption of nutrients; cathartic colon (syndrome resembling ulcerative colitis radiologically and pathologically) in chronic misuse; reddish discoloration in alkaline feces. **Skin:** dermatitis, pruritus.

♦ Available in U.S. and Canada. ♦♦ Available in Canada only. All other products (no symbol) available in U.S. only. Italicized side effects are common or life-threatening.

INTERACTIONS	NURSING CONSIDERATIONS
	administration so that it doesn't interfere with scheduled activities or sleep. • Magnesium sulfate is more potent than other saline laxatives. • Before giving for constipation, determine if patient has adequate fluid intake, exercise, and diet. Tell him that dietary sources of bulk include bran and other cereals, fresh fruit, and vegetables. • Magnesium may accumulate in renal insufficiency. • Chilling before use may make magnesium citrate more palatable. • Monitor serum electrolytes during prolonged use. • Frequent or prolonged use as a laxative may cause dependence.
None significant.	• Contraindicated in abdominal pain, nausea, vomiting, or other symptoms of appendicitis or acute surgical abdomen; and in intestinal obstruction or ulceration, disabling adhesion, or difficulty swallowing. • Laxative effect usually takes 12 to 24 hours, but may be delayed 3 days. • Tell patient to take drug with at least 8 oz (240 ml) of pleasant-tasting liquid to mask grittiness. • Especially useful in postpartum constipation, debilitated patients, chronic laxative abuse, irritable bowel syndrome, diverticular disease, colostomies, and to empty colon before barium enema examinations. • Use for short-term treatment. • Before giving for constipation, determine if patient has adequate fluid intake, exercise, and diet. Tell him that dietary sources of bulk include bran and other cereals, fresh fruit, and vegetables. • Not absorbed systemically; nontoxic. • Bulk laxative; increases bulk and water content of stool. • Instruct patient to notify doctor in 1 week about response to therapy.
None significant.	• Contraindicated in abdominal pain, nausea, vomiting, or other symptoms of appendicitis or acute surgical abdomen; in fecal impaction, intestinal obstruction or perforation. Use cautiously in young children; in elderly or debilitated patients due to susceptibility to lipid pneumonitis through aspiration, absorption, and transport from intestinal mucosa; in rectal bleeding. Enema contraindicated in children under 2 years. • Don't give drug with meals or immediately after, as it delays passage of food from stomach. More active on an empty stomach. • A lubricant laxative. • Give with fruit juices or carbonated drinks to disguise taste. • Use when patient needs to ease the strain of evacuation. • Before giving for constipation, determine if patient has adequate fluid intake, exercise, and diet. Tell him that dietary sources of bulk include bran and other cereals, fresh fruit, and vegetables.
None significant.	• Contraindicated in abdominal pain, nausea, vomiting, or other symptoms of appendicitis or acute surgical abdomen; in fecal impaction, intestinal obstruction or perforation. Use cautiously in rectal bleeding. • Laxative effect may last up to 3 to 4 days. • Produces semisolid stool within 6 to 8 hours, with little or no griping. Time drug administration so that it doesn't interfere with scheduled activities or sleep. • Warn patient with rash to avoid sun and discontinue use. • Before giving for constipation, determine if patient has adequate fluid intake, exercise, and diet. Tell him that dietary sources of bulk include bran and other cereals, fresh fruit, and vegetables.

(continued on following page)

NAME	INDICATIONS & DOSAGE	SIDE EFFECTS
phenolphthalein *(continued)*		**Other:** laxative dependence in long-term or excessive use.
psyllium Effersyllium Instant Mix, Konsyl, L.A. Formula, Metamucil♦, Metamucil Instant Mix♦, Modane Bulk, Mucillium, Mucilose, Plain Hydrocil, Siblin♦, Syllact	*Constipation; bowel management—* **Adults:** 1 to 2 rounded teaspoonfuls P.O. in full glass of liquid daily, b.i.d., or t.i.d., followed by second glass of liquid; or 1 packet P.O. dissolved in water daily, b.i.d., or t.i.d. **Children over 6 years:** 1 level teaspoonful P.O. in ½ glass of liquid h.s.	**GI:** nausea, vomiting, diarrhea, all after excessive use; esophageal, gastric, small intestinal, or colonic strictures when drug taken in dry form; abdominal cramps, especially in severe constipation.
senna Black Draught, Glysennid, Senokot, X-Prep	*Acute constipation, preparation for bowel or rectal examination—* **Adults:** Dosage range for Senokot: 1 to 8 tablets P.O.; ½ to 4 teaspoonfuls of granules added to liquid; 1 to 2 suppositories h.s.; 1 to 4 teaspoonfuls syrup h.s. Black Draught: 7.5 to 15 ml. **Children over 27 kg:** ½ adult dose of tablets, granules, or syrup (except Black Draught tablets and granules not recommended for children). **Children 1 month to 1 year:** 1.25 to 2.5 ml Senokot syrup P.O. h.s. X-Prep used solely as single dose for preradiographic bowel evacuation. Give ¾ oz powder dissolved in juice or 2.5 oz liquid between 2 and 4 p.m. on day before X-ray procedure. May be given in divided doses for elderly or debilitated patients.	**GI:** *nausea;* vomiting; diarrhea; loss of normal bowel function in excessive use; *abdominal cramps,* especially in severe constipation; malabsorption of nutrients; cathartic colon (syndrome resembling ulcerative colitis radiologically in chronic misuse; may cause constipation after catharsis); yellow, yellow-green cast feces, diarrhea in nursing infants of mothers on senna; darkened pigmentation of rectal mucosa in long-term use, which is usually reversible within 4 to 12 months after stopping drug. **GU:** red-pink discoloration in alkaline urine; yellow-brown color to acid urine. **Metabolic:** hypokalemia, protein enteropathy, electrolyte imbalance with excessive use. **Other:** laxative dependence in long-term or excessive use.

♦ Available in U.S. and Canada. ♦♦ Available in Canada only. All other products (no symbol) available in U.S. only. Italicized side effects are common or life-threatening.

INTERACTIONS	NURSING CONSIDERATIONS
	• May discolor alkaline urine red-pink and acidic urine yellow-brown. • Drug is available in many dosage forms. Most popular over-the-counter laxative; a frequent constituent of chewing gum and chocolate laxatives. Stimulant laxative, class of laxative most abused.
None significant.	• Contraindicated in abdominal pain, nausea, vomiting, or other symptoms of appendicitis; and in intestinal obstruction or ulceration, disabling adhesion, or difficulty swallowing. • Metamucil Instant Mix (effervescent form) contains a significant amount of sodium and should not be used for patients on sodium-restricted diets. • Mix with at least 8 oz (240 ml) of cold, pleasant-tasting liquid to mask grittiness, and stir only a few seconds. Patient should drink it immediately or mixture will congeal. Follow with additional glass of liquid. • Use for short-term treatment. Don't use for maintenance. • Frequent use of laxatives can cause drug dependence for evacuation. • Before giving for constipation, determine if patient has adequate fluid intake, exercise, and diet. Tell him that dietary sources of bulk include bran and other cereals, fresh fruit, and vegetables. • Laxative effect usually seen in 12 to 24 hours, but may be delayed 3 days. • Popular bulk laxative; increases bulk and water content of stool. • Highly refined, purified vegetable mucilloid; from seeds of plantago plant. • Not absorbed systemically; nontoxic. Especially useful in postpartum constipation, debilitated patients, chronic laxative abuse, irritable bowel syndrome, diverticular disease, and in combination with other laxatives to empty colon before barium enema examinations.
None significant.	• Contraindicated in ulcerative bowel lesions; in nausea, vomiting, abdominal pain, or other symptoms of appendicitis or acute surgical abdomen; in fecal impaction, intestinal obstruction, or perforation. • Use for short-term treatment. • More potent than cascara sagrada. Acts in 6 to 10 hours. X-Prep gives thorough, strong bowel action beginning in 6 hours. • Most recommended stimulant laxative. • Before giving for constipation, determine if patient has adequate fluid intake, exercise, and diet. Tell him that dietary sources of bulk include bran and other cereals, fresh fruit, and vegetables. • After X-Prep liquid is taken, diet should be confined to clear liquids.

NAME	INDICATIONS & DOSAGE	SIDE EFFECTS
sodium biphosphate Enemeez, Fleet Enema♦, Phospho-Soda, Saf-Tip Phosphate Enema, Travad Enema♦ **sodium phosphate** Sal-Hepatica	*Constipation*— **Adults:** 5 to 20 ml liquid P.O. with water; or 4 g powder P.O. dissolved in warm water; or 20 to 46 ml solution mixed with 4 oz cold water; or 2 to 4.5 oz enema.	**GI:** *abdominal cramping.* **Metabolic:** fluid and electrolyte disturbances (hypernatremia, hyperphosphatemia) if used daily. **Other:** laxative dependence in long-term or excessive use.

♦ Available in U.S. and Canada. ♦♦ Available in Canada only. All other products (no symbol) available in U.S. only. Italicized side effects are common or life-threatening.

PATIENT-TEACHING AID

FIBER CONTENT OF SOME COMMON FOODS

	GRAMS OF CRUDE FIBER PER ½ CUP		GRAMS OF CRUDE FIBER PER ½ CUP
Bran flakes (100% bran)	2.2	Peanuts, with skins	2.7
Bran flakes (40% bran)	1.0	Almonds, with skins	2.2
Raisin bran	0.8	Pecans	1.3
Puffed wheat	0.6	Peanut butter (2 tbsp)	0.7
Shredded wheat	0.6	Whole-grain bread (1 slice)	0.4
Sunflower seeds (kernels)	1.1	Bran muffin (1 muffin)	0.7
Sesame seeds	1.8	Fresh fruit, with skin (1 average)	1.5
Pumpkin seeds (kernels)	0.5	Fresh fruit, without skin	1.0
English walnuts	1.2	Raw vegetables	1.1

Note: Several methods are used today to compute the fiber content of foods, so values may vary. The crude fiber values listed here are provided only as a guideline.

INTERACTIONS	NURSING CONSIDERATIONS
None significant.	• Contraindicated in abdominal pain, nausea, vomiting, or other symptoms of appendicitis or acute surgical abdomen; in intestinal obstruction or perforation; edema; congestive heart failure; megacolon; impaired renal function; and in patients on salt-restricted diets. • Available in oral and rectal forms. • Before giving for constipation, determine if patient has adequate fluid intake, exercise, and diet. Tell him that dietary sources of bulk include bran and other cereals, fresh fruit, and vegetables. • Saline laxative; up to 10% of sodium content may be absorbed. • Enema form elicits response in 5 to 10 minutes. • Used in preparation for barium enema and for fecal impaction.

PATIENT-TEACHING AID

HOW TO PREVENT OR RELIEVE CONSTIPATION

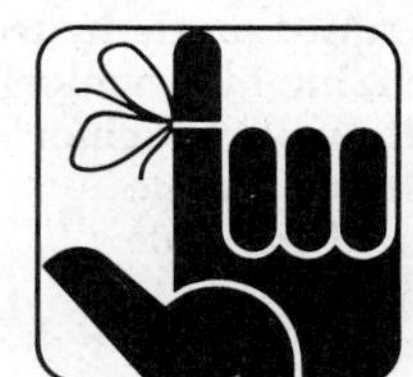

Dear Patient:

You can prevent or relieve constipation by following these suggestions:

• Get sufficient rest—at least 6 hours a night.

• Incorporate moderate exercise into your daily routine. Bicycling, swimming, or even walking will do; just don't be sedentary. Exercise improves muscle tone.

• Establish a regular pattern for bathroom visits; in the morning after breakfast is a good time. Allow enough time for elimination, and don't ignore the urge to defecate. Be aware of your own routine; a *daily* bowel movement isn't essential.

• Drink at least 8 glasses of liquid every day. Fluids help keep the intestinal contents in a semisolid state for easier passage. Before breakfast or in the evening, try drinking hot or cold water, or prune juice for bowel stimulation.

• Include in your diet enough fiber to contribute bulk to the intestines and induce peristalsis. The richest sources of fiber are bran and whole-grain cereals. But be careful: eating too much bran can cause an irritated bowel in some persons. Look for breakfast cereals with the word bran in their titles or, better yet, read the ingredients panel for fiber content: low fiber—0.3 to 1 gram; moderate fiber—1.1 to 2 grams; high fiber—2.1 to 4.2 grams. Some cereals to include in your diet are oatmeal, rolled oats, bran flakes, granola, grape nuts, shredded wheat, wheat flakes, and brown rice. Whole wheat and whole rye are good bread choices.

• Use fat-containing foods, such as bacon, butter, cream, and oil, in moderation. They produce sufficient bulk but sometimes cause diarrhea. If you're on a low-fat diet, you should avoid these foods anyway.

• Include an abundance of raw and cooked vegetables and fruit in your diet, for example, carrots, apples, oranges, celery, lettuce, stewed fruit, and potatoes cooked in skins (eat potato skins). These are high in dietary fiber.

• Avoid highly refined, low-fiber foods, such as white rice, cream of wheat, farina, pastries made from bleached flour, pies, cakes, macaroni, spaghetti, noodles, and ice cream.

• If you have any problems or questions, don't hesitate to call your doctor.

Emetics and antiemetics

apomorphine hydrochloride
benzquinamide hydrochloride
buclizine hydrochloride
cyclizine hydrochloride
cyclizine lactate
dimenhydrinate
diphenidol
ipecac syrup
meclizine hydrochloride
prochlorperazine edisylate
prochlorperazine maleate
scopolamine
thiethylperazine maleate
trimethobenzamide hydrochloride

Emetics (apomorphine and ipecac) are organic compounds used in emergencies to remove poisons from the stomach. They induce vomiting and prevent extensive absorption. Although emetics should be given immediately, they may still be useful even if administration is delayed. However, they should not be used after ingestion of corrosives such as lye since further injury may result. The use of emetics, along with symptomatic and supportive care, can be lifesaving.

Antiemetics (the remaining drugs listed) relieve nausea and vomiting. They are clearly indicated whenever vomiting is severe enough to produce significant fluid, electrolyte, and nutrient losses. By preventing violent retching, they minimize injury to the esophagus and disruption of suture lines (as after intraocular surgery). However, over-the-counter antiemetics can be overused and abused.

Major uses

Rx

- Emetics induce vomiting after ingestion of toxic substances.
- Antiemetics are used to prevent and treat nausea, vomiting, and dizziness.

Mechanism of action

- Apomorphine acts directly on the chemoreceptor trigger zone in the medulla oblongata to induce vomiting.
- Ipecac syrup induces vomiting by acting locally on the gastric mucosa and centrally on the chemoreceptor trigger zone.
- Benzquinamide and trimethobenzamide may act on the chemoreceptor trigger zone to inhibit nausea and vomiting, but this is not certain.
- Buclizine, cyclizine, dimenhydrinate, and meclizine (antihistamine antiemetics) may affect neural pathways originating in the labyrinth to inhibit nausea and vomiting, but the exact mechanism of action is unknown.
- Diphenidol influences the chemoreceptor trigger zone to inhibit nausea and vomiting.
- Prochlorperazine and thiethylperazine (phenothiazine antiemetics) also act on the chemoreceptor trigger zone to inhibit nausea and vomiting, and in larger doses partially depress the vomiting center as well.
- Scopolamine reduces the excitability of labyrinth receptors, depressing conduction in vestibular pathways.

AN ALTERNATIVE FOR MOTION SICKNESS: SCOPOLAMINE COMES IN A TRANSDERMAL PATCH

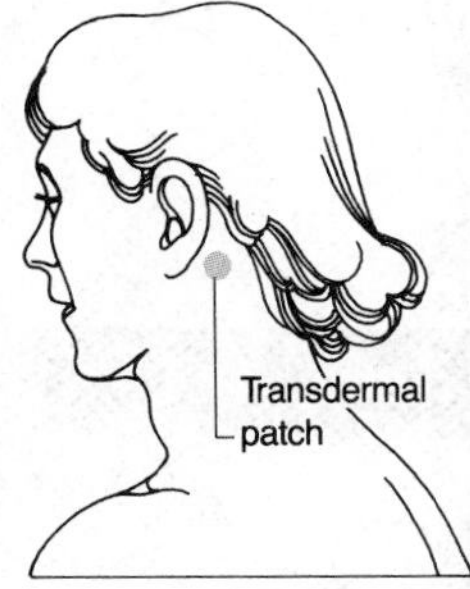
Transdermal
patch

The more than 9 million persons who suffer from motion sickness now have another way to prevent it. Transderm-V (scopolamine), the first FDA-approved transdermal system, consists of a small patch that's worn behind the ear for sustained release of scopolamine. Although the anticholinergic scopolamine isn't new, the transdermal route of administration is.

Why the transdermal route for motion sickness?

- The group of nerve fibers in the inner ear's vestibular apparatus helps people maintain balance. But for some, motion increases the activity of these fibers, causing dizziness, nausea, and vomiting. Transderm-V helps reduce the activity of these inner ear fibers.
- The patch releases minute amounts of scopolamine that permeate the intact skin at a preprogrammed rate, minimizing side effects. Scopolamine is directly adsorbed into the bloodstream, quickly achieving and maintaining an optimal dose for up to 72 hours. This prevents the nausea and vomiting of motion sickness.
- The patch is a flexible, adhesive disk of four layers, as shown in the illustration.

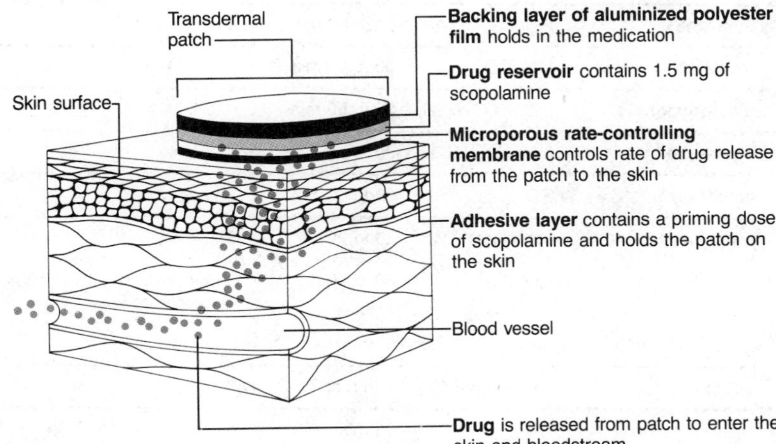
Transdermal
patch
Skin surface
Backing layer of aluminized polyester film holds in the medication
Drug reservoir contains 1.5 mg of scopolamine
Microporous rate-controlling membrane controls rate of drug release from the patch to the skin
Adhesive layer contains a priming dose of scopolamine and holds the patch on the skin
Blood vessel
Drug is released from patch to enter the skin and bloodstream

- The priming dose of scopolamine rapidly brings the blood level to the required steady-state level. Over the 3-day lifetime of the patch, the medication is delivered at a nearly constant rate from the patch to the skin to the blood.
- By diffusion, the drug passes through the membrane from the higher concentration inside the reservoir to the lower concentration outside the reservoir.
- The amount of drug delivered in the diffusion process is regulated by the membrane thickness, surface area and composition, and by the drug concentration on each side of the membrane.

Nursing considerations

Scopolamine should be used with caution in patients with glaucoma, pyloric obstruction, or urinary bladder neck obstruction. Some users experience dry mouth. However, drowsiness, which commonly occurs with higher doses of motion-sickness drugs, is minimized.

Transdermal administration systems have enormous potential, including treatment of such conditions as angina, high blood pressure, and asthma.

THERAPEUTIC ACTIVITY

THERAPEUTIC ACTIVITY OF EMETICS AND ANTIEMETICS

DRUG	ROUTE	ONSET	DURATION
Emetics			
apomorphine	parenteral	5 to 15 min	*
ipecac syrup	P.O.	20 to 30 min	*
Antiemetics			
benzquinamide	parenteral	15 to 30 min	3 to 4 hr
buclizine	P.O.	30 to 60 min	4 to 6 hr
cyclizine	I.M., P.O.	30 to 60 min	4 to 6 hr
dimenhydrinate	I.M., P.O., rectal	30 to 60 min	4 to 6 hr
diphenidol	parenteral, P.O.	30 to 40 min	4 to 6 hr
meclizine	P.O.	30 to 60 min	8 to 24 hr
prochlorperazine	parenteral	10 to 20 min	3 to 4 hr
	P.O.	30 to 40 min	3 to 4 hr (tablet) 10 to 12 hr (extended-release form)
	rectal	1 hr	3 to 4 hr
scopolamine	transdermal	2 to 8 hr	72 hr
thiethylperazine	P.O.	30 min	4 hr
trimethobenzamide	parenteral	15 to 35 min	2 to 3 hr
	P.O., rectal	10 to 40 min	3 to 4 hr

*Data not relevant

Absorption, distribution, metabolism, and excretion

• Apomorphine is poorly absorbed orally but well absorbed when administered by I.M. or subcutaneous injection. It is metabolized in the liver and excreted by the kidneys.

• Ipecac syrup is absorbed through the gastrointestinal tract; its metabolism and route of excretion, however, are unknown.

• Benzquinamide is rapidly absorbed after I.M. injection and rapidly distributed in body tissues, with highest concentration in the liver and kidneys. It is metabolized in the liver and elim-

ARE MARIJUANA DERIVATIVES USEFUL AS ANTIEMETICS?

Anecdotal accounts that smoking marijuana prior to cancer chemotherapy treatments prevented nausea and vomiting led to the study of cannabinoid antiemetic properties. Investigational studies did indeed show that marijuana derivatives and synthetic tetrahydrocannabinol (THC) successfully reduce severe nausea and vomiting associated with chemotherapy. In several clinical studies, THC relieved chemotherapy-induced nausea and vomiting better than a placebo and equal to or better than prochlorperazine.

However, many patients experienced side effects, such as drowsiness, dry mouth, dizziness, decreased coordination, blurred vision, and decreased concentration. A few patients experienced depression, euphoria, tachycardia, and anxiety, but most patients preferred these side effects to chemotherapy-induced nausea and vomiting.

inated in urine and feces.

- Buclizine, cyclizine, dimenhydrinate, and meclizine are well absorbed after either oral or parenteral administration. They are widely distributed in the tissues, metabolized in the liver, and excreted by the kidneys.
- Diphenidol is well absorbed after being given orally, distributed to most body tissues, and metabolized in the liver. It's eliminated in urine and feces.
- Prochlorperazine and thiethylperazine are well absorbed when given orally, parenterally, or rectally. Widely distributed, they are metabolized in the liver and eliminated either in urine or—through the bile—in feces.
- Scopolamine is completely and evenly absorbed transdermally (see illustration on p. 645). The drug is widely distributed and excreted unchanged in urine.
- Trimethobenzamide is well distributed to tissues, metabolized in the liver, and eliminated as both unchanged drug and metabolites in urine and feces.

Onset and duration

The table opposite summarizes the therapeutic activity of the emetics and antiemetics.

Combination products

None.

NAME	INDICATIONS & DOSAGE	SIDE EFFECTS
apomorphine hydrochloride Controlled Substance Schedule II	*To induce vomiting in poisoning*— **Adults:** 2 to 10 mg S.C. preceded by 200 to 300 ml water. Don't repeat. **Children over 1 year:** 0.07 mg/kg S.C. preceded by up to 2 glasses of water. **Children under 1 year:** 0.07 mg/kg S.C. preceded by ½ to 1 glass of water.	**CNS:** *depression, euphoria,* restlessness, tremors. **CV:** *acute circulatory failure in elderly or debilitated patients,* tachycardia. **Other:** *depressed respiratory center in large or repeated doses.*
benzquinamide hydrochloride Emete-Con	*Nausea and vomiting associated with anesthesia and surgery*— **Adults:** 50 mg I.M. (0.5 mg/kg to 1 mg/kg). May repeat in 1 hour, and thereafter q 3 to 4 hours, p.r.n.; or 25 mg (0.2 mg/kg to 0.4 mg/kg) I.V. as single dose, administered slowly.	**CNS:** *drowsiness,* fatigue, insomnia, restlessness, headache, excitation, tremors, twitching, dizziness. **CV:** sudden rise in blood pressure and transient arrhythmias (premature atrial and ventricular contractions, atrial fibrillation) after I.V. administration; hypertension; hypotension. **EENT:** dry mouth, salivation, blurred vision. **GI:** anorexia, nausea. **Skin:** urticaria, rash. **Other:** muscle weakness, flushing, hiccups, sweating, chills, fever. May mask signs of overdose of toxic agents or underlying conditions (intestinal obstruction, brain tumor).
buclizine hydrochloride Bucladin-S, Softran	*Motion sickness (prevention)*— **Adults:** 50 mg P.O. at least ½ hour before beginning travel. If needed, may repeat another 50 mg P.O. after 4 to 6 hours. *Nausea (treatment)*— **Adults:** 50 mg P.O., up to 150 mg P.O. daily in severe cases. Maintenance dose is 50 mg b.i.d.	**CNS:** *drowsiness,* headache, dizziness, jitters. **EENT:** blurred vision, dry mouth. **GU:** urinary retention. **Other:** may mask symptoms of ototoxicity, intestinal obstruction, or brain tumor.

◆ Available in U.S. and Canada. ◆◆ Available in Canada only. All other products (no symbol) available in U.S. only. Italicized side effects are common or life-threatening.

INTERACTIONS	NURSING CONSIDERATIONS
None significant.	• Contraindicated in patients with hypersensitivity to narcotics; impending shock; corrosive poisoning; narcosis resulting from opiates, barbiturates, alcohol, or other CNS depressants; and in patients too inebriated to stand unaided. Use cautiously in children and in patients who are debilitated, have cardiac decompensation, or are predisposed to nausea and vomiting. • Don't give after ingestion of petroleum distillates (for example, kerosene, gasoline) or volatile oils; retching and vomiting may cause aspiration and lead to bronchospasm, pulmonary edema, or aspiration pneumonitis. Vegetable oil will delay absorption of these substances. • Don't give after ingestion of caustic substances, such as lye; additional injury to the esophagus and mediastinum can occur. • Keep narcotic antagonists, such as naloxone, available to help stop vomiting and to alleviate drowsiness. • If delay in giving emetic is expected, give activated charcoal P.O. immediately. When absorbable poison is ingested, give activated charcoal P.O. immediately after apomorphine hydrochloride. • Vomiting occurs in 5 to 10 minutes in adults. If vomiting doesn't occur within 15 minutes, gastric lavage should begin. Apomorphine HCl is emetic of choice when rapid removal of poisons is necessary, and when identification of enteric-coated tablets or other ingested toxic material in vomitus is important. Stomach contents are usually expelled completely; vomitus may also contain material from upper portion of intestinal tract. • Don't administer if solution for injection is discolored or if precipitate is present.
None significant.	• I.V. use contraindicated in cardiovascular disease. Don't give I.V. within 15 minutes of preanesthetic or cardiovascular drugs. • Give I.M. injections in large muscle mass. Use deltoid area only if well developed. Be sure to aspirate syringe for I.M. injection to avoid inadvertent intravenous injection. • Reconstituted solution stable for 14 days at room temperature. Store dry powder and reconstituted solution in light-resistant container. • Monitor blood pressure frequently. • Excellent antiemetic if prochlorperazine (Compazine) is contraindicated.
None significant.	• Warn patient against driving and other activities that require alertness until CNS response to drug is established. • Tablets may be placed in mouth and allowed to dissolve without water. May also be chewed or swallowed whole.

NAME	INDICATIONS & DOSAGE	SIDE EFFECTS
cyclizine hydrochloride **cyclizine lactate** Marezine, Marzine♦♦	*Motion sickness (prevention and treatment)*— **Adults:** 50 mg P.O. (hydrochloride) ½ hour before travel, then q 4 to 6 hours, p.r.n., to maximum of 200 mg daily; or 50 mg I.M. (lactate) q 4 to 6 hours, p.r.n. *Postoperative vomiting (prevention)*— **Adults:** 50 mg I.M. (lactate) preoperatively or 20 to 30 minutes before expected termination of surgery; then postoperatively 50 mg I.M. (lactate) q 4 to 6 hours, p.r.n.; or 100 mg rectally (hydrochloride) q 4 to 6 hours. *Motion sickness and postoperative vomiting*— **Children 6 to 12 years:** 3 mg/kg (lactate) I.M. divided t.i.d., or 25 mg (hydrochloride) P.O. q 4 to 6 hours p.r.n. to a maximum of 75 mg daily.	**CNS:** *drowsiness,* dizziness, auditory and visual hallucinations. **CV:** hypotension. **EENT:** blurred vision, dry mouth. **GI:** constipation. **GU:** urinary retention. **Other:** may mask symptoms of ototoxicity, brain tumor, or intestinal obstruction.
dimenhydrinate Dimate, Dimen, Dimentabs, Dipendrate, Dramaject, Dramamine♦, Dramamine Junior, Dramocen, Dymenate, Eldodram, Gravol♦♦, Hydrate, Hypo-emesis, Marmine, Nauseal♦♦, Nauseatol♦♦, Novodimenate♦♦, Ram, Reidamine, Signate, Travamine♦♦, Trav-Arex, Traveltabs, Vertiban, Wehamine	*Nausea, vomiting, dizziness of motion sickness (treatment and prevention)*— **Adults:** 50 mg P.O. q 4 hours, or 100 mg q 4 hours if drowsiness is not objectionable; or 100 mg rectally daily or b.i.d. if oral route is not practical; or 50 mg I.M., p.r.n.; or 50 mg I.V. diluted in 10 ml NaCl solution, injected over 2 minutes. **Children:** 5 mg/kg P.O. or I.M. or rectally, divided q.i.d. Maximum 300 mg daily.	**CNS:** *drowsiness,* headache, incoordination, dizziness. **CV:** palpitations, hypotension. **EENT:** blurred vision, tinnitus, dry mouth and respiratory passages. **Other:** may mask symptoms of ototoxicity, brain tumor, or intestinal obstruction.
diphenidol Vontrol♦	*Peripheral (labyrinthine) dizziness; nausea and vomiting*— **Adults:** 25 to 50 mg P.O. q 4 hours, p.r.n., or 20 to 40 mg deep I.M. injection (for rapid control of acute symptoms), then another 20 mg I.M. after 1 hour if symptoms persist. Thereafter 20 to 40 mg I.M. q 4 hours, p.r.n., or 20 mg I.V. injected directly through venoclysis already in operation (for rapid control	**CNS:** drowsiness, dizziness, *confusion.* **CV:** transient hypotension; auditory and visual hallucinations, disorientation occur within 3 days of starting drug; subside within 3 days after stopping drug. **GI:** dry mouth, nausea, indigestion, heartburn. **Skin:** urticaria. **Other:** antiemetic effect may mask signs of overdose of drugs,

♦ Available in U.S. and Canada. ♦♦ Available in Canada only. All other products (no symbol) available in U.S. only. Italicized side effects are common or life-threatening.

INTERACTIONS	NURSING CONSIDERATIONS
None significant.	• Use cautiously in patients with glaucoma, GU or GI obstruction, and in elderly males with possible prostatic hypertrophy. • Warn patient against driving and other activities that require alertness until CNS response to drug is determined. • Classified as an antihistamine. • Store in cool place. When stored at room temperature, injection may turn slightly yellow, but this color change does not indicate loss of potency.
None significant.	• Use cautiously in seizures, narrow-angle glaucoma, enlargement of prostate gland. • Undiluted solution is irritating to veins; may cause sclerosis. • Classified as an antihistamine. • Warn patient against driving and other activities that require alertness until CNS response to drug is determined. • May mask ototoxicity of aminoglycoside antibiotics. • Avoid mixing parenteral preparation with other drugs; incompatible with many solutions. See Chapter 6, UNDERSTANDING INTRAVENOUS SOLUTION COMPATIBILITY.
None significant.	• Contraindicated in anuria. Use cautiously in glaucoma, pyloric stenosis, pylorospasm, obstructive lesions of GI or GU tract, prostatic hypertrophy, or organic cardiospasm. • I.V. use contraindicated in children and in patients with sinus tachycardia. • Don't give subcutaneously. Administer deep I.M. • Drug should be stopped if auditory or visual hallucinations, or disorientation or confusion occurs. • Closely supervise patient. Patients are usually hospitalized when receiving this drug. Monitor intake and output; report any changes. • Treatment of toxicity is symptomatic and supportive. • Used in Ménière's disease, following middle and inner ear surgery,

(continued on following page)

NAME	INDICATIONS & DOSAGE	SIDE EFFECTS
diphenidol *(continued)*	of acute symptoms). May inject another 20 mg I.V. after 1 hour if symptoms persist, then switch to P.O. or I.M. route. Total daily dosage should not exceed 300 mg. *Nausea and vomiting—* **Children:** 0.9 mg/kg P.O. or rectally, or 0.4 mg/kg I.M. Give children's doses no more frequently than q 4 hours unless symptoms persist after 1 dose. An oral or I.M. dose may be repeated after 1 hour. Thereafter, doses may be given p.r.n. Maximum children's dose 5.5 mg/kg P.O. daily; or 3.3 mg/kg I.M. daily.	or may obscure diagnosis of intestinal obstruction, brain tumor, or other conditions.
ipecac syrup	*To induce vomiting in poisoning—* **Adults:** 15 ml P.O., followed by 200 to 300 ml of water. **Children 1 year or older:** 15 ml P.O., followed by about 200 ml of water or milk. **Children under 1 year:** 5 to 10 ml P.O., followed by about 200 ml of water or milk. May repeat dose once after 20 minutes, if necessary.	**CV:** *cardiac arrhythmias, atrial fibrillation, or fatal myocarditis* if drug is absorbed (e.g., if patient doesn't vomit within 30 minutes) or after ingestion of excessive dose.
meclizine hydrochloride Antivert♦, Bonamine♦♦, Bonine, Lamine, Roclizine, Vertrol, Wehvert	*Dizziness—* **Adults:** 25 to 100 mg P.O. daily in divided doses. Dose varies with patient response. *Motion sickness—* **Adults:** 25 to 50 mg P.O. 1 hour before travel, repeated daily for duration of journey.	**CNS:** *drowsiness,* fatigue. **EENT:** dry mouth, blurred vision. **Other:** may mask symptoms of ototoxicity, brain tumor, or intestinal obstruction.
prochlorperazine edisylate **prochlorperazine maleate** Compazine, Stemetil♦♦	*Preoperative nausea control—* **Adults:** 5 to 10 mg I.M. 1 to 2 hours before induction of anesthetic, repeat once in 30 minutes, if necessary; or 5 to 10 mg I.V. 15 to 30 minutes before induction of anesthetic (repeat once if necessary); or	**Blood:** *transient leukopenia, agranulocytosis.* **CNS:** *extrapyramidal reactions (high incidence),* sedation (low incidence), pseudoparkinsonism, EEG changes, dizziness. **CV:** *orthostatic hypotension,* tachycardia, EKG changes.

♦ Available in U.S. and Canada. ♦♦ Available in Canada only. All other products (no symbol) available in U.S. only. Italicized side effects are common or life-threatening.

INTERACTIONS	NURSING CONSIDERATIONS
	labyrinthine disturbances, and to control nausea and vomiting associated with infectious disease, malignancies, radiation sickness, general anesthetics, and antineoplastic agents.
Activated charcoal: neutralized emetic effect. Don't give together but may give activated charcoal after vomiting has occurred.	• Contraindicated in semicomatose or unconscious patients, or those with severe inebriation, convulsions, shock, loss of gag reflex. • Don't give after ingestion of petroleum distillates (for example, kerosene, gasoline) or volatile oils; retching and vomiting may cause aspiration and lead to bronchospasm, pulmonary edema, or aspiration pneumonitis. Vegetable oil will delay absorption of these substances. • Don't give after ingestion of caustic substances, such as lye; additional injury to the esophagus and mediastinum can occur. • Clearly indicate ipecac *syrup,* not single word "ipecac," to avoid confusion with fluidextract. Fluidextract is 14 times more concentrated and if advertently used instead of syrup may cause death. • Induces vomiting within 30 minutes in more than 90% of patients; average time usually less than 20 minutes. • Stomach is usually emptied completely; vomitus may contain some intestinal material as well. • In antiemetic toxicity, ipecac syrup is usually effective if less than 1 hour has passed since ingestion of antiemetic. • Recommend that 1 ounce of syrup be readily available in the home when child becomes 1 year old for immediate use in case of emergency. • No systemic toxicity with doses of 30 ml or less. • If two doses do not induce vomiting, gastric lavage is necessary.
None significant.	• Warn patient against driving and other activities that require alertness until CNS response to drug is determined. • Antihistamine with a slower onset and longer duration of action than other antihistamine antiemetics.
Anticholinergics, including antidepressant and anti-Parkinson agents: increased anticholinergic activity, aggravated Parkinson-like symptoms. Use to-	• Contraindicated in phenothiazine hypersensitivity, coma, depression, CNS depression, bone marrow depression, subcortical damage; during pediatric surgery, use of spinal or epidural anesthetic or adrenergic blocking agents, alcohol usage. Use with caution in combination with other CNS depressants; in hepatic disease, arteriosclerosis or cardiovascular disease (may cause sudden drop in blood pressure), exposure to extreme heat or cold (including antipyretic therapy), respiratory disorders, hypocalcemia, vomiting in children,

(continued on following page)

NAME	INDICATIONS & DOSAGE	SIDE EFFECTS
prochlorperazine *(continued)*	20 mg/liter isotonic solution by I.V. infusion, added to infusion 15 to 30 minutes before induction. Maximum parenteral dose 40 mg daily. *Severe nausea, vomiting—* **Adults:** 5 to 10 mg P.O. t.i.d. or q.i.d.; or 15 mg sustained-release form P.O. on arising; or 10 mg sustained-release form P.O. q 12 hours; or 25 mg rectally b.i.d. or 5 to 10 mg I.M. injected deeply into upper outer quadrant of gluteal region. Repeat q 3 to 4 hours, p.r.n. **Children 18 to 39 kg:** 2.5 mg P.O. or rectally t.i.d.; or 5 mg P.O. or rectally b.i.d. Maximum 15 mg daily; or 0.132 mg/kg deep I.M. injection. (Control usually obtained with 1 dose.) **Children 14 to 17 kg:** 2.5 mg P.O. or rectally b.i.d. or t.i.d. Maximum 10 mg daily; or 0.132 mg/kg deep I.M. injection. (Control usually obtained with 1 dose.) **Children 9 to 13 kg:** 2.5 mg P.O. or rectally daily or b.i.d. Maximum 7.5 mg daily; or 0.132 mg/kg deep I.M. injection. (Control usually obtained with 1 dose.)	**EENT:** *ocular changes, blurred vision.* **GI:** *dry mouth, constipation.* **GU:** *urinary retention,* dark urine, menstrual irregularities, gynecomastia, inhibited ejaculation. **Hepatic:** *cholestatic jaundice.* **Metabolic:** hyperprolactinemia. **Skin:** *mild photosensitivity,* dermal allergic reactions, *exfoliative dermatitis.* **Other:** weight gain, increased appetite.
scopolamine Transderm-V	*Prevention of nausea and vomiting associated with motion sickness—* **Adults:** One Transderm-V system (a circular flat unit) programmed to deliver 0.5 mg scopolamine over 3 days (72 hours), applied to the skin behind the ear several hours before the antiemetic is required. Not recommended for children.	**CNS:** *drowsiness,* restlessness, disorientation, confusion. **EENT:** *dry mouth,* transient impairment of eye accommodation.
thiethylperazine maleate Torecan♦	*Nausea, vomiting—* **Adults:** 10 mg P.O., I.M., or rectally daily, b.i.d. or t.i.d.	**Blood:** *transient leukopenia, agranulocytosis.* **CNS:** *extrapyramidal reactions (high incidence),* sedation (low incidence), pseudoparkinsonism, EEG changes, dizziness.

♦ Available in U.S. and Canada. ♦♦ Available in Canada only. All other products (no symbol) available in U.S. only. Italicized side effects are common or life-threatening.

INTERACTIONS	NURSING CONSIDERATIONS
gether cautiously. *Antacids:* inhibited absorption of oral phenothiazines. Separate antacid and phenothiazine dosage by at least 2 hours. *Barbiturates:* may decrease phenothiazine effect. Monitor patient for decreased antiemetic effect.	convulsive disorders or severe reactions to insulin or electroshock therapy, suspected brain tumor or intestinal obstruction, glaucoma, or prostatic hypertrophy; in acutely ill or dehydrated children; and in elderly or debilitated patients. • Store in light-resistant container. Slight yellowing does not affect potency; discard very discolored solutions. • Since drug has a very long duration of action, timed-release capsules have no significant advantage over ordinary oral dosage forms. • Use only when vomiting can't be controlled by other measures, or when only a few doses are required. If more than 4 doses needed in 24-hour period, notify doctor. • Not effective in motion sickness. • To prevent contact dermatitis, avoid getting concentrate or injection solution on hands or clothing. • Dilute oral concentrate with tomato or fruit juice, milk, coffee, carbonated beverage, tea, water, soup, or pudding. • Monitor CBC and liver function studies during prolonged therapy. Warn patients to wear protective clothing when exposed to sunlight. • Watch for orthostatic hypotension. • Do not give subcutaneously or mix in syringe with another drug. Give deep I.M. • For toxicity, see APPENDIX, *Drug Toxicities.*
None significant.	• Use cautiously in patients with glaucoma, pyloric obstruction, or urinary bladder neck obstruction. • Wash and dry hands thoroughly before applying the system on dry skin behind the ear. After removing the system, discard it, then wash hands and application site thoroughly. • If the system becomes displaced, remove and replace it with another system on a fresh skin site in the postauricular area. • A patient brochure is available with the product; tell patient to request it from the pharmacist. • Warn patient against driving and other activities that require alertness until response to drug is determined. • Sugarless hard candy may help minimize dry mouth. • Transderm-V is effective if applied 2 to 3 hours before experiencing motion but is more effective if used 12 hours before. Therefore, advise patient to apply system the night before a planned trip. • Transdermal method of administration releases a controlled therapeutic amount of scopolamine.
Anticholinergics, including antidepressants and anti-Parkinson agents: increased anticholinergic activity, aggra-	• Contraindicated in severe CNS depression, hepatic disease, coma, phenothiazine hypersensitivity. • Don't give I.V. • For nausea and vomiting associated with anesthesia and surgery, give deep I.M. injection on or shortly before terminating anesthesia. • Possibly effective in dizziness; not effective in motion sickness.

(continued on following page)

NAME	INDICATIONS & DOSAGE	SIDE EFFECTS
thiethylperazine maleate *(continued)*		**CV:** *orthostatic hypotension,* tachycardia, EKG changes. **EENT:** *ocular changes, blurred vision.* **GI:** *dry mouth, constipation.* **GU:** *urinary retention,* dark urine, menstrual irregularities, gynecomastia, inhibited ejaculation. **Hepatic:** *cholestatic jaundice.* **Metabolic:** hyperprolactinemia. **Skin:** *mild photosensitivity,* dermal allergic reactions, *exfoliative dermatitis.* **Other:** weight gain, increased appetite.
trimethobenzamide hydrochloride Tigan	*Nausea and vomiting (treatment)*— **Adults:** 250 mg P.O. t.i.d. or q.i.d.; or 200 mg I.M. or rectally t.i.d. or q.i.d. *Postoperative nausea and vomiting (prevention)*— **Adults:** 200 mg I.M. or rectally (single dose) before or during surgery; may repeat 3 hours after termination of anesthesia, p.r.n. **Children 13 to 40 kg:** 100 to 200 mg P.O. or rectally t.i.d. or q.i.d. **Children under 13 kg:** 100 mg rectally t.i.d. or q.i.d. Limited to prolonged vomiting of known etiology.	**CNS:** drowsiness, dizziness (in large doses). **CV:** hypotension. **GI:** diarrhea, exaggeration of preexisting nausea (in large doses). **Hepatic:** *liver toxicity.* **Local:** pain, stinging, burning, redness, swelling at I.M. injection site. **Skin:** skin hypersensitivity reactions. **Other:** antiemetic effect may mask signs of overdosage of toxic agents, or intestinal obstruction, brain tumor, or other conditions.

INTERACTIONS	NURSING CONSIDERATIONS
vated Parkinson-like symptoms. Use together cautiously. *Antacids:* inhibited absorption of oral phenothiazines. Separate antacid and phenothiazine dosage by at least 2 hours. *Barbiturates:* may decrease phenothiazine effect. Monitor for decreased antiemetic effect.	• Use only when vomiting can't be controlled by other measures, or when only a few doses are required. • Warn patient about hypotension. Advise him to stay in bed for 1 hour after receiving the drug. • If drug gets on skin, wash off at once to prevent contact dermatitis. • For toxicity, see APPENDIX, *Drug Toxicities*.
None significant.	• Contraindicated in children with viral illness (a possible cause of vomiting in children); may contribute to the development of Reye's syndrome, a potentially fatal acute childhood encephalopathy, characterized by fatty degeneration of the liver. • Suppositories contraindicated in hypersensitivity to benzocaine hydrochloride or similar local anesthetic. • Stop drug if allergic skin reaction occurs. • Give I.M. dose by deep injection into upper outer quadrant of gluteal region to reduce pain and local irritation. • Warn patient of the possibility of drowsiness and dizziness, and caution him against driving or other activities requiring alertness until CNS response to drug is determined. • Store suppositories in refrigerator. • Has little or no value in preventing motion sickness; limited value as antiemetic.

50 Gastrointestinal anticholinergics

Belladonna alkaloids
atropine sulfate
belladonna alkaloids
belladonna leaf
levorotatory alkaloids of belladonna
l-hyoscyamine sulfate

Quaternary anticholinergics
anisotropine methylbromide
clidinium bromide
diphemanil methylsulfate
glycopyrrolate
hexocyclium methylsulfate
homatropine methylbromide
isopropamide iodide
mepenzolate bromide
methantheline bromide
methscopolamine bromide
oxyphenonium bromide
propantheline bromide
tridihexethyl chloride

Tertiary synthetics (antispasmodics)
dicyclomine hydrochloride
methixene hydrochloride
oxyphencyclimine hydrochloride
thiphenamil hydrochloride

(All drugs are listed in alphabetical order in the tables that follow.)

Gastrointestinal (GI) anticholinergics may be used to relieve peptic ulcer pain; we lack evidence, however, that they heal peptic ulcers. Anticholinergics inhibit GI smooth-muscle contraction and delay gastric emptying, thus enhancing the action of antacids. The anticholinergics should not be the sole basis of treatment, but rather part of a total therapeutic program.

Major uses

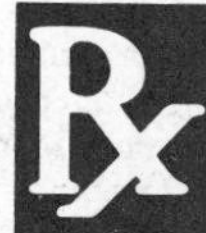

GI anticholinergics are therapeutic adjuncts for pain associated with peptic ulcers. They are also used to treat irritable colon (mucous colitis, spastic colon, and acute enterocolitis), other functional GI disorders, and neurogenic bowel disturbances, including splenic flexure syndrome and neurogenic colon.

Mechanism of action

• Belladonna alkaloids and quaternary anticholinergics block the actions of acetylcholine on the vagus nerve. (This blocking mechanism is known as competitive inhibition.) They decrease GI motility and inhibit gastric acid secretion.
• Tertiary synthetics exert a nonspecific direct spasmolytic action on smooth muscle. They also possess local anesthetic properties that may be partly responsible for the spasmolysis.

Absorption, distribution, metabolism, and excretion

• Belladonna alkaloids and tertiary synthetics are rapidly absorbed after oral administration. Because they readily cross the blood-brain barrier, they cause significant central nervous system (CNS) side effects. They are

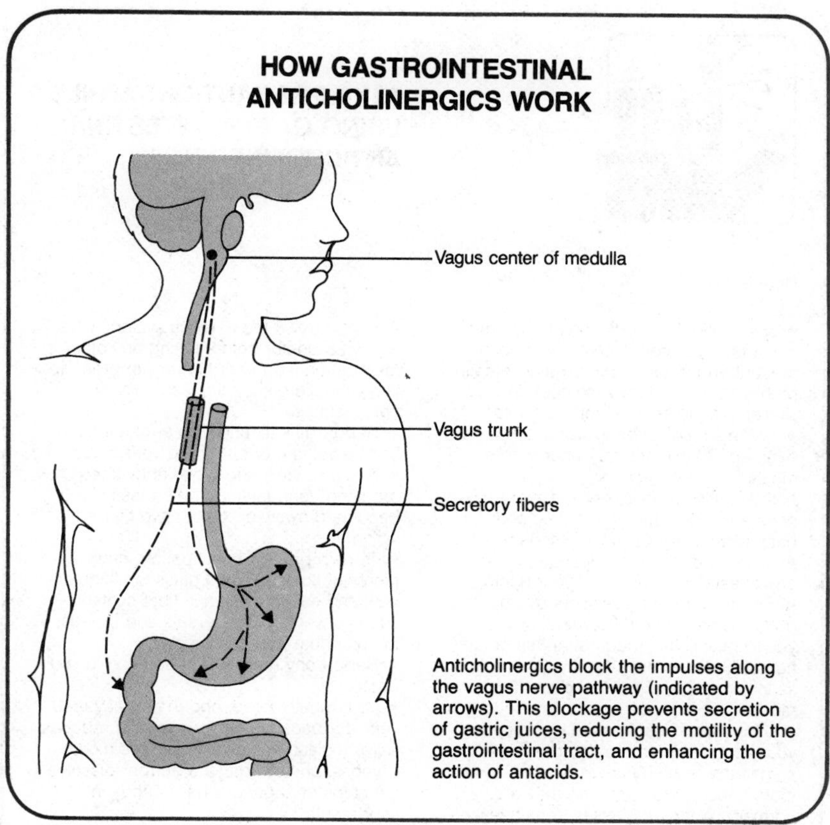

metabolized in the liver and eliminated both in urine and—through the bile—in feces.

HOW GASTROINTESTINAL ANTICHOLINERGICS WORK
Vagus center of medulla
Vagus trunk
Secretory fibers
Anticholinergics block the impulses along the vagus nerve pathway (indicated by arrows). This blockage prevents secretion of gastric juices, reducing the motility of the gastrointestinal tract, and enhancing the action of antacids.

• Quaternary anticholinergics are poorly and unreliably absorbed after oral administration. Since they *do not* cross the blood-brain barrier, their CNS side effects are negligible.

Onset and duration

Parenteral GI anticholinergics have a quicker onset and shorter duration than oral forms. Onset is usually 30 to 60 minutes, and duration 4 to 6 hours after oral administration.

• Belladonna alkaloids' effects usually last about 4 hours.

• Effects of the quaternary anticholinergics (except isopropamide) and the tertiary synthetics (except oxyphencyclimine) last 6 hours.

• Isopropamide and oxyphencyclimine have durations as long as 12 hours.

Combination products

BARBIDONNA ELIXIR: atropine sulfate 0.034 mg/5 ml, phenobarbital 21.6 mg/5 ml, hyoscyamine hydrobromide or sulfate 0.174 mg/5 ml, hyoscine hydrobromide 0.01 mg/5 ml, and alcohol 15%.

BARBIDONNA TABLETS: atropine sulfate 0.025 mg, hyoscine hydrobromide 0.0074 mg, hyoscyamine hydrobromide or sulfate 0.1286 mg, and phenobarbital 16 mg.

BARBIDONNA #2 TABLETS: atropine sulfate 0.025 mg, hyoscine hydrobromide 0.0074 mg, hyoscyamine hydrobromide or sulfate 0.1286 mg, and phenobarbital 32 mg.

BELLADENAL TABLETS♦: L-alkaloids of

PATIENT-TEACHING AID

TAKE PRECAUTIONS WHILE USING GASTROINTESTINAL ANTICHOLINERGICS

Dear Patient:

• Don't give this medication to others or use it for other conditions. It has been prescribed for your current gastrointestinal problem only. If a family member develops similar symptoms, contact the doctor.
• For this medication to work, take it as directed, 30 minutes to 1 hour before meals.
• If you miss a dose, don't take the missed dose and don't double the next one; go back to your regular dosing schedule. Also, don't change the dosage. If you have any questions, check with your doctor.
• Be careful not to become overheated during exercise or in hot weather while you're taking this medication, since heatstroke may develop. Hot baths or saunas may make you feel dizzy. This medication reduces your tolerance to heat, since it makes you perspire less, causing your body temperature to increase.
• This medication may make your eyes more sensitive to light than they are normally. Wear sunglasses to help lessen the discomfort from bright light.
• This medication increases the effects of alcoholic beverages and certain drugs that slow down the nervous system. Check with your doctor before taking any other medication—prescription or nonprescription—for allergies, pain, insomnia, or nervousness.
• Report difficult urination or changes in urinary volume or pattern to your doctor.
• Avoid driving and other activities requiring coordination or alertness if you become drowsy, dizzy, or have blurred vision.
• To help prevent constipation, drink plenty of fluids (8 to 10 glasses of liquid/day) and eat foods high in fiber content, such as whole-grain cereals and breads, to contribute bulk to your diet.
• Report any rash or skin eruption to your doctor.
• Your mouth, nose, and throat may feel very dry because this medication reduces salivary gland secretion. To relieve mouth dryness, chew sugarless gum or dissolve ice chips or sugarless hard candy in your mouth.
• If you want more information about this medication, don't hesitate to check with your doctor, nurse, or pharmacist.

belladonna 0.25 mg and phenobarbital 50 mg.
BENTYL WITH PHENOBARBITAL SYRUP: dicyclomine hydrochloride 10 mg/5 ml, phenobarbital 15 mg/5 ml, and alcohol 19%.
BENTYL 10 MG WITH PHENOBARBITAL CAPSULES: dicyclomine hydrochloride 10 mg and phenobarbital 15 mg.
BENTYL 20 MG WITH PHENOBARBITAL TABLETS: dicyclomine hydrochloride 20 mg and phenobarbital 15 mg.
BUTIBEL ELIXIR: belladonna extract 15 mg/5 ml, butabarbital sodium 15 mg/5 ml, and alcohol 7%.
BUTIBEL TABLETS: belladonna extract 15 mg and butabarbital sodium 15 mg.
CANTIL WITH PHENOBARBITAL TABLETS: mepenzolate bromide 25 mg and phenobarbital 16 mg.
CHARDONNA-2: belladonna extract 15 mg and phenobarbital 15 mg.
COMBID SPANSULES♦: isopropamide iodide 5 mg and prochlorperazine maleate 10 mg.
DARICON PB TABLETS: oxyphencyclimine hydrochloride 5 mg and phenobarbital 15 mg.

DONNATAL ELIXIR♦: atropine sulfate 0.0194 mg/5 ml, hyoscine hydrobromide 0.0065 mg/5 ml, alcohol 23%, hyoscyamine hydrobromide or sulfate 0.1037 mg/5 ml and phenobarbital 16 mg/5 ml.

DONNATAL EXTENTABS♦: atropine sulfate 0.0582 mg, hyoscine hydrobromide 0.0195 mg, hyoscyamine sulfate 0.3111 mg, and phenobarbital 48.6 mg.

DONNATAL TABLETS AND CAPSULES♦: atropine sulfate 0.0194 mg, hyoscine hydrobromide 0.0065 mg, hyoscyamine hydrobromide or sulfate 0.1037 mg, and phenobarbital 16 mg.

DONNATAL #2 TABLETS: atropine sulfate 0.0194 mg, hyoscine hydrobromide 0.0065 mg, hyoscyamine hydrobromide or sulfate 0.1037 mg, and phenobarbital 32.4 mg.

ENARAX 5 TABLETS: oxyphencyclimine hydrochloride 5 mg and hydroxyzine hydrochloride 25 mg.

ENARAX 10 TABLETS: oxyphencyclimine hydrochloride 10 mg and hydroxyzine hydrochloride 25 mg.

HYBEPHEN ELIXIR: atropine sulfate 0.0233 mg/5 ml, hyoscine hydrobromide 0.0094 mg/5 ml, hyoscyamine hydrobromide or sulfate 0.1277 mg/5 ml, phenobarbital 15 mg/5 ml, and alcohol 16.5%.

KINESED TABLETS: atropine sulfate 0.02 mg, hyoscine hydrobromide 0.007 mg, hyoscyamine hydrobromide or sulfate 0.1 mg, and phenobarbital 16 mg.

LIBRAX CAPSULES: clidinium bromide 2.5 mg and chlordiazepoxide hydrochloride 5 mg.

MILPATH 200 TABLETS: tridihexethyl chloride 25 mg and meprobamate 200 mg.

MILPATH 400 TABLETS: tridihexethyl chloride 25 mg and meprobamate 400 mg.

PATHIBAMATE 200 TABLETS: tridihexethyl chloride 25 mg and meprobamate 200 mg.

PATHIBAMATE 400 TABLETS: tridihexethyl chloride 25 mg and meprobamate 400 mg.

PATHILON WITH PHENOBARBITAL TABLETS: tridihexethyl chloride 25 mg and phenobarbital 15 mg.

PRO-BANTHINE WITH PHENOBARBITAL TABLETS♦: propantheline bromide 15 mg and phenobarbital 15 mg.

ROBINUL PH TABLETS♦: glycopyrrolate 1 mg in addition to phenobarbital 16.2 mg.

ROBINUL PH FORTE TABLETS♦: glycopyrrolate 2 mg and phenobarbital 16.2 mg.

VALPIN 50-PB TABLETS: anisotropine methylbromide 50 mg and phenobarbital 15 mg.

VISTRAX 10 TABLETS: oxyphencyclimine hydrochloride 10 mg and hydroxyzine hydrochloride 25 mg.

NAME	INDICATIONS & DOSAGE	SIDE EFFECTS
anisotropine methylbromide Valpin 50	*Adjunctive treatment of peptic ulcer—* **Adults:** 50 mg P.O. t.i.d. To be effective should be titrated to individual patient needs.	**CNS:** headache, insomnia, drowsiness, dizziness, *confusion or excitement in elderly patients,* nervousness, weakness. **CV:** *palpitations,* tachycardia. **EENT:** *blurred vision,* mydriasis, increased ocular tension, cycloplegia, photophobia. **GI:** *dry mouth,* dysphagia, heartburn, loss of taste, nausea, vomiting, *paralytic ileus, constipation.* **GU:** *urinary hesitancy and retention,* impotence. **Skin:** urticaria, decreased sweating and possible anhidrosis, other dermal manifestations. **Other:** fever, allergic reactions. Overdosage may cause curare-like symptoms.
atropine sulfate	*Adjunctive therapy in peptic ulcers, irritable bowel syndrome, neurogenic bowel disturbances, and functional gastrointestinal disorders—* **Adults:** 0.4 to 0.6 mg P.O. q 4 to 6 hours. **Children:** the following dosages P.O. q 4 to 6 hours: 3 to 7 kg—0.1 mg ($^1/_{600}$ gr) 8 to 11 kg—0.15 mg ($^1/_{400}$ gr) 11 to 18 kg—0.2 mg ($^1/_{300}$ gr) 18 to 30 kg—0.3 mg ($^1/_{200}$ gr) 30 to 41 kg—0.4 mg ($^1/_{150}$ gr) over 41 kg—0.4 to 0.6 mg ($^1/_{150}$ to $^1/_{100}$ gr)	**CNS:** headache, insomnia, drowsiness, dizziness, *confusion or excitement in elderly patients,* nervousness, weakness. **CV:** *palpitations,* tachycardia. **EENT:** *blurred vision,* mydriasis, increased ocular tension, cycloplegia, photophobia. **GI:** *dry mouth,* dysphagia, heartburn, loss of taste, nausea, vomiting, paralytic ileus. **GU:** *urinary hesitancy and retention,* impotence. **Skin:** urticaria, decreased sweating or anhidrosis, other dermal manifestations. **Other:** fever, allergic reactions. Overdosage may cause curare-like symptoms.
belladonna alkaloids	*Adjunctive therapy in gastric, peptic, duodenal, or intestinal ulcers to control excess motor activity, hyperirritability or spasm of the gastrointestinal tract—* **Adults:** 0.4 to 0.8 mg (timed-release capsules) P.O. q 12 hours.	**CNS:** headache, insomnia, drowsiness, dizziness, *confusion or excitement in elderly patients,* nervousness, weakness. **CV:** *palpitations,* tachycardia. **EENT:** *blurred vision,* mydriasis, increased ocular tension, cycloplegia, photophobia. **GI:** *dry mouth,* dysphagia, heartburn, loss of taste. **GU:** *urinary hesitancy and retention,* impotence. **Skin:** urticaria, decreased sweating or anhidrosis, other dermal manifestations.

INTERACTIONS	NURSING CONSIDERATIONS
None significant.	• Contraindicated in narrow-angle glaucoma, obstructive uropathy, obstructive disease of the GI tract, severe ulcerative colitis, myasthenia gravis, hypersensitivity to anticholinergics, paralytic ileus, intestinal atony, unstable cardiovascular status in acute hemorrhage, and toxic megacolon. Use cautiously in autonomic neuropathy, hyperthyroidism, coronary artery disease, cardiac arrhythmias, congestive heart failure, hypertension, hiatal hernia associated with reflux esophagitis, hepatic or renal disease, ulcerative colitis, or in patients over age 40 because of increased incidence of glaucoma. • Use with caution in hot or humid environments. Drug-induced heatstroke can develop. • Give 30 minutes to 1 hour before meals. • Administer smaller doses to the elderly. • Monitor patient's vital signs and urinary output carefully. • Instruct patient to avoid driving and other hazardous activities if he is drowsy, dizzy, or has blurred vision; to drink plenty of fluids to help prevent constipation; to report any skin rash or local eruption. • Gum or sugarless hard candy may relieve mouth dryness. • For toxicity, see APPENDIX, *Drug Toxicities*.
None significant.	• Contraindicated in narrow-angle glaucoma, obstructive uropathy, obstructive disease of GI tract, severe ulcerative colitis, myasthenia gravis, hypersensitivity to anticholinergics, paralytic ileus, intestinal atony, unstable cardiovascular status in acute hemorrhage, toxic megacolon. Use cautiously in autonomic neuropathy, hyperthyroidism, coronary artery disease, cardiac arrhythmias, congestive heart failure, hypertension, hiatal hernia associated with reflux esophagitis, hepatic or renal disease, ulcerative colitis, or in patients over age 40 because of increased incidence of glaucoma. • Use with caution in hot or humid environments. Drug-induced heatstroke can develop. • Give 30 minutes to 1 hour before meals and at bedtime. Bedtime dose can be larger; give 2 hours after last meal of day. • Administer smaller doses to the elderly. • Monitor patient's vital signs and urinary output carefully. • Instruct patient to avoid driving and other hazardous activities if he is drowsy, dizzy, or has blurred vision; to drink plenty of fluids to help prevent constipation; to report any skin rash. • Gum, sugarless hard candy, or pilocarpine syrup may relieve mouth dryness. • Other anticholinergic drugs may increase vagal blockage. • For toxicity, see APPENDIX, *Drug Toxicities*.
None significant.	• Contraindicated in narrow-angle glaucoma, obstructive uropathy, obstructive disease of GI tract, severe ulcerative colitis, myasthenia gravis, hypersensitivity to anticholinergics, paralytic ileus, intestinal atony, unstable cardiovascular status in acute hemorrhage, toxic megacolon. Use cautiously in autonomic neuropathy, hyperthyroidism, coronary artery disease, cardiac arrhythmias, congestive heart failure, hypertension, hiatal hernia with reflux esophagitis, hepatic or renal disease, ulcerative colitis, or in patients over age 40 because of increased incidence of glaucoma. • Use with caution in hot or humid environments. Drug-induced heatstroke can develop. • Administer smaller doses to the elderly. • Instruct patient to avoid driving and other hazardous activities if he is drowsy, dizzy, or has blurred vision; to drink plenty of fluids to help prevent constipation; and to report any skin rash.

(continued on following page)

NAME	INDICATIONS & DOSAGE	SIDE EFFECTS
belladonna alkaloids *(continued)*		**Other:** fever, allergic reactions. Overdosage may cause curare-like symptoms.
belladonna leaf (used to prepare extract, fluidextract, and tincture) Belladonna Tincture USP, Belladonna Fluidextract	*Adjunctive therapy for peptic ulcer, irritable bowel syndrome, functional gastrointestinal disorders, and neurogenic bowel disturbances—* **Adults:** 10.8 to 21.6 mg P.O. t.i.d. or q.i.d. of the extract; 0.06 ml P.O. t.i.d. or q.i.d. of the fluidextract; 0.6 to 1 ml t.i.d. or q.i.d. of tincture.	**CNS:** headache, insomnia, drowsiness, dizziness, *confusion or excitement in elderly patients,* nervousness, weakness. **CV:** *palpitations,* tachycardia. **EENT:** *blurred vision,* mydriasis, increased ocular tension, cycloplegia, photophobia. **GI:** *dry mouth,* dysphagia, heartburn, loss of taste, *constipation,* nausea, vomiting. **GU:** *urinary hesitancy and retention,* impotence. **Skin:** urticaria, decreased sweating or anhidrosis, other dermal manifestations. **Other:** fever, allergic reactions. Overdosage may cause curare-like symptoms.
clidinium bromide Quarzan	*Adjunctive therapy for peptic ulcers—* Dosage should be individualized according to severity of symptoms and occurrence of side effects. **Adults:** 2.5 to 5 mg P.O. t.i.d. or q.i.d. before meals and at bedtime. **Geriatric or debilitated patients:** 2.5 mg P.O. t.i.d. before meals.	**CNS:** headache, insomnia, drowsiness, dizziness, *confusion or excitement in elderly patients,* nervousness, weakness. **CV:** *palpitations,* tachycardia. **EENT:** *blurred vision,* mydriasis, increased ocular tension, cycloplegia, photophobia. **GI:** *dry mouth,* dysphagia, heartburn, loss of taste, nausea, vomiting, *paralytic ileus, constipation.* **GU:** *urinary hesitancy and retention,* impotence. **Skin:** urticaria, decreased sweating or anhidrosis, other dermal manifestations. **Other:** fever, allergic reactions. Overdosage may cause curare-like symptoms.
dicyclomine hydrochloride Antispas, Bentyl, Bentylol♦♦, Cyclobec♦♦, Dibent, Dicen, Formulex♦♦, Menospasm♦♦, Nospaz, Or-Tyl, Rocyclo, Rotyl HCl,	*Adjunctive therapy for peptic ulcers and other functional gastrointestinal disorders—* **Adults:** 10 to 20 mg P.O. t.i.d. or q.i.d.; 20 mg I.M. q 4 to 6 hours. **Children:** 10 mg P.O. t.i.d. or q.i.d. *Infant colic—* **Infants:** 5 mg P.O. t.i.d. or q.i.d.	**CNS:** *headache,* insomnia, drowsiness, *dizziness.* **CV:** *palpitations,* tachycardia. **GI:** nausea, *constipation,* vomiting, *paralytic ileus.* **GU:** urinary hesitancy and retention, impotence. **Skin:** urticaria, decreased sweating or anhidrosis, other dermal manifestations. **Other:** fever, allergic reactions.

♦ Available in U.S. and Canada. ♦♦ Available in Canada only. All other products (no symbol) available in U.S. only. Italicized side effects are common or life-threatening.

INTERACTIONS	NURSING CONSIDERATIONS
	• Monitor patient's vital signs and urinary output carefully. • For toxicity, see APPENDIX, *Drug Toxicities*.
None significant.	• Contraindicated in narrow-angle glaucoma, obstructive uropathy, obstructive disease of GI tract, severe ulcerative colitis, myasthenia gravis, hypersensitivity to anticholinergics, paralytic ileus, intestinal atony, unstable cardiovascular status in acute hemorrhage, and toxic megacolon. Use cautiously in autonomic neuropathy, hyperthyroidism, coronary artery disease, cardiac arrhythmias, congestive heart failure, hypertension, hiatal hernia associated with reflux esophagitis, hepatic or renal disease, ulcerative colitis, or in patients over age 40 because of increased incidence of glaucoma. • Give 30 minutes to 1 hour before meals and at bedtime. Bedtime dose can be larger and should be given at least 2 hours after last meal of day. • Administer smaller doses to the elderly. • Use with caution in hot or humid environments. Drug-induced heatstroke can develop. • Monitor patient's vital signs and urinary output carefully. • Instruct patient to avoid driving and other hazardous activities if he is drowsy, dizzy, or has blurred vision; to drink plenty of fluids to help prevent constipation; to report any skin rash. • Gum or sugarless hard candy may relieve mouth dryness. • For toxicity, see APPENDIX, *Drug Toxicities*.
None significant.	• Contraindicated in narrow-angle glaucoma, obstructive uropathy, obstructive disease of GI tract, severe ulcerative colitis, myasthenia gravis, hypersensitivity to anticholinergics, paralytic ileus, intestinal atony, unstable cardiovascular status in acute hemorrhage, and toxic megacolon. Use cautiously in autonomic neuropathy, hyperthyroidism, coronary artery disease, cardiac arrhythmias, congestive heart failure, hypertension, hiatal hernia associated with reflux esophagitis, hepatic or renal disease, ulcerative colitis, or in patients over age 40 because of increased incidence of glaucoma. • Give 30 minutes to 1 hour before meals and at bedtime. Bedtime dose can be larger; give 2 hours after last meal of day. • Administer smaller doses to the elderly. • Use with caution in hot or humid environments. Drug-induced heatstroke may develop. • Monitor patient's vital signs and urinary output carefully. • Instruct patient to avoid driving and other hazardous activities if he is drowsy, dizzy, or has blurred vision; to drink plenty of fluids to help prevent constipation; and to report any skin rash or local eruption. • Gum or sugarless hard candy may relieve mouth dryness. • For toxicity, see APPENDIX, *Drug Toxicities*.
None significant.	• Contraindicated in obstructive uropathy, obstructive disease of GI tract, severe ulcerative colitis, myasthenia gravis, hypersensitivity to anticholinergics, paralytic ileus, intestinal atony, unstable cardiovascular status in acute hemorrhage, and toxic megacolon. Use cautiously in autonomic neuropathy, narrow-angle glaucoma, hyperthyroidism, coronary artery disease, cardiac arrhythmias, congestive heart failure, hypertension, hiatal hernia associated with reflux esophagitis, hepatic or renal disease, ulcerative colitis. • Use with caution in hot or humid environments. Drug-induced heatstroke can develop. • Give 30 minutes to 1 hour before meals and at bedtime. Bedtime

(continued on following page)

NAME	INDICATIONS & DOSAGE	SIDE EFFECTS
dicyclomine hydrochloride *(continued)* Stannitol, Viscerol♦♦	Always adjust dosage according to patient's needs and response.	Overdosage may cause curare-like symptoms.
diphemanil methylsulfate Prantal	*Adjunctive therapy in gastric hypersecretion associated with duodenal ulcer*— **Adults:** 100 to 200 mg P.O. q 4 to 6 hours, between meals (initial dose). Daily dosage should be adjusted according to response and tolerance. Maintenance dose: 50 to 100 mg q 4 to 6 hours.	**CNS:** headache, insomnia, drowsiness, dizziness, *confusion or excitement in elderly patients,* nervousness, weakness. **CV:** *palpitations,* tachycardia. **EENT:** *blurred vision,* mydriasis, increased ocular tension, cycloplegia, photophobia. **GI:** *dry mouth,* dysphagia, *constipation,* heartburn, loss of taste, nausea, vomiting, *paralytic ileus.* **GU:** *urinary hesitancy and retention,* impotence. **Skin:** urticaria, decreased sweating, anhidrosis, other dermal manifestations. **Other:** fever, allergic reactions. Overdosage may cause curare-like symptoms.
glycopyrrolate Robinul♦, Robinul Forte♦	*Adjunctive therapy in peptic ulcers and other gastrointestinal disorders*— **Adults:** 1 to 2 mg P.O. t.i.d. or 0.1 mg I.M. t.i.d. or q.i.d. Dosage should be individualized.	**CNS:** headache, insomnia, drowsiness, dizziness, *confusion or excitement in elderly patients,* nervousness, weakness. **CV:** *palpitations,* tachycardia. **EENT:** *blurred vision,* mydriasis, increased ocular tension, cycloplegia, photophobia. **GI:** *dry mouth,* dysphagia, *constipation,* heartburn, loss of taste, nausea, vomiting, *paralytic ileus.* **GU:** *urinary hesitancy and retention,* impotence. **Skin:** urticaria, decreased sweating or anhidrosis, other dermal manifestations. **Other:** fever, allergic reactions. Overdosage may cause curare-like symptoms.
hexocyclium methylsulfate Tral	*Adjunctive therapy in peptic ulcer and other gastrointestinal disorders*— **Adults:** 25 mg q.i.d. before meals and h.s.	**CNS:** headache, insomnia, drowsiness, dizziness, *confusion or excitement in elderly patients,* nervousness, weakness. **CV:** *palpitations,* tachycardia.

♦ Available in U.S. and Canada. ♦♦ Available in Canada only. All other products (no symbol) available in U.S. only. Italicized side effects are common or life-threatening.

INTERACTIONS	NURSING CONSIDERATIONS
	dose can be larger and should be given at least 2 hours after last meal of day. • Administer smaller doses to the elderly. • Monitor patient's vital signs and urinary output carefully. • Instruct patient to avoid driving and other hazardous activities if he is drowsy, dizzy, or has blurred vision; to drink plenty of fluids to help prevent constipation; and to report any skin rash. • Gum or sugarless hard candy may relieve mouth dryness. • A synthetic tertiary derivative that is relatively free of atropine-like side effects. • For toxicity, see APPENDIX, *Drug Toxicities*.
None significant.	• Contraindicated in narrow-angle glaucoma, obstructive uropathy, obstructive disease of GI tract, severe ulcerative colitis, myasthenia gravis, hypersensitivity to anticholinergics, paralytic ileus, intestinal atony, unstable cardiovascular status in acute hemorrhage, and toxic megacolon. Use cautiously in autonomic neuropathy, hyperthyroidism, coronary artery disease, cardiac arrhythmias, congestive heart failure, hypertension, hiatal hernia associated with reflux esophagitis, hepatic or renal disease, ulcerative colitis, or in patients over age 40 because of increased incidence of glaucoma. • Use with caution in hot or humid environments. Drug-induced heatstroke can develop. • Give 30 minutes to 1 hour before meals and at bedtime. Bedtime dose can be larger and should be given at least 2 hours after last meal of day. • Administer smaller doses to the elderly. • Monitor patient's vital signs and urinary output carefully. • Instruct patient to avoid driving and other hazardous activities if he is drowsy, dizzy, or has blurred vision; to drink plenty of fluids to help prevent constipation; and to report any skin rash. • Gum or sugarless hard candy may relieve mouth dryness. • For toxicity, see APPENDIX, *Drug Toxicities*.
None significant.	• Contraindicated in narrow-angle glaucoma, obstructive uropathy, obstructive disease of GI tract, severe ulcerative colitis, myasthenia gravis, hypersensitivity to anticholinergics, paralytic ileus, intestinal atony, unstable cardiovascular status in acute hemorrhage, and toxic megacolon. Use cautiously in autonomic neuropathy, hyperthyroidism, coronary artery disease, cardiac arrhythmias, congestive heart failure, hypertension, hiatal hernia associated with reflux esophagitis, hepatic or renal disease, ulcerative colitis, or in patients over age 40 because of increased incidence of glaucoma. • Use with caution in hot or humid environments. Drug-induced heatstroke can develop. • Administer 30 minutes to 1 hour before meals. • Administer smaller doses to the elderly. • Monitor patient's vital signs and urinary output carefully. • Instruct patient to avoid driving and other hazardous activities if he is drowsy, dizzy, or has blurred vision; to drink plenty of fluids to help prevent constipation; to report any skin rash. • Gum or sugarless hard candy may relieve mouth dryness. • For toxicity, see APPENDIX, *Drug Toxicities*.
None significant.	• Contraindicated in narrow-angle glaucoma, obstructive uropathy, obstructive disease of GI tract, severe ulcerative colitis, myasthenia gravis, hypersensitivity to anticholinergics, paralytic ileus, intestinal atony, unstable cardiovascular status in acute hemorrhage, toxic megacolon. Use cautiously in autonomic neuropathy, hyperthyroid-

(continued on following page)

NAME	INDICATIONS & DOSAGE	SIDE EFFECTS
hexocyclium methylsulfate *(continued)*		**EENT:** *blurred vision,* mydriasis, increased ocular tension, cycloplegia, photophobia. **GI:** *dry mouth,* dysphagia, heartburn, loss of taste, nausea, *constipation,* vomiting, *paralytic ileus.* **GU:** *urinary hesitancy and retention,* impotence. **Skin:** urticaria, decreased sweating or anhidrosis, other dermal manifestations. **Other:** fever, allergic reactions. Overdosage may cause curare-like symptoms.
homatropine methylbromide Ru-Spas No. 2, Sed-Tens SE	*Treatment of gastrointestinal spasm, hyperchlorhydria, and other mild spastic conditions of the bile ducts and gallbladder*— **Adults:** 2.5 to 5 mg t.i.d. to q.i.d. before meals and h.s.	**CNS:** headache, insomnia, drowsiness, dizziness, *confusion or excitement in elderly patients,* nervousness, weakness. **CV:** *palpitations,* tachycardia. **EENT:** *blurred vision,* mydriasis, increased ocular tension, cycloplegia, photophobia. **GI:** *dry mouth,* dysphagia, *constipation,* heartburn, loss of taste, nausea, vomiting, *paralytic ileus.* **GU:** *urinary hesitancy and retention,* impotence. **Skin:** urticaria, decreased sweating or anhidrosis, other dermal manifestations. **Other:** fever, allergic reactions. Overdosage may cause curare-like symptoms.
isopropamide iodide Darbid♦	*Adjunctive therapy for peptic ulcer, irritable bowel syndrome*— **Adults, and children over 12 years:** 5 mg P.O. q 12 hours. Some patients may require 10 mg or more b.i.d. Dose should be individualized to patient's need.	**CNS:** headache, insomnia, drowsiness, dizziness, *confusion or excitement in elderly patients,* nervousness, weakness. **CV:** *palpitations,* tachycardia. **EENT:** *blurred vision,* mydriasis, increased ocular tension, cycloplegia, photophobia. **GI:** *dry mouth,* dysphagia, heartburn, loss of taste, nausea, vomiting, *constipation, paralytic ileus.* **GU:** *urinary hesitancy and retention,* impotence. **Skin:** urticaria, decreased sweating or anhidrosis, other dermal manifestations, iodine skin rash.

♦ Available in U.S. and Canada. ♦♦ Available in Canada only. All other products (no symbol) available in U.S. only. Italicized side effects are common or life-threatening.

INTERACTIONS	NURSING CONSIDERATIONS
	ism, coronary artery disease, cardiac arrhythmias, congestive heart failure, hypertension, hiatal hernia associated with reflux esophagitis, hepatic or renal disease, ulcerative colitis, or in patients over age 40 because of increased incidence of glaucoma. • Use with caution in hot or humid environments. Drug-induced heatstroke can develop. • Give 30 minutes to 1 hour before meals and at bedtime. Bedtime dose can be larger and should be given at least 2 hours after last meal of day. • Administer smaller doses to the elderly. • Monitor patient's vital signs and urinary output carefully. • Instruct patient to avoid driving and other hazardous activities if he is drowsy, dizzy, or has blurred vision; to drink plenty of fluids to help prevent constipation; and to report any skin rash. • Gum or sugarless hard candy may relieve mouth dryness. • Tablets contain tartrazine dye. May cause allergy in susceptible patients. • For toxicity, see APPENDIX, *Drug Toxicities*.
None significant.	• Contraindicated in narrow-angle glaucoma, obstructive uropathy, obstructive disease of GI tract, severe ulcerative colitis, myasthenia gravis, hypersensitivity to anticholinergics, paralytic ileus, intestinal atony, unstable cardiovascular status in acute hemorrhage, and toxic megacolon. Use cautiously in autonomic neuropathy, hyperthyroidism, coronary artery disease, cardiac arrhythmias, congestive heart failure, hypertension, hiatal hernia associated with reflux esophagitis, hepatic or renal disease, ulcerative colitis, or in patients over age 40 because of increased incidence of glaucoma. • Use with caution in hot or humid environments. Drug-induced heatstroke can develop. • Give 30 minutes to 1 hour before meals and at bedtime. Bedtime dose can be larger and should be given at least 2 hours after last meal of day. • Administer smaller doses to the elderly. • Monitor patient's vital signs and urinary output carefully. • Instruct patient to avoid driving and other hazardous activities if he is drowsy, dizzy, or has blurred vision; to drink plenty of fluids to help prevent constipation; and to report any skin rash. • Gum or sugarless hard candy may relieve mouth dryness. • For toxicity, see APPENDIX, *Drug Toxicities*.
None significant.	• Contraindicated in narrow-angle glaucoma, obstructive uropathy, obstructive disease of GI tract, severe ulcerative colitis, myasthenia gravis, hypersensitivity to anticholinergics, paralytic ileus, intestinal atony, unstable cardiovascular status in acute hemorrhage, toxic megacolon. Use cautiously in autonomic neuropathy, hyperthyroidism, coronary artery disease, cardiac arrhythmias, congestive heart failure, hypertension, hiatal hernia associated with reflux esophagitis, hepatic or renal disease, ulcerative colitis, or in patients over age 40 because of increased incidence of glaucoma. • Use with caution in hot or humid environments. Drug-induced heatstroke can develop. • Give 30 minutes to 1 hour before meals and at bedtime. Bedtime dose can be larger and should be given at least 2 hours after the last meal of the day. • Administer smaller doses to the elderly. • Monitor patient's vital signs and urinary output carefully.

(continued on following page)

NAME	INDICATIONS & DOSAGE	SIDE EFFECTS
isopropamide iodide *(continued)*		**Other:** fever, allergic reactions. Overdosage may cause curare-like symptoms.
levorotatory alkaloids of belladonna (as maleate salts) Bellafoline	*Adjunctive therapy for peptic ulcer, irritable bowel syndrome, and functional gastrointestinal disorders—* **Adults:** 0.25 to 0.5 mg P.O. t.i.d.; or 0.125 to 0.5 mg S.C. daily or b.i.d. **Children over 6 years:** 0.125 to 0.25 mg P.O. t.i.d.	**CNS:** headache, insomnia, drowsiness, dizziness, *confusion or excitement in elderly patients,* nervousness, weakness. **CV:** *palpitations,* tachycardia. **EENT:** *blurred vision,* mydriasis, increased ocular tension, cycloplegia, photophobia. **GI:** *dry mouth,* dysphagia, heartburn, loss of taste, *constipation, paralytic ileus.* **GU:** *urinary hesitancy and retention,* impotence. **Skin:** urticaria, decreased sweating or anhidrosis, other dermal manifestations. **Other:** fever, allergic reactions. Overdosage may cause curare-like symptoms.
l-hyoscyamine sulfate Anaspaz, Levsin♦, Levsinex, Levsinex Time Caps	*Treatment of gastrointestinal tract disorders due to spasm; adjunctive therapy for peptic ulcers—* **Adults:** 0.125 to 0.25 mg P.O. t.i.d. or q.i.d. before meals and at bedtime; sustained-release form 0.375 mg P.O. q 12 hours; or 0.25 to 0.5 mg (1 or 2 ml) I.M., I.V., or S.C. q 6 hours. (Substitute oral medication when symptoms are controlled.) **Children 2 to 10 years:** ½ adult dose P.O. **Children under 2 years:** ¼ adult dose P.O.	**CNS:** headache, insomnia, drowsiness, dizziness, *confusion or excitement in elderly patients,* nervousness, weakness. **CV:** *palpitations,* tachycardia. **EENT:** *blurred vision,* mydriasis, increased ocular tension, cycloplegia, photophobia. **GI:** *dry mouth,* dysphagia, *constipation,* heartburn, loss of taste, nausea, vomiting, *paralytic ileus.* **GU:** *urinary hesitancy and retention,* impotence. **Skin:** urticaria, decreased sweating or anhidrosis, other dermal manifestations. **Other:** fever, allergic reactions. Overdosage may cause curare-like symptoms.
mepenzolate bromide Cantil	*Adjunctive therapy in treating peptic ulcer, irritable bowel syndrome, and neurologic bowel disturbances—* **Adults:** 25 to 50 mg P.O. q.i.d. with meals and at bedtime. Ad-	**CNS:** headache, insomnia, drowsiness, dizziness, *confusion or excitement in elderly patients,* nervousness, weakness. **CV:** *palpitations,* tachycardia. **EENT:** *blurred vision,* mydriasis,

♦ Available in U.S. and Canada. ♦♦ Available in Canada only. All other products (no symbol) available in U.S. only. Italicized side effects are common or life-threatening.

INTERACTIONS	NURSING CONSIDERATIONS
	• Instruct patient to avoid driving and other hazardous activities if he is drowsy, dizzy, or has blurred vision; to drink plenty of fluids to help prevent constipation; and to report any skin rash. • Gum or sugarless hard candy may relieve mouth dryness. • Single dose produces 10- to 12-hour antisecretory effect and gastrointestinal antispasmodic effect. • Discontinue 1 week before thyroid function tests. • For toxicity, see APPENDIX, *Drug Toxicities*.
None significant.	• Contraindicated in narrow-angle glaucoma, obstructive uropathy, obstructive disease of GI tract, severe ulcerative colitis, myasthenia gravis, hypersensitivity to anticholinergics, paralytic ileus, intestinal atony, unstable cardiovascular status in acute hemorrhage, and toxic megacolon. Use cautiously in autonomic neuropathy, hyperthyroidism, coronary artery disease, cardiac arrhythmias, congestive heart failure, hypertension, hiatal hernia associated with reflux esophagitis, hepatic or renal disease, ulcerative colitis, or in patients over age 40 because of increased incidence of glaucoma. • Use with caution in hot or humid environments. Drug-induced heatstroke can develop. • Administer 30 minutes to 1 hour before meals. • Administer smaller doses to the elderly. • Monitor patient's vital signs and urinary output carefully. • Instruct patient to avoid driving and other hazardous activities if he is drowsy, dizzy, or has blurred vision; to drink plenty of fluids to help prevent constipation; to report any skin rash. • Gum or sugarless hard candy may relieve mouth dryness. • For toxicity, see APPENDIX, *Drug Toxicities*.
None significant.	• Contraindicated in narrow-angle glaucoma, obstructive uropathy, obstructive disease of GI tract, severe ulcerative colitis, myasthenia gravis, hypersensitivity to anticholinergics, paralytic ileus, intestinal atony, unstable cardiovascular status in acute hemorrhage, toxic megacolon. Use cautiously in autonomic neuropathy, hyperthyroidism, coronary artery disease, cardiac arrhythmias, congestive heart failure, hypertension, hiatal hernia associated with reflux esophagitis, hepatic or renal disease, ulcerative colitis, or in patients over age 40 because of the increased incidence of glaucoma. • Use with caution in hot or humid environments. Drug-induced heatstroke can develop. • Give 30 minutes to 1 hour before meals and at bedtime. Bedtime dose can be larger and should be given at least 2 hours after the last meal of the day. • Administer smaller doses to the elderly. • Monitor patient's vital signs and urinary output carefully. • Instruct patient to avoid driving and other hazardous activities if he is drowsy, dizzy, or has blurred vision; to drink plenty of fluids to help prevent constipation; and to report any skin rash. • Gum or sugarless hard candy may relieve mouth dryness. • For toxicity, see APPENDIX, *Drug Toxicities*.
None significant.	• Contraindicated in narrow-angle glaucoma, obstructive uropathy, obstructive disease of GI tract, severe ulcerative colitis, myasthenia gravis, hypersensitivity to anticholinergics, paralytic ileus, intestinal atony, unstable cardiovascular status in acute hemorrhage, toxic megacolon. Use cautiously in autonomic neuropathy, hyperthyroidism, coronary artery disease, cardiac arrhythmias, congestive heart

(continued on following page)

NAME	INDICATIONS & DOSAGE	SIDE EFFECTS
mepenzolate bromide *(continued)*	just dosage to individual patient's needs.	increased ocular tension, cycloplegia, photophobia. **GI:** *dry mouth,* dysphagia, heartburn, loss of taste, nausea, *constipation,* vomiting, *paralytic ileus.* **GU:** *urinary hesitancy and retention,* impotence. **Skin:** urticaria, decreased sweating or anhidrosis, other dermal manifestations. **Other:** fever, allergic reactions. Overdosage may cause curare-like symptoms.
methantheline bromide Banthine	*Adjunctive therapy in peptic ulcer, pylorospasm, spastic colon, biliary dyskinesia, pancreatitis, and certain forms of gastritis—* **Adults:** 50 to 100 mg P.O. q 6 hours. **Children over 1 year:** 12.5 to 50 mg P.O. q.i.d. **Infants under 1 year:** 12.5 to 25 mg P.O. q.i.d.	**CNS:** headache, insomnia, drowsiness, dizziness, *confusion or excitement in elderly patients,* nervousness, weakness. **CV:** *palpitations,* tachycardia. **EENT:** *blurred vision,* mydriasis, increased ocular tension, cycloplegia, photophobia. **GI:** *dry mouth,* dysphagia, *constipation,* heartburn, loss of taste, nausea, vomiting, *paralytic ileus.* **GU:** *urinary hesitancy and retention,* impotence. **Skin:** urticaria, decreased sweating or anhidrosis, other dermal manifestations. **Other:** fever, allergic reactions. Overdosage may cause curare-like symptoms.
methixene hydrochloride Trest♦	*Adjunctive treatment of gastrointestinal disorders associated with hypermotility or spasm—* **Adults:** 1 or 2 mg P.O. t.i.d.	**CNS:** *headache,* insomnia, drowsiness, *dizziness.* **CV:** *palpitations,* tachycardia. **EENT:** *blurred vision,* mydriasis, increased ocular tension, cycloplegia, photophobia. **GI:** *constipation,* nausea, vomiting, *paralytic ileus.* **GU:** urinary hesitancy and retention, impotence. **Skin:** urticaria, decreased sweating or anhidrosis, other dermal manifestations. **Other:** fever, allergic reactions. Overdosage may cause curare-like symptoms.

♦ Available in U.S. and Canada. ♦♦ Available in Canada only. All other products (no symbol) available in U.S. only. Italicized side effects are common or life-threatening.

INTERACTIONS	NURSING CONSIDERATIONS
	failure, hypertension, hiatal hernia associated with reflux esophagitis, hepatic or renal disease, ulcerative colitis, or in patients over age 40 because of increased incidence of glaucoma. • Use with caution in hot or humid environments. Drug-induced heatstroke can develop. • Give with meals and at bedtime. • Administer smaller doses to the elderly. • Monitor patient's vital signs and urinary output carefully. • Instruct patient to avoid driving and other hazardous activities if he is drowsy, dizzy, or has blurred vision; to drink plenty of fluids to help prevent constipation; and to report any skin rash. • Gum or sugarless hard candy may relieve mouth dryness. • For toxicity, see APPENDIX, *Drug Toxicities*.
None significant.	• Contraindicated in narrow-angle glaucoma, obstructive uropathy, obstructive disease of GI tract, severe ulcerative colitis, myasthenia gravis, hypersensitivity to anticholinergics, paralytic ileus, intestinal atony, unstable cardiovascular status in acute hemorrhage, toxic megacolon. Use cautiously in autonomic neuropathy, hyperthyroidism, coronary artery disease, cardiac arrhythmias, congestive heart failure, hypertension, hiatal hernia associated with reflux esophagitis, hepatic or renal disease, ulcerative colitis, or in patients over age 40 because of the increased incidence of glaucoma. • Use with caution in hot or humid environments. Drug-induced heatstroke can develop. • Give 30 minutes to 1 hour before meals and at bedtime. Bedtime dose can be larger and should be given at least 2 hours after the last meal of the day. • Administer smaller doses to the elderly. • If patient is also taking antihistamines, he may experience increased dryness of mouth. • Monitor patient's vital signs and urinary output carefully. • Instruct patient to avoid driving and other hazardous activities if he is drowsy, dizzy, or has blurred vision; to drink plenty of fluids to help prevent constipation; and to report any skin rash. • Gum or sugarless hard candy may relieve mouth dryness. • Therapeutic effects appear in 30 to 45 minutes; persist for 4 to 6 hours after oral administration. • For toxicity, see APPENDIX, *Drug Toxicities*.
None significant.	• Contraindicated in narrow-angle glaucoma, obstructive uropathy, obstructive disease of GI tract, severe ulcerative colitis, myasthenia gravis, hypersensitivity to anticholinergics, paralytic ileus, intestinal atony, unstable cardiovascular status in acute hemorrhage, toxic megacolon. Use cautiously in autonomic neuropathy, hyperthyroidism, coronary artery disease, cardiac arrhythmias, congestive heart failure, hypertension, hiatal hernia associated with reflux esophagitis, hepatic or renal disease, ulcerative colitis, or in patients over age 40 because of the increased incidence of glaucoma. • Use with caution in hot or humid environment. Drug-induced heatstroke could develop. • Administer 30 minutes to 1 hour before meals. • Administer smaller doses to the elderly. • Monitor patient's vital signs and urinary output. • Instruct patient to avoid driving and other hazardous activities if he is drowsy, dizzy, or has blurred vision; to drink plenty of fluids to help prevent constipation; and to report any skin rash. • Gum or sugarless hard candy may relieve mouth dryness.

(continued on following page)

NAME	INDICATIONS & DOSAGE	SIDE EFFECTS
methixene hydrochloride *(continued)*		
methscopolamine bromide Pamine♦, Scoline	*Adjunctive therapy in peptic ulcer—* **Adults:** 2.5 to 5 mg ½ hour before meals and h.s.	**CNS:** headache, insomnia, dizziness, *confusion or excitement in elderly patients,* nervousness, weakness. **CV:** *palpitations,* tachycardia. **EENT:** *blurred vision,* mydriasis, increased ocular tension, cycloplegia, photophobia. **GI:** *dry mouth,* dysphagia, *constipation,* heartburn, loss of taste, nausea, vomiting, *paralytic ileus.* **GU:** *urinary hesitancy and retention,* impotence. **Skin:** urticaria, decreased sweating or anhidrosis, other dermal manifestations. **Other:** fever, allergic reactions. Overdosage may cause curare-like symptoms.
oxyphencyclimine hydrochloride Daricon♦	*Adjunctive treatment of peptic ulcer—* **Adults:** 10 mg b.i.d. in the morning and h.s., or 5 mg b.i.d. or t.i.d.	**CNS:** *headache,* insomnia, drowsiness, *dizziness.* **CV:** *palpitations,* tachycardia. **EENT:** *blurred vision,* mydriasis, increased ocular tension, cycloplegia, photophobia. **GI:** *constipation,* nausea, vomiting, *paralytic ileus.* **GU:** urinary hesitancy and retention, impotence. **Skin:** urticaria, decreased sweating or anhidrosis, other dermal manifestations. **Other:** fever, allergic reactions. Overdosage may cause curare-like symptoms.
oxyphenonium bromide Antrenyl	*Adjunctive treatment of peptic ulcer—* **Adults:** 10 mg P.O. q.i.d. for several days, then reduced according to patient response.	**CNS:** headache, insomnia, drowsiness, dizziness, *confusion or excitement in elderly patients,* nervousness, weakness. **CV:** *palpitations,* tachycardia. **EENT:** *blurred vision,* mydriasis, increased ocular tension, cycloplegia, photophobia. **GI:** *dry mouth,* dysphagia, *constipation,* heartburn, loss of taste,

♦ Available in U.S. and Canada. ♦♦ Available in Canada only. All other products (no symbol) available in U.S. only. Italicized side effects are common or life-threatening.

INTERACTIONS	NURSING CONSIDERATIONS
	• Synthetic tertiary derivative that is relatively free of atropine-like side effects. • For toxicity, see APPENDIX, *Drug Toxicities*.
None significant.	• Contraindicated in narrow-angle glaucoma, obstructive uropathy, obstructive disease of GI tract, severe ulcerative colitis, myasthenia gravis, hypersensitivity to anticholinergics, paralytic ileus, intestinal atony, unstable cardiovascular status in acute hemorrhage, toxic megacolon. Use cautiously in autonomic neuropathy, hyperthyroidism, coronary artery disease, cardiac arrhythmias, congestive heart failure, hypertension, hiatal hernia associated with reflux esophagitis, hepatic or renal disease, ulcerative colitis, or in patients over age 40 because of increased incidence of glaucoma. • Use with caution in hot or humid environments. Drug-induced heatstroke can develop. • Give 30 minutes to 1 hour before meals and at bedtime. Bedtime dose can be larger and should be given at least 2 hours after the last meal of the day. • Administer smaller doses to the elderly. • Monitor patient's vital signs and urinary output carefully. • Instruct patient to avoid driving and other hazardous activities if he is drowsy, dizzy, or has blurred vision; to drink plenty of fluids to help prevent constipation; and to report any skin rash. • Gum or sugarless hard candy may relieve mouth dryness. • For toxicity, see APPENDIX, *Drug Toxicities*.
None significant.	• Contraindicated in narrow-angle glaucoma, obstructive uropathy, obstructive disease of GI tract, severe ulcerative colitis, myasthenia gravis, hypersensitivity to anticholinergics, paralytic ileus, intestinal atony, unstable cardiovascular status in acute hemorrhage, toxic megacolon. Use cautiously in autonomic neuropathy, hyperthyroidism, coronary artery disease, cardiac arrhythmias, congestive heart failure, hypertension, hiatal hernia associated with reflux esophagitis, hepatic or renal disease, ulcerative colitis, or in patients over age 40 because of increased incidence of glaucoma. • Use with caution in hot or humid environments. Drug-induced heatstroke can develop. • Give 30 minutes to 1 hour before breakfast and at bedtime. • Administer smaller doses to the elderly. • Monitor patient's vital signs and urinary output carefully. • Instruct patient to avoid driving and other hazardous activities if he is drowsy, dizzy, or has blurred vision; to drink plenty of fluids to help prevent constipation; and to report any skin rash. • Gum or sugarless hard candy may relieve mouth dryness. • Synthetic tertiary derivative that is relatively free of atropine-like side effects. • For toxicity, see APPENDIX, *Drug Toxicities*.
None significant.	• Contraindicated in narrow-angle glaucoma, obstructive uropathy, obstructive disease of GI tract, severe ulcerative colitis, myasthenia gravis, hypersensitivity to anticholinergics, paralytic ileus, intestinal atony, unstable cardiovascular status in acute hemorrhage, toxic megacolon. Use cautiously in autonomic neuropathy, hyperthyroidism, coronary artery disease, cardiac arrhythmias, congestive heart failure, hypertension, hiatal hernia associated with reflux esophagitis, hepatic or renal disease, ulcerative colitis, or in patients over age 40 because of increased incidence of glaucoma. • Use with caution in hot or humid environments. Drug-induced

(continued on following page)

NAME	INDICATIONS & DOSAGE	SIDE EFFECTS
oxyphenonium bromide *(continued)*		nausea, vomiting, *paralytic ileus.* **GU:** *urinary hesitancy and retention,* impotence. **Skin:** urticaria, decreased sweating or anhidrosis, other dermal manifestations. **Other:** fever, allergic reactions. Overdosage may cause curare-like symptoms.
propantheline bromide Banlin♦♦, Norpanth, Pro-Banthine♦, Propanthel♦♦, Robantaline, Ropanth	*Adjunctive treatment of peptic ulcer and irritable bowel syndrome, and other gastrointestinal disorders—* **Adults:** 15 mg P.O. t.i.d. before meals, and 30 mg at bedtime up to 60 mg q.i.d. For elderly patients, 7.5 mg P.O. t.i.d. before meals. When oral dosage is not possible, 30 mg I.M. or I.V. q 6 hours, depending on individual response. Maintenance dose 15 mg I.M. q 6 hours.	**CNS:** headache, insomnia, drowsiness, dizziness, *confusion or excitement in elderly patients,* nervousness, weakness. **CV:** *palpitations,* tachycardia. **EENT:** *blurred vision,* mydriasis, increased ocular tension, cycloplegia, photophobia. **GI:** *dry mouth,* dysphagia, constipation, heartburn, loss of taste, nausea, vomiting, paralytic ileus. **GU:** *urinary hesitancy and retention,* impotence. **Skin:** urticaria, decreased sweating or anhidrosis, other dermal manifestations. **Other:** fever, allergic reactions. Overdosage may cause curare-like symptoms.
thiphenamil hydrochloride Trocinate	*Hypermotility and spasm of the gastrointestinal tract—* **Adults:** initially, 400 mg P.O. repeated in 4 hours, usually to maximum of 4 doses. Maintenance dose may be given at a reduced frequency of dosage.	**CNS:** headache, insomnia, drowsiness, dizziness, *confusion or excitement in elderly patients,* nervousness, weakness. **CV:** *palpitations,* tachycardia. **EENT:** *blurred vision,* mydriasis, increased ocular tension, cycloplegia, photophobia. **GI:** *dry mouth,* dysphagia, *constipation,* heartburn, loss of taste, nausea, vomiting, *paralytic ileus.* **GU:** *urinary hesitancy and retention,* impotence. **Skin:** urticaria, decreased sweating or anhidrosis, other dermal manifestations. **Other:** fever, allergic reactions. Overdosage may cause curare-like symptoms.
tridihexethyl chloride Pathilon	*Adjunctive treatment of peptic ulcer, irritable bowel syndrome, and other gastrointestinal disorders—*	**CNS:** headache, insomnia, drowsiness, dizziness, *confusion or excitement in elderly patients,* nervousness, weakness.

♦ Available in U.S. and Canada. ♦♦ Available in Canada only. All other products (no symbol) available in U.S. only. Italicized side effects are common or life-threatening.

INTERACTIONS	NURSING CONSIDERATIONS
	heatstroke can develop. • Give 30 minutes to 1 hour before meals and at bedtime. Bedtime dose can be larger and should be given at least 2 hours after the last meal of the day. • Administer smaller doses to the elderly. • Monitor patient's vital signs and urinary output. • Instruct patient to avoid driving and other hazardous activities if he is drowsy, dizzy, or has blurred vision; to drink plenty of fluids to help prevent constipation; and to report any skin rash. • Gum or sugarless hard candy may relieve mouth dryness. • For toxicity, see APPENDIX, *Drug Toxicities*.
None significant.	• Contraindicated in narrow-angle glaucoma, obstructive uropathy, obstructive disease of GI tract, severe ulcerative colitis, myasthenia gravis, hypersensitivity to anticholinergics, paralytic ileus, intestinal atony, unstable cardiovascular status in acute hemorrhage, toxic megacolon. Use cautiously in autonomic neuropathy, hyperthyroidism, coronary artery disease, cardiac arrhythmias, congestive heart failure, hypertension, hiatal hernia associated with reflux esophagitis, hepatic or renal disease, ulcerative colitis, or in patients over age 40 because of the increased incidence of glaucoma. • Use with caution in hot or humid environments. Drug-induced heatstroke can develop. • Give 30 minutes to 1 hour before meals and at bedtime. Bedtime dose can be larger; give 2 hours after the last meal of the day. • Administer smaller doses to the elderly. • Monitor patient's vital signs and urinary output carefully. • Instruct patient to avoid driving and other hazardous activities if he is drowsy, dizzy, or has blurred vision; to drink plenty of fluids to help prevent constipation; and to report any skin rash. • Gum or sugarless hard candy may relieve mouth dryness. • For toxicity, see APPENDIX, *Drug Toxicities*.
None significant.	• Contraindicated in narrow-angle glaucoma, obstructive uropathy, obstructive disease of GI tract, severe ulcerative colitis, myasthenia gravis, hypersensitivity to anticholinergics, paralytic ileus, intestinal atony, unstable cardiovascular status in acute hemorrhage, toxic megacolon. Use cautiously in autonomic neuropathy, hyperthyroidism, coronary artery disease, cardiac arrhythmias, congestive heart failure, hypertension, hiatal hernia associated with reflux esophagitis, hepatic or renal disease, ulcerative colitis, or in patients over age 40 because of increased incidence of glaucoma. • Use with caution in hot or humid environments. Drug-induced heatstroke can develop. • Administer smaller doses to the elderly. • Monitor patient's vital signs and urinary output carefully. • Instruct patient to avoid driving and other hazardous activities if he is drowsy, dizzy, or has blurred vision; to drink plenty of fluids to help prevent constipation; and to report any skin rash. • Gum or sugarless hard candy may relieve mouth dryness. • For toxicity, see APPENDIX, *Drug Toxicities*.
None significant.	• Contraindicated in narrow-angle glaucoma, obstructive uropathy, obstructive disease of GI tract, severe ulcerative colitis, myasthenia gravis, hypersensitivity to anticholinergics, paralytic ileus, intestinal atony, unstable cardiovascular status in acute hemorrhage, toxic

(continued on following page)

NAME	INDICATIONS & DOSAGE	SIDE EFFECTS
tridihexethyl chloride *(continued)*	**Adults:** initially, 25 to 50 mg P.O. t.i.d. before meals, and 50 mg h.s., increased to 75 mg q.i.d., if needed. With sustained-release capsules, 75 mg q 12 or q 6 hours. Maintenance dose usually half the therapeutic dose. Parenteral use: 10 to 20 mg I.V., I.M., or S.C. q 6 hours. Change to oral as soon as possible.	**CV:** *palpitations,* tachycardia. **EENT:** *blurred vision,* mydriasis, increased ocular tension, cycloplegia, photophobia. **GI:** *dry mouth,* dysphagia, *constipation,* heartburn, loss of taste, nausea, vomiting, *paralytic ileus.* **GU:** *urinary hesitancy and retention,* impotence. **Skin:** urticaria, decreased sweating or anhidrosis, other dermal manifestations. **Other:** fever, allergic reactions. Overdosage may cause curare-like symptoms.

◆ Available in U.S. and Canada. ◆◆ Available in Canada only. All other products (no symbol) available in U.S. only. Italicized side effects are common or life-threatening.

INTERACTIONS	NURSING CONSIDERATIONS
	megacolon. Use cautiously in autonomic neuropathy, hyperthyroidism, coronary artery disease, cardiac arrhythmias, congestive heart failure, hypertension, hiatal hernia associated with reflux esophagitis, hepatic or renal disease, ulcerative colitis, or in patients over age 40 because of increased incidence of glaucoma. • Use with caution in hot or humid environments. Drug-induced heatstroke can develop. • Give 30 minutes to 1 hour before meals and at bedtime. Bedtime dose can be larger and should be given at least 2 hours after the last meal of the day. • Administer smaller doses to the elderly. • Monitor patient's vital signs and urinary output carefully. • Instruct patient to avoid driving and other hazardous activities if he is drowsy, dizzy, or has blurred vision; to drink plenty of fluids to help prevent constipation; and to report any skin rash. • Gum or sugarless hard candy may relieve mouth dryness. • For toxicity, see APPENDIX, *Drug Toxicities*.

51 Miscellaneous gastrointestinal drugs

choline
cimetidine
dexpanthenol
metoclopramide hydrochloride
sucralfate

The miscellaneous gastrointestinal (GI) drugs include lipotropic substances (choline), the histamine (H_2)-receptor antagonist cimetidine, the oral antiulcer drug sucralfate, the smooth-muscle relaxant dexpanthenol, and metoclopramide.

Major uses

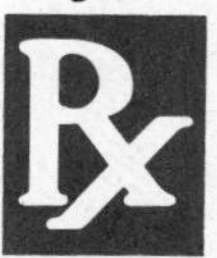

- Choline is essential for normal transport of lipids from the liver to the tissues and is used to treat hepatic fat-transport disorders.
- Cimetidine is used to treat pathologic hypersecretory conditions, such as Zollinger-Ellison syndrome, and duodenal ulcer.
- Dexpanthenol is used prophylactically immediately after major abdominal surgery to reduce the risk of paralytic ileus. It is also used to treat intestinal atony (which can cause abdominal distention), postpartum or postoperative retention of gas, and postoperative delay in resumption of intestinal motility.
- Metoclopramide facilitates small-bowel intubation and aids in radiologic examination. It is also used to treat diabetic gastroparesis.
- Sucralfate is used to treat duodenal ulcers.

Mechanism of action

- Choline promotes phospholipid turnover and enhances fat transport from the liver to the tissues, decreasing the liver's fat content.
- Cimetidine competitively inhibits the action of histamine at receptor sites of the parietal cells, decreasing gastric acid secretion.
- Dexpanthenol both stimulates and restores tone to intestinal smooth muscles.
- Metoclopramide stimulates motility of the upper GI tract by antagonizing dopamine's action.
- Sucralfate adheres to and protects the ulcer surface.

Absorption, distribution, metabolism, and excretion

- Choline is incompletely absorbed after oral administration since much of it is destroyed in the stomach by gastric acid. It is metabolized by the intestinal flora and eliminated in feces.
- Cimetidine is rapidly absorbed in the upper portion of the small intestine, widely distributed to all body tissues, metabolized in the liver, and excreted in urine.
- Dexpanthenol is given parenterally. It's completely absorbed, widely distributed, and converted in the blood to the active metabolite pantothenic acid. Most of the pantothenic acid is excreted unchanged in urine.
- Metoclopramide is immediately absorbed, widely distributed, metabolized in the liver, and excreted in urine.

UNDERSTANDING CIMETIDINE, THE *OTHER* ANTIHISTAMINE

When you hear the word antihistamine, you usually think of runny noses, clogged sinuses, and hay fever. But there's an antihistamine available that won't do a thing for your patient's allergy.

The *other* antihistamine—cimetidine (Tagamet)—decreases gastric acid secretion, providing excellent therapy for your patient with ulcers.

Two types of antihistamines

Antihistamines (technically referred to as histamine antagonists) were developed *to negate the effects of histamines.* Histamines, which occur naturally in our bodies,

- dilate capillaries and increase capillary permeability
- constrict bronchial smooth muscle in the lungs, and
- increase gastric acid secretion.

When classic antihistamines were developed in 1937, researchers initially thought these drugs would not only relieve allergy symptoms and inhibit histamine-induced smooth-muscle contraction in the lungs but would solve the problem of increased gastric acid secretion as well.

But classic antihistamines were ineffective in controlling gastric acid secretion, that is, they could not block the action of histamine in the stomach. Researchers then hypothesized that *more than one type of histamine receptor must exist.*

Two types of receptors

Physiologic substances (such as histamines) interact with cells to produce an anticipated response (such as increased gastric acid secretion). This response occurs at a specific site called the *receptor.* A drug (such as cimetidine) can modify the physiologic response by blocking the action of the physiologic substance. This drug is known as the *antagonist;* the physiologic substance, the *agonist* (see Chapter 1, PHARMACOLOGY FOR NURSES, for more information on agonists and antagonists).

After years of study, researchers determined that indeed at least two different histamine receptors exist, each responding to its specific histamine antagonist. This is why classic antihistamines won't affect your patient's ulcers and cimetidine doesn't alleviate allergies.

H_1 and H_2 receptor antagonists

Classic antihistamines are labeled H_1 receptor antagonists and their receptors, H_1 receptors. Cimetidine is labeled an H_2 receptor antagonist; its receptors, H_2 receptors. Cimetidine is the only antihistamine currently marketed that effectively decreases gastric acid secretion.

Several other H_2 receptor antagonists have been studied, but thus far have proved ineffective, of low potency, or toxic.

- Sucralfate is only minimally absorbed and is excreted unchanged in the urine.

Onset and duration

- Choline's onset and duration of action are unknown.
- Cimetidine blood levels peak within 75 minutes after oral or parenteral administration. The drug has a half-life of about 2 hours. Its therapeutic action lasts 4 to 5 hours after oral or parenteral administration of 300 mg.
- Dexpanthenol may take 72 hours or longer to be effective. Its action can last 4 to 12 hours.
- Metoclopramide acts within 1 to 3 minutes, and its effect lasts 1 to 2 hours after I.V. administration. After oral administration, it takes effect within 30 minutes; its action lasts 4 to 6 hours.
- Sucralfate begins to act within 1 hour; peak occurs in 1 to 3 hours and duration is 4 to 6 hours.

Combination products

GERIPLEX: choline 20 mg, vitamin A 5,000 units, vitamin E 5 units, vitamin B_1 5 mg, vitamin B_2 5 mg, vitamin B_3 15 mg, vitamin B_{12} 2 mcg, vitamin C 50 mg, iron 6 mg, calcium 59 mg, and phosphorus 46 mg.

METHISCHOL: choline 115 mg, inositol 83 mg, methionine 110 mg, vitamin B_1 3 mg, vitamin B_2 3 mg, vitamin B_3 10 mg, vitamin B_5 2 mg, vitamin B_6 2 mg, vitamin B_{12} 2 mcg, desiccated liver 56 mg, and liver concentrate 30 mg.

NAME	INDICATIONS & DOSAGE	SIDE EFFECTS
choline	*Hepatic disorders and disturbed fat metabolism—* **Adults and children:** 650 to 750 mg P.O. daily.	**CNS:** dizziness. **GI:** irritation if taken on an empty stomach, nausea. **Metabolic:** ketosis after excessive dosages. **Other:** breath and body odor smelling like dead fish.
cimetidine Tagamet♦	*Duodenal ulcer (short-term treatment)—* **Adults, and children over 16 years:** 300 mg P.O. q.i.d. with meals and h.s. for maximum therapy of 8 weeks. When healing occurs, stop treatment or give bedtime dose only to control nocturnal hypersecretion. Parenteral: 300 mg diluted to 20 ml with 0.9% normal saline solution or other compatible I.V. solution by I.V. push over 1 to 2 minutes q 6 hours. Or 300 mg diluted in 100 ml 5% dextrose solution or other compatible I.V. solution by I.V. infusion over 15 to 20 minutes q 6 hours. Or 300 mg I.M. q 6 hours (no dilution necessary). To increase dose, give 300 mg doses more frequently to maximum daily dose of 2,400 mg. *Duodenal ulcer prophylaxis—* **Adults, and children over 16 years:** 400 mg P.O. h.s. *Pathologic hypersecretory conditions (such as Zollinger-Ellison syndrome, systemic mastocytosis, and multiple endocrine adenomas)—* **Adults, and children over 16 years:** 300 mg P.O. q.i.d. with meals and h.s.; adjust to individual needs. Maximum daily dose 2,400 mg. Parenteral: 300 mg diluted to 20 ml with 0.9% normal saline solution or other compatible I.V. solutions by I.V. push over 1 to 2 minutes q 6 hours. Or 300 mg diluted in 100 ml 5% dextrose	**Blood:** *agranulocytosis*, neutropenia, *thrombocytopenia, aplastic anemia.* **CNS:** mental confusion, dizziness, headaches. **CV:** bradycardia. **GI:** mild and transient diarrhea, perforation of chronic peptic ulcers after abrupt cessation of drug. **GU:** interstitial nephritis, *transient elevations in BUN and serum creatinine*, reduced sperm count. **Hepatic:** jaundice. **Skin:** acne-like rash, urticaria, *exfoliative dermatitis.* **Other:** hypersensitivity, muscle pain, mild gynecomastia after use longer than 1 month (but no change in endocrine function).

INTERACTIONS	NURSING CONSIDERATIONS
None significant.	• Foods supplying choline include egg yolk, beef liver, legumes, vegetables, and milk. Average diet contains from 500 to 900 mg per day. • Lipotropic agent. • Used in many multivitamin preparations, but there is no evidence supplemental choline intake is more beneficial for long periods than an adequate diet. • Synthesized by the body from serine, with methionine acting as a methyl-donor in the reaction. • Choline is no longer considered effective in treatment of hepatic disorders or disorders of lipid transport or metabolism. • Investigative use in treatment of tardive dyskinesia: restores cholinergic tone and decreases choreic movements. Oral choline elevates brain choline and acetylcholine (the cholinergic neurotransmitter of the cholinergic nervous system) levels and restores cholinergic tone. • Lecithin (available in health food stores) is a source of choline.
Antacids: interfere with absorption of cimetidine. Separate cimetidine and antacids by at least 1 hour if possible.	• Maintenance dosing for more than 12 months cannot be recommended. Long-term effects are not known. • I.M. route of administration may be painful. • I.V. solutions compatible for dilution with cimetidine: 0.9% sodium chloride solution, 5% and 10% dextrose (and combinations of these) solutions, lactated Ringer's solution, and 5% sodium bicarbonate injection. Do not dilute with sterile water for injection. • Hemodialysis reduces blood levels of cimetidine. Schedule cimetidine dose at end of hemodialysis treatment. • Up to 10 g overdosage has been reported without untoward effects. • Effectiveness in treatment of gastric ulcers not as great as in duodenal ulcer. Cimetidine may prove useful but is still unapproved in pancreatic insufficiency, short-bowel syndrome, psoriasis, prevention and treatment of GI bleeding, relief of symptoms and acid sensitivity in reflux esophagitis, and prevention of gastric inactivation of oral enzyme preparations by gastric acid and pepsin. • Best to administer with meals in order to maintain blood levels. • Large parenteral doses should be avoided in asthmatics. • Elderly patients more susceptible to cimetidine-induced mental confusion. Dose should be decreased in elderly and in patients with renal insufficiency. • I.V. cimetidine often used in critically ill patients prophylactically to prevent GI bleeding. • When administering cimetidine I.V. in 100 ml of diluent solution, do not infuse so rapidly that circulatory overload is produced. • Available in liquid form (300 mg/5 ml). • Tablets available in two strengths: 200 mg (SKF T12) and 300 mg (SKF T13). Both tablets are pale green. Identify tablet when obtaining a drug history.

(continued on following page)

NAME	INDICATIONS & DOSAGE	SIDE EFFECTS
cimetidine *(continued)*	solution or other compatible I.V. solution by I.V. infusion over 15 to 20 minutes q 6 hours. To increase dose, give 300 mg doses more frequently to maximum daily dose of 2,400 mg.	
dexpanthenol Ilopan♦, Intrapan, Motilyn♦♦, Tonestat	*Postoperative abdominal distention (resulting from flatus retention)—* **Adults and children:** 250 to 500 mg I.M., repeat in 2 hours and again q 6 hours until distention is relieved. May require therapy for 48 to 72 hours or longer. Or, 500 mg infused slow I.V. drip in glucose or lactated Ringer's solution. *Treatment and postoperative prevention of paralytic ileus—* **Adults and children:** 500 mg I.M., repeat in 2 hours; then q 4 to 6 hours until distention is relieved. May require therapy for 48 to 72 hours or longer.	**Blood:** prolonged bleeding time. **GI:** excessive passage of flatus with increased doses or prolonged use, increased frequency of bowel movements, hyperperistalsis.
metoclopramide hydrochloride Maxeran♦♦, Reglan♦	*To facilitate small-bowel intubation and to aid in radiologic examinations—* **Adults:** 10 mg (2 ml) I.V. as a single dose over 1 to 2 minutes. **Children 6 to 14 years:** 2.5 to 5 mg (0.5 to 1 ml). **Children under 6 years:** 0.1 mg/kg. *Delayed gastric emptying secondary to diabetic gastroparesis—* **Adults:** 10 mg P.O. 30 minutes before meals and at bedtime for 2 to 8 weeks, depending on response.	**CNS:** restlessness, *drowsiness,* fatigue, *lassitude,* insomnia, headache, dizziness, extrapyramidal symptoms. **GI:** nausea, bowel disturbances.
sucralfate Carafate	*Short-term (up to 8 weeks) treatment of duodenal ulcer—* **Adults:** 1 g P.O. q.i.d. 1 hour before meals and at bedtime.	**CNS:** dizziness, sleepiness. **GI:** *constipation,* nausea, gastric discomfort, diarrhea.

INTERACTIONS	NURSING CONSIDERATIONS
None significant.	• Contraindicated in hemophilia because bleeding time is prolonged. • Don't administer full-strength solution I.V.; always dilute. • Dexpanthenol use shouldn't delay treatment of mechanical ileus if present. • A smooth-muscle stimulant; used postoperatively against delayed resumption of intestinal motility. Also used as adjunctive treatment of peripheral neuritis and lupus erythematosus. • Hypokalemia may cause a decreased response. If this occurs, potassium supplements should be started. Increased doses of dexpanthenol may be needed. • May also be useful during laxative withdrawal after long-term use. • Wait 12 hours after giving parasympathomimetics before starting dexpanthenol.
Anticholinergics, narcotic analgesics: antagonize effects of metoclopramide. Use together cautiously.	• Contraindicated whenever stimulation of GI motility might be dangerous (hemorrhage, obstruction, perforation), and in pheochromocytoma and epilepsy. • Speeds gastric emptying by stimulating smooth muscle in upper GI tract. • If I.V. injection is too rapid, a transient but intense feeling of anxiety and restlessness occurs, followed by drowsiness. • Warn patient to avoid activities requiring alertness for 2 hours after taking each dose. • Give oral form with meals. • Injectable form may be useful as an antiemetic following chemotherapy.
Antacids: May decrease binding of drug to gastroduodenal mucosa, impairing effectiveness. Don't give within 30 minutes of each other.	• No known contraindications. • Symptomatic improvement doesn't preclude possibility of gastric cancer. • Drug is minimally absorbed. Incidence of side effects is low. • Tell patient for best results to take sucralfate on an empty stomach (1 hour before each meal and at bedtime). • Pain and ulcer symptoms may subside within first few weeks of therapy. However, for complete healing, be sure patient continues on prescribed regimen. • Monitor for severe, persistent constipation. • Studies suggest that drug's as effective as cimetidine in healing duodenal ulcers. • Drug has been used to treat gastric ulcers, but effectiveness of this use is still under investigation. • Drug contains aluminum, but isn't classified as an antacid.

VIII Hormonal Agents

52 Corticosteroids

Glucocorticoids
beclomethasone dipropionate
betamethasone
betamethasone acetate and betamethasone sodium phosphate
betamethasone disodium phosphate
betamethasone sodium phosphate
cortisone acetate
dexamethasone
dexamethasone acetate
dexamethasone sodium phosphate
fluprednisolone
hydrocortisone
hydrocortisone acetate
hydrocortisone retention enema
hydrocortisone sodium phosphate
hydrocortisone sodium succinate
meprednisone
methylprednisolone
methylprednisolone acetate
methylprednisolone sodium succinate
paramethasone acetate
prednisolone
prednisolone acetate
prednisolone sodium phosphate
prednisolone tebutate
prednisone
triamcinolone
triamcinolone acetonide
triamcinolone diacetate
triamcinolone hexacetonide

Mineralocorticoids
desoxycorticosterone acetate
desoxycorticosterone pivalate
fludrocortisone acetate

Corticosteroids are hormones produced naturally by the adrenal cortex. The corticosteroids described in this chapter are organic or synthetic compounds used to treat adrenocortical disorders, produce immunosuppression, and reduce inflammation. Corticosteroids are divided into three groups on the basis of their primary physiologic actions:

- *Glucocorticoids* produce organic effects regulating carbohydrate, fat, and protein metabolism; they also have anti-inflammatory activity.
- *Mineralocorticoids* produce inorganic effects regulating electrolyte and water metabolism.
- *Adrenal androgens and estrogens* produce sex hormonal effects. (For a complete discussion of these, see Chapter 53, ANDROGENS AND ANABOLIC STEROIDS, and Chapter 55, ESTROGENS.)

Major uses

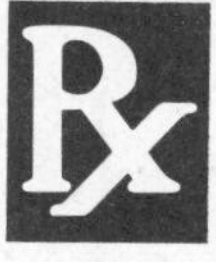

- Glucocorticoids have several uses, including:
  —treatment of adrenal insufficiency (Addison's disease)
  —treatment of hypercalcemia resulting from breast cancer, multiple myeloma, sarcoidosis, or vitamin D intoxication (but not hyperparathyroidism)
  —topical treatment of dermatologic and ocular inflammations, such as exfoliative dermatitis, uncontrollable eczema, cutaneous sarcoidosis, and Stevens-Johnson syndrome
  —systemic or inhalation therapy for

PATHWAY OF CORTICOSTEROID PRODUCTION

Adequate blood concentrations of corticosteroids *inhibit* CRF and ACTH secretion by a negative feedback mechanism. (CRF is secreted in a diurnal rhythm.) Abnormally low corticosteroid blood levels *stimulate* CRF and ACTH activity by positive feedback responses. Above-normal ACTH levels can also inhibit CRF release.

ACTH blood levels peak around 3 to 6 a.m., then ebb around 10 p.m. Corticosteroid blood levels peak around 4 to 10 a.m. and ebb around midnight.

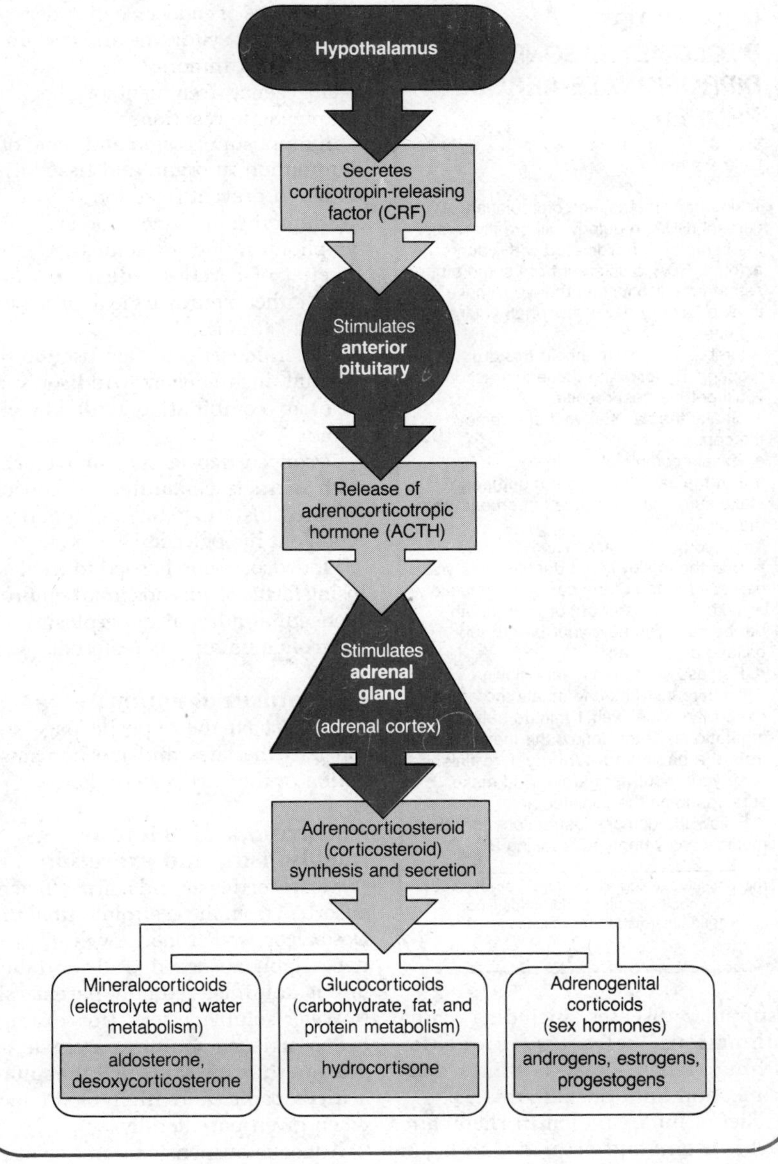

PATIENT-TEACHING AID

HOW TO USE BECLOMETHASONE DIPROPIONATE AEROSOL PROPERLY

Dear Patient:

Taking beclomethasone dipropionate aerosol (BDA) regularly will greatly reduce the symptoms associated with your asthma. BDA is different from some other asthma medications in that you'll have to take it every day, even when you're feeling fine.

First, learn how to inhale this drug properly. By following these instructions, you'll get the best results:

- Shake the canister well and remove the cap.
- Exhale completely.
- Put the canister in your mouth, and make sure your tongue is underneath the mouthpiece.
- Tilt your head back slightly.
- Breathe in slowly but deeply while you depress the top of the canister completely.
- Take the canister out of your mouth, but be sure you hold your breath for as long as you can.
- Release your breath very slowly.

If you're instructed to inhale the aerosol more than once, wait 1 minute between inhalations. Then, follow the instructions from the beginning. When you're finished, rinse your mouth or gargle. And make sure you keep the canister clean.

Follow the doctor's instructions for other medications when you're taking BDA.

respiratory diseases, including status asthmaticus, refractory bronchial asthma, berylliosis, Löffler's syndrome, and lipid pneumonitis
—relief of inflammation in rheumatic fever, rheumatoid arthritis, collagen diseases (systemic lupus erythematosus, dermatomyositis, and periarteritis nodosa), and nephrotic syndrome. (They do not affect the progression of these diseases.)
—suppression of inflammatory reaction in allergic dermatoses, food and drug allergies, asthma, ulcerative colitis, and vasculitis
—diagnosis of endocrine disorders such as Cushing's syndrome and certain adrenocortical tumors
—emergency treatment of shock and anaphylactic reactions
—immunosuppression and relief of inflammation in organ and tissue transplants to prevent rejection
—adjunctive treatment of leukemias, lymphomas, and myelomas
—relief of cerebral edema resulting from either neurosurgical procedures or brain tumors.

- Mineralocorticoids are used to treat adrenal insufficiency (Addison's disease) in combination with glucocorticoids.

Desoxycorticosterone, supplemented with extracts containing adrenocortical steroids, may be therapeutic for recurrent hypoglycemia.

Fludrocortisone is used to treat salt-losing forms of adrenogenital syndrome (congenital adrenal hyperplasia) after electrolyte balance is restored.

Mechanism of action

The chart on the opposite page summarizes the sites and mechanisms of action of the corticosteroids.

Absorption, distribution, metabolism, and excretion

- Most corticosteroids are efficiently absorbed from the gastrointestinal tract. Desoxycorticosterone, however, is not dependably absorbed orally and therefore is administered only parenterally.
- Water-soluble esters (for example, hydrocortisone sodium succinate and dexamethasone sodium phosphate) achieve rapid and high blood levels when given parenterally.
- Aqueous suspensions and solutions

CORTICOSTEROIDS: HOW THEY WORK

CLASSIFICATION	WHAT IS INFLUENCED	MECHANISM OF ACTION
Adrenal androgens and estrogens	Primary and secondary sex organs	Sex hormonal effects
Glucocorticoids	Fat metabolism	Induce lipogenesis, increasing adipose tissue formation; in high doses, cause fat redistribution with loss of fat from extremities and accumulation in neck, cheeks, and back.
	Protein metabolism	Increase protein catabolism, decrease use of amino acids for protein synthesis, and convert amino acids to glucose, resulting in accelerated protein breakdown and muscle weakness and wasting. Interference with wound healing, suppression of immune response, temporary growth arrest, and osteoporosis may also be related to protein catabolism.
	Carbohydrate metabolism	Convert amino acids to glucose and decrease peripheral utilization of glucose, raising blood glucose level, which in turn triggers insulin release from the pancreas. Prolonged glucocorticoid treatment in patients with controlled diabetes may result in resistance to exogenous insulin and necessitate adjustment of insulin levels.
	Inflammatory process	Interfere with histamine synthesis; inhibit fibroblast formation, collagen disposition, and capillary proliferation; inhibit microvascular dilation and increased capillary permeability in response to tissue injury; block plasma exudation, migration of polymorphonuclear leukocytes into inflamed area, and phagocytosis; stabilize cell membrane and inhibit release of proteolytic enzymes, preventing normal inflammatory response; exert antilymphocytic action in treatment of some neoplasms.
	Miscellaneous	Potentiate vasoconstricting effect of norepinephrine in treatment of shock; suppress pituitary ACTH release, leading to adrenocortical suppression; lower blood calcium levels by antagonizing vitamin D effects on calcium absorption from the bowel and by decreasing calcium reabsorption from bone in multiple myeloma.
Mineralocorticoids	Kidneys	Increase sodium reabsorption and potassium and hydrogen secretion at distal segment of renal tubules.
	Blood volume	Secondary to the increased sodium retention, there's a corresponding increase in water retention. This results in increased plasma volume and elevated blood pressure.

RECOGNIZING AND COMBATTING CUSHINGOID SYMPTOMS

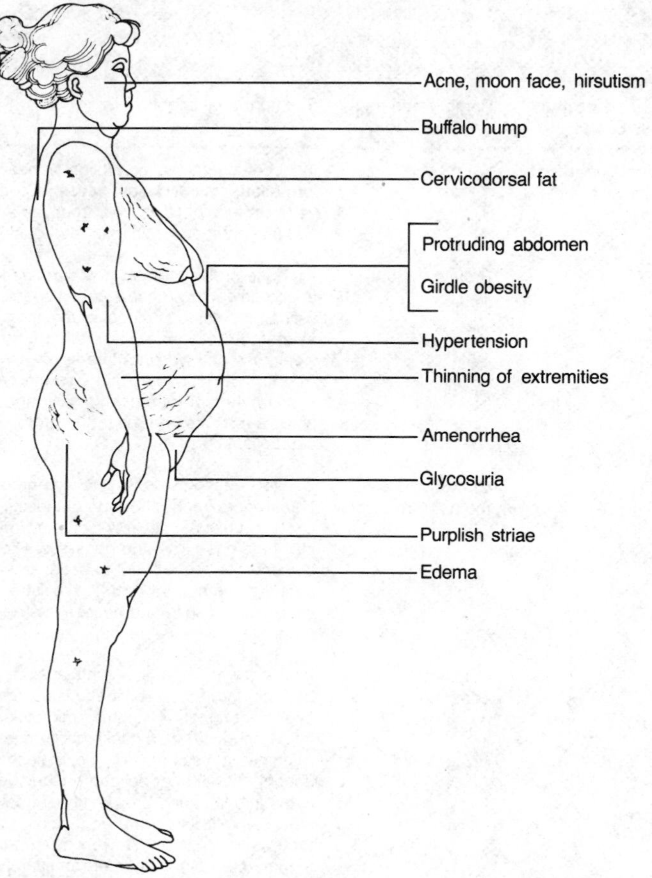

Prolonged corticosteroid therapy may cause the side effect of cushingoid syndrome, a peculiar type of obesity in which fat is distributed in pads between the shoulders—creating a buffalo hump—and around the waist—creating a girdle of fat.

RECOGNITION

- Observe the patient for cushingoid symptoms. In addition to those listed with the illustration, look for muscle weakness, wasting tissue, hyperglycemia, renal disorders, mental changes ranging from euphoria to depression, and lowered resistance to infection.
- Report your observations to the doctor.

NURSING CONSIDERATIONS

- Because adrenal hormones are excreted in urine, collect all urine for hormone analysis.
- Record food and fluid intake.
- Keep track of the patient's emotional state, and record the types of situations that disturb him.
- Relieve emotional stress by keeping the patient well informed. For example, tell the woman with distressing hirsutism and a tendency toward masculinization that these changes will disappear after the treatment.

RELATIVE POTENCY OF SELECTED GLUCOCORTICOIDS

DRUG	ANTI-INFLAMMATORY POTENCY (in mg equivalent to 5 mg prednisone)	MINERALOCORTICOID POTENCY (salt-retaining potency)	DURATION
betamethasone	0.6	0	48 hr or more
cortisone acetate	25	1	12 hr or less
dexamethasone	0.75	0	48 hr or more
fluprednisolone	2	1	12 hr or less
hydrocortisone	20	1	12 hr or less
meprednisone	4	0	24 to 36 hr
methylprednisolone	4	0.5	24 to 36 hr
paramethasone	2	0	24 to 36 hr
prednisolone	5	0.8	24 to 36 hr
prednisone	5	0.8	24 to 36 hr
triamcinolone	4	0	24 to 36 hr

Short-term therapy (less than 7 days) with moderate doses (40 mg or less) of prednisone or equivalent produces few side effects and may be abruptly discontinued. Long-term (more than 1 week) or high-dose therapy must be discontinued gradually or acute adrenal insufficiency may result.

To minimize adrenal insufficiency, administer the daily dose before 9 a.m.

in oil are slowly absorbed by I.M. injection.

- Corticosteroids are rapidly distributed to all body tissues, metabolized in the liver, and excreted in urine.

Onset and duration

- Oral corticosteroids usually begin to act within 6 hours.
- Aqueous suspensions and solutions in oil have slow onset after I.M. administration; they produce low, prolonged blood levels (days to weeks).
- Aqueous solutions given I.V. have a rapid onset.
- Implanted compressed pellets (desoxycorticosterone acetate) provide 6 to 8 months of steroid therapy.
- Some glucocorticoids (for example, betamethasone and dexamethasone) have a prolonged duration of action (more than 48 hours).

Because they have such a long duration of action, they should not be used in alternate-day therapy. (See *What You Should Know About Alternate-day Steroid Therapy*, p. 708.)

Combination products

None.

NAME	INDICATIONS & DOSAGE	SIDE EFFECTS
beclomethasone dipropionate Beclovent♦ Vanceril♦	*Steroid-dependent asthma—* **Adults:** 2 to 4 inhalations t.i.d. or q.i.d. Maximum 20 inhalations daily. **Children 6 to 12 years:** 1 to 2 inhalations t.i.d. or q.i.d. Maximum 10 inhalations daily.	**EENT:** hoarseness, fungal infections of mouth and throat. **GI:** dry mouth.
betamethasone Betnelan♦♦, Celestone♦ **betamethasone acetate and betamethasone sodium phosphate** Celestone Soluspan♦ **betamethasone disodium phosphate** Betnesol♦♦ **betamethasone sodium phosphate** Celestone Phosphate	*Severe inflammation or immunosuppression—* **Adults:** 0.6 to 7.2 mg P.O. daily; or 0.5 to 9 mg (sodium phosphate) I.M., I.V., or into joint or soft tissue daily; or 1.5 to 12 mg (sodium phosphate-acetate suspension) into joint or soft tissue q 1 to 2 weeks, p.r.n.	Most side effects of corticosteroids are dose- or duration-dependent. **CNS:** *euphoria, insomnia,* psychotic behavior, pseudotumor cerebri. **CV:** *congestive heart failure,* hypertension, edema. **EENT:** cataracts, glaucoma. **GI:** *peptic ulcer,* gastrointestinal irritation, increased appetite. **Metabolic:** *possible hypokalemia, hyperglycemia and carbohydrate intolerance,* growth suppression in children. **Skin:** delayed wound healing, acne, various skin eruptions. **Other:** muscle weakness, pancreatitis, hirsutism, susceptibility to infections. Acute adrenal insufficiency may follow increased stress (infection, surgery, trauma) or abrupt withdrawal after long-term therapy. **Withdrawal symptoms:** rebound inflammation, fatigue, weakness, arthralgia, fever, dizziness, lethargy, depression, fainting, orthostatic hypotension, dyspnea, anorexia, hypoglycemia. *Sudden withdrawal may be fatal.*
cortisone acetate Cortistan, Cortone Acetate♦	*Adrenal insufficiency, allergy, inflammation—* **Adults:** 25 to 300 mg P.O. or I.M. daily or on alternate days. Doses highly individualized, depending on severity of disease.	Most side effects of corticosteroids are dose- or duration-dependent. **CNS:** *euphoria, insomnia,* psychotic behavior, pseudotumor cerebri. **CV:** *congestive heart failure,* hypertension, edema. **EENT:** cataracts, glaucoma. **GI:** *peptic ulcer,* gastrointestinal

♦ Available in U.S. and Canada. ♦♦ Available in Canada only. All other products (no symbol) available in U.S. only. Italicized side effects are common or life-threatening.

INTERACTIONS	NURSING CONSIDERATIONS
None significant.	• Contraindicated in status asthmaticus. Not for asthma controlled by bronchodilators or other noncorticosteroids, or for nonasthmatic bronchial diseases. • Oral therapy should be tapered slowly. Acute adrenal insufficiency and death have occurred in asthmatics who changed abruptly from oral corticosteroids to beclomethasone. • During times of stress (trauma, surgery, infection) systemic corticosteroids may be needed to prevent adrenal insufficiency in previously steroid-dependent patients. • Instruct patient to carry a card indicating his need for supplemental systemic glucocorticoids during stress. • Patient requiring bronchodilator should use it several minutes before beclomethasone. • Don't store near heat or open flame. • Glucocorticoid with potent anti-inflammatory action. • Oral fungal infections can be prevented by following inhalations with glass of water.
Barbiturates, phenytoin, rifampin: decreased corticosteroid effect. Corticosteroid dose may need to be increased. *Indomethacin, aspirin:* increased risk of GI distress and bleeding. Give together cautiously.	• Contraindicated in systemic fungal infections. Use cautiously in patients with GI ulceration or renal disease, hypertension, osteoporosis, varicella, vaccinia, exanthema, diabetes mellitus, Cushing's syndrome, thromboembolic disorders, seizures, myasthenia gravis, congestive heart failure, tuberculosis, ocular herpes simplex, hypoalbuminemia, emotional instability, or psychotic tendencies. • Don't use for alternate-day therapy. • Adrenal suppression may last up to 1 year after drug stopped. Gradually reduce drug dosage after long-term therapy. Tell patient not to stop drug abruptly or without doctor's consent. • Always titrate to lowest effective dose. • To prevent muscle atrophy, give by deep I.M. injection. • Monitor blood and urine sugars, along with serum potassium, regularly. • Teach patients about the effects and side effects of the medication. Warn patients who are on long-term therapy about cushingoid symptoms. • Observe for signs of infection, especially after steroid withdrawal. Tell patients to report slow healing. • Instruct patient to carry a card indicating his need for supplemental glucocorticoids during stress. • Give with milk or food to reduce gastric irritation. • Glucocorticoid with little mineralocorticoid effect. • Watch for additional potassium depletion from diuretics and amphotericin B. • Immunizations may show decreased antibody response. • Obtain baseline weight before starting therapy, and weigh patient daily; report any sudden weight gain to doctor. • Check for glycosuria. (Use glucose oxidase reagent sticks instead of tablets.)
Barbiturates, phenytoin, rifampin: decreased corticosteroid effect. Corticosteroid dose may need to be increased. *Indomethacin, aspirin:* increased risk of GI distress and	• Contraindicated in systemic fungal infections. Use cautiously in patients with GI ulceration or renal disease, hypertension, osteoporosis, varicella, vaccinia, exanthema, diabetes mellitus, Cushing's syndrome, thromboembolic disorders, seizures, myasthenia gravis, congestive heart failure, tuberculosis, ocular herpes simplex, hypoalbuminemia, emotional instability, or psychotic tendencies. • Gradually reduce drug dosage after long-term therapy. Tell patient not to discontinue drug abruptly or without doctor's consent. • Always titrate to lowest effective dose.

(continued on following page)

NAME	INDICATIONS & DOSAGE	SIDE EFFECTS
cortisone acetate *(continued)*		irritation, increased appetite. **Metabolic:** *possible hypokalemia, hyperglycemia and carbohydrate intolerance,* growth suppression in children. **Skin:** delayed wound healing, acne, various skin eruptions. **Local:** atrophy at I.M. injection sites. **Other:** muscle weakness, pancreatitis, hirsutism, susceptibility to infections. Acute adrenal insufficiency may follow increased stress (infection, surgery, trauma) or abrupt withdrawal after long-term therapy. **Withdrawal symptoms:** rebound inflammation, fatigue, weakness, arthralgia, fever, dizziness, lethargy, depression, fainting, orthostatic hypotension, dyspnea, anorexia, hypoglycemia. *Sudden withdrawal may be fatal.*
desoxycorticosterone acetate Doca Acetate, Percorten Acetate **desoxycorticosterone pivalate** Percorten Pivalate	*Adrenal insufficiency (partial replacement), salt-losing adrenogenital syndrome—* **Adults:** 2 to 5 mg (acetate) I.M. daily; or 25 to 100 mg (pivalate) I.M. q 4 weeks. Or implant 1 pellet for each 0.5 mg of the daily injected maintenance dose. Pellets last for 8 to 12 months.	**CV:** *sodium and water retention,* hypertension, cardiac hypertrophy, edema. **Metabolic:** *hypokalemia.*
dexamethasone Decadron♦, Dexasone♦♦, Dexone, Dezone, Hexadrol, SK-Dexamethasone **dexamethasone acetate** Decadron-LA, Decameth-LA, Dexacen-LA, Dexasone-LA **dexamethasone sodium phosphate** Decadron Phosphate, Decaject, Decameth, Delladec, Dexacen-4,	*Cerebral edema—* **Adults:** initially, 10 mg (phosphate) I.V., then 4 to 6 mg I.M. q 6 hours for 2 to 4 days, then taper over 5 to 7 days. **Children:** 0.2 mg/kg P.O. daily in divided doses. *Inflammatory conditions, allergic reactions, neoplasias—* **Adults:** 0.25 to 4 mg P.O. b.i.d., t.i.d., or q.i.d.; or 4 to 16 mg (acetate) I.M. into joint or soft tissue q 1 to 3 weeks; or 0.8 to 1.6 mg (acetate) into lesions q 1 to 3 weeks. *Shock—* **Adults:** 1 to 6 mg/kg (phosphate) I.V. single dose; or 40 mg	Most side effects of corticosteroids are dose- or duration-dependent. **CNS:** *euphoria, insomnia,* psychotic behavior, pseudotumor cerebri. **CV:** *congestive heart failure,* hypertension, edema. **EENT:** cataracts, glaucoma. **GI:** *peptic ulcer,* gastrointestinal irritation, increased appetite. **Metabolic:** *possible hypokalemia, hyperglycemia and carbohydrate intolerance,* growth suppression in children. **Skin:** delayed wound healing, acne, various skin eruptions. **Local:** atrophy at I.M. injection sites.

♦ Available in U.S. and Canada. ♦♦ Available in Canada only. All other products (no symbol) available in U.S. only. Italicized side effects are common or life-threatening.

INTERACTIONS	NURSING CONSIDERATIONS
bleeding. Give together cautiously.	• Patient may need salt-restricted diet and potassium supplement. • I.M. route causes slow onset of action. Don't use in acute conditions where rapid effect required. May use on a b.i.d. schedule matching diurnal variation. • Glucocorticoid with potent mineralocorticoid effect; report sudden weight gain or edema to doctor. • Observe for signs of infection, especially after steroid withdrawal. Tell patients to report slow healing. • Drug of choice for replacement therapy in adrenal insufficiency. • Not used for alternate-day therapy. • Monitor serum electrolytes and blood and urine sugars. • Warn patients on long-term therapy about cushingoid symptoms. • Give with milk or food to reduce gastric irritation. • Instruct patient to carry a card indicating his need for supplemental glucocorticoids during stress. • Not for I.V. use. • Watch for additional potassium depletion from diuretics and amphotericin B. • Immunizations may show decreased antibody response.
None significant.	• Contraindicated in hypertension, congestive heart failure, cardiac disease. Use cautiously in Addison's disease. Patients may have exaggerated side effects. • Has no anti-inflammatory effect. • Most potent mineralocorticoid. Has little glucocorticoid effect. • Use with glucocorticoid for full treatment of adrenal insufficiency. • Report significant weight gain, edema, hypertension, or cardiac symptoms to doctor. Drug may have to be stopped. • Injection is sesame oil solution. Withdraw dose with 19G needle, but give with 23G needle. Inject in upper, outer quadrant of buttocks. Not for I.V. use. • Monitor sodium and potassium levels, fluid intake. Patient may need salt-restricted diet, potassium supplement. • Watch for additional potassium depletion from diuretics and amphotericin B.
Barbiturates, phenytoin, rifampin: decreased corticosteroid effect. Corticosteroid dose may need to be increased. *Indomethacin, aspirin:* increased risk of GI distress and bleeding. Give together cautiously.	• Contraindicated in systemic fungal infections and for alternate-day therapy. Use cautiously in patients with GI ulceration or renal disease, hypertension, osteoporosis, varicella, vaccinia, exanthema, diabetes mellitus, Cushing's syndrome, thromboembolic disorders, seizures, myasthenia gravis, metastatic cancer, congestive heart failure, tuberculosis, ocular herpes simplex, hypoalbuminemia, emotional instability or psychotic tendencies, and in children. • Gradually reduce drug dosage after long-term therapy. Tell patient not to discontinue drug abruptly or without doctor's consent. • Always titrate to lowest effective dose. • Monitor patient's weight, blood pressure, serum electrolytes. • Instruct patient to carry a card indicating his need for supplemental systemic glucocorticoids during stress, especially as dose is decreased. • Teach patient signs of early adrenal insufficiency: fatigue, muscular weakness, joint pain, fever, anorexia, nausea, dyspnea, dizziness, fainting. • May mask or exacerbate infections.

(continued on following page)

NAME	INDICATIONS & DOSAGE	SIDE EFFECTS
dexamethasone *(continued)* Dexasone, Dexon, Dexone, Dezone, Hexadrol Phosphate♦, Savacort-D, Solurex	I.V. q 2 to 6 hours, p.r.n. *Dexamethasone suppression test—* 0.5 mg P.O. q 6 hours for 48 hours.	**Other:** muscle weakness, pancreatitis, hirsutism, susceptibility to infections. Acute adrenal insufficiency may follow increased stress (infection, surgery, trauma) or abrupt withdrawal after long-term therapy. **Withdrawal symptoms:** rebound inflammation, fatigue, weakness, arthralgia, fever, dizziness, lethargy, depression, fainting, orthostatic hypotension, dyspnea, anorexia, hypoglycemia. *Sudden withdrawal may be fatal.*
fludrocortisone acetate Florinef♦	*Adrenal insufficiency (partial replacement), salt-losing adrenogenital syndrome—* **Adults:** 0.1 to 0.2 mg P.O. daily.	**CV:** *sodium and water retention,* hypertension, cardiac hypertrophy, edema. **Metabolic:** hypokalemia.
fluprednisolone Alphadrol	*Severe inflammation—* **Adults:** 2.5 to 30 mg P.O. daily divided t.i.d. or q.i.d. **Children:** 0.07 to 1 mg/kg P.O. daily divided t.i.d. or q.i.d., or 2.5 to 30 mg/m² divided t.i.d. or q.i.d.	Most side effects of corticosteroids are dose- or duration-dependent. **CNS:** *euphoria, insomnia,* psychotic behavior, pseudotumor cerebri. **CV:** *congestive heart failure,* hypertension, edema. **EENT:** cataracts, glaucoma. **GI:** *peptic ulcer,* gastrointestinal irritation, increased appetite. **Metabolic:** *possible hypokalemia, hyperglycemia and carbohydrate intolerance,* growth suppression in children. **Skin:** delayed wound healing, acne, various skin eruptions. **Other:** muscle weakness, pancreatitis, hirsutism, susceptibility to infections. Acute adrenal insufficiency with increased stress (infection, surgery, trauma) or abrupt cessation of long-term therapy. **Withdrawal symptoms:** rebound inflammation, fatigue, weakness, arthralgia, fever, dizziness, lethargy, depression, fainting, orthostatic hypotension, dyspnea, anorexia, hypoglycemia. *Sudden withdrawal may be fatal.*

INTERACTIONS	NURSING CONSIDERATIONS
	• Watch for depression or psychotic episodes, especially in high-dose therapy. • Inspect patient's skin for petechiae. Warn patient about easy bruising. • Patients with diabetes may need increased insulin; monitor urine for sugar. • Monitor growth in infants and children on long-term therapy. • Give I.M. injection deep into gluteal muscle. Avoid subcutaneous injection, as atrophy and sterile abscesses may occur. • Give P.O. dose with food when possible. • Warn patients on long-term therapy about cushingoid symptoms. • Watch for additional potassium depletion from diuretics and amphotericin B. • Immunizations may show decreased antibody response. • Follow your hospital's guidelines when performing dexamethasone suppression test.
None significant.	• Contraindicated in hypertension, congestive heart failure, cardiac disease. Use cautiously in Addison's disease. • Monitor patient's blood pressure, serum electrolytes. Weigh patient daily; report sudden weight gain to doctor. • Warn patient that mild peripheral edema is common. • Unless contraindicated, give salt-restricted diet rich in potassium and protein. Potassium supplement may be needed. • Has potent mineralocorticoid effects. Little glucocorticoid effect with usual doses. • Used with cortisone or hydrocortisone in adrenal insufficiency. • Watch for additional potassium depletion from diuretics and amphotericin B.
Barbiturates, phenytoin, rifampin: decreased corticosteroid effect. Corticosteroid dose may need to be increased. *Indomethacin, aspirin:* increased risk of GI distress and bleeding. Give together cautiously.	• Contraindicated in systemic fungal infections. Use cautiously in patients with GI ulceration or renal disease, hypertension, osteoporosis, varicella, vaccinia, exanthema, diabetes mellitus, Cushing's syndrome, thromboembolic disorders, seizures, myasthenia gravis, metastatic cancer, congestive heart failure, tuberculosis, ocular herpes simplex, hypoalbuminemia, emotional instability or psychotic tendencies, and in children. • Gradually reduce drug dosage after long-term therapy. Tell patient not to discontinue drug abruptly or without doctor's consent. • Always titrate to lowest effective dose. • Glucocorticoid with moderate mineralocorticoid effect. • Monitor patient's weight, blood pressure, serum electrolytes. • May mask or exacerbate infections. • Instruct patient to carry a card identifying his need for supplemental systemic glucocorticoids during stress. • Teach patient signs of early adrenal insufficiency: fatigue, muscular weakness, joint pain, fever, anorexia, nausea, dyspnea, dizziness, fainting. • Watch for depression or psychotic episodes, especially in high-dose therapy. • Inspect patient's skin for petechiae. Warn patient about easy bruising. • Patients with diabetes may need increased insulin dose; monitor urine for sugar. • Monitor growth in infants and children on long-term therapy. • Unless contraindicated, give salt-restricted diet rich in potassium and protein. Potassium supplement may be needed. • Give P.O. dose with food when possible, especially if GI irritation occurs. • Warn patients on long-term therapy about cushingoid symptoms.

(continued on following page)

NAME	INDICATIONS & DOSAGE	SIDE EFFECTS
fluprednisolone *(continued)*		
hydrocortisone Cortef♦, Hydrocortone♦ **hydrocortisone acetate** Cortef Acetate, Cortril Acetate, Hydrocortone Acetate **hydrocortisone retention enema** Cortenema, Rectoid **hydrocortisone sodium phosphate** Hydrocortone Phosphate **hydrocortisone sodium succinate** A-Hydrocort, S-Cortilean♦♦, Solu-Cortef♦, Solu-Ject♦♦	*Severe inflammation, adrenal insufficiency—* **Adults:** 5 to 30 mg P.O. b.i.d., t.i.d., or q.i.d. (as much as 80 mg P.O. q.i.d. may be given in acute situations); or initially, 100 to 250 mg (succinate) I.M. or I.V., then 50 to 100 mg I.M., as indicated; or 15 to 240 mg (phosphate) I.M. or I.V. q 12 hours; or 5 to 75 mg (acetate) into joints and soft tissue. Dose varies with size of joint. Often local anesthetics are injected with dose. *Shock—* **Adults:** 500 mg to 2 g (succinate) q 2 to 6 hours. **Children:** 0.16 to 1 mg/kg (phosphate or succinate) I.M. or I.V. b.i.d. or t.i.d. *Adjunctive treatment of ulcerative colitis and proctitis—* **Adults:** 1 enema (100 mg) nightly for 21 days.	Most side effects of corticosteroids are dose- or duration-dependent. **CNS:** *euphoria, insomnia,* psychotic behavior, pseudotumor cerebri. **CV:** *congestive heart failure,* hypertension, edema. **EENT:** cataracts, glaucoma. **GI:** *peptic ulcer,* gastrointestinal irritation, increased appetite. **Metabolic:** *possible hypokalemia, hyperglycemia and carbohydrate intolerance,* growth suppression in children. **Skin:** delayed wound healing, acne, various skin eruptions. **Other:** muscle weakness, pancreatitis, hirsutism, susceptibility to infections. Acute adrenal insufficiency may occur with increased stress (infection, surgery, trauma) or abrupt withdrawal after long-term therapy. **Withdrawal symptoms:** rebound inflammation, fatigue, weakness, arthralgia, fever, dizziness, lethargy, depression, fainting, orthostatic hypotension, dyspnea, anorexia, hypoglycemia. *Sudden withdrawal may be fatal.*
meprednisone Betapar	*Severe inflammation—* **Adults:** 4 to 15 mg P.O. b.i.d., t.i.d., or q.i.d.	Most side effects of corticosteroids are dose- or duration-dependent. **CNS:** *euphoria, insomnia,* psychotic behavior, pseudotumor cerebri. **CV:** *congestive heart failure,* hypertension, edema. **EENT:** cataracts, glaucoma. **GI:** *peptic ulcer,* gastrointestinal irritation, increased appetite. **Metabolic:** *possible hypokalemia, hyperglycemia and carbohydrate*

INTERACTIONS	NURSING CONSIDERATIONS
	• Watch for additional potassium depletion from diuretics and amphotericin B. • Immunizations may show decreased antibody response. • Not for alternate-day therapy.
Barbiturates, phenytoin, rifampin: decreased corticosteroid effect. Corticosteroid dose may need to be increased. *Indomethacin, aspirin:* increased risk of GI distress and bleeding. Give together cautiously.	• Contraindicated in systemic fungal infections. Use cautiously in patients with GI ulceration or renal disease, hypertension, osteoporosis, varicella, vaccinia, exanthema, diabetes mellitus, Cushing's syndrome, thromboembolic disorders, seizures, myasthenia gravis, metastatic cancer, congestive heart failure, tuberculosis, ocular herpes simplex, hypoalbuminemia, emotional instability or psychotic tendencies, and in children. • Gradually reduce drug dosage after long-term therapy. Tell patient not to discontinue drug abruptly or without doctor's consent. • Always titrate to lowest effective dose. • Glucocorticoid and mineralocorticoid effect. • Monitor patient's weight, blood pressure, serum electrolytes. • May mask or exacerbate infections. • Stress (fever, trauma, surgery, emotional problems) may increase adrenal insufficiency. Dose may have to be increased. • Instruct patient to carry a card identifying his need for supplemental systemic glucocorticoids during stress. • Teach patient signs of early adrenal insufficiency: fatigue, muscular weakness, joint pain, fever, anorexia, nausea, dyspnea, dizziness, fainting. • Watch for depression or psychotic episodes, especially in high-dose therapy. • Inspect patient's skin for petechiae. Warn patient about easy bruising. • Patients with diabetes may need increased insulin; monitor urine for sugar. • Monitor growth in infants and children on long-term therapy. • Give I.M. injection deep into gluteal muscle. Avoid subcutaneous injection as atrophy and sterile abscesses may occur. • Unless contraindicated, give salt-restricted diet rich in potassium and protein. Potassium supplement may be needed. Watch for additional potassium depletion from diuretics and amphotericin B. • Give P.O. dose with food when possible. • Warn patients on long-term therapy about cushingoid symptoms. • Acetate form for I.M. use only. • Enema may produce same systemic effects as other forms of hydrocortisone. If enema therapy must exceed 21 days, discontinue gradually by reducing administration to every other night for 2 or 3 weeks. • Immunizations may show decreased antibody response. • Do not confuse Solu-Cortef with Solu-Medrol. • Not for alternate-day therapy.
Barbiturates, phenytoin, rifampin: decreased corticosteroid effect. Corticosteroid dose may need to be increased. *Indomethacin, aspirin:* increased risk of GI distress and bleeding. Give together cautiously.	• Contraindicated in systemic fungal infections. Use cautiously in patients with GI ulceration or renal disease, hypertension, osteoporosis, varicella, vaccinia, exanthema, diabetes mellitus, Cushing's syndrome, thromboembolic disorders, seizures, myasthenia gravis, metastatic cancer, congestive heart failure, tuberculosis, ocular herpes simplex, hypoalbuminemia, emotional instability or psychotic tendencies. • Gradually reduce drug dosage after long-term therapy. Tell patient not to discontinue drug abruptly or without doctor's consent. • Always titrate to lowest effective dose. • Glucocorticoid with little mineralocorticoid effect. • Monitor patient's weight, blood pressure, serum electrolytes.

(continued on following page)

NAME	INDICATIONS & DOSAGE	SIDE EFFECTS
meprednisone *(continued)*		*intolerance,* growth suppression in children. **Skin:** delayed wound healing, acne, various skin eruptions. **Other:** muscle weakness, pancreatitis, hirsutism, susceptibility to infections. Acute adrenal insufficiency may occur with increased stress (infection, surgery, trauma) or abrupt withdrawal after long-term therapy. **Withdrawal symptoms:** rebound inflammation, fatigue, weakness, arthralgia, fever, dizziness, lethargy, depression, fainting, orthostatic hypotension, dyspnea, anorexia, hypoglycemia. *Sudden withdrawal may be fatal.*
methylprednisolone Medrol♦ **methylprednisolone acetate** Depo-Medrol♦, D-Med, Medralone, Methydrol-40, Pre-Dep, Rep-Pred **methylprednisolone sodium succinate** A-Methapred, Solu-Medrol♦	*Severe inflammation or immunosuppression*— **Adults:** 2 to 60 mg P.O. in 4 divided doses; or 40 to 80 mg (acetate) daily, I.M. or 10 to 250 mg (succinate) I.M. or I.V. q 4 hours; or 4 to 30 mg (acetate) into joints and soft tissue, p.r.n. **Children:** 117 mcg to 1.66 mg/kg (succinate) I.V. in 3 or 4 divided doses. *Shock*—100 to 250 mg (succinate) I.V. at 2- to 6-hour intervals.	Most side effects of corticosteroids are dose- or duration-dependent. **CNS:** *euphoria, insomnia,* psychotic behavior, pseudotumor cerebri. **CV:** *congestive heart failure,* hypertension, edema. **EENT:** cataracts, glaucoma. **GI:** *peptic ulcer,* gastrointestinal irritation, increased appetite. **Metabolic:** *possible hypokalemia, hyperglycemia and carbohydrate intolerance,* growth suppression in children. **Skin:** delayed wound healing, acne, various skin eruptions. **Other:** muscle weakness, pancreatitis, hirsutism, susceptibility to infections. Acute adrenal insufficiency may occur with increased stress (infection, surgery, trauma) or abrupt withdrawal after long-term therapy. **Withdrawal symptoms:** rebound inflammation, fatigue, weakness, arthralgia, fever, dizziness, lethargy, depression, fainting, orthostatic hypotension, dyspnea, anorexia, hypoglycemia. *Sudden withdrawal may be fatal.*

♦ Available in U.S. and Canada. ♦♦ Available in Canada only. All other products (no symbol) available in U.S. only. Italicized side effects are common or life-threatening.

INTERACTIONS	NURSING CONSIDERATIONS
	• May mask or exacerbate infections. Tell patient to report slow healing. • Instruct patient to carry a card identifying his need for supplemental systemic glucocorticoids during stress. • Useful in rheumatoid and collagen diseases. • Teach patient signs of early adrenal insufficiency: fatigue, muscular weakness, joint pain, fever, anorexia, nausea, dyspnea, dizziness, fainting. • Watch for depression or psychotic episodes, especially in high-dose therapy. • Patients with diabetes may need increased insulin; monitor urine for sugar. • Monitor growth in infants and children on long-term therapy. • Unless contraindicated, give salt-restricted diet rich in potassium and protein. Potassium supplement may be needed. Watch for additional potassium depletion from diuretics and amphotericin B. • Give P.O. dose with food when possible, especially if GI irritation occurs. • Warn patients on long-term therapy about cushingoid symptoms. • Immunizations may show decreased antibody response. • Not for alternate-day therapy.
Barbiturates, phenytoin, rifampin: decreased corticosteroid effect. Corticosteroid dose may need to be increased. *Indomethacin, aspirin:* increased risk of GI distress and bleeding. Give together cautiously.	• Contraindicated in systemic fungal infections. Use cautiously in patients with GI ulceration or renal disease, hypertension, osteoporosis, varicella, vaccinia, exanthema, diabetes mellitus, Cushing's syndrome, thromboembolic disorders, seizures, myasthenia gravis, metastatic cancer, congestive heart failure, tuberculosis, ocular herpes simplex, hypoalbuminemia, emotional instability, or psychotic tendencies. • Gradually reduce drug dosage after long-term therapy. Tell patient not to discontinue drug abruptly or without doctor's consent. • Always titrate to lowest effective dose. • Glucocorticoid with little mineralocorticoid effect. • Discard reconstituted solutions after 48 hours. • Don't use acetate salt when immediate onset of action needed. • Dermal atrophy may occur with large doses of acetate salt. Use multiple small injections into lesions. • Monitor weight, blood pressure, serum electrolytes, sleep patterns. Euphoria may initially interfere with sleep, but patient generally adjusts to the medication after 1 to 3 weeks. • May mask or exacerbate infections. • Instruct patient to carry a card identifying his need for supplemental systemic glucocorticoids during stress. • Teach patient signs of early adrenal insufficiency: fatigue, muscular weakness, joint pain, fever, anorexia, nausea, dyspnea, dizziness, fainting. • Watch for depression or psychotic episodes, especially in high-dose therapy. • Patients with diabetes may need increased insulin; monitor urine for sugar. • Give I.M. injection deep into gluteal muscle. Avoid subcutaneous injection as atrophy and sterile abscesses may occur. • Unless contraindicated, give salt-restricted diet rich in potassium and protein. Potassium supplement may be needed. Watch for additional potassium depletion from diuretics and amphotericin B. • Give P.O. dose with food when possible. • Give I.V. dose slowly over 1 minute; in shock, give massive I.V. doses over 3 to 15 minutes to prevent cardiac arrhythmias and circulatory collapse.

(continued on following page)

NAME	INDICATIONS & DOSAGE	SIDE EFFECTS
methylprednisolone *(continued)*		
paramethasone acetate Haldrone	*Inflammatory conditions—* **Adults:** 0.5 to 6 mg P.O. t.i.d. or q.i.d. **Children:** 58 to 800 mcg/kg daily divided t.i.d. or q.i.d.	Most side effects of corticosteroids are dose- or duration-dependent. **CNS:** *euphoria, insomnia,* psychotic behavior, pseudotumor cerebri. **CV:** *congestive heart failure,* hypertension, edema. **EENT:** cataracts, glaucoma. **GI:** *peptic ulcer,* gastrointestinal irritation, increased appetite. **Metabolic:** *possible hypokalemia, hyperglycemia and carbohydrate intolerance,* growth suppression in children. **Skin:** delayed wound healing, acne, various skin eruptions. **Other:** muscle weakness, pancreatitis, hirsutism, susceptibility to infections. Acute adrenal insufficiency may occur with increased stress (infection, surgery, trauma) or abrupt withdrawal after long-term therapy. **Withdrawal symptoms:** rebound inflammation, fatigue, weakness, arthralgia, fever, dizziness, lethargy, depression, fainting, orthostatic hypotension, dyspnea, anorexia, hypoglycemia. *Sudden withdrawal may be fatal.*
prednisolone Cordrol, Delta-Cortef♦, Predoxine, Ropredlone, Ster 5, Sterane **prednisolone acetate** **prednisolone sodium phosphate** **prednisolone tebutate** Hydeltra-TBA, Metalone-TBA	*Severe inflammation or immunosuppression—* **Adults:** 2.5 to 15 mg P.O. b.i.d., t.i.d., or q.i.d.; 2 to 30 mg I.M. (acetate, phosphate), or I.V. (phosphate) q 12 hours; or 2 to 30 mg (phosphate) into joints, lesions, and soft tissue; or 4 to 40 mg (tebutate) into joints and lesions; or 0.25 to 1 ml (acetate-phosphate suspension) into joints weekly, p.r.n.	Most side effects of corticosteroids are dose- or duration-dependent. **CNS:** *euphoria, insomnia,* psychotic behavior, pseudotumor cerebri. **CV:** *congestive heart failure,* hypertension, edema. **EENT:** cataracts, glaucoma. **GI:** *peptic ulcer,* gastrointestinal irritation, increased appetite. **Metabolic:** *possible hypokalemia, hyperglycemia and carbohydrate intolerance,* growth suppression in children. **Skin:** delayed wound healing, acne, various skin eruptions. **Other:** muscle weakness, pancreatitis, hirsutism, susceptibility to infections. Acute adrenal insufficiency may occur with increased stress (infection, surgery, trauma)

INTERACTIONS	NURSING CONSIDERATIONS
	• Warn patients on long-term therapy about cushingoid symptoms. • Acetate form not for I.V. use. • Do not confuse Solu-Medrol with Solu-Cortef. • Immunizations may show decreased antibody response. • May be used for alternate-day therapy.
Barbiturates, phenytoin, rifampin: decreased corticosteroid effect. Corticosteroid dose may need to be increased. *Indomethacin, aspirin:* increased risk of GI distress and bleeding. Give together cautiously.	• Contraindicated in systemic fungal infections and alternate-day therapy. Use cautiously in patients with GI ulceration or renal disease, hypertension, osteoporosis, varicella, vaccinia, exanthema, diabetes mellitus, Cushing's syndrome, thromboembolic disorders, seizures, myasthenia gravis, metastatic cancer, congestive heart failure, tuberculosis, ocular herpes simplex, hypoalbuminemia, emotional instability, or psychotic tendencies. • Gradually reduce drug dosage after long-term therapy. Tell patient not to discontinue drug abruptly or without doctor's consent. • Always titrate to lowest effective dose. • Glucocorticoid with little mineralocorticoid effect. • Monitor patient's weight, blood pressure, serum electrolytes. • May mask or exacerbate infections. • Instruct patient to carry a card identifying his need for supplemental systemic glucocorticoids during stress. • Teach patient signs of early adrenal insufficiency: fatigue, muscular weakness, joint pain, fever, anorexia, nausea, dyspnea, dizziness, fainting. • Watch for depression or psychotic episodes, especially in high-dose therapy. • Patients with diabetes may need increased insulin; monitor urine for sugar. • Monitor growth in infants and children on long-term therapy. • Unless contraindicated, give salt-restricted diet rich in potassium and protein. Potassium supplement may be needed. Watch for additional potassium depletion from diuretics and amphotericin B. • Give P.O. dose with food when possible, especially if GI irritation occurs. • Warn patients on long-term therapy about cushingoid symptoms. • Immunizations may show decreased antibody response.
Barbiturates, phenytoin, rifampin: decreased corticosteroid effect. Corticosteroid dose may need to be increased. *Indomethacin, aspirin:* increased risk of GI distress and bleeding. Give together cautiously.	• Contraindicated in systemic fungal infections. Use cautiously in patients with GI ulceration or renal disease, hypertension, osteoporosis, varicella, vaccinia, exanthema, diabetes mellitus, Cushing's syndrome, thromboembolic disorders, seizures, myasthenia gravis, metastatic cancer, congestive heart failure, tuberculosis, ocular herpes simplex, hypoalbuminemia, emotional instability, or psychotic tendencies. • Gradually reduce drug dosage after long-term therapy. Tell patient not to discontinue drug abruptly or without doctor's consent. • Always titrate to lowest effective dose. • Glucocorticoid with slight mineralocorticoid action. • Prednisolone salts (acetate, sodium phosphate, and tebutate) are used parenterally less often than other corticosteroids that have more potent anti-inflammatory action. • May use for alternate-day therapy. • Monitor patient's weight, blood pressure, serum electrolytes. • May mask or exacerbate infections. Tell patient to report slow healing. • Instruct patient to carry a card identifying his need for supplemental systemic glucocorticoids during stress. • Warn patients on long-term therapy about cushingoid symptoms. • Teach patient signs of early adrenal insufficiency: fatigue, muscular

(continued on following page)

NAME	INDICATIONS & DOSAGE	SIDE EFFECTS
prednisolone *(continued)*		or abrupt withdrawal after long-term therapy. **Withdrawal symptoms:** rebound inflammation, fatigue, weakness, arthralgia, fever, dizziness, lethargy, depression, fainting, orthostatic hypotension, dyspnea, anorexia, hypoglycemia. *Sudden withdrawal may be fatal.*
prednisone Colisone♦♦, Deltasone♦, Fernisone, Meticorten, Orasone, Paracort♦, Prednicen-M, SK-Prednisone, Sterapred	*Severe inflammation or immunosuppression—* **Adults:** 2.5 to 15 mg P.O. b.i.d., t.i.d., or q.i.d. Maintenance dose given once daily or every other day. **Children:** 0.14 to 2 mg/kg daily P.O. divided q.i.d.	Most side effects of corticosteroids are dose- or duration-dependent. **CNS:** *euphoria, insomnia,* psychotic behavior, pseudotumor cerebri. **CV:** *congestive heart failure,* hypertension, edema. **EENT:** cataracts, glaucoma. **GI:** *peptic ulcer,* gastrointestinal irritation, increased appetite. **Metabolic:** *possible hypokalemia, hyperglycemia and carbohydrate intolerance,* growth suppression in children. **Skin:** delayed wound healing, acne, various skin eruptions. **Other:** muscle weakness, pancreatitis, hirsutism, susceptibility to infections. Acute adrenal insufficiency may occur with increased stress (infection, surgery, trauma) or abrupt withdrawal after long-term therapy. **Withdrawal symptoms:** rebound inflammation, fatigue, weakness, arthralgia, fever, dizziness, lethargy, depression, fainting, orthostatic hypotension, dyspnea, anorexia, hypoglycemia. *Sudden withdrawal may be fatal.*
triamcinolone Aristocort♦, Cino, Kenacort♦, Spencort, Tricilone **triamcinolone acetonide** Kenalog♦	*Severe inflammation or immunosuppression—* **Adults:** 4 to 48 mg P.O. daily divided b.i.d., t.i.d., or q.i.d., or 40 mg I.M. (diacetate or acetonide) weekly; or 5 to 48 mg (diacetate or acetonide) into lesions; or 2 to 40 mg (diacetate or acetonide) into joints and soft tissue; or up to 0.5 mg (hexace-	Most side effects of corticosteroids are dose- or duration-dependent. **CNS:** *euphoria, insomnia,* psychotic behavior, pseudotumor cerebri. **CV:** *congestive heart failure,* hypertension, edema. **EENT:** cataracts, glaucoma. **GI:** *peptic ulcer,* gastrointestinal irritation, increased appetite.

♦ Available in U.S. and Canada. ♦♦ Available in Canada only. All other products (no symbol) available in U.S. only. Italicized side effects are common or life-threatening.

INTERACTIONS	NURSING CONSIDERATIONS
	weakness, joint pain, fever, anorexia, nausea, dyspnea, dizziness, fainting. • Watch for depression or psychotic episodes, especially in high-dose therapy. • Patients with diabetes may need increased insulin; monitor urine for sugar. • Give I.M. injection deep into gluteal muscle. Avoid subcutaneous injection, as atrophy and sterile abscesses may occur. • Unless contraindicated, give salt-restricted diet rich in potassium and protein. Potassium supplement may be needed. Watch for additional potassium depletion from diuretics and amphotericin B. • Give P.O. dose with food when possible, to reduce GI irritation. • Acetate form not for I.V. use. • Immunizations may show decreased antibody response.
Barbiturates, phenytoin, rifampin: decreased corticosteroid effect. Corticosteroid dose may need to be increased. *Indomethacin, aspirin:* increased risk of GI distress and bleeding. Give together cautiously.	• Contraindicated in systemic fungal infections. Use cautiously in patients with GI ulceration or renal disease, hypertension, osteoporosis, varicella, vaccinia, exanthema, diabetes mellitus, Cushing's syndrome, thromboembolic disorders, seizures, myasthenia gravis, metastatic cancer, congestive heart failure, tuberculosis, ocular herpes simplex, hypoalbuminemia, emotional instability, or psychotic tendencies. • Gradually reduce drug dosage after long-term therapy. Tell patient not to discontinue drug abruptly or without doctor's consent. • Always titrate to lowest effective dose. • Monitor patient's blood pressure, sleep patterns, serum potassium levels. • Weigh patient daily; report sudden weight gain to doctor. • May mask or exacerbate infections. Tell patient to report slow healing. • Instruct patient to carry a card identifying his need for supplemental systemic glucocorticoids during stress. • Teach patient signs of early adrenal insufficiency: fatigue, muscular weakness, joint pain, fever, anorexia, nausea, dyspnea, dizziness, fainting. • Watch for depression or psychotic episodes, especially in high-dose therapy. • Patients with diabetes may need increased insulin; monitor urine for sugar. • Monitor growth in infants and children on long-term therapy. • Give salt-restricted diet rich in potassium and protein. Potassium supplement may be needed. Watch for additional potassium depletion from diuretics and amphotericin B. • Unless contraindicated, give P.O. dose with food when possible, to reduce GI irritation. • May use for alternate-day therapy. • Warn patients on long-term therapy about cushingoid symptoms. • Immunizations may show decreased antibody response.
Barbiturates, phenytoin, rifampin: decreased corticosteroid effect; dose may need to be increased. *Indomethacin, aspirin:* increased risk of GI distress and bleeding. Give together cautiously.	• Contraindicated in systemic fungal infections. Use cautiously in patients with GI ulceration or renal disease, hypertension, osteoporosis, varicella, vaccinia, exanthema, diabetes mellitus, Cushing's syndrome, thromboembolic disorders, seizures, myasthenia gravis, metastatic cancer, congestive heart failure, tuberculosis, ocular herpes simplex, hypoalbuminemia, emotional instability, or psychotic tendencies. • Gradually reduce drug dosage after long-term therapy. Tell patient not to discontinue drug abruptly or without doctor's consent. • Always titrate to lowest effective dose.

(continued on following page)

NAME	INDICATIONS & DOSAGE	SIDE EFFECTS
triamcinolone *(continued)* **triamcinolone diacetate** Amcort, Aristocort Parenteral Forte, Cenocort Forte, Cino-40, Tracilon, Triam-Forte, Tristoject **triamcinolone hexacetonide** Aristospan♦	tonide) per square inch of affected skin intralesional; or 2 to 20 mg (hexacetonide) intra-articular or intrasynovial into soft tissue or into joint or lesion. Often, a local anesthetic is injected into the joint with triamcinolone.	**Metabolic:** *possible hypokalemia, hyperglycemia and carbohydrate intolerance,* growth suppression in children. **Skin:** delayed wound healing, acne, various skin eruptions. **Other:** muscle weakness, pancreatitis, hirsutism, susceptibility to infections. Acute adrenal insufficiency may occur with increased stress (infection, surgery, trauma) or abrupt withdrawal after long-term therapy. **Withdrawal symptoms:** rebound inflammation, fatigue, weakness, arthralgia, fever, dizziness, lethargy, depression, fainting, orthostatic hypotension, dyspnea, anorexia, hypoglycemia. *Sudden withdrawal may be fatal.*

♦ Available in U.S. and Canada. ♦♦ Available in Canada only. All other products (no symbol) available in U.S. only. Italicized side effects are common or life-threatening.

QUESTIONS & ANSWERS

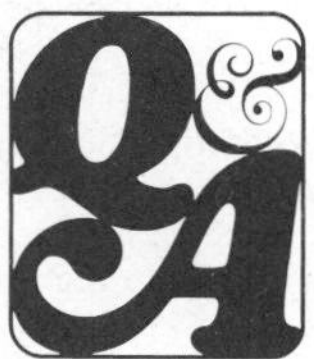

WHAT YOU SHOULD KNOW ABOUT ALTERNATE-DAY STEROID THERAPY

What's the rationale for alternate-day therapy?

Your patient can avoid the complications of long-term steroid therapy by having alternate-day therapy prescribed for him. With this method of steroid administration, your patient will receive his entire 48-hour dose at one time.

Long-term glucocorticoid therapy suppresses the hypothalamic-pituitary-adrenal (HPA) axis, which causes most of your patient's side effects. Administering glucocorticoids on alternate days allows his body to rest and gives the HPA axis a chance to recover.

How will the doctor initiate alternate-day therapy?

First, if your patient's receiving multiple daily doses, the doctor will order the glucocorticoid to be given in one daily dose. Then in a few days, he'll prescribe a 48-hour dose that will be given at one time. For example, if your patient's receiving 5 mg of prednisone twice daily, the new order will be for 10 mg once daily. Then it'll change to 20 mg every other day.

What time of day is best for administration?

The body's endogenous level of glucocorticoids is highest in the morning (between 6 and 9 a.m.) and lowest in the evening (between 9 p.m. and midnight). Since the idea is to simulate the body's natural glucocorticoid production, you should administer the drug between 7 and 8 a.m. in order to obtain maximum benefit. This schedule causes less HPA suppression, hence, fewer side effects.

INTERACTIONS	NURSING CONSIDERATIONS
	• Monitor patient's weight, blood pressure, serum electrolytes. • May mask or exacerbate infections. Tell patient to report slow healing. • Instruct patient to carry a card identifying his need for supplemental systemic glucocorticoids during stress. • Teach patient signs of early adrenal insufficiency: fatigue, muscular weakness, joint pain, fever, anorexia, nausea, dyspnea, dizziness, fainting. • Watch for depression or psychotic episodes, especially in high-dose therapy. • Patients with diabetes may need increased insulin; monitor urine for sugar. • Give I.M. injection deep into gluteal muscle. Avoid subcutaneous injection, as atrophy and sterile abscesses may occur. • Unless contraindicated, give salt-restricted diet rich in potassium and protein. Potassium supplement may be needed. Watch for additional potassium depletion from diuretics and amphotericin B. • Give P.O. dose with food when possible, to reduce GI irritation. • Glucocorticoid with very little mineralocorticoid effect. • Discard unused diluted suspension within 7 days. • Don't use diluents that contain preservatives. Flocculation may occur. • Warn patients on long-term therapy about cushingoid symptoms. • Immunizations may show decreased antibody response. • Not for alternate-day therapy. • No forms for I.V. use. Hexacetonide not for I.V. or I.M. use.

Will alternate-day therapy work for all patients?

Unfortunately, no. Alternate-day therapy works well for patients who have asthma, systemic lupus erythematosus, uveitis, nephrotic syndrome, and for some dermatoses. It's especially heartening to watch asthmatic children whose growth has been suppressed by glucocorticoids resume normal growth patterns after beginning alternate-day therapy.

In some patients, however, disease symptoms reappear toward the end of the 48-hour period. Increasing the dose or resuming once-daily therapy usually eliminates this problem.

Alternate-day therapy does *not* work well for patients with rheumatoid arthritis and ulcerative colitis. And the doctor won't attempt alternate-day therapy in patients with diseases such as leukemia and hemolytic anemia.

Why are only certain glucocorticoids used for alternate-day therapy?

Doctors usually prescribe only prednisone, prednisolone, and methylprednisolone because these glucocorticoids suppress the HPA axis for no more than 24 to 36 hours. Longer-acting drugs such as dexamethasone defeat the purpose of alternate-day therapy. And shorter-acting drugs such as hydrocortisone provide an inadequate therapeutic effect.

How can I help my patient comply with an alternate-day regimen?

Advise your patient to mark off every odd or even day on his calendar and to keep the calendar next to his medicine cabinet. Remind him that following this regimen will make his glucocorticoid side effects more bearable. If he happens to miss a day, advise him to call his doctor right away.

Sometimes the larger dose can cause gastrointestinal (GI) upset; if so, tell your patient to take his dose right after breakfast. If this doesn't ease the gastrointestinal discomfort, he may need to take an antacid. But, generally, if your patient didn't experience GI upset before starting alternate-day therapy, he probably won't have any GI problems with his new schedule.

Androgens and anabolic steroids

danazol
ethylestrenol
fluoxymesterone
methandrostenolone
methyltestosterone
nandrolone decanoate
nandrolone phenpropionate
oxandrolone
oxymetholone
stanozolol
testosterone
testosterone cypionate
testosterone enanthate
testosterone propionate

Androgens (danazol, fluoxymesterone, methyltestosterone, and testosterone and its salts) include both the organic and the synthetic steroids that stimulate growth of the male accessory sex organs, promoting development of secondary sex characteristics such as facial and body hair, deep voice, and skeletal muscle. Testosterone, the primary natural androgen in humans, is produced by the interstitial cells of the testes under the stimulation of luteinizing hormone (LH) from the pituitary. A smaller amount of testosterone is secreted by the adrenal cortex in both sexes and by the ovaries in females.

Anabolic steroids (ethylestrenol, methandrostenolone, nandrolone decanoate, nandrolone phenpropionate, oxandrolone, oxymetholone, and stanozolol) are synthetic compounds structurally related to testosterone. They promote tissue-building and reverse tissue-depleting processes. They have an advantage over testosterone, its esters, and synthetic androgens when anabolic rather than androgenic activity is desired. Despite their preponderant anabolic properties, their residual androgenic activity may produce some virilization in female patients if large doses are administered for long periods.

Major uses

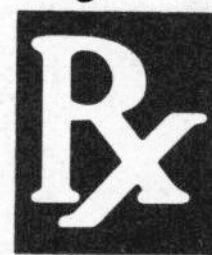

• *Androgens in androgen-deficient males* combat hypogonadism of either primary origin (for example, Klinefelter's syndrome or myotonic dystrophy) or secondary origin (for example, pituitary tumors or pituitary insufficiency, and selective gonadotropin deficiencies, such as eunuchoidism).

They're also used to treat oligospermia and impotence.

• *Androgens in women* prevent postpartum breast pain and engorgement in non–breast-feeding mothers (lactation is not suppressed).

They may also palliate androgen-responsive, advanced inoperable breast cancer in patients who have been in menopause for more than 1 year but less than 5 years, or who have an estrogen-dependent tumor.

They're also used to treat certain gynecologic conditions (for example, uterine hemorrhage, dysmenorrhea, and menopausal syndrome).

Danazol, a synthetic androgen, is therapeutic for fibrocystic breast disease. It is also used to treat refractory endometriosis.

- Anabolic steroids promote weight gain in patients who are underweight due to predisposing catabolic states. An adequate dietary regimen should be established to maximize tissue-building.

Anabolic steroids also correct corticosteroid catabolism and reverse the profound negative nitrogen balance that occurs in corticosteroid therapy.

As adjunctive therapy, they may be effective in senile and postmenopausal osteoporosis as well as refractory anemias associated with chronic disease.

Mechanism of action

- Androgens are simply exogenous replacements that stimulate target tissues to develop normally in androgen-deficient males.
- Anabolic steroids stimulate cellular protein synthesis in debilitated patients. The resulting positive nitrogen balance promotes anabolism. Anabolic steroids also promote a sense of well-being in debilitated patients. This may encourage the patient to eat more and gain weight.

They improve calcium balance and decrease bone resorption. They also enhance erythropoiesis by stimulating secretion of renal or extrarenal erythropoietin and by directly stimulating heme synthesis, an action potentiated by erythropoietin.

Absorption, distribution, metabolism, and excretion

- Testosterone and its derivatives are well absorbed from the gastrointestinal tract. However, since most of these drugs undergo rapid degradation in the liver (because of first-pass effect), they are not effective when given orally. Administering testosterone buccally or sublingually circumvents the drug's hepatic degradation.
- Methyltestosterone and fluoxymesterone resist hepatic metabolism because they are alkylated in the 17-alpha position and are therefore the only orally active agents.
- Testosterone cypionate and enanthate are dissolved in oil and injected intramuscularly.
- All androgens and anabolic steroids are metabolized in the liver and excreted primarily by the kidneys.

Onset and duration

- Onset of the androgens and anabolic steroids is difficult to determine because subjective response varies. Hematologic and other objective responses are not apparent for at least 3 months.
- Nandrolone decanoate and phenpropionate given I.M. have durations of 3 to 4 weeks and 1 to 2 weeks, respectively.
- Testosterone cypionate and enanthate have effects that last as long as 4 weeks.
- Testosterone propionate dissolved in oil has a shorter action than the other two ester analogs; however, its 2- to 3-day duration supplies the effect of daily injections of testosterone alone.
- Subcutaneous implantation of testosterone pellets prolongs action up to 6 months.

Combination products

DELADUMONE INJECTION (oil)♦: testosterone enanthate 90 mg, estradiol valerate 4 mg, and chlorobutanol 0.5%.

DEPO-TESTADIOL (oil): testosterone cypionate 50 mg, estradiol cypionate 2 mg, and chlorobutanol 0.5%.

DITATE-DS: estradiol valerate 8 mg and testosterone enanthate 180 mg.

FORMATRIX: conjugated estrogens 1.25 mg, methyltestosterone 10 mg, and ascorbic acid 400 mg.

GYNETONE .02: ethinyl estradiol 0.02 mg and methyltestosterone 5 mg.

GYNETONE .04: ethinyl estradiol 0.04 mg and methyltestosterone 10 mg.

LACTOSTAT (oil)♦♦: testosterone enanthate benzilic acid hydrazone 300 mg, estradiol dienanthate 15 mg, and estradiol benzoate 6 mg.

PREMARIN WITH METHYLTESTOSTERONE♦: conjugated estrogens 0.625 mg and methyltestosterone 5 mg.

NAME	INDICATIONS & DOSAGE	SIDE EFFECTS
danazol Cyclomen♦♦, Danocrine	*Endometriosis—* **Women:** 400 mg P.O. b.i.d. uninterrupted for 3 to 6 months; may continue for 9 months. *Fibrocystic breast disease—* **Women:** 100 to 400 mg P.O. daily uninterrupted for 2 to 6 months.	**Androgenic:** acne, edema, *weight gain, hirsutism,* hoarseness, clitoral enlargement, *decrease in breast size,* changes in libido, male-pattern baldness, *oiliness of skin or hair.* **CNS:** dizziness, headache, sleep disorders, fatigue, tremor, irritability, excitation, lethargy, mental depression, chills, paresthesias. **CV:** elevated blood pressure. **EENT:** visual disturbances. **GI:** gastric irritation, nausea, vomiting, diarrhea, constipation, change in appetite. **GU:** hematuria. **Hepatic:** jaundice. **Hypoestrogenic:** flushing; sweating; vaginitis, including itching, dryness, burning, and vaginal bleeding; nervousness, emotional lability. **Other:** muscle cramps or spasms.
ethylestrenol Maxibolin♦	*Promote weight gain and combat tissue depletion, refractory anemias, catabolic effects of corticosteroid therapy, osteoporosis, prolonged immobilization, and debilitated states—* **Adults:** 4 to 8 mg P.O. daily, reduced to minimum levels at first evidence of clinical response. **Children:** 1 to 3 mg P.O. daily; highly individualized. A single course of therapy in both adults and children should not exceed 6 weeks; may be reinstituted after 4-week interval.	**Androgenic:** in females—*acne, edema, oily skin, weight gain, hirsutism, hoarseness,* clitoral enlargement, changes in libido. In males—prepubertal: premature epiphyseal closure, acne, priapism, growth of body and facial hair, phallic enlargement; postpubertal: testicular atrophy, oligospermia, decreased ejaculatory volume, impotence, gynecomastia, epididymitis. **CV:** edema. **GI:** gastroenteritis, nausea, vomiting, diarrhea, constipation, change in appetite. **GU:** bladder irritability. **Hepatic:** jaundice. **Hypoestrogenic:** in females—flushing; sweating; vaginitis with itching, drying, burning, or bleeding; menstrual irregularities. **Other:** hypercalcemia.

♦ Available in U.S. and Canada. ♦♦ Available in Canada only. All other products (no symbol) available in U.S. only. Italicized side effects are common or life-threatening.

INTERACTIONS	NURSING CONSIDERATIONS
None significant.	• Contraindicated in patients with undiagnosed abnormal genital bleeding; impaired renal, cardiac, or hepatic function. Use cautiously in patients with epilepsy or migraine headache. • Use with diet high in calories and protein unless contraindicated. • Monitor closely for signs of virilization. Some androgenic effects, such as deepening of voice, may not be reversible upon discontinuation of drug. • Instruct patient to wear cotton underwear only. • Washing after intercourse is recommended to decrease the risk of vaginitis.
None significant.	• Contraindicated in patients with prostatic hypertrophy with obstruction; carcinoma of male breast; hypercalcemia; prostatic cancer; cardiac, hepatic, or renal decompensation; nephrosis; and in premature infants. Use cautiously in prepubertal males; patients with diabetes or coronary disease; patients taking ACTH, corticosteroids, or anticoagulants. • Hypercalcemia symptoms may be difficult to distinguish from symptoms of condition being treated unless anticipated and thought of as a symptom cluster. Hypercalcemia is particularly likely to occur in patients with metastatic breast cancer and may indicate bone metastases. • Stop therapy if female patient reports menstrual irregularities. • Watch for signs of virilization; may be irreversible despite prompt discontinuation of therapy. Doctor must decide if benefits outweigh effects. • Closely monitor boys under 7 years for precocious development of male sexual characteristics. • In children: therapy should be preceded by X-ray of wrist bones to establish level of bone maturation. During treatment, bone maturation may proceed more rapidly than linear growth; dosage should be intermittent and X-rays taken periodically. • Edema is generally controllable with salt restriction and/or diuretics. Monitor weight routinely. • Watch for symptoms of jaundice. Dose adjustment may reverse condition. Periodic liver function studies are recommended. • Observe patient on concomitant anticoagulant therapy for ecchymotic areas, petechiae, or abnormal bleeding. Monitor prothrombin time. • Watch for symptoms of hypoglycemia in patients with diabetes. Dosage of antidiabetic drug may need adjustment. • Use with diet high in calories and protein unless contraindicated. • Anabolic steroids may alter many laboratory studies during therapy and for 2 to 3 weeks after therapy is stopped.

NAME	INDICATIONS & DOSAGE	SIDE EFFECTS
fluoxymesterone Android-F, Halotestin♦, Oratestin♦♦, Oratestryl	*Hypogonadism and impotence due to testicular deficiency*— **Adults:** 2 to 10 mg P.O. daily. *Palliation of breast cancer in women*—15 to 30 mg P.O. daily in divided doses. All dosages should be individualized and reduced to minimum when effect is noted. *Postpartum breast engorgement*— 2.5 mg P.O. followed by 5 to 10 mg daily for 5 days.	**Androgenic:** in females—*acne, edema, oily skin, weight gain, hirsutism, hoarseness,* clitoral enlargement, change in libido. In males—prepubertal: premature epiphyseal closure, acne, priapism, growth of body and facial hair, phallic enlargement; postpubertal: testicular atrophy, oligospermia, decreased ejaculatory volume, impotence, gynecomastia, epididymitis. **CV:** edema. **GI:** gastroenteritis, nausea, vomiting, constipation, change in appetite, diarrhea. **GU:** bladder irritability. **Hepatic:** jaundice. **Hypoestrogenic:** in females—flushing; sweating; vaginitis with itching, drying, burning, or bleeding; menstrual irregularities; emotional lability. **Other:** hypercalcemia.
methandrostenolone Danabol♦♦, Dianabol	*Senile and postmenopausal osteoporosis*— **Adults:** initially 5 mg P.O. daily. Maintenance 2.5 to 5 mg P.O. daily. *Anabolic effect*— **Adults:** 5 to 10 mg P.O. daily. *Severe debilitation*— **Adults:** 10 to 20 mg P.O. daily for 3 weeks, reduced to 5 to 10 mg P.O. daily for maintenance. *Severe maturational delay when growth hormone is unavailable*— **Children:** (postpubertal) up to 0.05 mg/kg P.O. daily. Intermittent therapy is recommended in prolonged use.	**Androgenic:** in females—*acne, edema, oily skin, weight gain, hirsutism, hoarseness,* clitoral enlargement, changes in libido. In males—prepubertal: premature epiphyseal closure, acne, priapism, growth of body and facial hair, phallic enlargement; postpubertal: testicular atrophy, oligospermia, decreased ejaculatory volume, impotence, gynecomastia, epididymitis. **CV:** edema. **EENT:** burning of tongue. **GI:** gastroenteritis, nausea, vomiting, change in appetite, diarrhea, anorexia, constipation. **GU:** bladder irritability. **Hepatic:** jaundice. **Hypoestrogenic:** in females—flushing; sweating; vaginitis with itching, drying, burning, or bleeding; menstrual irregularities. **Other:** hypercalcemia.

INTERACTIONS	NURSING CONSIDERATIONS
None significant.	• Contraindicated in patients with prostatic hypertrophy with obstruction; carcinoma of male breast; prostatic cancer; cardiac, hepatic, or renal decompensation; nephrosis; hypercalcemia; and in premature infants. Use cautiously in prepubertal males; patients with diabetes or coronary disease; and patients taking ACTH, corticosteroids, or anticoagulants. • Hypercalcemia symptoms may be difficult to distinguish from symptoms associated with condition being treated unless anticipated and thought of as a symptom cluster. Hypercalcemia is particularly likely to occur in patients with metastatic breast cancer and may indicate bone metastases. • Explain to patient on drug for palliation of breast cancer that virilization usually occurs at dosage used. Give emotional support. Tell patient to report androgenic effects immediately. Stopping drug will prevent further androgenic changes but will probably not reverse those already existing. • When used in breast cancer, subjective effects may not be seen for about 1 month; objective symptoms not for 3 months. • Discontinue use if female patient reports menstrual irregularities. • Edema is generally controllable with salt restriction and/or diuretics. Monitor weight routinely. • Watch for symptoms of jaundice. Dose adjustment may reverse condition. Periodic liver function studies are recommended. • Observe patient on concomitant anticoagulant therapy for ecchymotic areas, petechiae, or abnormal bleeding. Monitor prothrombin time. • Watch for symptoms of hypoglycemia in patients with diabetes. Dosage of antidiabetic drug may need adjustment. • Use with diet high in calories and protein unless contraindicated.
None significant.	• Contraindicated in patients with prostatic hypertrophy with obstruction, carcinoma of male breast, prostatic cancer; cardiac, hepatic, or renal decompensation; nephrosis; and in premature infants. Use cautiously in prepubertal males; patients with diabetes or coronary disease; patients taking ACTH, corticosteroids, or anticoagulants. • Hypercalcemia symptoms may be difficult to distinguish from symptoms of condition being treated unless anticipated and thought of as a cluster. Hypercalcemia is particularly likely to occur with metastatic breast cancer and may indicate bone metastases. Therapy should be discontinued. • Discontiue use if female patient reports menstrual irregularities. • Watch closely for signs of virilization; they may be irreversible despite prompt discontinuation of therapy. • In children, therapy should be preceded by X-ray of wrist bones to establish level of bone maturation. During treatment, bone maturation may proceed more rapidly than linear growth; dosage should be intermittent and X-rays taken periodically. • Edema is generally controllable with salt restriction and/or diuretics. Monitor weight routinely. • Watch for symptoms of jaundice. Dose adjustment may reverse condition. Periodic liver function studies are recommended. • Watch for ecchymotic areas, petechiae, or abnormal bleeding in patients on concomitant anticoagulant therapy. Monitor prothrombin time. • Watch for symptoms of hypoglycemia in patients with diabetes. Dosage of antidiabetic drug may need adjustment. • May lower fasting blood sugar in both diabetic and nondiabetic patients. • Erroneously thought to enhance athletic ability. • Anabolic steroids may alter many laboratory studies during therapy and for 2 to 3 weeks after therapy is stopped.

NAME	INDICATIONS & DOSAGE	SIDE EFFECTS
methyltestosterone Android-5, Android-10, Metandren♦, Oreton-Methyl, Testred, Virilon	**Adults:** *Breast engorgement of non–breast-feeding mothers*—80 mg P.O. daily, or 40 mg buccal daily for 3 to 5 days. *Breast cancer in women 1 to 5 years postmenopausal*—200 mg P.O. daily; or 100 mg buccal daily. *Eunuchoidism and eunuchism, male climacteric symptoms*—10 to 40 mg P.O. daily; or 5 to 20 mg buccal daily. *Postpubertal cryptorchidism*—30 mg P.O. daily; or 15 mg buccal daily.	**Androgenic:** in females—*acne, edema, oily skin, weight gain, hirsutism, hoarseness,* clitoral enlargement, changes in libido. In males—prepubertal: premature epiphyseal closure, acne, priapism, growth of body and facial hair, phallic enlargement; postpubertal: testicular atrophy, oligospermia, decreased ejaculatory volume, impotence, gynecomastia, epididymitis. **CV:** edema. **GI:** gastroenteritis, constipation, nausea, vomiting, diarrhea, change in appetite. **GU:** bladder irritability. **Hepatic:** jaundice. **Hypoestrogenic:** in females—flushing; sweating; vaginitis with itching, drying, burning, or bleeding; menstrual irregularities. **Local:** irritation of oral mucosa with buccal administration. **Other:** hypercalcemia.
nandrolone decanoate Deca-Durabolin♦, Deca-Hybolin **nandrolone phenpropionate** Anabolin, Anorolone, Durabolin♦, Nandrolin	*Severe debility or disease states, refractory anemias (decanoate)*— **Adults:** 100 to 200 mg I.M. weekly. Therapy should be intermittent. *Tissue-building (decanoate)*— **Adults:** 50 to 100 mg I.M. q 3 to 4 weeks. **Children 2 to 13 years:** 25 to 50 mg I.M. q 3 to 4 weeks. *Severe debility or disease states (phenpropionate)*— **Adults:** 50 to 100 mg I.M. weekly. **Children 2 to 13 years:** 12.5 to 25 mg I.M. q 2 to 4 weeks. **Children under 2 years:** 12.5 mg I.M. q 2 to 4 weeks. Therapy should be intermittent, based on therapeutic response. *Tissue building and/or erythropoietic effects (phenpropionate)*— **Adults:** 25 to 50 mg I.M. weekly.	**Androgenic:** in females—*acne, edema, oily skin, weight gain, hirsutism, hoarseness,* clitoral enlargement, decreased or increased libido. In males—prepubertal: premature epiphyseal closure, acne, priapism, growth of body and facial hair, phallic enlargement; postpubertal: testicular atrophy, oligospermia, decreased ejaculatory volume, impotence, gynecomastia, epididymitis. **CV:** edema. **GI:** gastroenteritis, nausea, vomiting, diarrhea, change in appetite. **GU:** bladder irritability. **Hepatic:** jaundice. **Hypoestrogenic:** in females—flushing; sweating; vaginitis with itching, drying, burning, or bleeding; menstrual irregularities with large doses. **Local:** pain at injection site, induration. **Other:** hypercalcemia, hypercalciuria.

INTERACTIONS	NURSING CONSIDERATIONS
None significant.	• Contraindicated in women of childbearing potential (possible masculinization of female infant); in elderly, asthenic males who may react adversely to androgen overstimulation; in hypercalcemia; cardiac, hepatic, or renal decompensation; prostatic or breast cancer in males; benign prostatic hypertrophy with obstruction; conditions aggravated by fluid retention; hypertension; and in premature infants. Use cautiously in myocardial infarction or coronary artery disease. • Treatment of breast cancer usually restricted to patients 1 to 5 years postmenopausal. • Edema is generally controllable with salt restriction and/or diuretics. • Periodic serum cholesterol and calcium determinations, and cardiac and liver function studies recommended. Watch closely for jaundice. • In metastatic breast cancer, hypercalcemia may indicate progression of bone metastases. Report signs of hypercalcemia. • Therapeutic response in breast cancer is usually apparent within 3 months. Therapy should be stopped if signs of disease progression appear. • Enhances hypoglycemia; teach patient signs of hypoglycemia, and instruct him to report immediately if they occur. • Watch for ecchymoses, petechiae, and abnormal bleeding in patients receiving concomitant anticoagulants. • Promptly report signs of virilization in females. • Use with diet high in calories and protein unless contraindicated. • Buccal tablets twice as potent as oral tablets. Tell patient to avoid eating, drinking, chewing, or smoking while buccal tablet is in place, and that tablet is not to be swallowed. Tablet requires 30 to 60 minutes to dissolve. Instruct patient to change tablet absorption site with each dose to minimize risk of buccal irritation.
None significant.	• Contraindicated in patients with prostatic hypertrophy with obstruction; male breast and prostatic cancer; cardiac, hepatic, or renal decompensation; nephrosis; and in premature infants. Use cautiously in prepubertal males; patients with diabetes or coronary disease; patients taking ACTH, corticosteroids, or anticoagulants. • Inject drug deep I.M., preferably into upper outer quadrant of gluteal muscle in adults. • Monitor serum cholesterol in cardiac patients. • Hypercalcemia is most likely to occur in patients with mammary carcinoma; these patients should have quantitative urinary and serum calcium level determinations. • Discontinue use if female patient reports menstrual irregularities. • Watch for signs of virilization; they may be irreversible despite prompt discontinuation of therapy. • Closely observe boys under 7 years for precocious development of male sexual characteristics. • In children, therapy should be preceded by X-ray of wrist bones to establish level of bone maturation. During treatment, bone maturation may proceed more rapidly than linear growth; dosage should be intermittent and X-rays taken periodically. • Edema is generally controllable with salt restrictions and/or diuretics. • Watch for symptoms of jaundice. Dose adjustment may reverse condition. Periodic liver function studies are recommended. • Observe patients receiving concomitant anticoagulant therapy for ecchymotic areas, petechiae, or abnormal bleeding. Monitor prothrombin time. • Watch for symptoms of hypoglycemia in patients with diabetes. Dosage of antidiabetic drug may need adjustment.

(continued on following page)

NAME	INDICATIONS & DOSAGE	SIDE EFFECTS
nandrolone *(continued)*		
oxandrolone Anavar	*To combat catabolic effects of corticosteroid therapy, osteoporosis, prolonged immobilization and debilitated states—* **Adults:** 2.5 mg P.O. b.i.d., t.i.d., or q.i.d.; up to 20 mg daily for 2 to 4 weeks. **Children:** 0.25 mg/kg daily P.O. for 2 to 4 weeks. Continuous therapy should not exceed 3 months.	**Androgenic:** in females—*acne, edema, oily skin, weight gain, hirsutism, hoarseness,* clitoral enlargement, decreased or increased libido. In males—prepubertal: premature epiphyseal closure, acne, priapism, growth of body and facial hair, phallic enlargement; postpubertal: testicular atrophy, oligospermia, decreased ejaculatory volume, impotence, gynecomastia, epididymitis. **CV:** edema. **GI:** gastroenteritis, nausea, vomiting, constipation or diarrhea, change in appetite. **GU:** bladder irritability. **Hepatic:** jaundice. **Hypoestrogenic:** in females—flushing; sweating; vaginitis with itching, drying, burning, or bleeding; menstrual irregularities. **Other:** hypercalcemia.
oxymetholone Adroyd♦, Anadrol-50, Anapolon 50♦♦	*Aplastic anemia—* **Adults and children:** 1 to 5 mg/kg P.O. daily. Dose highly individualized; response not immediate. Trial of 3 to 6 months required. *Osteoporosis, catabolic conditions—* **Adults:** 5 to 15 mg P.O. daily, or up to 30 mg P.O. daily. **Children over 6 years:** up to 10 mg P.O. daily. **Children under 6 years:** 1.25 mg P.O. daily or up to q.i.d. Continuous therapy should not exceed 30 days in children; 90 days in any patient.	**Androgenic:** in females—*acne, edema, oily skin, weight gain, hirsutism, hoarseness,* clitoral enlargement, decreased or increased libido, male-pattern hair loss. In males—prepubertal: premature epiphyseal closure, acne, priapism, growth of body and facial hair, phallic enlargement; postpubertal: testicular atrophy, oligospermia, decreased ejaculatory volume, impotence, gynecomastia, epididymitis. **CV:** edema. **GI:** gastroenteritis, nausea, vomiting, constipation, diarrhea, change in appetite. **GU:** bladder irritability. **Hepatic:** jaundice.

INTERACTIONS	NURSING CONSIDERATIONS
	• Use with diet high in calories and protein unless contraindicated. • Erroneously thought to enhance athletic ability. • Considered an adjunctive therapy. • Anabolic steroids may alter many laboratory studies during therapy and for 2 to 3 weeks after therapy is stopped.
None significant.	• Contraindicated in patients with prostatic hypertrophy with obstruction; prostatic and male breast cancer; cardiac, hepatic, or renal decompensation; nephrosis; and in premature infants. Use cautiously in prepubertal males; patients with diabetes or coronary disease; patients taking ACTH, corticosteroids, or anticoagulants. • Hypercalcemia symptoms may be difficult to distinguish from symptoms of condition being treated unless anticipated and thought of as a cluster. Hypercalcemia most likely to occur with metastatic breast cancer and may indicate bone metastases. • Discontinue use if female patient reports menstrual irregularities. • Watch for signs of virilization; may be irreversible despite prompt discontinuation of therapy. Doctor must decide if benefits outweigh effects. • Boys under 7 years should be closely observed for precocious development of male sexual characteristics. • In children, therapy should be preceded by X-ray of wrist bones to establish level of bone maturation. During treatment, bone maturation may proceed more rapidly than linear growth; dosage should be intermittent and X-rays taken periodically. • Edema is generally controllable with salt restriction and/or diuretics. Monitor weight routinely. • Watch for symptoms of jaundice. Dose adjustment may reverse condition. Periodic liver function studies are recommended. • Observe patient on concomitant anticoagulant therapy for ecchymotic areas, petechiae, or abnormal bleeding. Monitor prothrombin time. • Watch for symptoms of hypoglycemia in patients with diabetes. Change of dosage of antidiabetic drug may be required. • Use with diet high in calories and protein unless contraindicated. • Erroneously thought to enhance athletic ability. • Anabolic steroids may alter many laboratory studies during therapy and for 2 to 3 weeks after therapy is stopped.
None significant.	• Contraindicated in patients with prostatic hypertrophy with obstruction; prostatic and male breast cancer; cardiac, hepatic, or renal decompensation; nephrosis; and in premature infants. Use cautiously in prepubertal males; patients with diabetes or coronary diseases; patients taking ACTH, corticosteroids, or anticoagulants. • Hypercalcemia symptoms may be difficult to distinguish from symptoms of condition being treated unless anticipated and thought of as a cluster. Hypercalcemia most likely to occur in metastatic breast cancer and may indicate bone metastases. • Supportive treatment of anemias (transfusions, correction of iron, folic acid, vitamin B_{12}, or pyridoxine deficiency). Give 3 to 6 months for response. • Effects in osteoporosis usually seen in 4 to 6 weeks. • Discontinue use if female patient reports menstrual irregularities. • Watch for signs of virilization; may be irreversible despite prompt stopping of therapy. Doctor must decide if benefits outweigh effects. • Boys under 7 years should be closely observed for precocious development of male sexual characteristics. • In children, therapy should be preceded by X-ray of wrist bones to

(continued on following page)

NAME	INDICATIONS & DOSAGE	SIDE EFFECTS
oxymetholone *(continued)*		**Hypoestrogenic:** in females—flushing; sweating; vaginitis with itching, drying, burning, or bleeding; menstrual irregularities. **Other:** hypercalcemia.
stanozolol Winstrol♦	*To increase hemoglobin in some cases of aplastic anemia—* **Adults:** 2 mg P.O. t.i.d. **Children 6 to 12 years:** up to 2 mg P.O. t.i.d. **Children under 6 years:** 1 mg P.O. b.i.d. Therapy should be intermittent.	**Androgenic:** in females—*acne, edema, oily skin, weight gain, hirsutism, hoarseness,* clitoral enlargement, decreased or increased libido. In males— prepubertal: premature epiphyseal closure, acne, priapism, growth of body and facial hair, phallic enlargement; postpubertal: testicular atrophy, oligospermia, decreased ejaculatory volume, impotence, gynecomastia, epididymitis. **CV:** edema. **GI:** gastroenteritis, nausea, vomiting, constipation, diarrhea, change in appetite. **GU:** bladder irritability. **Hypoestrogenic:** in females—flushing; sweating; vaginitis with itching, drying, burning or bleeding; menstrual irregularities. **Other:** hypercalcemia.
testosterone Android-T, Andronaq, Histerone, Malogen♦, Oreton, Testaqua, Testoject	*Eunuchoidism, eunuchism, male climacteric symptoms—* **Adults:** 10 to 25 mg I.M. 2 to 5 times weekly; or 2 to 6 pellets (75 mg each) implanted subcutaneously q 3 to 6 months.	**Androgenic:** in females—*acne, edema, oily skin, weight gain, hirsutism, hoarseness,* clitoral enlargement, decreased or increased libido. In males—prepubertal: premature epiphyseal closure,

♦ Available in U.S. and Canada. ♦♦ Available in Canada only. All other products (no symbol) available in U.S. only. Italicized side effects are common or life-threatening.

INTERACTIONS	NURSING CONSIDERATIONS
	establish level of bone maturation. During treatment, bone maturation may proceed more rapidly than linear growth; dosage should be intermittent and X-rays taken periodically. Epiphyseal development may continue 6 months after stopping therapy. • Edema is generally controllable with salt restriction and/or diuretics. Monitor weight routinely. • Watch for symptoms of jaundice. Dose adjustment may reverse condition. Periodic liver function studies are recommended. • Observe patient on concomitant anticoagulant therapy for ecchymotic areas, petechiae, or abnormal bleeding. Monitor prothrombin time. • Watch for symptoms of hypoglycemia in patients with diabetes. Change of dosage in antidiabetic drug may be required. • Use with diet high in calories and protein unless contraindicated. • Erroneously thought to enhance athletic ability. • Anabolic steroids may alter many laboratory studies during therapy and for 2 to 3 weeks after therapy is stopped.
None significant.	• Contraindicated in patients with prostatic hypertrophy with obstruction; prostatic and male breast cancer; cardiac, hepatic, or renal decompensation; nephrosis; and in premature infants. Use cautiously in prepubertal males; patients with diabetes or coronary disease; patients taking ACTH, corticosteroids, or anticoagulants. • Hypercalcemia symptoms may be difficult to distinguish from symptoms of condition being treated unless anticipated and thought of as a cluster. Hypercalcemia most likely to occur in metastatic breast cancer and may indicate bone metastases. • Discontinue use if female patient reports menstrual irregularities. • Smaller dose (2 mg b.i.d.) is used in females to avoid virilization. Watch for these side effects; may be irreversible despite prompt stopping of therapy. Doctor must decide if benefits outweigh effects. • Boys under 7 years should be closely observed for precocious development of male sexual characteristics. • In children, therapy should be preceded by X-ray of wrist bones to establish level of bone maturation. During treatment, bone maturation may proceed more rapidly than linear growth; dosage should be intermittent and X-rays taken periodically. • Edema is generally controllable with salt restriction and/or diuretics. Monitor weight routinely. • Watch for symptoms of jaundice. Dose adjustment may reverse condition. Periodic liver function studies are recommended. • Observe patient on concomitant anticoagulant therapy for ecchymotic areas, petechiae, or abnormal bleeding. Monitor prothrombin time. • Watch for symptoms of hypoglycemia in patients with diabetes. Change of dosage of antidiabetic drug may be required. • Use with diet high in calories and protein unless contraindicated. • Administer before or with meals to minimize GI distress. • Monitor serum cholesterol in cardiac patients. • Erroneously thought to enhance athletic ability. • Anabolic steroids may alter many laboratory studies during therapy and for 2 to 3 weeks after therapy is stopped.
None significant.	• Contraindicated in women of childbearing potential (possible masculinization of female infant); in elderly, asthenic males who may react adversely to androgen overstimulation; in hypercalcemia; cardiac, hepatic, or renal decompensation; prostatic or breast cancer in males; benign prostatic hypertrophy with obstruction; conditions aggravated by fluid retention; hypertension; and in premature infants.

(continued on following page)

NAME	INDICATIONS & DOSAGE	SIDE EFFECTS
testosterone *(continued)*	*Breast engorgement of non–breast-feeding mothers*—25 to 50 mg I.M. daily for 3 to 4 days, starting at delivery. *Breast cancer in women 1 to 5 years postmenopausal*—100 mg I.M. 3 times weekly as long as improvement maintained.	acne, priapism, growth of body and facial hair, phallic enlargement; postpubertal: testicular atrophy, oligospermia, decreased ejaculatory volume, impotence, gynecomastia, epididymitis. **CV:** edema. **GI:** gastroenteritis, nausea, vomiting, constipation, diarrhea, change in appetite. **GU:** bladder irritability. **Hepatic:** jaundice. **Hypoestrogenic:** in females—flushing; sweating; vaginitis with itching, drying, burning, or bleeding; menstrual irregularities. **Local:** pain at injection site, induration, irritation and sloughing with pellet implantation, edema. **Other:** hypercalcemia.
testosterone cypionate Andro-Cyp, Androgen-860, Depotest, Depo-Test, Depo-Testosterone♦, D-Test, Durandro, Duratest, Jactatest, Malogen Cyp **testosterone enanthate** Android-T, Andryl, Arderone, Delatestryl♦, Everone, Malogen LA, Malogex♦♦, Span-Test, Testate, Testone LA, Testostroval-P.A. **testosterone propionate** Androlan, Androlin, Malogen in Oil♦♦, Oreton Propionate, Testex, Vulvan	*Eunuchism, eunuchoidism, deficiency after castration and male climacteric*— **Adults:** 200 to 400 mg (cypionate or enanthate) I.M. q 4 weeks. *Oligospermia*— **Adults:** 100 to 200 mg (cypionate or enanthate) I.M. q 4 to 6 weeks for development and maintenance of testicular function. *Eunuchism and eunuchoidism, male climacteric, impotence*— **Adults:** 10 to 25 mg (propionate) I.M. 2 to 4 times weekly; or 5 to 20 mg buccal daily (strictly individualized). *Breast engorgement of non–breast-feeding mothers*—40 mg (propionate) buccal daily, for 3 to 5 days starting at delivery. *Metastatic breast cancer in women*—50 to 100 mg (propionate) I.M. 3 times weekly; or 100 mg buccal daily as long as improvement maintained. *Postpubertal cryptorchidism*—15 mg (propionate) buccal daily.	**Androgenic:** in females—*acne, edema, oily skin, weight gain, hirsutism, hoarseness,* clitoral enlargement, changes in libido. In males—prepubertal: premature epiphyseal closure, acne, priapism, growth of body and facial hair, phallic enlargement; postpubertal: testicular atrophy, oligospermia, decreased ejaculatory volume, impotence, gynecomastia, epididymitis. **CV:** edema. **GI:** gastroenteritis, nausea, vomiting, constipation, diarrhea, change in appetite. **GU:** bladder irritability. **Hepatic:** jaundice. **Local:** pain at injection site, induration, postinjection furunculosis. **Other:** hypercalcemia.

INTERACTIONS	NURSING CONSIDERATIONS
	Use cautiously in patients with myocardial infarction or coronary artery disease, and in prepubertal males. • Periodic liver function studies should be performed. • In metastatic breast cancer, hypercalcemia usually indicates progression of bone metastases. Report signs of hypercalcemia. • Therapeutic response in breast cancer is usually apparent within 3 months. Stop therapy if signs of disease progression appear. • Enhances hypoglycemia; tell patient to report signs of hyperinsulinism. • Instruct males to report priapism, reduced ejaculatory volume, and gynecomastia. Withdraw drug if these occur. • Report signs of virilization in females; reevaluate treatment. • Monitor prepubertal males by X-ray for rate of bone maturation. • Edema is generally controllable with salt restriction and/or diuretics. Monitor weight routinely. • Use with diet high in calories and protein unless contraindicated. • Inject deep into upper outer quadrant of gluteal muscle. • Watch for irritation and sloughing with pellet implantation. • Watch for ecchymotic areas, petechiae, or abnormal bleeding in patients on concomitant anticoagulant therapy. Monitor prothrombin time. • Implantation of pellets may take place in doctor's office in a minor surgical procedure with aseptic precautions observed. • Many laboratory studies may be altered during therapy and for 2 to 3 weeks after therapy is stopped.
None significant.	• Contraindicated in women of childbearing potential (possible masculinization of female infant); in patients with hypercalcemia; cardiac, hepatic, or renal decompensation; prostatic or breast cancer in males; benign prostatic hypertrophy with obstruction; conditions aggravated by fluid retention; hypertension; elderly, asthenic males who may react adversely to androgen overstimulation; and in premature infants. Use cautiously in patients with myocardial infarction or coronary artery disease, and in prepubertal males. • Periodic liver function studies should be performed. • In metastatic breast cancer, hypercalcemia usually indicates progression of bone metastases. Report signs of hypercalcemia. • Response in breast cancer is usually apparent within 3 months. Stop therapy if signs of disease progression appear. • Enhances hypoglycemia; teach patient signs of hypoglycemia, and instruct him to report immediately if they occur. • Instruct males to report priapism, reduced ejaculatory volume, and gynecomastia. Withdraw drug. • Watch for signs of ecchymoses, petechiae with concomitant anticoagulant therapy. Monitor prothrombin time. • Inject deep into upper outer quadrant of gluteal muscle. Report soreness at site; possibility of postinjection furunculosis. • Report signs of virilization in females; reevaluate treatment. • Monitor prepubertal males by X-ray for rate of bone maturation. • Edema is generally controllable with salt restriction and/or diuretics. Monitor weight routinely. • Use with diet high in calories and protein unless contraindicated. • Good oral hygiene decreases possibility of irritation from buccal tablet. Patient shouldn't eat, drink, chew, or smoke while tablet is in place. • May alter many laboratory studies during therapy and for 2 to 3 weeks after therapy is stopped.

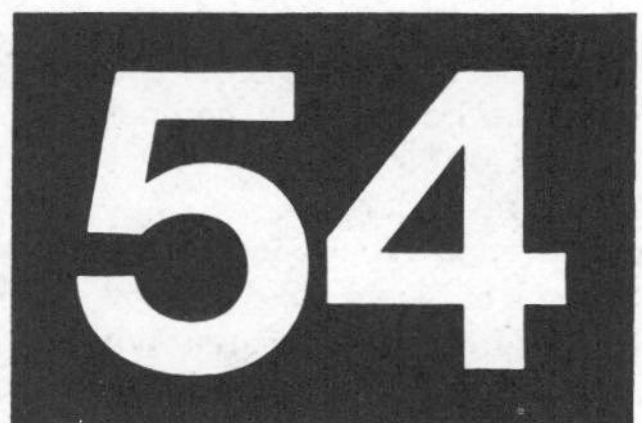

Oral contraceptives

estrogen with progestogen

Oral contraceptives are one of the most popular and effective forms of birth control used today. Although they're convenient to use, they may produce serious side effects in women predisposed to certain risk factors.

Currently, two recognized classes of oral contraceptives are being marketed: an estrogen-progestogen combination and a progestogen-only "minipill." The combination tablet contains a synthetic estrogen compound (ethinyl estradiol or mestranol) and a synthetic progestogen (ethynodiol diacetate, norethindrone, norethindrone acetate, norethynodrel, or norgestrel). It is taken for 21 days of the menstrual cycle (usually days 5 through 24). Natural steroids aren't used because large doses are required to achieve the same pharmacologic effect as the synthetics.

The progestogen-only pill contains either norethindrone or norgestrel and is taken once daily every day of the menstrual cycle. (For complete infor-

QUESTIONS & ANSWERS

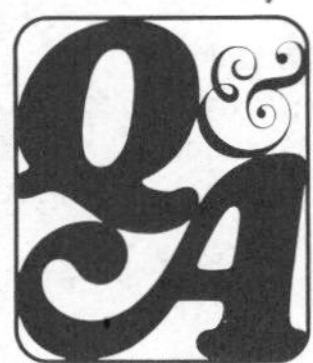

MINIMIZING THROMBOEMBOLIC COMPLICATIONS

Are thromboembolic complications less prevalent with low-dose estrogen oral contraceptive use?

Studies show that thromboembolic complications—venous thrombosis and stroke—are more prevalent in women who take high-dose estrogen oral contraceptives. In fact, in one study the incidence of venous thrombosis decreased 25% in women who changed from high-dose (75 to 100 mcg) to low-dose (50 mcg) estrogen oral contraceptives.

Since thromboembolic complications were initially observed in 1970, researchers have recommended using the lowest estrogen content possible to prevent thromboembolic disease yet maintain contraceptive effectiveness.

Today, the trend is to reduce the estrogen content even further—from 50 to 30 mcg. The results appear beneficial since contraceptive effectiveness has not been significantly decreased.

So, encourage your patients who use oral contraceptives to ask their doctors about changing to low-dose estrogen oral contraceptives. They may reduce their risk of thromboembolic complications and still receive effective therapy.

mation on progestogen-only contraceptives, see Chapter 56, PROGESTOGENS.)

The minipill is not widely used because it frequently causes menstrual irregularities. Although slightly less effective than the combination product, it may suffice for the patient who has to avoid the use of estrogen or for whom pregnancy is not life-threatening.

In choosing an appropriate oral contraceptive, the doctor must weigh the side effects of the high-dose combinations against the possibly weaker action of the low-dose combinations. In general, the more estrogen and progestogen in the preparation, the more serious, frequent, and fast-acting the side effects. The lower the hormonal concentration, the less effective the preparation, especially in a woman taking drugs that increase metabolism and thus lower the blood levels of estrogens. A woman who misses taking a pill may have a greater risk of failure with a low-dose than with a high-dose preparation.

Generally, oral contraceptives that contain the smallest effective quantity of hormone and produce the fewest side effects are preferable. This usually means a product with 50 mcg or less of estrogen.

PATIENT-TEACHING AID

CHOOSING A METHOD OF CONTRACEPTION

Dear Patient:

Before you decide on a method of contraception, ask your doctor to explain the advantages and disadvantages of each method. Since each woman's contraceptive needs vary, your doctor can help by properly assessing your life-style, answering your questions, and considering your needs.

If you choose an oral contraceptive, follow these guidelines:

- Determine that oral contraceptives are safe for you. Your doctor is the best person to help you make this decision. Always remain under a doctor's care while you're on the pill. *Remember:* if you have thromboembolic disease, you *should not* take the pill.
- Take the medication as prescribed. If you miss *one* pill, take it as soon as you remember. If you miss *two* consecutive pills, take two pills a day for the next two days. If you miss *three or more* consecutive pills, stop treatment and use another contraceptive for the rest of the cycle (month). Then, begin again, according to your doctor's directions.
- Remember to use an alternate method of contraception for the first 7 days after you begin taking the pill. Also, if you stop taking the pill for any reason, use an alternate contraceptive method.
- Call your doctor if you notice any side effects like nausea, headache, dizziness, or swelling.
- Recognize that the pill increases your susceptibility to vaginal infections. Call your doctor if you notice any vaginal discharge, itching, or pain.
- Schedule a Pap test semiannually and a complete physical examination yearly.
- Contact your doctor if you miss your menstrual period. If you miss two consecutive periods, your doctor may advise you to stop taking the pill until he can determine whether or not you may be pregnant.
- Consult your doctor if you wish to discontinue therapy, especially if you plan to become pregnant. He may advise you not to become pregnant for 2 or more months *after* discontinuing the pill.

Major uses

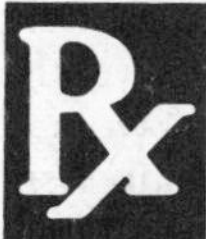

Oral contraceptives are used to prevent pregnancy. High-dose estrogen-progestogen combinations are usually used to treat such menstrual cycle disorders as endometriosis and hypermenorrhea.

Estrogen with progestogen is also commonly used to treat hormone-induced acne, but it's often ineffective.

Mechanism of action

Oral contraceptives inhibit ovulation through a negative feedback mechanism directed at the hypothalamus. They may also prevent transport of the ovum through the fallopian tubes.

- Estrogen suppresses secretion of follicle-stimulating hormone, blocking follicular development and ovulation.
- Progestogen suppresses luteinizing hormone secretion so ovulation can't occur even if the follicle develops. Progestogen thickens cervical mucus, which interferes with sperm migration, and causes endometrial changes that prevent implantation of the fertilized ovum.

Absorption, distribution, metabolism, and excretion

Oral contraceptives are rapidly and completely absorbed from the gastrointestinal tract and distributed to all body tissues. They are metabolized in the liver and excreted in urine.

Onset and duration

As contraceptives begun on day 5 of the menstrual cycle, these drugs theoretically provide complete protection, if taken on schedule. But, alternative protection is recommended for at least the first 7 days of therapy since ovulation and conception are still possible during this time.

Duration of effect is about 1 day; hence strict compliance is necessary to ensure effectiveness. For complex endocrine, metabolic, and acne disorders, several months of treatment may be needed to obtain a satisfactory response.

UNDERSTANDING THE MENSTRUAL CYCLE

The menstrual cycle works by a series of hormonal peaks and valleys. One cycle usually takes about 28 days and is regulated by negative and positive feedback mechanisms.

Menstrual (preovulatory) phase
The menstrual cycle starts with menstruation. (The first day of menstruation is considered day 1 of the cycle.) At the beginning of the cycle, low levels of estrogen and progesterone in the bloodstream stimulate the hypothalamus to secrete gonadotropin-releasing hormones (GnRH). These releasing hormones stimulate the anterior pituitary to secrete luteinizing hormone (LH) and follicle-stimulating hormone (FSH). LH output begins to increase soon after FSH begins to rise.

Follicular phase and ovulation
LH and FSH act on the ovarian follicle, which secretes estrogen. The rising production of estrogen from the follicle has a *negative feedback* (decreasing) effect on FSH and a *positive feedback* (increasing) effect on LH. During this time, the follicle matures and ovulation occurs.

Postovulatory (luteal) phase
After ovulation, LH converts the now-ruptured follicle to a corpus luteum. The corpus luteum secretes lutein which contains both estrogen and progesterone, the latter having a *negative feedback* on LH production.

Progesterone secretion prepares the body for pregnancy. If pregnancy does not occur, the negative feedback effect of progesterone on LH production has an adverse effect on the corpus luteum, which becomes less responsive to the effects of LH as it ages. Without continuous LH stimulation, the corpus luteum further ages and regresses, and estrogen and progesterone production decreases until hormone levels are no longer adequate to maintain the endometrium, which is then shed as the menstrual flow.

As estrogen and progesterone levels fall, the hypothalamus is stimulated, causing the cycle to begin again. (For more information on progesterone, see Chapter 56, PROGESTOGENS.)

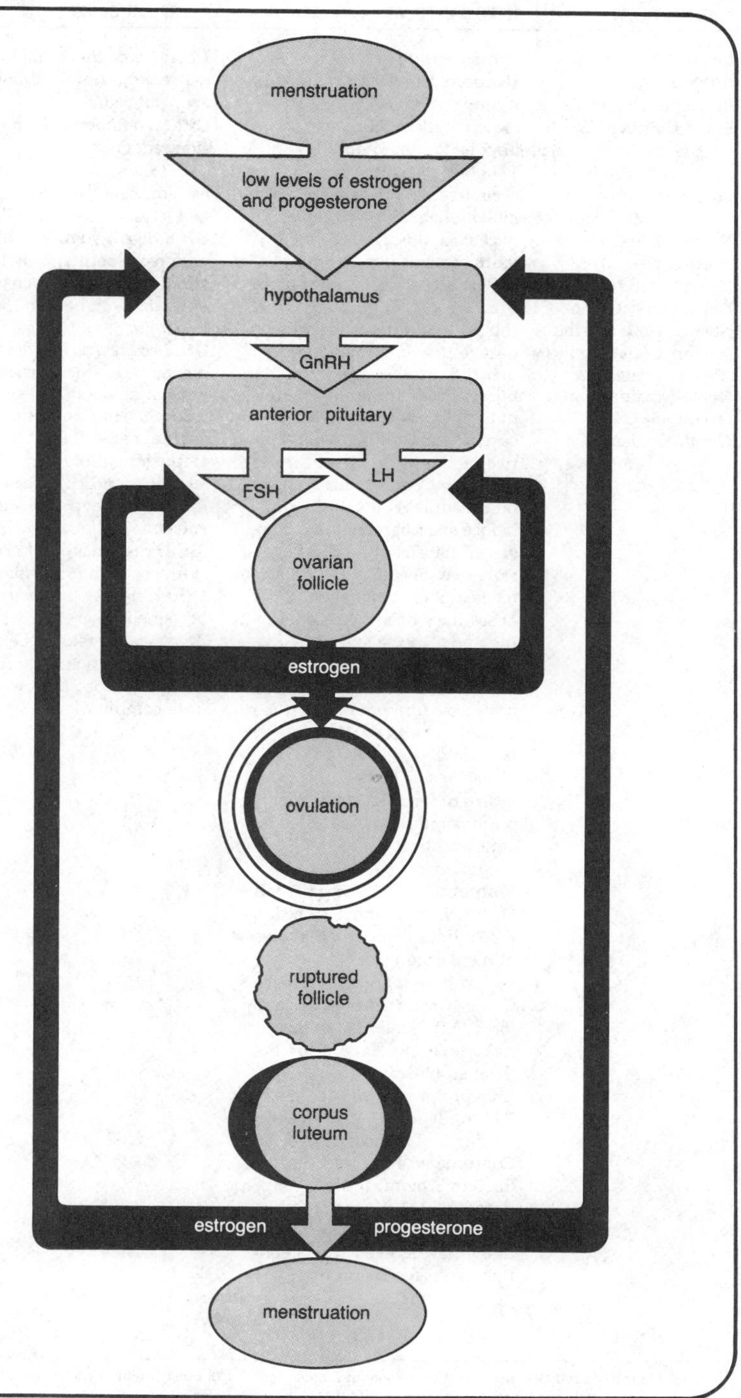
menstruation
low levels of estrogen and progesterone
hypothalamus
GnRH
anterior pituitary
FSH
LH
ovarian follicle
estrogen
ovulation
ruptured follicle
corpus luteum
estrogen
progesterone
menstruation

NAME	INDICATIONS & DOSAGE	SIDE EFFECTS
estrogen with progestogen Brevicon, Demulen♦, Enovid, Enovid-E, Loestrin 1/20, Loestrin 1.5/30♦, Lo/Ovral, Min-Ovral♦♦, Modicon, Norinyl 1 + 50♦, Norinyl 1 + 80♦, Norinyl 2 mg♦, Norlestrin♦, Ortho-Novum 1/50♦, Ortho-Novum 1/80♦, Ortho-Novum 2 mg♦, Ortho-Novum 10 mg, Ovcon 35, Ovcon 50, Ovral, Ovulen♦	*Contraception—* **Women:** 1 tablet P.O. daily, beginning on day 5 of menstrual cycle (first day of menstrual flow is day 1). With 20- and 21-tablet packages, new dosing cycle begins 7 days after last tablet taken. With 28-tablet packages, dosage is 1 tablet daily without interruption; extra tablets are placebos or contain iron. If only 1 or 2 doses are missed, dosage may continue on schedule. If 3 or more doses are missed, remaining tablets in monthly package must be discarded and another contraceptive method substituted. If next menstrual period doesn't begin on schedule, rule out pregnancy before starting new dosing cycle. If menstrual period begins, start new dosing cycle 7 days after last tablet was taken. If all doses have been taken on schedule and 1 menstrual period is missed, continue dosing cycle. If 2 consecutive menstrual periods are missed, pregnancy test is required before new dosing cycle is started. *Hypermenorrhea—* **Women:** use high-dose combinations only. Dose same as for contraception. *Endometriosis—* **Women:** Cyclic therapy: 1 tablet Ortho-Novum 10 mg P.O. daily for 20 days from day 5 to day 24 of menstrual cycle. Suppressive therapy: 1 tablet Ortho-Novum 10 mg P.O. daily for 3 to 9 months. May increase to 20 to 30 mg daily if breakthrough bleeding occurs. Enovid 5 mg or 10 mg—1 tablet P.O. daily for 2 weeks starting on day 5 of menstrual cycle. Continue without interruption for 6 to 9 months, increasing dose by 5 to 10 mg q 2 weeks, up to 20 mg daily. Up to 40 mg daily may be needed if breakthrough bleeding occurs.	**CNS:** *headache, dizziness,* depression, libido changes, lethargy, migraine. **CV:** *thromboembolism,* hypertension, edema. **EENT:** worsening of myopia or astigmatism, intolerance to contact lenses. **GI:** *nausea,* vomiting, abdominal cramps, bloating, diarrhea, constipation, anorexia, changes in appetite, weight gain, *bowel ischemia.* **GU:** *breakthrough bleeding,* dysmenorrhea, amenorrhea, cervical erosion or abnormal secretions, enlargement of uterine fibromas, vaginal candidiasis. **Hepatic:** gallbladder disease, cholestatic jaundice, liver tumors. **Metabolic:** hyperglycemia, hypercalcemia, folic acid deficiency. **Skin:** rash, acne, seborrhea, oily skin, erythema multiforme. **Other:** *breast tenderness,* enlargement, secretion. Adverse effects may be more serious, frequent, and rapid in onset with high-dose than with low-dose combinations.

INTERACTIONS	NURSING CONSIDERATIONS
Ampicillin, tetracycline, barbiturates, anticonvulsants, rifampin: may diminish contraceptive effectiveness. Use supplemental form of contraception.	• Contraindicated in thromboembolic disorders, cerebrovascular or coronary artery disease, myocardial infarction, known or suspected cancer of breasts or reproductive organs, benign or malignant liver tumors, undiagnosed abnormal vaginal bleeding, known or suspected pregnancy, lactation; and in adolescents with incomplete epiphyseal closure. Also contraindicated in women 35 years or older who smoke more than 15 cigarettes a day, and in all women over 40 years. Use cautiously in patients with hypertension, depression, migraine, epilepsy, asthma, diabetes, amenorrhea, scanty or irregular periods, fibrocystic breast disease, family history (mother, grandmother, sister) of breast or genital tract cancer, renal or gallbladder disease. Report development or worsening of these conditions. Prolonged therapy inadvisable in women who plan to become pregnant. • If one menstrual period is missed and tablets have been taken on schedule, tell patient to continue pills. If two consecutive periods are missed, tell patient to stop drug and to have pregnancy test. Progestogens may cause birth defects if taken early in pregnancy. • Missed doses in midcycle greatly increase likelihood of pregnancy. • Warn patient that headache, nausea, dizziness, breast tenderness, spotting, and breakthrough bleeding are common at first and should diminish after 3 to 6 dosing cycles (months). However, breakthrough bleeding in patients taking high-dose estrogen-progestogen combinations for menstrual disorders may need dosage adjustment. • Warn patient to report immediately abdominal pain; numbness, stiffness, or pain in legs or buttocks; pressure or pain in chest; shortness of breath; severe headache; visual disturbances, such as blind spots, blurriness, or flashing lights; undiagnosed vaginal bleeding or discharge; two consecutive missed menstrual periods; lumps in the breast; swelling of hands or feet; severe pain in the abdomen. • Tell patient to take tablets at same time each day; nighttime dosing may reduce nausea and headaches. • Stress importance of semiannual Pap test and complete annual physical examination while taking this drug. • Warn the patient of signs and symptoms of gallbladder disease. • Warn the patient of possible delay in achieving pregnancy when pill is discontinued. • Teach the patient how to perform a breast self-examination. • Advise the patient of increased risks associated with simultaneous use of cigarettes and oral contraceptives. • Many laboratory tests are affected by oral contraceptives; some include: increase in serum bilirubin, alkaline phosphatase, SGOT, SGPT, and protein-bound iodine; decrease in glucose tolerance and urinary excretion of 17-hydroxycorticosteroids (17-OHCS). • Estrogens and progestogens may alter glucose tolerance, thus changing requirements for antidiabetic drugs. • Instruct patient to weigh herself at least twice a week and to report any sudden weight gain or edema to doctor. • Many doctors recommend women not become pregnant within 2 months after stopping the pill. Advise patient to ask her doctor how soon pregnancy may be attempted after hormonal therapy. • Advise patient not to take same drug for longer than 18 months without consulting doctor. • Many doctors advise women on the pill for extended time (5 years or more) to stop drug and use other birth control methods in order to periodically reassess patient while off hormone therapy. • Oral contraceptive use increases risk of cardiovascular disorders and may increase risk of developing certain cancers. See Chapter 55, ESTROGENS.

55 Estrogens

chlorotrianisene
dienestrol
diethylstilbestrol
diethylstilbestrol diphosphate
esterified estrogens
estradiol
estradiol cypionate
estradiol valerate
estrogenic substances, conjugated
estrone
ethinyl estradiol
quinestrol

Estrogens are organic compounds that occur naturally in humans and animals; they are also produced synthetically. They can be chemically classified as either steroidal or nonsteroidal estrogens.

Steroidal estrogens include all natural estrogens (estradiol, estriol, and estrone), esters of natural estrogens (estradiol cypionate, estradiol valerate, and esterified estrogens), a conjugate of natural estrogens (conjugated estrogenic substances, and a semisynthetic estrogen (ethinyl estradiol).

Nonsteroidal estrogens comprise the synthetic estrogens (chlorotrianisene, dienestrol, diethylstilbestrol, diethylstilbestrol diphosphate, and quinestrol).

Estrogens have been traditionally described as agents that produce estrus, whether or not they are derived from the ovaries. Secreted mainly by the ovarian follicles, they are also secreted in large amounts by the placenta, in smaller quantities by the testes, and—in both sexes—by the adrenal cortex.

The reproductive physiochemistry of estrogens in women parallels that of testosterone in men. Estrogens promote growth and development of the vagina, uterus, and fallopian tubes; enlargement of the breasts; molding of the body contours; and closure of the epiphyses of the long bones. They also promote growth of axillary and pubic hair, and pigmentation of the skin of the nipples and genital region. They stimulate estrus and produce changes in the genital tract and mammary glands during pregnancy.

Metabolic activities of estrogens occur in three areas: Estrogens reduce blood cholesterol by altering lipid metabolism, exert a protein anabolic action, and promote sodium and water retention.

Major uses

Rx

Estrogens have the following uses:

- As replacement therapy, they're used in menopause, pituitary failure to stimulate development of secondary sex characteristics, and postoperative radical hysterectomy.

They are used to treat atrophic changes in the lower genital tract (as in atrophic vaginitis or pruritus vulvae), which are caused by chronic estrogen deficiency.

They can also initiate menstrual periods and relieve secondary amenorrhea (as in female hypogonadism, female castration, and primary ovarian failure).

- They relieve postpartum breast engorgement.
- They are used in the palliation and inhibition of androgen-dependent primary tumors with soft-tissue metastases (for example, inoperable cancer of the prostate and breast in males, inoperable postmenopausal breast carcinoma).
- They provide contraception (in combination with progestogen). Their use as a contraceptive is described in greater detail in Chapter 54, ORAL CONTRACEPTIVES.

Mechanism of action

- Estrogens replace endogenous hormones to maintain normal hormonal balance.
- They suppress lactation by inhibiting prolactin secretion from the anterior pituitary.
- They antagonize the action of androgens that stimulate growth of tumor tissue.
- As oral contraceptives, estrogens suppress gonadotropin output from the anterior pituitary by a negative feedback effect. (Their mechanism of action is described in greater detail in Chapter 54.)

Absorption, distribution, metabolism, and excretion

Estrogens are readily absorbed from the gastrointestinal tract, distributed to all body tissues, metabolized in the liver, and excreted primarily in urine. Small amounts are also eliminated—through the bile—in feces.

- Estradiol is rapidly metabolized (oxidized) in the liver to estrone, which is subsequently converted to estriol.
- Ethinyl estradiol is well absorbed when given orally. Most of it is metabolized in the liver. Because metabolism is slow, the drug retains its high intrinsic potency.

Onset and duration

- Estrogens begin to act immediately.
- Oral estrogens (except chlorotrianisene) have a short duration of action; daily doses are usually needed.

Chlorotrianisene is a long-acting drug because it's stored in and released only gradually from adipose tissue.

- Parenteral estrogens have a longer duration of action than the oral preparations; their effect may last several days.

Combination products

MENRIUM 5-2♦: chlordiazepoxide 5 mg and esterified estrogens 0.2 mg.
MENRIUM 5-4♦: chlordiazepoxide 5 mg and esterified estrogens 0.4 mg.
MENRIUM 10-4♦: chlordiazepoxide 10 mg and esterified estrogens 0.4 mg.
MILPREM-200: conjugated estrogens 0.45 mg and meprobamate 200 mg.
MILPREM-400: conjugated estrogens 0.45 mg and meprobamate 400 mg.
PMB 200: conjugated estrogens 0.45 mg and meprobamate 200 mg.
PMB 400: conjugated estrogens 0.45 mg and meprobamate 400 mg.
See Chapter 54 for oral contraceptives and other estrogen combinations.

NAME	INDICATIONS & DOSAGE	SIDE EFFECTS
chlorotrianisene Tace♦	**Men:** *Prostatic cancer*—12 to 25 mg P.O. daily. **Non–breast-feeding mothers:** *Postpartum breast engorgement*—72 mg P.O. b.i.d. for 2 days; or 50 mg q 6 hours for 6 doses; or 12 mg q.i.d. for 7 days. Start dosing within 8 hours after delivery. **Women:** *Menopausal symptoms*—12 to 25 mg P.O. daily for 30 days or cyclic (3 weeks on, 1 week off). *Female hypogonadism*—12 to 25 mg P.O. for 21 days, followed by 1 dose of progesterone 100 mg I.M. or 5 days of oral progestogen given concurrently with last 5 days of chlorotrianisene (i.e., medroxyprogesterone 5 to 10 mg). *Atrophic vaginitis*—12 to 25 mg P.O. daily for 30 to 60 days.	**CNS:** headache, dizziness, chorea, migraine, depression, libido changes. **CV:** thrombophlebitis; *thromboembolism;* hypertension; edema; *increased risk of stroke, pulmonary embolism, and myocardial infarction.* **EENT:** worsening of myopia or astigmatism, intolerance to contact lenses. **GI:** *nausea,* vomiting, abdominal cramps, bloating, diarrhea, constipation, anorexia, increased appetite, excessive thirst, weight changes. **GU:** *in females*—breakthrough bleeding, altered menstrual flow, dysmenorrhea, amenorrhea, cervical erosion or abnormal secretions, enlargement of uterine fibromas, vaginal candidiasis; *in males—gynecomastia, testicular atrophy, impotence.* **Hepatic:** cholestatic jaundice. **Metabolic:** hyperglycemia, hypercalcemia, folic acid deficiency. **Skin:** melasma, urticaria, acne, seborrhea, oily skin, hirsutism or loss of hair. **Other:** leg cramps, purpura, breast changes (tenderness, enlargement, secretion).
dienestrol Dienestrol cream♦ Available in combination with sulfanilamide and aminacrine as AVC/Dienestrol, cream or suppositories	**Postmenopausal women:** *Atrophic vaginitis and kraurosis vulvae*—1 to 2 applicatorfuls of cream daily for 2 weeks, then half that dose for 2 more weeks; or 1 to 2 vaginal suppositories daily for 1 month, as directed. *Atrophic and senile vaginitis and kraurosis vulvae when complicated by infection*—1 applicatorful AVC/Dienestrol cream intravaginally daily or b.i.d. for 1 to 2 weeks, then every other day for 1 to 2 weeks.	**GU:** vaginal discharge; with excessive use, uterine bleeding. **Local:** increased discomfort, burning sensation. Systemic effects possible. **Other:** breast tenderness.
diethylstilbestrol DES, Stilbestrol, Stibilium♦♦ **diethylstilbestrol diphosphate** Honvol♦♦, Stilphostrol	**Women:** *Atrophic vaginitis or kraurosis vulvae*—0.1 to 1 mg as suppository daily for 10 to 14 days concurrently with oral therapy; or up to 5 mg weekly as suppository. *Hypogonadism, castration, pri-*	**CNS:** headache, dizziness, chorea, depression, lethargy. **CV:** *thrombophlebitis; thromboembolism;* hypertension; edema; *increased risk of stroke, pulmonary embolism, and mycardial infarction.* **EENT:** worsening of myopia or

♦ Available in U.S. and Canada. ♦♦ Available in Canada only. All other products (no symbol) available in U.S. only. Italicized side effects are common or life-threatening.

INTERACTIONS	NURSING CONSIDERATIONS
None significant.	• Contraindicated in thrombophlebitis or thromboembolic disorders; cancer of breast, reproductive organs, or genitalia; undiagnosed abnormal genital bleeding. Use cautiously in patients with hypertension, asthma, mental depression, bone diseases, blood dyscrasias, gallbladder disease, migraine, seizures, diabetes mellitus, amenorrhea, heart failure, hepatic or renal dysfunction, and family history (mother, grandmother, sister) of breast or genital tract cancer. Development or worsening of these conditions may require discontinuation of the drug. • FDA regulations require that female patients receive package insert explaining possible estrogen side effects before first dose. Provide verbal explanation also. • Warn patient to report immediately: abdominal pain; pain, numbness, or stiffness in legs or buttocks; pressure or pain in chest; shortness of breath; severe headaches; visual disturbances, such as blind spots, flashing lights, blurriness; vaginal bleeding or discharge; breast lumps; swelling of hands or feet; yellow skin and sclera; dark urine; and light-colored stools. • Tell male patients on long-term therapy about possible gynecomastia and impotence, which will disappear when therapy is terminated. • Not used for menstrual disorders because duration of action is very long. • Pathologist should be advised of estrogen therapy when specimen is sent. • Patients with diabetes should report positive urine tests so antidiabetic medication dose can be adjusted. • Teach female patients how to perform routine breast self-examination. • Explain to patient on cyclic therapy for postmenopausal symptoms that although withdrawal bleeding may occur during week off drug, fertility has not been restored. Pregnancy is not possible since she has not ovulated.
None significant.	• Contraindicated in thrombophlebitis or thromboembolic disorders; cancer of breasts, reproductive organs, or genitals; undiagnosed abnormal genital bleeding. Use cautiously in menstrual irregularities or endometriosis. • Prolonged therapy with estrogen-containing products is contraindicated. • Systemic reactions possible with normal intravaginal use. Monitor closely. • Warn patient not to exceed the prescribed dose. • Withdrawal bleeding may occur if estrogen is suddenly stopped. • Teach patient how to insert suppositories or cream.
None significant.	• Contraindicated in thrombophlebitis or thromboembolic disorders; undiagnosed abnormal genital bleeding. Use cautiously in patients with hypertension, asthma, mental depression, bone disease, migraine headaches, seizures, blood dyscrasias, diabetes mellitus, gallbladder disease, amenorrhea, heart failure, hepatic or renal dysfunction, and family history (mother, grandmother, sister) of breast or genital tract cancer. Development or worsening of these conditions may necessitate discontinuation of the drug.

(continued on following page)

NAME	INDICATIONS & DOSAGE	SIDE EFFECTS
diethylstilbestrol *(continued)*	*mary ovarian failure*—0.2 to 0.5 mg P.O. daily. *Menopausal symptoms*—0.1 to 2 mg P.O. daily in cycles of 3 weeks on and 1 week off. *Postcoital contraception ("morning-after pill")*—25 mg P.O. b.i.d. for 5 days, starting within 72 hours after coitus. *Postpartum breast engorgement*—5 mg P.O. daily or t.i.d. up to total dose of 30 mg. **Men:** *Prostatic cancer*—1 to 3 mg P.O. daily, initially; may be reduced to 1 mg P.O. daily, or 5 mg I.M. twice weekly initially, followed by up to 4 mg I.M. twice weekly. Or 50 to 200 mg (diphosphate) P.O. t.i.d.; or 0.25 to 1 g I.V. daily for 5 days, then once or twice weekly. **Men and postmenopausal women:** *Breast cancer*—15 mg P.O. daily.	astigmatism, intolerance to contact lenses. **GI:** *nausea,* vomiting, abdominal cramps, bloating, diarrhea, constipation, anorexia, increased appetite, excessive thirst, weight changes. **GU:** *in females*—breakthrough bleeding, altered menstrual flow, dysmenorrhea, amenorrhea, cervical erosion, altered cervical secretions, enlargement of uterine fibromas, vaginal candidiasis, loss of libido; *in males:*—gynecomastia, testicular atrophy, impotence. **Hepatic:** cholestatic jaundice. **Metabolic:** hyperglycemia, hypercalcemia, folic acid deficiency. **Skin:** melasma, urticaria, acne, seborrhea, oily skin, hirsutism or loss of hair. **Other:** leg cramps, breast tenderness or enlargement.
esterified estrogens Amnestrogen, Climestrone♦♦, Estabs, Estratab, Evex, Femogen, Menest, Menotrol♦♦, Ms-Med, Neo-Estrone♦♦	**Men:** *Prostatic cancer*—1.25 to 2.5 mg P.O. t.i.d. **Men and postmenopausal women:** *Breast cancer*—10 mg P.O. t.i.d. for 3 or more months. **Women:** *Hypogonadism, castration, primary ovarian failure*—2.5 mg daily to t.i.d. in cycles of 3 weeks on, 1 week off. *Menopausal symptoms*—average 0.3 to 3.75 mg P.O. daily in cycles of 3 weeks on, 1 week off.	**CNS:** headache, dizziness, chorea, depression, libido changes, lethargy. **CV:** thrombophlebitis; *thromboembolism;* hypertension; edema; *increased risk of stroke, pulmonary embolism, and myocardial infarction.* **EENT:** worsening of myopia or astigmatism, intolerance to contact lenses. **GI:** *nausea,* vomiting, abdominal cramps, bloating, diarrhea, constipation, anorexia, increased appetite, weight changes. **GU:** *in females*—breakthrough bleeding, altered menstrual flow, dysmenorrhea, amenorrhea, cervical erosion, altered cervical secretions, enlargement of uterine fibromas, vaginal candidiasis; *in males*—gynecomastia, testicular

♦ Available in U.S. and Canada. ♦♦ Available in Canada only. All other products (no symbol) available in U.S. only. Italicized side effects are common or life-threatening.

INTERACTIONS	NURSING CONSIDERATIONS
	• FDA regulations require that all female patients receive package insert explaining possible estrogen side effects before first dose. Provide verbal explanation also. • Only the 25-mg tablet is approved by FDA as the "morning-after pill." To be effective, it must be taken within 72 hours after coitus. • Warn patient to stop taking drug immediately if she becomes pregnant, since it can affect the fetus adversely. • Warn patient to report immediately: abdominal pain; pain, numbness, or stiffness in legs or buttocks; pressure or pain in chest; shortness of breath; severe headache; visual disturbances, such as blind spots, flashing lights, or blurriness; vaginal bleeding or discharge; breast lumps; sudden weight gain; swelling of hands or feet; yellow sclera or skin; dark urine or light-colored stools. • Pathologist should be advised of estrogen therapy when specimen sent. • Patients with diabetes should report positive urine tests so antidiabetic medication dose can be adjusted. • High incidence of gross nonmalignant genital changes in offspring of women taking drug during pregnancy. Female offspring have higher than normal risk of developing cervical and vaginal adenocarcinoma. Male offspring may have higher than normal risk of developing testicular tumors. • Increased number of cardiovascular deaths reported in men taking diethylstilbestrol tablet (5 mg daily) for prostatic cancer over long period. This effect not associated with 1-mg daily dose. • Reassure male patients on estrogen therapy that side effects such as gynecomastia and impotence will disappear when therapy ends. • Teach female patients how to perform routine breast self-examination. • Explain to patient on cyclic therapy for postmenopausal symptoms that although withdrawal bleeding may occur during week off drug, fertility has not been restored. Pregnancy is not possible since she has not ovulated. • Use of estrogens associated with increased risk of endometrial cancer. Possible increased risk of breast cancer.
None significant.	• Contraindicated in thrombophlebitis or thromboembolic disorders; undiagnosed abnormal genital bleeding. Use cautiously in patients with history of hypertension, mental depression, gallbladder disease, migraine headaches, seizures, diabetes mellitus, amenorrhea, or family history (mother, grandmother, sister) of breast or genital tract cancer. Development or worsening of these conditions may require discontinuation of the drug. • FDA regulations require that female patients receive package insert explaining possible estrogen side effects before first dose. Provide verbal explanation also. • Warn patient to report immediately: abdominal pain; pain, numbness, or stiffness in legs or buttocks; pressure or pain in chest; shortness of breath; severe headaches; visual disturbances, such as blind spots, flashing lights, or blurriness; vaginal bleeding or discharge; breast lumps; swelling of hands or feet; yellow skin or sclera; dark urine or light-colored stools. • Pathologist should be advised of estrogen therapy when specimen sent. • Patients with diabetes should report positive urine tests so antidiabetic medication dose can be adjusted. • Explain to patient on cyclic therapy for postmenopausal symptoms that although she may experience withdrawal bleeding during week

(continued on following page)

NAME	INDICATIONS & DOSAGE	SIDE EFFECTS
esterified estrogens *(continued)*		atrophy, impotence. **Hepatic:** cholestatic jaundice. **Metabolic:** hyperglycemia, hypercalcemia, folic acid deficiency. **Skin:** melasma, rash, acne, hirsutism or hair loss, seborrhea, oily skin. **Other:** breast changes (tenderness, enlargement, secretion).
estradiol Estrace♦, Progynon **estradiol cypionate** Depo-Estradiol Cypionate, Depogen, D-Est 5, Dura-Estrin, E-lonate P.A., Estro-Cyp, Estroject-L.A. **estradiol valerate** Ardefem, Delestrogen♦♦, Dioval♦, Duragen, Estate, Estradiol L.A., Estraval-P.A., Rep Estra, Repo-Estro Med, Reposo-E, Retestrin, Valergen	**Women:** *Menopausal symptoms, hypogonadism, castration, primary ovarian failure*—1 to 2 mg P.O. daily, in cycles of 21 days on and 7 days off, or cycles of 5 days on and 2 days off; or 0.2 to 1 mg I.M. weekly. *Kraurosis vulvae*—1 to 1.5 mg I.M. once or more per week. *Menopausal symptoms*—1 to 5 mg (cypionate) I.M. q 3 to 4 weeks. Or 5 to 20 mg (valerate) I.M., repeated once after 2 to 3 weeks *Postpartum breast engorgement*—10 to 25 mg (valerate) I.M. at end of first stage of labor. **Men:** *Prostatic cancer*—25 mg S.C. pellet implants (Progynon) q 3 to 4 months, or 50 mg q 4 to 6 months. Or 30 mg (valerate) I.M. q 1 to 2 weeks.	**CNS:** headache, dizziness, chorea, depression, libido changes, lethargy. **CV:** thrombophlebitis, *thromboembolism,* hypertension, edema. **EENT:** worsening of myopia or astigmatism, intolerance to contact lenses. **GI:** *nausea,* vomiting, abdominal cramps, bloating, diarrhea, constipation, anorexia, increased appetite, weight changes. **GU:** *in females*—breakthrough bleeding, altered menstrual flow, dysmenorrhea, amenorrhea, cervical erosion, altered cervical secretions, enlargement of uterine fibromas, vaginal candidiasis; *in males*—gynecomastia, testicular atrophy, impotence. **Hepatic:** cholestatic jaundice. **Metabolic:** hyperglycemia, hypercalcemia, folic acid deficiency. **Skin:** melasma, urticaria, acne, seborrhea, oily skin, hirsutism or hair loss. **Other:** breast changes (tenderness, enlargement, secretion), leg cramps.
estrogenic substances, conjugated Estrocon, Menotab, Ovest, Premarin♦, Sodestrin-H	**Women:** *Abnormal uterine bleeding (hormonal imbalance)*—25 mg I.V. or I.M. Repeat in 6 to 12 hours. *Breast cancer (at least 5 years after menopause)*—10 mg P.O. t.i.d. for 3 months or more. *Castration, primary ovarian failure, and osteoporosis*—	**CNS:** headache, dizziness, chorea, depression, libido changes, lethargy. **CV:** thrombophlebitis; *thromboembolism;* hypertension; edema; *increased risk of stroke, pulmonary embolism, and myocardial infarction.* **EENT:** worsening of myopia or

♦ Available in U.S. and Canada. ♦♦ Available in Canada only. All other products (no symbol) available in U.S. only. Italicized side effects are common or life-threatening.

INTERACTIONS	NURSING CONSIDERATIONS
	off drug, fertility has not been restored. Pregnancy cannot occur since she has not ovulated. • Teach female patients how to perform routine breast self-examination. • Reassure male patients on estrogen therapy that side effects such as gynecomastia and impotence will disappear when therapy ends.
None significant.	• Contraindicated in thrombophlebitis or thromboembolic disorders; cancer of breast, reproductive organs; undiagnosed abnormal genital bleeding. Use cautiously in patients with hypertension, mental depression, bone diseases, blood dyscrasias, migraine headaches, seizures, diabetes mellitus, amenorrhea, heart failure, hepatic or renal dysfunction, or family history (mother, grandmother, sister) of breast or genital tract cancer. Development or worsening of these conditions may necessitate discontinuation of the drug. • FDA regulations require that female patients receive package insert explaining possible estrogen side effects before first dose. Provide verbal explanation also. • Warn patient to report immediately: abdominal pain; pain, numbness, or stiffness in legs or buttocks; pressure or pain in chest; shortness of breath; severe headaches; visual disturbances, such as blind spots, flashing lights, or blurriness; vaginal bleeding or discharge; breast lumps; swelling of hands or feet; yellow skin or sclera; dark urine or light-colored stools. • Risk of endometrial cancer is increased in postmenopausal women who take estrogens for more than 1 year. • Patients with diabetes should report positive urine tests so antidiabetic medication dose can be adjusted. • Pathologist should be advised of estrogen therapy when specimen sent. • Estradiol available as aqueous suspension or solution in peanut oil. • Estradiol cypionate available as solution in cottonseed oil or vegetable oil. • Estradiol valerate available as solution in castor oil, sesame oil, and vegetable oil. Check for allergy. • Before injection, make sure drug is well dispersed in solution by rolling vial between palms. Inject deep I.M. into large muscle. • Reassure male patient that possible side effects of gynecomastia and impotence disappear after termination of therapy. • Teach female patients how to perform routine breast self-examination. • Explain to patient on cyclic therapy for postmenopausal symptoms that although withdrawal bleeding may occur during week off drug, fertility has not been reinstated. Pregnancy cannot occur since she has not ovulated.
None significant.	• Contraindicated in thrombophlebitis or thromboembolic disorders; undiagnosed abnormal genital bleeding. Use cautiously in hypertension, gallbladder disease, bone diseases, blood dyscrasias, migraine headaches, seizures, diabetes mellitus, amenorrhea, heart failure, hepatic or renal dysfunction, or family history (mother, grandmother, sister) of breast or genital tract cancer. Development or worsening of these conditions may require discontinuation of the drug. • FDA regulations require that female patients receive package insert explaining possible estrogen side effects before first dose. Provide ver-

(continued on following page)

NAME	INDICATIONS & DOSAGE	SIDE EFFECTS
estrogenic substance conjugated *(continued)*	1.25 mg P.O. daily in cycles of 3 weeks on, 1 week off. *Hypogonadism*—2.5 mg P.O. b.i.d. or t.i.d. for 20 consecutive days each month. *Menopausal symptoms*—0.3 to 1.25 mg P.O. daily in cycles of 3 weeks on, 1 week off. *Postpartum breast engorgement*— 3.75 mg P.O. q 4 hours for 5 doses or 1.25 mg q 4 hours for 5 days. **Men:** *Prostatic cancer*—1.25 to 2.5 mg P.O. t.i.d.	astigmatism, intolerance to contact lenses. **GI:** *nausea,* vomiting, abdominal cramps, bloating, diarrhea, constipation, anorexia, increased appetite, weight changes. **GU:** *in females*—breakthrough bleeding, altered menstrual flow, dysmenorrhea, amenorrhea, cervical erosion, altered cervical secretions, enlargement of uterine fibromas, vaginal candidiasis; *in males*—gynecomastia, testicular atrophy, impotence. **Hepatic:** cholestatic jaundice. **Metabolic:** hyperglycemia, hypercalcemia, folic acid deficiency. **Skin:** melasma, urticaria, acne, seborrhea, oily skin, flushing (when given rapidly I.V.), hirsutism or loss of hair. **Other:** breast changes (tenderness, enlargement, secretion), leg cramps.
estrone Foygen, Gravigen, Ogen♦, Theelin	**Women:** *Atrophic vaginitis*—0.2 mg intravaginal suppository daily or apply cream to vagina once nightly. *Hypogonadism, castration, ovarian failure*—1.25 to 7.5 mg P.O. daily for 20 consecutive days each month; or 0.1 to 2 mg I.M. weekly. *Menopausal symptoms*— 0.625 to 5 mg P.O. daily in cycle of 3 weeks on, 1 week off; or 0.1 to 0.5 mg I.M. 2 to 3 times weekly. **Men:** *Prostatic cancer*—2 to 4 mg I.M. 2 to 3 times weekly.	**CNS:** headache, dizziness, chorea, depression, libido changes, lethargy. **CV:** thrombophlebitis, *thromboembolism,* hypertension, edema. **EENT:** worsening of myopia or astigmatism, intolerance to contact lenses. **GI:** *nausea,* vomiting, abdominal cramps, bloating, diarrhea, constipation, anorexia, increased appetite, weight changes. **GU:** *in females*—breakthrough bleeding, altered menstrual flow, dysmenorrhea, amenorrhea, cervical erosion, altered cervical secretions, enlargement of uterine fibromas, vaginal candidiasis; *in males*—gynecomastia, testicular atrophy, impotence. **Hepatic:** cholestatic jaundice. **Metabolic:** hyperglycemia, hypercalcemia, folic acid deficiency. **Skin:** melasma, urticaria, acne, seborrhea, oily skin, hirsutism or hair loss. **Other:** breast changes (tenderness, enlargement, secretion), leg cramps.

INTERACTIONS	NURSING CONSIDERATIONS
	bal explanation also. • Warn patient to report immediately: abdominal pain; pain, numbness, or stiffness in legs or buttocks; pressure or pain in chest; shortness of breath; severe headaches; visual disturbances, such as blind spots, flashing lights, or blurriness; vaginal bleeding or discharge; breast lumps; swelling of hands or feet; yellow skin or sclera; dark urine or light-colored stools. • I.M. or I.V. use preferred for rapid treatment of dysfunctional uterine bleeding or reduction of surgical bleeding. • Refrigerate before reconstituting. Agitate gently after adding diluent. • Pathologist should be advised of estrogen therapy when specimen sent. • Patients with diabetes should report positive urine tests so antidiabetic medication dose can be adjusted. • Use associated with increased risk of endometrial cancer. Possible increased risk of breast cancer. • Teach female patients how to perform routine breast self-examination. • Explain to patient on cyclic therapy for postmenopausal symptoms that although withdrawal bleeding may occur during week off drug, fertility has not been restored. Pregnancy cannot occur since she has not ovulated. • Reassure male patients that possible side effects of gynecomastia and impotence disappear after termination of therapy.
None significant.	• Contraindicated in thrombophlebitis or thromboembolic disorders; cancer of breast or reproductive organs; undiagnosed abnormal genital bleeding. Use cautiously in patients with hypertension, mental depression, migraine headaches, seizures, diabetes mellitus, amenorrhea, hepatic or renal dysfunction, or family history (mother, grandmother, sister) of breast or genital tract cancer. Development or worsening of these conditions may necessitate discontinuation of drug. • I.V. use contraindicated. • FDA regulations require that female patients receive package insert explaining possible estrogen side effects before first dose. Provide verbal explanation also. • Warn patient to report immediately: abdominal pain; pain, numbness, or stiffness in legs or buttocks; pressure or pain in chest; shortness of breath; severe headaches; visual disturbances, such as blind spots, flashing lights, or blurriness; vaginal bleeding or discharge; breast lumps; swelling of hands or feet. • Oil preparation may become cloudy if chilled. Warm solution until clear before use. Also available in aqueous suspension. • Pathologist should be advised of estrogen therapy when specimen is sent. • Patients with diabetes should report positive urine test so antidiabetic medication dose can be adjusted. • Teach female patients how to perform routine breast self-examination. • Use of estrogens associated with increased risk of endometrial cancer. Possible increased risk of breast cancer. • Explain to patient on cyclic therapy for postmenopausal symptoms that although withdrawal bleeding may occur during week off drug, fertility has not been restored. Pregnancy cannot occur since she has not ovulated. • Reassure male patients that possible side effects of gynecomastia and impotence disappear after termination of therapy.

NAME	INDICATIONS & DOSAGE	SIDE EFFECTS
ethinyl estradiol Estinyl♦, Feminone	**Women:** *Breast cancer (at least 5 years after menopause)*—1 mg P.O. t.i.d. *Hypogonadism*—0.05 mg daily to t.i.d. for 2 weeks a month, followed by 2 weeks progesterone therapy; continue for 3 to 6 monthly dosing cycles, followed by 2 months off. *Menopausal symptoms*—0.02 to 0.05 mg P.O. daily for cycles of 3 weeks on, 1 week off. *Postpartum breast engorgement*— 0.5 to 1 mg P.O. daily for 3 days, then taper over 7 days to 0.1 mg and discontinue. **Men:** *Prostatic cancer*—0.15 to 2 mg P.O. daily.	**CNS:** headache, dizziness, chorea, depression, libido changes, lethargy. **CV:** thrombophlebitis, *thromboembolism,* hypertension, edema. **EENT:** worsening of myopia or astigmatism, intolerance to contact lenses. **GI:** *nausea,* vomiting, abdominal cramps, bloating, diarrhea, constipation, anorexia, increased appetite, weight changes. **GU:** *in females*—breakthrough bleeding, altered menstrual flow, dysmenorrhea, amenorrhea, cervical erosion, altered cervical secretions, enlargement of uterine fibromas, vaginal candidiasis; *in males*—gynecomastia, testicular atrophy, impotence. **Hepatic:** cholestatic jaundice. **Metabolic:** hyperglycemia, hypercalcemia, folic acid deficiency. **Skin:** melasma, urticaria, acne, seborrhea, oily skin, hirsutism or hair loss. **Other:** breast changes (tenderness, enlargement, secretion), leg cramps.
quinestrol Estrovis	**Women:** *Moderate to severe vasomotor symptoms associated with menopause, and for atrophic vaginitis, kraurosis vulvae, female hypogonadism, female castration, and primary ovarian failure*—100-mcg tablet once daily for 7 days, followed by 100 mcg weekly as maintenance dose beginning 2 weeks after start of treatment. Dosage may be increased to 200 mcg weekly.	**CNS:** headache, dizziness, chorea, migraine, depression, libido changes. **CV:** thrombophlebitis; *thromboembolism;* hypertension; edema; *increased risk of stroke, pulmonary embolism, and myocardial infarction.* **EENT:** worsening of myopia or astigmatism, intolerance to contact lenses. **GI:** *nausea,* vomiting, abdominal cramps, bloating, diarrhea, constipation, anorexia, increased appetite, excessive thirst, weight changes. **GU:** breakthrough bleeding, altered menstrual flow, dysmenorrhea, amenorrhea, cervical erosion or abnormal secretions, enlargement of uterine fibromas, vaginal candidiasis. **Hepatic:** cholestatic jaundice. **Metabolic:** hyperglycemia, hypercalcemia, folic acid deficiency. **Skin:** melasma, urticaria, acne, seborrhea, oily skin, hirsutism or

INTERACTIONS	NURSING CONSIDERATIONS
None significant.	• Contraindicated in thrombophlebitis or thromboembolic disorders; undiagnosed abnormal genital bleeding. Use cautiously in patients with hypertension, mental depression, bone diseases, migraine headaches, seizures, blood dyscrasias, diabetes mellitus, amenorrhea, heart failure, hepatic or renal dysfunction, or family history (mother, grandmother, sister) of breast or genital tract cancer. Development or worsening of these conditions may necessitate discontinuation of drug. • FDA regulations require that female patients receive package insert explaining possible estrogen side effects before first dose. Provide verbal explanation also. • Warn patient to report immediately: abdominal pain; pain, numbness, or stiffness in legs or buttocks; pressure or pain in chest; shortness of breath; severe headaches; visual disturbances, such as blind spots, flashing lights, or blurriness; vaginal bleeding or discharge; breast lumps; swelling of hands or feet; yellow skin or sclera; dark urine or light-colored stools. • Pathologist should be advised of estrogen therapy when specimen sent. • Patients with diabetes should report positive urine test so antidiabetic medication dose can be adjusted. • Teach female patients how to perform routine breast self-examination. • Use of estrogens associated with increased risk of endometrial cancer. Possible increased risk of breast cancer. • Explain to patient on cyclic therapy for postmenopausal symptoms that although withdrawal bleeding may occur during week off drug, fertility has not been restored. Pregnancy cannot occur since she has not ovulated. • Reassure male patients that possible side effects of gynecomastia and impotence disappear after termination of therapy.
None significant.	• Contraindicated in thrombophlebitis or thromboembolic disorders; cancer of breast or reproductive organs; undiagnosed abnormal genital bleeding. Use cautiously in patients with hypertension, mental depression, migraine headaches, seizures, diabetes mellitus, amenorrhea, hepatic or renal dysfunction, or family history (mother, grandmother, sister) of breast or genital tract cancer. Development or worsening of these may necessitate discontinuation of the drug. • FDA regulations require that female patients receive package insert explaining possible estrogen side effects before first dose. Provide verbal explanation also. • Warn patient to report immediately: abdominal pain; pain, numbness, or stiffness in legs or buttocks; pressure or pain in chest; shortness of breath; severe headaches; visual disturbances, such as blind spots, flashing lights, or blurriness; vaginal bleeding or discharge; breast lumps; swelling of hands or feet; yellow skin or sclera; dark urine or light-colored stools. • Pathologist should be advised of estrogen therapy when specimen is sent. • Patients with diabetes should report positive urine test so antidiabetic medication dose can be adjusted. • Attempts to discontinue medication should be made at 3- to 6-month intervals. • Similar in effectiveness to conjugated estrogens in treatment of postmenopausal symptoms. Biggest advantage is that quinestrol can be taken once a week. • Use of estrogens associated with increased risk of endometrial cancer. Possible increased risk of breast cancer.

(continued on following page)

NAME	INDICATIONS & DOSAGE	SIDE EFFECTS
quinestrol *(continued)*		loss of hair. **Other:** leg cramps, purpura, breast changes (tenderness, enlargement, secretion).

♦ Available in U.S. and Canada. ♦♦ Available in Canada only. All other products (no symbol) available in U.S. only.

NURSING TIPS

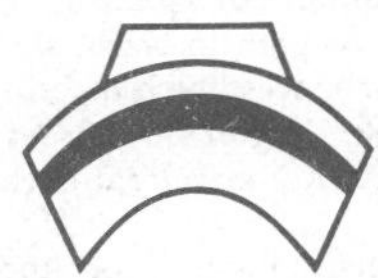

PROVIDING SUPPORT FOR PATIENTS ON ESTROGEN THERAPY

- Encourage your patient to report any discomforting side effects, such as:
—mood changes, especially depression
—thrombophlebitis (warmth or pain in the calf)
—excessive fluid retention
—jaundice
—excessive nausea and vomiting
—dizziness and frequent headaches (which point to elevated blood pressure)
—loss of scalp hair
—hirsutism
—indigestion after eating fatty foods, or stomach pain.
- Stress the need for your patient to visit her gynecologist regularly—at least once a year. (Visits should include a pelvic examination, a Pap test, and a breast examination.)
- Show her how to perform a breast self-examination and advise her to do this monthly.
- Explain that bleeding after estrogen withdrawal is expected. Inform the postmenopausal woman her bleeding is pseudomenstruation and does not mean fertility has been restored.
- Instruct a patient with diabetes to make frequent urine checks for sugar and acetone.
- Although there's some controversy concerning estrogen's link to cancer (see opposite page), encourage your patient to discuss her concerns with her doctor. Stress the need for follow-up examinations to carefully monitor this risk.

As you probably know, estrogen—specifically diethylstilbestrol—is used to *treat* some cancers. Be sure to explain this mode of therapy to your patient.

INTERACTIONS	NURSING CONSIDERATIONS
	• Explain to patients on replacement therapy for postmenopausal symptoms that although menstrual-like bleeding or spotting may occur, fertility has not been restored. • Teach female patients how to perform breast self-examination. • Reassure male patients that possible side effects of gynecomastia and impotence disappear after termination of therapy.

DRUG ALERT

KNOW THE FACTS ABOUT ESTROGEN AND CANCER

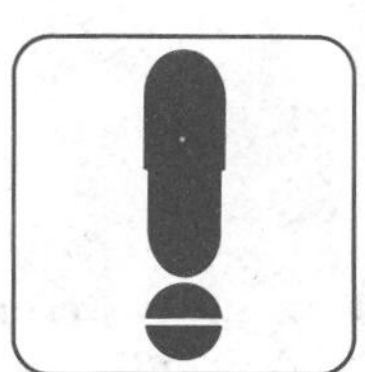

According to the Food and Drug Administration (FDA), the incidence of endometrial cancer has risen dramatically since 1969. This increase is probably linked to the growing use of estrogens in the last decade.

Substitute estrogens—that is, estrogen replacement therapy (ERT)—can be given as a woman's natural estrogen level decreases. Advocates of ERT claim a marked control of the physical and emotional symptoms of menopause with this treatment.

But opponents cite the side effects of estrogen therapy (vaginal bleeding, breast tenderness, nausea, vomiting, abdominal bloating, and uterine cramps) and its association with cancer in estrogen-dependent tissue, such as the endometrium and the breast. The FDA warns that menopausal and postmenopausal women who take estrogen increase their risk of developing endometrial cancer.

The FDA also suggests that when estrogens are used to treat menopausal symptoms, the lowest dose that will control symptoms should be ordered, and therapy should be discontinued as soon as possible.

Three important findings can serve as cautionary guidelines for your patient:

- The increased risk of endometrial cancer is proportional to the duration of estrogen use. (The reported risk increases with use over a period of 5 years or longer. For patients taking estrogen for 5 years or more, the relative risk is 15 times greater. In patients who've taken estrogen for 1 year or less, the risk is considered to be double that of the population at large.)
- Use of cyclic therapy or progestins for 7 days each month is thought not to protect a woman meaningfully from the risk of endometrial cancer.
- The risk is greatly reduced if the lowest possible dose is prescribed.

If your patient does agree to receive ERT, she must be monitored regularly to detect possible cancer in its earliest, asymptomatic stages. ERT is *contraindicated* in pregnant women and those with histories of breast or genital tract cancer. It's used with caution in women with histories of these cancers in their immediate families. *Note:* There's no evidence at present that natural estrogens are more or less hazardous than synthetic estrogens if given in equivalent doses.

56 Progestogens

dydrogesterone
hydroxyprogesterone caproate
medroxyprogesterone acetate
norethindrone
norethindrone acetate
norgestrel
progesterone

The natural hormone progesterone and its synthetic derivatives are called progestogens or progestins; they produce the characteristic endometrial changes that favor pregnancy (gestation). Progesterone is secreted mainly by the corpus luteum after ovulation (during the last half of the menstrual cycle). Large amounts, however, are also secreted by the placenta. Smaller quantities are produced by both the mature follicle before ovulation (during the first half of the menstrual cycle) and the adrenal cortex.

Progestogens trigger glandular and vascular development, which results in the endometrial swelling essential for implantation of the fertilized ovum. If implantation doesn't occur, the sharp drop in the progesterone level at the end of the menstrual cycle helps start menstruation.

Progestogens also relax uterine smooth muscle. During pregnancy, increased progesterone secretion prevents premature uterine contractions and allows the pregnancy to continue to term. Along with estrogen, progestogens aid growth and development of the alveolar duct system in the mammary glands.

Progestogens also promote protein catabolism and sodium and water retention.

Major uses

Rx Progestogens relieve dysfunctional uterine bleeding, amenorrhea, and dysmenorrhea.

- Norethindrone and norethindrone acetate are used to treat endometriosis.
- Norethindrone, norethindrone acetate, and norgestrel are used alone or in combination with estrogens in oral contraceptives.

Mechanism of action

- Progestogens mimic the body's production of progesterone to reestablish a normal menstrual cycle in patients with amenorrhea.
- They promote glandular and vascular development of the endometrium by restoring progesterone levels.
- Progestogens suppress ovulation possibly by inhibiting pituitary gonadotropin secretion. They also form a thick cervical mucus that is relatively impermeable to sperm.

Absorption, distribution, metabolism, and excretion

Progestogens are rapidly absorbed, distributed to all tissues, metabolized in the liver, and excreted in urine.

Onset and duration

Onset and duration vary with the dis-

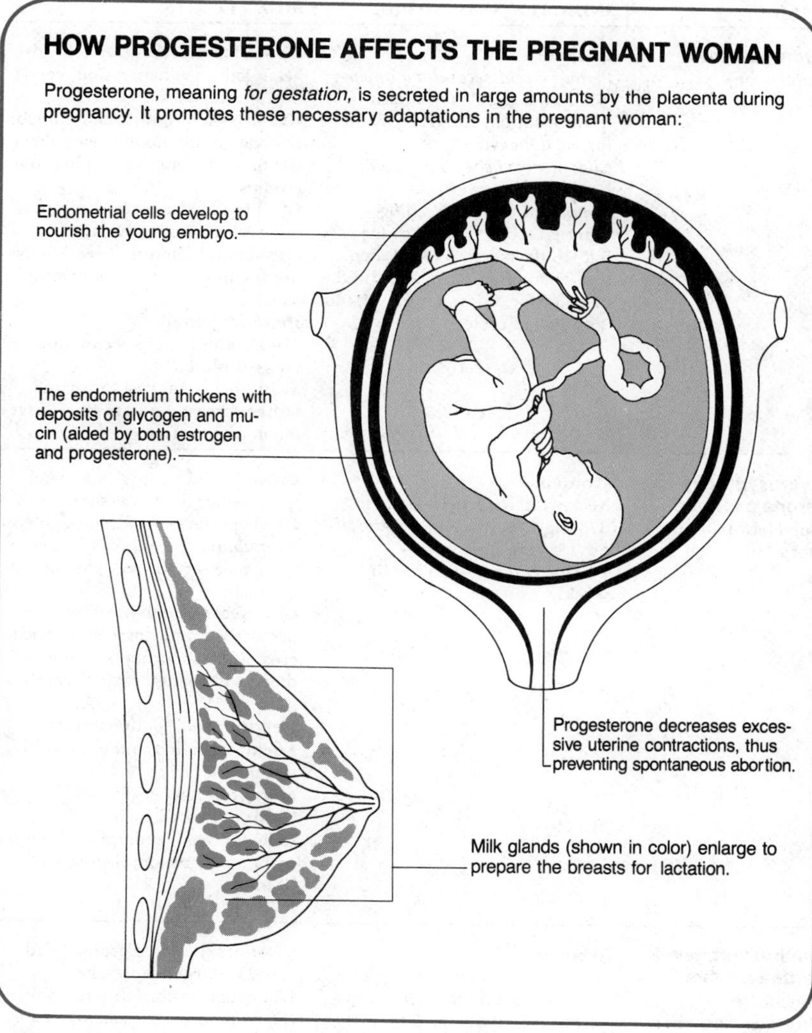

order, the progestogen given, and use of an estrogen (that is, whether the progestogen is administered with, after, or without an estrogen). Generally, however, onset is fastest when estrogens are given first; duration is longest when the slow-release ("depot") forms (injection in oil, for example) are used.

HOW PROGESTERONE AFFECTS THE PREGNANT WOMAN
Progesterone, meaning for gestation, is secreted in large amounts by the placenta during pregnancy. It promotes these necessary adaptations in the pregnant woman:
Endometrial cells develop to nourish the young embryo.
The endometrium thickens with deposits of glycogen and mucin (aided by both estrogen and progesterone).
Progesterone decreases excessive uterine contractions, thus preventing spontaneous abortion.
Milk glands (shown in color) enlarge to prepare the breasts for lactation.

Combination products

See Chapter 54, ORAL CONTRACEPTIVES, for combination products.

NAME	INDICATIONS & DOSAGE	SIDE EFFECTS
dydrogesterone Duphaston♦	**Women:** *Primary and secondary amenorrhea*—5 mg P.O. b.i.d. or q.i.d. from day 15 to day 25 of menstrual cycle. *Oligomenorrhea*—5 mg P.O. b.i.d. for 5 days. *Abnormal uterine bleeding*—5 mg P.O. b.i.d. or q.i.d. for 5 to 10 days before usual menses. Thereafter, 5 mg P.O. b.i.d. to q.i.d. for 5 days on the 21st to 25th day of cycle.	**CNS:** dizziness, migraine headache, lethargy, depression, cerebral thrombosis. **CV:** hypertension, thrombophlebitis, edema, *pulmonary embolism.* **GI:** nausea, vomiting, abdominal cramps. **GU:** breakthrough bleeding, dysmenorrhea, amenorrhea; cervical erosion and abnormal secretions; uterine fibromas; vaginal candidiasis. **Hepatic:** jaundice. **Metabolic:** hyperglycemia, decreased libido. **Skin:** melasma, rash, pruritus. **Other:** breast tenderness, enlargement, or secretion.
hydroxyprogesterone caproate Curretab, Delalutin♦, Dura-Lutin	**Women:** *Menstrual disorders*—125 to 375 mg I.M. q 4 weeks. Stop after 4 cycles. *Uterine cancer*—1 to 5 g I.M. weekly.	**CNS:** dizziness, migraine headache, lethargy, depression. **CV:** hypertension, thrombophlebitis, *pulmonary embolism, edema.* **GI:** nausea, vomiting, abdominal cramps. **GU:** breakthrough bleeding, dysmenorrhea, amenorrhea; cervical erosion or abnormal secretions; uterine fibromas; vaginal candidiasis. **Hepatic:** cholestatic jaundice. **Local:** irritation and pain at injection site. **Metabolic:** hyperglycemia. **Skin:** melasma, rash. **Other:** breast tenderness, enlargement, or secretion; decreased libido.
medroxyprogesterone acetate Amen, Depo-Provera♦, Provera♦	**Women:** *Abnormal uterine bleeding due to hormonal imbalance*—5 to 10 mg P.O. daily for 5 to 10 days beginning on the 16th day of cycle. If patient has received estrogen—10 mg P.O. daily for 10 days beginning on 16th day of cycle. *Secondary amenorrhea*—5 to 10 mg P.O. daily for 5 to 10 days.	**CNS:** dizziness, migraine headache, lethargy, depression. **CV:** hypertension, thrombophlebitis, *pulmonary embolism, edema.* **GI:** nausea, vomiting, abdominal cramps. **GU:** breakthrough bleeding, dysmenorrhea, amenorrhea; cervical erosion or abnormal secretions; uterine fibromas, vaginal candidiasis. **Hepatic:** cholestatic jaundice. **Metabolic:** hyperglycemia, decreased libido. **Skin:** melasma, rash. **Other:** breast tenderness, enlargement, or secretion.

INTERACTIONS	NURSING CONSIDERATIONS
None significant.	• Contraindicated in thromboembolic disorders, breast cancer, undiagnosed abnormal vaginal bleeding, missed abortion, pregnancy, hepatic dysfunction. Use cautiously when diabetes mellitus, seizure disorder, migraine, cardiac or renal disease, asthma, or mental illness is present. • FDA regulations require that before receiving first dose patients read package insert explaining possible progestogen side effects. Provide verbal explanation also. Patient should report any unusual symptoms immediately and should stop drug and call doctor if visual disturbances or migraine occurs. • Don't use as test for pregnancy; drug may cause birth defects and masculinization of female fetus. • Preliminary estrogen treatment is usually needed in menstrual disorders. • Not approved by FDA for use as contraceptive in United States. • Teach the patient how to perform a breast self-examination. • This drug does not inhibit ovulation.
None significant.	• Contraindicated in thromboembolic disorders, breast cancer, undiagnosed abnormal vaginal bleeding, severe hepatic disease, missed abortion, or pregnancy. Use cautiously when diabetes mellitus, seizure disorder, migraine, cardiac or renal disease, asthma, or mental illness is present. • FDA regulations require that before receiving first dose patients read package insert explaining possible progestogen side effects. Provide verbal explanation also. Patient should report any unusual symptoms immediately and should stop drug and call doctor if visual disturbances or migraine occurs. • Don't use as test for pregnancy; drug may cause birth defects and masculinization of female fetus. • Warn patient that edema and weight gain are likely. • Give oil solutions (sesame oil and castor oil) deep I.M. in gluteal muscle. • Preliminary estrogen treatment is usually needed in menstrual disorders. • Effect lasts 7 to 14 days. • For I.M. use only. • Teach patient how to perform a breast self-examination.
None significant.	• Contraindicated in thromboembolic disorders, breast cancer, undiagnosed abnormal vaginal bleeding, pregnancy, missed abortion, hepatic dysfunction. Use cautiously when diabetes mellitus, seizure disorder, migraine, cardiac or renal disease, asthma, or mental illness is present. • FDA regulations require that before receiving first dose patients read package insert explaining possible progestogen side effects. Provide verbal explanation also. Patient should report any unusual symptoms immediately and should stop drug and call doctor if visual disturbances or migraine occurs. • Don't use as test for pregnancy; drug may cause birth defects and masculinization of female fetus. • Teach patient how to perform a breast self-examination.

NAME	INDICATIONS & DOSAGE	SIDE EFFECTS
norethindrone Norlutin♦, Nor-Q.D.	**Women:** *Amenorrhea; abnormal uterine bleeding*—5 to 20 mg P.O. daily on days 5 to 25 of menstrual cycle. *Endometriosis*—10 mg P.O. daily for 14 days, then increase by 5 mg P.O. daily q 2 weeks up to 30 mg daily.	**CNS:** dizziness, migraine headache, lethargy, depression. **CV:** hypertension, thrombophlebitis, *pulmonary embolism, edema.* **GI:** nausea, vomiting, abdominal cramps. **GU:** breakthrough bleeding, dysmenorrhea, amenorrhea; cervical erosion or abnormal secretions; uterine fibromas; vaginal candidiasis. **Hepatic:** cholestatic jaundice. **Metabolic:** hyperglycemia, decreased libido. **Skin:** melasma, rash. **Other:** breast tenderness, enlargement, or secretion.
norethindrone acetate Norlutate♦	**Women:** *Amenorrhea, abnormal uterine bleeding*—2.5 to 10 mg P.O. daily on days 5 to 25 of menstrual cycle. *Endometriosis*—5 mg P.O. daily for 14 days, then increase by 2.5 mg daily q 2 weeks up to 15 mg daily.	**CNS:** dizziness, migraine headache, lethargy, depression. **CV:** hypertension, thrombophlebitis, *pulmonary embolism, edema.* **GI:** nausea, vomiting, abdominal cramps. **GU:** breakthrough bleeding, dysmenorrhea, amenorrhea; cervical erosion or abnormal secretions; uterine fibromas; vaginal candidiasis. **Hepatic:** cholestatic jaundice. **Metabolic:** hyperglycemia, decreased libido. **Skin:** melasma, rash. **Other:** breast tenderness, enlargement, or secretion.
norgestrel Ovrette	**Women:** *Contraception*—1 tablet P.O. daily.	**CNS:** cerebral thrombosis or hemorrhage, migraine headache, lethargy, depression. **CV:** hypertension, thrombophlebitis, *pulmonary embolism, edema.* **GI:** nausea, vomiting, abdominal cramps, gallbladder disease. **GU:** *breakthrough bleeding, change in menstrual flow,* dysmenorrhea, spotting, amenorrhea; cervical erosion, vaginal candidiasis. **Hepatic:** cholestatic jaundice. **Skin:** melasma, rash. **Other:** breast tenderness, enlargement, or secretion.

INTERACTIONS	NURSING CONSIDERATIONS
None significant.	• Contraindicated in thromboembolic disorders, breast cancer, undiagnosed abnormal vaginal bleeding, severe hepatic disease, missed abortion, or pregnancy. Use cautiously when diabetes mellitus, seizure disorder, migraine, cardiac or renal disease, asthma, or mental illness is present. • Don't use as test for pregnancy; drug may cause birth defects and masculinization of female fetus. • FDA regulations require that before receiving first dose patients read package insert explaining possible progestogen side effects. Provide verbal explanation also. Patient should report any unusual symptoms immediately and should stop drug and call doctor if visual disturbances or migraine occurs. • Watch patient carefully for signs of edema. • Preliminary estrogen treatment is usually needed in menstrual disorders. • Teach the patient how to perform a breast self-examination.
None significant.	• Contraindicated in thromboembolic disorders, breast cancer, undiagnosed abnormal vaginal bleeding, severe hepatic disease, missed abortion, or pregnancy. Use cautiously when diabetes mellitus, seizure disorder, migraine, cardiac or renal disease, asthma, or mental illness is present. • FDA regulations require that before receiving first dose patients read package insert explaining possible progestogen side effects. Provide verbal explanation also. Patient should report any unusual symptoms immediately and should stop drug and call doctor if visual disturbances or migraine occurs. • Don't use as test for pregnancy; drug may cause birth defects and masculinization of female fetus. • Preliminary estrogen treatment is usually needed in menstrual disorders. • Twice as potent as norethindrone. • Teach patient how to perform a breast self-examination.
None significant.	• Contraindicated in thromboembolic disorders, breast cancer, undiagnosed abnormal vaginal bleeding, severe hepatic disease, missed abortion, or pregnancy. Use cautiously when diabetes mellitus, seizure disorder, migraine, cardiac or renal disease, asthma, or mental illness is present. • FDA regulations require that before receiving first dose patients read package insert explaining possible progestogen effects. Provide verbal explanation also. Patient should report any unusual symptoms immediately and should stop drug and call doctor if visual disturbances, migraine, or numbness or tingling in limbs occurs. • Tell patient to take pill every day even if menstruating. Pill should be taken at the same time every day. • Progestogen-only oral contraceptive known as "minipill." • Teach the patient how to perform a breast self-examination. • Women using oral contraceptives should be advised of the increased risk of serious cardiovascular side effects associated with heavy cigarette smoking (15 or more cigarettes per day). These risks are quite marked in women over 35 years. • Risk of pregnancy increases with each tablet missed. A patient who misses one tablet should take it as soon as she remembers; she should then take the next tablet at the regular time. A patient who misses two tablets should take one as soon as she remembers and

(continued on following page)

NAME	INDICATIONS & DOSAGE	SIDE EFFECTS
norgestrel *(continued)*		
progesterone Profac-O, Progelan, Progestasert♦, Progestilin♦♦, Progestin	**Women:** *Amenorrhea*—5 to 10 mg I.M. daily for 6 to 8 days. *Dysfunctional uterine bleeding*—5 to 10 mg I.M. daily for 6 doses. *Contraception (as an intrauterine device)*—Progestasert system inserted into uterine cavity. Replace after 1 year.	**CNS:** dizziness, migraine headache, lethargy, depression. **CV:** hypertension, thrombophlebitis, *pulmonary embolism, edema.* **GI:** nausea, vomiting, abdominal cramps. **GU:** breakthrough bleeding, dysmenorrhea, amenorrhea; cervical erosion or abnormal secretions; uterine fibromas; vaginal candidiasis. **Hepatic:** cholestatic jaundice. **Local:** pain at injection site. **Metabolic:** hyperglycemia, decreased libido. **Skin:** melasma, rash. **Other:** breast tenderness, enlargement, or secretion.

♦ Available in U.S. and Canada. ♦♦ Available in Canada only. All other products (no symbol) available in U.S. only. Italicized side effects are common or life-threatening.

PROGESTERONE'S EFFECT ON THE MENSTRUAL CYCLE

Progesterone secretion peaks from ovulation to the middle of the secretory, or luteal, phase of the menstrual cycle (days 14 to 24). The elevated progesterone level inhibits gonadotropin secretion by a negative feedback mechanism. This causes involution of the corpus luteum, a decrease in ovarian hormone levels, and finally, menstrual bleeding.

KEY TO PHASES OF THE MENSTRUAL CYCLE:

A = menstrual phase

B = follicular phase

C = ovulation (about day 14—midcycle)

D = luteal phase

Adapted with permission from Donald Woodruff, *Novak's Gynecological and Obstetric Pathology* (Philadelphia: W.B. Saunders Co., 1979).

INTERACTIONS	NURSING CONSIDERATIONS
	then take the next regular dose at the usual time; she should use a nonhormonal method of contraception in addition to norgestrel until 14 tablets have been taken. A patient who misses three or more tablets should discontinue the drug and use a nonhormonal method of contraception until after her menses. If her menstrual period does not occur within 45 days, pregnancy testing is necessary. • Instruct the patient to report immediately excessive bleeding or bleeding between menstrual cycles.
None significant.	• Contraindicated in thromboembolic disorders, breast cancer, undiagnosed abnormal vaginal bleeding, severe hepatic disease, or missed abortion. Use cautiously when diabetes mellitus, seizure disorder, migraine, cardiac or renal disease, asthma, or mental illness is present. • FDA regulations require that before receiving first dose patients read package insert explaining possible progestogen side effects. Provide verbal explanation also. Patient should report any unusual symptoms immediately and should stop drug and call doctor if visual disturbances or migraine occurs. • Give oil solutions (peanut oil or sesame oil) deep I.M. • A progesterone-containing IUD (Progestasert) available that releases 65 mcg progesterone daily for 1 year. • Instruct patient with Progestasert IUD how to check for proper IUD placement. Also, advise patient that she may experience cramps for several days after insertion and menstrual periods may be heavier. Patient should report excessively heavy menses and bleeding between menses to the doctor. • Tell patient with Progestasert IUD that the progesterone supply is depleted in 1 year and the device must be changed. Pregnancy risk increases after 1 year if patient relies on progesterone-depleted device for contraception. • Patients considering IUD contraception should be advised of side effects, including uterine perforation, increased risk of infection, pelvic inflammatory disease, ectopic pregnancy, abdominal cramping, increased menstrual flow, and expulsion of the device. • Preliminary estrogen treatment is usually needed in menstrual disorders. • Teach the patient how to perform a breast self-examination.

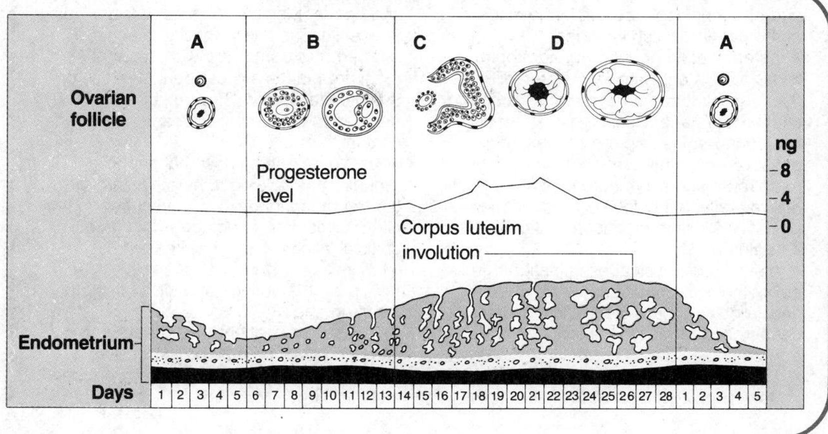

57 Gonadotropins

chorionic gonadotropin, human menotropins

Gonadotropins are hormones that stimulate both male and female gonads. Human chorionic gonadotropin (HCG) originates in the placenta. Human menopausal gonadotropin (HMG or menotropins) is an extract of both luteinizing hormone (LH) and follicle-stimulating hormone (FSH), two gonadotropins that originate in the pituitary gland.

HCG and HMG are the only commercially available gonadotropins. They're purified preparations obtained from the urine of pregnant and postmenopausal women, respectively.

LH and FSH are only available investigationally.

EVALUATING AND SUPPORTING PATIENTS ON INFERTILITY THERAPY

Gonadotropins are used to induce ovulation in anovulatory women. When ovulatory dysfunction has been demonstrated, gonadotropins are initially given in sufficient doses to induce follicular growth and maturation.

Before treatment, a thorough gynecologic and endocrinologic evaluation is made of the patient, which includes:

- determination of urine gonadotropin levels to rule out primary ovarian failure. (Urine gonadotropin levels vary according to a woman's age. Gonadotropin hormone secretion begins at puberty, signaling onset of sexual maturation. Normally, gonadotropin secretion increases at a steady rate, as reflected in total urine gonadotropin levels, until menopause and then it begins to decline.)
- meticulous physical examination to rule out pathologic conditions of the uterus and fallopian tubes, pregnancy, endometrial cancer, and other organic causes of abnormal bleeding.
- similar evaluation of the patient's sexual partner. (Approximately 15% of all couples face infertility, from multiple causes. In the population at large, more female abnormalities than male abnormalities are responsible for infertility.)

Before treatment

- Provide your patient with the support she needs. Many women appear anxious and tense. The natural desire to achieve motherhood combined with societal pressure places a great deal of stress on the infertile woman. The patient who decides to *discontinue* therapy also needs special support.
- Let your patient know that support groups are available to help her through the trauma of infertility. Counsel her on her alternatives, which include adoption or artificial insemination, if her partner is infertile.
- Explain the actions and side effects of the drug she's taking.
- Advise your patient that gonadotropin-induced ovulation may be expensive, difficult to achieve, and likely to produce multiple birth.

Major uses

HCG and HMG induce ovulation in infertile women when anovulation is not due primarily to ovarian failure.

• HCG is used to treat cryptorchidism not due to anatomic obstruction. Stimulation of androgen secretion by HCG leads to the development of secondary sex characteristics and may promote testicular descent.

• HCG is also therapeutic for hypogonadism secondary to pituitary deficiency in males.

• HMG, administered to women without primary ovarian failure, mimics FSH in inducing follicular growth, and LH in aiding follicular maturation.

Mechanism of action

• HCG, when given on the day after the last dose of HMG, serves as a substitute for LH to stimulate ovulation of an HMG-prepared follicle.

• HCG also promotes secretion of gonadal steroid hormones by stimulating production of androgen by the interstitial cells of the testes (Leydig's cells).

Absorption, distribution, metabolism, and excretion

Gonadotropins are administered I.M. because oral doses are destroyed by digestive enzymes. They're distributed throughout the body, with highest concentrations in the ovaries and testes.

• HCG is partly degraded in the body but is largely excreted in urine.

• HMG is not excreted and is believed to undergo total degradation in the body.

Onset and duration

Gonadotropin blood levels peak 6 hours after injection.

Duration of action varies widely, as the half-lives of these agents range from 4 to 70 hours.

QUESTIONS & ANSWERS

NEWS ON CANCER TREATMENT AND GONADAL DYSFUNCTION

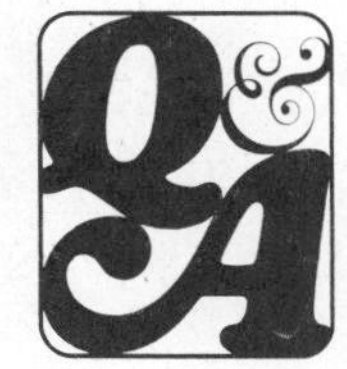

Can cancer treatment in children lead to gonadal dysfunction?

Recent studies suggest that radiation therapy and chemotherapy may affect gonadal tissues in prepubertal and pubertal children. *The severity of the effects is probably sex- and age-dependent.* Because of their different patterns of development, males and females are more sensitive to these effects at different ages.

From age 6 on, estrogen levels in females rise; large follicles and granulosa cells increase in number. In 10- to 14-year-old males, adult spermatocytes and androgen-producing Leydig's cells enter the phase of rapid proliferation and growth. During these metabolically active periods, cancer chemotherapy, radiation therapy, and particularly the combination of these treatments can be detrimental. Chemotherapy alone is usually less damaging than when combined with radiation therapy.

Adverse effects in females include histologic damage in the ovaries, absence of menarche, and secondary amenorrhea; in males, reduced spermatogenesis, raised FSH and LH concentrations, and lowered testosterone concentrations indicating failure of the Leydig's cells.

Although long-term studies are needed to clearly define the risk of permanent gonadal damage, reassure the parents of childhood cancer patients that results of studies on the hazards to offspring are, so far, optimistic. Offspring of young patients who underwent cancer treatment had no more abortions, stillbirths, cancer, or major chronic disease than the normal population.

NAME	INDICATIONS & DOSAGE	SIDE EFFECTS
chorionic gonadotropin, human Android HCG, Antuitrin-S♦, A.P.L.♦, Chorex, Follutein, Glukor, Gonadex, Libigen, Pregnyl, Stemultrolin	*Anovulation and infertility*— **Women:** 10,000 units I.M. 1 day after last dose of menotropins. *Hypogonadism*— **Men:** 500 to 1,000 units I.M. 3 times weekly for 3 weeks, then twice weekly for 3 weeks; or 4,000 units I.M. 3 times weekly for 6 to 9 months, then 2,000 units 3 times weekly for 3 more months. *Nonobstructive cryptorchidism*— **Boys 4 to 9 years:** 5,000 units I.M. every other day for 4 doses.	**CNS:** headache, fatigue, irritability, restlessness, depression. **GU:** early puberty (growth of testes, penis, pubic and axillary hair; voice change; down on upper lip; growth of body hair). **Local:** *pain at injection site.* **Other:** gynecomastia, edema.
menotropins Pergonal	*Anovulation*— **Women:** 75 IU (international units) each FSH (follicle-stimulating hormone) and LH (luteinizing hormone) I.M. daily for 9 to 12 days, followed by 10,000 units chorionic gonadotropin I.M. 1 day after last dose of menotropins. Repeat for 1 to 3 menstrual cycles until ovulation occurs. *Infertility with ovulation*— 75 IU each of FSH and LH I.M. daily for 9 to 12 days, followed by 10,000 units chorionic gonadotropin I.M. 1 day after last dose of menotropins. Repeat for 2 menstrual cycles and then increase to 150 IU each FSH and LH I.M. daily for 9 to 12 days, followed by 10,000 units chorionic gonadotropin I.M. 1 day after last dose of menotropins. Repeat for 2 menstrual cycles. Menotropins are available in ampuls containing 75 IU each FSH and LH.	**Blood:** hemoconcentration with fluid loss into abdomen. **GI:** nausea, vomiting, diarrhea. **GU:** *ovarian enlargement with pain and abdominal distention,* multiple births, ovarian hyperstimulation syndrome (sudden ovarian enlargement, ascites with or without pain, or pleural effusion). **Other:** fever.

INTERACTIONS	NURSING CONSIDERATIONS
None significant.	• Contraindicated in pituitary hypertrophy or tumor, prostatic cancer, and early puberty (usual onset between 10 and 13 years of age). Use cautiously in epilepsy, migraine, asthma, cardiac or renal disease. • Not for obesity control. • When used with menotropins to induce ovulation, multiple births possible. • In infertility, encourage daily intercourse from day before chorionic gonadotropin is given until ovulation occurs. • Inspect genitalia of boys for signs of early puberty. Notify doctor, who may discontinue drug if early puberty occurs.
None significant.	• Contraindicated in high urinary gonadotropin levels, thyroid or adrenal dysfunction, pituitary tumor, abnormal uterine bleeding, ovarian cysts or enlargement, and pregnancy. • Tell patient that there is a possibility of multiple births. • In infertility, encourage daily intercourse from day before chorionic gonadotropin is given until ovulation occurs. • Reconstitute with 1 to 2 ml sterile saline injection. Use immediately.

Antidiabetic agents and glucagon

acetohexamide
chlorpropamide
glucagon
insulins
tolazamide
tolbutamide

Antidiabetic drugs supply exogenous insulin or stimulate production of endogenous insulin in patients with diabetes mellitus. Endogenous insulin, produced by beta cells of the pancreatic islets of Langerhans, and commercial insulin, obtained from beef and pork pancreases, *lower* glucose levels.

Synthetic antidiabetic drugs (sulfonylureas including acetohexamide, chlorpropamide, tolazamide, and tolbutamide) are given orally to stimulate insulin secretion in patients with diabetes who have some beta-cell function. They have no value in patients with no functional beta-cell tissue.

Glucagon, a hormone normally produced by alpha cells of the pancreatic islets, *raises* blood glucose levels by stimulating glycogenolysis and glyconeogenesis. It thus reverses insulin-induced hypoglycemia in patients with adequate hepatic glycogen stores.

Major uses

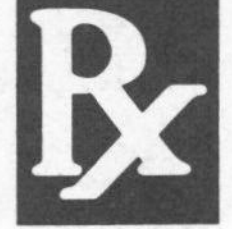

• Glucagon is used in emergencies to reverse insulin-induced hypoglycemia in patients with diabetes mellitus.

• Insulin supplements or replaces endogenous insulin in the treatment of

NURSING TIPS

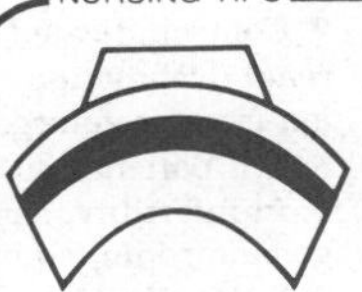

TIPS ON THE NEW INSULINS

Before 1972, most insulins were only 92% pure. The impurities contributed to the major side effect of insulin therapy—lipodystrophy—and to insulin allergy. But in 1972, insulins that were almost 99% pure were developed. These new insulins are available in beef, pork, and beef-pork combination form.

If your patient calls to say he's sweating, has a headache, and feels shaky and irritable, ask him if he's had his insulin order refilled recently. Chances are he's received new insulin and is experiencing the classic symptoms of hypoglycemia. Why? Since the new form contains fewer impurities, your patient may be receiving more insulin per dose than he's used to. Tell him to contact his doctor, who may decrease the dose.

If your patient does develop hypoglycemia with the new insulin, he'll probably get it with the first dose or within the first few weeks of taking it. To alert patients to this possibility, some insulin manufacturers have supplied community pharmacists with patient-teaching aids that describe the new insulin and warn patients to check with their doctors before taking the first dose of new insulin.

Your patient's changeover to new insulin will probably be uneventful. But if he does have problems, reassure him they're easy to correct.

THE SOMOGYI EFFECT AND HOW TO CONTROL IT

The Somogyi effect, or "bouncing," is a rebound hyperglycemic response. This effect can be caused by taking too much insulin, by not eating regularly, or by exercising more than usual.

The body reacts to hypoglycemia by increasing the liver's production of glucose. The following hormones stimulate this increased production and provide peripheral resistance to insulin:

- Growth hormone, secreted by the anterior pituitary, increases blood glucose by decreasing the uptake of glucose by the cells.
- Cortisol, secreted by the adrenal cortex, stimulates glyconeogenesis and produces hyperglycemia by decreasing glucose transport and utilization.
- Epinephrine, secreted by the adrenal medulla, increases glycogenolysis.

However, these hormonal effects may overshoot the body's need for glucose and cause the rebound hyperglycemia seen in the Somogyi effect.

To control the Somogyi effect, split the NPH insulin dosage. As shown in this chart, the single dosage program causes hypoglycemia the afternoon of the first day. The rebound effect then causes hyperglycemia the following morning. The split dosage program corrects these undesirable effects.

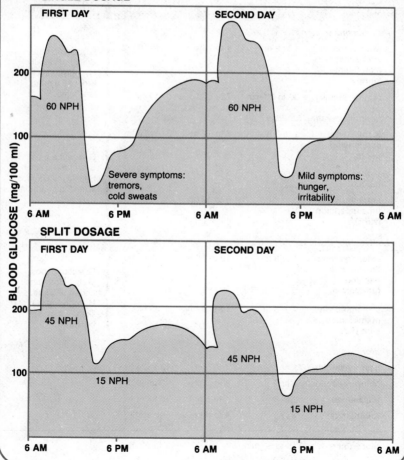

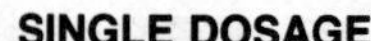

diabetes mellitus, especially the juvenile-onset (insulin-dependent) form. It's used in maturity-onset (non–insulin-dependent) diabetes mellitus if oral sulfonylureas are ineffective.

• Sulfonylureas are used to treat maturity-onset diabetes mellitus that is inadequately controlled by diet alone.

Chlorpropamide is also used to treat diabetes insipidus.

THERAPEUTIC ACTIVITY

THERAPEUTIC ACTIVITY OF ANTIDIABETIC DRUGS AND GLUCAGON

DRUG	ONSET	PEAK	DURATION	REMARKS
Rapid-acting insulins				
prompt insulin zinc suspension (semilente)	1 to 2 hr	4 to 7 hr	12 to 16 hr	Glycosuria most likely nocturnally. Hypoglycemia most likely 10 a.m. to lunchtime.
regular insulin	30 to 60 min	2 to 3 hr	5 to 7 hr	
Intermediate-acting insulins				
insulin zinc suspension (lente)	1 to 2 hr	8 to 12 hr	24 to 28 hr	Glycosuria most likely before lunch. Hypoglycemia most likely 3 p.m. to dinnertime.
globin zinc insulin	2 hr	8 to 16 hr	18 to 24 hr	
isophane insulin suspension (NPH)	1 to 2 hr	8 to 12 hr	24 to 28 hr	
Long-acting insulins				
extended insulin zinc suspension (ultralente)	4 to 8 hr	18 to 24 hr	> 36 hr	Glycosuria most likely before lunch and at bedtime. Hypoglycemia most likely 2 a.m. to breakfast.
protamine zinc insulin suspension (PZI)	4 to 8 hr	14 to 24 hr	> 36 hr	
Sulfonylureas				
acetohexamide	1 hr	4 to 5 hr	12 to 24 hr	
chlorpropamide	1 hr	3 to 6 hr	40 to 60 hr	
tolazamide	4 to 6 hr	4 to 6 hr	10 to 14 hr	
tolbutamide	1 hr	4 to 6 hr	6 to 12 hr	
glucagon	15 to 30 min	—	1 to 1½ hr	

INSULIN NEEDS DURING PREGNANCY

As you can see from the graph, during the first trimester of pregnancy, insulin needs usually decrease by one third. In fact, hypoglycemic reactions can be the first indication of pregnancy.

In the second trimester, insulin requirements rise to 66% above the prepregnancy dose, and by the last trimester the need for insulin is twice the prepregnancy dose.

For about 5 days after delivery, most mothers have a temporary remission in their diabetes. Their need for insulin drops to about two thirds their prepregnancy dose. But within 6 weeks, they usually return to their normal insulin dose.

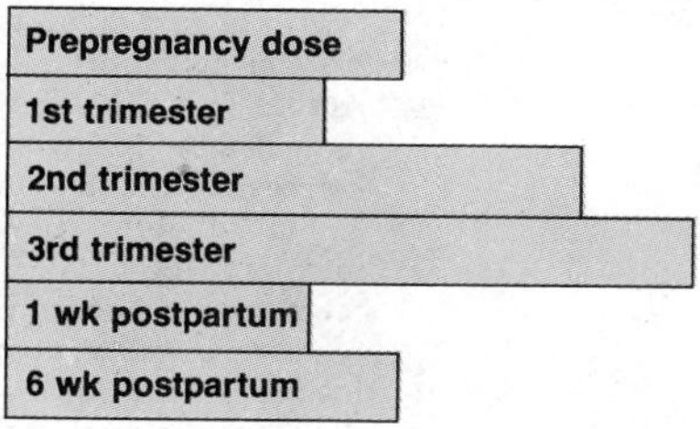

Prepregnancy dose
1st trimester
2nd trimester
3rd trimester
1 wk postpartum
6 wk postpartum

Mechanism of action

• Glucagon raises blood glucose levels by promoting catalytic depolymerization of hepatic glycogen to glucose.

• Insulin increases glucose transport across muscle and fat-cell membranes to reduce blood glucose levels. It promotes conversion of glucose to its storage form, glycogen; triggers amino acid uptake and conversion to protein in muscle cells and inhibits protein degradation; stimulates triglyceride formation and inhibits release of free fatty acids from adipose tissue; and stimulates lipoprotein lipase activity, which converts circulating lipoproteins to fatty acids.

• Sulfonylureas stimulate insulin release from the pancreatic beta cells and reduce glucose output by the liver.

Chlorpropamide also exerts an antidiuretic effect in patients with pituitary-deficient diabetes insipidus.

Absorption, distribution, metabolism, and excretion

• Glucagon is rapidly absorbed after parenteral administration, metabolized mainly in the liver, and excreted in urine.

• Insulin, because it is destroyed in the gastrointestinal tract, is generally administered by subcutaneous injection. It is absorbed directly from the injection site into the bloodstream. Absorption rate depends on insulin type, concentration, dose, volume, vascularity at the injection site, and the patient's physical activity pattern. Vigorous exercise, for example, accelerates absorption and metabolism from an injection in the thigh but not from an injection in the arm.

Insulin is distributed throughout extracellular fluid and metabolized in the liver (primary site) and in the kidneys and muscles (secondary sites). Only small quantities of insulin are excreted in urine.

• Of the sulfonylureas, acetohexamide and tolazamide are metabolized to active metabolites and excreted in urine.

Chlorpropamide is excreted in urine, primarily unchanged.

Tolbutamide is metabolized to inactive metabolites and excreted in urine.

Onset and duration

The chart opposite shows the onset, peak, and duration of these drugs.

Combination products

Drugs are usually available only as individual components.

NAME	INDICATIONS & DOSAGE	SIDE EFFECTS
acetohexamide Dimelor♦♦, Dymelor	*Stable, maturity-onset nonketotic diabetes mellitus uncontrolled by diet alone and previously untreated—* **Adults:** initially, 250 mg P.O. daily before breakfast; may increase dose q 5 to 7 days (by 250 to 500 mg) as needed to maximum 1.5 g daily, divided b.i.d. to t.i.d. before meals. *To replace insulin therapy*—if insulin dose is less than 20 units daily, insulin may be stopped and oral therapy started with 250 mg P.O. daily, before breakfast, increased as above if needed. If insulin dose is 20 to 40 units daily, start oral therapy with 250 mg P.O. daily, before breakfast, while reducing insulin dose 25% to 30% daily or every other day, depending on response to oral therapy.	**Blood:** *bone marrow aplasia.* **GI:** nausea, heartburn, vomiting. **Metabolic:** sodium loss, *hypoglycemia.* **Skin:** rash, pruritus, facial flushing. **Other:** hypersensitivity reactions.
chlorpropamide Chloromide♦♦, Chloronase♦♦, Diabinese♦, Novopropamide♦♦, Stabinol♦♦	*Stable, maturity-onset nonketotic diabetes mellitus uncontrolled by diet alone and previously untreated—* **Adults:** 250 mg P.O. daily with breakfast or in divided doses if GI disturbances occur. First dosage increase may be made after 5 to 7 days due to extended duration of action, then dose may be increased q 3 to 5 days by 50 to 125 mg, if needed, to maximum 750 mg daily. Start with dose of 100 to 125 mg in older patients. *To change from insulin to oral therapy*—if insulin dose less than 40 units daily, insulin may be stopped and oral therapy started as above. If insulin dose is 40 units or more daily, start oral therapy as above with insulin dose reduced 50%. Further insulin reductions should be made according to the patient's response.	**Blood:** *bone marrow aplasia.* **GI:** nausea, heartburn, vomiting. **GU:** tea-colored urine. **Metabolic:** prolonged hypoglycemia, *dilutional hyponatremia.* **Skin:** rash, pruritus, facial flushing. **Other:** *hypersensitivity reactions.*

♦ Available in U.S. and Canada. ♦♦ Available in Canada only. All other products (no symbol) available in U.S. only. Italicized side effects are common or life-threatening.

INTERACTIONS	NURSING CONSIDERATIONS
Alcohol, corticosteroids, dextrothyroxine, estrogens, glucagon, rifampin, thiazide diuretics, thyroxine: decreased hypoglycemic response. Monitor blood glucose. *Anabolic steroids, clofibrate, guanethidine, halofenate, MAO inhibitors, phenylbutazone, salicylates, sulfonamides, oral anticoagulants:* increased hypoglycemic activity. Monitor blood glucose. *Metoprolol, propranolol, clonidine:* prolonged hypoglycemic effect and masked symptoms of hypoglycemia. Use together cautiously.	• Contraindicated in treatment of juvenile, growth-onset, brittle, and severe diabetes; in diabetes mellitus adequately controlled by diet; and in maturity-onset diabetes complicated by ketosis, acidosis, diabetic coma, Raynaud's gangrene, renal or hepatic impairment, thyroid or other endocrine dysfunction. Use cautiously in patients with sulfonamide hypersensitivity. • Instruct patient about nature of the disease; importance of following therapeutic regimen and adhering to specific diet, weight reduction, exercise, personal hygiene, and avoiding infection; how and when to test for glycosuria and ketonuria; recognition of hypoglycemia and hyperglycemia. • Be sure patient knows that the therapy relieves symptoms but doesn't cure the disease. • Patient transferring from another oral sulfonylurea antidiabetic drug usually needs no transition period. • Monitor patient transferring from insulin therapy to an oral antidiabetic for urine glucose and ketones at least t.i.d., before meals; emphasize the need for a double-voided specimen. Patient may require hospitalization during transition. • During periods of increased stress, such as infection, fever, surgery, or trauma, patient may require insulin therapy. Monitor patient closely for hyperglycemia in these situations. • Advise patient to avoid moderate to large intake of alcohol; disulfiram reaction possible. • For toxicity, see APPENDIX, *Drug Toxicities.*
Alcohol, corticosteroids, dextrothyroxine, glucagon, rifampin, thiazide diuretics: decreased hypoglycemic response. Monitor blood glucose. *Anabolic steroids, chloramphenicol, clofibrate, guanethidine, halofenate, MAO inhibitors, phenylbutazone, salicylates, sulfonamides, oral anticoagulants:* increased hypoglycemic activity. Monitor blood glucose. *Metoprolol, propranolol, clonidine:* prolonged hypoglycemic effect and masked symptoms of hypoglycemia. Use together cautiously.	• Contraindicated in the treatment of juvenile, growth-onset, brittle, and severe diabetes; in diabetes mellitus adequately controlled by diet; and in maturity-onset diabetes complicated by fever, ketosis, acidosis, diabetic coma, major surgery, severe trauma, Raynaud's gangrene, renal or hepatic impairment, thyroid or other endocrine dysfunction. Use cautiously in patients with sulfonamide hypersensitivity. • Instruct patient about nature of the disease; importance of following therapeutic regimen and adhering to specific diet, weight reduction, exercise, personal hygiene, avoiding infection; how and when to test for glycosuria and ketonuria; and recognition of and intervention for hypoglycemia and hyperglycemia. • Side effects, especially hypoglycemia, may be more frequent or severe than with some other sulfonylurea drugs (acetohexamide, tolazamide, and tolbutamide) because of its long duration of effect (36 hours). • If hypoglycemia occurs, patient should be monitored closely for a minimum of 3 to 5 days. • Patient transferring from another oral sulfonylurea antidiabetic drug usually needs no transition period. • Patient may require hospitalization during transition from insulin therapy to an oral antidiabetic. Monitor patient for urine glucose and ketones at least t.i.d., before meals; emphasize the need for a double-voided specimen. • Drug may accumulate in patients with renal insufficiency. • Advise patient to avoid moderate to large intake of alcohol; disulfiram reaction possible. • Watch for signs of impending renal insufficiency, such as dysuria, anuria, and hematuria, and report them to the doctor immediately. • For toxicity, see APPENDIX, *Drug Toxicities.*

NAME	INDICATIONS & DOSAGE	SIDE EFFECTS
glucagon	*Coma of insulin-shock therapy—* **Adults:** 0.5 to 1 mg S.C., I.M., or I.V. 1 hour after coma develops; may repeat within 25 minutes, if necessary. In very deep coma, also give glucose 10% to 50% I.V. for faster response. When patient responds, give additional carbohydrate immediately. *Severe insulin-induced hypoglycemia during diabetic therapy—* **Adults and children:** 0.5 to 1 mg S.C., I.M., or I.V.; may repeat q 20 minutes for 2 doses, if necessary. If coma persists, give glucose 10% to 50% I.V.	**GI:** nausea, vomiting. **Other:** hypersensitivity.
insulins **regular insulin** Actrapid, Beef Regular Iletin II (acid neutral CZI), Insulin-Toronto (beef or pork)♦♦, Pork Regular Iletin II **regular insulin concentrated** Regular (concentrated) Iletin **prompt insulin zinc suspension** Semilente Iletin, Semilente Insulin♦, Semitard **isophane insulin suspension (NPH)** Beef NPH Iletin II, Lentard, NPH Iletin, NPH Insulin♦♦, Pork NPH Iletin II **insulin zinc suspension** Beef Lente Iletin, Lente Iletin, Lente Insulin♦, Pork Lente Iletin II	*Diabetic ketoacidosis (use regular insulin only)—* **Adults:** 25 to 150 units I.V. stat, then additional doses may be given q 1 hour based on blood sugar levels until patient is out of acidosis; then give S.C. q 6 hours thereafter. Alternative dosage schedule: 50 to 100 units I.V. and 50 to 100 units S.C. stat; additional doses may be given q 2 to 6 hours based on blood sugar levels; or 0.33 units/kg I.V. bolus, followed by 7 to 10 units/hour I.V. by continuous infusion. Continue infusion until blood sugar drops to 250 mg%, then start S.C. insulin q 6 hours. **Children:** 0.5 to 1 unit/kg divided into 2 doses, 1 given I.V. and the other S.C., followed by 0.5 to 1 unit/kg I.V. q 1 to 2 hours; or 0.1 unit/kg I.V. bolus, then 0.1 unit/kg/hour continuous I.V. infusion until blood sugar drops to 250 mg%, then start S.C. insulin. Preparation of infusion: add 100 units regular insulin and 1 g albumin to 100 ml of 0.9% saline solution. Insulin concentration will be 1 unit/ml. (The albumin will adsorb to plastic, preventing loss of the insulin to plastic.) *Ketosis-prone and juvenile-onset diabetes mellitus, diabetes mellitus inadequately controlled by*	**Metabolic:** *hypoglycemia, hyperglycemia (rebound, or Somogyi, effect).* **Skin:** urticaria. **Local:** *lipoatrophy, lipohypertrophy,* itching, swelling, redness, stinging, warmth at site of injection. **Other:** *anaphylaxis.*

♦ Available in U.S. and Canada. ♦♦ Available in Canada only. All other products (no symbol) available in U.S. only. Italicized side effects are common or life-threatening.

INTERACTIONS	NURSING CONSIDERATIONS
Phenytoin: inhibited glucagon-induced insulin release. Use cautiously.	• Use glucagon only under medical supervision. • Hypoglycemic juvenile or unstable diabetics usually do not respond to glucagon. Give dextrose I.V. instead. • It is vital to arouse the patient from coma as quickly as possible and to give additional carbohydrates orally to prevent secondary hypoglycemic reactions. • For I.V. drip infusion, glucagon is compatible with dextrose solution but forms a precipitate in chloride solutions. • Instruct the patient and family in proper glucagon administration, recognition of hypoglycemia, and urgency of calling doctor immediately in emergencies. • May be used as diagnostic aid in radiologic examination of the stomach, duodenum, small bowel, and colon when a hypotonic state is advantageous. • May be stored for 3 months at 2° to 15° C. (35.6° to 59° F.) after reconstitution.
Metoprolol, propranolol: hyperglycemia or hypoglycemia may occur. Symptoms of hypoglycemia may be masked. Use together cautiously. *Alcohol, corticosteroids, dextrothyroxine, estrogens, glucagon, rifampin, thiazide diuretics, thyroxine:* decreased insulin response. Monitor blood glucose. *Anabolic steroids, clofibrate, guanethidine, halofenate, MAO inhibitors, phenylbutazone, salicylates, sulfonamides, oral anticoagulants:* increased insulin response. Monitor for blood glucose.	• Use only regular insulin in patients with circulatory collapse, diabetic ketoacidosis, or hyperkalemia. Do not use regular insulin concentrated, I.V. Do not use intermediate- or long-acting insulins for coma or other emergency requiring rapid drug action. • During 1980, more purified forms of insulin became available. (These are called "new" insulin and are so labeled.) These new, highly purified forms may require dosage adjustment in patients previously stabilized on insulin. Patient should be made aware of this. Observe closely until dosage is established. • Accuracy of measurement is very important, especially with regular insulin concentrated. Aids such as magnifying sleeve, dose magnifier, or cornwall syringe may help improve accuracy. • With regular insulin concentrated, a deep secondary hypoglycemic reaction may occur 18 to 24 hours after injection. • Regular, and intermediate- and long-acting insulins may be mixed to meet the patient's needs. All insulins should be of the same concentration. • Store insulin in cool area. Refrigeration desirable but not essential, except with regular insulin concentrated. • Don't use insulin that has changed color. • Check expiration date on vial before using contents. • Administration route is subcutaneous because absorption rate and pain are less than with I.M. injections. Ketosis-prone juvenile-onset, severely ill, and newly diagnosed diabetics with very high blood sugar levels may require hospitalization and I.V. treatment with regular fast-acting insulin. Ketosis-resistant diabetics may be treated as outpatients with intermediate-acting insulin and instructions on how to alter dosage according to self-performed urine or blood glucose determinations. Some patients, primarily pregnant or brittle diabetics, may perform fingerstick blood glucose tests at home. • Press but do not rub site after injection. Rotate injection sites. Chart sites to avoid overuse of one area. However, unstable diabetics may achieve better control if injection site is rotated within same anatomic region. • To mix insulin suspension, swirl vial gently or rotate between palms or between palm and thigh. Don't shake vigorously: this causes bubbling and air in syringe. • Insulin requirements increase, sometimes drastically, in pregnant diabetics, then decline immediately postpartum.

(continued on following page)

NAME	INDICATIONS & DOSAGE	SIDE EFFECTS
insulins *(continued)* **globin zinc insulin** **protamine zinc insulin suspension (PZI)** Beef Protamine Zinc Iletin II, Pork Protamine Zinc Iletin II, Protamine Zinc Iletin **extended insulin zinc suspension** Ultralente Iletin, Ultralente Insulin♦, Ultratard	*diet and oral hypoglycemics*— **Adults and children:** therapeutic regimen prescribed by doctor and adjusted according to patient's blood and urine glucose concentrations.	
tolazamide Tolinase	*Stable, maturity-onset nonketotic diabetes mellitus uncontrolled by diet alone and previously untreated*— **Adults:** initially, 100 mg P.O. daily with breakfast if fasting blood sugar (FBS) under 200 mg%; or 250 mg if FBS is over 200 mg%. May adjust dose at weekly intervals by 100 to 250 mg. Maximum dose 500 mg b.i.d. before meals. **Elderly or debilitated patients:** increase dose by 50 to 125 mg at weekly intervals. *To change from insulin to oral therapy*—if insulin dose under 20 units daily, insulin may be stopped and oral therapy started at 100 mg P.O. daily with breakfast. If insulin dose is 20 to 40 units daily, insulin may be stopped and oral therapy started at 250 mg P.O. daily with breakfast. If insulin dose is over 40 units daily, decrease insulin dose 50% and start oral therapy	**Blood:** *bone marrow aplasia.* **GI:** nausea, vomiting. **Metabolic:** hypoglycemia. **Skin:** rash, urticaria, facial flushing. **Other:** hypersensitivity reactions.

INTERACTIONS	NURSING CONSIDERATIONS
	• Be sure the patient knows that therapy relieves symptoms but doesn't cure the disease. • Dosage is always expressed in USP units. • Tell patient about the nature of disease, the importance of following the therapeutic regimen and specific diet, weight reduction, exercise, personal hygiene, avoiding infection, and timing of injection and eating. Emphasize that meals must not be omitted. Teach that urine tests are essential guides to dosage and success of therapy; important to recognize hypoglycemic symptoms because insulin-induced hypoglycemia is hazardous and may cause brain damage if prolonged; most side effects are self-limiting and temporary. • Advise patient to wear medical ID always; to carry ample insulin supply and syringes on trips; to have carbohydrates (lump of sugar or candy) on hand for emergency; to take note of time zone changes for dose schedule when traveling. • Marijuana use may increase insulin requirements. • U-80 strength no longer certified by Food and Drug Administration. Instruct patient in use of U-100 strength. • Some patients may develop insulin resistance and require large insulin doses to control symptoms of diabetes. U-500 insulin is available for such patients as Purified Pork Iletin Regular Insulin, U500. Although every pharmacy may not normally stock it, it is readily available. Patient should notify pharmacist several days before refill of prescription is needed. Nurse should give hospital pharmacy sufficient notice before needing to refill in-house prescription. Never store U-500 insulin in same area with other insulin preparations due to danger of severe overdose if given accidentally to other patients. U-500 insulin must be administered with a U-100 syringe since no syringes are made for this drug. • For toxicity, see APPENDIX, *Drug Toxicities*.
Alcohol, corticosteroids, dextrothyroxine, estrogens, glucagon, rifampin, thiazide diuretics, thyroxine: decreased hypoglycemic response. Monitor blood glucose. *Anabolic steroids, clofibrate, guanethidine, halofenate, MAO inhibitors, phenylbutazone, salicylates, sulfonamides, oral anticoagulants:* increased hypoglycemic activity. Monitor blood glucose. *Metoprolol, propranolol, clonidine:* prolonged hypoglycemic effect and masked symptoms of hypoglycemia. Use together cautiously.	• Contraindicated in juvenile, growth-onset, and severe diabetes mellitus; diabetes mellitus adequately controlled by diet or in maturity-onset diabetes mellitus complicated by fever, ketosis, acidosis, or coma; major surgery; severe trauma; Raynaud's gangrene; renal or hepatic impairment; thyroid or other endocrine dysfunction. Use cautiously in patients with sulfonamide hypersensitivity and in elderly, debilitated, or malnourished patients. • Instruct patient about nature of disease; importance of following therapeutic regimen and specific diet, weight reduction, exercise, personal hygiene, avoiding infection; how and when to test for glycosuria and ketonuria; and recognition of hypoglycemia and hyperglycemia. • Be sure patient knows that therapy relieves symptoms but doesn't cure disease. • Patient transferring from another oral sulfonylurea antidiabetic drug usually needs no transition period. • Patient transferring from insulin therapy to an oral hypoglycemic should test urine for glucose and ketones at least t.i.d., before meals; emphasize the need for a double-voided specimen. Hospitalization may be required during the transition. • Advise patient to avoid moderate to large intake of alcohol; disulfiram reaction possible. • For toxicity, see APPENDIX, *Drug Toxicities*.

(continued on following page)

NAME	INDICATIONS & DOSAGE	SIDE EFFECTS
tolazamide *(continued)*	at 250 mg P.O. daily with breakfast. Increase doses as above.	
tolbutamide Mellitol♦♦, Mobenol♦♦, Neo-Dibetic♦♦, Novobutamide♦♦, Oramide♦♦, Orinase♦, SK-Tolbutamide, Tolbutone♦♦	*Stable, maturity-onset nonketotic diabetes mellitus uncontrolled by diet alone and previously untreated*— **Adults:** initially, 1 to 2 g P.O. daily as single dose or divided b.i.d. to t.i.d. May adjust dose to maximum 3 g daily. *To change from insulin to oral therapy*—if insulin dose is under 20 units daily, insulin may be stopped and oral therapy started at 1 to 2 g daily. If insulin dose is 20 to 40 units daily, insulin dose is reduced 30% to 50% and oral therapy started as above. If insulin dose is over 40 units daily, insulin dose is decreased 20% and oral therapy started as above. Further reductions in insulin dose are based on patient's response to oral therapy.	**Blood:** *bone marrow aplasia.* **GI:** nausea, heartburn. **Metabolic:** hypoglycemia. **Skin:** rash, pruritus, facial flushing. **Other:** hypersensitivity reactions.

♦ Available in U.S. and Canada. ♦♦ Available in Canada only. All other products (no symbol) available in U.S. only. Italicized side effects are common or life-threatening.

INTERACTIONS	NURSING CONSIDERATIONS
Alcohol, corticosteroids, dextrothyroxine, estrogens, glucagon, rifampin, thiazide diuretics, thyroxine: decreased hypoglycemic response. Monitor blood glucose. *Anabolic steroids, chloramphenicol, clofibrate, guanethidine, halofenate, MAO inhibitors, phenylbutazone, salicylates, sulfonamides, oral anticoagulants:* increased hypoglycemic activity. Monitor blood glucose. *Metoprolol, propranolol, clonidine:* prolonged hypoglycemic effect and masked symptoms of hypoglycemia. Use together cautiously.	• Contraindicated in juvenile, growth-onset, brittle, and severe diabetes; diabetes mellitus adequately controlled by diet or in maturity-onset diabetes mellitus complicated by fever, ketosis, acidosis, or coma; major surgery; severe trauma; Raynaud's gangrene; renal or hepatic impairment; thyroid or other endocrine dysfunction; pregnancy. Use cautiously in patients with sulfonamide hypersensitivity. • Instruct patient about nature of disease; importance of following therapeutic regimen and specific diet, weight reduction, exercise, personal hygiene, and avoiding infection; how and when to test for glycosuria and ketonuria; and recognition of hypoglycemia and hyperglycemia. • Be sure patient knows that therapy relieves symptoms but doesn't cure disease. • Patient transferring from another oral sulfonylurea antidiabetic drug usually needs no transition period. • Patient transferring from insulin therapy to an oral hypoglycemic should test urine for glucose and ketones at least t.i.d., before meals; emphasize the need for a double-voided specimen. Hospitalization may be required during the transition. • Advise patient to avoid moderate to large intake of alcohol: disulfiram reaction possible. • For toxicity, see APPENDIX, *Drug Toxicities.*

59 Thyroid hormones

levothyroxine sodium (T_4 or L-thyroxine sodium)
liothyronine sodium (T_3)
liotrix
thyroglobulin
thyroid USP (desiccated)
thyrotropin (thyroid-stimulating hormone or TSH)

The thyroid preparations described in this chapter are used as replacement therapy in patients with diminished or absent thyroid function.

Thyroid hormones are produced and stored in the follicles of the thyroid gland. Their synthesis and release are regulated by *thyrotropin,* also known as thyroid-stimulating hormone (TSH), which is secreted by the anterior pituitary gland. Increased blood levels of thyroid hormones inhibit release of pituitary TSH. Through this negative feedback mechanism, they homeostatically control further increases in thyroid hormone.

Thyroid extract is the prototype of the substances used to treat hypothyroidism. This substance, the desiccated thyroid gland of animals, contains T_3 (liothyronine) and T_4 (tetraiodothyronine or thyroxine), as well as other organic materials. *Thyroglobulin* is a purified extract of a hog's thyroid gland that is standardized on the basis of iodine content and metabolic activity. Thyroid USP (desiccated) is a cleaned, dried, and powdered thyroid gland obtained from animal (usually hog) sources.

Major uses

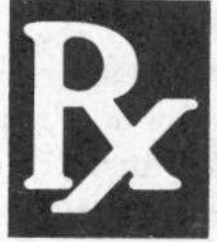

Thyroid hormones prevent goiter and hypothyroidism in patients receiving antithyroid drugs for thyrotoxicosis. They are also used to treat confirmed hypothyroidism and supply replacement therapy in primary and secondary myxedema, myxedema coma, cretinism, and simple nontoxic goiter.

• Thyroglobulin and thyroid USP are used to treat certain thyrotropin-dependent carcinomas of the thyroid.

• Thyrotropin is used in combination with radioactive iodine in treatment of thyroid tumors and is also used in differential diagnosis of subclinical hypothyroidism and low thyroid reserve.

Mechanism of action

Thyroid hormones stimulate the metabolism of all body tissues by accelerating the rate of cellular oxidation. They enhance carbohydrate and protein biosynthesis by glyconeogenesis, which increases the mobilization and utilization of glycogen stores. They also affect lipid metabolism by decreasing cholesterol levels in the liver and blood.

• Thyrotropin stimulates the uptake of radioactive iodine in patients with thyroid carcinoma. It also promotes thyroid hormone production by the anterior pituitary.

Absorption, distribution, metabolism, and excretion

• Levothyroxine, liothyronine, thyro-

globulin, and thyroid USP are efficiently absorbed from the gastrointestinal tract. Liothyronine is better absorbed, however, than levothyroxine.
• Levothyroxine, well distributed to all body tissues, is partially metabolized in the liver. Both the metabolite and the unchanged hormone are passed into the bile. The metabolite is eliminated in feces; the small amount of free levothyroxine is recycled to the liver.
• Liothyronine's metabolism is unclear. Liothyronine releases iodine into the body tissues. The thyroid then uses this iodine for synthesis of additional levothyroxine and liothyronine. Some of the iodine released by liothyronine is either excreted in urine or eliminated through the bile in feces.

Onset and duration

• Full onset of levothyroxine, liotrix, thyroglobulin, and thyroid USP takes 1 to 3 weeks, although a response may be noted after several days.
• Levothyroxine generally has the slowest onset (several days), and a half-life of 6½ days. It has a long duration: its action may persist for weeks after therapy is terminated.
• Liothyronine has a relatively rapid onset of action (a few hours), and its half-life is less than 3 days. Its action persists for several days.

Combination products

EUTHROID-½: levothyroxine sodium 30 mcg and liothyronine sodium 7.5 mcg.
EUTHROID-1: levothyroxine sodium 60 mcg and liothyronine sodium 15 mcg.
EUTHROID-2: levothyroxine sodium 120 mcg and liothyronine sodium 30 mcg.
EUTHROID-3: levothyroxine sodium 180 mcg and liothyronine sodium 45 mcg.
THYROLAR-¼: levothyroxine sodium 12.5 mcg and liothyronine sodium 3.1 mcg.
THYROLAR-½♦: levothyroxine sodium 25 mcg and liothyronine sodium 6.25 mcg.
THYROLAR-1♦: levothyroxine sodium 50 mcg and liothyronine sodium 12.5 mcg.
THYROLAR-2♦: levothyroxine sodium 100 mcg and liothyronine sodium 25 mcg.
THYROLAR-3♦: levothyroxine sodium 150 mcg and liothyronine sodium 37.5 mcg.

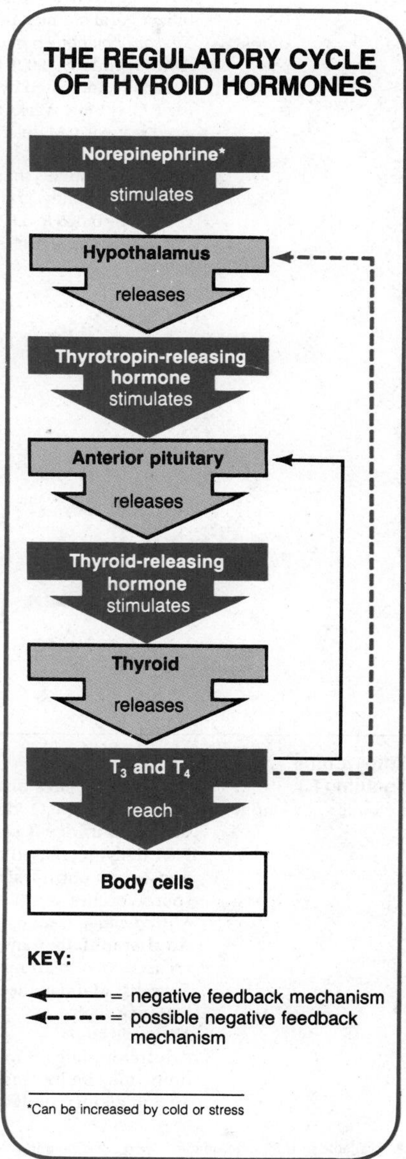

NAME	INDICATIONS & DOSAGE	SIDE EFFECTS
levothyroxine sodium (T_4 or L-thyroxine sodium) Eltroxin♦♦, Levoid, Levothroid, LTS, Noroxine, Synthroid♦	*Cretinism in children younger than 1 year*—initially, 0.025 to 0.05 mg P.O. daily, increased by 0.05 mg P.O. q 2 to 3 weeks to total daily dose 0.1 to 0.4 mg P.O. *Myxedema coma*— **Adults:** 0.2 to 0.5 mg I.V. If no response in 24 hours, additional 0.1 to 0.3 mg I.V. After condition stabilized, oral maintenance. *Thyroid hormone replacement*— **Adults:** initially, 0.025 to 0.1 mg P.O. daily, increased by 0.05 to 0.1 mg P.O. q 1 to 4 weeks until desired response. Maintenance dose 0.1 to 0.4 mg daily. **Children:** initially, maximum 0.05 mg P.O. daily, gradually increased by 0.025 to 0.05 mg P.O. q 1 to 4 weeks until desired response.	Side effects of thyroid hormones are extensions of their pharmacologic properties and reflect patient sensitivity to them. Signs of overdosage: **CNS:** *nervousness, insomnia, tremor.* **CV:** *tachycardia, palpitations, arrhythmias, angina pectoris,* hypertension. **GI:** change in appetite, nausea, diarrhea. **Other:** headache, leg cramps, weight loss, sweating, heat intolerance, fever, menstrual irregularities.
liothyronine sodium (T_3) Cytomel♦, Cytomine	*Cretinism*— **Children 3 years and older:** 50 to 100 mcg P.O. daily. **Children under 3 years:** 5 mcg P.O. daily, increased by 5 mcg q 3 to 4 days until desired response occurs. *Myxedema*— **Adults:** initially 5 mcg daily, increased by 5 to 10 mcg q 1 or 2 weeks. Maintenance dose 50 to 100 mcg daily. *Nontoxic goiter*— **Adults:** initially, 5 mcg P.O. daily; may be increased by 12.5 to 25 mcg daily q 1 to 2	Side effects of thyroid hormones are extensions of their pharmacologic properties and reflect patient sensitivity to them. **CNS:** hyperirritability, *nervousness, insomnia,* twitching, *tremors,* headache. **CV:** increased cardiac output, *tachycardia,* cardiac arrhythmias, *angina pectoris,* increased blood pressure, *cardiac decompensation and collapse.* **GI:** diarrhea, abdominal cramps, vomiting. **Other:** weight loss, heat intolerance, hyperhidrosis, menstrual ir-

♦ Available in U.S. and Canada. ♦♦ Available in Canada only. All other products (no symbol) available in U.S. only. Italicized side effects are common or life-threatening.

INTERACTIONS	NURSING CONSIDERATIONS
Cholestyramine: levothyroxine absorption impaired. Separate doses by 4 to 5 hours. *I.V. phenytoin:* free thyroid released. Monitor for tachycardia.	• Contraindicated in myocardial infarction, thyrotoxicosis (except with antithyroid drugs), or uncorrected adrenal insufficiency (thyroid hormones increase tissue demand for adrenocortical hormone and may cause acute adrenal crisis). Use with extreme caution in angina pectoris, hypertension, or other cardiovascular disorders; renal insufficiency; or ischemic states. • Use carefully in myxedema; patients are unusually sensitive to thyroid hormone. Dose varies widely among patients; start at lowest and titrate in higher doses according to patient's symptoms and laboratory data until euthyroid state is reached. • Rapid replacement in patients with arteriosclerosis may precipitate angina, coronary occlusion, or stroke. Use cautiously in such patients. • In patients with coronary artery disease who must receive thyroid, observe carefully for possible coronary insufficiency if catecholamines must be given. • Potentially dangerous; not indicated to relieve vague symptoms such as physical and mental sluggishness, irritability, depression, nervousness, ill-defined pains; to treat obesity in euthyroid persons; to treat metabolic insufficiency not associated with thyroid insufficiency; or to treat menstrual disorders or male infertility, unless associated with hypothyroidism. • When changing from levothyroxine to liothyronine, stop levothyroxine and begin liothyronine. Increase in small increments after residual effects of levothyroxine have disappeared. When changing from liothyronine to levothyroxine, start levothyroxine several days before withdrawing liothyronine to avoid relapse. • Warn patient to tell doctor at once if chest pain (especially in elderly), palpitations, sweating, nervousness, or other signs of overdosage occur. Also notify doctor immediately if any signs of aggravated cardiovascular disease develop (chest pain, dyspnea, tachycardia). • Tell patient to take thyroid hormones regularly, at the same time each day, to maintain constant hormone levels. • Suggest morning dosage to prevent insomnia. • Monitor pulse rate, blood pressure. • Protect from moisture and light. Prepare I.V. dose immediately before injection. • Thyroid hormones alter thyroid function test results. Monitor prothrombin time; patients taking these hormones usually require less anticoagulant. Alert patients to report unusual bleeding and bruising. • Patients taking levothyroxine who need to have radioactive iodine uptake studies must discontinue drug 4 weeks before test.
Cholestyramine: liothyronine absorption impaired. Separate doses by 4 to 5 hours. *I.V. phenytoin:* free thyroid released. Monitor for tachycardia.	• Contraindicated in myocardial infarction, thyrotoxicosis (except with antithyroid drugs), or uncorrected adrenal insufficiency (thyroid hormones increase tissue demand for adrenocortical hormone and may cause acute adrenal crisis). Use with extreme caution in angina pectoris, hypertension, or other cardiovascular disorders; renal insufficiency; or ischemic states. • Rapid replacement in patients with arteriosclerosis may precipitate angina, coronary occlusion, or stroke. Use cautiously in such patients. • In patients with coronary artery disease who must receive thyroid, observe carefully for possible coronary insufficiency if catecholamines must be given. • Use carefully in myxedema; patients are unusually sensitive to thyroid hormone. • Potentially dangerous; not indicated to relieve vague symptoms, such as physical and mental sluggishness, irritability, depression, nervousness, and ill-defined aches and pains; to treat obesity in eu-

(continued on following page)

NAME	INDICATIONS & DOSAGE	SIDE EFFECTS
liothyronine sodium (T_3) *(continued)*	weeks. Usual maintenance dose 75 mcg daily. **Elderly:** initially, 5 mcg P.O. daily, increased by 5-mcg increments at weekly intervals until desired response. **Children:** initially, 5 mcg P.O. daily, increased by 5-mcg increments at weekly intervals until desired response. *Thyroid hormone replacement*— **Adults:** initially, 25 mcg P.O. daily, increased by 12.5 to 25 mcg q 1 to 2 weeks until satisfactory response. Usual maintenance dose 25 to 75 mcg daily.	regularities; in infants and children—accelerated rate of bone maturation.
liotrix Euthroid, Thyrolar♦	*Hypothyroidism*—dosages must be individualized to approximate the deficit in the patient's thyroid secretion. **Adults and children:** initially, 15 to 30 mg P.O. daily, increasing by 15 to 30 mg q 1 to 2 weeks to desired response; increments in children's dose q 2 weeks. **Elderly:** initially, 15 to 30 mg. Usual adult dose doubled q 6 to 8 weeks to desired response.	Side effects of thyroid hormones are extensions of their pharmacologic properties and reflect patient sensitivity to them. **CNS:** hyperirritability, *nervousness, insomnia,* twitching, *tremors.* **CV:** increased cardiac output, *tachycardia,* cardiac arrhythmia, *angina pectoris,* increased blood pressure, *cardiac decompensation and collapse.* **GI:** diarrhea, abdominal cramps, vomiting. **Other:** weight loss, menstrual irregularities, heat intolerance, hyperhidrosis; infants and children—accelerated rate of bone maturation.

♦ Available in U.S. and Canada. ♦♦ Available in Canada only. All other products (no symbol) available in U.S. only. Italicized side effects are common or life-threatening.

INTERACTIONS	NURSING CONSIDERATIONS
	thyroid persons; to treat metabolic insufficiency; or to treat menstrual disorders or male infertility, unless associated with hypothyroidism. • When changing from levothyroxine to liothyronine, stop levothyroxine and begin liothyronine. Increase in small increments after residual effects of levothyroxine have disappeared. When changing from liothyronine to levothyroxine, start levothyroxine several days before withdrawing liothyronine to avoid relapse. • Warn patient to tell doctor at once if chest pain (especially in elderly), palpitations, sweating, nervousness, or other signs of overdosage occur. Also notify doctor immediately if any signs of aggravated cardiovascular disease develop (chest pain, dyspnea, tachycardia). • Tell patient to take thyroid hormones regularly, at the same time each day, to maintain constant hormone levels. • Suggest morning dosage to prevent insomnia. • Monitor pulse rate, blood pressure. • Thyroid hormones alter thyroid function tests. Monitor prothrombin time; patients taking these hormones may require less anticoagulant. Alert patients to report unusual bleeding and bruising. • Patients taking liothyronine who need to have radioactive iodine uptake studies must discontinue drug 7 to 10 days before test.
Cholestyramine: liotrix absorption impaired. Separate doses by 4 to 5 hours. *I.V. phenytoin:* free thyroid released. Monitor for tachycardia.	• Contraindicated in myocardial infarction, thyrotoxicosis (except with antithyroid drugs), or uncorrected adrenal insufficiency (thyroid hormones increase tissue demand for adrenocortical hormone and may cause acute adrenal crisis). Use with extreme caution in angina pectoris, hypertension, or other cardiovascular disorders; renal insufficiency; or ischemic states. • Rapid replacement in patients with arteriosclerosis may precipitate angina, coronary occlusion, or stroke. Use cautiously in such patients. • Use carefully in myxedema; patients are unusually sensitive to thyroid hormone. • In patients with coronary artery disease who must receive thyroid, observe carefully for possible coronary insufficiency if catecholamines must be given. Also observe carefully during surgery, since cardiac arrhythmias can be precipitated. • Potentially dangerous; not indicated to relieve vague symptoms, such as physical and mental sluggishness, irritability, depression, nervousness, ill-defined pains; to treat obesity in euthyroid persons; to treat metabolic insufficiency not associated with thyroid insufficiency; or to treat menstrual disorders or male infertility, unless associated with hypothyroidism. • Tell patient to take thyroid hormones regularly, at the same time each day, preferably before breakfast, to maintain constant hormone levels. • Warn patient to tell doctor at once if chest pain (especially in elderly), palpitations, sweating, nervousness, or other signs of overdosage occur. Also notify doctor immediately if any signs of aggravated cardiovascular disease develop (chest pain, dyspnea, tachycardia). • The two commercially prepared liotrix drugs contain different amounts of each ingredient; do not change from one brand to the other without considering the differences in potency: Thyrolar-½ contains 25 mcg T_4 and 6.25 mcg T_3; Euthroid-½ contains 30 mcg T_4 and 7.5 mcg T_3. • Monitor pulse rate, blood pressure. • Protect from heat, light, moisture. • Thyroid hormones alter thyroid function test results. Monitor prothrombin time; patients taking these hormones usually require less anticoagulant. Alert patients to report unusual bleeding and bruising.

NAME	INDICATIONS & DOSAGE	SIDE EFFECTS
thyroglobulin Proloid♦	*Cretinism and juvenile hypothyroidism—* **Children 1 year and older:** dosage may approach adult dose (60 to 180 mg P.O. daily), depending on response. **Children 4 to 12 months:** 60 to 80 mg P.O. daily. **Children 1 to 4 months:** initially, 15 to 30 mg P.O. daily, increased at 2-week intervals. Usual maintenance dose 30 to 45 mg P.O. daily. *Hypothyroidism or myxedema—* **Adults:** initially, 15 to 30 mg P.O. daily, increased by 15 to 30 mg at 2-week intervals until desired response. Usual maintenance dose 60 to 180 mg P.O. daily, as a single dose. **Elderly:** initially 7.5 to 15 mg P.O. daily; the dose is doubled at 6- to 8-week intervals until desired response is obtained.	Side effects of thyroid hormones are extensions of their pharmacologic properties and reflect patient sensitivity to them. **CNS:** hyperirritability, *nervousness, insomnia,* twitching, *tremors,* headache. **CV:** increased cardiac output, *tachycardia,* cardiac arrhythmias, *angina pectoris,* increased blood pressure, *cardiac decompensation and collapse.* **GI:** diarrhea, abdominal cramps, vomiting. **Other:** weight loss, heat intolerance, hyperhidrosis, menstrual irregularities; in infants and children—accelerated rate of bone maturation.
thyroid USP (desiccated) Dathroid, Delcoid, S-P-T, Thyrar, Thyro-Teric	*Adult hypothyroidism—* **Adults:** initially, 60 mg P.O. daily, increased by 60 mg q 30 days until desired response. Usual maintenance dose 60 to 180 mg P.O. daily, as a single dose. **Elderly:** 7.5 to 15 mg P.O. daily; dose is doubled at 6- to 8-week intervals. *Adult myxedema—* **Adults:** 16 mg P.O. daily. May double dose q 2 weeks to maximum 120 mg. *Cretinism and juvenile hypothyroidism—* **Children 1 year and older:** dosage may approach adult dose (60 to 180 mg) daily, depending on response. **Children 4 to 12 months:** 30 to 60 mg P.O. daily. **Children 1 to 4 months:** initially, 15 to 30 mg P.O. daily, increased at 2-week intervals. Usual maintenance dose 30 to 45 mg P.O. daily.	Side effects of thyroid hormones are extensions of their pharmacologic properties and reflect patient sensitivity to them. **CNS:** *hyperirritability, nervousness, insomnia,* twitching, tremors, headache. **CV:** increased cardiac output, *tachycardia,* cardiac arrhythmias, *angina pectoris,* increased blood pressure, *cardiac decompensation and collapse.* **GI:** diarrhea, abdominal cramps, vomiting. **Other:** weight loss, heat intolerance, hyperhidrosis, menstrual irregularities; in infants and children—accelerated rate of bone maturation.

INTERACTIONS	NURSING CONSIDERATIONS
Cholestyramine: thyroglobulin absorption impaired. Separate doses by 4 to 5 hours. *I.V. phenytoin:* free thyroid released. Monitor for tachycardia.	• Contraindicated in myocardial infarction, thyrotoxicosis (except with antithyroid drugs), or uncorrected adrenal insufficiency (thyroid hormones increase tissue demand for adrenocortical hormone and may cause acute adrenal crisis). Use with extreme caution in angina pectoris, hypertension, or other cardiovascular disorders; renal insufficiency; or ischemic states. • In patients with coronary artery disease who must receive thyroid, observe carefully for possible coronary insufficiency if catecholamines must be given. • Use carefully in myxedema; patients are unusually sensitive to thyroid hormone. • Potentially dangerous; not indicated to relieve vague symptoms, such as physical and mental sluggishness, irritability, depression, nervousness, and ill-defined pains; to treat obesity in euthyroid persons; to treat metabolic insufficiency not associated with thyroid insufficiency; or to treat menstrual disorders or male infertility, unless associated with hypothyroidism. • Tell patient to take thyroid hormones regularly, at the same time each day, to maintain constant hormone levels. • Warn patient to tell doctor at once if chest pain (especially in elderly), palpitations, sweating, nervousness, or other signs of overdosage occur. Also notify doctor immediately if any signs of aggravated cardiovascular disease develop (chest pain, dyspnea, tachycardia). • Suggest morning dosage to prevent insomnia. • Monitor pulse rate, blood pressure. • Thyroid hormones alter thyroid function test results. Monitor prothrombin time; patients taking these hormones usually require less anticoagulant. Alert patients to report unusual bleeding and bruising.
Cholestyramine: thyroid absorption impaired. Separate doses by 4 to 5 hours. *I.V. phenytoin:* free thyroid released. Monitor for tachycardia.	• Contraindicated in myocardial infarction, thyrotoxicosis (except with antithyroid drugs), or uncorrected adrenal insufficiency (thyroid hormones increase tissue demand for adrenocortical hormone and may cause acute adrenal crisis). Use with extreme caution in angina pectoris, hypertension, or other cardiovascular disorders; renal insufficiency; or ischemic states. • Use carefully in myxedema; patients are unusually sensitive to thyroid hormone. • In patients with coronary artery disease who must receive thyroid, observe carefully for possible coronary insufficiency if catecholamines must be given. • Potentially dangerous; not indicated to relieve vague symptoms, such as physical and mental sluggishness, irritability, or depression; to treat obesity in euthyroid persons; to treat metabolic insufficiency not associated with thyroid insufficiency; or to treat menstrual disorders or male infertility, unless associated with hypothyroidism. • Tell patient to take thyroid hormones regularly, at the same time each day, to maintain constant hormone levels. • Warn patient to tell doctor at once if chest pain (especially in elderly), palpitations, sweating, nervousness, or other signs of overdosage occur. Also notify doctor immediately if any signs of aggravated cardiovascular disease develop (chest pain, dyspnea, tachycardia). • Suggest morning dosage to prevent insomnia. • Monitor pulse rate and blood pressure. • In children, sleeping pulse rate and basal morning temperature are guides to treatment. • Thyroid hormones alter thyroid function test results. Monitor prothrombin time; patients taking these hormones usually require less anticoagulant. Alert patients to report unusual bleeding and bruising.

NAME	INDICATIONS & DOSAGE	SIDE EFFECTS
thyrotropin Thyrotron♦♦, Thytropar♦	*Diagnosis of thyroid cancer remnant with ^{131}I after surgery*—10 international units I.M. or S.C. for 3 to 7 days. *Differential diagnosis of primary and secondary hypothyroidism*—10 units I.M. or S.C. for 1 to 3 days. *In PBI or ^{131}I uptake determinations for differential diagnosis of subclinical hypothyroidism or low thyroid reserve*—10 units I.M. or S.C. *Therapy for thyroid carcinoma (local or metastatic) with ^{131}I*—10 units I.M. or S.C. for 3 to 8 days. *To determine thyroid status of patient receiving thyroid*—10 units I.M. or S.C. for 1 to 3 days.	**CNS:** headache. **CV:** *tachycardia,* atrial fibrillation, *angina pectoris, congestive failure,* hypotension. **GI:** nausea, vomiting. **Other:** thyroid hyperplasia (large doses), fever, menstrual irregularities, allergic reactions (postinjection flare, urticaria, *anaphylaxis).*

♦ Available in U.S. and Canada. ♦♦ Available in Canada only. All other products (no symbol) available in U.S. only. Italicized side effects are common or life-threatening.

THERAPEUTIC EFFECTIVENESS OF THYROID HORMONES

DRUG	EQUIVALENT DOSE	CONTENTS	RELATIVE DURATION
levothyroxine	100 mcg	T_4	Long (once-daily dosing possible)
liothyronine	25 mcg	T_3	Short (multiple doses must be given daily)
liotrix	Either Euthroid-1 or Thyrolar-1	T_4 and T_3 in 4:1 ratio	Intermediate
thyroglobulin	65 mg	T_4 and T_3 in 2.5:1 ratio	Intermediate
thyroid USP	65 mg	T_4 and T_3 in variable ratios	Intermediate

(For liotrix, thyroglobulin and thyroid USP: Those with higher T_4 concentration are longer-acting; those with lower T_4 concentration are shorter-acting.)

INTERACTIONS	NURSING CONSIDERATIONS
None significant.	• Contraindicated in coronary thrombosis, untreated Addison's disease. Use cautiously in angina pectoris, heart failure, hypopituitarism, adrenocortical suppression. • Purified thyrotropic hormone (TSH) is isolated from bovine anterior pituitary. It stimulates the formation and secretion of thyroid hormone and increases thyroidal uptake of iodine: May cause thyroid hyperplasia. • Diagnostic use: to identify subclinical hypothyroidism or low thyroid reserve, to evaluate need for thyroid therapy, to distinguish between primary and secondary hypothyroidism, and to detect thyroid remnants and metastases of thyroid carcinoma. • Therapeutic use: management of certain types of thyroid carcinoma and resulting metastases, and in conjunction with radioactive ^{131}I to enhance uptake of ^{131}I by the thyroid. • Three-day dosage schedule may be used in long-standing pituitary myxedema or with prolonged use of thyroid medication. • For treatment of anaphylaxis, see inside front cover.

PATIENT-TEACHING AID

CONTROLLING YOUR HYPOTHYROIDISM

Dear Patient:

The doctor has prescribed medication to *replace* your missing thyroid hormone. So your hypothyroidism can be controlled if you take your medication regularly.

The thyroid hormone replacement acts like normal thyroid hormone. The doctor may start with small amounts, then gradually increase the dose until your thyroid levels are normal. Your symptoms, therefore, may disappear slowly.

You can help the doctor assess your hormonal status by telling him how you feel. For example, if you notice your heart rate is faster, or if you feel nervous, sweaty, and hot, or have muscle tremors, call your doctor. These symptoms may mean you're receiving too much thyroid medication.

If you begin to feel increasingly tired, weak, and constipated, or if you're more sensitive to cold and your face looks puffy, you could be getting too little thyroid hormone, so again, call the doctor.

After the doctor's determined the correct dose of thyroid medication for you, you can live your life normally, with no restrictions on diet or activities. But remember, hypothyroidism is almost always a lifelong disease; stopping your medication for long periods could cause your symptoms to reappear. Set aside a regular time for taking your daily medication; if you tie it in with a regular activity, such as breakfast, it'll become more of a habit.

If you change doctors or if another doctor is treating a different disorder, make sure he knows you're taking a thyroid medication. You may also want to carry a medical identification card in your wallet about your thyroid medication.

Thyroid hormone antagonists

iodine
methimazole
propylthiouracil (PTU)
radioactive iodine (sodium iodide)^{131}I

Thyroid hormone antagonists, or antithyroid agents, are used to treat hyperthyroidism. Some antagonists, such as iodine and the thionamines (methimazole and propylthiouracil), have reversible effects and may be used in a young patient or one in whom hyperthyroidism is not necessarily permanent. They do not permanently affect the thyroid gland, but control hormone production until spontaneous remission of hyperthyroidism occurs.

Radiation therapy (with radioactive iodine) and thyroidectomy (partial or total) are definitive treatments for hyperthyroidism. Both procedures are reserved for adult patients who may not respond to milder agents. Unfortunately, radiation therapy and surgical treatment carry a long-term risk of hypothyroidism. For more information on these treatments, see chart on pp. 780 and 781.

Major uses

• Iodine, methimazole, and propylthiouracil are used to treat hyperthyroidism (Graves' disease, multinodular goiter, and thyroiditis) in children, pregnant women, patients in whom thyroidectomy is contraindicated, and those in whom the condition is not necessarily permanent. These agents also help prepare patients for thyroidectomy and are effective for thyrotoxic crisis.

• Iodine combats lethal thyrotoxic crisis in adults and neonates. It is used preoperatively to decrease vascularity of the thyroid gland.

• Radioactive iodine is usually therapeutic for hyperthyroidism in adults when surgical treatment is contraindicated. However, it is not used in pregnant women.

Radioactive iodine is also used as a diagnostic tracer in thyroid function disorders and as a therapeutic adjunct after thyroidectomy for thyroid cancer. It causes ablation of any residual thyroid tissue. It can also be used to treat thyroid-cancer metastases.

Mechanism of action

• Iodine inhibits thyroid hormone formation by blocking iodotyrosine and iodothyronine synthesis. It also limits iodide transport into the thyroid gland and blocks thyroid hormone release.

• Radioactive iodine limits thyroid hormone secretion by destroying thyroid tissue. The affinity of thyroid tissue for radioactive iodine facilitates uptake of the drug by cancerous thyroid tissue that has metastasized to other sites in the body.

• The thionamines inhibit oxidation of iodine in the thyroid gland, blocking iodine's ability to combine with tyrosine to form thyroxine. They may also prevent the coupling of monoiodotyrosine and diiodotyrosine to form thyroxine and triiodothyronine.

Absorption, distribution, metabolism, and excretion

• Methimazole and propylthiouracil are readily absorbed from the gastrointestinal tract and metabolized in the liver. Their metabolites are excreted in urine; however, 35% of propylthiouracil is excreted unchanged.
• Radioactive iodine in high concentrations is trapped in the thyroid gland within 30 minutes of oral administration and incorporated into the thyroid follicles; it is excreted in urine.

Onset and duration

• Radioactive iodine's action may not begin for weeks, so be alert for temporary but potentially serious thyrotoxic reactions that may occur during the first few days of treatment. Radioactive iodine has a half-life of 8 days.
• The thionamines' onset may not be apparent for days or weeks—until the stored supply of thyroid hormones is depleted. The half-life of propylthiouracil is 2 hours; that of methimazole, 6 to 9 hours. After correction of the abnormally high metabolic rate (as in hyperthyroidism), the half-lives of these drugs may increase, necessitating lower doses. Patients with severe hyperthyroidism respond most rapidly, usually within 1 or 2 days.

Combination products

None.

PATIENT-TEACHING AID

PREVENTING NECK STRAIN AFTER THYROIDECTOMY

Dear Patient:

After your thyroidectomy, to prevent strain on your neck muscles when rising to a sitting position, support your head with a pillow and put your hands together behind your head (as shown).

TREATMENTS FOR HYPERTHYROIDISM: DISTINGUISHING FACTORS

TREATMENT	INDICATIONS
Thyroid hormone antagonists (antithyroid drugs)	• Patients in whom spontaneous remission is expected or thyroidectomy is contraindicated; children, adults under age 35, pregnant women • Presurgical control • Adjunct with radioactive iodine while patient awaits effects of radiation • Thyrotoxic crisis • Long-term suppression of hyperthyroid function • Progressive exophthalmos • Multinodular goiter • Thyrocardiac disease
Surgery	• Failure of drug treatment • Toxic uninodular goiter • Large multinodular gland which doesn't regress with oral therapy • Esophageal obstruction • Possible malignancy
Radioactive iodine	• Elderly or debilitated adults who are not good candidates for surgery • Failure of drug treatment • Adjunct for ablation of residual thyroid tissue after thyroidectomy for cancer • Recurring hyperthyroidism after surgery • Persistent hyperthyroidism • Small thyroid • Diffuse goiter • Toxic uninodular goiter • Multinodular goiter • Metastatic thyroid cancer lesions • Thyrocardiac disease

CONTRAINDICATIONS	DISADVANTAGES
• None	• Poor compliance • Drug toxicity (especially hematologic) • Possible hypothyroidism after therapy
• Medical risks to surgery (such as diabetes, heart disease) • Small thyroid • Uncontrolled thyrotoxicosis • Severe or progressive exophthalmos • Thyrocardiac disease	• Long-term potential for hypothyroidism • Possible recurrent hyperthyroidism • Risk of surgical complications (such as damage to recurrent laryngeal nerve)
• Pregnancy and lactation • Under age 35 unless patient has special indications, such as severe heart disease, cancer	• Necessary avoidance of pregnancy for 1 year after treatment • Questionable safety in children • Possible hypothyroidism • Difficulty in establishing safe but effective dose • Delayed action • Possible genetic damage from small but definite radiation dose to gonads (especially when abdominal and testicular metastatic thyroid cancer lesions are present) • Possible increased risk of leukemia later in life for patients receiving doses high enough to cause thyroid ablation in cancer treatment

NAME	INDICATIONS & DOSAGE	SIDE EFFECTS
iodine Potassium Iodide Solution, USP; Sodium Iodide, USP; Strong Iodine Solution, USP (Lugol's Solution), containing 5% iodine and 10% potassium iodide	*Preparation for thyroidectomy—* **Adults and children:** Strong Iodine Solution, USP, 0.1 to 0.3 ml P.O. t.i.d., or Potassium Iodide Solution, USP, 5 drops in water P.O. t.i.d. after meals for 2 to 3 weeks before surgery. *Thyrotoxic crisis—* **Adults and children:** Strong Iodine Solution, USP, 1 ml in water P.O. t.i.d. after meals in refractory cases; Sodium Iodide, USP, 250 to 500 mg (or up to 2 g) daily, slow I.V. infusion with antithyroid drugs and propranolol.	**EENT:** acute rhinitis, inflammation of salivary glands, periorbital edema, conjunctivitis, hyperemia. **GI:** burning, irritation, *nausea,* vomiting, *metallic taste.* **Skin:** acneiform rash, mucous membrane ulceration. **Other:** fever, frontal headache; with I.V. use (sodium iodide): acute iodism, *colloidoclastic shock,* pulmonary edema.
methimazole Tapazole	*Hyperthyroidism—* **Adults:** 5 mg P.O. t.i.d. if mild; 10 to 15 mg P.O. t.i.d. if moderately severe; and 20 mg P.O. t.i.d. if severe. Continue until patient euthyroid, then start maintenance dose of 5 mg daily to t.i.d. Maximum dose 150 mg daily. **Children:** 0.4 mg/kg/day divided q 8 hours. Continue until patient euthyroid, then start maintenance dose of 0.2 mg/kg/day divided q 8 hours. *Preparation for thyroidectomy—* **Adults and children:** same doses as for hyperthyroidism until patient is euthyroid; then iodine may be added for 10 days before surgery. *Thyrotoxic crisis—* **Adults and children:** same doses as for hyperthyroidism, with concomitant iodine therapy and propranolol.	**Blood:** *agranulocytosis,* leukopenia, granulopenia, thrombocytopenia (appear to be dose-related). **CNS:** headache, drowsiness, vertigo. **GI:** diarrhea, nausea, vomiting (may be dose-related). **Hepatic:** jaundice. **Skin:** rash, urticaria, skin discoloration. **Other:** arthralgia, myalgia, salivary gland enlargement, loss of taste, drug fever, lymphadenopathy.
propylthiouracil (PTU) Propyl-Thyracil♦♦	*Hyperthyroidism—* **Adults:** 100 mg P.O. t.i.d.; up to 300 mg q 8 hours have been used in severe cases. Continue until patient euthyroid, then start maintenance dose of 100 mg daily to t.i.d. **Children over 10 years:** 100 mg P.O. t.i.d. Continue until patient euthyroid, then start maintenance dose of 25 mg t.i.d. to 100 mg b.i.d. **Children 6 to 10 years:** 50 to 150 mg P.O. divided q 8 hours. *Preparation for thyroidectomy—*	**Blood:** *agranulocytosis,* leukopenia, thrombocytopenia (appear to be dose-related). **CNS:** headache, drowsiness, vertigo. **EENT:** visual disturbances. **GI:** diarrhea, *nausea, vomiting* (may be dose-related). **Hepatic:** jaundice. **Skin:** rash, urticaria, skin discoloration, pruritus. **Other:** arthralgia, myalgia, salivary gland enlargement, loss of taste, drug fever, lymphadenopathy.

♦ Available in U.S. and Canada. ♦♦ Available in Canada only. All other products (no symbol) available in U.S. only. Italicized side effects are common or life-threatening.

INTERACTIONS	NURSING CONSIDERATIONS
Lithium carbonate: hypothyroidism may occur. Use with caution.	• Contraindicated in tuberculosis, iodide hypersensitivity, hyperkalemia; after meals that contain excessive starch; in laryngeal edema, swelling of salivary glands. • Generally use I.V. route only if patient is vomiting or cannot receive anything by mouth. Some prefer I.V. route to prevent GI side effects, especially during critical time at beginning of treatment. • Dilute oral doses in water, milk, fruit juice, and give after meals to prevent gastric irritation, to hydrate the patient, and to mask the very salty taste. • Tell patient to ask the doctor about using iodized salt and eating shellfish during treatment. Iodine-rich foods may not be permitted. • Warn the patient that sudden withdrawal may precipitate thyroid storm. • Store in light-resistant container. • Give iodides through straw to avoid tooth discoloration. • Usually given with other antithyroid drugs.
None significant.	• Use cautiously in pregnancy. Pregnant women may require less drug as pregnancy progresses. Monitor thyroid function studies closely. Thyroid may be added to regimen. Drugs may be stopped during last few weeks of pregnancy. • Watch for signs of hypothyroidism (mental depression; cold intolerance; hard, nonpitting edema). Dose may need to be adjusted. • Monitor CBC periodically to detect impending leukopenia, thrombocytopenia, and agranulocytosis. • Warn patient to report immediately: fever, sore throat, or mouth sores (possible signs of developing agranulocytosis). Agranulocytosis can develop too rapidly to be detected by periodic blood cell counts. Tell patient also to immediately report skin eruptions (sign of hypersensitivity). • Drug should be stopped if severe rash or enlarged cervical lymph nodes develop. • Tell patient to ask doctor about using iodized salt and eating shellfish during treatment. • Warn patient against over-the-counter cough medicines; many contain iodine. • Give with meals to reduce GI side effects. • Store in light-resistant container.
None significant.	• Use cautiously in pregnancy. Pregnant women may require less drug as pregnancy progresses. Monitor thyroid function studies closely. Thyroid may be added to regimen. Drugs may be stopped during last few weeks of pregnancy. • Watch for signs of hypothyroidism (mental depression; cold intolerance; hard, nonpitting edema). Dose may need to be adjusted. • Monitor CBC periodically to detect impending leukopenia, thrombocytopenia, and agranulocytosis. • Stop drug if severe rash or enlarged cervical lymph nodes develop. • Warn patient to report immediately: fever, sore throat, or mouth sores (possible signs of developing agranulocytosis). Agranulocytosis can develop too rapidly to be detected by periodic blood cell counts. Tell patient also to report immediately skin eruptions (sign of hypersensitivity). • Tell patient to ask doctor about using iodized salt and eating shell-

(continued on following page)

NAME	INDICATIONS & DOSAGE	SIDE EFFECTS
propylthiouracil *(continued)*	**Adults and children:** same doses as for hyperthyroidism, then iodine may be added 10 days before surgery. *Thyrotoxic crisis—* **Adults and children:** same doses as for hyperthyroidism, with concomitant iodine therapy and propranolol.	
radioactive iodine (sodium iodide) ^{131}I	*Hyperthyroidism—* **Adults:** usual dose is 4 to 10 millicuries P.O. Dose based on estimated weight of thyroid gland and thyroid uptake. Treatment may be repeated after 6 weeks, according to serum thyroxine levels. *Thyroid cancer—* **Adults:** 50 to 150 millicuries P.O. Dose based on estimated malignant thyroid tissue and metastatic tissue as determined by total body scan. Dose may be repeated according to clinical status.	**EENT:** *feeling of fullness in neck,* metallic taste, "radiation mumps." **Endocrine:** hypothyroidism, radiation thyroiditis. **GU:** possible increased risk of birth defects in offspring after sufficient ^{131}I dose for thyroid ablation following cancer surgery. **Other:** possible increased risk of developing leukemia later in life after sufficient ^{131}I dose for thyroid ablation following cancer surgery.

INTERACTIONS	NURSING CONSIDERATIONS
	fish during treatment. • Warn patient against over-the-counter cough medicines; many contain iodine. • Give with meals to reduce GI side effects. • Store in light-resistant container.
Lithium carbonate: hypothyroidism may occur. Use with caution.	• Contraindicated in pregnancy and lactation unless used to treat thyroid cancer. • Stop all antithyroid medications, thyroid preparations, and iodine-containing preparations 1 week before ^{131}I dose. If medications are not stopped, patient may receive thyroid-stimulating hormone for 3 days before ^{131}I dose. When treating women of childbearing age, give dose during menstruation or within 7 days after menstruation. • After therapy for hyperthyroidism, patient should not resume antithyroid drugs, but should continue propranolol or other drugs used to treat symptoms of hyperthyroidism until onset of full ^{131}I effect (usually 6 weeks). • Monitor thyroid function with serum thyroxine levels. • After dose for hyperthyroidism, patient's urine and saliva are slightly radioactive for 24 hours; vomitus is highly radioactive for 6 to 8 hours. Institute full radiation precautions during this time. Instruct patient to use appropriate disposal methods when coughing and expectorating. • After dose for thyroid cancer, patient's urine, saliva, and perspiration remain radioactive for 3 days. Isolate patient and observe the following precautions: pregnant personnel should not take care of patient; disposable eating utensils and linens should be used; instruct patient to save all urine in lead containers for 24 to 48 hours so amount of radioactive material excreted can be determined. Patient should drink as much fluid as possible for 48 hours after drug administration to facilitate excretion. Limit contact with patient to 30 minutes per shift per person the first day. May increase time to 1 hour second day and longer on third day. • If patient is discharged less than 7 days after ^{131}I dose for thyroid cancer, warn him to avoid close, prolonged contact with small children (for example, holding children on lap), and instruct him not to sleep in same room with spouse for 7 days after treatment due to increased risk of thyroid cancer in persons exposed to ^{131}I. Tell patient he may use same bathroom facilities as rest of family. However, pets should not be allowed to drink from toilet for 7 days (increased risk of thyroid cancer).

Pituitary hormones

corticotropin (ACTH)
cosyntropin
desmopressin acetate
lypressin
somatotropin (human growth hormone)
vasopressin (antidiuretic hormone)
vasopressin tannate

The pituitary hormones fall into three groups according to use: Corticotropin and cosyntropin are used to diagnose primary adrenal insufficiency; somatotropin spurs growth in patients with pituitary growth deficiency; and vasopressin and its synthetic derivatives desmopressin acetate and lypressin regulate water balance in patients with diabetes insipidus. All these hormones are either natural pituitary extracts or synthetic derivatives.

The pituitary gland is the most complex endocrine structure in the body. Its two major divisions are the anterior lobe (adenohypophysis) and the posterior lobe (neurohypophysis). Except for melanocyte-stimulating hormone—which is not commercially available—and somatotropin, the anterior lobe secretes tropic (primary) hormones that activate other organs (target glands) to secrete their characteristic hormones, called genic (secondary) hormones (see diagram on pp. 788 to 789).

Extract from the posterior lobe may be divided into two active components: vasopressin (primarily associated with pressor and antidiuretic activities) and oxytocin (primarily associated with pronounced uterine-contracting and milk-releasing action). (See Chapter 106, OXYTOCICS, for a detailed description of oxytocin.)

Major uses

Rx

- Corticotropin and cosyntropin act as screening agents for primary adrenal insufficiency.
- Desmopressin, lypressin, and vasopressin combat symptoms of central diabetes insipidus.
- Somatotropin is used to treat growth impairment due to growth hormone deficiency.

Mechanism of action

- Corticotropin and cosyntropin, by replacing the body's own tropic hormone, stimulate the adrenal cortex to secrete its entire spectrum of hormones.
- Desmopressin, lypressin, and vasopressin increase the permeability of the renal tubular epithelium to adenosine monophosphate and water; the epithelium promotes reabsorption of water and produces a concentrated urine (antidiuretic hormone effect).
- Lypressin and vasopressin cause contraction of smooth muscle in the vascular bed (vasopressor effect). Vasopressin also causes contraction of smooth muscle in the gastrointestinal (GI) tract.
- Somatotropin stimulates linear growth in patients with pituitary growth deficiency by various mechanisms.

PATIENT-TEACHING AID

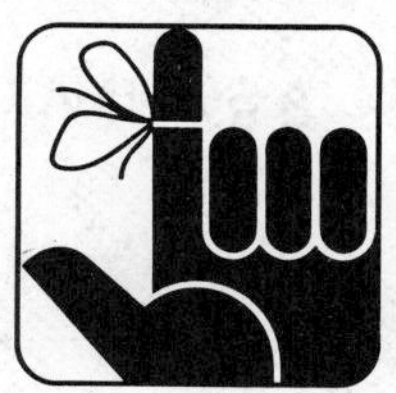

HOW TO USE LYPRESSIN NASAL SPRAY

Dear Patient:

Frequent urination and thirstiness are signs of diabetes insipidus. Your doctor has prescribed lypressin, a nasal spray that treats this condition.

You may regulate the dosage according to your needs. Spray the medication as directed in one or both nostrils. Take an extra dose at bedtime if you are urinating frequently at night. If the usual dosage is inadequate, use the medication more often; don't increase the number of sprays each time you use it.

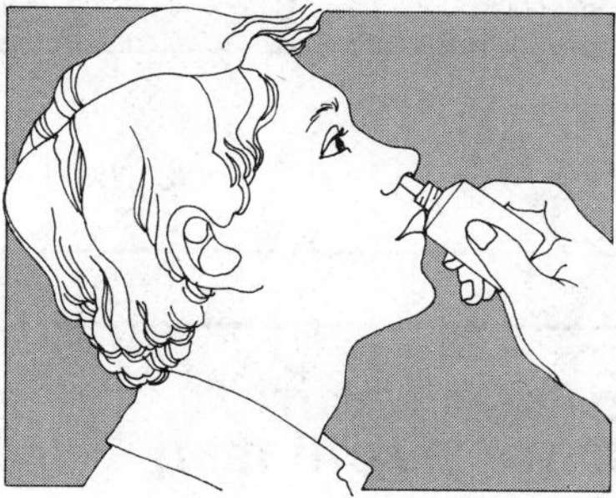

Here's how to spray the medication most effectively:

1. Before you begin, read the medication label carefully, so you know the exact amount of medication to administer. Make sure you have tissues handy. Then, sit upright, with your head tilted back.

2. Now, place the tip of the squeeze bottle about ½″ (1 cm) inside your nostril. Point it straight up your nose, toward the inner corner of your eye. Don't angle the squeeze bottle downward, or the medication will run down your throat.

Without inhaling, squeeze the bottle once, quickly and firmly. Use just enough force to coat the inside of your nose with medication. Too much force may send the medicine into your sinuses and give you a headache. Then, spray again, if the instructions on the label order it. Repeat the procedure in the other nostril.

3. Keep your head tilted back for several minutes, so the medication has time to work. Avoid blowing your nose while you wait.

These include facilitating intracellular transport of amino acids; increasing intestinal absorption and urinary excretion of calcium; increasing renal tubular reabsorption of phosphorus and decreasing that of calcium; promoting synthesis of collagen and chondroitin, which form cartilage; and inhibiting intracellular glucose metabolism.

Absorption, distribution, metabolism, and excretion

- Corticotropin is destroyed in the GI tract after oral administration but is well absorbed parenterally. The parenteral form is well distributed and inactivated in body tissues and excreted in urine.
- Cosyntropin is destroyed by the proteolytic enzymes of the GI tract and so must be given either I.M. or I.V. It is inactivated in the tissues and excreted in urine.
- Desmopressin and lypressin, because they are inactivated in the GI tract by the enzyme trypsin, are given

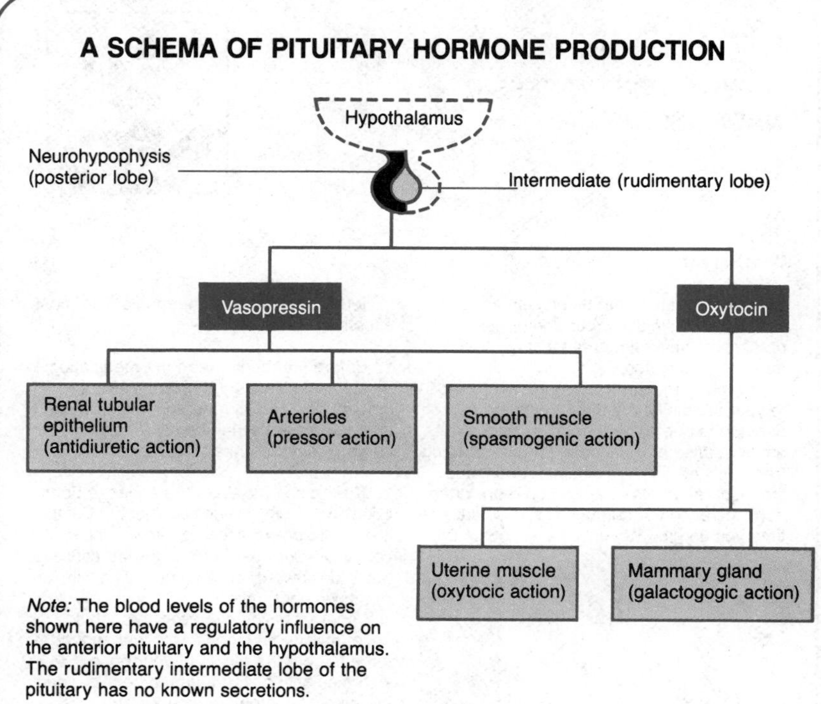

Note: The blood levels of the hormones shown here have a regulatory influence on the anterior pituitary and the hypothalamus. The rudimentary intermediate lobe of the pituitary has no known secretions.

WHAT YOU SHOULD KNOW ABOUT THE COSYNTROPIN TEST (RAPID ACTH TEST)

The cosyntropin test helps identify adrenal insufficiency. Using a synthetic duplication of the biologically active part of the ACTH molecule, this test provides faster results and causes fewer allergic reactions than the 8-hour ACTH stimulation test, which uses natural ACTH from animal sources.

Patient preparation
Explain the purpose of the test to your patient beforehand. He may have to fast for 10 to 12 hours and rest for 30 minutes before the 1-hour test. Also, he shouldn't take ACTH or steroid medications before the test.

Test procedures
Draw a preinjection blood sample (5 ml) into a heparinized tube. Then, inject 250 mcg (0.25 mg) of cosyntropin I.V. or I.M. (Determinations are more accurate with I.V. administration.) Draw two more samples (5 ml each) 30 and 60 minutes after the injection. Handle the samples gently to prevent hemolysis.

After the test, observe your patient for possible allergic reactions, such as hives, itching, or tachycardia.

Test results
In patients with Addison's disease (primary adrenal hypofunction), cortisol levels remain low. In patients with hypopituitarism (secondary adrenal hypofunction), baseline values of cortisol double.

A patient's failure to observe dietary, medication, and activity restrictions may cause inaccurate results. Certain drugs—such as estrogens, amphetamines, and lithium—alter cortisol levels. Also, radioactive scans performed within 1 week before the test may alter test results.

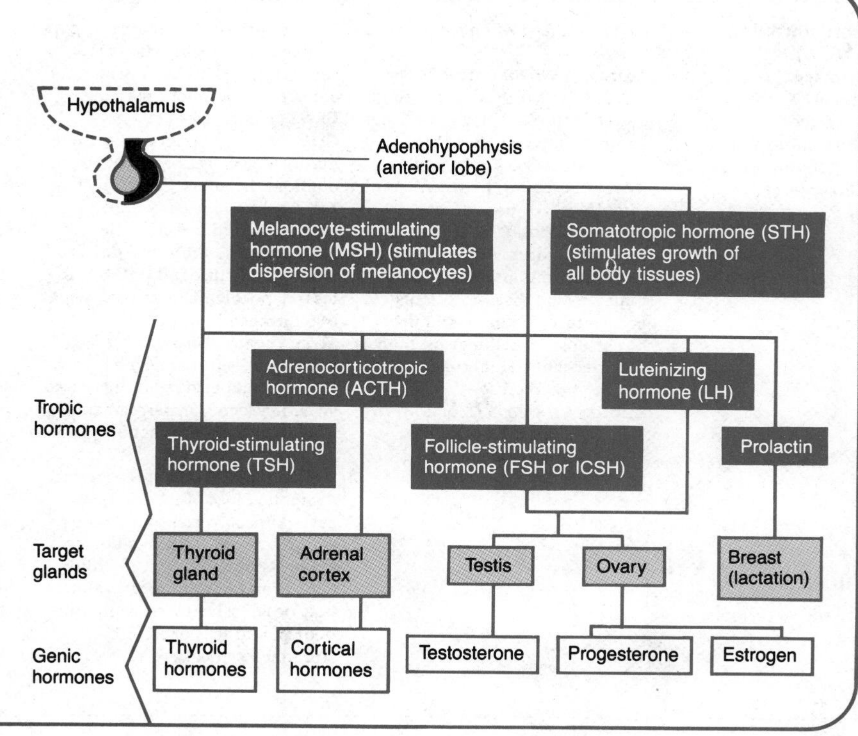

intranasally. Absorption through the nasal mucosa is adequate but decreases in nasal congestion, rhinitis, and upper respiratory tract infection.

Desmopressin and lypressin are distributed throughout the extracellular fluid, metabolized in the liver and kidneys, and excreted in urine.

• Somatotropin is destroyed in the GI tract after oral administration but is well distributed to the body tissues after I.M. administration. It is metabolized in the liver and excreted in urine.

• Vasopressin tannate in oil is absorbed more slowly than the aqueous solution. Vasopressin is distributed throughout the extracellular fluid, metabolized in the liver and kidneys, and excreted in urine.

Onset and duration

• Corticotropin begins to work within 5 minutes and lasts 3 to 25 hours, depending on dose and route of administration.

• Cosyntropin, as reflected by plasma cortisol levels, has an onset within 5 minutes, peaks within 1 hour, and lasts 4 hours.

• Desmopressin and lypressin take effect within 1 hour. Desmopressin peaks in 1 to 5 hours and lasts 8 to 20 hours. Lypressin lasts 3 to 8 hours.

• Somatotropin takes effect immediately; its action lasts several days.

• Vasopressin (aqueous solution) goes to work within 1 hour and lasts 2 to 8 hours when given subcutaneously, and 6 to 12 hours when given I.V.

• Vasopressin tannate becomes effective within 1 hour and lasts 48 to 72 hours after I.M. injection.

Combination products

None.

NAME	INDICATIONS & DOSAGE	SIDE EFFECTS
corticotropin (ACTH) Acthar♦, Acton "X"♦♦, Cortigel-80, Cortrophin Gel, Cortrophin Zinc, Duracton♦♦, H.P. Acthar Gel	*Diagnostic test of adrenocortical function—* **Adults:** up to 80 units I.M. or S.C. in divided doses; or a single dose of repository form; or 10 to 25 units (aqueous form) in 500 ml dextrose 5% in water I.V. over 8 hours, between blood samplings. Individual dosages generally vary with adrenal glands' sensitivity to stimulation as well as with specific disease. Infants and younger children require larger doses per kilogram than do older children and adults. *For therapeutic use—* **Adults:** 40 units S.C. or I.M. in 4 divided doses (aqueous); 40 units q 12 to 24 hours (gel or repository form).	**CNS:** *convulsions, dizziness,* papilledema, headache, *euphoria, insomnia,* mood swings, personality changes, depression, psychosis. **EENT:** cataracts, glaucoma. **GI:** *peptic ulcer with perforation and hemorrhage,* pancreatitis, abdominal distention, ulcerative esophagitis, nausea, vomiting. **GU:** menstrual irregularities. **Metabolic:** *sodium and fluid retention,* calcium and potassium loss, hypokalemic alkalosis, negative nitrogen balance. **Skin:** *impaired wound healing,* thin fragile skin, petechiae, ecchymoses, facial erythema, increased sweating, acne, hyperpigmentation, allergic skin reactions, hirsutism. **Other:** muscle weakness, steroid myopathy, loss of muscle mass, osteoporosis, vertebral compression fractures, cushingoid state, suppression of growth in children, *activation of latent diabetes mellitus,* progressive increase in antibodies, and loss of ACTH stimulatory effect.
cosyntropin Cortrosyn♦, Synacthen Depot♦♦	*Diagnostic test of adrenocortical function—* **Adults and children:** 0.25 to 1 mg I.M. or I.V. (unless label prohibits I.V. administration) between blood samplings. **Children younger than 2 years:** 0.125 mg I.M. or I.V.	**Skin:** pruritus. **Other:** flushing.
desmopressin acetate DDAVP	*Nonnephrogenic diabetes insipidus, temporary polyuria and polydipsia associated with pituitary trauma—* **Adults:** 0.1 to 0.4 ml intranasally daily in 1 to 3 doses. Adjust morning and evening doses separately for adequate diurnal rhythm of water turnover. **Children 3 months to 12 years:** 0.05 to 0.3 ml intranasally daily in 1 or 2 doses.	**CNS:** headache. **CV:** slight rise in blood pressure at high dosage. **EENT:** nasal congestion, rhinitis. **GI:** nausea. **GU:** vulval pain. **Other:** flushing.
lypressin Diapid	*Nonnephrogenic diabetes insipidus—* **Adults and children:** 1 or 2 sprays (approximately 2 USP	**CNS:** headache, dizziness. **EENT:** nasal congestion or ulceration, irritation, pruritus of nasal passages, rhinorrhea, and

♦ Available in U.S. and Canada. ♦♦ Available in Canada only. All other products (no symbol) available in U.S. only. Italicized side effects are common or life-threatening.

INTERACTIONS	NURSING CONSIDERATIONS
None significant.	• Contraindicated in scleroderma, osteoporosis, systemic fungal infections, ocular herpes simplex, recent surgery, peptic ulcer, congestive heart failure, hypertension, sensitivity to pork products, concomitant smallpox vaccination, adrenocortical hyperfunction or primary insufficiency, or Cushing's syndrome; patients being immunized; latent tuberculosis or tuberculin reactivity; hypothyroidism; cirrhosis; infection (use anti-infective therapy during and after ACTH treatment); acute gouty arthritis (limit ACTH treatment to a few days, and use conventional therapy during and for several days after ACTH treatment); emotional instability; diabetes; abscess; pyogenic infections; renal insufficiency; myasthenia gravis. • ACTH treatment should be preceded by verification of adrenal responsiveness and test for hypersensitivity and allergic reactions. • Oral agents are preferred for long-term therapy. • Unusual stress may require additional use of rapidly acting corticosteroids. When possible, gradually reduce ACTH dosage to smallest effective dose to minimize induced adrenocortical insufficiency. Reinstitute therapy if stressful situation (trauma, surgery, severe illness) occurs shortly after stopping drug. • Watch neonates of ACTH-treated mothers for signs of hypoadrenalism. • Counteract edema by low-sodium, high-potassium intake; nitrogen loss by high-protein diet; and psychotic changes by reducing ACTH dosage or administering sedatives. • ACTH may mask signs of chronic disease and decrease host resistance and ability to localize infection. • Note and record weight changes, fluid exchange, and resting blood pressures until minimal effective dose is achieved. • Refrigerate reconstituted solution and use within 24 hours. • If administering gel, warm it to room temperature, draw into large needle, give slowly deep I.M. with 21G or 22G needle. Warn patient that injection is painful.
None significant.	• Use cautiously in hypersensitivity to natural corticotropin. • Drug is synthetic duplication of the biologically active part of the ACTH molecule. It is less likely to produce sensitivity than natural ACTH from animal sources.
None significant.	• Use with caution in patients with coronary artery insufficiency or hypertensive cardiovascular disease. • Adjust fluid intake to reduce risk of water intoxication and sodium depletion, especially in very young or old patients. • Titrate dosage to allow patient sufficient sleep. • Give intranasally only. • Overdose may cause oxytocic or vasopressor activity. Withhold drug until effects subside. Furosemide may be used if fluid retention is excessive. • Not effective in nephrogenic diabetes insipidus. • Teach patient correct method of administration.
None significant.	• Use with caution in patients with coronary artery disease. • Particularly useful if diabetes insipidus is unresponsive to other therapy, or if antidiuretic hormones of animal origin cause adverse reactions.

(continued on following page)

NAME	INDICATIONS & DOSAGE	SIDE EFFECTS
lypressin *(continued)*	posterior pituitary pressor units per spray) in either or both nostrils q.i.d. and an additional dose at bedtime, if needed, to prevent nocturia. If usual dosage is inadequate, increase frequency rather than number of sprays.	conjunctivitis. **GI:** heartburn due to drip of excess spray into pharynx, abdominal cramps, frequent bowel movements. **GU:** possible transient fluid retention due to overdose. **Skin:** hypersensitivity reaction.
somatotropin (human growth hormone) Asellacrin, Crescormon	*Growth failure due to pituitary growth hormone deficiency—* **Children:** 2 IU (1 ml) I.M. 3 times weekly, with a minimum of 48 hours between injections. Double dose if growth doesn't exceed 1 inch in 6 months, or recheck diagnosis.	**GU:** excess calcium in urine. **Metabolic:** hyperglycemia.
vasopressin Pitressin Synthetic♦ **vasopressin tannate** Pitressin Tannate	*Nonnephrogenic, nonpsychogenic diabetes insipidus—* **Adults:** 5 to 10 units I.M. or S.C. b.i.d. to q.i.d., p.r.n.; or intranasally (spray or cotton balls) in individualized doses, based on response. For chronic therapy, inject 2.5 to 5 units Pitressin Tannate in oil suspension I.M. or S.C. every 2 to 3 days. **Children:** 2.5 to 10 units I.M. or S.C. b.i.d. to q.i.d., p.r.n.; or intranasally (spray or cotton balls) in individualized doses. For chronic therapy, inject 1.25 to 2.5 units Pitressin Tannate in oil suspension I.M. or S.C. every 2 to 3 days. *Postoperative abdominal distention—* **Adults:** 5 units (aqueous) I.M. initially, then q 3 to 4 hours, increasing dose to 10 units, if needed. Reduce dose for children proportionately. *To expel gas before abdominal X-ray—* **Adults:** inject 10 units S.C. at 2 hours, then again at 30 minutes before X-ray. *Upper GI tract hemorrhage (intra-arterial)—* **Adults:** 0.2 to 0.4 units/minute. Do not use Tannate in oil suspension.	**CNS:** tremor, dizziness, headache. **CV:** *angina in patients with vascular disease,* vasoconstriction. Large doses may cause hypertension, electrocardiographic changes. **GI:** abdominal cramps, nausea, vomiting, diarrhea, intestinal hyperactivity. **GU:** uterine cramps, anuria. **Skin:** circumoral pallor. **Other:** water intoxication (drowsiness, listlessness, headache, confusion, weight gain), hypersensitivity reactions (urticaria, angioneurotic edema, bronchoconstriction, fever, rash, wheezing, dyspnea, *anaphylaxis),* sweating.

♦ Available in U.S. and Canada. ♦♦ Available in Canada only. All other products (no symbol) available in U.S. only. Italicized side effects are common or life-threatening.

INTERACTIONS	NURSING CONSIDERATIONS
	• Nasal congestion, allergic rhinitis, or upper respiratory infections may diminish drug absorption and require larger dose or adjunctive therapy. • Inadvertent inhalation of spray may cause tightness in chest, coughing, and transient dyspnea. • Test patients sensitive to antidiuretic hormone for sensitivity to lypressin. • To administer a uniform, well-diffused spray, hold bottle upright with patient in vertical position holding head upright. • Instruct the patient to carry the medication with him at all times because of its fairly short duration.
None significant.	• Contraindicated in patients with closed epiphyses or intracranial lesions. Use with caution in patients with diabetes or family history of diabetes mellitus. Regular testing for glycosuria should be done. • Subcutaneous administration not recommended. • Concurrent thyroid hormone or androgen therapy may accelerate epiphyseal closure and limit duration of somatotropin treatment. • Monitor bone age progression annually. • Store powder at or below room temperature. • Reconstitute with 5 ml of bacteriostatic water per 10-IU vial. Refrigerate unused portion; discard after 1 month. Rotate injection sites.
Lithium, demeclocycline: reduced antidiuretic activity. Use together cautiously. *Chlorpropamide:* increased antidiuretic response. Use together cautiously.	• Contraindicated in chronic nephritis with nitrogen retention. Use cautiously in children, elderly persons, pregnant women, and patients with epilepsy, migraine, asthma, cardiovascular disease, or fluid overload. • Never inject vasopressin tannate in oil I.V. • Never inject during first stage of labor; may cause ruptured uterus. • Monitor specific gravity of urine. Monitor intake and output to aid evaluation of drug effectiveness. • Place tannate in oil in warm water for 10 to 15 minutes. Then shake thoroughly to make suspension uniform before withdrawing I.M. injection dose. Small brown particles must be seen in suspension. Use absolutely dry syringe to avoid dilution. • Give with 1 to 2 glasses of water to reduce side effects and to improve therapeutic response. • To prevent possible convulsions, coma, and death, observe patient closely for early signs of water intoxication. • Overhydration more likely with long-acting tannate oil suspension than with aqueous vasopressin solution. • Use minimum effective dose to reduce side effects. • May be used for transient polyuria due to antidiuretic hormone deficiency related to neurosurgery or head injury. • Synthetic desmopressin is sometimes preferred because of longer duration and less frequent side effects. • Question the patient with abdominal distention about passage of flatus and stool. • Monitor blood pressure of patient on vasopressin twice daily. Watch for excessively elevated blood pressure or lack of response to drug, which may be indicated by hypotension. • Use to expel gas before abdominal X-ray. To increase effectiveness, give enema before first dose, if ordered. • For treatment of anaphylaxis, see inside front cover.

Parathyroid and parathyroid-like agents

calcitonin (Salmon)
calcitriol
dihydrotachysterol (AT-10)
etidronate disodium
parathyroid hormone (PTH)

For information on calcifediol, see APPENDIX, *New Drugs*.

The major regulatory hormone of the parathyroid glands is parathyroid hormone (PTH); its secretion is indirectly related to the concentration of calcium ions in the blood. In humans, the serum calcium level is regulated within narrow limits (10 ± 1 mg/100 ml). A decrease in this concentration stimulates release of endogenous PTH that in turn lowers serum phosphate and raises serum calcium concentrations.

Calcitonin is a hormone secreted by the parafollicular cells of the thyroid gland. It immediately lowers higher-than-normal serum calcium levels.

Calcitriol and dihydrotachysterol, the activated forms of vitamin D, are like PTH in that they stimulate transport of calcium from bone to blood, raising serum calcium and lowering PTH.

Etidronate, a synthetic compound, acts primarily on the bones to lower serum calcium levels, but it has little effect on PTH levels.

The body has an exceptional capacity to ensure normal serum calcium levels. Normally, calcium homeostasis is regulated by the kidneys and gastrointestinal (GI) tract. Alternative regulating mechanisms may maintain homeostasis levels at the expense of bone.

Major uses

℞

- Calcitonin reduces serum calcium levels in acute hypercalcemia.
- Calcitonin and etidronate combat Paget's disease (osteitis deformans).
- Calcitriol is used to treat hypocalcemia in patients undergoing hemodialysis.
- Dihydrotachysterol is effective against hypocalcemia in renal failure.
- PTH is used in the diagnosis of hypoparathyroidism.

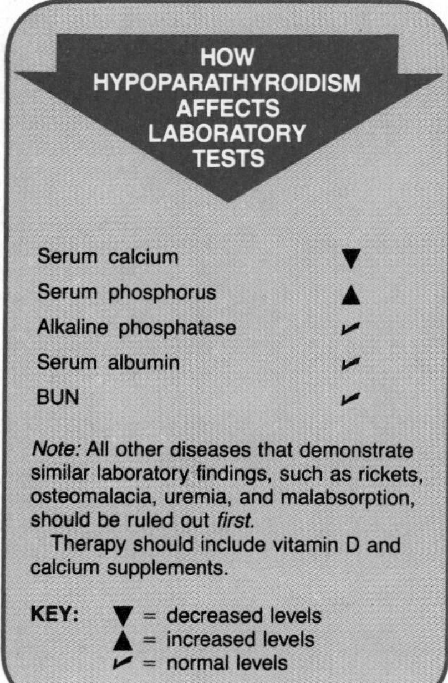

HOW HYPOPARATHYROIDISM AFFECTS LABORATORY TESTS
Serum calcium ▼
Serum phosphorus ▲
Alkaline phosphatase ✓
Serum albumin ✓
BUN ✓
Note: All other diseases that demonstrate similar laboratory findings, such as rickets, osteomalacia, uremia, and malabsorption, should be ruled out *first*.
Therapy should include vitamin D and calcium supplements.
KEY: ▼ = decreased levels
▲ = increased levels
✓ = normal levels

• Dihydrotachysterol and PTH combat hypocalcemia associated with hypoparathyroidism.

Mechanism of action

• Calcitonin and etidronate decrease osteoclastic activity by inhibiting osteocytic osteolysis. They also decrease mineral release and matrix or collagen breakdown in bone.
• Calcitriol and dihydrotachysterol stimulate calcium absorption from the GI tract and promote secretion of calcium from bone to blood, thereby raising serum calcium levels; they may also increase urinary excretion of inorganic phosphate.
• PTH enhances phosphate excretion by inhibiting renal tubular reabsorption of phosphate, mobilizing bone calcium and increasing GI absorption of calcium.

THYROIDECTOMY? CHECK POSTOPERATIVELY

In 100 patients with thyroidectomies, you may see one case of post-thyroidectomy hypoparathyroidism. The incidence of hypoparathyroidism is especially high in patients who have had radical thyroidectomy for cancer. Symptoms begin about 24 hours after surgery. To detect this disorder, watch for:

• Chvostek's or Trousseau's sign
• hypocalcemia
• dystonia
• choreoathetoid movement
• grand mal seizures
• tetany
• paresthesias (especially circumoral)
• impaired cognitive function
• depression
• psychological changes (especially in older patients) such as irritability and emotional lability.

Absorption, distribution, metabolism, and excretion

• Calcitonin and PTH are well absorbed after subcutaneous or I.M. administration. Because they're destroyed in the GI tract, they must be given parenterally. Calcitonin is metabolized by the kidneys and excreted in urine.
• Calcitriol, dihydrotachysterol, and etidronate are absorbed from the GI tract. Calcitriol and dihydrotachysterol are metabolized in the liver and eliminated—through the bile—in feces. Etidronate, as the unchanged drug, is primarily excreted in the urine; a small amount, however, is eliminated in feces.

Onset and duration

• Calcitonin's onset after I.V. administration is 15 minutes; its duration is 30 minutes to 12 hours. After I.M. or subcutaneous injection, onset is 4 hours and duration is 8 to 24 hours.
• Calcitriol becomes effective in about 2 hours. Maximal hypercalcemic effect of calcitriol occurs in 10 hours. Duration of action of this activated vitamin D is about 3 to 5 days.
• Dihydrotachysterol begins to work several hours after administration. Maximal hypercalcemic effect of this drug occurs within 1 week if a loading dose is used and within 2 weeks if a loading dose is not used. Serum calcium level drops markedly within 4 to 5 days after therapy is stopped, and the drug's effect completely disappears after 2 weeks.
• Etidronate begins to work after 1 to 3 months. Maximal therapeutic activity occurs in about 6 months.
• PTH, after I.M. or subcutaneous injection, raises serum calcium level within 4 hours; the level peaks in 12 to 18 hours. Duration of action is 20 to 24 hours.

After I.V. administration, PTH begins to work within 15 minutes, and serum calcium level rises in 1 hour. Duration of action is much shorter with I.V. administration than with the I.M. or subcutaneous form.

Combination products

None.

NAME	INDICATIONS & DOSAGE	SIDE EFFECTS
calcitonin (Salmon) Calcimar♦	*Paget's disease of bone (osteitis deformans)*— **Adults:** initially, 100 MRC units daily, S.C. or I.M. Maintenance: 50 to 100 units daily or every other day. *Hypercalcemia*— **Adults:** 100 to 400 MRC units I.M. once or twice daily.	**CNS:** headaches. **GI:** transient nausea with or without vomiting, diarrhea. **GU:** transient diuresis. **Metabolic:** hyperglycemia. **Local:** inflammation at injection site, skin rashes. **Other:** *facial flushing;* hypocalcemia; swelling, tingling, and tenderness of hands; unusual taste sensation; *anaphylaxis.*
calcitriol (1,25-dihydroxy-cholecalciferol) Rocaltrol	*Management of hypocalcemia in patients undergoing chronic dialysis*— **Adults:** initially, 0.25 mcg daily. Dosage may be increased by 0.25 mcg/day at 2- to 4-week intervals. Maintenance: 0.25 mcg every other day up to 0.5 to 1.25 mcg daily.	*Vitamin D intoxication associated with hypercalcemia:* **CNS:** headache, somnolence. **EENT:** conjunctivitis, photophobia, rhinorrhea. **GI:** nausea, vomiting, constipation, metallic taste, dry mouth. **GU:** polyuria. **Other:** weakness, bone and muscle pain.
dihydrotachysterol (AT-10) Hytakerol♦	*Familial hypophosphatemia*— **Adults and children:** 0.5 to 2 mg P.O. daily. Maintenance: 0.3 to 1.5 mg daily.	*Vitamin D intoxication associated with hypercalcemia:* **CNS:** headache, somnolence. **EENT:** conjunctivitis, photopho-

INTERACTIONS	NURSING CONSIDERATIONS
None significant.	• Contraindicated in allergy to gelatin diluent used to prepare drug. Not recommended for women who are or may become pregnant. Safe use in children not established. • Periodic serum alkaline phosphatase and 24-hour urine hydroxyproline levels should be determined to evaluate drug effect. • Skin test is usually done before beginning therapy. • Systemic allergic reactions possible since hormone is protein. Keep epinephrine on hand when giving parathyroid hormone. • Patients with good initial clinical response to calcitonin who suffer relapse should be evaluated for antibody formation response to the hormone protein. • Tell patient in whom calcitonin loses its hypocalcemic activity that further medication or increased dosages will be of no value. • Teach patient aseptic method of preparing and administering injection, and stress the importance of rotating injection sites. • Facial flushing and warmth occur in 20% to 30% of all patients within minutes of injection; usually last about 1 hour. Reassure patient that this is a transient effect. • Observe patient for signs of hypocalcemic tetany during therapy (muscle twitching, tetanic spasms, and convulsions if hypocalcemia is severe). • Monitor calcium levels closely. Watch for signs of hypercalcemic relapse: bone pain, renal calculi, polyuria, anorexia, nausea, vomiting, thirst, constipation, lethargy, bradycardia, muscle hypotonicity, pathologic fracture, psychosis, and coma. • Periodic examinations of urine sediment advisable. • Actually derived from the thyroid gland, not the parathyroid. • Refrigerate solution. • For treatment of anaphylaxis, see inside front cover.
None significant.	• Contraindicated in hypercalcemia or vitamin D toxicity. Withhold all preparations containing vitamin D. Not recommended in breast-feeding mothers. Use cautiously in patients on digitalis; hypercalcemia may precipitate cardiac arrhythmias. • Monitor serum calcium; serum calcium times serum phosphate should not exceed 70. During titration, determine serum levels twice weekly. If hypercalcemia occurs, discontinue, but resume after serum calcium level returns to normal. Patient should receive adequate daily intake of calcium, 1,000 mg RDA. • Protect from heat and light. • Tell patient to adhere to diet and calcium supplementation and avoid nonprescription drugs, especially vitamin D–containing multivitamins. • Patients should not use magnesium-containing antacids or candy-type antacids, especially Rolaids or Tums, while taking this drug. • Patients should report to doctor immediately any of the following symptoms: weakness, nausea, vomiting, dry mouth, constipation, muscle or bone pain, or metallic taste—early symptoms of vitamin D intoxication. • Tell patient that, although this drug is a vitamin, it must not be taken by anyone for whom it was not prescribed due to its potentially serious toxicities. • Most potent form of vitamin D available.
None significant.	• Contraindicated in hypercalcemia, hypocalcemia associated with renal insufficiency and hyperphosphatemia, renal stones, hypersensitivity to vitamin D, and in breast-feeding mothers. • Monitor serum and urine calcium levels. Watch for signs of hyper-

(continued on following page)

NAME	INDICATIONS & DOSAGE	SIDE EFFECTS
dihydrotachysterol *(continued)*	*Hypocalcemia associated with hypoparathyroidism and pseudohypoparathyroidism*— **Adults:** initially, 0.8 to 2.4 mg P.O. daily for several days. Maintenance: 0.2 to 2 mg daily, as required for normal serum calcium levels. Average dose 0.6 mg daily. **Children:** initially, 1 to 5 mg for several days. Maintenance: 0.5 to 1.5 mg daily, as required for normal serum calcium levels. *Renal osteodystrophy in chronic uremia*— **Adults:** 0.1 to 0.6 mg P.O. daily.	bia, rhinorrhea. **GI:** nausea, vomiting, constipation, metallic taste, dry mouth. **GU:** polyuria. **Other:** weakness, bone and muscle pain.
etidronate disodium Didronel	*Symptomatic Paget's disease*— **Adults:** 5 mg/kg/day P.O. as a single dose 2 hours before a meal with water or juice. Patient should not eat for 2 hours after dose. May give up to 10 mg/kg/day in severe cases. Maximum dose 20 mg/kg/day. *Heterotrophic ossification in spinal cord injuries*— **Adults:** 20 mg/kg/day for 2 weeks, then 10 mg/kg/day for 10 weeks. Total treatment period 12 weeks.	**GI:** (seen most frequently at 20 mg/kg/day) diarrhea, increased frequency of bowel movements, nausea. **Other:** increased or recurrent bone pain at pagetic sites, pain at previously asymptomatic sites, increased risk of fracture, elevated serum phosphate.
parathyroid hormone (PTH) Para-thor-mone, Paroidin	*Acute hypoparathyroidism with tetany*— **Adults:** 20 to 40 units S.C., I.M., or I.V. q 12 hours. **Infants:** (with transient congenital idiopathic true hypoparathyroidism) 25 to 50 units I.M. q 12 hours for 1 to 3 days.	**Allergic:** *anaphylactic reactions* (parathyroid hormone is a foreign protein). **CNS:** headache, vertigo. **GI:** anorexia, nausea, vomiting, abdominal cramps, diarrhea. **Other:** hypercalcemia (muscle weakness, bone and flank pain), lethargy, tinnitus, ataxia.

◆ Available in U.S. and Canada. ◆◆ Available in Canada only. All other products (no symbol) available in U.S. only. Italicized side effects are common or life-threatening.

INTERACTIONS	NURSING CONSIDERATIONS
	calcemia. • Adequate dietary calcium intake is necessary; usually supplemented with 10 to 15 g oral calcium lactate or gluconate daily. • Report hypercalcemia reactions to doctor. Early signs of hypercalcemia include thirst, headache, vertigo, tinnitus, anorexia. • 1 mg equal to 120,000 units ergocalciferol (vitamin D_2). • Store in tightly closed, light-resistant containers. Don't refrigerate.
None significant.	• Use cautiously in enterocolitis, impaired renal function. • Therapy should not last more than 6 months. After 3 months, resume if needed. Don't give longer than 3 months at doses above 10 mg/kg/day. • Don't give drug with food, milk, or antacids; may reduce absorption. • Monitor renal function before and during therapy. • Monitor drug effect by serum alkaline phosphatase and urinary hydroxyproline excretion (both lowered if therapy effective). • Tell patient that improvement may not occur for up to 3 months but may continue for months after drug is stopped. Stress importance of good nutrition, especially diet high in calcium and vitamin D.
None significant.	• Contraindicated in hypercalcemia, hypercalciuria, and tetany unrelated to parathyroid failure; and by I.V. administration when serum calcium levels are above normal. Use cautiously in sarcoidosis, renal or cardiac disease, and in digitalized patients. • Rarely used because calcium salts often effective alone. • Subcutaneous injections may produce moderate inflammatory reaction. • Therapy lasts only a few days; patients may soon become refractory to treatment due to parathyroid-initiated production of antihormone antibodies. • If given I.V., skin-test for sensitivity. If positive, desensitize patient. • Keep epinephrine injection on hand when giving parathyroid hormone. • Monitor serum calcium and serum phosphate levels, intake and output. • Know and watch for signs of hypoparathyroidism and calcium deficiency. Test for Chvostek's and Trousseau's signs. Watch for drug-induced hypercalcemia. • Use seizure precautions in patients with calcium deficiency: padded rails, soft light, no irritating noises until normal calcium level is restored. • Do not dilute with saline solution, as a precipitate will form. • Store ampuls at 2° to 8° C. (36° to 46° F.); do not freeze. • For treatment of anaphylaxis, see inside front cover.

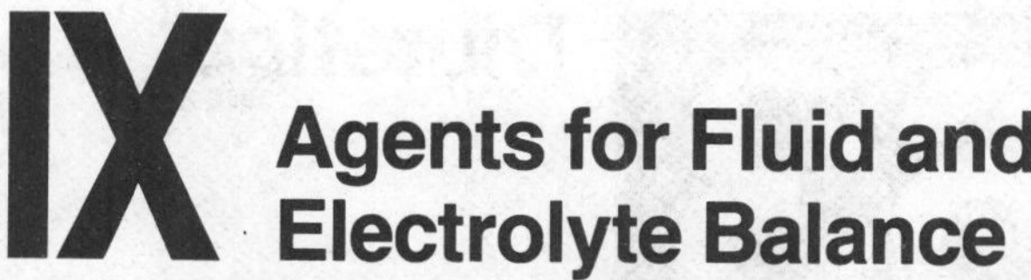

IX Agents for Fluid and Electrolyte Balance

Diuretics

Thiazide diuretics
bendroflumethiazide
benzthiazide
chlorothiazide
cyclothiazide
hydrochlorothiazide
hydroflumethiazide
methyclothiazide
polythiazide
trichlormethiazide

Thiazide-like diuretics
chlorthalidone
metolazone
quinethazone

Loop diuretics
ethacrynate sodium
ethacrynic acid
furosemide

Carbonic anhydrase inhibitors
acetazolamide
acetazolamide sodium
dichlorphenamide
ethoxzolamide
methazolamide

Miscellaneous diuretics
mannitol
mercaptomerin sodium
spironolactone
triamterene
urea

(The diuretics are listed in alphabetical order in the tables that follow. For information on amiloride, see APPENDIX, *New Drugs*.)

Diuretics reduce the body's total volume of water and salt by increasing their urinary excretion. This occurs mainly because diuretics impair sodium chloride reabsorption in the renal tubules. Diuretics can be classified according to chemical structure (thiazide and thiazide-like drugs), location of salt- and water-depleting effect on the kidney's nephrons (loop diuretics), and pharmacologic activity (carbonic anhydrase inhibitors and miscellaneous drugs with other mechanisms).

Major uses

The matrix on the opposite page indicates the major uses of the diuretics.

Mechanism of action

• The thiazide and thiazide-like diuretics increase urinary excretion of sodium and water by inhibiting sodium reabsorption in the cortical diluting site of the ascending loop of Henle. They also increase urinary excretion of chloride, potassium, and—to a lesser extent—bicarbonate ions.
• Loop diuretics inhibit reabsorption of sodium and chloride at the proximal portion of the ascending loop of Henle, enhancing water excretion. These very potent diuretics can be effective in patients with markedly reduced glomerular filtration rates (in whom other diuretics usually fail).
• Carbonic anhydrase inhibitors, by enzymatic blocking, promote renal excretion of sodium, potassium, bicarbonate, and water. Bicarbonate-ion excretion makes the urine alkaline; blood bicarbonate levels are accord-

Rx MAJOR USES OF DIURETICS

	thiazide diuretics	thiazide-like diuretics	loop diuretics	carbonic anhydrase inhibitors	mannitol	mercaptomerin	spironolactone	triamterene	urea
Treatment of essential hypertension	•	•	•			•	•	•	
Treatment of edema associated with congestive heart failure, cirrhosis of liver, and renal disease	•	•	•			•	•	•	
Treatment of pulmonary edema			•						
Reduction of intracranial pressure in hydrocephalus				•	•				•
Reduction of intraocular pressure				•	•				•
Treatment of open-angle glaucoma (as adjunct)				•					
Prophylaxis for epilepsy (as adjunct)				•					
Treatment of primary aldosteronism							•		
Potentiation of effects of mercurial diuretics				•					

ingly reduced, leading to metabolic acidosis. In this condition, the carbonic anhydrase inhibitors become less effective as diuretics. (Carbonic anhydrase inhibitors also decrease secretion of aqueous humor in the eye, thereby lowering intraocular pressure, but this mechanism is unrelated to their diuretic action.)

• Among miscellaneous diuretics, mannitol increases the osmotic pressure of glomerular filtrate, inhibiting tubular reabsorption of water and electrolytes.

Mercaptomerin works mainly in the ascending limb of the loop of Henle where the mercuric (Hg^{++}) ion interferes with renal tubular transport of chloride. During the ensuing diuresis, sodium, chloride, and water are excreted without profound potassium depletion. Diuresis is enhanced by acidifying agents.

Spironolactone antagonizes the hormone aldosterone at the distal tubule, increasing excretion of sodium and water but sparing potassium.

Triamterene depresses sodium reabsorption and potassium secretion by direct action on the distal segment of the uriniferous tubule. This reduces potassium excretion.

Urea rapidly increases blood tonicity, which results in passage of fluid from the tissue (including the brain) to the blood.

Absorption, distribution, metabolism, and excretion

• Thiazides and thiazide-like diuretics are all well absorbed from the gastrointestinal (GI) tract, well distributed

COMPARING THIAZIDE AND THIAZIDE-LIKE DIURETICS

DIURETIC	EQUIVALENT DOSE (mg)	MAXIMUM DAILY DOSE (mg)	DURATION OF ACTION (hr)
Thiazide			
bendroflumethiazide	5	20	18 to 24
benzthiazide	50	200	12 to 18
chlorothiazide	500	1,000	6 to 12
cyclothiazide	2	6	24 to 36
hydrochlorothiazide	50	200	12
hydroflumethiazide	50	200	10 to 12
methyclothiazide	5	10	24
polythiazide	2	4	24 to 36
trichlormethiazide	2	4	24
Thiazide-like			
chlorthalidone	50	200	48 to 72
metolazone	5	20	12 to 24
quinethazone	50	200	18 to 24

Many thiazides have been developed since chlorothiazide (Diuril) was introduced in 1958. Chemical derivatives of the thiazides are known as thiazide-like diuretics. Closely related pharmacologically, thiazides and thiazide-like diuretics are used to treat edema and essential hypertension.

All have similar mechanisms of action and side effects, as well as similar therapeutic effects, under most clinical conditions. Their durations of action, however, may differ. Those that act for 24 hours can be given once daily, promoting patient compliance.

to the body tissues, and excreted primarily unchanged in urine.

- Among loop diuretics ethacrynic acid is rapidly absorbed after oral administration, metabolized in the liver, and excreted by the kidneys. Ethacrynate sodium is administered parenterally. Its metabolism and excretion are the same as ethacrynic acid's.

Furosemide is partially (about 60%) absorbed from the GI tract; a small amount is metabolized. Both metabolite and unchanged drug are excreted in urine.

- Carbonic anhydrase inhibitors are absorbed from the GI tract after oral administration and are distributed throughout body tissue.

Acetazolamide is excreted unchanged in urine, but other carbonic anhydrase inhibitors are partially metabolized and eliminated in both urine and feces.

- Among miscellaneous diuretics, mannitol remains in the extracellular fluid, is filtered by the glomeruli, and is excreted unchanged in urine.

Mercaptomerin is completely absorbed after I.M. or subcutaneous injection, distributed mainly to the kidneys, metabolized in the liver, and excreted almost entirely in urine.

Spironolactone is absorbed from the GI tract, distributed to body tissues, metabolized in the liver, and eliminated in both urine and feces.

Triamterene is absorbed from the GI tract, partially bound to plasma proteins, distributed to body tissues, and rapidly excreted unchanged in urine.

Urea is well absorbed after oral administration, but it's seldom given orally because of its unpleasant taste. After I.V. administration, it's distributed to intracellular and extracellular fluids, including cerebrospinal fluid. It's hydrolyzed in the GI tract by bacterial ureases and excreted by the kidneys.

Onset and duration

- Thiazides and thiazide-like diuretics begin to act 1 to 2 hours after oral

DIURETICS: PRINCIPAL SITES OF ACTION

Diuretics increase the urinary excretion of water and salt by impairing sodium chloride reabsorption in the renal tubules.

NEPHRON UNIT

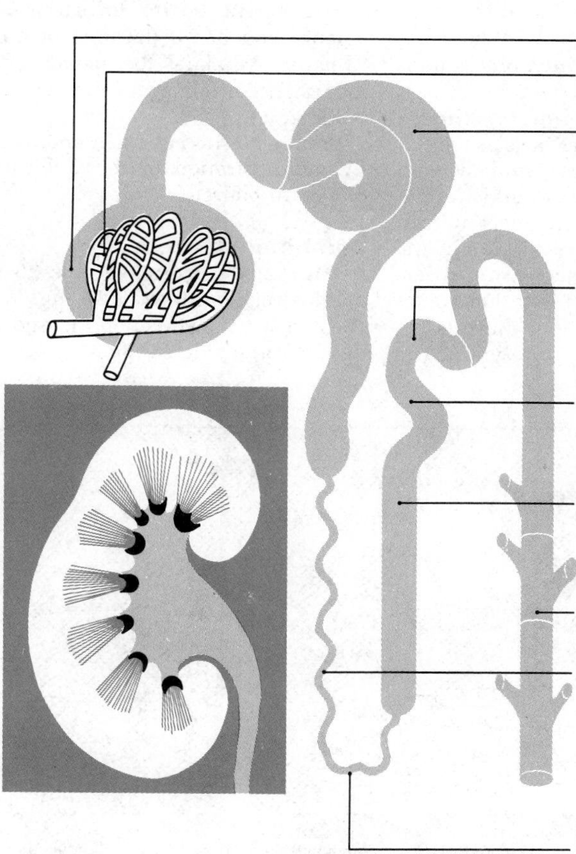

Bowman's capsule
Glomerulus
Proximal convoluted tubule *(carbonic anhydrase inhibitors, mannitol, urea)*
Distal convoluted tubule *(spironolactone, triamterene)*
Renal cortical diluting site *(thiazides, thiazide-like diuretics)*
Ascending loop *(loop diuretics, mercaptomerin sodium)*
Collecting tubule duct
Descending loop
Loop of Henle

administration. Most of them have a duration of action of 12 to 24 hours, but several act as long as 36 to 72 hours (see chart, above left). Intravenous chlorothiazide takes effect within 15 minutes after administration and has a duration of 2 hours.

• Among loop diuretics, ethacrynic acid begins to act 30 minutes after oral administration and has a duration of up to 12 hours. Ethacrynate sodium, after I.V. administration, begins to act within 5 minutes. Its duration is 2 hours.

Furosemide, after oral administration, begins to act in 30 to 60 minutes and has a duration of 6 to 8 hours. After I.V. administration, its onset occurs within 5 minutes, and it has a duration of 2 hours. After I.M. injection, it begins to act within 30 minutes and has a duration of 6 to 8 hours.

• Carbonic anhydrase inhibitors begin to act 1 to 3 hours after oral administration and have a duration of 8 to 12 hours. Acetazolamide (timed-release form), however, acts as long as 24 hours, and methazolamide acts up to 18 hours. After I.V. administration, acetazolamide has an onset within 2 minutes and a duration of 4 to 5 hours.

• Among miscellaneous diuretics, mannitol begins to act 15 to 30 minutes after I.V. administration; diuresis occurs in 1 to 3 hours. Duration is 4 to 6 hours, but it may reduce cerebrospinal fluid pressure for up to 8 hours.

Mercaptomerin begins to act 1 to 3 hours after I.M. or subcutaneous injection; its duration is 12 to 24 hours.

Spironolactone's onset occurs gradually over 2 to 3 days, but a loading dose may be used for faster effect. The drug continues to act for 2 to 3 days.

Triamterene begins to act in 2 to 4 hours and has a duration of up to 24 hours. Maximal therapeutic effect may not occur during the first few days of therapy.

Urea begins to act 1 to 2 hours after I.V. administration and has a duration of 3 to 10 hours.

Combination products

ALDACTAZIDE♦: spironolactone 25 mg and hydrochlorothiazide 25 mg.

DYAZIDE♦: triamterene 50 mg and hydrochlorothiazide 25 mg.

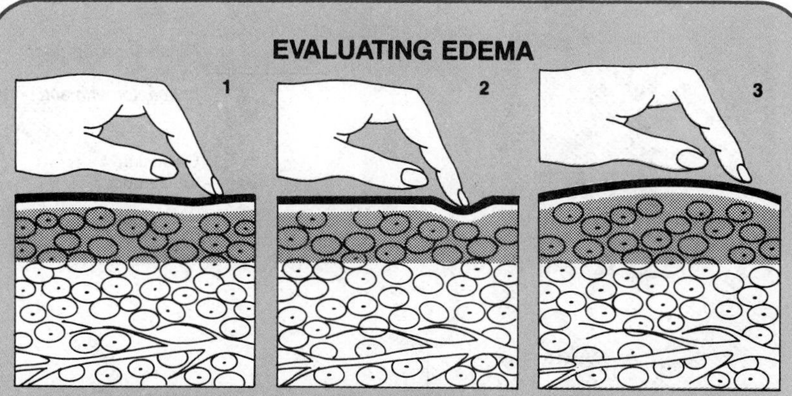

An adult patient can accumulate up to 4.5 kg (10 lb) of fluid before a pit can be detected. The skin pits against a bony surface, such as the subcutaneous aspect of the tibia, fibula, sacrum, or sternum. Pitting edema is evaluated on a 4-point scale: from +1 (a barely detectable pit, illustration 1) to +4 (a deep and persistent pit, approximately 1″ or 25.4 mm deep, illustration 2).

Edema can become so severe that pitting is not possible: the tissue becomes so full that fluid can't be displaced. Subcutaneous tissue becomes fibrotic; as a result, the surface tissue feels rock hard. In time, this condition can develop into brawny edema (illustration 3). For example, a patient who has had a mastectomy and whose axillary nodes have been removed may develop brawny edema in her affected arm. The patient's skin looks like a pig's skin, and her arm feels hard or gelatinous. Brawny edema can also indicate lymphatic obstruction. Protect all edematous extremities from injury. Edema makes the skin prone to sloughing and ulceration.

PATIENT-TEACHING AID

GUIDE TO POTASSIUM-RICH FOODS

Dear Patient:

If your doctor has ordered potassium-depleting diuretics, he may ask you to increase your dietary intake of potassium. Symptoms of lowered potassium include muscle cramps (especially in the legs), muscle weakness, paralysis, spasms, and dizziness when standing up quickly. If these symptoms persist after adding potassium to your diet, consult the doctor.

MEATS	mg per 100g (3½ oz)
Beef	370
Chicken	411
Lamb	290
Liver	380
Pork	326
Turkey	411
Veal	500

FRUITS	mg per 100 g
Apricots	281
Bananas	370
Dates	648
Figs	152
Nectarines	294
Oranges	200
Peaches	202
Plums	299
Prunes	262
Raisins	355

FISH	mg per 100 g
Bass	256
Flounder	342
Haddock	348
Halibut	525
Oysters	203
Perch	284
Salmon	421
Sardines, canned	590
Scallops	476
Tuna	301

VEGETABLES	mg per 100 g
Asparagus	238
Brussel sprouts	295
Cabbage	233
Carrots	341
Endive	294
Lima beans	394
Peppers	213
Potatoes	407
Radishes	322
Spinach	324
Sweet potatoes	300

MISCELLANEOUS	mg per 100 g
Gingersnap cookies	462
Graham crackers	384
Oatmeal cookies (with raisins	370
Ice milk	195
Milk, dry (nonfat solids)	1,745
Molasses (light)	917
Peanuts	674
Peanut butter	670

JUICES	mg per 100 g
Orange, fresh or	200
reconstituted	186
Tomato	227

NAME	INDICATIONS & DOSAGE	SIDE EFFECTS
acetazolamide Acetazolam♦♦, Diamox♦, Diamox Sequels♦, Hydrazol **acetazolamide sodium** Diamox Parenteral♦	*Narrow-angle glaucoma—* **Adults:** 250 mg q 4 hours; or 250 mg b.i.d. P.O., I.M., or I.V. for short-term therapy. *Edema, in congestive heart failure—* **Adults:** 250 to 375 mg P.O., I.M., or I.V. daily in a.m. **Children:** 5 mg/kg daily in a.m. *Epilepsy—* **Children:** 8 to 30 mg/kg daily P.O., I.M., or I.V. in divided doses. *Open-angle glaucoma—* **Adults:** 250 mg daily to 1 g P.O., I.M., or I.V. divided q.i.d.	**Blood:** *aplastic anemia,* hemolytic anemia, leukopenia. **CNS:** drowsiness, paresthesias. **EENT:** transient myopia. **GI:** nausea, vomiting, anorexia. **GU:** crystalluria, renal calculi. **Metabolic:** *hyperchloremic acidosis,* hypokalemia, asymptomatic hyperuricemia **Skin:** rash.
bendroflumethiazide Naturetin♦	*Edema, hypertension—* **Adults:** 5 to 20 mg P.O. daily or b.i.d. in divided doses. **Children:** initially, 0.1 to 0.4 mg/kg daily in 1 or 2 doses. Maintenance: 0.05 to 0.1 mg/kg daily in 1 or 2 doses.	**Blood:** *aplastic anemia, agranulocytosis,* leukopenia, thrombocytopenia. **CV:** *volume depletion and dehydration,* orthostatic hypotension. **GI:** anorexia, nausea, pancreatitis. **Hepatic:** hepatic encephalopathy. **Metabolic:** *hypokalemia, asymptomatic hyperuricemia, hyperglycemia and impairment of glucose tolerance,* fluid and electrolyte imbalances including dilutional hyponatremia and hypochloremia, metabolic alkalosis, hypercalcemia, gout. **Skin:** dermatitis, photosensitivity, rash. **Other:** hypersensitivity reactions such as pneumonitis and vasculitis.
benzthiazide Aquapres, Aqua-Scrip, Aquasec, Aquatag, Diretic, Exna♦, Hydrex, Lemazide, Marazide, Proaqua, Rid-ema, S-Aqua, Urazide	*Edema—* **Adults:** 50 to 200 mg P.O. daily or in divided doses. **Children:** 1 to 4 mg/kg daily in 3 divided doses. *Hypertension—* **Adults:** 50 mg P.O. daily b.i.d., t.i.d., or q.i.d., adjusted to patient's response.	**Blood:** *aplastic anemia, agranulocytosis,* leukopenia, thrombocytopenia. **CV:** *volume depletion and dehydration,* orthostatic hypotension. **GI:** anorexia, nausea, pancreatitis. **Hepatic:** hepatic encephalopathy. **Metabolic:** *hypokalemia, asymptomatic hyperuricemia, hypergly-*

♦ Available in U.S. and Canada. ♦♦ Available in Canada only. All other products (no symbol) available in U.S. only. Italicized side effects are common or life-threatening.

INTERACTIONS	NURSING CONSIDERATIONS
None significant.	• Contraindicated in long-term therapy for chronic noncongestive narrow-angle glaucoma; also in depressed sodium or potassium serum levels, renal or hepatic disease or dysfunction, adrenal gland failure, and hyperchloremic acidosis. Use cautiously in respiratory acidosis, emphysema, chronic pulmonary disease, or patients receiving other diuretics. • Monitor intake/output and electrolytes, especially serum potassium. When used in diuretic therapy, consult with doctor and dietitian to provide high-potassium diet. • Weigh patient daily. Rapid weight loss may cause hypotension. • Diuretic effect decreased when acidosis occurs but can be reestablished by withdrawing drug for several days and then restarting, or by using intermittent administration schedules. • Reconstitute 500-mg vial with at least 5 ml sterile water for injection. Use within 24 hours of reconstitution. • I.M. injection painful because of alkalinity of solution. Direct I.V. administration preferred (100 to 500 mg/minute). • Elderly patients are especially susceptible to excessive diuresis. • May cause false-positive urine protein tests by alkalinizing the urine. • A carbonic anhydrase inhibitor. Its acidotic effects limit usefulness for daily treatment of edema.
Cholestyramine, colestipol: intestinal absorption of thiazides decreased. Keep doses as separate as possible. *Diazoxide:* increased antihypertensive, hyperglycemic, hyperuricemic effects. Use together cautiously.	• Contraindicated in anuria and in hypersensitivity to other thiazides or other sulfonamide-derived drugs. Use cautiously in severe renal disease and impaired hepatic function. • Monitor intake/output, weight, and serum electrolytes regularly. Monitor serum creatinine and BUN levels regularly. Not effective if these levels are more than twice normal. • Monitor serum potassium levels; consult with doctor and dietitian to provide high-potassium diet. Watch for signs of hypokalemia (for example, muscle weakness, cramps). Patients on digitalis have an increased risk of digitalis toxicity due to potassium-depleting side effect of this diuretic. May use with potassium-sparing diuretic to prevent potassium loss. • Foods rich in potassium include citrus fruits, bananas, tomatoes, dates, and apricots. • Monitor blood sugar. Check insulin requirements in patients with diabetes. May treat severe hyperglycemia with oral antidiabetic agents. • Monitor blood uric acid levels, especially in patients with a history of gout. • Give in a.m. to prevent nocturia. • Elderly patients are especially susceptible to excessive diuresis. • In hypertension, therapeutic response may be delayed several days. • A thiazide diuretic. • Thiazides should be discontinued before tests for parathyroid function are performed.
Cholestyramine, colestipol: intestinal absorption of thiazides decreased. Keep doses as separate as possible. *Diazoxide:* increased antihypertensive, hyperglycemic,	• Contraindicated in anuria; hypersensitivity to other thiazides or other sulfonamide-derived drugs. Use cautiously in severe renal disease, impaired hepatic function. • Monitor intake/output, weight, and serum electrolytes regularly. Monitor serum potassium levels; consult with doctor and dietitian to provide high-potassium diet. Watch for signs of hypokalemia (for example, muscle weakness, cramps). Patients on digitalis have an increased risk of digitalis toxicity due to the potassium-depleting side effect of this diuretic. May use with potassium-sparing diuretic to

(continued on following page)

NAME	INDICATIONS & DOSAGE	SIDE EFFECTS
benzthiazide *(continued)*		*cemia and impairment of glucose tolerance,* fluid and electrolyte imbalances including dilutional hyponatremia and hypochloremia, metabolic alkalosis, hypercalcemia, gout. **Skin:** dermatitis, photosensitivity, rash. **Other:** hypersensitivity reactions such as pneumonitis and vasculitis.
chlorothiazide Diuril♦, Ro-Chlorozide, SK-Chlorothiazide	*Diuresis—* **Children over 6 months:** 20 mg/kg P.O. or I.V. daily in divided doses. **Children under 6 months:** may require 30 mg/kg P.O. or I.V. daily in 2 divided doses. *Edema, hypertension—* **Adults:** 500 mg to 2 g P.O. or I.V. daily or in 2 divided doses.	**Blood:** *aplastic anemia, agranulocytosis,* leukopenia, thrombocytopenia. **CV:** *volume depletion and dehydration,* orthostatic hypotension. **GI:** anorexia, nausea, pancreatitis. **Hepatic:** hepatic encephalopathy. **Metabolic:** *hypokalemia, asymptomatic hyperuricemia, hyperglycemia and impairment of glucose tolerance,* fluid and electrolyte imbalances including dilutional hyponatremia and hypochloremia, metabolic alkalosis, hypercalcemia, gout. **Skin:** dermatitis, photosensitivity, rash. **Other:** hypersensitivity reactions such as pneumonitis and vasculitis.
chlorthalidone Hygroton♦, Novothalidone♦♦, Uridon♦♦	*Edema, hypertension—* **Adults:** 25 to 100 mg P.O. daily, or 100 mg 3 times weekly or on alternate days. Occasionally, up to 200 mg daily may be needed. **Children:** 2 mg/kg P.O. 3 times weekly.	**Blood:** *aplastic anemia, agranulocytosis,* leukopenia, thrombocytopenia. **CV:** *volume depletion and dehydration,* orthostatic hypotension. **GI:** anorexia, nausea, pancreatitis. **Hepatic:** hepatic encephalopathy. **Metabolic:** *hypokalemia, asymptomatic hyperuricemia, hyperglycemia and impairment of glucose*

INTERACTIONS	NURSING CONSIDERATIONS
hyperuricemic effects. Use together cautiously.	prevent potassium loss. • Foods rich in potassium include citrus fruits, bananas, tomatoes, dates, and apricots. • Monitor serum creatinine and BUN levels regularly. Not effective if these levels are more than twice normal. • Monitor blood sugar. Check insulin requirements in patients with diabetes. May treat severe hyperglycemia with oral antidiabetic agents. • Monitor blood uric acid levels, especially in patients with a history of gout. • Give in a.m. to prevent nocturia. • Elderly patients are especially susceptible to excessive diuresis. • In hypertension, therapeutic response may be delayed several days. • A thiazide diuretic.
Cholestyramine, colestipol: intestinal absorption of thiazides decreased. Keep doses as separate as possible. *Diazoxide:* increased antihypertensive, hyperglycemic, hyperuricemic effects. Use together cautiously.	• Contraindicated in anuria; hypersensitivity to other thiazides or other sulfonamide-derived drugs; impaired hepatic function; progressive hepatic disease. Use cautiously in severe renal disease. • Monitor intake/output, weight, and serum electrolytes regularly. • Monitor potassium levels; consult with doctor and dietitian to provide high-potassium diet. Watch for signs of hypokalemia (for example, muscle weakness, cramps). Patients on digitalis have an increased risk of digitalis toxicity due to the potassium-depleting effect of the diuretic. May use with potassium-sparing diuretic to prevent potassium loss. • Foods rich in potassium include citrus fruits, tomatoes, bananas, dates, and apricots. • Monitor blood sugar. Check insulin requirements in patients with diabetes. May treat severe hyperglycemia with oral antidiabetic agents. • Monitor serum creatinine and BUN levels regularly. Not effective if these levels are more than twice normal. • Monitor blood uric acid levels, especially in patients with a history of gout. • Watch for decreased calcium excretion, progressive renal impairment. • Only injectable thiazide. For I.V. use only—not I.M. or subcutaneous. Reconstitute with 18 ml of sterile water for injection/500 mg vial. May store reconstituted solutions at room temperature up to 24 hours. Compatible with intravenous dextrose or sodium chloride solutions. • Avoid I.V. infiltration; can be very painful. • Give in a.m. to prevent nocturia. • In hypertension, therapeutic response may be delayed several days. • Elderly patients are especially susceptible to excessive diuresis. • A thiazide diuretic. • The only thiazide available in liquid form. • Thiazides should be stopped before tests for parathyroid function are performed.
Cholestyramine, colestipol: intestinal absorption of thiazides decreased. Keep doses as separate as possible. *Diazoxide:* increased antihypertensive, hyperglycemic, hyperuricemic ef-	• Contraindicated in anuria; hypersensitivity to thiazides or other sulfonamide-derived drugs. Use cautiously in severe renal disease, progressive hepatic disease, impaired hepatic function. • Monitor intake/output, weight, and serum electrolytes regularly. • Monitor serum potassium levels; consult with doctor and dietitian to provide high-potassium diet. Watch for signs of hypokalemia (for example, muscle weakness, cramps). Patients on digitalis have an increased risk of digitalis toxicity due to the potassium-depleting effect on this diuretic. May use with potassium-sparing diuretic to prevent potassium loss.

(continued on following page)

NAME	INDICATIONS & DOSAGE	SIDE EFFECTS
chlorthalidone *(continued)*		*tolerance,* fluid and electrolyte imbalances including dilutional hyponatremia and hypochloremia, metabolic alkalosis, hypercalcemia, gout. **Skin:** dermatitis, photosensitivity, rash. **Other:** hypersensitivity reactions such as pneumonitis and vasculitis.
cyclothiazide Anhydron	*Edema—* **Adults:** 1 to 2 mg P.O. daily. May be used on alternate days as maintenance dose. **Children:** 0.02 to 0.04 mg/kg P.O. daily. *Hypertension—* **Adults:** 2 mg P.O. daily; up to 2 mg b.i.d. or t.i.d.	**Blood:** *aplastic anemia, agranulocytosis,* leukopenia, thrombocytopenia. **CV:** *volume depletion and dehydration,* orthostatic hypotension. **GI:** anorexia, nausea, pancreatitis. **Hepatic:** hepatic encephalopathy. **Metabolic:** *hypokalemia, asymptomatic hyperuricemia, hyperglycemia and impairment of glucose tolerance,* fluid and electrolyte imbalances including dilutional hyponatremia and hypochloremia, metabolic alkalosis, hypercalcemia, gout. **Skin:** dermatitis, photosensitivity, rash. **Other:** hypersensitivity reactions such as pneumonitis and vasculitis.
dichlorphenamide Daranide♦, Oratrol	*Adjunct in glaucoma—* **Adults:** initially, 100 to 200 mg P.O., followed by 100 mg q 12 hours until desired response obtained. Maintenance: 25 to 50 mg P.O. daily b.i.d. or t.i.d. Give miotics concomitantly.	**Blood:** *aplastic anemia,* hemolytic anemia, leukopenia. **CNS:** drowsiness, paresthesias. **EENT:** transient myopia. **GI:** nausea, vomiting, anorexia. **GU:** crystalluria, renal calculi. **Metabolic:** *hyperchloremic acidosis,* hypokalemia, asymptomatic hyperuricemia. **Skin:** rash.
ethacrynate sodium Sodium Edecrin	*Acute pulmonary edema—* **Adults:** 50 to 100 mg of etha-	**Blood:** *agranulocytosis,* thrombocytopenia.

♦ Available in U.S. and Canada. ♦♦ Available in Canada only. All other products (no symbol) available in U.S. only. Italicized side effects are common or life-threatening.

INTERACTIONS	NURSING CONSIDERATIONS
fects. Use together cautiously.	• Focds rich in potassium include citrus fruits, tomatoes, bananas, dates, and apricots. • Monitor serum creatinine and BUN levels regularly. Not effective if these levels are more than twice normal. • Monitor blood uric acid levels, especially in patients with a history of gout. • Monitor blood sugar. Check insulin requirements in patients with diabetes. May treat severe hyperglycemia with oral antidiabetic agents. • In hypertension, therapeutic response may be delayed several days. • Give in a.m. to prevent nocturia. • Elderly patients are especially susceptible to excessive diuresis. • A thiazide-like diuretic.
Cholestyramine, colestipol: intestinal absorption of thiazides decreased. Keep doses as separate as possible. *Diazoxide:* increased antihypertensive, hyperglycemic, hyperuricemic effects. Use together cautiously.	• Contraindicated in anuria; hypersensitivity to other thiazides or other sulfonamide-derived drugs. Use cautiously in severe renal disease, impaired hepatic function, progressive hepatic disease. • Monitor intake/output, weight, and serum electrolytes regularly. • Monitor serum potassium levels; consult with doctor and dietitian to provide high-potassium diet. Watch for signs of hypokalemia (for example, muscle weakness, cramps). Patients on digitalis have an increased risk of digitalis toxicity due to the potassium-depleting effect of this diuretic. May use with potassium-sparing diuretic to prevent potassium loss. • Foods rich in potassium include citrus fruits, tomatoes, bananas, dates, and apricots. • Monitor blood sugar. Check insulin requirements in patients with diabetes. May treat severe hyperglycemia with oral antidiabetic agents. • Monitor serum creatinine and BUN levels regularly. Not effective if these levels are more than twice normal. • Monitor blood uric acid levels, especially in patients with a history of gout. • In hypertension, therapeutic response may be delayed several days. • Give in a.m. to prevent nocturia. • Elderly patients are especially susceptible to excessive diuresis. • A thiazide diuretic.
None significant.	• Contraindicated in hepatic insufficiency, renal failure, adrenocortical insufficiency, hyperchloremic acidosis, depressed sodium or potassium levels, severe pulmonary obstruction with inability to increase alveolar ventilation, Addison's disease. Long-term use contraindicated in severe, absolute, or chronic noncongestive narrow-angle glaucoma. Use cautiously in respiratory acidosis, monitoring blood pH and blood gases. • Monitor electrolytes, especially serum potassium in initial treatment. Usually no problem in long-term glaucoma therapy unless risk for hypokalemia from other causes; potassium supplements may be necessary. • May cause false-positive results in urine protein tests. • Anticipate that drug will be given every day for glaucoma but intermittently for edema. • Evaluate patient with glaucoma for eye pain to make sure drug is effective in decreasing intraocular pressure. • A carbonic anhydrase inhibitor.
Aminoglycoside antibiotics: potentiated	• Contraindicated in patients with anuria and in infants. Use cautiously in electrolyte abnormalities. If electrolyte imbalance, azo-

(continued on following page)

NAME	INDICATIONS & DOSAGE	SIDE EFFECTS
ethacrynate sodium *(continued)* **ethacrynic acid** Edecrin♦	crynate sodium I.V. slowly over several minutes. *Edema—* **Adults:** 50 to 200 mg P.O. daily. Refractory cases may require up to 200 mg b.i.d. **Children:** initial dose 25 mg P.O., cautiously, increased in 25 mg increments daily until desired effect is obtained.	**CV:** *volume depletion and dehydration, orthostatic hypotension.* **EENT:** transient deafness with too rapid I.V. injection. **GI:** abdominal discomfort and pain, diarrhea. **Metabolic:** *hypokalemia; hypochloremic alkalosis; asymptomatic hyperuricemia; fluid and electrolyte imbalances including dilutional hyponatremia and hypochloremia, hypocalcemia, hypomagnesemia;* hyperglycemia and impairment of glucose tolerance. **Skin:** dermatitis.
ethoxzolamide Cardrase, Ethamide	*Edema (from congestive heart failure)—* **Adults:** 62.5 to 125 mg P.O. daily in a.m. for 3 consecutive days each week or every other day. Refractory cases may require 250 mg/day. *Glaucoma—* **Adults:** 62.5 to 250 mg P.O. b.i.d., t.i.d., or q.i.d. Give miotics concomitantly.	**Blood:** *aplastic anemia,* hemolytic anemia, leukopenia. **CNS:** drowsiness, paresthesias. **EENT:** transient myopia. **GI:** nausea, vomiting, anorexia. **GU:** crystalluria, renal calculi. **Metabolic:** *hyperchloremic acidosis,* hypokalemia, asymptomatic hyperuricemia. **Skin:** rash.
furosemide Lasix♦, Novosemide♦♦, Uritol♦♦	*Acute pulmonary edema—* **Adults:** 40 mg I.V. injected slowly; then 40 mg I.V. in 1 to 1½ hours if needed. *Edema—* **Adults:** 20 to 80 mg P.O. daily in a.m., second dose can be given in 6 to 8 hours; carefully titrated up to 600 mg daily if needed; or 20 to 40 mg I.M. or I.V. Increase by 20 mg q 2 hours until desired response is achieved. I.V. dose should be given slowly over 1 to 2 minutes.	**Blood:** *agranulocytosis,* thrombocytopenia. **CV:** *volume depletion and dehydration, orthostatic hypotension.* **EENT:** transient deafness with too rapid I.V. injection. **GI:** abdominal discomfort and pain. **Metabolic:** *hypokalemia; hypochloremic alkalosis; asymptomatic hyperuricemia, fluid and electrolyte imbalances including dilutional hyponatremia and hypochloremia, hypocalcemia,*

♦ Available in U.S. and Canada. ♦♦ Available in Canada only. All other products (no symbol) available in U.S. only. Italicized side effects are common or life-threatening.

INTERACTIONS	NURSING CONSIDERATIONS
ototoxic side effects of both ethacrynic acid and aminoglycosides. Use together cautiously.	temia, or oliguria develops, may require discontinuing drug. • Monitor intake/output, weight, and serum electrolytes regularly. • Monitor serum potassium levels; consult with doctor and dietitian to provide high-potassium diet. Watch for signs of hypokalemia (e.g., muscle weakness, cramps). • Foods rich in potassium include citrus fruits, tomatoes, bananas, dates, and apricots. • Patients also on digitalis have an increased risk of digitalis toxicity due to the potassium-depleting effect of this diuretic. • I.V. injection painful; may cause thrombophlebitis. Don't give subcutaneously or I.M. Give slowly through tubing of running infusion over several minutes. • Salt and potassium chloride supplement may be needed during therapy. • Reconstitute vacuum vial with 50 ml of 5% dextrose injection or NaCl injection. Discard unused solution after 24 hours. Don't use cloudy or opalescent solutions. • Elderly patients are especially susceptible to excessive diuresis. • Give P.O. doses in a.m. to prevent nocturia. • Severe diarrhea may necessitate discontinuing drug. • Monitor blood uric acid levels, especially in patients with history of gout. • May potentiate effects of the anticoagulant warfarin; carefully monitor patients receiving both drugs. • A loop diuretic, especially strong.
None significant.	• Contraindicated in hyperchloremic acidosis, renal failure, hepatic insufficiency, adrenal failure, depressed sodium or potassium blood levels, and long-term therapy for chronic noncongestive narrow-angle glaucoma. Use with caution in advanced pulmonary disease, respiratory acidosis, and concomitantly with other diuretics. • Monitor electrolytes, especially serum potassium; consult with doctor and dietitian to provide high-potassium diet. Monitor intake/output and weight. • May cause false-positive results in urine protein tests. • Watch for dehydration, especially in elderly patients. • Anticipate that drug will be given every day for glaucoma but intermittently for edema. Caution patient to comply with prescribed dosage and schedule to lessen chance of metabolic acidosis. • Carefully evaluate the patient with glaucoma for eye pain to make sure drug is effective in decreasing intraocular pressure. • A carbonic anhydrase inhibitor. When used on a daily basis for edema, its acidotic effects limit its usefulness.
Aminoglycoside antibiotics: potentiated ototoxicity. Use together cautiously. *Chloral hydrate:* sweating, flushing with I.V. furosemide. Observe patient. *Clofibrate:* enhanced furosemide effects. Use cautiously. *Indomethacin:* inhibited response. Use cautiously.	• Use cautiously in cardiogenic shock complicated by pulmonary edema, anuria, hepatic coma, or electrolyte imbalances. Drug is not routinely administered to women of childbearing age because its safety in pregnancy hasn't been established. • Potent loop diuretic; can lead to profound water and electrolyte depletion. Monitor blood pressure and pulse rate during rapid diuresis. • Sulfonamide-sensitive patients may have allergic reactions to furosemide. • If oliguria or azotemia develops or increases, may require stopping drug. • Monitor serum electrolytes, BUN, and CO_2 frequently. • Monitor serum potassium levels. Watch for signs of hypokalemia (for example, muscle weakness, cramps). Patients also on digitalis have an increased risk of digitalis toxicity due to the potassium-

(continued on following page)

NAME	INDICATIONS & DOSAGE	SIDE EFFECTS
furosemide *(continued)*	**Infants and children:** 2 mg/kg daily; dose increased by 1 to 2 mg/kg in 6 to 8 hours if needed; carefully titrated up to 6 mg/kg daily if needed. *Hypertensive crisis, acute renal failure—* **Adults:** 100 to 200 mg I.V. over 1 to 2 minutes. *Chronic renal failure—* **Adults:** initially, 80 mg P.O. daily. Increase by 80 to 120 mg daily until desired response is achieved.	*hypomagnesemia;* hyperglycemia and impairment of glucose tolerance. **Skin:** dermatitis.
hydrochlorothiazide Chlorzide, Diuchlor-H♦♦, Diu-Scrip, Esidrix♦, Hydrid♦♦, HydroAquil♦♦, Hydro Diuril♦, Hydromal, Hydro-Z-25, Hydro-Z-50, Hydrozide♦♦, Hyperetic, Kenazide, Lexor, Neo-Codema♦♦, Novohydrazide♦♦, Oretic, Ro-Hydrazide, Thiuretic, Urozide♦♦, Zide	*Edema—* **Adults:** initially, 25 to 100 mg P.O. daily or intermittently for maintenance to minimize electrolyte imbalance. **Children over 6 months:** 2.2 mg/kg P.O. daily divided b.i.d. **Children under 6 months:** up to 3.3 mg/kg P.O. daily divided b.i.d. *Hypertension—* **Adults:** 25 to 100 mg P.O. daily or divided dosage. Daily dosage increased or decreased according to blood pressure.	**Blood:** *aplastic anemia, agranulocytosis,* leukopenia, thrombocytopenia. **CV:** *volume depletion and dehydration,* orthostatic hypotension. **GI:** anorexia, nausea, pancreatitis. **Hepatic:** hepatic encephalopathy. **Metabolic:** *hypokalemia, asymptomatic hyperuricemia, hyperglycemia and impairment of glucose tolerance,* fluid and electrolyte imbalances including dilutional hyponatremia and hypochloremia, metabolic alkalosis, hypercalcemia, gout. **Skin:** dermatitis, photosensitivity, rash.

♦ Available in U.S. and Canada. ♦♦ Available in Canada only. All other products (no symbol) available in U.S. only. Italicized side effects are common or life-threatening.

INTERACTIONS	NURSING CONSIDERATIONS
	depleting effect of this diuretic. • Consult with doctor and dietitian to provide high-potassium diet. • Foods rich in potassium include citrus fruits, tomatoes, bananas, dates, and apricots. • Monitor blood sugar levels in patients with diabetes. May treat severe hyperglycemia with oral antidiabetic agents. • Monitor blood uric acid levels, especially in patients with a history of gout. • Give I.V. doses over 1 to 2 minutes. For doses over 100 mg, give at 10 mg/minute to prevent tinnitus associated with rapid infusion of large doses. In decreased renal function, give I.V. doses at rate of 10 mg/minute or less. • Don't use parenteral route in infants and children unless oral dosage form is not practical. • I.M. injection causes transient pain; moderate by using "Z" track to limit leakage into subcutaneous tissues. • Give P.O. and I.M. preparations in a.m. to prevent nocturia. Give second doses in early afternoon. • Elderly patients are especially susceptible to excessive diuresis, with potential for circulatory collapse and thromboembolic complications. • Store tablets in light-resistant container to prevent discoloration (doesn't affect potency). Don't use discolored (yellow) injectable preparation. Oral furosemide solution should be stored in the refrigerator to ensure stability of the drug. • Promotes calcium excretion. I.V. furosemide often used to treat hypercalcemia. • Advise patients taking furosemide to stand slowly to prevent dizziness, and to limit alcohol intake and strenuous exercise in hot weather since these exacerbate orthostatic hypotension. • Advise patients to report immediately ringing in ears, severe abdominal pain, or sore throat and fever; may indicate furosemide toxicity. • Discourage patients receiving furosemide therapy at home from storing different types of medication in the same container. This increases the risk of drug errors, especially for patients taking both furosemide and digoxin, since the most popular strengths of these drugs pills are white tablets approximately equal in size. • To prepare parenteral furosemide for I.V. infusion, mix drug with 5% dextrose in water, 0.9% sodium chloride solution, or lactated Ringer's solution. Use prepared infusion solution within 24 hours.
Cholestyramine, colestipol: intestinal absorption of thiazides decreased. Keep doses as separate as possible. *Diazoxide:* increased antihypertensive, hyperglycemic, hyperuricemic effects. Use together cautiously.	• Contraindicated in anuria; hypersensitivity to other thiazides or other sulfonamide derivatives. Use cautiously in severe renal disease, impaired hepatic function, progressive hepatic disease. • Monitor intake/output, weight, and serum electrolytes regularly. • Monitor serum potassium levels; consult with doctor and dietitian to provide high-potassium diet. Watch for hypokalemia (for example, muscle weakness, cramps). Patients also on digitalis have an increased risk of digitalis toxicity due to the potassium-depleting effect of this diuretic. May use with potassium-sparing diuretic to prevent potassium loss. • Foods rich in potassium include citrus fruits, tomatoes, bananas, dates, and apricots. • Monitor serum creatinine and BUN levels regularly. Not effective if these levels are more than twice normal. • Monitor blood uric acid levels, especially in patients with a history of gout. • Check insulin requirements in patients with diabetes. May treat se-

(continued on following page)

NAME	INDICATIONS & DOSAGE	SIDE EFFECTS
hydrochlorothiazide *(continued)*		**Other:** hypersensitivity reactions such as pneumonitis and vasculitis.
hydroflumethiazide Diucardin♦, Saluron	*Edema—* **Adults:** 25 mg to 200 mg P.O. daily in divided doses. Maintenance doses may be on intermittent or alternate-day schedule. **Children:** 1 mg/kg P.O. daily. *Hypertension—* **Adults:** 50 to 100 mg P.O. daily or b.i.d.	**Blood:** *aplastic anemia, agranulocytosis,* leukopenia, thrombocytopenia. **CV:** *volume depletion and dehydration,* orthostatic hypotension. **GI:** anorexia, nausea, pancreatitis. **Hepatic:** hepatic encephalopathy. **Metabolic:** *hypokalemia, asymptomatic hyperuricemia, hyperglycemia and impairment of glucose tolerance,* fluid and electrolyte imbalances including dilutional hyponatremia and hypochloremia, metabolic alkalosis, hypercalcemia, gout. **Skin:** dermatitis, photosensitivity, rash. **Other:** hypersensitivity reactions such as pneumonitis and vasculitis.
mannitol Osmitrol♦	**Adults, and children over 12 years:** *Test dose for marked oliguria or suspected inadequate renal function*—200 mg/kg or 12.5 g as a 15% or 20% solution I.V. over 3 to 5 minutes. Response adequate if 30 to 50 ml urine/hour is excreted over 2 to 3 hours. *Treatment of oliguria*—50 to 100 g I.V. as a 15% to 20% solution over 90 minutes to several hours. *Prevention of oliguria or acute renal failure*—50 to 100 g I.V. of a concentrated (5% to 25%) solution. Exact concentration is determined by fluid requirements. *Edema*—100 g as a 10% to 20% solution over 2- to 6-hour period. *To reduce intraocular pressure or intracranial pressure*—1.5 to 2 g/kg as a 15% to 25% solution I.V. over 30 to 60 minutes. *To promote diuresis in drug intoxication*—5% to 10% solution continuously up to 200 g I.V.,	**CNS:** rebound increase in intracranial pressure 8 to 12 hours after diuresis, headache, confusion. **CV:** *transient expansion of plasma volume during infusion causing circulatory overload and pulmonary edema,* tachycardia, angina-like chest pain. **EENT:** blurred vision, rhinitis. **GI:** thirst, nausea, vomiting. **GU:** urinary retention. **Metabolic:** *fluid and electrolyte imbalances, water intoxication, cellular dehydration.*

INTERACTIONS	NURSING CONSIDERATIONS
	vere hyperglycemia with oral antidiabetic agents. • In hypertension, therapeutic response may be delayed several days. • Give in a.m. to prevent nocturia. • Elderly patients are especially susceptible to excessive diuresis. • A thiazide diuretic.
Cholestyramine, colestipol: intestinal absorption of thiazides decreased. Keep doses as separate as possible. *Diazoxide:* increased antihypertensive, hyperglycemic, hyperuricemic effects. Use together cautiously.	• Contraindicated in anuria; hypersensitivity to other thiazides or other sulfonamide-derived drugs. Use cautiously in severe renal disease, impaired hepatic function, progressive hepatic disease. • Monitor intake/output, weight, and serum electrolytes regularly. • Monitor serum potassium levels; consult with doctor and dietitian to provide high-potassium diet. Food rich in potassium include citrus fruits, tomatoes, bananas, dates, and apricots. Watch for hypokalemia (for example, muscle weakness, cramps). May use with potassium-sparing diuretic to prevent potassium loss. Patients also on digitalis have an increased risk of digitalis toxicity due to the potassium-depleting effects of this diuretic. • Monitor serum creatinine and BUN levels regularly. Not effective if these levels are more than twice normal. • Monitor blood uric acid levels, especially in patients with history of gout. • Check insulin requirements in patients with diabetes. May treat severe hyperglycemia with oral antidiabetic agents. • Give in a.m. to prevent nocturia. • In hypertension, therapeutic response may be delayed several days. • Elderly patients are especially susceptible to excessive diuresis. • A long-acting thiazide diuretic.
None significant.	• Contraindicated in anuria, severe pulmonary congestion, frank pulmonary edema, severe congestive heart disease, severe dehydration, metabolic edema, progressive renal disease or dysfunction, progressive heart failure during administration, active intracranial bleeding except during craniotomy. • Monitor vital signs (including CVP) at least hourly; intake/output hourly (report increasing oliguria). Monitor daily: weight, renal function, fluid balance, serum and urine sodium and potassium levels. • Solution often crystallizes, especially at low temperatures. To redissolve, warm bottle in hot water bath, shake vigorously. Cool to body temperature before giving. Concentrations greater than 15% have greater tendency to crystallize. Do not use solution with undissolved crystals. • Infusions should always be given I.V. via an in-line filter. • Avoid infiltration; observe for inflammation, edema, potential necrosis. • For maximum pressure reduction before surgery, give 1 to 1½ hours preoperatively. • Can be used to measure glomerular filtration rate. • Give frequent mouth care or fluids as permitted to relieve thirst. • Foley catheter is inserted in comatose or incontinent patients because therapy is based on strict evaluation of intake and output. In patients with Foley catheters, use an hourly urometer collection bag to facilitate accurate evaluation of output. • An osmotic diuretic.

(continued on following page)

NAME	INDICATIONS & DOSAGE	SIDE EFFECTS
mannitol *(continued)*	while maintaining 100 to 500 ml urinary output/hour and a positive fluid balance.	
mercaptomerin sodium Thiomerin Sodium♦	*Edema*— **Adults:** 125 to 250 mg I.M. or S.C. daily. Maintenance with 1 to 2 times weekly dose. **Children:** 125 mg/m² I.M.	**Blood:** *agranulocytosis*, leukopenia. **CNS:** dizziness, confusion, headache. **CV:** volume depletion and dehydration, orthostatic hypotension. **Metabolic:** *fluid and electrolyte imbalances including dilutional hyponatremia and hypochloremia, metabolic alkalosis*, asymptomatic hyperuricemia. **Local:** pain on injection. **Other:** signs of mercury toxicity (albuminuria, hematuria, renal casts, stomatitis, metallic taste, colitis).
methazolamide Neptazane	*Glaucoma (open-angle, or preoperatively in obstructive or narrow-angle)*— **Adults:** 50 to 100 mg b.i.d. or t.i.d.	**Blood:** *aplastic anemia*, hemolytic anemia, leukopenia. **CNS:** drowsiness, paresthesias. **EENT:** transient myopia. **GI:** nausea, vomiting, anorexia. **GU:** crystalluria, renal calculi. **Metabolic:** *hyperchloremic acidosis*, hypokalemia, asymptomatic hyperuricemia. **Skin:** rash.
methyclothiazide Aquatensen, Duretic♦♦, Enduron	*Edema, hypertension*— **Adults:** 2.5 to 10 mg P.O daily.	**Blood:** *aplastic anemia, agranulocytosis*, leukopenia, thrombocytopenia. **CV:** *volume depletion and dehydration*, orthostatic hypotension. **GI:** anorexia, nausea, pancreatitis. **Hepatic:** hepatic encephalopathy. **Metabolic:** *hypokalemia, asymptomatic hyperuricemia, hyperglycemia and impairment of glucose tolerance*, fluid and electrolyte imbalances including dilutional hyponatremia and hypochloremia, metabolic alkalosis, hypercalcemia, gout. **Skin:** dermatitis, photosensitivity, rash. **Other:** hypersensitivity reactions such as pneumonitis and vasculitis.

INTERACTIONS	NURSING CONSIDERATIONS
None significant.	• Contraindicated in renal insufficiency, acute or subacute nephritis. Use cautiously in impaired hepatic function. • Rarely used; agents available with less severe side effects. • Mercurial diuretic. Test for mercury hypersensitivity with 0.5 ml 24 hours before initiating therapy. Watch for signs of mercurialism. • Monitor urine for albumin, blood cells, and casts. Regularly monitor weight and serum electrolyte levels, especially potassium. Consult with doctor and dietitian to provide high-potassium diet. • Give in a.m. for diuresis within 1 to 2 hours. • Rotate site of injections, massage gently; avoid edematous or adipose tissue, areas of poor circulation. Do not use I.V. route. • Good oral hygiene important to limit or prevent stomatitis. • Elderly patients are more susceptible to excessive dehydration with potential for circulatory collapse or thromboembolic phenomena.
None significant.	• Contraindicated in severe or absolute glaucoma; for long-term use in chronic noncongestive narrow-angle glaucoma; in patients with depressed sodium or potassium serum levels, renal or hepatic disease or dysfunction, adrenal gland dysfunction, and hyperchloremic acidosis. Use cautiously in respiratory acidosis, emphysema, chronic pulmonary disease. • Monitor intake/output, weight, and serum electrolytes frequently. • May cause false-positive urine protein tests by alkalinizing urine. • A carbonic anhydrase inhibitor. • Elderly patients are especially susceptible to excessive diuresis. • Diuretic effect decreases in acidosis. • Anticipate that drug will be given every day for glaucoma but intermittently for edema. Caution patient to comply with prescribed dosage and schedule to lessen risk of metabolic acidosis. • Carefully evaluate the patient with glaucoma for eye pain to make sure drug is effective in decreasing intraocular pressure.
Cholestyramine, colestipol: intestinal absorption of thiazides decreased. Keep doses as separate as possible. *Diazoxide:* increased antihypertensive, hyperglycemic, hyperuricemic effects. Use together cautiously.	• Contraindicated in renal decompensation; anuria; hypersensitivity to other thiazides or other sulfonamide-derived drugs. Use cautiously in potassium depletion, renal disease or dysfunction, impaired hepatic function, progressive hepatic disease. • Monitor intake/output, weight, and serum electrolytes regularly. • Monitor serum potassium levels; consult with doctor and dietitian to provide high-potassium diet. For foods rich in potassium see p. 807. Watch for hypokalemia (for example, muscle weakness, cramps). Patients also on digitalis have an increased risk of digitalis toxicity due to the potassium-depleting effect of this diuretic. • Check insulin requirements in patients with diabetes. May treat severe hyperglycemia with oral antidiabetic agents. • Monitor serum creatinine and BUN levels regularly. Not effective if these levels are more than twice normal. • Monitor blood uric acid levels, especially in patients with a history of gout. • In hypertension, therapeutic response may be delayed several days. • Give in a.m. to prevent nocturia. • Elderly patients are especially susceptible to excessive diuresis.

NAME	INDICATIONS & DOSAGE	SIDE EFFECTS
metolazone Diulo, Zaroxolyn♦	*Edema (heart failure)—* **Adults:** 5 to 10 mg P.O. daily. *Edema (renal disease)—* **Adults:** 5 to 20 mg P.O. daily. *Hypertension—* **Adults:** 2.5 to 5 mg P.O. daily. Maintenance dose determined by patient's blood pressure.	**Blood:** *aplastic anemia, agranulocytosis,* leukopenia, thrombocytopenia. **CV:** *volume depletion and dehydration,* orthostatic hypotension. **GI:** anorexia, nausea, pancreatitis. **Hepatic:** hepatic encephalopathy. **Metabolic:** *hypokalemia, asymptomatic hyperuricemia, hyperglycemia and impairment of glucose tolerance,* fluid and electrolyte imbalances including dilutional hyponatremia and hypochloremia, metabolic alkalosis, hypercalcemia, gout. **Skin:** dermatitis, photosensitivity, rash. **Other:** hypersensitivity reactions such as pneumonitis and vasculitis.
polythiazide Renese♦	*Hypertension—* **Adults:** 2 to 4 mg P.O. daily. *Edema (heart failure, renal failure)—* **Adults:** 1 to 4 mg P.O. daily.	**Blood:** *aplastic anemia, agranulocytosis,* leukopenia, thrombocytopenia. **CV:** *volume depletion and dehydration,* orthostatic hypotension. **GI:** anorexia, nausea, pancreatitis. **Hepatic:** hepatic encephalopathy. **Metabolic:** *hypokalemia, asymptomatic hyperuricemia, hyperglycemia and impairment of glucose tolerance,* fluid and electrolyte imbalances including dilutional hyponatremia and hypochloremia, metabolic alkalosis, hypercalcemia, gout. **Skin:** dermatitis, photosensitivity, rash. **Other:** hypersensitivity reactions such as pneumonitis and vasculitis.
quinethazone Aquamox♦♦, Hydromox	*Edema—* **Adults:** 50 to 100 mg P.O. daily or 50 mg P.O. b.i.d. Occasionally, up to 150 to 200 mg P.O. daily may be needed.	**Blood:** *aplastic anemia, agranulocytosis,* leukopenia, thrombocytopenia. **CV:** *volume depletion and dehydration,* orthostatic hypotension. **GI:** anorexia, nausea, pancreatitis. **Hepatic:** *hepatic encephalopathy.* **Metabolic:** *hypokalemia, asymptomatic hyperuricemia, hyperglycemia and impairment of glucose tolerance,* fluid and electrolyte imbalances including dilutional hyponatremia and hypochloremia,

INTERACTIONS	NURSING CONSIDERATIONS
Cholestyramine, colestipol: intestinal absorption of thiazides decreased. Keep doses as separate as possible. *Diazoxide:* increased antihypertensive, hyperglycemic, hyperuricemic effects. Use together cautiously.	• Contraindicated in anuria; hepatic coma or precoma; hypersensitivity to thiazides or other sulfonamide-derived drugs. Use cautiously in hyperuricemia or gout and severely impaired renal function. • Monitor intake/output, weight, and serum electrolytes regularly. • Monitor serum potassium levels; consult with doctor and dietitian to provide high-potassium diet. Foods rich in potassium include citrus fruits, tomatoes, bananas, dates, and apricots. Watch for hypokalemia (for example, muscle weakness, cramps). Patients also on digitalis may have an increased risk of digitalis toxicity due to the potassium-depleting effect of this diuretic. May use with potassium-sparing diuretic to prevent potassium loss. • Check insulin requirements in patients with diabetes. May treat severe hyperglycemia with oral antidiabetic agents. • Monitor blood uric acid levels, especially in patients with a history of gout. • In hypertension, therapeutic response may be delayed several days. • Give in a.m. to prevent nocturia. • Elderly patients are especially susceptible to excessive diuresis. • A thiazide-related diuretic. However, unlike thiazide diuretics, metolazone is effective in patients with decreased renal function. • Used as an adjunct in furosemide-resistant edema.
Cholestyramine, colestipol: intestinal absorption of thiazides decreased. Keep doses as separate as possible. *Diazoxide:* increased antihypertensive, hyperglycemic, hyperuricemic effects. Use together cautiously.	• Contraindicated in anuria; hypersensitivity to other thiazides or other sulfonamide-derived drugs. Use cautiously in severe renal disease, impaired hepatic function, allergies. • Monitor intake/output, weight, and serum electrolytes regularly. • Monitor serum potassium levels; consult with doctor and dietitian to provide high-potassium diet. Foods rich in potassium include citrus fruits, tomatoes, bananas, dates, and apricots. Watch for hypokalemia (for example, muscle weakness, cramps). Patients also on digitalis may have an increased risk of digitalis toxicity due to the potassium-depleting effect of this diuretic. May use with potassium-sparing diuretic to prevent potassium loss. • Monitor serum creatinine and BUN levels regularly. Not effective if these levels are more than twice normal. • Monitor blood uric acid levels, especially in patients with a history of gout. • Check insulin requirements in patients with diabetes. May treat severe hyperglycemia with oral antidiabetic agents. • In hypertension, therapeutic response may be delayed several days. • Give in a.m. to prevent nocturia. • Elderly patients are especially susceptible to excessive diuresis. • A long-acting thiazide diuretic.
Cholestyramine, colestipol: intestinal absorption of thiazides decreased. Keep doses as separate as possible. *Diazoxide:* increased antihypertensive, hyperglycemic, hyperuricemic effects. Use together cautiously.	• Contraindicated in anuria; hypersensitivity to quinethazones, thiazides, or other sulfonamide-derived drugs. Use cautiously in severe renal disease, impaired hepatic function, allergies. • Monitor intake/output, weight, and serum electrolytes regularly. • Monitor serum potassium levels; consult with doctor and dietitian to provide high-potasium diet. Foods rich in potassium include citrus fruits, tomatoes, bananas, dates, and apricots. Watch for hypokalemia (for example, muscle weakness, cramps). Patients also on digitalis have an increased risk of digitalis toxicity due to the potassium-depleting effect of this diuretic. May use with potassium-sparing diuretic to prevent potassium loss. • Monitor serum creatinine and BUN levels regularly. Not effective if these levels are more than twice normal.

(continued on following page)

NAME	INDICATIONS & DOSAGE	SIDE EFFECTS
quinethazone *(continued)*		metabolic alkalosis, hypercalcemia, gout. **Skin:** dermatitis, photosensitivity, rash. **Other:** hypersensitivity reactions such as pneumonitis and vasculitis.
spironolactone Aldactone♦, Altex	*Edema—* **Adults:** 25 to 200 mg P.O. daily in divided doses. **Children:** initially, 3.3 mg/kg P.O. daily in divided doses. *Hypertension—* **Adults:** 50 to 100 mg P.O. daily in divided doses. *Treatment of diuretic-induced hypokalemia—* **Adults:** 25 to 100 mg P.O. daily when oral potassium supplements are considered inappropriate. *Detection of primary hyperaldosteronism—* **Adults:** 400 mg P.O. daily for 4 days (short test) or for 3 to 4 weeks (long test). If hypokalemia and hypertension are corrected, a presumptive diagnosis of primary hyperaldosteronism is made.	**CNS:** headache. **GI:** anorexia, nausea, diarrhea. **Metabolic:** *hyperkalemia,* dehydration, hyponatremia, transient rise in BUN, acidosis. **Skin:** urticaria. **Other:** gynecomastia in males, breast soreness and menstrual disturbances in females.
triamterene Dyrenium♦	*Diuresis—* **Adults:** initially, 100 mg P.O. b.i.d. after meals. Total daily dosage should not exceed 300 mg.	**Blood:** megaloblastic anemia related to low folic acid levels. **CNS:** dizziness. **CV:** hypotension. **EENT:** sore throat. **GI:** dry mouth, nausea, vomiting. **Metabolic:** *hyperkalemia,* dehydration, hyponatremia, transient rise in BUN, acidosis. **Skin:** photosensitivity, rash. **Other:** *anaphylaxis,* muscle cramps.
trichlormethiazide Diurese, Metahydrin, Naqua, Rochlomethiazide, Trichlorex	*Edema—* **Adults:** 1 to 4 mg P.O. daily or in 2 divided doses. *Hypertension—* **Adults:** 2 to 4 mg P.O. daily.	**Blood:** *aplastic anemia, agranulocytosis,* leukopenia, thrombocytopenia. **CV:** *volume depletion and dehydration,* orthostatic hypotension. **GI:** anorexia, nausea, pancreatitis. **Hepatic:** hepatic encephalopathy. **Metabolic:** *hypokalemia, asymptomatic hyperuricemia, hyperglycemia and impairment of glucose*

♦ Available in U.S. and Canada. ♦♦ Available in Canada only. All other products (no symbol) available in U.S. only. Italicized side effects are common or life-threatening.

INTERACTIONS	NURSING CONSIDERATIONS
	• Check insulin requirements in patients with diabetes. May treat severe hyperglycemia with oral antidiabetic agents. • Monitor blood uric acid levels, especially in patients with a history of gout. • In hypertension, therapeutic response may be delayed several days. • Give in a.m. to prevent nocturia. • Elderly patients are especially susceptible to excessive diuresis. • A long-acting sulfonamide similar to thiazide diuretics.
Aspirin: possible blocked spironolactone effect. Watch for diminished spironolactone response.	• Contraindicated in anuria, acute or progressive renal insufficiency, hyperkalemia. Use cautiously in fluid or electrolyte imbalances, impaired renal function, and hepatic disease. • Monitor serum potassium levels, electrolytes, intake/output, weight, and blood pressure regularly. • Potassium-sparing diuretic; useful as an adjunct to other diuretic therapy. Less potent diuretic than thiazide and loop types. Diuretic effect delayed 2 to 3 days when used alone. • Maximum antihypertensive response may be delayed up to 2 weeks. • Warn patient to avoid excessive ingestion of potassium-rich foods. • Elderly patients are more susceptible to excessive diuresis. • Protect drug from light. • Breast cancer reported in some patients taking spironolactone, but cause-and-effect relationship not confirmed. Warn against taking drug indiscriminately. • Give with meals to enhance absorption. • Concomitant potassium supplement can lead to serious hyperkalemia.
None significant.	• Contraindicated in anuria, severe or progressive renal disease or dysfunction, severe hepatic disease, hyperkalemia. Use cautiously in impaired hepatic function, diabetes mellitus, pregnancy, or lactation. • Watch for blood dyscrasias. • Monitor BUN and serum potassium, electrolytes. • A potassium-sparing diuretic, useful as an adjunct to other diuretic therapy. Less potent than thiazides and loop diuretics. Full diuretic effect delayed 2 to 3 days. • Warn patients to avoid excessive ingestion of potassium-rich foods. • Give medication after meals to prevent nausea. • Should be withdrawn gradually to prevent excessive rebound potassium excretion. • Concomitant potassium supplement can lead to serious hyperkalemia. • Concomitant use of spironolactone is not recommended.
Cholestyramine, colestipol: intestinal absorption of thiazides decreased. Keep doses as separate as possible. *Diazoxide:* increased antihypertensive, hyperglycemic, hyperuricemic ef-	• Contraindicated in anuria; hypersensitivity to other thiazides or other sulfonamide-derived drugs. Use cautiously in severe renal disease, impaired hepatic function. • Monitor intake/output, weight, and electrolytes regularly. • Monitor serum potassium levels; consult with doctor and dietitian to provide high-potassium diet. Foods rich in potassium include citrus fruits, tomatoes, bananas, dates, and apricots. Watch for hypokalemia (for example, muscle weakness, cramps). Patients also on digitalis have an increased risk of digitalis toxicity due to the potassium-depleting effect of this diuretic. May use with potassium-

(continued on following page)

NAME	INDICATIONS & DOSAGE	SIDE EFFECTS
trichlormethiazide *(continued)*		*tolerance,* fluid and electrolyte imbalances including dilutional hyponatremia and hypochloremia, metabolic alkalosis, hypercalcemia, gout. **Skin:** dermatitis, photosensitivity, rash. **Other:** hypersensitivity reactions such as pneumonitis and vasculitis.
urea (carbamide) Ureaphil	*Intracranial or intraocular pressure—* **Adults:** 1 to 1.5 g/kg as a 30% solution by slow I.V. infusion over 1 to 2.5 hours. **Children over 2 years:** 0.5 to 1.5 g/kg slow I.V. infusion. **Children under 2 years:** as little as 0.1 g/kg slow I.V. infusion. To prepare 135 ml 30% solution, mix contents of 40-g vial of urea with 105 ml dextrose 5% or 10% in water or 10% invert sugar in water. Each ml of 30% solution provides 300 mg urea. Maximum adult dose 4 ml per minute.	**CNS:** *headache.* **CV:** tachycardia, volume expansion. **GI:** *nausea, vomiting.* **Metabolic:** sodium and potassium depletion. **Local:** irritation or necrotic sloughing may occur with extravasation.

INTERACTIONS	NURSING CONSIDERATIONS
fects. Use together cautiously.	sparing diuretic to prevent potassium loss. • Monitor serum creatinine and BUN levels regularly. Not effective if these levels are more than twice normal. • Check insulin requirements in patients with diabetes. May treat severe hyperglycemia with oral antidiabetic agents. Monitor blood sugar. • Monitor blood uric acid levels, especially in patients with a history of gout. • In hypertension, therapeutic response may be delayed several days. • Give in a.m. to prevent nocturia. • Elderly patients are especially susceptible to excessive diuresis. • A long-acting thiazide diuretic.
None significant.	• Contraindicated in severely impaired renal function, marked dehydration, frank hepatic failure, active intracranial bleeding. Use cautiously in pregnancy, lactation, cardiac disease, hepatic impairment, or sickle cell damage with CNS involvement. • Avoid rapid I.V. infusion; may cause hemolysis or increased capillary bleeding. Avoid extravasation; may cause reactions ranging from mild irritation to necrosis. • Don't administer through the same infusion as blood. • Don't infuse into leg veins; may cause phlebitis or thrombosis, especially in the elderly. • Watch for hyponatremia or hypokalemia (muscle weakness, lethargy); may indicate electrolyte depletion before serum levels are reduced. • Maintain adequate hydration; monitor fluid and electrolyte balance. • In renal disease, monitor BUN frequently. • Indwelling urethral catheter should be used in comatose patients to assure bladder emptying. Use an hourly urometer collection bag to facilitate accurate evaluation of diuresis. • If satisfactory diuresis does not occur in 6 to 12 hours, urea should be discontinued and renal function reevaluated. • Use freshly reconstituted urea only for I.V. infusion; solution becomes ammonia upon oxidation when standing. • Use within minutes of reconstitution.

NURSING TIP

ADMINISTERING FUROSEMIDE AS AN INFUSION

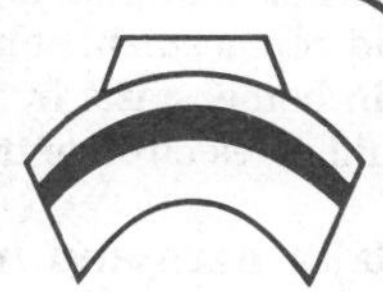

Furosemide is given as an infusion only when very large doses are ordered.
To prepare parenteral furosemide as an infusion, mix it with 5% dextrose in water, sodium chloride 0.9%, or lactated Ringer's solution. Don't mix it with strongly acidic solutions, such as those containing ascorbic acid, tetracycline, or norepinephrine, because a precipitate may form. Use the prepared infusion within 24 hours.

Since furosemide injection is available in only 20- and 100-mg ampuls, opening many ampuls to prepare a large dose may create glass particles. Filter the furosemide with a needle filter to keep glass from entering the solution.

Electrolytes and replacement solutions

calcium chloride
calcium gluceptate
calcium gluconate
calcium lactate
dextrans (low molecular weight)
dextrans (high molecular weight)
hetastarch
magnesium sulfate
potassium acetate
potassium bicarbonate
potassium chloride
potassium gluconate
potassium phosphate
Ringer's injection
Ringer's injection, lactated
sodium chloride

Maintaining proper fluid and electrolyte balance is one of the most critical goals of total patient care. Electrolytes and replacement solutions help maintain homeostasis by replacing specific fluid or electrolyte deficiencies.

Major uses and mechanism of action

Rx Electrolytes and replacement solutions replace and maintain specific anion or cation levels.

- Dextrans and hetastarch are mainly used to expand plasma volume and provide fluid replacement.

Absorption, distribution, metabolism, and excretion

- All electrolytes and replacement solutions are immediately absorbed by the I.V. route. All these preparations (except calcium salts) are excreted by the kidneys.
- Oral forms of calcium are readily absorbed from the duodenum and proximal jejunum at pH 5.0 to 7.0, if parathyroid hormone and vitamin D levels are adequate. Calcium salts are eliminated mainly in feces and to a lesser degree in urine.
- Potassium is slowly but completely absorbed from the gastrointestinal tract.

Onset and duration

- Calcium, when given I.V., raises blood levels immediately; levels return to normal in 30 minutes to 2 hours.
- Dextrans and hetastarch expand plasma volume several minutes after the infusion ends; maximal duration of action is 24 hours.
- Magnesium sulfate's onset occurs 30 minutes after I.V. administration; 1 hour after I.M. administration. Duration is 3 to 4 hours by either route.
- Potassium's onset and duration vary according to the form used. Oral sugar-coated tablets containing potassium chloride embedded in a wax matrix release the drug slowly (1 to 2 hours); doses are repeated every 8 to 12 hours. Liquid potassium preparations are absorbed much faster than the tablets (usually within 30 minutes) and are also excreted faster.

  I.V. potassium chloride is infused directly into the systemic circulation. Excretion of I.V. potassium is rapid.
- Ringer's injection solution and sodium chloride solutions replace elec-

trolytes as soon as they're infused into the bloodstream. Requirements for repeated doses vary greatly from patient to patient.

Combination products

BI-K: 20 mEq potassium (as potassium gluconate and potassium citrate) per 15 ml.

CALCIUM-SANDOZ FORTE♦♦: calcium lactate-gluconate 2.94 g, calcium carbonate 0.3 g, elemental sodium 275.8 mg; provides 500 mg elemental calcium.

DUO-K: 20 mEq potassium, 3.4 mEq chloride (from potassium gluconate and potassium chloride).

GRAMCAL♦♦: calcium lactate-gluconate 3,080 mg, calcium carbonate 1,500 mg, and potassium 390 mg; provides 1,000 mg of elemental calcium.

HEATROL: 635 mg sodium chloride, 40 mg potassium chloride, 31.5 mg calcium phosphate tribasic, and 9 mg magnesium carbonate.

KAOCHLOR-EFF:20 mEq potassium, 20 mEq chloride (from potassium chloride, potassium citrate, potassium bicarbonate, and betaine hydrochloride).

KEFF: 20 mEq each potassium and chloride (potassium chloride, potassium carbonate, potassium bicarbonate, and betaine hydrochloride).

KLORVESS: 20 mEq each potassium and chloride (from potassium chloride, potassium bicarbonate, and l-lysine monohydrochloride).

KOLYUM: 20 mEq potassium, 3.4 mEq chloride (from potassium gluconate and potassium chloride).

NEUTRA-PHOS: phosphorus 250 mg, sodium 164 mg, potassium 278 mg (from dibasic and monobasic sodium and potassium phosphate).

OSTO-K: 1 mEq (39 mg) potassium (from chloride, citrate, and gluconate) and 10 mg vitamin C.

POTASSIUM-SANDOZ♦♦: potassium chloride 600 mg and potassium bicarbonate 400 mg (provides 12 mEq potassium and 8 mEq chloride).

POTASSIUM TRIPLEX: 45 mEq potassium (from potassium acetate, potassium bicarbonate, and potassium citrate) per 15 ml.

TRIKATES: 45 mEq potassium (from potassium acetate, potassium bicarbonate, and potassium citrate) per 15 ml.

TWIN-K: 20 mEq potassium (as potassium gluconate and potassium citrate).

NURSING TIP

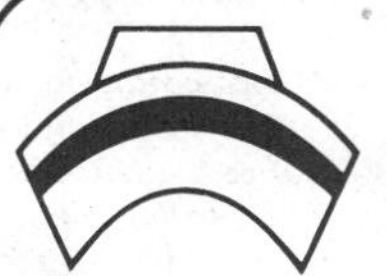

WHAT YOU SHOULD KNOW ABOUT TREATING HYPOKALEMIA

Hypokalemia occurs when a patient's serum potassium level falls below 3.5 mEq/liter. The most common cause of hypokalemia is drug therapy, particularly the use of diuretics. Both thiazide and loop diuretics cause mild to moderate hypokalemia in many patients.

When hypokalemia occurs, it's often accompanied by hypochloremic alkalosis. Therefore, potassium chloride (KCl) oral solution is usually prescribed, although it's not very palatable. You can suggest mixing it with beverages (see *Guide for Potassium Mixing,* p. 841), but if your patient still can't tolerate any of the products, slow-release preparations, such as Slow-K and Kaon-Cl, are available. These preparations contain KCl in a wax matrix. However, these are more expensive than most forms of liquid KCl and may cause small bowel ulceration.

Some doctors advocate potassium-rich foods, such as bananas and orange juice, as the sole source of potassium replacement. But these natural sources of potassium are expensive, high in calories and sugar, and usually adequate only for very mild cases.

Salt substitutes containing KCl may be an effective dietary supplement for a hypokalemic patient, but they should be used sparingly when taken with other forms of potassium.

Some doctors use potassium-sparing diuretics, such as triamterene and spironolactone, which cause potassium to be retained rather than excreted.

NAME	INDICATIONS & DOSAGE	SIDE EFFECTS
calcium chloride **calcium gluceptate** **calcium gluconate** **calcium lactate**	*Hypocalcemia, hypocalcemic tetany, hypocalcemia during exchange transfusions, cardiac resuscitation for inotropic effect when epinephrine has failed; magnesium intoxication; hypoparathyroidism*— **Adults and children:** initially 500 mg to 1 g elemental calcium I.V., with further dosage based on serum calcium determinations. Dosage with calcium chloride (1 g [10 ml] yields 13.5 mEq Ca^{++}): *Magnesium intoxication*— **Adults and children:** initially 500 mg I.V., with further doses based on calcium and magnesium determination. *Cardiac arrest*—0.5 to 1 g I.V., not to exceed 1 ml/minute; or 200 to 800 mg into the ventricular cavity. *Hypocalcemia*—500 mg to 1 g I.V. at intervals of 1 to 3 days. Dosage with calcium gluconate (1 g [10 ml] yields 4.5 mEq Ca^{++}): *Hypocalcemia*— **Adults:** 500 mg to 1 g I.V., repeated q 1 to 3 days p.r.n. as determined by serum calcium. **Children:** 500 mg/kg I.V. daily. Rate of infusion should not exceed 0.5 ml/minute. Dosage with calcium gluceptate (1.1 g [5 ml] yields 4.5 mEq Ca^{++}) and calcium salts (18 mg [1 ml] yields 0.898 mEq Ca^{++}): *Hypocalcemia*— **Adults:** initially 5 to 20 ml I.V., with further doses based on serum calcium determinations. If I.V. injection is impossible, 2 to 5 ml I.M. Average adult oral dose, 1 to 2 g/day P.O. in divided doses, t.i.d. or q.i.d. Average oral dose for children, 45 to 65 mg/kg P.O. daily, in divided doses, t.i.d. or q.i.d. *During exchange transfusions*— **Adults and children:** 0.5 ml I.V. after each 100 ml blood exchanged.	**CNS:** from I.V. use, tingling sensations, sense of oppression or heat waves; with rapid I.V. injection, syncope. **CV:** mild fall in blood pressure; with rapid I.V. injection, vasodilation, *bradycardia, cardiac arrhythmias, and cardiac arrest.* **GI:** with oral ingestion, irritation, hemorrhage, *constipation;* with I.V. administration, chalky taste; with oral calcium chloride, gastrointestinal hemorrhage, nausea, vomiting, thirst, abdominal pain. **GU:** hypercalcemia, polyuria, renal calculi. **Skin:** local reaction if calcium salts given I.M.: burning, necrosis, sloughing of tissue, cellulitis, soft-tissue calcification. **Local:** with S.C. injection, pain and irritation; *with I.V., venous irritation.*

INTERACTIONS	NURSING CONSIDERATIONS
Cardiotonic glycosides: increased digitalis toxicity; administer calcium very cautiously (if at all) to digitalized patients.	• Contraindicated in ventricular fibrillation, hypercalcemia, renal calculi. Use cautiously in patients with sarcoidosis and renal or cardiac disease, and in digitalized patients. Use calcium chloride cautiously in cor pulmonale, respiratory acidosis, or respiratory failure. • Monitor EKG when giving calcium I.V. Such injections should not exceed 0.7 to 1.5 mEq/minute. Stop if patient complains of discomfort. Following I.V. injection, patient should remain recumbent for a short while. • I.M. injection should be given in the gluteal region in adults; lateral thigh in infants. I.M. route used only in emergencies when no I.V. route available. • Monitor blood calcium levels frequently. Report abnormalities. • Hypercalcemia may result after large doses in chronic renal failure. • I.V. route generally recommended in children, but not by scalp vein (can cause tissue necrosis). • Solutions should be warmed to body temperature before administration. • Calcium chloride and calcium gluconate should be given I.V. only. • Severe necrosis and sloughing of tissues follow extravasation. Calcium gluconate is less irritating to veins and tissues than calcium chloride. • If gastrointestinal upset occurs, give oral calcium products 1 to 1½ hours after meals. • Oxalic acid (found in rhubarb and spinach), phytic acid (in bran and whole cereals), and phosphorus (in milk and dairy products) may interfere with absorption of calcium. • Crash carts usually contain both gluconate and chloride. Make sure doctor specifies form he wants administered.

NAME	INDICATIONS & DOSAGE	SIDE EFFECTS
dextrans (low molecular weight dextrans) Dextran 40, Gentran 40, LMVD, Rheomacrodex♦	*Plasma volume expansion*— Dosage of 10% solution by I.V. infusion depends on amount of fluid loss. First 500 ml of Dextran 40 may be infused rapidly with central venous pressure monitoring. Infuse remaining dose slowly. Total daily dose not to exceed 2 g/kg body weight. If therapy continued past 24 hours, do not exceed 1 g/kg daily. Continue for no longer than 5 days. *Reduction of blood sludging*— 500 ml of 10% solution by I.V. infusion.	**Blood:** *decreased level of hemoglobin and hematocrit;* with higher doses, increased bleeding time. **GI:** nausea, vomiting. **GU:** tubular stasis and blocking, increased viscosity of urine. **Hepatic:** increased SGPT and SGOT levels. **Skin:** hypersensitivity reaction, urticaria. **Other:** *anaphylaxis.*
dextrans (high molecular weight dextrans) Dextran 70, Dextran 75♦, Gentran 75, Macrodex♦	*Plasma expander*— **Adults:** usual dose 30 g (500 ml of 6% solution) I.V. In emergency situations, may be administered at rate of 1.2 to 2.4 g (20 to 40 ml) per minute. In normovolemic or nearly normovolemic patients, rate of infusion should not exceed 240 mg (4 ml) per minute. Total dose during first 24 hours not to exceed 1.2 g/kg; actual dose depends on amount of fluid loss and resultant hemoconcentration, and must be determined for each patient.	**Blood:** *decreased level of hemoglobin and hematocrit;* with doses of 15 ml/kg body weight, prolonged bleeding time and significant suppression of platelet function. **GI:** nausea, vomiting. **GU:** increased specific gravity and viscosity of urine, tubular stasis and blocking. **Hepatic:** increased SGPT and SGOT levels. **Skin:** hypersensitivity reaction, urticaria. **Other:** fever, arthralgia, nasal congestion, *anaphylaxis.*

INTERACTIONS	NURSING CONSIDERATIONS
None significant.	• Contraindicated in marked hemostatic defects; marked cardiac decompensation or pulmonary edema; renal disease with severe oliguria or anuria; or extreme dehydration. Use cautiously in active hemorrhage; may cause additional blood loss. Evaluate patient's hydration status before administration. • Hazardous when given to patients with heart failure, especially if in saline solution. Use dextrose solution instead. • Works as plasma expander via colloidal osmotic effect, thereby drawing fluid from interstitial to intravascular space. Provides plasma expansion slightly greater than volume infused. Watch for circulatory overload, rise in central venous pressure readings. • Monitor urine flow rate during administration. If oliguria or anuria occurs or is not relieved by infusion, stop dextran and give osmotic diuretic. • Hydration should be assessed before starting therapy; otherwise, use urine or serum osmolarity because urine specific gravity is affected by urine dextran concentration. • Check hemoglobin and hematocrit; don't allow to fall below 30% by volume. • Draw blood samples *before* starting infusion. • Observe patient closely during early phase of infusion: most anaphylactoid reactions occur during this time. • May interfere with analysis of blood grouping, crossmatching, bilirubin, blood glucose, and protein. • Store at constant 25° C. (77° F.). May precipitate in storage, but can be heated to dissolve if necessary. • For treatment of anaphylaxis, see inside front cover.
None significant.	• Contraindicated in marked hemostatic defects; marked cardiac decompensation or pulmonary edema; renal disease with severe oliguria or anuria; and extreme dehydration. Use cautiously in active hemorrhage; may cause additional blood loss. • Hazardous when given to patients with heart failure, especially if in saline solution. Use dextrose solution instead. • Works as plasma expander via colloidal osmotic effect, thereby drawing fluid from interstitial to intravascular space. Provides plasma expansion slightly greater than volume infused. Watch for circulatory overload. • Monitor urine flow rate during administration. If oliguria or anuria occurs or is not relieved by infusion, stop dextran and give osmotic diuretic. • Hydration should be assessed before starting therapy; otherwise, use urine or serum osmolarity because urine specific gravity is affected by the urine dextran concentration. • Check hemoglobin and hematocrit; don't allow to fall below 30% by volume. • Draw blood samples *before* starting infusion. • Observe patient closely during early phase of infusion: most anaphylactoid reactions occur during this time. • May interfere with analysis of blood grouping, crossmatching, bilirubin, blood glucose, and protein. • May precipitate in storage, but can be heated to dissolve if necessary. • Dextran 70 and Dextran 75 can be used interchangeably. Both differ significantly from Dextran 40—do not interchange. • For treatment of anaphylaxis, see inside front cover.

NAME	INDICATIONS & DOSAGE	SIDE EFFECTS
hetastarch Hespan, Volex	*Plasma expander—* **Adults:** 500 to 1,000 ml I.V. dependent on amount of blood lost and resultant hemoconcentration. Total dosage usually not to exceed 1,500 ml/day. Up to 20 ml/kg/hour may be used in hemorrhagic shock.	**CNS:** headaches. **CV:** peripheral edema of lower extremities. **EENT:** periorbital edema. **GI:** nausea, vomiting. **Skin:** urticaria. **Other:** wheezing, mild fever.
magnesium sulfate	*Hypomagnesemia—* **Adults:** 1 g, or 8.12 mEq, of 50% solution (2 ml) I.M. q 6 hours for 4 doses, depending on serum magnesium level. *Severe hypomagnesemia (serum magnesium 0.8 mEq/liter or less, with symptoms)—*6 g, or 50 mEq, of 50% solution I.V. in 1 liter of solution over 4 hours. Subsequent doses depend on serum magnesium levels. *Magnesium supplementation in hyperalimentation—* **Adults:** 8 to 24 mEq/day added to hyperalimentation solution. **Children over 6 years:** 2 to 10 mEq/day added to hyperalimentation solution. Each 2 ml of 50% solution contains 1 g, or 8.12 mEq, magnesium sulfate.	**CNS:** toxicity: weak or absent deep-tendon reflexes, flaccid paralysis, hypothermia, drowsiness, respiratory depression or paralysis; hypocalcemia (perioral paresthesias, twitching, carpopedal spasm, tetany, and seizures). **CV:** slow, weak pulse; cardiac arrhythmias (hypocalcemia); hypotension. **Skin:** flushing, sweating.
potassium acetate	*Potassium replacement—*I.V. should be used for life-threatening hypokalemia or when oral replacement not feasible. Give no more than 20 mEq/hour in concentration of 40 mEq/liter or less. Total 24-hour dose should not exceed 150 mEq (3 mEq/kg in children). Potassium replacement should be done with EKG monitoring and frequent serum K^+ determinations. *Prevention of hypokalemia—* **Adults and children:** 20 mEq P.O. daily, in divided doses b.i.d., t.i.d., or q.i.d. *Potassium depletion—* **Adults and children:** usual dose 40 to 100 mEq P.O. daily, in divided doses b.i.d., t.i.d., or q.i.d.	*Signs of hyperkalemia—* **CNS:** paresthesias of the extremities, listlessness, mental confusion, weakness or heaviness of legs, flaccid paralysis. **CV:** *peripheral vascular collapse with fall in blood pressure, cardiac arrhythmias,* heart block, possible cardiac arrest, EKG changes (prolonged P-R intervals; wide QRS; ST segment depression; tall, tented T waves). **GI:** nausea, vomiting, abdominal pain, diarrhea, bowel ulceration. **GU:** oliguria. **Skin:** cold skin, gray pallor.

♦ Available in U.S. and Canada. ♦♦ Available in Canada only. All other products (no symbol) available in U.S. only. Italicized side effects are common or life-threatening.

INTERACTIONS	NURSING CONSIDERATIONS
None significant.	• Contraindicated in severe bleeding disorders or with severe congestive heart failure and renal failure with oliguria and anuria. • To avoid circulatory overload, monitor patients with impaired renal function carefully. • Discontinue if allergic or sensitivity reactions occur. If necessary, administer an antihistamine. • Hetastarch is *not* a substitute for blood or plasma. • Available in 500 ml I.V. infusion bottles.
None significant.	• Contraindicated in impaired renal function, myocardial damage, heart block, and in actively progressing labor. Use parenteral magnesium with extreme caution in patients receiving digitalis preparations. Treating magnesium toxicity with calcium in such patients could cause serious alterations in cardiac conduction; heart block may result. • Maximum infusion rate 150 mg/minute. Rapid drip causes feeling of heat. • Keep I.V. calcium available to reverse magnesium intoxication. • Monitor vital signs every 15 minutes when giving I.V. for severe hypomagnesemia. Watch for respiratory depression and signs of heart block. Respirations should be more than 16/minute before dose is given. • Monitor intake/output. Output should be 100 ml or more during 4-hour period before dose. • Test knee jerk and patellar reflexes before each additional dose. If absent, give no more magnesium until reflexes return; otherwise, patient may develop temporary respiratory failure and need cardiopulmonary resuscitation or I.V. administration of calcium. • Check magnesium levels after repeated doses. • After giving to toxemic mothers within 24 hours before delivery, watch newborn for signs of magnesium toxicity, including neuromuscular and respiratory depression.
None significant.	• Contraindicated in severe renal impairment with oliguria, anuria, azotemia, and untreated Addison's disease; acute dehydration, hyperkalemia, hyperkalemic form of familial periodic paralysis, and conditions associated with extensive tissue breakdown. Use cautiously in patients with cardiac disease, patients receiving potassium-sparing diuretics, and those with renal impairment. • During therapy, monitor EKG, serum potassium level, renal function, BUN, serum creatinine, and intake/output. Never give potassium postoperatively until urine flow is established. • Give slowly as diluted solution; potentially fatal hyperkalemia may result from too rapid infusion. • Parenteral potassium given by infusion only; never I.V. push or I.M. • Observe for pain and redness at infusion site. Large-bore needle reduces local irritation. • Watch for signs of GI ulceration: obstruction, hemorrhage, pain, distention, severe vomiting, bleeding. • Reconstitute potassium acetate powder with liquids; give after meals with a full glass of water or fruit juice to minimize GI irritation. • To prevent serious hyperkalemia, potassium deficits must be replaced gradually.

NAME	INDICATIONS & DOSAGE	SIDE EFFECTS
potassium bicarbonate K-Lyte, K-Lyte DS	*Hypokalemia*— 25 mEq or 50 mEq tablet dissolved in water 1 to 4 times a day.	**CNS:** paresthesias of the extremities, listlessness, mental confusion, weakness or heaviness of legs, flaccid paralysis. **CV:** *cardiac arrhythmias,* EKG changes (prolonged P-R interval; wide QRS; ST segment depression; tall, tented T waves). **GI:** *nausea, vomiting, abdominal pain,* diarrhea, ulcerations, hemorrhage, obstruction, perforation.
potassium chloride K-Lor, K-Lyte/Cl, K-10♦, Kaochlor S-F 10%, Kaochlor 10%, Kaon, Kaon-Cl, Kaon-Cl 20%, Kato Powder, KayCiel♦, Klor-10%, Kloride, Klorvess, Klotrix, K Tab, Pfiklor, SK-Potassium Chloride, Slow K♦	*Hypokalemia*— 40 to 100 mEq P.O. divided into 3 to 4 doses daily for treatment; 20 mEq for prevention. Further dose based on serum potassium determinations. I.V. route when oral replacement not feasible or when hypokalemia life-threatening. Usual dose 20 mEq/hour in concentration of 40 mEq/liter or less. Total daily dose not to exceed 150 mEq (3 mEq/kg in children). Potassium replacement should be done only with EKG monitoring and frequent serum K^+ determinations.	*Signs of hyperkalemia:* **CNS:** paresthesias of the extremities, listlessness, mental confusion, weakness or heaviness of limbs, flaccid paralysis. **CV:** *peripheral vascular collapse with fall in blood pressure, cardiac arrhythmias, heart block, possible cardiac arrest,* EKG changes (prolonged P-R interval; wide QRS; ST segment depression; tall, tented T waves). **GI:** *nausea, vomiting, abdominal pain,* diarrhea, GI ulcerations (possible stenosis, hemorrhage, obstruction, perforation). **GU:** oliguria. **Skin:** cold skin, gray pallor.
potassium gluconate Kalinate Elixir, Kaon Liquid, Kaon Tablets♦, Potassium Rougier♦♦	*Hypokalemia*—40 to 100 mEq P.O. divided into 3 to 4 doses daily for treatment; 20 mEq/day for prevention. Further dose based on serum potassium determinations.	**CNS:** paresthesias of the extremities, listlessness, mental confusion, weakness or heaviness of legs, flaccid paralysis. **CV:** cardiac arrhythmias, EKG changes (prolonged P-R interval; wide QRS; ST segment depression; tall, tented T waves). **GI:** *nausea, vomiting, abdominal pain,* diarrhea, GI ulcerations with oral products (especially

♦ Available in U.S. and Canada. ♦♦ Available in Canada only. All other products (no symbol) available in U.S. only. Italicized side effects are common or life-threatening.

INTERACTIONS	NURSING CONSIDERATIONS
None significant.	• Contraindicated in severe renal impairment with oliguria, anuria, azotemia, and untreated Addison's disease; also in acute dehydration, hyperkalemia, hyperkalemic familial periodic paralysis, and conditions associated with extensive tissue breakdown. Use with caution in cardiac disease and patients receiving potassium-sparing diuretics. • Monitor serum potassium level, BUN, serum creatinine, and intake/output. • Never switch potassium products without a doctor's order. • Dissolve potassium bicarbonate tablets in 6 to 8 ounces of cold water. • Have patient take with meals and sip slowly over a 5- to 10-minute period. • Potassium bicarbonate cannot be given instead of potassium chloride. • Potassium bicarbonate does not correct hypochloremic alkalosis. • Available in lime and orange flavors. Check for patient's flavor preference.
None significant.	• Contraindicated in severe renal impairment with oliguria, anuria, azotemia, and untreated Addison's disease; also in acute dehydration, hyperkalemia, hyperkalemic form of familial periodic paralysis, conditions associated with extensive tissue breakdown. Use with caution in cardiac disease, patients receiving potassium-sparing diuretics. • Potassium should not be given during immediate postoperative period until urine flow is established. • Parenteral potassium given by infusion only; never I.V. push or I.M. • Give slowly as dilute solution; potentially fatal hyperkalemia may result from too rapid infusion. • Give oral potassium supplements with extreme caution because its many forms deliver varying amounts of potassium. Never switch products without a doctor's order. Tell the doctor if patient tolerates one product better than another. • Sugar-free liquid available (Kaochlor S-F 10%). • Have patient sip liquid potassium slowly to minimize GI irritation. • Give with or after meals with full glass of water or fruit juice to lessen GI distress. • Make sure powders are completely dissolved before giving. • Enteric-coated tablets not recommended due to potential GI bleeding and small-bowel ulcerations. • Tablets in wax matrix sometimes lodge in esophagus and cause ulceration in cardiac patients who have esophageal compression due to enlarged left atrium. In such patients and in those with esophageal stasis or obstruction, use liquid form. • Often used orally with diuretics that cause potassium excretion. Potassium chloride most useful since diuretics waste chloride ion. Hypokalemic alkalosis treated best with potassium chloride. • Monitor EKG, serum potassium levels, and other electrolytes during therapy.
None significant.	• Contraindicated in severe renal impairment with oliguria, anuria, azotemia, and untreated Addison's disease; also in acute dehydration, hyperkalemia, hyperkalemic form of familial periodic paralysis, and conditions associated with extensive tissue breakdown. Use with caution in patients with cardiac disease, and in those receiving potassium-sparing diuretics. • Monitor serum potassium level, BUN, serum creatinine, and intake/output. • Give oral potassium supplements with extreme caution because their many forms deliver varying amounts of potassium. Never switch products without doctor's order. If one product is tolerated better

(continued on following page)

NAME	INDICATIONS & DOSAGE	SIDE EFFECTS
potassium gluconate *(continued)*		enteric-coated tablets); ulcerations may be accompanied by stenosis, hemorrhage, obstruction, perforation.
potassium phosphate	*Hypokalemia*—I.V. should be used when oral replacement not feasible or when hypokalemia life-threatening. Dosage up to 20 mEq/hour in concentration of 60 mEq/liter or less. Total daily dose not to exceed 150 mEq. Should be done only with EKG monitoring and frequent serum K^+ determinations. Average P.O. dose: 40 to 100 mEq. *Hypophosphatemia*—3 mM/ml is administered I.V. after diluting in a larger volume of fluid. Dosage is adjusted according to individual needs of patient.	*Signs of hyperkalemia*— **CNS:** paresthesias of the extremities, listlessness, mental confusion, weakness or heaviness of legs, flaccid paralysis; hypocalcemia—perioral paresthesias, twitching, carpopedal spasm, tetany, and seizures. **CV:** *peripheral vascular collapse with fall in blood pressure, cardiac arrhythmias, heart block, possible cardiac arrest,* EKG changes (prolonged P-R interval; wide QRS; ST segment depression; tall, tented T waves). **GI:** nausea, vomiting, abdominal pain, diarrhea. **GU:** oliguria. **Skin:** cold skin, gray pallor. **Other:** soft-tissue calcification.
Ringer's injection	*Fluid and electrolyte replacement*— **Adults and children:** dose highly individualized, but generally 1.5 to 3 liters (2% to 6% body weight) infused I.V. over 18 to 24 hours.	**CV:** fluid overload.
Ringer's injection, lactated (Hartmann's solution, Ringer's lactate solution)	*Fluid and electrolyte replacement*— **Adults and children:** dose highly individualized, but generally 1.5 to 3 liters (2% to 6% body weight) infused I.V. over 18 to 24 hours.	**CV:** fluid overload.
sodium chloride	*Highly individualized fluid and electrolyte replacement in hyponatremia due to electrolyte loss or in severe salt depletion*— 400 ml of 3% or 5% solutions	**CV:** aggravation of congestive heart failure; edema and pulmonary edema if too much given or given too rapidly. **Metabolic:** hypernatremia and

INTERACTIONS	NURSING CONSIDERATIONS
	than another, tell doctor so brand and dosage can be changed. • Have patient sip liquid potassium slowly to minimize GI irritation. • Give with or after meals with full glass of water or fruit juice to lessen GI distress. • Potassium gluconate does not correct hypokalemic hypochloremic alkalosis. • Enteric-coated tablets not recommended due to potential for GI bleeding and small-bowel ulcerations. • Monitor EKG, serum potassium, and other electrolytes during therapy.
None significant.	• Contraindicated in severe renal impairment with oliguria, anuria, azotemia, and untreated Addison's disease; also in acute dehydration, hyperkalemia, hyperkalemic form of familial periodic paralysis, extensive tissue damage, and hypocalcemia. Use with caution in patients with cardiac disease, and in those receiving potassium-sparing diuretics. • Never give potassium postoperatively until urine flow is established. • Monitor EKG for indications of tissue potassium levels; plasma potassium and calcium levels as well as BUN and creatinine for renal function; inorganic phosphorus levels; intake/output. • Give slowly as dilute solution; potentially fatal hyperkalemia may result from too rapid an infusion. • Parenteral potassium given by infusion only; never I.V. push or I.M. • Reconstitute powder in juice. Give after meals.
None significant.	• Contraindicated in renal failure, except as emergency volume expander. Use cautiously in congestive heart failure, circulatory insufficiency, renal dysfunction, hypoproteinemia, or pulmonary edema. • Ringer's injection contains sodium, 147 mEq/liter; potassium, 4 mEq/liter; calcium, 4.5 mEq/liter; and chloride, 155.5 mEq/liter. This electrolyte content is insufficient for treating severe electrolyte deficiencies, although it does provide electrolytes in levels approximately equal to those of the blood. • May be given with dextrose infusion, other carbohydrates, or sodium lactate.
None significant.	• Contraindicated in renal failure, except as emergency volume expander. Use cautiously in congestive heart failure, circulatory insufficiency, renal dysfunction, hypoproteinemia, and pulmonary edema. • Ringer's injection, lactated, contains sodium, 130 mEq/liter; potassium, 4 mEq/liter; calcium, 2.7 mEq/liter; chloride, 109.7 mEq/liter; and lactate, 27 mEq/liter. • Approximates more closely the electrolyte concentration in blood plasma than Ringer's injection. • May be given with dextrose infusion.
None significant.	• Use with caution in congestive heart failure, circulatory insufficiency, renal dysfunction, hypoproteinemia. • Infuse 3% and 5% solutions very slowly and with caution to avoid pulmonary edema. Use only for critical situations. Observe patient constantly.

(continued on following page)

NAME	INDICATIONS & DOSAGE	SIDE EFFECTS
sodium chloride *(continued)*	only with frequent electrolyte determination and only if given slow I.V.; *with 0.45% solution:* 3% to 8% of body weight, according to deficiencies, over 18 to 24 hours; *with 0.9% solution:* 2% to 6% of body weight, according to deficiencies, over 18 to 24 hours. *Management of "heat cramp" due to excessive perspiration*— **Adults:** 1 g P.O. with every glass of water.	aggravation of existing acidosis with excessive infusion; serious electrolyte disturbance, loss of potassium.

INTERACTIONS	NURSING CONSIDERATIONS
	• Concentrates available for addition to parenteral nutrient solutions. Don't confuse these small volumes of parenterals with sodium chloride injection isotonic 0.9%. *Read label carefully.* • Monitor serum electrolytes during therapy.

PATIENT-TEACHING AID

GUIDE FOR POTASSIUM MIXING

Dear Patient:

Your doctor has prescribed a potassium supplement as part of your therapy. This product should be mixed with water or fruit juice. Or try these combinations for flavor variety.

THE BRAZILIAN
1 or 2 tablespoonfuls of potassium chloride oral solution *or* 1 packet of potassium chloride powder; 1 cup of coffee (with cream and/or sugar, if desired). Stir to mix.

HAWAIIAN DELIGHT
1 or 2 tablespoonfuls of potassium chloride oral solution *or* 1 packet of potassium chloride powder; 180 to 210 ml (6 to 7 oz) of pineapple juice (canned or frozen); crushed ice. Stir to mix.

THE ZINGER
1 or 2 tablespoonfuls of potassium chloride oral solution *or* 1 packet of potassium chloride powder; 210 to 240 ml (7 to 8 oz) of lemon-lime carbonated beverage (such as 7-Up or Sprite); ice cubes. Stir gently.

THE SLIM JIM
1 or 2 tablespoonfuls of potassium chloride oral solution *or* 1 packet of potassium chloride powder; 210 to 240 ml (7 to 8 oz) of sugar-free cola-flavored beverage (such as Diet Pepsi or Tab); crushed ice or ice cubes. Stir gently.

THE STARTER
1 or 2 tablespoonfuls of potassium chloride oral solution *or* 1 packet of potassium chloride powder; 210 ml (7 oz) of grapefruit juice or orange juice (fresh, frozen, or reconstituted); crushed ice. Stir to mix.

THE PSEUDO BRAZILIAN
1 or 2 tablespoonfuls of potassium chloride oral solution *or* 1 packet of potassium chloride powder; 1 cup of decaffeinated coffee (with cream and/or sugar, if desired). Stir to mix.

THE OCEAN SPRAY
1 or 2 tablespoonfuls of potassium chloride oral solution *or* 1 packet of potassium chloride powder; 180 to 240 ml (6 to 8 oz) of cranberry juice. Stir to mix.

Recipes developed by Roxane Laboratories, Inc.

Potassium-removing resin

sodium polystyrene sulfonate

Potassium-removing resin is used to lower dangerously elevated serum potassium levels.

This drug is generally used, in conjunction with other modes of therapy, to treat renal failure. It is too slow acting to be used alone or in an emergency hyperkalemic situation.

Major uses

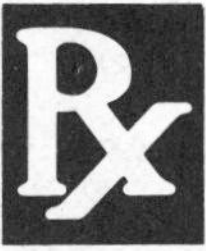

Potassium-removing resin is used to treat hyperkalemia. It is effective in *chronic* renal failure.

Because sodium polystyrene sulfonate is relatively slow acting and gives a variable response, it should not be used as primary treatment of either acute renal failure or burns with rapid tissue breakdown.

Mechanism of action

The potassium-removing resin exchanges sodium ions for potassium ions in the intestine: 1 g of sodium polystyrene sulfonate is exchanged for 0.5 to 1 mEq of potassium. The resin is then eliminated. Much of the exchange capacity is used for cations other than potassium (calcium and magnesium) and possibly for fats and proteins.

Absorption, distribution, metabolism, and excretion

The potassium-removing resin is distributed through the intestine (especially the large intestine) and eliminated in feces.

Onset and duration

- Intestinal ion exchange requires about 6 hours.
- Action of the potassium-removing resin is slow, unpredictable, and variable. Because therapeutic effect isn't evident for 2 to 24 hours, sodium polystyrene sulfonate is most useful when either potassium levels aren't life-threatening or other measures (such as glucose-insulin infusions) have reduced the immediate danger of hyperkalemia.

Combination products

None.

MANAGING HYPERKALEMIA

It's time to watch dietary potassium when serum potassium concentrations rise above 5.5 mEq/liter, causing severe muscle weakness, paralysis, abdominal distention, diarrhea, oliguria, and anuria.

You can expect potassium excess (hyperkalemia) to develop in patients with inadequate renal function; adrenocortical insufficiency; increased potassium load, as in severe tissue damage, metabolic acidosis, or overtreatment with potassium salts; and in patients taking potassium-sparing diuretics.

One way to control hyperkalemia is to limit dietary intake of potassium. Use the patient-teaching aid for a low-potassium diet as a guide for your patients in measuring and minimizing potassium intake.

PATIENT-TEACHING AID

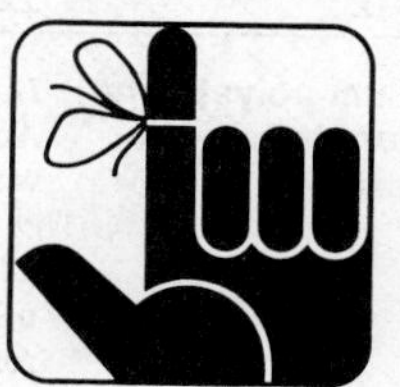

SUGGESTIONS FOR A LOW-POTASSIUM DIET

Dear Patient:

The doctor has asked you to go on a low-potassium diet because your body retains too much of this mineral. Here's a list showing the amount of potassium in 100-gram portions (approximately 3½ oz) of some foods you can eat. Buy or borrow a food scale to weigh your portions.

Avoid high-potassium foods, such as milk, potatoes and potato chips, bananas, dried fruit, catsup, pickles, nuts, chocolate, and peanut butter. Limit your intake of meats and eggs. You can reduce the potassium content of vegetables by boiling them for a long period in large amounts of water. Keep track of what you eat, and be sure the total daily amount of potassium doesn't exceed your doctor's recommendation (usually 2 grams or 2,000 milligrams).

DAIRY PRODUCTS	**mg/100 g**
Cheese, cheddar	82
Cheese, cream	85
Eggs	98
Butter	23

FRUITS AND VEGETABLES	
Applesauce	65
Blueberries	81
Cranberry juice	10
Pears, canned	84
Pineapple, canned	96
Beans, snap	95
Corn, canned	97
Peas, canned	96

MEAT, FISH, POULTRY	**mg/100 g**
	approx. 350

BREAD AND CEREAL	
Rice	28
Noodles	44
Macaroni	61
Bread, cracked wheat	134
Bread, white	105
Bread, rye	115
Oatmeal	61
Cornflakes	120
Corn grits	11
Farina	188

NAME	INDICATIONS & DOSAGE	SIDE EFFECTS
sodium polystyrene sulfonate Kayexalate♦	*Hyperkalemia—* **Adults:** 15 g daily to q.i.d. in water or sorbitol (3 to 4 ml/g of resin). **Children:** 1 g of resin for each mEq of potassium to be removed. Oral administration preferred since drug should remain in intestine for at least 6 hours; otherwise, consider nasogastric administration. Nasogastric administration: mix dose with appropriate medium: aqueous suspension or diet appropriate for renal failure; instill in plastic tube. Rectal administration: **Adults:** 30 to 50 g/100 ml of sorbitol q 6 hours as warm emulsion deep into sigmoid colon (20 cm). In persistent vomiting or paralytic ileus, high retention enema of sodium polystyrene sulfonate (30 g) suspended in 200 ml of 10% methylcellulose, 10% dextrose, or 25% sorbitol solution.	**GI:** *constipation,* fecal impaction (in elderly), anorexia, gastric irritation, nausea, vomiting, *diarrhea (with sorbitol emulsions).* **Other:** *hypokalemia,* hypocalcemia, hypomagnesemia, sodium retention.

♦ Available in U.S. and Canada. ♦♦ Available in Canada only. All other products (no symbol) available in U.S. only. Italicized side effects are common or life-threatening.

GLUCOSE + INSULIN: ANOTHER TREATMENT FOR HYPERKALEMIA

If your patient's hyperkalemia is severe and doesn't respond to other forms of treatment, the doctor may order an infusion of glucose and insulin to lower your patient's serum potassium. This method drives glucose and potassium from serum into the cells, where the glucose is stored as glycogen.

Here are some points to remember for these infusions:

- Usual dosage range is 1 unit of insulin for every 2 to 4 g of glucose.
- Over 30 to 60 minutes, infuse 200 to 300 ml of a 50% glucose solution containing 30 to 50 units of regular insulin. This should produce a 1 to 2 mEq/liter reduction in serum potassium for about 12 to 24 hours.
- Then, continue the glucose-insulin infusion at a slower rate, and titrate against the serum potassium level.
- Sodium bicarbonate—usually 2 to 4 ampuls (1 ampul = 44 mEq)—may be used with glucose-insulin therapy. It's usually added to the glucose-insulin solution, or infused with glucose while insulin is injected. Its action raises blood pH, creating alkalosis, which aids potassium transfer into cells in exchange for hydrogen. The excess sodium also promotes potassium excretion.
- Glucose-insulin therapy and alkali treatments begin to take effect within 30 minutes.
- The volume of fluid needed for this treatment could aggravate edema in patients with oliguria, heart failure, or hypertension. Alternate therapy may be preferable.
- Glucose-insulin therapy results are only temporary and must be followed by dialysis to correct the condition. When dialysis isn't feasible, Kayexalate may be administered.

INTERACTIONS	NURSING CONSIDERATIONS
Antacids and laxatives (nonabsorbable cation-donating type, including magnesium hydroxide): systemic alkalosis, reduced potassium exchange capability. Don't use together.	• Use with caution in elderly patients and those on digitalis therapy, with severe congestive heart failure, severe hypertension, and marked edema. • Treatment may result in potassium deficiency. Monitor serum potassium at least once daily. Usually stopped when potassium level is reduced to 4 or 5 mEq/liter. Watch for other signs of hypokalemia: irritability, confusion, cardiac arrhythmias, EKG changes, severe muscle weakness and sometimes paralysis, and digitalis toxicity in digitalized patients. • Monitor for symptoms of other electrolyte deficiencies (magnesium, calcium) since drug is nonselective. Monitor serum calcium determination in patients receiving sodium polystyrene therapy for more than 3 days. Supplementary calcium may be needed. • Watch for sodium overload. About ⅓ of resin's sodium is retained. • Use only fresh suspensions. Stir just before use. Discard unused portions after 24 hours. • Do not heat resin. This will impair effectiveness of drug. • Mix only with water or sorbitol. Chill oral suspension to improve taste. • Consider solid form. Resin cookie recipe is available; perhaps pharmacist or dietitian can supply. • Watch for constipation in oral or nasogastric administration. Use sorbitol (10 to 20 ml of 70% syrup every 2 hours as needed) to produce 1 or 2 watery stools daily. • If hyperkalemia is severe, more drastic modalities should be added; for example, dextrose 50% with regular insulin I.V. push. Do not depend solely on polystyrene resin to lower serum potassium levels in severe hyperkalemia.

TIPS FOR GIVING A KAYEXALATE ENEMA

• Mix polystyrene resin only with water and sorbitol. Do not use other vehicles, such as mineral oil, to prevent impactions. Ion exchange requires an aqueous medium, and sorbitol prevents impaction.

• Prevent fecal impaction in the elderly by administering resin rectally rather than orally. Give a cleansing enema first. Explain to the patient the necessity of retaining the Kayexalate enema. Retention for 6 to 10 hours is ideal, but 30 to 60 minutes is acceptable.

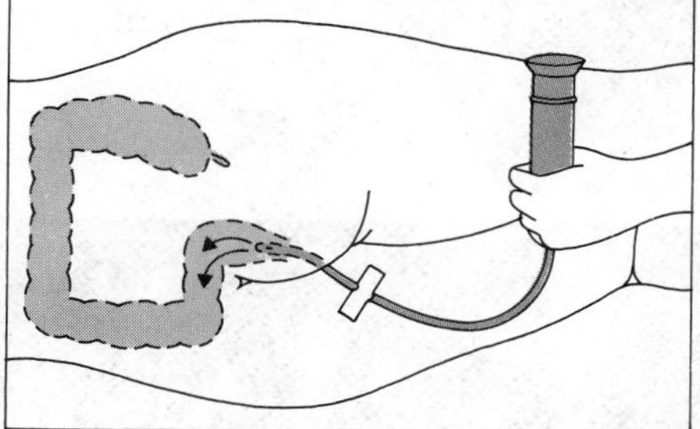

• Make sure the mixture is at body temperature to ensure patient comfort and to avoid stimulating peristalsis. But don't heat resin, as this impairs the drug's effectiveness.

• With the patient in Sims's position, insert a 28 French rubber catheter or a rectal tube about 10 cm (4") into the patient's sigmoid colon. Tape the tube in place.

• Agitate resin emulsion gently during administration to prevent settling.

• After administration, flush the tubing with 50 ml of water to ensure full delivery of medication to the patient.

• If back leakage occurs, place the patient in knee-chest position or elevate his hips.

• To help the patient with poor sphincter control retain the enema, consider using (if hospital policy permits) a Foley catheter with a 30-ml balloon inflated distal to the anal sphincter.

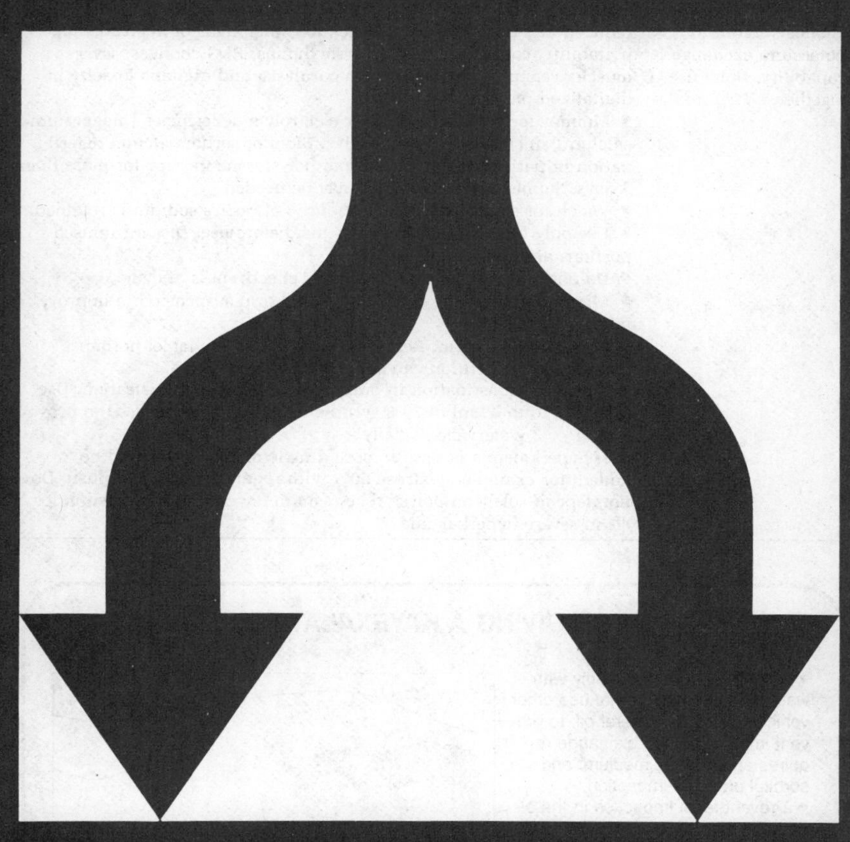

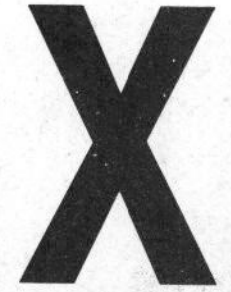

Hematologic Agents

66 Hematinics

ferrocholinate
ferrous fumarate
ferrous gluconate
ferrous sulfate
iron dextran

Hematinics are iron-containing compounds that increase both the hemoglobin level and the number of red blood cells. Iron is necessary for formation of hemoglobin, which transports oxygen within the red blood cells from the lungs to the tissues. Iron deficiency, reflected by decreased hemoglobin synthesis and decreased red cell production, may result from blood loss, or inadequate iron intake during accelerated growth or pregnancy. Although many expensive forms of iron therapy are available, ferrous sulfate is the cheapest and most effective.

COMPARING ORAL IRON SALTS

Different oral iron salts contain different amounts of available iron, so they're not interchangeable in treating iron deficiencies. Here are the percentages of elemental iron contained in oral preparations:

IRON SALT	ELEMENTAL IRON (%)
ferrous fumarate	33
ferrous gluconate	12
ferrous sulfate, dried	30
ferrous sulfate, hydrous	20
ferrocholinate	12

Major uses

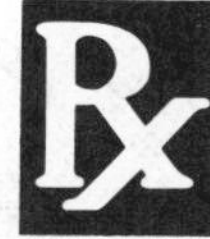

Iron preparations supplement depleted stores, thereby arresting anemia. As a daily dietary supplement, 10 to 18 mg of elemental iron for adults and 4 to 8 mg for children are sufficient. Patients with iron deficiency may require 90 to 200 mg of elemental iron daily. (See accompanying chart for percentage of elemental iron in various iron salts.)

Mechanism of action

After absorption into the blood, iron is immediately bound to transferrin. Transferrin carries iron to bone marrow, where it's used to synthesize hemoglobin. Some iron is also used to synthesize myoglobin or other nonhemoglobin heme units.

Absorption, distribution, metabolism, and excretion

- The absorption of iron is complex and influenced by many factors, including the iron salt given, iron stores in the body, degree of erythropoiesis, drug dose, and diet.

Absorption occurs mainly in the duodenum after oral administration, although a small amount is typically absorbed as well in the proximal jejunum. Healthy persons absorb about 10% of the iron present in their diets,

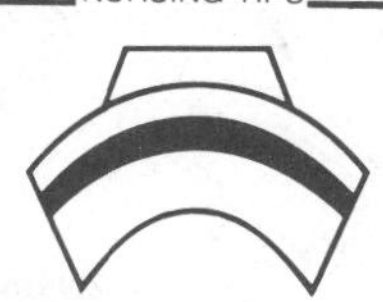

NEW THINKING ABOUT PARENTERAL IRON

A patient with uncomplicated iron deficiency anemia usually responds to oral iron salts. But if your patient has a severe case—caused by acute peptic ulcer, malabsorption syndrome, colitis or enteritis, or bowel resection—he needs parenteral iron.

Here's why: Oral iron salts contain only 12% to 33% elemental iron. The large amount of oral iron needed to replace severely depleted stores could cause extreme nausea and vomiting. Parenteral iron neatly avoids gastrointestinal distress. Iron dextran (Imferon and others), with 50 mg of elemental iron/ml, is the most common form for parenteral use. The preferred method of administration has traditionally been I.M., using the Z-track technique, but many doctors are now favoring the I.V. route.

A rationale for I.V.

Disadvantages of I.M. injections include pain and discoloration at the injection site (although using the Z-track method and changing needles before injection minimize discoloration). And since no more than 2 ml (100 mg) of iron dextran should be administered in one I.M. site, your patient might need as many as 20 injections to complete a single course of therapy.

Many doctors now specify iron dextran by I.V. infusion. It's relatively painless, compared to I.M. injection, and one infusion replaces the patient's entire iron deficit.

The incidence of allergic reactions, once thought more common with I.V. administration, is about the same for both I.V. and I.M. But the I.V. route may be safer, because you can stop the infusion immediately if your patient reacts to the iron. An infusion does risk phlebitis, however. To reduce this risk, the doctor may order the iron dextran given by direct I.V. push at a rate no faster than 50 mg/minute (1 ml/minute).

Both forms of parenteral iron can cause vomiting, chills, fever, headache, joint pain, and urticaria. Patients with asthma or who are allergy-prone may show hypersensitivity.

Preparing an I.V. infusion

Dilute the iron dextran with 500 to 1,000 ml of normal saline solution. (Don't use 5% dextrose in water; it increases the risk of phlebitis.) Infuse the first few milliliters slowly, at 10 drops/minute, so you can watch for an allergic reaction. After 10 to 15 minutes, administer the solution at a rate no faster than 60 drops/minute. Depending on the amount of iron to be given, the infusion may last up to 10 hours. But an infusion completed in less than 5 hours reduces the risk of phlebitis.

One brand for I.V. use

Only Imferon brand of iron dextran, available in 2-ml and 5-ml ampuls without preservatives, is currently acceptable for I.V. administration. Other brands available in 10-ml multidose vials contain phenol, a potentially toxic preservative.

Monitoring patient response

Check the results of your patient's laboratory tests. His reticulocyte count should start to climb by the fourth day of treatment, peak within 7 to 12 days, then return to normal 1 week later. More subtle signs include increased appetite and activity, improved color, and faster wound healing (when applicable). Hemoglobin level starts to increase within 2 weeks and should reach a normal level in 2 months.

whereas patients with iron deficiency may absorb as much as 30% of dietary iron in an attempt to replace body stores of this element.

When given therapeutically, the ferrous form of iron is better absorbed orally than the ferric form. Patients with iron deficiency absorb as much as 60% of an iron dose. When total body stores of iron are large, absorption is diminished.

After I.M. injection, 60% of the iron is absorbed after 3 days and up to 90% is absorbed after 1 to 3 weeks.

When administered I.V., all the iron is absorbed immediately.

- Iron is distributed in the bone marrow (2,400 mg) and in the liver (800 mg

NURSING TIPS

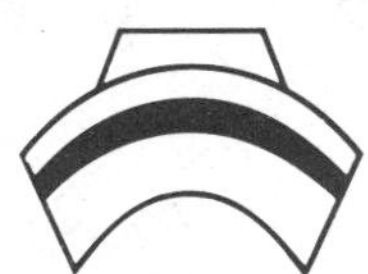

ADDING IRON TO YOUR PATIENT'S DIET

If your patient's suffering from an iron deficiency, use this list to help him develop a menu of iron-rich foods to replenish his body's stores. Advise him that cooking in cast-iron pots and pans instead of aluminum or stainless steel increases the amount of iron he ingests, particularly if he's cooking something acidic like spaghetti sauce or apple butter. And if the doctor has prescribed an iron supplement, tell your patient that he can increase its effectiveness by taking it with orange or other citrus juice, since these facilitate iron absorption.

FOOD SOURCE (Serving Size)	IRON (mg)
Fish and shellfish	
Clams, soft, raw, meat only (4 large)	3.4
Clams, canned (½ cup)	4.1
Cod, raw, dehydrated (3½ oz)	3.6
Mussels (3½ oz)	3.4
Oysters, raw (5 to 8 medium)	7.2
Oysters, fried (1 serving)	8.1
Sardines, canned in oil (8 medium)	3.5
Meats	
Bacon, Canadian, raw (¼ lb)	3.7
Beef, chuck, stew meat, raw (¼ lb)	3.7
Corned, canned (3 slices)	3.7
Dried or chipped (3 oz)	4.3
Hamburger, cooked, medium (¼ lb)	3.3
Porterhouse, broiled steak (½ lb)	3.8
Rib steak, cooked (½ lb)	3.6
Round, broiled (½ lb)	6.1
Rump, pot roasted (½ lb)	3.8
Sirloin, broiled (½ lb)	4.8
T-bone steak (½ lb)	3.6
Heart, average, braised (⅓ heart with gravy)	4.6
Kidney, beef (3 slices)	7.9
Pork (3 slices)	8.0
Sheep (3 slices)	9.2
Lamb, chop, cooked (3½ oz)	3.0
Liver, beef, raw (3½ oz)	6.6
Calf, raw (3½ oz)	10.6
Chicken, raw (2 large)	7.4
Lamb, raw (2 slices)	12.6
Pork, raw (2 slices)	18.0
Liverwurst, liver sausage (3½ slices)	5.4
Pork, blade, cooked (3½ oz)	3.7
Tenderloin, roasted (3½ oz)	4.7
Veal, arm steak, cooked (3½ oz)	3.8
Cutlet, round, cooked (3½ oz)	4.2
Poultry and game	
Chicken, broiler, fried (½ bird)	3.5
Duck, roasted (3 slices)	5.8
Goose, domestic, cooked (3 slices)	4.6
Pheasant, raw (3½ oz)	3.7
Quail, raw (3½ oz)	3.8
Turkey, roasted (3 slices)	5.1
Venison, fresh, cooked (3 slices)	7.8
Vegetables	
Beans, chickpeas, or garbanzos (½ cup)	6.9
Common, white (½ cup)	7.8
Cowpeas, mature seeds, dry, raw (½ cup)	5.8
Lima (⅝ cup)	7.8
Red (½ cup)	6.9
Peas, common (½ cup)	5.1
Soybeans (½ cup)	8.4
Pinto beans (½ cup)	6.4
Fruits	
Apricots, dried, uncooked (17 large halves)	5.5
Mangoes, raw (½ medium)	50.0
Prunes, dehydrated (8 large)	4.4
Raisins, dried, seedless (⅝ cup)	3.5
Fruit juices	
Prune juice, canned (¾ cup)	7.4
Nuts and nut products	
Almonds, dried, unblanched (⅔ cup)	4.4
Cashews, roasted (1 cup)	3.8
Peanuts, roasted with skin (3½ oz)	3.4
Peanut butter (1 cup)	4.9
Walnuts, black (3½ oz)	6.0

Adapted from Robert Peter Knott, "Iron Therapy," *pharmindex*, 22:1:13, January 1980, with permission from the publisher.

HOW TO INJECT IRON SOLUTIONS

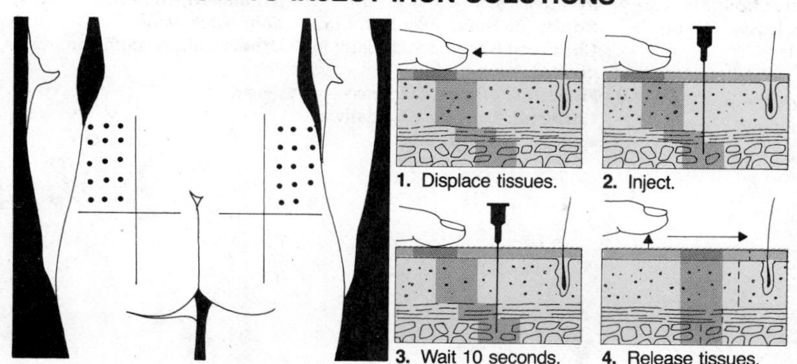
1. Displace tissues.
2. Inject.
3. Wait 10 seconds.
4. Release tissues.

For I.M. injections of iron solutions, use the Z-track technique to prevent subcutaneous irritation and discoloration from leaking medication. Follow these guidelines:

- Choose a 19G or 20G, 2″ or 3″ needle, depending on the patient's size.
- After drawing up the solution, allow 0.5 cc of air into the syringe. Then change to a fresh needle to prevent tracking iron solution through to subcutaneous tissue.
- Select an injection site in the upper outer quadrant of buttocks only. If the patient is standing, have him bear weight on the leg opposite the site; if he's in bed, place him in lateral position, with injection site up.
- Displace the skin, fat, and muscle at the site firmly to one side. Cleanse the area and insert the needle.
- Aspirate to check for entry into a blood vessel. Inject the medication and the air bubble in the syringe slowly.
- Wait 10 seconds, pull the needle straight out, and release the tissues to seal off the needle track.
- Apply direct pressure to the site, but don't massage it. To increase the absorption rate, encourage physical activity, like walking. But caution your patient against exercising vigorously for 15 to 30 minutes, and against wearing tight-fitting clothes that could force medication into subcutaneous tissue and cause irritation.
- For subsequent injections, alternate buttocks.

in males, 300 mg in females). The remainder is bound to plasma proteins and contained in muscles (myoglobin) and certain enzymes.

- Iron metabolism is a closed system: the body conserves and reuses most of the iron that's liberated by hemoglobin destruction.
- Elimination of iron is minimal; 500 mcg to 2 mg are lost daily, primarily as cells exfoliated from the skin, gastrointestinal mucosa, nails, and hair. Only trace amounts of iron are secreted in bile or excreted in sweat. Women normally lose 12 to 30 mg of iron during each menstrual period.

Onset and duration

With therapeutic doses of iron salts, symptoms of iron deficiency usually improve within 2 to 3 days. Peak reticulocytosis (formation of young red cells) occurs in 5 to 10 days, and hemoglobin level rises after 2 to 4 weeks. Normal hemoglobin values are usually attained in 2 months, unless blood loss continues.

Combination products

FERMALOX: ferrous sulfate 200 mg, and magnesium hydroxide and dried aluminum hydroxide gel 200 mg.
FEROCYL: iron (as fumarate) 50 mg and docusate sodium 100 mg.
FER-REGULES: iron (as fumarate) 150 mg and docusate sodium 100 mg.
FERRO-SEQUELS: iron (as fumarate) 50 mg and docusate sodium 100 mg.
SIMRON: iron (as gluconate) 10 mg and polysorbate 20, 400 mg.

NAME	INDICATIONS & DOSAGE	SIDE EFFECTS
ferrocholinate Chel-Iron, Firon, Kelex	*Iron deficiency—* **Adults:** 333-mg tablet P.O. t.i.d. **Children:** 6 mg/kg P.O. daily in divided doses t.i.d. *Prevention of iron deficiency—* **Children:** 1 mg/kg P.O. daily as single or divided dose.	**GI:** *nausea,* vomiting, *constipation, black stools.* **Other:** stained tooth enamel.
ferrous fumarate Eldofe, F&B Caps, Farbegen, Feco-T, Feostat, Feroton♦♦, Ferranol, Ferrofume♦♦, Fersamal♦♦, Fumasorb, Fumerin, Hematon♦♦, Hemocyte, Ircon, Laud-Iron, Maniron, Novofumar♦♦, Palafer♦♦, Palmiron, Span-FF, Toleron	*Iron deficiency states—* **Adults:** 200 mg P.O. daily t.i.d. or q.i.d.	**GI:** *nausea,* vomiting, *constipation, black stools.* **Other:** stained tooth enamel.
ferrous gluconate Entron, Fergon♦, Ferralet, Ferrous-G, Fertinic♦♦, Novoferrogluc♦♦	*Iron deficiency—* **Adults:** 200 to 600 mg P.O., t.i.d. **Children 6 to 12 years:** 300 to 900 mg P.O. daily. **Children under 6 years:** 100 to 300 mg P.O. daily. 1 tablet contains 320 mg ferrous gluconate (37 mg elemental iron). 5 ml of elixir contains 300 mg ferrous gluconate (35 mg elemental iron).	**GI:** *nausea,* vomiting, *constipation, black stools.* **Other:** elixir may stain teeth.

♦ Available in U.S. and Canada. ♦♦ Available in Canada only. All other products (no symbol) available in U.S. only. Italicized side effects are common or life-threatening.

INTERACTIONS	NURSING CONSIDERATIONS
Antacids, cholestyramine resin, pancreatic extracts, vitamin E: decreased iron absorption. Separate doses if possible. *Chloramphenicol:* watch for delayed response to iron therapy. *Vitamin C:* may increase iron absorption. Beneficial drug interaction.	• Contraindicated in hemosiderosis, hemochromatosis, and hemolytic anemia. Usually contraindicated in peptic ulcer or ulcerative colitis. Use cautiously on long-term basis. • GI upset related to dose. Between-meal dosing preferable, but can be given with some foods although absorption may be decreased. Enteric-coated products reduce GI upset but also reduce amount of iron absorbed. • Iron is toxic; parents should be aware of iron poisoning in children. • Dilute liquid preparations in juice (preferably orange juice) or water, but not in milk or antacids. Give tablets with orange juice to promote iron absorption. • To avoid staining teeth, give liquid iron preparations with glass straw. • Check for constipation; record color and amount of stool. Teach dietary measures for preventing constipation. • Monitor hemoglobin and reticulocyte counts periodically during therapy.
Antacids, cholestyramine resin, pancreatic extracts, vitamin E: decreased iron absorption. Separate doses if possible. *Chloramphenicol:* watch for delayed response to iron therapy. *Vitamin C:* may increase iron absorption. Beneficial drug interaction.	• Contraindicated in peptic ulcer, regional enteritis, ulcerative colitis, hemosiderosis, and hemochromatosis. Use cautiously on long-term basis and in patients with anemia. • GI upset related to dose. Between-meal dosing preferable, but can be given with some foods although absorption may be decreased. Enteric-coated products reduce GI upset but also reduce amount of iron absorbed. • Iron is toxic; parents should be aware of iron poisoning in children. • Tablets may be given with juice or water, but not in milk or antacids. Give with orange juice to promote iron absorption. • To avoid staining teeth, give liquid iron preparations with glass straw. • Check for constipation; record color and amount of stool. Teach dietary measures for preventing constipation. • Monitor hemoglobin and reticulocyte counts during therapy. • Combination products—Simron, Ferro-Sequels, Ferocyl, Fer-Regules—contain stool softeners to help prevent constipation. Fermalox contains antacids to help relieve GI upset, if present; don't use this product unless absolutely necessary because of decreased iron absorption.
Antacids, cholestyramine resin, pancreatic extracts, vitamin E: decreased iron absorption. Separate doses if possible. *Chloramphenicol:* watch for delayed response to iron therapy. *Vitamin C:* may increase iron absorption. Beneficial drug interaction.	• Contraindicated in peptic ulcer, regional enteritis, ulcerative colitis, hemosiderosis, and hemochromatosis. Use cautiously on long-term basis and in patients with anemia. • GI upset related to dose. Between-meal dosing preferable, but can be given with some foods although absorption may be decreased. Enteric-coated products reduce GI upset but also reduce amount of iron absorbed. • Iron is toxic; parents should be aware of iron poisoning in children. • Dilute liquid preparations in juice (preferably orange juice) or water, but not in milk or antacids. Give tablets with orange juice to promote absorption. • To avoid staining teeth, give liquid iron preparations with glass straw. • Check for constipation; record color and amount of stool. Teach dietary measures for preventing constipation. • Monitor hemoglobin and reticulocyte counts during therapy.

NAME	INDICATIONS & DOSAGE	SIDE EFFECTS
ferrous sulfate Arne Modified Caps, Feosol, Fer-In-Sol♦, Fero-Grad♦♦, Fero-Gradumet, Ferolix, Ferospace, Ferralyn, Fesofor♦♦, Irospan, Mol-Iron, Novo-ferrosulfa♦♦, Slow-Fe♦♦, Telefon	*Iron deficiency—* **Adults:** 750 mg to 1.5 g P.O. daily divided t.i.d.; or 225 to 525 mg P.O. sustained-release preparations once daily or q 12 hours. **Children 6 to 12 years:** 600 mg P.O. daily in divided doses. *Prophylaxis for iron deficiency anemia—* **Pregnant women:** 300 to 600 mg P.O. daily in divided doses. **Premature or undernourished infants:** 3 to 6 mg/kg P.O. daily in divided doses.	**GI:** *nausea,* vomiting, *constipation, black stools.* **Other:** elixir may stain teeth.
iron dextran Hematran, Hydextran, Imferon♦, K-FeRON	*Iron deficiency anemia—* **Adults:** I.M. or I.V. injections of iron are advisable only for patients for whom oral administration is impossible or ineffective. Test dose (0.5 ml) required before administration. I.M. (by Z-track): inject 0.5 ml test dose. If no reactions, next daily dose should ordinarily not exceed 0.5 ml (25 mg) for infants under 5 kg; 1 ml (50 mg) for children under 9 kg; 2 ml (100 mg) for patients under 50 kg; 5 ml (250 mg) for patients over 50 kg. I.V. push: inject 0.5 ml test dose. If no reactions, within 2 to 3 days the dosage may be raised to 2 ml per day I.V., 1 ml/minute undiluted and infused slowly until total dose is achieved. No single dose should exceed 100 mg of iron. I.V. infusion: dosages are expressed in terms of elemental iron. Dilute in 250 to 1,000 ml of normal saline solution; dextrose increases local vein irritation. Infuse test dose of 25 mg slowly over 5 minutes. If no reaction occurs in 5 minutes, infusion may be started. Infuse total dose slowly over approximately 6 to 12 hours. 1 ml iron dextran = 50 mg elemental iron.	**CNS:** headache, transitory paresthesias, arthralgia, myalgia, dizziness, malaise, syncope. **CV:** *hypotensive reaction, peripheral vascular flushing with overly rapid I.V. administration, tachycardia.* **GI:** nausea, vomiting, metallic taste, transient loss of taste perception. **Local:** *soreness and inflammation at injection site (I.M.); brown skin discoloration at injection site (I.M.); local phlebitis at injection site (I.V.).* **Skin:** rash, urticaria. **Other:** *anaphylaxis.*

♦ Available in U.S. and Canada. ♦♦ Available in Canada only. All other products (no symbol) available in U.S. only. Italicized side effects are common or life-threatening.

INTERACTIONS	NURSING CONSIDERATIONS
Antacids, cholestyramine resin, pancreatic extracts, vitamin E: decreased iron absorption. Separate doses if possible. *Chloramphenicol:* watch for delayed response to iron therapy. *Vitamin C:* may increase iron absorption. Beneficial drug interaction.	• Contraindicated in peptic ulcer, ulcerative colitis, regional enteritis, hemosiderosis and hemochromatosis. Use cautiously on long-term basis and in patients with anemia. • GI upset related to dose. Between-meal dosing preferable, but can be given with some foods although absorption may be decreased. Enteric-coated products reduce GI upset but also reduce amount of iron absorbed. • Iron is toxic; parents should be aware of iron poisoning in children. • Dilute liquid preparations in juice or water, but not in milk or antacids. Dilute liquids in orange juice; give tablets with orange juice to promote iron absorption. • To avoid staining teeth, give liquid iron preparations with glass straw. • Check for constipation; record color and amount of stool. Teach dietary measures for preventing constipation. • Monitor hemoglobin and reticulocyte counts during therapy.
None significant.	• Contraindicated in all anemias other than iron deficiency anemia. Use with extreme caution in patients with impaired hepatic function and rheumatoid arthritis. • Monitor vital signs for drug reaction. Reactions are varied and severe, ranging from pain, inflammation, and myalgia to hypotension, shock, and death. • Inject deeply into upper outer quadrant of buttock—never into arm or other exposed area—with a 2″ to 3″ 19G or 20G needle. Use Z-track technique to avoid leakage into subcutaneous tissue and tattooing of skin. (See *How to Inject Iron Solutions,* p. 851.) • Hemoglobin concentration, hematocrit, and reticulocyte count should be determined periodically. • Use I.V. in these situations: insufficient muscle mass for deep intramuscular injection; impaired absorption from muscle due to stasis or edema; possibility of uncontrolled intramuscular bleeding from trauma (as may occur in hemophilia); and when massive and prolonged parenteral therapy is indicated (as may be necessary in cases of chronic substantial blood loss). • Patient should rest 15 to 30 minutes after I.V. administration. • Check hospital policy before administering I.V. In some hospitals, only doctor may administer iron I.V. • Not removed by hemodialysis. • For treatment of anaphylaxis, see inside front cover.

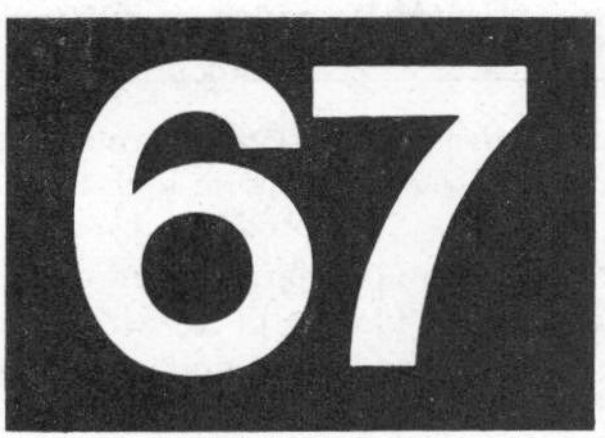

Anticoagulants and heparin antagonist

anisindione
dicumarol
heparin sodium
phenindione
phenprocoumon
protamine sulfate
warfarin potassium
warfarin sodium

Anticoagulants are given to patients at risk of developing clots (thromboses). These drugs are also used to prevent clot enlargement or fragmentation (thromboembolism).

Oral anticoagulants include the coumarin derivatives (dicumarol, phenprocoumon, warfarin potassium, and warfarin sodium) and the indandione derivatives (anisindione and phenindione). Heparin sodium, a parenteral anticoagulant, is antagonized by protamine sulfate.

Heparin, the coumarin derivatives, and the indandione derivatives impede clotting by preventing fibrin formation.

Major uses

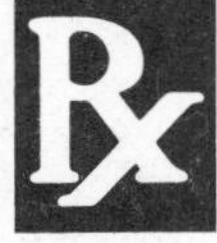

All anticoagulants are used to treat pulmonary emboli and deep vein thrombosis (DVT) and to reduce thrombus formation after myocardial infarction.

• Heparin is administered subcutaneously in low doses (minidoses) to prevent not only DVT but pulmonary embolism as well.

• Oral anticoagulants are also used in rheumatic heart disease with valvular damage and in atrial arrhythmias that obstruct hemodynamics.

• Protamine sulfate neutralizes the effects of heparin.

Mechanism of action

• Heparin accelerates formation of an antithrombin III-thrombin complex. It inactivates thrombin and prevents conversion of fibrinogen to fibrin.

• The oral anticoagulants inhibit vitamin K–dependent activation of clotting factors II, VII, IX, and X, which are formed in the liver.

• Protamine sulfate, a strong base, forms a physiologically inert complex with heparin sodium, a strong acid.

Absorption, distribution, metabolism, and excretion

• Heparin is not absorbed from the gastrointestinal (GI) tract and must be administered parenterally. Although absorption after subcutaneous injection varies greatly among patients, heparin is generally well absorbed and is usually administered by this route.

Heparin is distributed widely in the blood.

Although heparin's metabolism is not completely clear, most of the drug seems to be removed from circulation by the reticuloendothelial cells. However, some heparin is probably metabolized by the liver. A small fraction of the drug is excreted unchanged in urine.

• The oral anticoagulants anisindione, phenindione, phenprocoumon, and warfarin salts are well absorbed

UNDERSTANDING ANTICOAGULANT ACTION

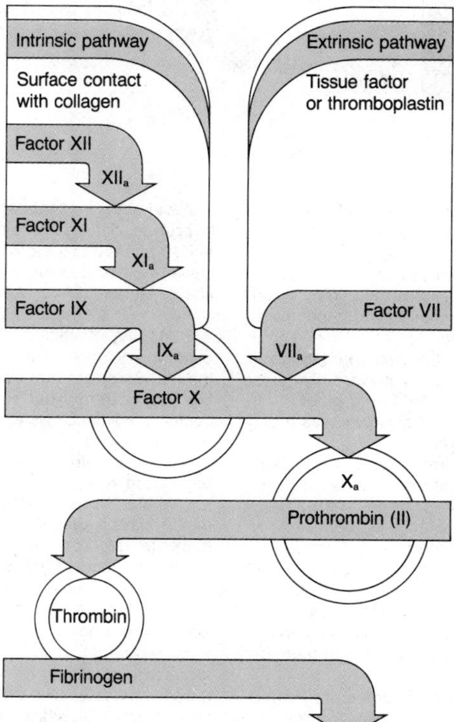

Coagulation results from the activation of a series of *factors*—a sequence known as a cascade. The process occurs by the intrinsic (intravascular) pathway and the extrinsic (extravascular) pathway. Both pathways are shown here.

The intrinsic pathway is started when Factor XII is disturbed (by coming in contact with collagen). This produces Factor XII_a (activated Factor XII) and the activation of Factor XI and Factor IX. Factor IX_a—with Factor VIII (as a cofactor) and phospholipids—then activates Factor X.

Factor X is also activated by the extrinsic pathway. As blood reaches the tissues, tissue factors or thromboplastin activate Factor VII. Factor VII_a then activates Factor X. As you can see, Factor X occupies a key position at the junction of the extrinsic and intrinsic pathways.

Coagulation then proceeds along a common pathway of more clotting factor activation. Factor X_a—with cofactor Factor V and phospholipids—converts prothrombin (Factor II) to thrombin. Thrombin converts fibrinogen to fibrin, forming a clot.

Thrombin also *increases* the activity of Factors V, VII_a, VIII, and X. So, if thrombin is inhibited, coagulation will be significantly affected. A naturally occurring protein, antithrombin III, neutralizes thrombin. Heparin acts by potentiating (increasing) the thrombin-neutralizing action of antithrombin III. Therefore, heparin's effect on the coagulation cascade is *multiple.*

Oral anticoagulants antagonize vitamin K, which is responsible for the formation of Factors II, VII, IX, and X from the liver.

Diagram adapted from the figure "The Coagulation System," in "Clinical Uses of Warfarin," *Drug Therapy,* January 1981. Used with permission of the publisher.

PATIENT-TEACHING AID

GUIDELINES FOR SUCCESSFUL ANTICOAGULANT THERAPY

Dear Patient:

Although you may be receiving heparin while in the hospital, your doctor will probably change the order to an oral anticoagulant before you are discharged. Since oral anticoagulants take time to work, probably you'll continue taking heparin as well for up to 5 days.

Oral anticoagulants affect your blood's clotting mechanism; they prevent dangerous clots from forming inside your blood vessels, but they don't dissolve clots that have already formed.

To get the most from your anticoagulant therapy, follow these instructions carefully:

- Tell the doctor if you've ever had any unusual reactions to anticoagulants.
- Don't take any other medications—including nonprescription medications, such as aspirin products, multiple vitamins, laxatives, and antacids—without asking the doctor first. Don't make substitutions in the medications he has given you permission to take.
- Tell the doctor if you become pregnant or are breast-feeding since oral anticoagulants may increase the risk of bleeding for you and your baby. Also, anticoagulants may cause birth defects if taken during the first 3 months of pregnancy.
- Don't use an intrauterine device while taking anticoagulants.
- Take your pills as ordered, at the same time every day. Don't skip a dose. If you miss a dose, take it as soon as possible; then resume your schedule. Never double a missed dose; *doubling the dose may cause bleeding.* Check with the doctor if you have any questions.
- The doctor will check your prothrombin (clotting) time regularly so that your dosage can be adjusted if necessary. This test measures the level of certain blood clotting factors necessary for coagulation. Your next appointment for this is ____________.
- Wear Medic Alert bracelet or carry identification card. Tell your dentist and other doctors you're taking anticoagulants.
- Avoid activities that can cause cuts or bruises; don't go barefoot.
- Use sharp items cautiously. Don't use power tools or a razor; try an electric shaver instead. Never trim corns, calluses, or nails with a sharp knife or razor.
- Don't play contact sports. If you have a minor injury, apply direct pressure to the cut. Be aware that clotting may take a little longer than usual. Report to the doctor any falls, blows to the body or head, or other injuries.
- Don't use bath oils. Place a nonslip bathmat in your tub.
- Use a soft-bristled toothbrush, and floss gently. Have a dental checkup regularly to ensure good oral hygiene.
- Ask the doctor if you can drink alcoholic beverages. Drinking too much alcohol may change the way this anticoagulant affects your body.
- Eat a normal, balanced diet, but avoid foods high in vitamin K—such as yellow and green vegetables, like broccoli—and foods high in fat, which increase the body's absorption of vitamin K. Check with the doctor if you can't eat for several days, or if you are vomiting or have continual diarrhea. These conditions decrease absorption of oral anticoagulants.
- Call the doctor if you notice color change in urine. Depending on your diet, urine may turn orange, but you may not be able to tell the difference between blood in urine and this normal coloration.
- Call the doctor if you notice any of the following symptoms: nosebleeds; bloody gums; red or brown urine; red or black bowel movements; cuts that won't stop bleeding; blood-tinged sputum; bruises; excessive menstrual flow; fever; rash; headaches; back or abdominal pain; dizziness, faintness, or unexplained weakness; hair loss; diarrhea; yellowing of skin or eyes; or sore mouth and throat.
- Tell the doctor if you have any concerns about taking this medication.

from the GI tract; dicumarol is incompletely absorbed.

Oral anticoagulants are 98% bound to plasma proteins, primarily albumin, and are widely distributed in body tissues.

They are largely metabolized in the liver, secreted into the bile as inactive metabolites, reabsorbed, and excreted in the urine.

- Protamine's metabolism and excretion are unclear.

Onset and duration

- Heparin sodium begins to act immediately, with peak effects occurring within minutes. Clotting time returns to normal within 2 to 6 hours.
- Oral anticoagulants are detectable in the blood within 1 hour after administration, and blood levels usually peak within 12 hours. However, oral anticoagulants require 1 to 3 days to produce therapeutic anticoagulation, even though they alter prothrombin time the first day of therapy. The average course of therapy is 3 to 6 months, but the anticoagulants should be used for the shortest period necessary. Durations vary from 1 to 14 days.
- Protamine sulfate neutralizes heparin within 5 minutes after I.V. administration.

Combination products

None.

THERAPEUTIC ACTIVITY

THERAPEUTIC ACTIVITY OF ORAL ANTICOAGULANTS

DRUG	PEAK PROTHROMBIN TIME	DURATION
anisindione	1 to 3 days	1 to 6 days
dicumarol	1 to 3 days	2 to 10 days
phenindione	½ to 3 days	1 to 5 days
phenprocoumon	1½ to 3 days	7 to 14 days
warfarin salts*	½ to 3 days	2 to 5 days

*Potassium and sodium salts

NAME	INDICATIONS & DOSAGE	SIDE EFFECTS
anisindione Miradon	*Treatment of pulmonary emboli; prevention and treatment of deep vein thrombosis, myocardial infarction, rheumatic heart disease with heart valve damage, atrial arrhythmias*— **Adults:** 300 mg P.O. first day, 200 mg P.O. second day, 100 mg P.O. third day. Maintenance dose: 25 to 250 mg daily based on prothrombin times.	**Blood:** *hemorrhage with excessive dosage, agranulocytosis,* leukopenia, leukocytosis, eosinophilia. **CNS:** headache. **CV:** myocarditis, tachycardia. **EENT:** conjunctivitis, blurred vision, paralysis of ocular accommodation. **GI:** diarrhea, sore mouth and throat. **GU:** *nephropathy with renal tubular necrosis,* albuminuria. **Hepatic:** jaundice. **Skin:** *rash, severe exfoliative dermatitis.* **Other:** *fever.*

◆ Available in U.S. and Canada. ◆◆ Available in Canada only. All other products (no symbol) available in U.S. only. Italicized side effects are common or life-threatening.

INTERACTIONS

Allopurinol, clofibrate, dextrothyroxine, thyroid drugs, heparin, anabolic steroids, disulfiram, para-aminosalicylic acid, glucagon, inhalation anesthetics, sulfonamides: increased prothrombin time. Monitor patient carefully. Consider anticoagulant dose reduction.

Ethacrynic acid, indomethacin, mefenamic acid, oxyphenbutazone, phenylbutazone, salicylates: increased prothrombin time; ulcerogenic effects. Don't use together.

Antipyrine, carbamazepine, antacids, griseofulvin, haloperidol, paraldehyde, rifampin: decreased prothrombin time. Monitor patient carefully.

Phenytoin, glutethimide, chloral hydrate, triclofos sodium, alcohol, diuretics: increased or decreased prothrombin time. Avoid use if possible, or monitor patient carefully.

Barbiturates: inhibition of hypoprothrombinemic effect of anticoagulants. If barbiturates are withdrawn, reduce anticoagulant dose; inhibition may last for weeks after anticoagulant is withdrawn, but fatal hemorrhage can occur when inhibiting effect disappears.

Cholestyramine: decreased response when administered too close together. Administer 6 hours after oral anticoagulants.

NURSING CONSIDERATIONS

- Contraindicated in hemophilia, thrombocytopenic purpura, leukemia with pronounced bleeding tendency, open wounds or ulcers, impaired hepatic or renal function, severe hypertension, acute nephritis, subacute bacterial endocarditis. Use cautiously in pregnancy or lactation, during menses, during use of any drainage tube in any orifice, and in any patient in whom slight bleeding is dangerous. Use with extreme caution (if at all) in psychiatric patients, debilitated patients, or cachectic patients.
- Use caution when adding or stopping any drug for patient receiving anticoagulants. May change the clotting status and result in hemorrhage.
- Fever and skin rash signal severe complications.
- Give drug at same time daily. Stress importance of complying with recommended dosage and keeping follow-up appointments. Patient should carry a card that identifies him as a potential bleeder.
- Regularly inspect patient for bleeding gums, bruises on arms or legs, petechiae, nosebleeds, melena, tarry stools, hematuria, hematemesis. Tell patient and family to watch for these signs and notify doctor immediately.
- Warn patient to avoid over-the-counter products containing aspirin, other salicylates, or any drugs that may interact with anisindione.
- Because onset of action is delayed, heparin sodium is often given during first few days of treatment. When heparin is being given simultaneously, don't draw blood for prothrombin time within 5 hours after I.V. heparin administration.
- Schedule doses according to prothrombin time (PT). Doctors usually try to maintain PT at 1.5 to 2 times normal. Numerical PT values depend on procedure and reagents used in individual laboratory.
- Tell patient to notify doctor if menses is heavier than usual. May require adjusting dose.
- Tell patient to use electric razor when shaving to avoid scratching skin, and to brush teeth with a soft toothbrush.
- Warn patient that alkaline urine may turn red-orange.
- Duration of action 1 to 6 days.
- Light to moderate alcohol intake does not significantly affect prothrombin time.
- For symptoms and treatment of toxicity, see APPENDIX, *Drug Toxicities*.

NAME	INDICATIONS & DOSAGE	SIDE EFFECTS
dicumarol Dufalone♦♦	*Treatment of pulmonary emboli; prevention and treatment of deep vein thrombosis, myocardial infarction, rheumatic heart disease with heart valve damage, atrial arrhythmias*— **Adults:** 200 to 300 mg P.O. on first day, 25 to 200 mg P.O. daily thereafter, based on prothrombin times.	**Blood:** *hemorrhage with excessive dosage,* leukopenia, *agranulocytosis.* **GI:** anorexia, nausea, vomiting, cramps, *diarrhea,* mouth ulcers. **GU:** hematuria. **Skin:** dermatitis, urticaria, alopecia, *rash.* **Other:** *fever.*

♦ Available in U.S. and Canada. ♦♦ Available in Canada only. All other products (no symbol) available in U.S. only. Italicized side effects are common or life-threatening.

INTERACTIONS	NURSING CONSIDERATIONS
Allopurinol, clofibrate, dextrothyroxine, thyroid drugs, heparin, anabolic steroids, disulfiram, para-aminosalicylic acid, glucagon, inhalation anesthetics, sulfonamides: increased prothrombin time. Monitor patient carefully. Consider anticoagulant dose reduction. *Ethacrynic acid, indomethacin, mefenamic acid, oxyphenbutazone, phenylbutazone, salicylates:* increased prothrombin time; ulcerogenic effects. Don't use together. *Antipyrine, carbamazepine, antacids, griseofulvin, haloperidol, paraldehyde, rifampin:* decreased prothrombin time. Monitor patient carefully. *Phenytoin, glutethimide, chloral hydrate, triclofos sodium:* increased or decreased prothrombin time. Avoid use if possible, or monitor patient carefully. *Barbiturates:* inhibition of hypoprothrombinemic effect of anticoagulants. If barbiturates are withdrawn, reduce anticoagulant dose; inhibition may last weeks after anticoagulant withdrawn, but fatal hemorrhage can occur when inhibiting effect disappears. *Cholestyramine:* decreased response when given too close together. Give 6 hours after oral anticoagulants.	• Contraindicated in hemophilia, thrombocytopenic purpura, leukemia with pronounced bleeding tendency, open wounds or ulcers, impaired hepatic or renal function, severe hypertension, acute nephritis, subacute bacterial endocarditis. Use cautiously in pregnancy or lactation, during menses, during use of any drainage tube, and in any patient in whom slight bleeding is dangerous. Use with extreme caution (if at all) in psychiatric patients, debilitated patients, or cachectic patients. • Use caution when adding or stopping any drug for patient receiving anticoagulants. May change the clotting status and result in hemorrhage. • Fever and skin rash signal severe complications. • Give drug at same time daily. Stress importance of complying with recommended dosage and keeping follow-up appointments. Patient should carry a card that identifies him as a potential bleeder. • Regularly inspect patient for bleeding gums, bruises on arms or legs, petechiae, nosebleeds, melena, tarry stools, hematuria, hematemesis. Tell patient and family to watch for these signs and notify doctor immediately. • Warn patient to avoid over-the-counter products containing aspirin, other salicylates, or drugs that may interact with dicumarol. • Because onset of action is delayed, heparin sodium is often given during first few days of treatment. When heparin is being given simultaneously, don't draw blood for prothrombin time within 5 hours after I.V. heparin administration. • Dose given depends on prothrombin time (PT). Doctors usually try to maintain PT at 1.5 to 2 times normal. PT values depend on procedure and reagents used in individual laboratory. • Tell patient to notify doctor if menses is heavier than usual. May require adjusting dose. • Tell patient to use electric razor when shaving to avoid scratching skin and to brush teeth with a soft toothbrush. • May turn alkaline urine red-orange. • Duration of action 2 to 10 days. • Light to moderate alcohol intake does not significantly affect prothrombin times. • For symptoms and treatment of toxicity, see APPENDIX, *Drug Toxicities*.

NAME	INDICATIONS & DOSAGE	SIDE EFFECTS
heparin sodium Hepalean♦♦, Heprinar, Lipo-Hepin, Liquaemin Sodium, Panheprin	*Treatment of deep vein thrombosis, myocardial infarction—* **Adults:** initially, 5,000 to 7,500 units I.V. push, then adjust dose according to PTT results and give dose I.V. q 4 hours (usually 4,000 to 5,000 units); or 5,000 to 7,500 units I.V. bolus, then 1,000 units/hour by I.V. infusion pump. Wait 8 hours following bolus dose, and adjust hourly rate according to PTT. *Treatment of pulmonary embolism—* **Adults:** initially, 7,500 to 10,000 units I.V. push, then adjust dose according to PTT results and give dose I.V. q 4 hours (usually 4,000 to 5,000 units); or 7,500 to 10,000 units I.V. bolus, then 1,000 units/ hour by I.V. infusion pump. Wait 8 hours following bolus dose, and adjust hourly rate according to PTT. *Prophylaxis of embolism—* **Adults:** 5,000 units S.C. q 12 hours. *Open heart surgery—* **Adults:** (total body perfusion) 150 to 300 units/kg continuous I.V infusion. *Treatment of pulmonary emboli; prevention and treatment of deep vein thrombosis—* **Children:** initially, 50 units/kg I.V. drip. Maintenance dose 100 units/kg I.V. drip q 4 hours. Constant infusion: 20,000 units/ m^2 daily. Dosages adjusted according to PTT. Heparin dosing is highly individualized, depending upon disease state, age, renal and hepatic status.	**Blood:** *hemorrhage with excessive dosage, overly prolonged clotting time, thrombocytopenia.* **Local:** irritation, mild pain. **Other:** hypersensitivity reactions including chills, fever, pruritus, rhinitis, burning of feet, conjunctivitis, lacrimation, arthralgia, urticaria.

INTERACTIONS	NURSING CONSIDERATIONS
Salicylates: increased anticoagulant effect. Don't use together. *Anticoagulants, oral:* additive anticoagulation. Monitor prothrombin time and partial thromboplastin time.	• Conditionally contraindicated in active bleeding; blood dyscrasias; or bleeding tendencies such as hemophilia, thrombocytopenia, or hepatic disease with hypoprothrombinemia; suspected intracranial hemorrhage; suppurative thrombophlebitis; inaccessible ulcerative lesions (especially of GI tract); open ulcerative wounds; extensive denudation of skin; ascorbic acid deficiency and other conditions causing increased capillary permeability; during or after brain, eye, or spinal cord surgery; during continuous tube drainage of stomach or small intestine; in subacute bacterial endocarditis; shock; advanced renal disease; threatened abortion; severe hypertension. Although the use of heparin is clearly hazardous in these conditions, a decision to use it depends on the comparative risk in failure to treat the coexisting thromboembolic disorder. • Use cautiously during menses; in mild hepatic or renal disease; alcoholism; in patients in occupations with the risk of physical injury; immediately postpartum; and in patients with history of allergies, asthma, or GI ulcers. • Monitor platelet counts regularly. Thrombocytopenia caused by heparin may be associated with arterial thrombosis. • Measure partial thromboplastin time (PTT) carefully and regularly. Anticoagulation present when PTT values are 1.5 to 2 times control values. • Drug requirements are higher in early phases of thrombogenic diseases and febrile states; lower when patient becomes stabilized. • Regularly inspect patient for bleeding gums, bruises on arms or legs, petechiae, nosebleeds, melena, tarry stools, hematuria, hematemesis. Tell patient and family to watch for these signs and notify doctor immediately. • Tell patient to avoid over-the-counter medications containing aspirin, other salicylates, or drugs that may interact with heparin. • Heparin comes in various concentrations. Check order and vial carefully. • Low-dose injections given sequentially between iliac crests in lower abdomen deep into subcutaneous fat. Inject drug slowly subcutaneously into fat pad. Leave needle in place for 10 seconds after injection; then withdraw needle. Alternate site every 12 hours—right for a.m., left for p.m. • Don't massage after subcutaneous injection. Watch for signs of bleeding at injection site. Rotate sites and keep accurate record. • Check constant I.V. infusions regularly, even when pumps are in good working order, to prevent overdosage or underdosage. • I.M. administration not recommended. • I.V. administration preferred because of long-term effect and irregular absorption when given subcutaneously. Whenever possible, administer I.V. heparin using infusion pump to provide maximum safety. • Concentrated heparin solutions (greater than 100 units/ml) can irritate blood vessels. • Place notice above patient's bed to inform I.V. team or lab personnel to apply pressure dressings after taking blood. • Avoid excessive I.M. injections of other drugs to prevent or minimize hematomas. If possible, don't give I.M. injections at all. • Elderly patients should usually start at lower doses. • When intermittent I.V. therapy is utilized, always draw blood ½ hour before next scheduled dose to avoid falsely elevated PTT. • Blood for PTT can be drawn any time after 8 hours of initiation of continuous I.V. heparin therapy. Never draw blood for PTT from the I.V. tubing of the heparin infusion, or from vein of infusion. Falsely

(continued on following page)

NAME	INDICATIONS & DOSAGE	SIDE EFFECTS
heparin sodium *(continued)*		
phenindione Danilone♦♦, Eridione, Hedulin	*Treatment of pulmonary emboli; prevention and treatment of deep vein thrombosis, myocardial infarction, rheumatic heart disease with heart valve damage, atrial arrhythmias*— **Adults:** 300 mg P.O. first day; 200 mg P.O. second day. Maintenance dose: 50 to 150 mg daily, based on prothrombin times.	**Blood:** *hemorrhage with excessive dosage, agranulocytosis,* leukopenia, leukocytosis, eosinophilia. **CNS:** headache. **CV:** myocarditis, tachycardia. **EENT:** conjunctivitis, blurred vision, paralysis of ocular accommodation. **GI:** diarrhea, sore mouth and throat. **GU:** *nephropathy with renal tubular necrosis,* albuminuria. **Hepatic:** jaundice. **Skin:** *rash, severe exfoliative dermatitis.* **Other:** *fever.*

♦ Available in U.S. and Canada. ♦♦ Available in Canada only. All other products (no symbol) available in U.S. only. Italicized side effects are common or life-threatening.

INTERACTIONS	**NURSING CONSIDERATIONS**
	elevated PTT will result. Always draw blood from opposite arm. • Give on time; try not to skip a dose. If I.V. is out, get it restarted as soon as possible, and reschedule dose immediately. • Never piggyback other drugs into an infusion line while heparin infusion is running. Many antibiotics and other drugs inactivate heparin. Never mix any drug with heparin in syringe when bolus therapy is used. • Abrupt withdrawal may cause increased coagulability. Usually, heparin therapy is followed by oral anticoagulants for prophylaxis. • For symptoms and treatment of toxicity, see APPENDIX, *Drug Toxicities*.
Allopurinol, clofibrate, dextrothyroxine, thyroid drugs, heparin, anabolic steroids, disulfiram, para-aminosalicylic acid, glucagon, inhalation anesthetics, sulfonamides: increased prothrombin time. Monitor patient carefully. Consider anticoagulant dose reduction. *Ethacrynic acid, indomethacin, mefenamic acid, oxyphenbutazone, phenylbutazone, salicylates:* increased prothrombin time; ulcerogenic effects. Don't use together. *Antipyrine, carbamazepine, antacids, griseofulvin, haloperidol, paraldehyde, rifampin:* decreased prothrombin time. Monitor patient carefully. *Phenytoin, glutethimide, chloral hydrate, triclofos sodium, alcohol, diuretics:* increased or decreased prothrombin time. Avoid use if possible, or monitor patient carefully. *Barbiturates:* inhibition of hypoprothrombinemic effect of anticoagulants. If barbiturates are withdrawn, reduce anticoagulant dose;	• Contraindicated in hemophilia, thrombocytopenic purpura, leukemia with pronounced bleeding tendency, open wounds or ulcers, impaired hepatic or renal function, severe hypertension, acute nephritis, and subacute bacterial endocarditis. Use cautiously in pregnancy or lactation, during menses, during use of any drainage tube in any orifice, and in any patient in whom slight bleeding is dangerous. Use with extreme caution (if at all) in psychiatric patients, debilitated patients, or cachectic patients. • Use caution when adding or stopping any drug. May cause alteration in clotting status and result in hemorrhage. • Fever and skin rash signal severe complications. • Give drug at same time daily. Stress importance of complying with recommended dosage and keeping follow-up appointments. Patient should carry a card that identifies him as a potential bleeder. • Regularly inspect patient for bleeding gums, bruises on arms or legs, petechiae, nosebleeds, melena, tarry stools, hematuria, hematemesis. Tell patient and family to watch for these signs and notify doctor immediately. • Warn patient to avoid over-the-counter products containing aspirin, salicylates, or other drugs that may interact with phenindione. • Because onset of action is delayed, heparin sodium is often given during first few days of treatment. When heparin is being given simultaneously, don't draw blood for prothrombin time within 5 hours after I.V. heparin administration. • Dose given depends on prothrombin time (PT). Doctors usually try to maintain PT at 1.5 to 2 times normal. Numerical PT values depend on procedure and reagents used in individual laboratory. • Tell patient to notify doctor if menses is heavier than usual. May require adjusting dose. • Tell patient to use electric razor when shaving to avoid scratching skin and to brush teeth with a soft toothbrush. • Warn patient that alkaline urine may turn red-orange. • Duration of action is 1 to 5 days. • Light to moderate alcohol intake does not significantly affect prothrombin time. • For symptoms and treatment of toxicity, see APPENDIX, *Drug Toxicities*.

(continued on following page)

NAME	INDICATIONS & DOSAGE	SIDE EFFECTS
phenindione *(continued)*		
phenprocoumon Liquamar, Marcumar♦♦	*Treatment of pulmonary emboli; prevention and treatment of deep vein thrombosis, myocardial infarction, rheumatic heart disease with heart valve damage, atrial arrhythmias—* **Adults:** initially, 24 mg P.O. Maintenance dose: 0.75 to 6 mg daily, based on prothrombin time.	**Blood:** *hemorrhage with excessive dosage, agranulocytosis,* leukopenia. **GI:** paralytic ileus and intestinal obstruction (both resulting from hemorrhage), nausea, vomiting, cramps, diarrhea, mouth ulcers. **GU:** nephropathy, hematuria. **Skin:** *rash,* alopecia, necrosis. **Other:** *fever.*

♦ Available in U.S. and Canada. ♦♦ Available in Canada only. All other products (no symbol) available in U.S. only. Italicized side effects are common or life-threatening.

INTERACTIONS	NURSING CONSIDERATIONS
inhibition may last weeks after anticoagulant withdrawn, but fatal hemorrhage can occur when inhibiting effect disappears. *Cholestyramine:* decreased response when administered too close together. Administer 6 hours after oral anticoagulants.	
Allopurinol, clofibrate, dextrothyroxine, thyroid drugs, heparin, anabolic steroids, disulfiram, para-aminosalicylic acid, glucagon, inhalation anesthetics, sulfinpyrazone, sulindac, sulfonamides: increased prothrombin time. Monitor patient carefully. Consider anticoagulant dose reduction. *Ethacrynic acid, indomethacin, mefenamic acid, oxyphenbutazone, phenylbutazone, salicylates:* increased prothrombin time; ulcerogenic effects. Don't use together. *Antipyrine, carbamazepine, antacids, griseofulvin, haloperidol, paraldehyde, rifampin:* decreased prothrombin time. Monitor patient carefully. *Phenytoin, glutethimide, chloral hydrate, triclofos sodium:* increased or decreased prothrombin time. Avoid use if possible, or monitor patient carefully. *Barbiturates:* inhibition of hypoprothrombinemic effect of anticoagulants. If	• Contraindicated in hemophilia, thrombocytopenic purpura, leukemia with pronounced bleeding tendency, open wounds or ulcers, impaired hepatic or renal function, severe hypertension, acute nephritis, and subacute bacterial endocarditis. Use cautiously in pregnancy or lactation, during menses, during use of any drainage tube in any orifice, and in any patient in whom slight bleeding is dangerous. Use with extreme caution (if at all) in psychiatric, debilitated, or cachectic patients. • Use caution when adding or stopping any drug for patient receiving anticoagulants. May change the clotting status and result in hemorrhage. • Fever and skin rash signal severe complications. • Give drug at same time daily. Stress importance of complying with recommended dosage and keeping follow-up appointments. Patient should carry a card that identifies him as a potential bleeder. • Regularly inspect patient for bleeding gums, bruises on arms or legs, petechiae, nosebleeds, melena, tarry stools, hematuria, hematemesis. Tell patient and family to watch for these signs and notify doctor immediately. • Warn patient to avoid over-the-counter products containing aspirin, other salicylates, or drugs that may interact with phenprocoumon. • Because onset of action is delayed, heparin sodium is often given during first few days of treatment. When heparin is being given simultaneously, don't draw blood for prothrombin time within 5 hours of I.V. heparin administration. • Dose given depends on prothrombin time (PT). Doctors usually try to maintain PT at 1.5 to 2 times normal. Numerical PT values depend on procedure and reagents used in individual laboratory. • Tell patient to notify doctor if menses is heavier than usual. May require adjusting dose. • Tell patient to use electric razor when shaving to avoid scratching skin and to brush teeth with a soft toothbrush. • Warn patient that alkaline urine may turn orange-red. • A coumarin derivative. • Duration of action is 7 to 14 days. • Light to moderate alcohol intake does not significantly affect prothrombin times. • For symptoms and treatment of toxicity, see APPENDIX, *Drug Toxicities.*

(continued on following page)

NAME	INDICATIONS & DOSAGE	SIDE EFFECTS
phenprocoumon *(continued)*		
protamine sulfate	*Heparin overdose—* **Adults:** dosage based on venous blood coagulation studies, generally 1 mg for each 78 to 95 units of heparin. Give diluted to 1% (10 mg/ml) slow I.V. injection over 1 to 3 minutes. Maximum 50 mg/10 minutes.	**CV:** fall in blood pressure, bradycardia. **Other:** transitory flushing, feeling of warmth, dyspnea.
warfarin potassium Athrombin-K♦ **warfarin sodium** Coumadin♦, Panwarfin, Warfilone Sodium♦♦, Warnerin Sodium♦♦	*Treatment of pulmonary emboli; prevention and treatment of deep vein thrombosis, myocardial infarction, rheumatic heart disease with heart valve damage, atrial arrhythmias—* **Adults:** 10 to 15 mg P.O. for 3 days, then dosage based on daily prothrombin times. Usual maintenance dose 2 to 10 mg P.O. daily. Alternate regimen: initially, 40 to 60 mg P.O. daily; then 2 to 10 mg daily based on PT determinations. Warfarin sodium also available for I.V. use (50 mg per vial). Reconstitute with sterile water for injection. I.V. form rarely used and may be in periodic short supply.	**Blood:** *hemorrhage with excessive dosage,* leukopenia. **GI:** paralytic ileus, intestinal obstruction (both resulting from hemorrhage), diarrhea, vomiting, cramps, nausea. **GU:** excessive uterine bleeding. **Skin:** dermatitis, urticaria, *rash,* necrosis, alopecia. **Other:** *fever.*

♦ Available in U.S. and Canada. ♦♦ Available in Canada only. All other products (no symbol) available in U.S. only. Italicized side effects are common or life-threatening.

INTERACTIONS	NURSING CONSIDERATIONS
barbiturates are withdrawn, reduce anticoagulant dose; inhibition may last for weeks after anticoagulant is withdrawn, but fatal hemorrhage can occur when inhibiting effect disappears. *Cholestyramine:* decreased response when administered too close together. Administer 6 hours after oral anticoagulants.	
None significant.	• Use cautiously in patients with allergy to fish or after cardiac surgery. • Doctor gives this drug. Should be given slowly to reduce side effects. Have equipment available to treat shock. • Monitor patient continually. Check vital signs frequently. • Watch for spontaneous bleeding (heparin "rebound"), especially in patients undergoing dialysis and those who have had cardiac surgery. • Protamine sulfate may act as anticoagulant in very high doses. • 1 mg of protamine neutralizes 78 to 95 units of heparin. • Heparin antagonist.
Allopurinol, clofibrate, dextrothyroxine, thyroid drugs, heparin, anabolic steroids, cimetidine, disulfiram, para-aminosalicylic acid, glucagon, inhalation anesthetics, sulfinpyrazone, sulindac, sulfonamides: increased prothrombin time. Monitor patient carefully. Consider anticoagulant dose reduction. *Ethacrynic acid, indomethacin, mefenamic acid, oxyphenbutazone, phenylbutazone, salicylates:* increased prothrombin time; ulcerogenic effects. Don't use together. *Griseofulvin, haloperidol, paraldehyde, rifampin:* decreased prothrombin time.	• Contraindicated in bleeding or hemorrhagic tendencies resulting from open wounds, visceral cancer, GI ulcers, severe hepatic or renal disease, severe uncontrolled hypertension, subacute bacterial endocarditis, vitamin K deficiency; after recent operations in eye, brain, or spinal cord. Use cautiously in diverticulitis, colitis, mild or moderate hypertension, mild or moderate hepatic or renal disease, lactation; in presence of drainage tubes in any orifice; with regional or lumbar block anesthesia; or in any condition increasing risk of hemorrhage. • Observe nursing infants of mothers on drug for unexpected bleeding. • PT determinations essential for proper control. High incidence of bleeding when PT exceeds 2.5 times control values. Doctors usually try to maintain PT at 1.5 to 2 times normal. • May divide large doses to reduce GI distress. • Give at same time daily. Stress importance of complying with recommended dosage and keeping follow-up appointments. Patient should carry a card that identifies him as a potential bleeder. • Elderly patients and patients with renal or hepatic failure are especially sensitive to warfarin effect. • Half-life of warfarin is 36 to 44 hours. • Warfarin effect can be neutralized by vitamin K injections. • Regularly inspect patient for bleeding gums, bruises on arms or legs, petechiae, nosebleeds, melena, tarry stools, hematuria, hematemesis. Tell patient and family to watch for these signs and notify doctor immediately. • Warn patient to avoid over-the-counter products containing aspirin, other salicylates, or drugs that may interact with warfarin salts. • Because onset of action is delayed, heparin sodium is often given during first few days of treatment. When heparin is being given simultaneously, don't draw blood for prothrombin time within 5 hours

(continued on following page)

NAME	INDICATIONS & DOSAGE	SIDE EFFECTS
warfarin *(continued)*		

♦ Available in U.S. and Canada. ♦♦ Available in Canada only. All other products (no symbol) available in U.S. only. Italicized side effects are common or life-threatening.

INTERACTIONS	NURSING CONSIDERATIONS
Monitor patient carefully. *Glutethimide, chloral hydrate, triclofos sodium:* increased or decreased prothrombin time. Avoid use if possible, or monitor patient carefully. *Barbiturates:* inhibition of hypoprothrombinemic effect of anticoagulants. If barbiturates are withdrawn, reduce anticoagulant dose; inhibition may last weeks after anticoagulant withdrawn, but fatal hemorrhage can occur when inhibiting effect disappears. *Cholestyramine:* decreased response when administered too close together. Administer 6 hours after oral anticoagulants.	of I.V. heparin administration. • Fever and skin rash signal severe complications. • Tell patient to notify doctor if menses is heavier than usual. May require adjusting dose. • Tell patient to use electric razor when shaving to avoid scratching skin and to brush teeth with a soft toothbrush. • Best oral anticoagulant when patient must receive antacids or phenytoin. • Light to moderate alcohol intake does not significantly affect prothrombin time. • Possibly effective in treatment of transient cerebral ischemic attacks. • For symptoms and treatment of toxicity, see APPENDIX, *Drug Toxicities*.

WHAT YOU SHOULD KNOW ABOUT INJECTING HEPARIN

To inject heparin, follow the usual procedure for any subcutaneous injection, except for these considerations:

- Use a ½″ 25G or 26G needle.
- Select an injection site on the patient's abdomen. The preferred site is between the iliac crests, as shown in this illustration. Remember, you must rotate injection sites. Study this illustration to determine which sites to choose.
- Pinch a ½″ (1.3 cm) fold of tissue between your thumb and forefinger, and insert the needle into the fold at a 90° angle. Using this technique will minimize heparin's irritating qualities. Applying ice to the site before injecting may help too. But don't apply it until you check your hospital's policy on this technique and have a doctor's order for it.
- Don't check for blood backflow. You could damage the tissue and cause a hematoma.
- Never massage the site after the injection. You could rupture the small blood vessels and cause a hematoma.

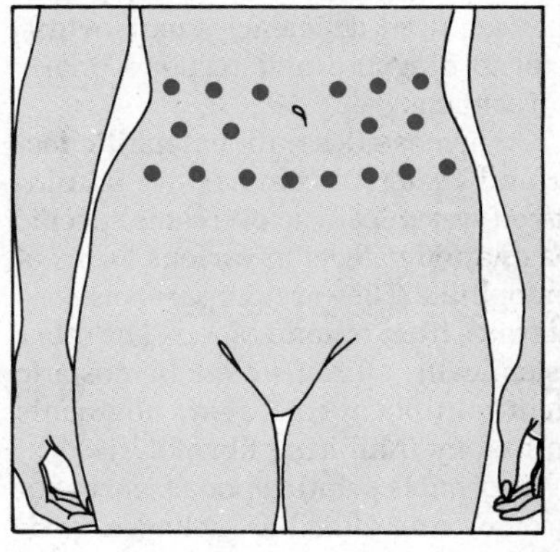

68 Hemostatics

absorbable gelatin sponge
aminocaproic acid
antihemophilic factor (AHF)
carbazochrome salicylate
Factor IX complex
microfibrillar collagen hemostat
negatol
oxidized cellulose
thrombin

Hemostatics, which arrest blood flow or reduce capillary bleeding, should be used cautiously to avoid the risk of redundant clotting. Although all these agents stop excessive bleeding, each has a specific indication in clotting. An accurate diagnosis of the cause of excessive bleeding should be established quickly. If the bleeding results from a specific hereditary deficiency (hemophilia A), diagnosis and treatment may be relatively simple; conversely, multiple acquired deficiencies may be difficult to diagnose and respond poorly to treatment.

The hemostatics antihemophilic factor and Factor IX complex are administered systemically to overcome specific coagulation defects in various forms of hemophilia. They are prepared as concentrates from human blood. The other systemically administered hemostatic agent, aminocaproic acid, augments clotting by inhibiting fibrinolysis.

Absorbable gelatin sponge, carbazochrome, microfibrillar collagen, oxidized cellulose, negatol, and thrombin are applied locally to control surface bleeding and capillary oozing.

Major uses

Rx

- Absorbable gelatin sponge, microfibrillar collagen hemostat, and oxidized cellulose are hemostatic adjuncts in various surgical procedures. Absorbable gelatin sponge also aids healing of decubitus ulcers.
- Aminocaproic acid is used to arrest excessive bleeding resulting from hyperfibrinolysis. It is also an antidote for streptokinase and urokinase toxicity.
- Antihemophilic factor corrects hemophilia A (Factor VIII deficiency).
- Carbazochrome salicylate corrects excessive capillary permeability during surgical treatment for conditions accompanied by excessive oozing.
- Factor IX complex, which contains factors II, VII, IX, and X, is used to treat hemophilia B (Factor IX deficiency, or Christmas disease) and also combats anticoagulant overdose.
- Negatol, which acts as a styptic and hemostatic, is used for oral ulcers and cervical bleeding.
- Thrombin controls bleeding from tissue parenchyma, cancellous bone, and dental sockets; during nasal and laryngeal surgical procedures, plastic surgery, and skin-grafting procedures; and in acute gastrointestinal hemorrhages.

Mechanism of action

- Absorbable gelatin sponge and oxidized cellulose absorb and hold many times their weight in blood. Absorbable gelatin sponge also provides a framework for growth of granulation tissue.

• Aminocaproic acid inhibits plasminogen activator substances. To a lesser degree, it blocks antiplasmin activity by inhibiting fibrinolysis.
• Antihemophilic factor and Factor IX complex directly replace deficient clotting factors.
• Carbazochrome salicylate decreases capillary permeability.
• Microfibrillar collagen hemostat attracts and aggregates platelets.
• Negatol is an astringent and protein denaturant.
• Thrombin clots to form fibrin in the presence of fibrinogen.

Absorption, distribution, metabolism, and excretion

• Aminocaproic acid is rapidly absorbed after oral administration and excreted mostly unmetabolized in urine.
• Antihemophilic factor and Factor IX complex are distributed to the plasma after I.V. administration. They are metabolized and excreted as normal physiologic substances.
• The topical agents aren't absorbed and therefore aren't distributed, metabolized, or excreted.

Onset and duration

• Aminocaproic acid begins to act almost immediately after oral or parenteral administration and reaches peak levels within 1 to 2 hours. Rapid excretion and short duration require either repeated oral doses at 1- to 2-hour intervals or continuous I.V. infusion.
• Antihemophilic factor and Factor IX complex begin to act immediately. Their durations are related to the level of factor deficiency and the presence of Factor VIII and Factor IX antibodies.
• Thrombin's onset and duration depend on concentration. For example, 5,000 units of thrombin/5 ml normal saline solution clot an equal volume of blood in less than 1 second and clot 1 liter of blood in less than 1 minute.
• Onset and duration of the other topical agents depend on the amount used, extent of blood saturation, and type of tissue bed.

HOW AMINOCAPROIC ACID AIDS CLOTTING

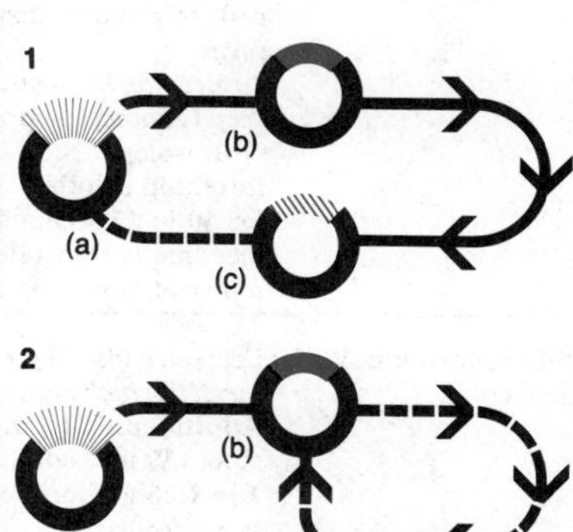

Here's what happens in the typical hemorrhagic process (illustration 1):
(a) Ruptured aneurysm results in bleeding.
(b) Bleeding stops. Clot seals the rupture, reinforcing aneurysm.
(c) In 7 to 10 days, fibrinolysis normally occurs, dissolving the clot and creating the danger of rebleed.

Aminocaproic acid counters fibrinolysis (illustration 2) in this way:
(a) Ruptured aneurysm results in bleeding.
(b) Bleeding stops. Clot seals the rupture, reinforcing the aneurysm. Some doctors use aminocaproic acid during the acute period, to maintain this seal. An antifibrinolytic agent, aminocaproic acid delays clot dissolution and may forestall a potential rebleed.

Remember these points when administering aminocaproic acid:
• If the patient is receiving the drug I.V., *don't infuse too rapidly.* Rapid infusion could result in bradycardia, hypotension, or arrhythmias. *Tip:* Use an I.V. infusion pump to control the rate of administration.
• Observe the patient receiving aminocaproic acid for side effects, such as generalized thrombosis, headache, hypotension, nausea, cramps, and diarrhea.
• Antifibrinolytic activity may increase the risk of thrombophlebitis and of pulmonary embolus.

Combination products

None.

NAME	INDICATIONS & DOSAGE	SIDE EFFECTS
absorbable gelatin sponge Gelfoam	**Adults:** *Decubitus ulcers*—place aseptically deep into ulcer. Don't disturb or remove; may add extra p.r.n. *To provide hemostasis in surgery (adjunct)*—apply saturated with isotonic NaCl injection or thrombin solution. Hold in place for 10 to 15 seconds. When bleeding is controlled, allow material to remain in place.	None reported.
aminocaproic acid Amicar♦	*Excessive bleeding resulting from hyperfibrinolysis*— **Adults:** initially, 5 g P.O. or slow I.V. infusion, followed by 1 to 1.25 g hourly until bleeding is controlled. Maximum dose 30 g daily.	**Blood:** generalized thrombosis. **CNS:** dizziness, malaise, headache. **CV:** hypotension, bradycardia, arrhythmia (with rapid I.V. infusion). **EENT:** tinnitus, nasal stuffiness, conjunctival suffusion. **GI:** nausea, cramps, diarrhea. **Skin:** rash. **Other:** malaise.
antihemophilic factor (AHF) Antihemophilic Globulin (AHG), Factorate, Hemofil, Humafac Koate, Profilate	*Hemophilia A (Factor VIII deficiency)*— **Adults and children:** 10 to 20 units/kg I.V. push or infusion q 8 to 24 hours. Maintenance doses may be less. Infusion rate usually 10 to 20 ml reconstituted solution per 3 minutes. Dosage varies with individual needs.	**CNS:** headache, paresthesias, clouding or loss of consciousness. **CV:** tachycardia, hypotension, possible intravascular hemolysis in patients with blood type A, B, or AB. **EENT:** disturbed vision. **GI:** nausea, vomiting. **Skin:** erythema, urticaria. **Other:** *chills, fever, backache, flushing,* constriction in chest; hypersensitivity.
carbazochrome salicylate Adrenosem Salicylate	*Surgery with excessive capillary bleeding or oozing*— **Adults, and children over 12 years:** 10 mg I.M. preoperatively on night before surgery and with on-call medication, and 5 mg P.O. or I.M. postoperatively q 2 to 4 hours. **Children under 12 years:** 5 mg I.M. preoperatively on night before surgery and with on-call medication, and 2.5 mg P.O. or I.M. postoperatively q 2 to 4 hours.	**Local:** pain at I.M. injection site.

♦ Available in U.S. and Canada. ♦♦ Available in Canada only. All other products (no symbol) available in U.S. only. Italicized side effects are common or life-threatening.

INTERACTIONS	NURSING CONSIDERATIONS
None significant.	• Contraindicated in frank infection, as sole hemostatic agent in abnormal bleeding, or in postpartum bleeding or hemorrhage. • Avoid overpacking when placed into body cavities or closed tissue spaces. • Systemically absorbed within 4 to 6 weeks; no need to remove.
Oral contraceptives: increased probability of hypercoagulability. Use together cautiously.	• Contraindicated in active intravascular clotting. Use cautiously in thrombophlebitis and cardiac, hepatic, or renal disease. • Monitor coagulation studies, heart rhythm, and blood pressure. Notify doctor of any change immediately. • Also used as antidote for streptokinase or urokinase toxicity; not beneficial in the treatment of thrombocytopenia. • Dilute solution with sterile water for injection, normal saline injection, 5% dextrose in water, or Ringer's injection.
None significant.	• Use cautiously in neonates, infants, and patients with hepatic disease because of susceptibility to hepatitis, which may be transmitted in antihemophilic factor. • Have blood typed and crossmatched to treat possible hemorrhage. • Monitor vital signs regularly. Take baseline pulse rate before I.V. administration. If pulse rate increases significantly, flow rate should be reduced or administration stopped. • Monitor patient for allergic reactions. • For I.V. use only. Use plastic syringe; drug may interact with glass syringe, causing binding of ground-glass surface. • Refrigerate concentrate until ready to use, but not after reconstituted. Refrigeration after reconstitution may cause the active ingredient to precipitate. Before reconstituting, concentrate and diluent bottles should be warmed to room temperature. To mix drug, gently roll vial between your hands. Reconstituted solution unstable; use within 3 hours. Store away from heat. Don't shake or mix with other I.V. solutions. • Monitor coagulation studies before and during therapy.
None significant.	• Contraindicated in hypersensitivity to salicylates. • Obtain patient history of allergies, especially to salicylates. • Has no effect on clotting time, prothrombin time, and vitamin K levels.

NAME	INDICATIONS & DOSAGE	SIDE EFFECTS
Factor IX complex Konyne, Proplex	*Factor IX deficiency (hemophilia B or Christmas disease), anticoagulant overdosage—* **Adults and children:** units required equal 0.6 × body weight in kg × percentage of desired increase of Factor IX level, by slow I.V. infusion or I.V. push. Dosage is highly individualized, depending on degree of deficiency, level of Factor IX desired, weight of patient, and severity of bleeding.	**CNS:** headache. **CV:** possible intravascular hemolysis in patients with blood types A, B, AB. **Other:** *transient fever, chills, flushing, tingling,* hypersensitivity.
microfibrillar collagen hemostat Avitene	*To provide hemostasis in surgery (adjunct)—* **Adults and children:** amount depends on severity of bleeding. Compress area with dry sponges. Apply drug directly to bleeding site for 1 to 5 minutes. Gently remove excess. Reapply if needed.	**Blood:** hematoma. **Local:** exacerbation of wound dehiscence, abscess formation, foreign body reaction, adhesion formation. **Other:** enhanced infection in contaminated wounds, mediastinitis, hypersensitivity.
negatol Negatan	*Cervical bleeding—* **Women:** apply 1-inch gauze dipped in 1:10 dilution of drug; insert in cervical canal. If tolerated, may increase to full-strength solution. Remove pack after 24 hours; give 2-quart douche of dilute negatol or vinegar. *Oral ulcers—* **Adults and children:** apply to dried lesion with applicator, leave for 1 minute, then neutralize with large amounts of water.	**Local:** *burning sensation.* **Skin:** erythema, superficial desquamation when applied to skin.
oxidized cellulose Oxycel♦, Surgicel	*To provide hemostasis in surgery (adjunct)—* **Adults and children:** apply with sterile technique, p.r.n. Remove after hemostasis, if possible, with dry sterile forceps. Leave in place if necessary.	**CNS:** headache when used as packing for epistaxis, or after rhinologic procedures or application to surface wounds. **EENT:** sneezing, epistaxis or stinging, burning when used as packing for rhinologic procedures; nasal membrane necrosis or septal perforation. **Local:** encapsulation of fluid, foreign body reaction, burning or stinging after application to surface wounds. **Other:** possible prolongation of drainage in cholecystectomies.

INTERACTIONS	NURSING CONSIDERATIONS
None significant.	• Contraindicated in hepatic disease, intravascular coagulation, or fibrinolysis. Use cautiously in neonates and infants because of susceptibility to hepatitis, which may be transmitted with Factor IX complex. • Have blood typed and crossmatched to treat possible hemorrhage. If given to patients with blood types A, B, AB, intravascular hemolysis may occur. • Observe patient for allergic reactions, and monitor vital signs regularly. • Avoid rapid infusion. If tingling sensation, fever, chills, or headache develops during I.V. infusion, decrease flow rate and notify the doctor. • Reconstitute with 20 ml sterile water for injection for each vial of lyophilized drug. Keep refrigerated until ready to use; warm to room temperature before reconstituting. Use within 3 hours of reconstitution. Unstable in solution. Don't shake, refrigerate, or mix reconstituted solution with other I.V. solutions. Store away from heat.
None significant.	• Contraindicated in closure of skin incisions; it may interfere with healing. • Not for injection. • Don't spill on nonbleeding surfaces. • Don't dilute. Always apply dry. • Adheres to wet gloves, instruments, or tissue surfaces. Handle and apply with smooth, dry forceps. Apply directly to source of bleeding.
None significant.	• Vaginal membrane turns grayish after vaginal use. • When used in vagina, patient should wear a perineal pad to prevent soiling of clothing. • When used for oral ulcers, may apply topical anesthetic first to prevent burning sensation. • Always clean and dry area to be treated. • Astringent, styptic, and protein denaturant; highly acidic.
None significant.	• Contraindicated in controlling hemorrhage from large arteries; in nonhemorrhagic, serous, oozing surfaces; in implantation in bone defects. • Don't pack or wad unless it will be removed after hemostasis. Don't apply too tightly when used as wrap sheet in vascular surgery. Apply loosely against bleeding surface. • Always remove after hemostasis when used in laminectomies or near optic nerve chain. • Don't autoclave this product. • Use only amount needed to produce hemostasis. Remove excess before surgical closure. • Use minimal amounts in urologic procedures. • In large wounds, don't overlap skin edges. • Use sterile technique to remove from open wounds after hemostasis. Don't remove without irrigating material first; otherwise, fresh bleeding may occur.

(continued on following page)

NAME	INDICATIONS & DOSAGE	SIDE EFFECTS
oxidized cellulose *(continued)*		
thrombin Fibrindex	*Bleeding from parenchymatous tissue, cancellous bone, dental sockets, nasal and laryngeal surgery, and in plastic surgery and skin-grafting procedures—* **Adults:** apply 100 units/ml of sterile isotonic NaCl solution or sterile distilled water to area where clotting needed (or may apply dry powder in bone surgery); in major bleeding, apply 1,000 to 2,000 units/ml sterile isotonic NaCl solution. Sponge blood from area before application, but avoid sponging area after application. *GI hemorrhage—* **Adults:** give 2 oz of milk, followed by 2 oz of milk containing 10,000 to 20,000 units thrombin. Repeat t.i.d. for 4 to 5 days or until bleeding is controlled.	**Systemic:** hypersensitivity and fever.

♦ Available in U.S. and Canada. ♦♦ Available in Canada only. All other products (no symbol) available in U.S. only. Italicized side effects are common or life-threatening.

PATIENT CARE

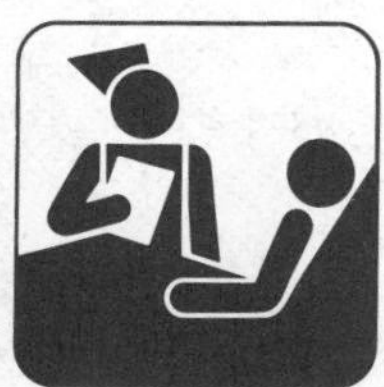

RELIEVING THE YOUNG HEMOPHILIAC'S ANXIETY

Because hemophilia is a chronic disease, the young patient is likely to remember past bleeding episodes and be very nervous. To counteract his anxiety, remain gentle, calm, and patient.

Don't confine the child to bed unnecessarily. If such confinement is really necessary, be creative in providing safe sensory stimuli. You can ensure safety and comfort by checking toys and padding the sides of the bed.

INTERACTIONS	NURSING CONSIDERATIONS
	• Don't moisten. Hemostatic effect is greater when applied dry. • Should not be used for permanent packing in fractures because it may result in cyst formation.
None significant.	• Contraindicated in hypersensitivity to thrombin or bovine products. • Obtain patient history of reactions to thrombin or bovine products. • Observe patient for allergic reactions, and monitor vital signs regularly. • Have blood typed and crossmatched to treat possible hemorrhage. • Don't inject topical thrombin or allow it to enter large blood vessels. I.V. injection may cause death because of severe intravascular clotting. • May be used with absorbable gelatin sponge but not with oxidized cellulose. Check sponge labeling before use. • Neutralize stomach acids before oral use in GI hemorrhage. • Keep refrigerated, preferably frozen, until ready to use. Unstable in solution. Use within 24 hours of reconstitution; discard after 48 hours. Store away from heat. • Broken down by diluted acid, alkali, and salts of heavy metals.

UNDERSTANDING INHERITANCE PATTERNS OF HEMOPHILIA

1

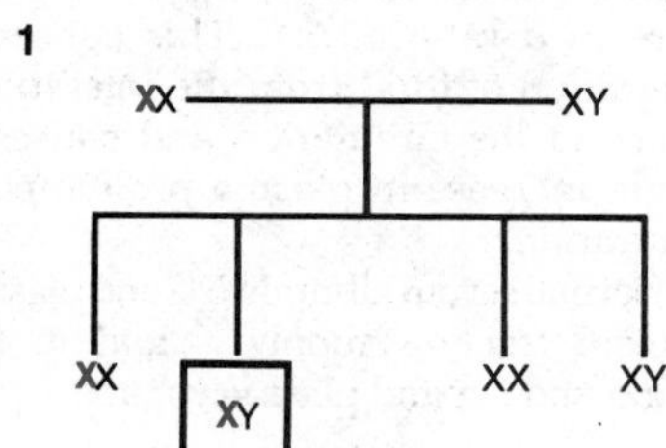

2

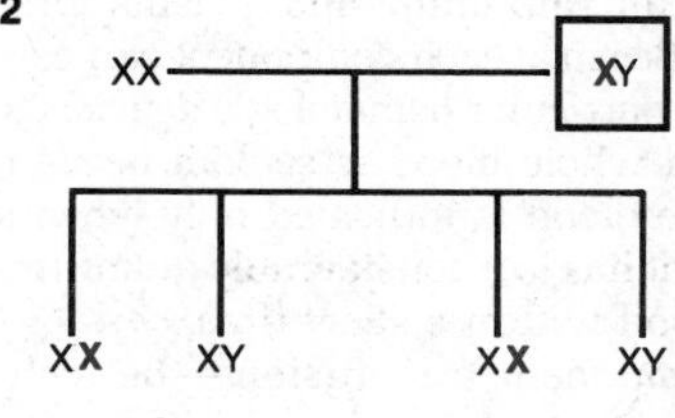

Illustration 1: A female carrier (XX) marries a normal male (XY). Their daughters have a 50% chance of being carriers (XX) and a 50% chance of being normal (XX). If the couple has sons, each son has a 50% chance of being hemophiliac (XY) and a 50% chance of being normal (XY).

Illustration 2: A normal female (XX) marries a hemophiliac (XY). All the daughters are carriers (XX) and all the sons are normal (XY).

69 Blood derivatives

normal serum albumin
plasma protein fraction

Normal serum albumin and plasma protein fraction are made from pooled normal human blood, plasma, or serum; albumin is also obtained from human placentas. Both preparations furnish means for stabilizing the body's hemodynamic mechanisms in hypovolemic shock or hypoproteinemia, or both.

Current techniques allow separation of freshly donated whole blood into its component fractions: human red cells (packed red cells), plasma, platelets, granulocytes, $Rh_o(D)$ immune human globulin, albumin, and plasma protein. Because each component can correct a particular hematologic deficiency, use of whole blood is seldom needed. Whole blood is indicated only when a patient has lost considerable quantities of blood within a short time.

Component transfusion—the technique of administering specific components rather than whole blood to a patient—has several advantages. In addition to providing deficiency-specific therapy, the technique expands the potential usefulness of a single blood donation and helps ease the chronic shortage of blood. The risk of viral hepatitis and exposure to sensitizing agents or drugs in blood are also reduced.

Major uses

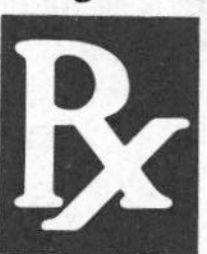

The blood derivatives act as plasma expanders in hypovolemic shock caused by burns, trauma, sepsis, or surgical procedures. They are also used to treat hypoproteinemia associated with malnutrition, toxemia of pregnancy, or prematurity.

• Normal serum albumin 25% is used to treat hypoproteinemia associated with hepatic cirrhosis and nephrotic syndrome.

Mechanism of action

• Normal serum albumin 25% furnishes an intravascular oncotic pressure in a ratio of 5:1. This causes a migration of fluid from the interstitial space to the circulation and causes a slight increase in plasma protein concentration.

• Normal serum albumin 5% and plasma protein fraction supply colloid to the blood and expand plasma volume.

Absorption, distribution, metabolism, and excretion

Since these blood derivatives are given only by the I.V. route, absorption is complete; they are rapidly distributed in the blood.

Onset and duration

Adequate patient response to normal serum albumin usually occurs within

HOW BURN DAMAGE AFFECTS FLUID BALANCE

Osmosis and diffusion maintain a delicate balance of body fluid distribution (70% intracellular fluid; 30% extracellular fluid, consisting of 6% in the plasma and 24% in the interstitial fluid) in the healthy adult.

With severe burn injury, huge amounts of fluids shift out of the blood into the interstitial space in the first 24 to 48 hours. This shift is called burn shock.

Burn damage increases capillary permeability. This increase and the inflammatory process cause the fluid leakage into the interstitial space. Since water, electrolyte, and albumin molecules are small, more of these are lost from the vascular space than blood cells (red, white, and platelets) or large protein molecules, like globulins, which remain in the vessels.

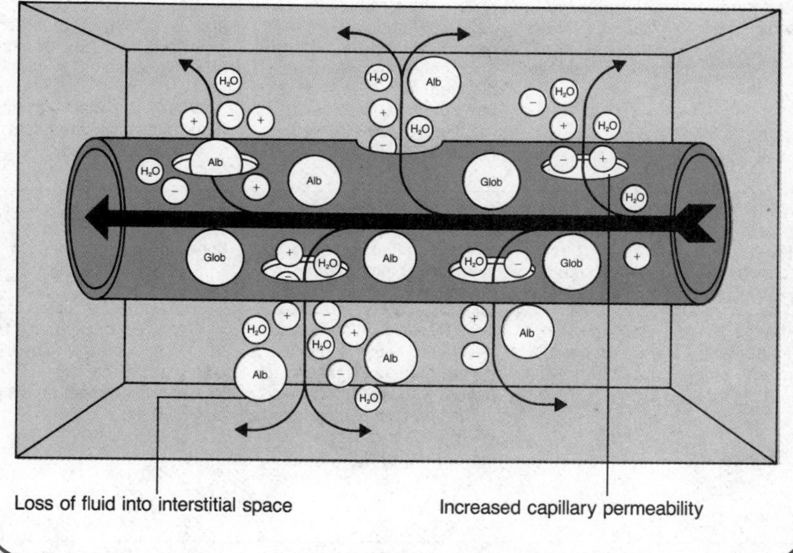

15 to 30 minutes. Duration of therapy with albumin and plasma protein fraction varies not only with the patient but also with the abnormality or condition that is being treated.

Combination products
None.

For guide to major blood components, see next page.

NURSE'S GUIDE TO MAJOR BLOOD COMPONENTS

TYPE	DESCRIPTION	INDICATIONS	CONTRAINDICATIONS
Whole blood	Blood complete with all plasma and cell constituents	• To restore adequate blood volume in hemorrhaging, trauma, or burn patients	• When the patient doesn't need volume increase and a specific component is available
Red blood cells (packed, frozen)	Whole blood with 80% of the supernatant plasma removed	• To correct red blood cell deficiency and improve oxygen-carrying capacity of blood • To transfuse organ transplant patients or to treat repeated febrile transfusion reactions (frozen-thawed RBCs)	• When the patient's anemic from a deficiency of the hematopoietic nutrients, for example, iron, vitamin B_{12}, or folic acid • When the patient's asymptomatic, but his hematocrit level must be raised
White blood cells (leukocyte concentrate)	Whole blood with RBCs and 80% of supernatant plasma removed	• To treat life-threatening granulocytopenia from intensive chemotherapy, especially infections that don't respond to antibiotics	• When the patient's health depends on the recovery of bone marrow functions
Plasma (fresh, fresh frozen)	Uncoagulated plasma separated from whole blood	• To treat a clotting factor deficiency, hypovolemia, or severe hepatic disease in a patient with limited synthesis of plasma coagulation factors • To prevent dilutional hypocoagulability	• When blood coagulation can be corrected with available specific therapy • When the patient needs only albumin
Platelets	Platelet sediment from platelet-rich plasma, resuspended in 30 to 50 ml of plasma	• To treat thrombocytopenia when bleeding is caused by the following: decreased platelet production, increased platelet destruction, functionally abnormal platelets, or massive transfusions of stored blood (dilutional thrombocytopenia)	• When bleeding's unrelated to decreased number of platelets or abnormal function of platelets • When the patient's suffering either from post-transfusion purpura or from thrombotic thrombocytopenic purpura
Plasma protein fraction	5% selected proteins solution pooled plasma in buffered, stabilized saline diluent	• To treat hypovolemic shock or hypoproteinemia • For initial treatment of shock in infants, or dehydration or electrolyte deficiencies in children	• When the patient has severe anemia, heart failure, or cardiac bypass
Normal serum albumin 5% **Normal serum albumin 25%**	Heat-treated, aqueous, chemically processed fraction of pooled plasma	• To treat shock • To prevent marked hemoconcentration • To maintain appropriate electrolyte balance • To treat hypoproteinemia • To treat hyperbilirubinemia in infants	• When the patient has severe anemia or heart failure

CROSS-MATCHING	SHELF LIFE	ADMINISTRATION TECHNIQUES	SPECIAL CONSIDERATIONS
Necessary	• 21 days at 5° C. (41° F.)	• Straight line set, Y-set, or microaggregate recipient set	• Although whole blood is seldom transfused, necessary components are extracted from it. • Plasma protein fraction or normal serum albumin given as volume expander until patient's component needs are known.
Necessary	• For stored fresh packed cells, 21 days; or 24 hours after opening • For stored frozen cells, 3 years; or 24 hours after thawing	• Straight line set, Y-set, or microaggregate recipient set	• RBCs have the same O_2-carrying capacity as whole blood without overload hazards. Their use avoids buildup of potassium and ammonia that can occur in stored blood plasma. Frozen-thawed RBCs are expensive.
Must be ABO compatible	• 24 hours after collection at 5° C. (41° F.)	• Straight line set with standard in-line filter. Dosage: 1 unit daily until infection clears (usually within 5 days).	• *Important:* Infusion induces fever and can cause mild hypertension, severe chills, disorientation, and hallucinations.
Unnecessary	• For fresh plasma, within 6 hours after collection • For fresh frozen plasma, 12 months at −18° C. (−0.4° F.) or 2 hours after thawing	• Any straight line set; administer as rapidly as possible	• Normal saline solution not needed for Y-set because the component contains no RBCs
Unnecessary (donor plasma and recipient's RBCs should be ABO compatible)	• Up to 72 hours after whole blood collection	• Syringe or component drip set only; give as rapidly as possible (uninterrupted) • Must use a nonwettable filter. • Dosage: 2 units/kg of body weight raise platelet count at least 50,000/mm^3	• Usually given when platelet count is below 10,000/mm^3 • With a history of side effects: give antihistamines before transfusion. Slow administration may prevent overload. • Least hazardous when given fresh
Unnecessary	• 5 years if refrigerated; 3 years at room temperature	• Any straight line set; rate and volume depend on the patient's condition and response	• Don't mix in same line with protein hydrolysates and alcohol solutions • Often used as volume expander while crossmatching is done
Unnecessary	• 5 years at 2° C. (35.6° F.); 3 years at room temperature	• Give undiluted, or diluted with saline or D5W. • In hypoproteinemia: administer slowly (1 to 3 ml/min) to prevent rapid volume expansion. • In shock: administer as rapidly as possible.	• Can't transmit hepatitis because it's heat-treated at 60° C. (140° F.) for 10 hours • Often given as a volume expander in place of whole blood while crossmatching is being completed

NAME	INDICATIONS & DOSAGE	SIDE EFFECTS
normal serum albumin 5% Albuconn 5%, Albuminar 5%, Albumisol 5%, Albuspan 5%, Albutein 5%, Buminate 5%, Plasbumin 5% **normal serum albumin 25%** Albuconn 25%, Albuminar 25%, Albumisol 25%, Buminate 25%, Plasbumin 25%	*Shock*— **Adults:** initially, 500 ml (5% solution) by I.V. infusion, repeat q 30 minutes, p.r.n. Dose varies with patient's condition and response. **Children:** 25% to 50% adult dose in nonemergency. *Hypoproteinemia*— **Adults:** 1,000 to 1,500 ml 5% solution by I.V. infusion daily, maximum rate 5 to 10 ml/minute; or 25 to 100 g 25% solution by I.V. infusion daily, maximum rate 3 ml/minute. Dose varies with patient's condition and response. *Burns*—dosage varies according to extent of burn and patient's condition. Generally maintain plasma albumin at 2 to 3 g/ 100 ml. *Hyperbilirubinemia*— **Infants:** 1 g albumin (4 ml 25%)/kg before transfusion.	**CV:** *vascular overload after rapid infusion,* hypotension, altered pulse rate. **GI:** increased salivation, nausea, vomiting. **Skin:** urticaria. **Other:** chills, fever, altered respiration.
plasma protein fraction Plasmanate, Plasmatein, Protenate	*Shock*— **Adults:** varies with patient's condition and response, but usual dose is 250 to 500 ml (12.5 to 25 g protein), usually not faster than 10 ml/minute. **Children:** 22 to 33 ml/kg I.V. infused at rate of 5 to 10 ml/ minute. *Hypoproteinemia*— **Adults:** 1,000 to 1,500 ml I.V. daily. Maximum infusion rate 8 ml/minute.	**CNS:** headache. **CV:** variable effects on blood pressure after rapid infusion or intra-arterial administration; *vascular overload after rapid infusion.* **GI:** nausea, vomiting, hypersalivation. **Skin:** erythema, urticaria. **Other:** flushing, chills, fever, back pain, dyspnea.

INTERACTIONS	NURSING CONSIDERATIONS
None significant.	• Contraindicated in severe anemia and heart failure. Use cautiously in low cardiac reserve, absence of albumin deficiency, and restricted salt intake. • Do not give more than 250 g in 48 hours. • Watch for hemorrhage or shock if used after surgery or injury. • Monitor vital signs carefully. • Watch for signs of vascular overload (heart failure or pulmonary edema). • Patient should be properly hydrated before infusion of solution. • Avoid rapid I.V. infusion. Specific rate is individualized according to patient's age, condition, diagnosis. • Dilute with sterile water for injection, 0.9% NaCl solution, or 5% dextrose injection. Use solution promptly; contains no preservatives. Discard unused solution. • Don't use cloudy solutions or those containing sediment. Solution should be clear amber color. • Freezing may cause bottle to break. Follow storage instructions on bottle. • One volume of 25% albumin is equivalent to five volumes of 5% albumin in producing hemodilution and relative anemia. • This product is very expensive, and random supply shortages occur often. • Monitor intake and output, hemoglobin, hematocrit, and serum protein and electrolytes during therapy.
None significant.	• Contraindicated in patients with severe anemia or heart failure, and in patients undergoing cardiac bypass. Use cautiously in hepatic or renal failure, low cardiac reserve, restricted salt intake. • Monitor blood pressure. Infusion should be slowed or stopped if hypotension suddenly occurs. • Vital signs should return to normal gradually; monitor hourly. • Watch for signs of vascular overload (heart failure or pulmonary edema). • Monitor intake and output. Watch for decreased urinary output. • Check expiration date on container before using. Discard solutions in containers that have been opened for more than 4 hours. Solution contains no preservatives. • Don't use solutions that are cloudy, contain sediment, or have been frozen. • If patient is dehydrated, give additional fluids either P.O. or I.V. • Do not give more than 250 g (5,000 ml 5%) in 48 hours. • Contains 130 to 160 mEq sodium/liter.

70 Thrombolytic enzymes

streptokinase
urokinase

Thrombolytic enzymes are effective in treating acute and extensive episodes of thrombotic disorders. Before administering these enzymes, however, be aware of the increased risk of hemorrhage that attends their use. Although major bleeding is a possible complication of treatment, bruising and oozing of blood at the incision site and surgical trauma are more likely. Because of the inherent risk of hemorrhage, thrombolytic enzyme therapy should be initiated only by doctors skilled in its use and under close laboratory monitoring.

Major uses

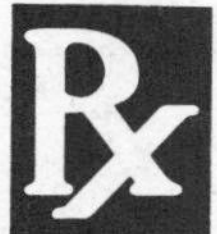

Streptokinase and urokinase are used to treat acute, massive pulmonary emboli. Streptokinase is also used to dissolve acute, extensive deep-vein thrombi and acute arterial thromboemboli.

Mechanism of action

Both streptokinase and urokinase activate plasminogen and convert it to plasmin, which degrades fibrin clots, fibrinogen, and other plasma proteins.

• Streptokinase activates plasminogen in a two-step process. Plasminogen and streptokinase form a complex that exposes the plasminogen-activating site. Plasminogen is converted to plasmin by cleavage of the peptide bond.

OCCLUSION: COMMON SITES AND SYMPTOMS

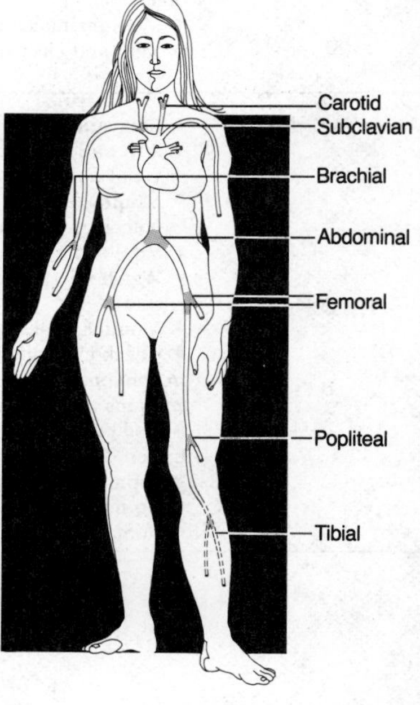

Thrombolytic enzymes are used to treat emboli that develop in these common sites. By watching for respiratory distress, pulse changes, temperature drops, and skin color changes from mottled to blue that appear distal to the site, you can help detect occlusive problems early and report them to the doctor.

HOW DRUGS ACTIVATE THE FIBRINOLYTIC SYSTEM

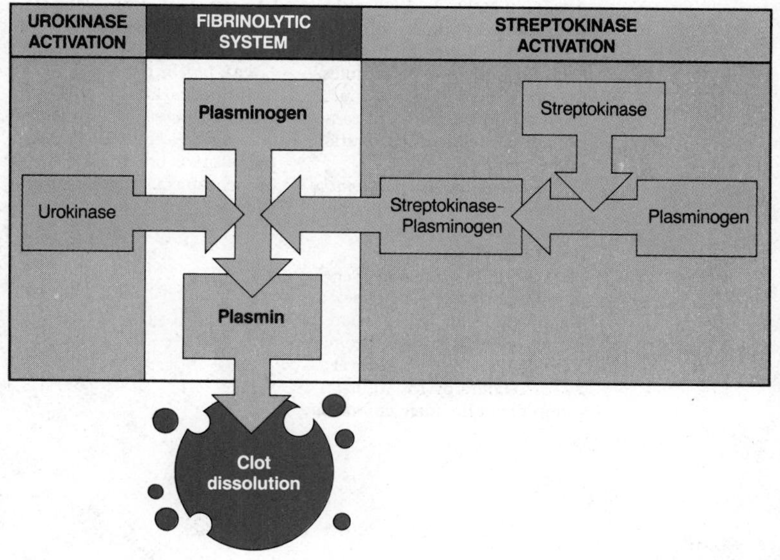

When blood begins to form a clot, the natural mechanism for dissolving this clot is also initiated.

The mechanism for dissolving clotted blood when it's no longer needed is called the fibrinolytic system. Its physiologic stimuli are kinases, activated Factor XII, and certain tissue activators. They activate plasminogen to form plasmin, the proteolytic enzyme that dissolves a clot's fibrin threads.

When undesirable clots form, the fibrinolytic system's anticoagulant action can be hastened with the thrombolytic drugs streptokinase and urokinase.

These drugs imitate the system's natural activators. Urokinase reacts directly with plasminogen to create the lysing agent plasmin; streptokinase joins plasminogen in a complex that then reacts with plasminogen to form plasmin. This activated plasmin then dissolves the clot.

Adapted with permission from Philip P. Gerbino and Sanford J. Shattil, "Prevention and Treatment of Pulmonary Embolism," *U.S. Pharmacist,* 5:5:H-1, May 1980.

- Urokinase activates plasminogen by directly cleaving peptide bonds at two different sites.

Absorption, distribution, metabolism, and excretion

Streptokinase and urokinase are administered only by I.V. infusion and are distributed throughout the body. Their metabolism and excretion have not been fully elucidated.

Onset and duration

Streptokinase and urokinase begin to act immediately. They must be infused at a constant dosage level to maintain therapeutic effectiveness. Their action ceases when the I.V. infusion is discontinued, but residual effects on coagulation may last as long as 12 hours.

Combination products

None.

NAME	INDICATIONS & DOSAGE	SIDE EFFECTS
streptokinase Kabikinase, Streptase	*Arteriovenous cannula occlusion—* **Adults:** 250,000 IU in 2 ml I.V. solution by I.V. pump infusion into each occluded limb of the cannula over 25 to 35 minutes. Clamp off cannula for 2 hours. Then aspirate contents of cannula; flush with saline solution and reconnect. *Venous thrombosis, pulmonary embolism, and arterial thrombosis and embolism—* **Adults:** loading dose: 250,000 IU I.V. infusion over 30 minutes. Sustaining dose: 100,000 IU/hour I.V. infusion for 72 hours for deep-vein thrombosis and 100,000 IU/hour over 24 to 72 hours by I.V. infusion pump for pulmonary embolism.	**Blood:** *bleeding, decreased hematocrit.* **CV:** transient lowering or elevation of blood pressure. **EENT:** periorbital edema. **Local:** *phlebitis at injection site.* **Skin:** urticaria. **Other:** *hypersensitivity to drug, anaphylaxis,* musculoskeletal pain, minor breathing difficulty, bronchospasms, angioneurotic edema.
urokinase Abbokinase, Breokinase, Win-Kinase	*Lysis of acute massive pulmonary emboli and lysis of pulmonary emboli accompanied by unstable hemodynamics—* **Adults:** for I.V. infusion only by constant infusion pump that will deliver a total volume of 195 ml. Priming dose: 4,400 IU/kg/hour of urokinase–normal saline solution admixture given over 10 minutes. Follow with 4,400 IU/kg/hour for 12 to 24 hours. Total volume	**Blood:** *bleeding, decreased hematocrit.* **Local:** *phlebitis at injection site.* **Other:** hypersensitivity (not as frequent as streptokinase), musculoskeletal pain, bronchospasm, *anaphylaxis.*

INTERACTIONS	NURSING CONSIDERATIONS
Anticoagulants: concurrent use of anticoagulants with streptokinase is not recommended. Reversing the effects of oral anticoagulants must be considered before beginning therapy, and heparin must be stopped and its effect allowed to diminish. *Aspirin, indomethacin, phenylbutazone, drugs affecting platelet activity:* increased risk of bleeding. Do not use together.	• Contraindicated in ulcerative wounds, active internal bleeding, and recent cerebrovascular accident; recent trauma with possible internal injuries; visceral or intracranial malignancy; ulcerative colitis; diverticulitis; severe hypertension; acute or chronic hepatic or renal insufficiency; uncontrolled hypocoagulation; chronic pulmonary disease with cavitation; subacute bacterial endocarditis or rheumatic valvular disease; recent cerebral embolism, thrombosis, or hemorrhage. Also contraindicated within 10 days after intra-arterial diagnostic procedure or any surgery, including liver or kidney biopsy, lumbar puncture, thoracentesis, paracentesis, or extensive or multiple cutdowns. • Use cautiously when treating arterial emboli that originate from left side of heart because of danger of cerebral infarction. • I.M. injections contraindicated during streptokinase therapy. • Before initiating therapy, draw blood to determine PTT and PT. Rate of I.V. infusion depends on thrombin time and streptokinase resistance. • If the patient has had either a recent streptococcal infection or recent treatment with streptokinase, a higher loading dose may be necessary. • Preparation of I.V. solution: reconstitute each vial with 5 ml sodium chloride for injection. Further dilute to 45 ml. Don't shake; roll gently to mix. Use within 24 hours. Store at room temperature in powder form; refrigerate after reconstitution. • Monitor patient for excessive bleeding; if evident, stop therapy. Pretreatment with heparin or drugs affecting platelets causes high risk of bleeding. • Have typed and crossmatched packed red cells and whole blood available to treat possible hemorrhage. • Keep aminocaproic acid available to treat bleeding. Corticosteroids are used to treat allergic reactions. • Before using streptokinase to clear an occluded arteriovenous cannula, try flushing with heparinized saline solution. • Bruising more likely during therapy; avoid unnecessary handling. • Keep venipuncture sites to a minimum; use pressure dressing on puncture sites for at least 15 minutes. • Monitor vital signs frequently. • Watch for signs of hypersensitivity. Notify doctor immediately. • Heparin by continuous infusion is usually started within an hour after stopping streptokinase. Use infusion pump to administer heparin. • Should be used only by doctors with wide experience in thrombotic disease management where clinical and laboratory monitoring can be performed. • For treatment of anaphylaxis, see inside front cover.
Anticoagulants: concurrent use of anticoagulants with urokinase is not recommended. Reversing the effects of oral anticoagulants must be considered before beginning therapy, and heparin must be stopped and its effect allowed to diminish. *Aspirin, indomethacin, phenylbutazone,*	• Contraindicated in ulcerative wounds, active internal bleeding, and cerebrovascular accident; recent trauma with possible internal injuries; visceral or intracranial malignancy; pregnancy and first 10 days postpartum; ulcerative colitis; diverticulitis; severe hypertension; acute or chronic hepatic or renal insufficiency; uncontrolled hypocoagulation; chronic pulmonary disease with cavitation; subacute bacterial endocarditis or rheumatic valvular disease; and recent cerebral embolism, thrombosis, or hemorrhage. Also contraindicated within 10 days after intra-arterial diagnostic procedure or any surgery, including liver or kidney biopsy, lumbar puncture, thoracentesis, paracentesis, or extensive or multiple cutdowns. • I.M. injections are contraindicated during urokinase therapy. • Preparation of I.V. solution: add 5.2 ml sterile water for injection to vial. Dilute further with 0.9% saline solution before infusion. Don't

(continued on following page)

NAME	INDICATIONS & DOSAGE	SIDE EFFECTS
urokinase *(continued)*	should not exceed 200 ml. Follow therapy with continuous I.V. infusion of heparin, then oral anticoagulants.	

♦ Available in U.S. and Canada. ♦♦ Available in Canada only. All other products (no symbol) available in U.S. only. Italicized side effects are common or life-threatening.

INTERACTIONS	NURSING CONSIDERATIONS
other drugs affecting platelet activity: increased risk of bleeding. Do not use together.	use bacteriostatic water for injection to reconstitute; it contains preservatives. • Monitor patient for bleeding. Pretreatment with drugs affecting platelets places patient at high risk of bleeding. • Have typed and crossmatched red cells and whole blood available to treat possible hemorrhage. • Keep aminocaproic acid available to treat bleeding. Corticosteroids are used to treat allergic reactions. • Watch for signs of hypersensitivity. Notify doctor immediately. • Monitor vital signs. • Keep venipuncture sites to a minimum; use pressure dressing on puncture sites for at least 15 minutes. • Heparin by continuous infusion usually started within an hour after urokinase has been stopped. Use infusion pump to administer heparin. • Bruising during therapy more likely; avoid unnecessary handling of patient. • Should be used only by doctors with wide experience in thrombotic disease management where clinical and laboratory monitoring can be performed. • For treatment of anaphylaxis, see inside front cover.

FACTORS AFFECTING THROMBOLYTIC ENZYME ACTIVITY

FACTOR	EFFECT
Thrombus location	Clots in small or totally occluded vessels are difficult to dissolve.
Thrombus duration	Clots more than 7 days old generally do not respond to this therapy.
Thrombus size	Complete clot dissolution is more difficult with large, extensive clots.
Activatibility of fibrinolytic system **Concentration of endogenous inhibitors** **Dysproteinemia**	If endogenous inhibitors are abnormally elevated, or the fibrinolytic system is dysfunctional, or abnormal proteins are present, it may be impossible to activate the fibrinolytic system adequately.
Plasminogen concentration in thrombus	High plasminogen concentration in the clot promotes complete dissolution of the thrombus.
Body temperature	Extremes in body temperature decrease efficiency of the fibrinolytic system.

Adapted from William R. Bell and Allen G. Meek, "Guidelines for the Use of Thrombolytic Agents," *The New England Journal of Medicine*, 301:23:1267, December 6, 1979. Used with permission of the publisher.

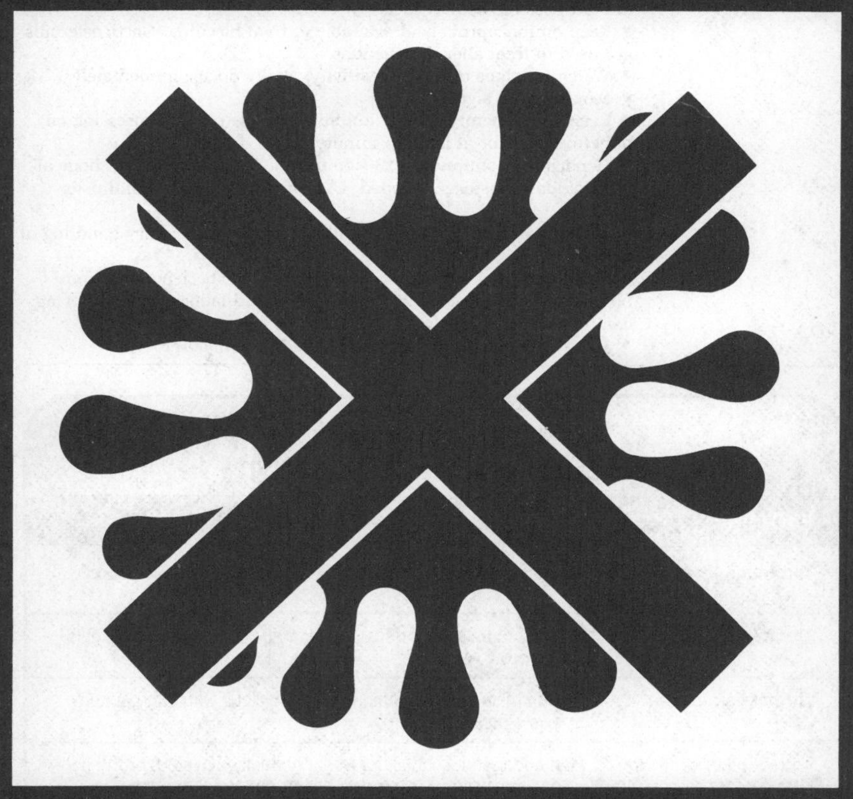

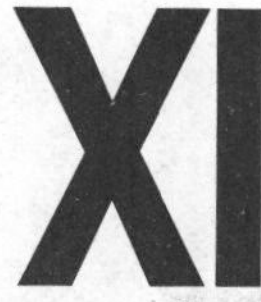

XI Antineoplastic Agents

71 Nursing implications of chemotherapy

Antineoplastic drugs destroy cancer cells by interfering with neoplastic cell growth and division. They block the supply or utilization of essential cellular building blocks or interrupt the process of cell division known as the cell cycle. The cell cycle consists of five specific phases (see *How Antimetabolites Affect the Cell Cycle,* p. 926). Antineoplastic drugs that destroy cells only at a specific point in the cell cycle are called cell cycle specific; those that affect the cells at any phase of the cell cycle are called cell cycle nonspecific.

Because of the toxic effects these drugs have on normal as well as cancerous cells, chemotherapy is most effective during the early stages of a tumor's growth, when fewer cancer cells are present. At this time, when the patient is not debilitated and overwhelmed by his disease, he is better able to combat the drug's toxic effects.

In a solid tumor, chemotherapy may be used with surgery and/or radiation therapy, usually after the tumor mass has been reduced. Therapy that combines antineoplastics and surgery is less successful when the malignancy is extensive or metastatic.

Chemotherapy alone is the treatment of choice in hematologic malignancies, such as leukemia or lymphatic tumors with no localized focus of disease. Chemotherapy has been successful in treating certain lymphatic and leukemic diseases, commonly producing remissions of many years. Thousands of children who would have died within a year of diagnosis more than 15 years ago have now reached adulthood disease-free due to advances in chemotherapy.

Adjuvant chemotherapy is often administered after surgery or radiation of the primary lesion—even to patients showing no clinical evidence of disease—to destroy any remaining cancer cells and prevent local or metastatic recurrent disease.

Combination therapy

In the early 1950s methotrexate and nitrogen mustard were the only antineoplastic agents used; combination therapy wasn't tried until the late 1960s. Today, more than 30 cancer chemotherapeutic drugs are available and more than 50 others are being investigated.

Drug therapy seldom comprises a single agent; most cancer chemotherapy regimens combine at least three drugs. Combination therapy can triple or quadruple single-agent response rates, while minimizing toxicity.

Drugs are combined to delay the development of neoplastic cells resistant to specific antineoplastics. Also, drugs that act in different parts of the cell cycle or by different mechanisms can be used together synergistically. Furthermore, the highest tolerable dose of each drug may be used if drugs with different, rather than overlapping, side effects are combined. An example is the combination of prednisone and vincristine in the treatment of acute

DETERMINING BODY SURFACE AREA FOR DOSAGE CALCULATIONS

Dosage is usually based on body surface area in square meters (m^2). Determine a patient's body surface area by using a nomogram based on the patient's height and body weight. Then, with careful mathematical calculation, obtain the dosage of the drug. Weigh the patient carefully, since dosage is based on lean (ideal) body weight or actual weight, whichever is less.

How to use the nomogram

By using a straight edge, connect the height (line on left) with the weight (line on right). Read the corresponding body surface area on the center line. For example, if your patient is 66″ (168 cm) tall and weighs 110 lb (50 kg), his body surface area is 1.55 m^2.

Height

cm 200, 195, 190, 185, 180, 175, 170, 165, 160, 155, 150, 145, 140, 135, 130, 125, 120, 115, 110, 105, cm 100

78 in, 76, 74, 72, 70, 68, 66, 64, 62, 60, 58, 56, 54, 52, 50, 48, 46, 44, 43, 42, 41, 40, 39 in

Body surface area

2.80 m^2, 2.70, 2.60, 2.50, 2.40, 2.30, 2.20, 2.10, 2.00, 1.90, 1.80, 1.70, 1.60, 1.50, 1.40, 1.30, 1.25, 1.20, 1.15, 1.10, 1.05, 1.00, 0.95, 0.90, 0.86 m^2

Weight

kg 150, 140, 130, 120, 110, 100, 90, 80, 75, 70, 65, 60, 55, 50, 45, 40, 35, kg 30

320 lb, 300, 280, 260, 240, 220, 200, 180, 160, 150, 140, 130, 120, 110, 100, 90, 85, 80, 75, 70, 66 lb

COMMON PROTOCOLS FOR COMBINATION CHEMOTHERAPY

HODGKIN'S DISEASE	
MOPP	(repeated every 28 days) mechlorethamine (Mustargen): 6 mg/m² I.V. push on days 1 and 8. vincristine (Oncovin): 1.4 mg/m² (2 mg maximum) I.V. on days 1 and 8. procarbazine (Matulane): 100 mg/m² daily P.O. for 14 days. prednisone: 40 mg/m² daily P.O. for 14 days.
(optional)	bleomycin (Blenoxane): 2 to 4 mg/m² I.V. on days 1 and 8.
ABVD	(repeated every 28 days) doxorubicin (Adriamycin): 25 mg/m² I.V. on days 1 and 14. bleomycin (Blenoxane): 10 mg/m² I.V. on days 1 and 14. vinblastine (Velban): 6 mg/m² I.V. on days 1 and 14. dacarbazine (DTIC): 150 mg/m² I.V. on days 1 to 5.
NON-HODGKIN'S LYMPHOMA	
COP	(repeated every 21 days) cyclophosphamide (Cytoxan): 800 mg/m² I.V. on day 1. vincristine (Oncovin): 1.4 mg/m² (2 mg maximum) I.V. on day 1. prednisone: 60 mg/m² P.O. on days 1 to 5.
CHOP	(repeated every 21 days) cyclophosphamide (Cytoxan): 750 mg/m² I.V. on day 1. *doxorubicin (Adriamycin): 50 mg/m² I.V. on day 1. vincristine (Oncovin): 1.4 mg/m² (2 mg maximum) I.V. on day 1. prednisone: 100 mg/m² P.O. on days 1 to 5.
(optional)	bleomycin (Blenoxane): 4 mg I.V. on days 1 and 8.
	*H is for hydroxyldaunorubicin, a chemical synonym for doxorubicin
LEUKEMIA	
OAP	(repeated according to the degree of bone marrow depression) vincristine (Oncovin): 1.4 mg/m² (2 mg maximum) I.V. on day 1. ara-C (Cytosar): 200 mg/m²/day for 5 days as continuous infusion. prednisone: 100 mg P.O. daily for 5 days.
COAP	(repeated according to the degree of bone marrow depression) cyclophosphamide (Cytoxan): 100 mg/m² I.V. daily for 5 days. vincristine (Oncovin): 1.4 mg/m² (2 mg maximum) I.V. on day 1. ara-C (Cytosar): 100 mg/m² for 5 days as continuous infusion. prednisone: 100 mg P.O. daily for 5 days.
Ad-OAP	(repeated according to the degree of bone marrow depression) doxorubicin (Adriamycin): 40 mg/m² I.V. on day 1. vincristine (Oncovin): 2 mg I.V. on day 1. ara-C (Cytosar): 70 mg/m²/day for 7 days as continuous infusion. prednisone: 100 mg P.O. daily for 5 days.
SOFT-TISSUE SARCOMA	
CY-VA-DIC	cyclophosphamide (Cytoxan): 500 mg/m² I.V. on day 1. vincristine (Oncovin): 1 mg/m² (maximum 1.5 mg) I.V. on days 1 and 5. doxorubicin (Adriamycin): 50 mg/m² I.V. on day 1. dacarbazine (DTIC): 250 mg/m² I.V. daily for 5 days.

lymphocytic leukemia (ALL) in children. When these medications are used together for the initial treatment of ALL, the complete remission (CR) rate is higher than 90%. If either prednisone or vincristine were used singly,

Because of continuing research, all dosages for chemotherapy are subject to change. The specific protocols used in your hospital may differ slightly. Always check the latest protocols or current literature for dosing information.

BREAST CARCINOMA	
FAC	(repeated every 22 days) 5-fluorouracil: 500 mg/m² I.V. on days 1 and 8. doxorubicin (Adriamycin): 50 mg/m² I.V. on day 1. cyclophosphamide (Cytoxan): 500 mg/m² I.V. on day 1.
Cooper regimen	5-fluorouracil: 12 mg/kg I.V. daily for 4 days, then 500 mg I.V. weekly. methotrexate: 25 to 50 mg I.V. weekly. vincristine (Oncovin): 0.035 mg/kg I.V. weekly. cyclophosphamide (Cytoxan): 2.5 mg/kg P.O. daily. prednisone: 0.75 mg/kg P.O. daily.
CAF	(repeated every 28 days) cyclophosphamide (Cytoxan): 100 mg/m² P.O. daily for 14 days. doxorubicin (Adriamycin): 30 mg/m² I.V. on days 1 and 8. 5-fluorouracil: 400 mg/m² I.V. on days 1 and 8.
CMF	(repeated every 28 days) cyclophosphamide (Cytoxan): 100 mg/m² P.O. daily for 14 days. methotrexate: 30 mg/m² I.V. on days 1 and 8. 5-fluorouracil: 400 mg/m² I.V. on days 1 and 8.
UPPER GASTROINTESTINAL TUMORS	
FAM	(repeated every 8 weeks) 5-fluorouracil: 600 mg/m² I.V. on days 1, 8, 28, and 35. doxorubicin (Adriamycin): 30 mg/m² I.V. on days 1 and 28. mitomycin (Mutomycin): 10 mg/m² I.V. on day 1.
TESTICULAR TUMORS	
VB-3	(repeated every 3 to 6 weeks) vinblastine (Velban): 0.2 to 0.4 mg/kg split into two doses. bleomycin (Blenoxane): 30 mg/day on days 2 to 6 as continuous infusion.
MULTIPLE MYELOMA	
VCAP	(repeated every 4 weeks) vincristine (Oncovin): 1 mg I.V. on day 1. cyclophosphamide (Cytoxan): 100 mg/m²/day P.O. on days 1 to 4. doxorubicin (Adriamycin): 25 mg/m² I.V. on day 2. prednisone: 60 mg/m²/day on days 1 to 4.
VBAP	(repeated every 3 weeks) vincristine (Oncovin): 1 mg I.V. on day 1. carmustine (BCNU): 30 mg/m² I.V. on day 2. doxorubicin (Adriamycin): 30 mg/m² I.V. on day 2. prednisone: 60 mg/m²/day P.O. on days 2 to 5.

the CR rate would be only about 50%.

In some cancers, such as leukemia, different antineoplastic agents are administered in a specific order to achieve optimal results. For instance, one drug may induce remission but not maintain it, so this drug is then followed by another more effective at maintaining the remission. Higher remission and survival rates are the goals of combination therapy.

Toxic effects of chemotherapy

Chemotherapy affects rapidly dividing cells. Unfortunately, the doses needed to obtain maximum therapeutic response are quite toxic. Actively dividing normal cells—such as bone marrow, skin, gastrointestinal (GI) mucosa, hair follicles, and fetal tissue—are most susceptible to toxicity.

Advise patients of the side effects that may occur with their medications and of the measures that can alleviate them. Patients should be able to recognize potentially life-threatening side effects. With close monitoring and good patient care, you can prevent or minimize many side effects and make your patients more comfortable.

The benefits of using chemotherapy in pregnant or lactating women should be weighed against the risks of probable teratogenicity, mutagenicity, and carcinogenicity in fetuses or infants. For the same reasons, some oncologists discourage men receiving chemotherapy from fathering children during treatment and for several months afterward. Most doctors advise women to avoid pregnancy during therapy.

Bone marrow depression

Bone marrow depression is usually the dose-limiting factor of an antineoplastic. Leukopenia and thrombocytopenia are indications of bone marrow depression. When a patient's WBC count falls below 4,000 cells/mm^3, the dosage of most antineoplastics is reduced by 50%. Further dosage reductions are made as subsequent counts drop. When the WBC count falls below 2,500 cells/mm^3, or the platelet count falls below 80,000 cells/mm^3, all drugs except bleomycin are sometimes withheld. After the bone marrow recovers (WBC more than 4,000 cells/mm^3 and platelet count more than 120,000 cells/mm^3), therapy is resumed.

Carefully monitor for bone marrow depression and remember to:

- Teach your patient how to read a thermometer. Instruct him to take his temperature at home once daily in the late afternoon and to report any temperature of 101° F. (38.3° C.) or higher to the doctor or nurse. Antipyretics, such as acetaminophen, mask fever and should not be taken unless ordered by the doctor.
- Tell your patient to avoid aspirin or any medication containing aspirin while on chemotherapy. Aspirin interferes with the clotting process.
- Stress the importance of reporting for scheduled blood counts. When the absolute granulocyte count falls below 1,000 cells/mm^3, your patient is in danger of infection.
- Prepare injection sites carefully with iodophor or similar solutions to help prevent infection.
- Question your patient carefully about signs of infection, such as increased temperature, cough, sore throat, mouth sores, and burning on urination. Immediately report these to the doctor.
- Avoid administering suppositories or I.M. injections and taking rectal temperatures if platelets fall below 50,000 cells/mm^3. When platelets are at this level, tell the patient to use an electric razor and soft-bristled toothbrush to prevent injuring skin, which could lead to bleeding.
- Tell your patient to report any signs of decreased platelet count, such as petechiae, ecchymoses, easy bruising, hematuria, bleeding from gums, or epistaxis. Antineoplastic destruction of platelets can cause spontaneous bleeding that is difficult to stop.
- Be especially careful to watch for bone marrow depression in a patient undergoing concurrent radiation therapy, which may potentiate the problem. Myelosuppression is generally cumulative with antineoplastic agents, so a patient usually doesn't tolerate subsequent courses of treatment as well as the first.

Nausea and vomiting

Nausea, vomiting, and anorexia are common side effects of most chemotherapeutic agents. Antineoplastics rapidly stimulate the brain's chemoreceptor trigger zone, which affects the vomiting center. Here are some guidelines for good patient care:

- Nausea and vomiting may increase with anxiety, so administer chemotherapy in a pleasant atmosphere.
- Maintain good hydration, especially before giving an antineoplastic. The patient may not be able to keep down food for several days after treatment, and dehydration must be prevented. Force 2 to 3 liters of fluid daily. Carbonated beverages, Popsicles, and gelatin desserts are usually well tolerated. Carbonated beverages may also reduce nausea.
- Observe for signs of dehydration: poor skin turgor, dryness; significant weight loss during treatment course; and signs of electrolyte imbalance. The patient may need supplemental I.V. therapy.
- When a fluid deficit is known, monitor vital signs closely.
- Watch for elevated BUN. Remnants of the neoplastic cells are excreted through the kidneys and may affect the patient's renal function.
- Record fluid intake and output. (Be sure to include emesis.) Drug excretion depends on good urine output.
- Apply lotion to dry skin and water-soluble lubricant to dry lips.
- Treat each patient individually. Some patients prefer a light meal before receiving chemotherapy, whereas others prefer not to eat.
- Giving an antiemetic and small amounts of bland food 30 to 60 minutes

LEGAL ADVICE

DON'T EXCEED THE BOUNDS OF NURSING

Dilemma: The pharmacy department has refused to prepare chemotherapeutic medications (including cyclophosphamide [Cytoxan], doxorubicin [Adriamycin], and vincristine [Oncovin]) because the pharmacists have heard these medications adversely affect the preparer's reproductive organs. As a result, the job has been delegated to nurses. Naturally, you and many of the other nurses aren't willing to prepare these drugs either.

Are chemotherapeutic medications dangerous to the preparer? Should a nurse ever prepare these toxic drugs?

These drugs are corrosive and therefore dangerous if accidently splashed on the skin or in the eyes. Preliminary studies have shown that those who prepare such drugs can exhibit urinary levels of the drug, drug side effects, and varying degrees of mutagenicity. The only way to absolutely prevent drug exposure and its undesirable effects during preparation is to prepare the drugs under a vertical flow laminar hood, which should be present in the pharmacy.

Therefore, the pharmacist—who is the expert in preparing and dispensing medications and who has access to the proper equipment—should dispense these drugs. As you know, chemotherapeutic drugs are so toxic that an error in dilution could be fatal to the patient.

Dispensing and labeling drugs are not nursing functions; these activities are generally performed by a pharmacist. If a patient were harmed, you could be charged with malpractice because you overstepped the bounds of your nursing responsibilities, as determined by your state or provincial nursing practice act.

If you're faced with such a dilemma, arrange a meeting with the nursing and the pharmacy committees to work it out. The resolution is crucial to your patients' well-being, your legal safety, and your professional livelihood.

PRECAUTIONS

PREVENTING EXTRAVASATION

When administering a vesicant, you can take precautions to prevent extravasation. For safe, effective chemotherapy, adhere strictly to proper intravenous administration techniques.

- Don't use existing I.V. lines. Make new venipunctures to ensure proper needle placement and vein patency.
- Select site carefully. Distal veins that allow for successive proximal venipunctures are preferred to major veins. However, to preclude tendon and nerve damage with possible extravasation, try to avoid the dorsum of the hand. Also, avoid the wrist and digits; they are difficult to immobilize.
- Venipuncture should be "clean." If probing is necessary, stop I.V. and start again.
- Start I.V. with 5% dextrose in water or normal saline solution.
- Tape needle securely; don't cover immediate I.V. site.
- Test for proper needle placement. Lower I.V. bottle for good blood return.
- Administer vesicant by slow I.V. push through a running I.V. or by small-volume infusion (50 to 100 ml).
- During administration, observe site for erythema or infiltration. Tell patient to report burning or stinging. Check for needle placement by lowering bottle to observe blood return. Follow drug administration with several ml of 5% dextrose in water or normal saline solution to rinse the drug from the vein and to preclude drug leakage when needle is removed.

before administering antineoplastics may help reduce nausea and vomiting. An antiemetic is more effective when given before rather than after chemotherapy. (Some oncologists request patients to start taking antiemetics 24 hours before treatment.)

- Call the doctor immediately if a patient vomits after receiving an antineoplastic drug orally; the drug may be lost and dosage may need to be adjusted.
- To speed recovery and lessen toxicity during the treatment course, encourage the patient to eat well and drink sufficient fluids despite anorexia. The dietitian may be able to work out a diet the patient likes. (He's most likely to accept food that does not have an overpowering aroma.) Suggest that the patient's family bring his favorite soups or stews, or other foods that can be warmed easily. Be flexible about mealtimes. Postpone care that may tire the patient until after he has eaten.
- If the patient develops a nutritional deficiency from chemotherapy, request some dietary supplements and ask the dietitian to add more calories and protein to the patient's menu. Freezing the supplements and serving them like ice cream in sundaes and milk shakes may make them more palatable.

Diarrhea and constipation

Diarrhea and constipation are GI side effects of some antineoplastic agents. Diarrhea is due to the direct irritation of bowel mucosa caused by the death of rapidly dividing cells that line the GI tract. Constipation is an early symptom of central nervous system toxicity (neurotoxicity) resulting from drug therapy. Diarrhea and constipation should be prevented if possible to avoid further irritation of the lower GI tract. Here's what you can do:

- Question the patient frequently about stools. If the patient has diarrhea, give small feedings and decrease roughage; if he is constipated, increase roughage in his diet. See that the doctor orders a laxative, antidiarrheal, or stool softener as needed.
- Be sure the patient has access to a bathroom. If he's too weak to walk, place a bedpan within his reach.
- After each bowel movement, the perianal area should be cleaned and dried. Protective cream should be applied to irritated skin.
- Observe the patient for dehydration. Body fluids and electrolytes are lost

WHAT TO DO WHEN EXTRAVASATION OCCURS

Extravasation—the escape of medication from the vein into surrounding tissue—occurs through a puncture in the vein wall or from leakage around the insertion site. The following antineoplastic drugs are vesicants that may seriously damage tissue if extravasation occurs: dactinomycin, daunorubicin, doxorubicin, mechlorethamine, mithramycin, mitomycin, vinblastine, vincristine, and vindesine.

CAUSES	SIGNS AND SYMPTOMS	TREATMENT
• Inappropriate site or equipment (such as needles or catheters) • Improper technique • Fragile veins • Accidental movement of needle or catheter	• Pain, burning, itching, stinging, or temperature changes. (These are first noticed by the patient. Always *listen* to the patient.) • Slight inflammation or swelling, which may proceed over several weeks to necrosis, ulceration, or sloughing, with severe pain • Absence of blood backflow. If a tourniquet's applied above the site, the infusion continues to run. • Sluggish flow rate	**1.** Stop I.V. and leave needle in place. This provides a path to infiltrated tissue and decreases need for more punctures. **2.** If hospital policy permits, infuse at least 10 to 50 ml of normal saline solution through retained line into infiltrated tissue to dilute drug's effects. **3.** Notify the doctor. **4.** *If doxorubicin (Adriamycin) is extravasated,* 5 ml of 8.4% sodium bicarbonate solution may be injected through the needle. Raising the pH may slow cell metabolism, and less damage may result.* **5.** *For all extravasated drugs,* 50 to 100 mg of hydrocortisone may be injected into area (immediately after sodium bicarbonate injection with Adriamycin extravasation) to reduce inflammation.† **6.** Remove I.V. **7.** *First 24 hours:* Pack area in ice for a 20-minute period every 4 hours. Ice causes vasoconstriction that may localize drug and slow cell metabolism. Don't leave ice on too long. **8.** *After 24 hours:* Apply warm compresses for a 20-minute period every 4 hours. **9.** With severe extravasation, plastic surgery or physical therapy may be needed.

* Use of sodium bicarbonate is controversial; this step may be omitted.
† Use of hydrocortisone is controversial; this step may be omitted.

with diarrhea. Monitor electrolytes.
• Encourage fluid intake. I.V. therapy may be needed to replace lost fluids.
• Record diarrhea as output. Avoid taking temperature rectally as this may further irritate rectal mucosa.

Alopecia

Alopecia is common with certain antineoplastic drugs, and many patients find it distressing. Antineoplastics damage hair follicles perhaps even more than they do malignant cells. With many drugs, a patient may lose some or all of his hair, including scalp hair, eyelashes, eyebrows, and underarm and pubic hair. Remember:
• If your patient is receiving a drug that generally causes alopecia, warn him that this side effect is likely. Reassure him that his hair should begin to grow back about 8 weeks after ther-

PATIENT CARE

WHEN A CANCER DIAGNOSIS IS MADE, YOUR PATIENT NEEDS YOUR SUPPORT

You are best qualified to give your patient psychological support. Why? You know him probably better than anyone else who comes in contact with him in the hospital. You are your patient's ally against disease as you interact with him, his doctors, and family members.

Ask the doctor what he's told your patient about his illness. When talking with your patient, reinforce the doctor's explanations as you try to clarify your patient's concerns. You might ask a family member or friend of the patient to help you discuss the doctor's explanations with the patient.

Ask your patient to write down his understanding of what the doctor has told him, and any questions he may have for the next time he sees the doctor. In a stressful situation, your patient may be emotionally overwhelmed and not understand the doctor's comments.

Some general nursing pointers

- *Listen* to your patient's concerns about his diagnosis and treatment; try to find out how he feels about his illness.
- Remember that the patient may direct his anger about his illness toward the nurse. This is a normal coping mechanism, and you should be understanding.
- Always be truthful and respect your patient's individuality.
- Allow your patient to come to terms with his illness at his own pace, even if it means that he copes by denial.
- If your patient is terminally ill, your emotional support and continued efforts to promote physical comfort will help him live with hope and die with dignity.

apy is stopped. With some drugs, new hair may grow even during maintenance therapy. However, the new hair may be a different texture or color. Suggest that the patient obtain a hairpiece, scarves, hats, or a ski cap before treatment begins.

- Hair loss usually begins several days after chemotherapy is given and may continue for several weeks.
- Once hair loss starts, some patients prefer to shave their heads rather than lose hair gradually.
- Some patients may experience hair thinning only.
- In most cases, ice bags and scalp tourniquets have not proven helpful in preventing hair loss. Also, they may counteract the chemotherapy's effectiveness in blood-borne tumors. Their use is therefore not appropriate for some tumors and in the presence of metastatic disease.

Stomatitis

Inflammation of the buccal mucosa may occur with most antineoplastics but is most commonly associated with the antimetabolites and antibiotics. Remember:

- The patient should have all dental work completed before beginning chemotherapy, to reduce possible infection or bleeding. Ill-fitting dentures are potentially irritating and should be replaced before therapy begins. Check denture fit periodically as patient's weight fluctuates.
- Encourage good mouth care before and during treatment to help prevent oral side effects. Mucosal deterioration begins when more than 6 hours pass without good mouth care. Patient should use soft rayon-tipped swabs for mouth care. (Lemon-glycerin swabs should not be used because they dry the mouth.)
- To prevent gum irritation, the patient should use a soft-bristled toothbrush and dental floss unless he has thrombocytopenia. If platelet count falls below 50,000 cells/mm^3, tell him to discontinue brushing and flossing and to use a mouth rinse frequently instead.
- Tell the patient to cleanse his mouth by rinsing with hydrogen peroxide and water (1:6 solution) three to four times daily.

HOW TO ANSWER YOUR PATIENTS' QUESTIONS ABOUT CHEMOTHERAPY

Before speaking to your patient about chemotherapy, assess his knowledge of his illness. He may not recognize or accept his illness as cancer. For instance, he may speak of "my tumor." Only after he himself tells you he has cancer should you use this word. If needed, modify the following answers to use the patient's own terms for his illness.

What is chemotherapy?

Chemotherapy literally means treatment with chemicals. However, it's commonly accepted to mean drug treatment of cancer.

Is there more than one type of chemotherapy?

Yes. Many drugs can be given many ways (orally, by injection into a muscle or subcutaneous tissue, or by intravenous infusion). One that is correct for you and your condition will be selected.

Will it hurt?

Not usually. However, with some intravenous drugs, you may experience a temporary burning or cold sensation. You will be told this beforehand, so you won't be alarmed if it happens.

How long will each treatment take?

This will depend on the kind and number of drugs. Some drugs are given directly into the vein; others are given with a running I.V. solution; still others are added to an I.V. solution and dripped in over a specified time. Ask your doctor or nurse how long the treatment will take.

Will I have to be hospitalized?

Most drugs can be given in your doctor's office or at a hospital's outpatient department. But if you are taking a drug that requires close medical supervision, you may have to be hospitalized.

How long will I have to take these drugs and how often?

Check with your doctor or nurse for a time estimate. Usually, the duration of treatment varies from several months to 2 years, depending on the type of cancer, the types and number of drugs, and your response to the drugs (including adverse reactions). Most drugs are given weekly or monthly. Between times, you may take an oral form at home.

Will I be sick when I have chemotherapy?

Everyone responds differently. With many of the drugs, you may experience nausea or vomiting. If you do, you will be given another drug to relieve it.

Will I be able to continue working or taking care of my family?

Again, this depends on the kind of cancer and response to treatment. You will probably be able to resume normal activities without problems. But if you feel a little tired after treatment, relax for the rest of the day.

May I have alcoholic drinks while I'm undergoing chemotherapy?

Usually, a cocktail or glass of wine will not be harmful, but ask your doctor.

Will my diet be restricted?

No. As long as you're not having any problems eating normally, continue to do so. If you have any problems, your doctor may suggest a diet change. You may tolerate chemotherapy better if you eat a light meal before and after the procedure. Also, increase your fluid intake by two to four glasses daily before, during, and after chemotherapy.

Should I discontinue other drugs I'm taking?

Tell your doctor about all other drugs you're taking, how much and how often. He needs to know this because some drugs can interfere with your chemotherapy. Examples of such drugs are anticoagulants, antibiotics, aspirin, barbiturates, diuretics, hormones, cough medicines, and medications for diabetes and high blood pressure. Your prescriptions should be adjusted as needed.

Is chemotherapy really worthwhile?

Patients *really do benefit* from chemotherapy with increased chances of survival and enhanced quality of life. Ultimately based on your condition and the kind of chemotherapy, only you and your family can decide how worthwhile it is for you.

• If the peroxide is irritating, the patient may rinse with normal saline solution alone or with 1 teaspoon baking soda mixed with 1 liter normal saline solution, four times daily.
• If pain is a problem, the doctor may prescribe Benylin Elixir and Kaopectate (1:1) to be used as a mouthwash every 4 hours.
• To further reduce discomfort, the patient may use Xylocaine Viscous as an oral rinse before he eats. Xylocaine Viscous 2% should be diluted with equal parts water when used for severe mucositis.
• The patient with candidiasis may use nystatin suspension (mouthwash), vaginal tablets as lozenges, or flavored nystatin ice pops.
• The patient may apply a water-soluble lubricant such as KY jelly to treat or prevent cracked, dry lips.
• Encourage soothing foods, such as milk products and Popsicles. The patient should avoid tart, spicy, or rough-textured foods if his mouth becomes irritated or inflamed. Ask the dietary staff to provide a soft, palatable diet to help prevent anorexia.
• Erythema of buccal mucosa may be an early symptom of bone marrow toxicity. Antineoplastic dosage should be lowered or the drug stopped to prevent oral ulceration. If stopped, therapy may be started again, at a lower dose, about 7 to 10 days after the ulcer heals.
• Tell the patient to report ulcerations to the doctor or nurse.

QUESTIONS & ANSWERS

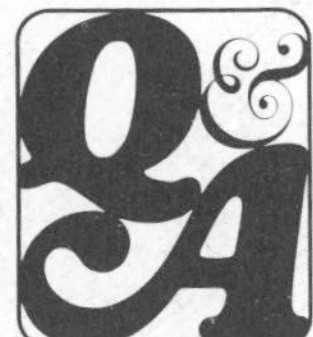

GIVE THE FACTS ABOUT LAETRILE

What should I tell my patients about laetrile?

The truth. Clinical trials concluded in 1981 by the National Cancer Institute and the FDA proved that laetrile is not effective in treating human cancer: There are no benefits, no cures; no delays in cancer progression; cancer-related symptoms are not suppressed. Life is not extended.

Earlier, numerous animal test studies had shown no benefits from laetrile in treating or preventing cancer.

Why, then, were clinical trials conducted?

Because laetrile had become a significant health issue. By 1980, 20 states had legalized the substance, and 50,000 to 70,000 Americans were taking laetrile regularly.

The trials included patients with a wide variety of common cancers who had exhausted available therapy or had cancer for which no effective treatment was available. Patients received laetrile I.V. for 21 days, then orally until their tumors began to grow again. Treatment also included a special diet, pancreatic enzymes, and large doses of vitamins.

After 3 months, cancer had progressed in 90% of the patients.

Misled by its supporters, thousands of Americans have been treated with laetrile; unfortunately, its use interferes with and delays competent diagnosis and proven treatment. This delay in seeking recognized therapy has cost many patients their lives.

Laetrile's supporters may not be deterred. But as a health-care professional, you can help overcome your patients' confusion by giving them the facts about laetrile and providing emotional support as they undergo scientifically validated treatment.

Adapted from "Laetrile: The Hollow Promise," *The Cancer Calendar,* May 1981, with permission from The Cancer Information Service, The Fox Chase Cancer Center, Philadelphia, Pa.

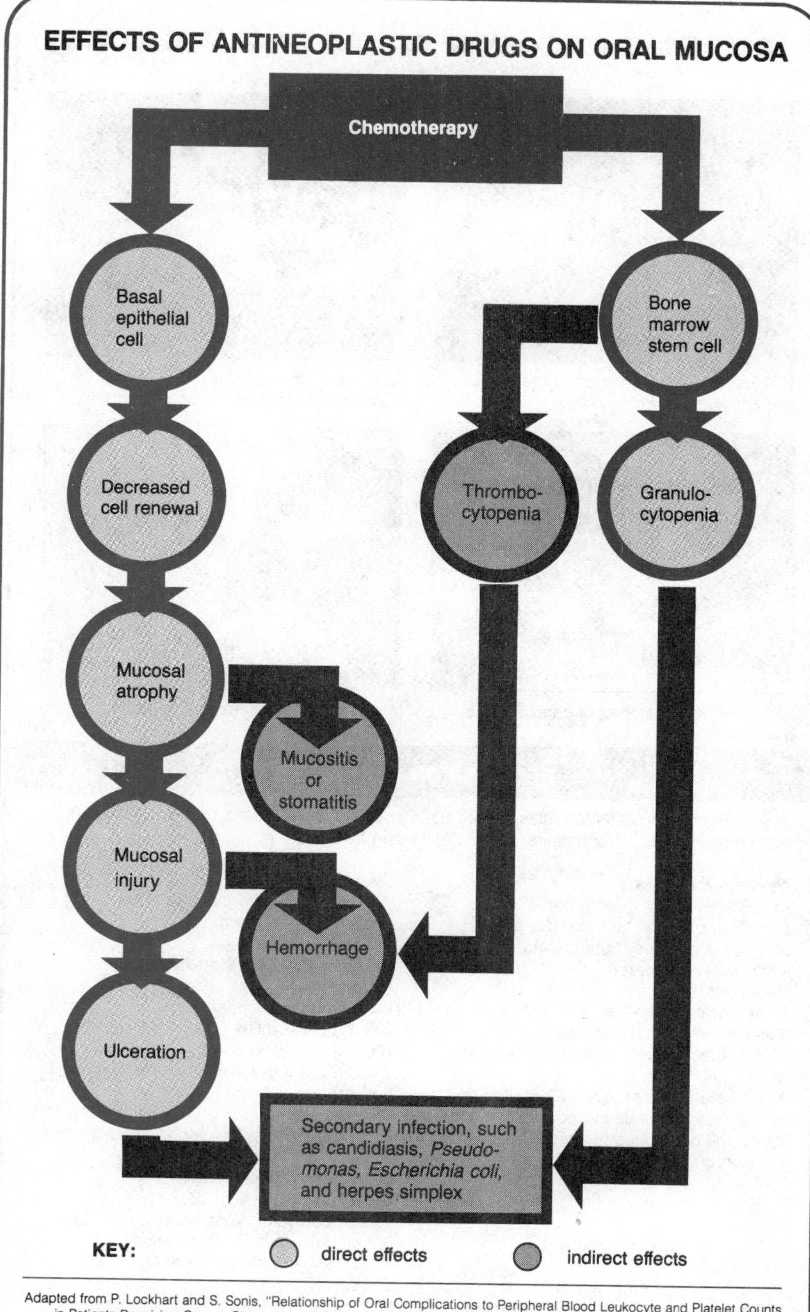

Adapted from P. Lockhart and S. Sonis, "Relationship of Oral Complications to Peripheral Blood Leukocyte and Platelet Counts in Patients Receiving Cancer Chemotherapy," *Oral Surgery, Oral Medicine, and Oral Pathology,* July 1979. Used with permission of C.V. Mosby Co. and the authors.

COMMON SECONDARY INFECTIONS OF ORAL MUCOSA

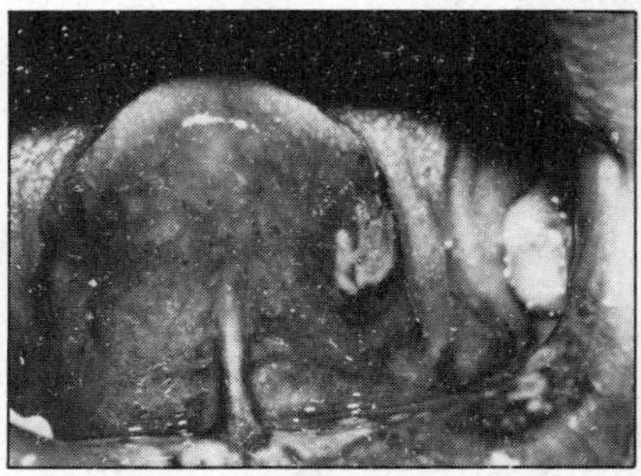

1. Mucositis and ulceration of the tongue and lips, various forms

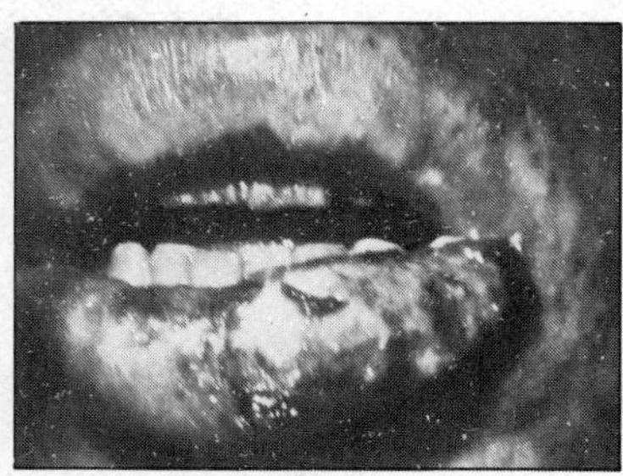

2. Signs of gram-negative infection *(Escherichia coli)* on the lip

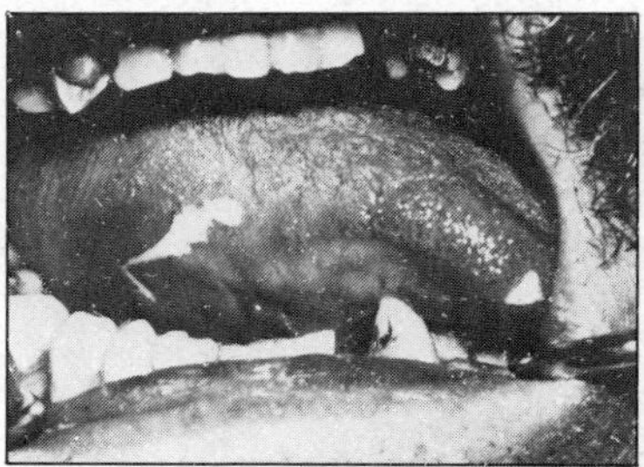

3. Pearly white patches of candidiasis on the tongue

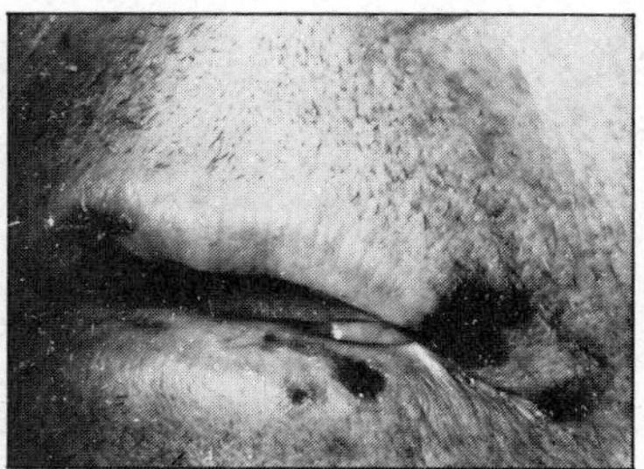

4. Herpes simplex lesion on the lip

RECIPES FOR ORAL CARE

The following stomatitis formulas can be used to treat the symptoms of chemotherapy's oral complications. Your hospital may have its own favorites.

Nystatin Ice Pops

Ingredients

60 million units nystatin powder
300 ml black cherry concentrate
1,800 ml sterile water

Directions

1. Mix nystatin powder with 300 ml of sterile water to make solution.
2. Add black cherry concentrate and stir well.
3. Add sterile water, q.s. to 1,800 ml.
4. Stir or shake well and pour into 30-ml unit-dose cups (makes 60 cups, 1 million units nystatin each).
5. Freeze.
6. Eat with a spoon q.i.d.

Cook's Stomatitis Ointment

Ingredients

120 g boric acid ointment 10%
120 g tetracaine (Pontocaine) ointment
30 drops peppermint oil

Directions

Mix thoroughly and place in ½-oz (14-g) ointment jars for p.r.n. use.

Dr. Marv Powell's Mouthwash

Ingredients

1.2 million units nystatin
500 mg tetracycline
100 mg hydrocortisone
q.s. 250 ml diphenhydramine (Benadryl elixir)

Directions

Mix thoroughly; swish and swallow q.i.d.

Dr. Sullivan's Mouthwash

Ingredients

16 ml neomycin 1% solution
3.2 ml polymyxin B 2% solution
32 oz (960 ml) sterile water

Directions

Mix medications with water, q.s. to 32 oz (960 ml); swish and swallow t.i.d. or q.i.d.

COMMON TERMS IN CANCER CARE

BLOOD-RELATED TERMS

Absolute granulocyte count: the number of granulocytes (mostly neutrophils) per mm^3. To calculate, multiply % Polys times WBC. For example, WBC = 5,000/mm^3 Polys = 60%: 5,000 × 60% = 3,000.

Leukopenia: decrease in circulating WBCs (leukocytes)

Nadir: point at which blood counts (WBC or platelets) reach their lowest level as a result of chemotherapy (usually 7 to 10 days after dose). The patient is then at greatest risk of developing complications, such as infections.

Neutropenia: decrease in circulating neutrophils

Neutrophils: (polymorphonuclear leukocytes, PMNs, or Polys): the most important type of white cell for fighting acute infections

Pancytopenia: decreased level of all blood components—WBC, platelets, granulocytes

Thrombocytopenia: decrease in circulating platelets

SIDE EFFECTS

Cystitis: inflammation of the urinary bladder. Bleeding may develop (hemorrhagic cystitis)

Extravasation: leakage of fluid (or drug) out of the vein into surrounding tissue

Myelosuppression: suppression of bone marrow function

Stomatitis: inflammation of mucous membranes of the mouth; often appears as white patches on oral mucosa

TYPES OF THERAPY

Adjuvant therapy: chemotherapy and radiation therapy used in addition to surgery even though there is no evidence of metastasis and the patient is asymptomatic

Immunotherapy: administration of preformed antibodies (serum or gamma globulin) to produce or enhance immunity

Supportive therapy: treatment given with systemic chemotherapy (steroids, radiation, antibiotics, blood, etc.)

RESPONSE RATE

Complete (CR): complete disappearance of all measurable and evaluable disease

Partial (PR): 50% decrease of all measurable and evaluable disease except for hepatomegaly, in which only a 30% decrease is needed

No change: less than 50% decrease in all measurable and evaluable disease

Progression: appearance of any new lesions, or increase by 25% of any previously measurable disease

Hyperuricemia

Hyperuricemia is a common problem in newly treated patients with hematologic malignancies, such as leukemia and lymphomas. Massive cell destruction releases purines, which convert to uric acid. The uric acid may precipitate into crystals in the kidneys and lead to renal failure. To minimize the risk of hyperuricemia:

- Force 3 liters of fluid daily.
- Monitor intake and output.
- Monitor serum uric acid and serum creatinine levels.
- Allopurinol prevents uric acid from forming. It should be ordered by the doctor and started 24 hours before chemotherapy is initiated and continued throughout treatment.

Advances in cancer therapy

Researchers are constantly refining protocols; developing new, more effective drugs and methods of administering them; and searching for new solutions to the cancer problem. Synthetic antineoplastics, Interferon research, intra-arterial chemotherapy, and immunotherapy are examples of these continuing efforts. In the next few pages, see short summaries of the latter two advances to increase and refine your understanding of cancer techniques.

RON BALLENTINE, PharmD

CARING FOR THE PATIENT ON INTRA-ARTERIAL CHEMOTHERAPY

Intra-arterial chemotherapy (IAC) is being more widely used every day at cancer centers across the country.

By this method, an antineoplastic drug is infused through a catheter in a major artery directly into a tumor—usually a localized, inoperable tumor in the liver, head, neck, or bones. A high concentration of the drug can be delivered to the tumor with relatively little dilution in the circulatory system and before its metabolism by the liver or kidneys.

Branches of the celiac artery are usually used to treat liver tumors, the most common tumor treated with IAC; the external carotid artery is used to treat head and neck tumors; and the internal carotid artery, to treat brain tumors.

Catheter placement pros and cons

Until recently, most arterial catheters were placed surgically. However, repeated catheterizations without the risks of surgery are now possible.

Most IAC patients who are to have angiographically placed catheters are hospitalized for about 5 days for catheter placement and chemotherapy administration. No general anesthetic is needed during insertion, and the patient usually has only moderate discomfort for a short time. After each IAC cycle, the catheter is removed and the patient sent home until the next cycle, when the process is repeated. In the meantime, he has no physical reminder of his disease.

Surgical placement results in a more permanent and stable positioning of the catheter. It's done through the gastroduodenal artery or the inferior epigastric artery. The catheter is then brought through a separate stab wound on the abdominal wall.

For long-term IAC, surgical placement is less expensive than angiographic placement, because patients can be treated as outpatients. Most can even continue working while receiving IAC. Each type of placement has important physiologic and psychosocial advantages, crucial to the overall treatment.

A simple, portable pump that the patient can wear is usually used for the chemotherapy infusion to maintain a slow, steady flow of medication to the tumor. An exciting new development is an implantable infusion pump, now available at some cancer centers. This pump is loaded by injecting through the abdomen into a port.

Angiographic catheterization

When an arterial catheter is placed angiographically, the patient's arterial anatomy is observed while the catheter is being inserted. Sometimes angiography shows that several arteries are supplying a tumor site or that the desired artery can't be infused without incidentally infusing other arteries. In either case, some of the arteries will be occluded by injecting Gelfoam or metal coils through the catheter. These materials lodge in the arteries so clots will form around them. (Sometimes merely occluding an artery causes tumor necrosis and shrinkage, without chemotherapy.)

If Gelfoam is used, it is absorbed by the body in several days, reestablishing the circulation. But if metal coils are used, the vascular occlusion is permanent.

Vascular occlusion may cause fever, generalized malaise, and pain in the area affected, until collateral circulation is established. The occlusion should be well documented in the patient's chart so staff members won't be unduly concerned if he shows any of these symptoms.

When the catheter has been positioned properly, the femoral or axillary insertion site is painted with tincture of benzoin, and a germicidal solution, such as povidone-iodine (Betadine), is applied. A transparent polyurethane dressing (Op-Site) is placed over the insertion site to anchor the catheter and provide a microbial barrier. The entire site is then covered with a sterile occlusive dressing. The catheter stopcock is taped away from the site, to further reduce tension on the catheter. All catheter connections and the catheter-infusion pump connection are securely taped to prevent accidental disconnection.

What to watch for

Displacement of the angiographically placed catheter tip is the most common complication of IAC. Check catheter placement daily either by X-ray or a nuclear-medicine flow study. If the catheter becomes displaced, it must be repositioned or removed.

Stay alert for signs that catheter displacement has caused the IAC infusion to reach the wrong organs. These signs include dyspepsia, excessive nausea, vomiting, diarrhea, gastritis, pain from peptic ulcers, or upper abdominal pain from pancreatitis. Temporarily stopping the drug and infusing heparinized saline solution

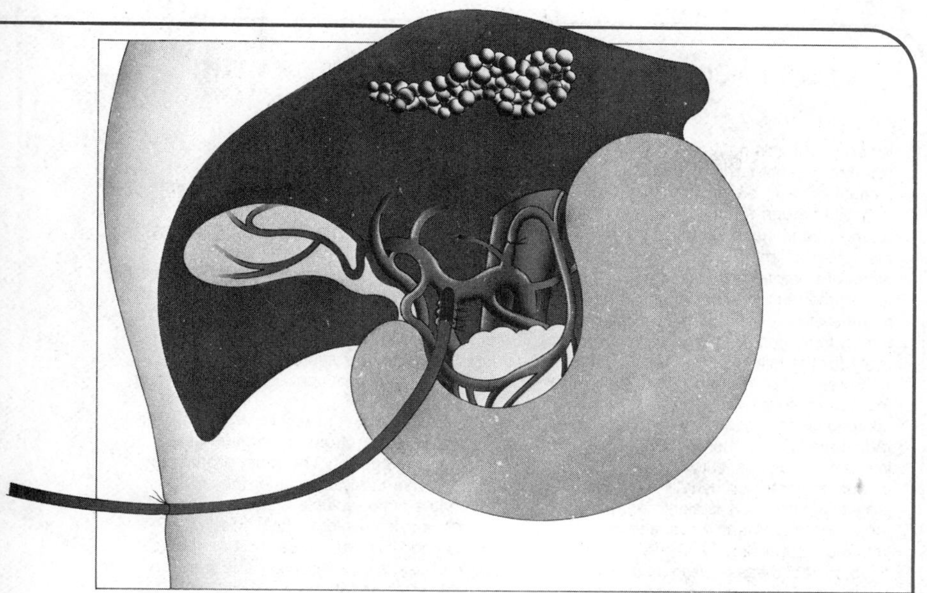

while giving antacids or cimetidine (Tagamet) will usually alleviate the discomfort.

If the patient complains of pain during the infusion, near the target organ, this may indicate a subintimal tear (separation of the intima and media of the arterial wall) caused by catheter manipulation during angiography. When this happens, the doctor usually postpones the infusion for 4 to 8 weeks, until healing occurs. Later, the healed tear may cause a pseudoaneurysm or arterial occlusion. Irregularities in the arterial wall can also be caused by a local reaction to the antineoplastic drugs.

You can usually prevent the potential complications of embolus and thrombus by providing vigorous anticoagulation therapy, as ordered. Administering 10,000 to 30,000 units of heparin intra-arterially every 24 hours produces a partial thromboplastin time 1½ times that of normal value, which is usually adequate prophylaxis. As an added precaution, the patient should be given 650 mg of aspirin twice daily to decrease platelet aggregation.

In the hospitalized patient, catheter occlusion is rare and preventable. When it does occur, the radiologist either removes the catheter or attempts to irrigate it. Patients generally can tolerate the injection of clotted materials into the liver. But if the catheter is in an artery supplying another organ, it should *not* be irrigated.

Surgical catheterization

If a patient is a candidate for long-term IAC, the doctor may recommend surgical placement of the catheter.

The doctor will probably use a Silastic (Intrasil) catheter. This type of catheter resists becoming brittle with age, and it can easily be repaired if it breaks externally.

If a clot should obstruct the catheter, it can usually be removed by infusing the fibrinolytic enzyme preparation urokinase (50,000 units/ml) in an amount equal to the catheter volume. Increasing the infusion pressure only slightly expands the catheter and allows the urokinase to flow around the clot, dissolving it.

Aspirate the clot as it dissolves, and repeat the process if necessary, always using the lowest infusion pressure possible to avoid rupturing the catheter. The relatively low dose of urokinase usually produces no side effects in patients other than a transient fever.

The portable infusion pump is selected on the basis of individual patient needs, cost, availability of medical supervision in the patient's home community, and IAC protocol requirements.

After surgical placement of the catheter, a heparinized saline solution is infused, using a large-volume infusion pump at about 1,000 ml/24 hours. This flow rate maintains catheter patency during the initial period of healing and possible rejection. About 7 or 8 days postoperatively, the patient can begin using a portable infusion pump. About 10 to 14 days postoperatively, he can begin chemotherapy, usually as an outpatient.

ENHANCING THE BODY'S IMMUNE SYSTEM WITH CANCER IMMUNOTHERAPY

When a patient's natural immunity has failed to prevent tumor development, immunotherapy is used to stimulate the natural immune response. It's used most often in combination with surgery, radiation therapy, or chemotherapy. These primary types of treatment destroy most of the tumor; then immunotherapy helps the immune system eliminate any remaining tumor. Immunotherapy may be used effectively for the following tasks:

- *To prevent or reverse natural or therapy-induced immunosuppression.* Conventional approaches to cancer therapy (surgery, radiotherapy, and chemotherapy) suppress immunity. Those patients with the greatest immunosuppression usually have the worst prognosis; prognosis is significantly better for patients who show resistance to immunosuppression.
- *To correct disease-associated immunodeficiency.* Many patients with cancer are thought to have some defect in the immune system. For example, patients having rare immunodeficiency diseases, such as ataxia telangiecstasia (a congenital immunologic disorder) and Bruton's disease (a sex-linked agammaglobulinemia), have increased incidence of tumor development.
- *To boost immunocompetency.* The relationship between immunocompetence and prognosis is well established. Among cancer patients whose disease is progressive, in vitro and in vivo analyses almost always show a decline in immune responsiveness. Because immune mechanisms are weakest and immunocompetence is poorest in childhood and old age, these are peak periods for malignancy to occur.

Types of immunotherapy

Active immunotherapy tries to stimulate the body's natural response against cancer cells with vaccines or other immunostimulants.

The most popular form of this immunotherapy is active nonspecific. This approach uses vaccines (most notably bacille Calmette Guérin [BCG] vaccine) and vaccine extracts to stimulate general immune responsiveness. BCG vaccine is an attenuated form of the *Mycobacterium bovis* that's been long used as a prophylaxis against tuberculosis. In the early 1960s, investigators noted fewer cases of leukemia in children who had been vaccinated with BCG for prevention of TB. BCG's main stimulatory effect is on the cellular immune response, specifically that of T cells, which are cancer fighters.

Active specific immunotherapy attempts to produce resistance to tumor growth by preimmunizing the patient with vaccine made from his own tumor. Cancer cells taken from the patient are modified in the laboratory and are injected into the patient. The resulting immune response is directed specifically at the tumor. Early therapeutic results indicate this approach may eventually prove to be the most successful form of immunotherapy.

Passive immunotherapy involves transfer of immune serum from an immune to a nonimmune patient. The most promising agent in use today is transfer factor, which is a water-soluble dialyzable extract of lymphocytes. Unfortunately, this immunity is short-lived because the transferred serum breaks down quickly and the patient eliminates it.

Adoptive immunotherapy is the transfer of live immune lymphocytes from a compatible donor to the patient with cancer. The lymphocytes are incubated in vitro with the patient's tumor cells to become sensitized. Then they're infused into the patient. Ultimately he'll accept these new immune cells and incorporate them into his immunologic defense.

Side effects

Immunotherapy doesn't produce the severe side effects associated with chemotherapy. It's not debilitating. These are the most common side effects:

- *Local reactions:* mild erythema and induration at the treatment site, pruritus, pustules, weeping patches, and possibly necrosis
- *Systemic reactions:* low-grade fever (temperature to 37.8° C [100° F.]) during the first 24 to 48 hours, chills, increased sweating, warm flushing, mild malaise, and local lymph node tenderness
- *Anaphylaxis:* may be mild, with fever and urticaria, but can be life-threatening, with dyspnea, cyanosis, hypotension, tachycardia, and convulsions.

The nurse's role

Managing an immunotherapy protocol is mainly a nursing task. Before, during, and after immunotherapy, you may be asked to help *assess* your patient's immune response. This includes collecting blood samples for laboratory analysis and administering and evaluating skin tests.

When you give a patient a skin test, encourage him to return to the clinic in 48 hours so the results can be interpreted. If he's unable to return, teach him how to check his injection site for redness, feel for thickness and swelling, and measure the reaction area. Ask him to phone you in 48 hours and report the results.

Patient teaching can reduce the patient's anxiety and encourage compliance. Be a good listener and show support as your patient reveals his concerns.

- Assess your patient's knowledge of immunotherapy and clarify misconceptions about how it differs from chemotherapy.
- Explain to the patient the purpose of skin and blood tests, in simple terms.
- When possible, include family members in patient teaching.

In some hospitals, you may be asked to *administer* immunotherapy by a variety of routes. For instance, you may give BCG vaccine intradermally, intravenously, or orally. (The doctor may give this drug intralesionally or intravesically.)

After treatment, your responsibility includes *direct nursing care* and *patient teaching.* If your patient is treated in the hospital, assess his reactions to treatment, minimize his discomfort, and try to prevent serious complications. Outpatients who receive immunotherapy need to know how their specific type of immunotherapy acts and the potential adverse effects that should be reported to the doctor.

How immunity develops

Immunity is an essential physiologic state. The key to immunity is the activity of white blood cells called lymphocytes. Two types of lymphocytes, T cells and B cells, are responsible for immunity. Although precursors of both T and B cells arise from the same source in the lymphocytic stem cells of the bone marrow, each develops differently and is responsible for a different type of immunity. The B-cell precursors develop in a source independent of the thymus (bursal equivalent). They yield B lymphocytes that provide antibody-mediated (humoral) immunity when stimulated by foreign antigens. The T-cell precursors migrate to the thymus gland and develop into T lymphocytes, which provide cell-mediated immunity when stimulated by foreign antigens. These sensitized T cells attack invading antigens and are capable of destroying foreign cells including tumor (cancer) cells. (See diagram.)

IMMUNE CELL DEVELOPMENT AND THEIR IMMUNE REACTIONS

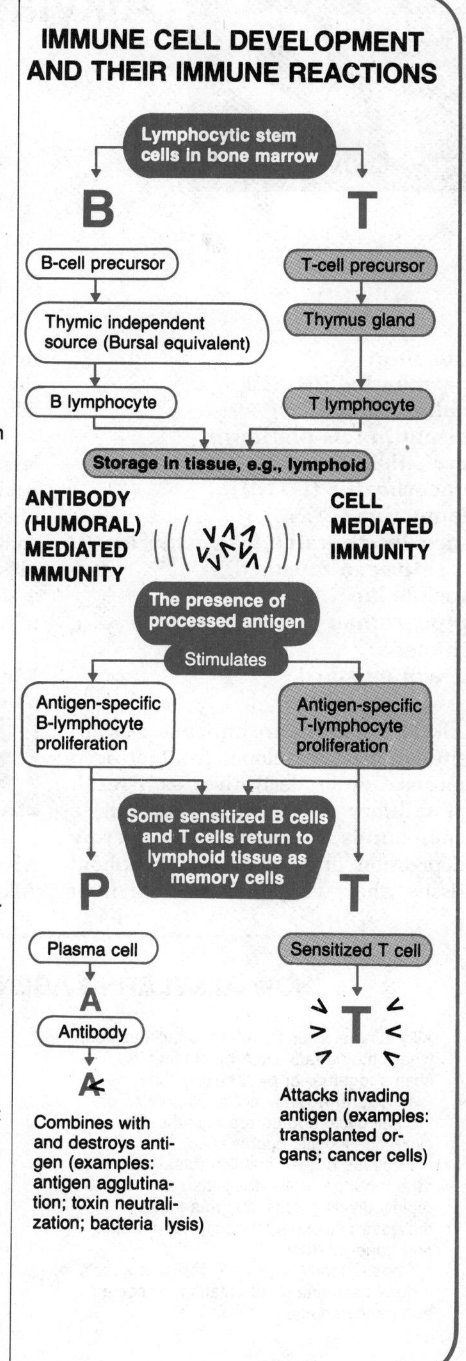

72 Alkylating agents

busulfan
carmustine (BCNU)
chlorambucil
cisplatin (cis-platinum)
cyclophosphamide
dacarbazine (DTIC)
lomustine (CCNU)
mechlorethamine hydrochloride (nitrogen mustard)
melphalan
pipobroman
thiotepa
uracil mustard

Alkylating agents are anticancer or antitumor drugs developed from nitrogen mustard or its derivatives as a result of military research. Because these compounds produce bone-marrow depression and atrophy of lymphoid tissue, they were first used to treat malignant lymphomas and leukemias. But since the introduction of mechlorethamine, the first nitrogen mustard, an intensive search for more potent and less toxic agents has been underway. Alkylating agents act during any phase of cellular activity, giving them an advantage over more specific antineoplastics, which are effective only during a single phase. This makes their toxicity nonspecific.

Major uses

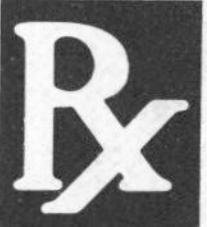

Alkylating agents are used to treat carcinomas, sarcomas, lymphomas, and leukemias. They're also used to treat polycythemia vera.

Mechanism of action

Alkylating agents cross-link strands of

HOW ALKYLATING AGENTS AFFECT DNA

Alkylating agents settle in the cell nucleus, where they attack DNA by binding its chains together or by breaking them apart (see diagram). They act at all phases of the cell cycle and so are called cell-cycle nonspecific agents.

Because of their inability to selectively attack cancer cells, they also affect other rapidly dividing cells, such as those in the gastrointestinal mucosa, hair follicles, and bone marrow.

Consequently, their common side effects include gastrointestinal irritation, alopecia, and pancytopenia.

Binding chains

Breaking chains

CISPLATIN: A BREAKTHROUGH FOR THE CANCER PATIENT

Cisplatin (Platinol) is a new and very effective intravenous drug for cancer. As the name implies, cisplatin (also called cis-platinum) is a derivative of the heavy metal platinum. Although it's officially approved to treat only testicular and ovarian tumors, you may also see cisplatin prescribed for both bladder and head and neck cancer, as well as for other primary tumors.

Cisplatin is especially effective because it works well together with other chemotherapeutic drugs. Before the advent of cisplatin, testicular and ovarian tumors resisted most attempts at chemotherapy. But when cisplatin is combined with vinblastine (Velban, Velbe) and bleomycin (Blenoxane) for testicular cancer, the response rate is between 84% and 100%. When combined with doxorubicin (Adriamycin) for ovarian cancer, the response rate is between 50% and 92%.

Common side effects

When cisplatin is given by I.V. push or by a rapid infusion (taking less than 2 hours), the patient will almost always experience severe nausea and vomiting. Symptoms usually begin within an hour. The vomiting usually subsides within 24 to 36 hours, but the patient may be nauseated for several days. When the doctor orders the infusion to run over a longer period, these symptoms are still present but are milder.

Administration tips

To prepare the drug for administration, reconstitute each vial with sterile water for injection. (Keep unreconstituted cisplatin refrigerated, but store the reconstituted drug at room temperature; if refrigerated, it may precipitate.) When adding the reconstituted cisplatin to the I.V. container, be sure to dilute it with either normal or half-normal saline solution to prolong the drug's stability. You don't have to protect the container from light when infusing.

Aluminum reacts with cisplatin, making cisplatin lose its potency. Therefore, don't use I.V. sets, catheters, or needles that contain aluminum when preparing or administering cisplatin.

DON'T USE THESE PRODUCTS WHEN PREPARING OR ADMINISTERING CISPLATIN

A partial list of aluminum-containing products

Disposable needles

Jelco disposable needle 22-1½"—
HRI 8003-002305 and
HRI 8003-002307

Monoject (Sherwood) #200 and #250 disposable needle 20-1"

I.V. administration sets

McGaw Disposable SECONDARY SET for use with ADDit I.V.®
Primary Sets V 1903

Travenol 2CO418 Add-A-Line™ secondary medication set, 86 cm (34") long

cellular DNA, causing an imbalance of growth that leads to cell death.

Absorption, distribution, metabolism, and excretion

Busulfan, chlorambucil, cyclophosphamide, lomustine, melphalan, pipobroman, and uracil mustard are absorbed from the gastrointestinal tract after oral administration. All other alkylating agents must be administered parenterally.

- All alkylating agents are distributed widely to body tissues. Carmustine, lomustine, and thiotepa diffuse into the cerebrospinal fluid and cross the blood-brain barrier.
- All alkylating agents except thiotepa are metabolized in the liver and excreted in the urine as either active or inactive metabolites. Thiotepa is excreted unchanged by the kidneys.

Onset and duration

Therapeutic activity varies with the alkylating agent, disease, and patient response.

Combination products

None.

NAME	INDICATIONS & DOSAGE	SIDE EFFECTS
busulfan Myleran♦	*Chronic myelocytic (granulocytic) leukemia—* **Adults:** 4 to 6 mg P.O. daily up to 8 mg P.O. daily until WBC falls to 10,000/mm³; stop drug until WBC rises to 50,000/mm³, then resume treatment as before; or 4 to 8 mg P.O. daily until WBC falls to 10,000 to 20,000/mm³, then reduce daily dose as needed to maintain WBC at this level (usually 2 mg daily). **Children:** 0.06 to 0.12 mg/kg or 2.3 to 4.6 mg/m²/day P.O.; adjust dose to maintain WBC at 20,000/mm³, but never less than 10,000/mm³.	**Blood:** WBC falling after about 10 days and continuing to fall for 2 weeks after stopping drug; *thrombocytopenia,* pancytopenia, anemia. **GI:** nausea, vomiting, diarrhea, cheilosis, glossitis. **GU:** amenorrhea, testicular atrophy, impotence. **Metabolic:** Addison-like wasting syndrome, profound hyperuricemia due to increased cell lysis. **Skin:** transient hyperpigmentation, anhidrosis. **Other:** gynecomastia; alopecia; *irreversible pulmonary fibrosis, commonly termed "busulfan lung."*
carmustine (BCNU) BiCNU♦	*Brain, colon, and stomach cancer; Hodgkin's disease; non-Hodgkin's lymphomas; melanomas; multiple myeloma; and hepatoma—* **Adults:** 100 mg/m² I.V. by slow infusion daily for 2 days; repeat q 6 weeks if platelets are above 100,000/mm³ and WBC is above 4,000/mm³. Dose is reduced 50% when WBC less than 2,000/mm³ and platelets less than 25,000/mm³. Alternate therapy: 200 mg/m² I.V. slow infusion as a single dose, repeated q 6 to 8 weeks; or 40 mg/m² I.V. slow infusion for 5 consecutive days, repeated q 6 weeks.	**Blood:** *cumulative bone marrow depression, delayed 4 to 6 weeks, lasting 1 to 2 weeks; leukopenia; thrombocytopenia.* **GI:** *nausea, which lasts 2 to 6 hours after giving (can be severe); vomiting.* **Hepatic:** hepatotoxicity. **Metabolic:** possible hyperuricemia in lymphoma patients when rapid cell lysis occurs. **Local:** *intense pain at infusion site.*
chlorambucil Leukeran♦	*Chronic lymphocytic leukemia, lymphosarcoma, giant follicular lymphoma, Hodgkin's disease, ovarian carcinoma, mycosis fungoides—* **Adults:** 0.1 to 0.2 mg/kg P.O. daily for 3 to 6 weeks, then adjust for maintenance (usually 2 mg daily). **Children:** 0.1 to 0.2 mg/kg/day or 4.5 mg/m²/day P.O. as single dose or in divided doses.	**Blood:** leukopenia, delayed up to 3 weeks, lasting up to 10 days after last dose; thrombocytopenia; anemia; myelosuppression (usually moderate, gradual, and rapidly reversible). **Metabolic:** hyperuricemia. **Skin:** *exfoliative dermatitis.* **Other:** allergic febrile reactions.

♦ Available in U.S. and Canada. ♦♦ Available in Canada only. All other products (no symbol) available in U.S. only. Italicized side effects are common or life-threatening.

INTERACTIONS	NURSING CONSIDERATIONS
None significant.	• Use cautiously in patients recently given other myelosuppressive drugs or radiation treatment, and in those with depressed neutrophil or platelet count. • Watch for signs of infection (fever, sore throat). • Warn patient that side effects may be delayed for 4 to 6 months. • Persistent cough, progressive dyspnea with alveolar exudate may result from drug toxicity, not pneumonia. • Monitor uric acid and CBC. • Patient response usually begins within 1 to 2 weeks (increased appetite, sense of well-being, decreased total leukocyte count, reduction in size of spleen). • Can cause false-positive cytology in all body secretions. • Anticoagulants should be used cautiously. Watch closely for signs of bleeding. • Avoid all I.M. injections when platelets are low.
None significant.	• To reduce pain on infusion, dilute further or slow infusion rate. • Warn patient to watch for signs of infection and bone marrow toxicity (fever, sore throat, anemia, fatigue, easy bruising, nose or gum bleeds, melena). Take temperature daily. • Monitor uric acid, CBC. • To reduce nausea, give antiemetic before administering. • Don't mix with other drugs during administration. • To reconstitute, dissolve 100 mg carmustine in 3 ml absolute alcohol. Dilute solution with 27 ml sterile water for injection. Resultant solution contains 3.3 mg carmustine/ml in 10% alcohol. Dilute in normal saline solution or dextrose 5% in water for I.V. infusion. Give at least 250 ml over 1 to 2 hours. • May store reconstituted solution in refrigerator for 24 hours. • If powder liquefies or appears oily, it is a sign of decomposition. Discard. • Can cause false-positive cytology in all body secretions. • To prevent hyperuricemia with resulting uric acid nephropathy, allopurinol may be used with adequate hydration and alkalinization of urine. Screen urine for stones. • Avoid contact with skin, as carmustine will cause a brown stain. If drug comes into contact with skin, wash off thoroughly. • Anticoagulants should be used cautiously. Watch closely for signs of bleeding. • Avoid all I.M. injections when platelets are low.
None significant.	• Myelosuppression reversible up to cumulative dose of 6.5 mg/kg. • Monitor uric acid, CBC. • To prevent hyperuricemia with resulting uric acid nephropathy, allopurinol may be used with adequate hydration and alkalinization of urine. Screen urine for stones. • Can cause false-positive cytology in all body secretions. • Avoid all I.M. injections when platelets are low. • Anticoagulants should be used cautiously. Watch closely for signs of bleeding.

NAME	INDICATIONS & DOSAGE	SIDE EFFECTS
cisplatin (cis-platinum) Platinol	*Adjunctive therapy in metastatic testicular cancer—* **Adults:** 20 mg/m² I.V. daily for 5 days. Repeat every 3 weeks for 3 cycles or longer. *Adjunctive therapy in metastatic ovarian cancer*—100 mg/m² I.V. Repeat every 4 weeks; or 50 mg/m² I.V. every 3 weeks with concurrent doxorubicin HCl therapy. Give as I.V. infusion in 2 liters normal saline solution with 37.5 g mannitol over 6 to 8 hours. *Note:* Prehydration and mannitol diuresis may reduce renal toxicity and ototoxicity significantly.	**Blood:** *reversible myelosuppression in 25% to 30% of patients, leukopenia, thrombocytopenia,* anemia; nadirs in circulating platelets and leukocytes on days 18 to 23, with recovery by day 39. **CNS:** peripheral neuritis, loss of taste, seizures. **EENT:** *tinnitus, hearing loss.* **GI:** *nausea, vomiting, beginning 1 to 4 hours after dose and lasting 24 hours; diarrhea.* **GU:** *more prolonged and severe renal toxicity with repeated courses of therapy.* **Other:** anaphylactoid reaction.
cyclophosphamide Cytoxan♦, Procytox♦♦	*Breast, colon, head, neck, lung, ovarian, and prostatic cancer; Hodgkin's disease; chronic lymphocytic leukemia; chronic myelocytic leukemia; acute lymphoblastic leukemia; neuroblastoma; retinoblastoma; non-Hodgkin's lymphomas; multiple myeloma; mycosis fungoides; sarcomas—* **Adults:** 40 to 50 mg/kg P.O. or I.V. in single dose or in 2 to 5 daily doses, then adjust for maintenance; or 2 to 4 mg/kg P.O. daily for 10 days, then adjust for maintenance. Maintenance dose 1.5 to 3 mg/kg/day P.O.; or 10 to 15 mg/kg q 7 to 10 days I.V.; or 3 to 5 mg/kg twice weekly I.V. **Children:** 2 to 8 mg/kg/day or 60 to 250 mg/m²/day P.O. or I.V. for 6 days (dose depends on susceptibility of neoplasm); divide oral dosages; give I.V. dosages once weekly. Maintenance dose 2 to 5 mg/kg or 50 to 150 mg/m² twice weekly P.O.	**Blood:** *leukopenia,* nadir between days 8 to 15, recovery in 17 to 28 days; thrombocytopenia; anemia. **CV:** *cardiotoxicity* (with very high doses and in combination with doxorubicin). **GI:** anorexia; *nausea and vomiting beginning within 6 hours, lasting 4 hours;* stomatitis; mucositis. **GU:** gonadal suppression (may be irreversible), *hemorrhagic cystitis,* bladder fibrosis, sterility, nephrotoxicity. **Metabolic:** hyperuricemia; syndrome of inappropriate ADH secretion (with high doses). **Other:** *alopecia in 50% of patients, especially with high doses;* secondary malignancies, *pulmonary fibrosis (high doses).*

INTERACTIONS	NURSING CONSIDERATIONS
None significant.	• Use cautiously in preexisting renal impairment, myelosuppression, and hearing impairment. • Hydrate patient with normal saline solution before giving drug. Maintain urine output of 100 ml/hour for 4 consecutive hours before therapy and for 24 hours after therapy. • Don't use aluminum needles for reconstitution or administration of cisplatin; a black precipitate may form. • Mannitol may be given as 12.5 g I.V. bolus before starting cisplatin infusion. Follow by infusion of mannitol at rate up to 10 g/hour p.r.n. to maintain urine output during and 6 to 24 hours after cisplatin infusion. • Do not repeat dose unless platelets are over 100,000/mm^3, WBC is over 4,000/mm^3, creatinine is under 1.5 mg%, or BUN is under 25 mg%. • Monitor CBC, platelets, and renal function studies before initial and subsequent doses. • Tell patient to report tinnitus immediately to prevent permanent hearing loss. Do audiometry before and during treatment. • Nausea and vomiting may be severe and protracted (up to 24 hours). Antiemetics can be started 24 hours before therapy. Monitor intake and output. Continue I.V. hydration until patient can tolerate adequate oral intake. • Reconstitute with sterile water for injection. Stable for 24 hours in normal saline solution at room temperature. Don't refrigerate. • Given with bleomycin and vinblastine for testicular cancer and with doxorubicin HCl for ovarian cancer. • Renal toxicity becomes more severe with repeated doses. Renal function must return to normal before next dose can be given. • Avoid all I.M. injections when platelets are low.
Corticosteroids, chloramphenicol: reduced activity of cyclophosphamide. Use cautiously. *Allopurinol:* may produce excessive cyclophosphamide effect. Monitor for enhanced toxicity.	• Use cautiously in severe leukopenia, thrombocytopenia, malignant cell infiltration of bone marrow, recent radiation therapy or chemotherapy, hepatic or renal disease. • Advise both male and female patients to practice contraception while taking this drug and for 4 months after; drug is potentially teratogenic. • Monitor uric acid, CBC, renal and hepatic functions. • To reduce nausea, give antiemetic before administering. • Push fluid (3 liters daily) to prevent hemorrhagic cystitis. Don't give drug at bedtime, since voiding is too infrequent to avoid cystitis. If hemorrhagic cystitis occurs, drug is stopped. Cystitis can occur months after therapy has been stopped. • Reconstituted solution is stable 6 days refrigerated or 24 hours at room temperature. • Can cause false-positive cytology in all body secretions. • Avoid all I.M. injections when platelets are low. • Can be given by direct I.V. push into a running I.V. line or by infusion in normal saline solution or dextrose 5% in water. • To prevent hyperuricemia with resulting uric acid nephropathy, keep patient well hydrated; alkalinize the urine. • Warn patient that alopecia is likely to occur. • Anticoagulants should be used cautiously. Watch closely for signs of bleeding. • Has been used successfully to treat many nonmalignant conditions.

NAME	INDICATIONS & DOSAGE	SIDE EFFECTS
dacarbazine (DTIC) DTIC-Dome♦	*Hodgkin's disease, metastatic malignant melanoma, neuroblastoma, sarcomas—* **Adults:** 2 to 4.5 mg/kg or 70 to 160 mg/m² I.V. daily for 10 days, then repeat q 4 weeks as tolerated; or 250 mg/m² I.V. daily for 5 days, repeated at 3-week intervals.	**Blood:** *WBC falling for up to 5 weeks, recovering in 2 weeks; thrombocytopenia.* **GI:** *severe nausea and vomiting begin within 1 to 3 hours in 90% of patients, last 1 to 12 hours; anorexia.* **Local:** severe pain if I.V. infiltrates or if solution is too concentrated; tissue damage. **Other:** *flu-like syndrome* (fever, malaise, myalgia beginning 7 days after treatment stopped and possibly lasting 7 to 21 days), alopecia.
lomustine (CCNU) CeeNU♦	*Brain, colon, lung, and renal cell cancer; Hodgkin's disease; lymphomas; melanomas; multiple myeloma—* **Adults and children:** 130 mg/m² P.O. as single dose q 6 weeks. Reduce dose according to bone marrow depression. Repeat doses should not be given until WBC is more than 4,000/mm³ and platelet count is more than 100,000/mm³.	**Blood:** *leukopenia, delayed up to 6 weeks, lasting 1 to 2 weeks; thrombocytopenia, delayed up to 4 weeks, lasting 1 to 2 weeks.* **GI:** *nausea and vomiting beginning within 4 to 5 hours, lasting 24 hours;* stomatitis. **Other:** alopecia.
mechlorethamine hydrochloride (nitrogen mustard) Mustargen♦	*Breast, lung, and ovarian cancer; Hodgkin's disease; non-Hodgkin's lymphomas; lymphosarcoma—* **Adults:** 0.4 mg/kg or 10 mg/m² I.V. as single or divided dose q 3 to 6 weeks. Give through running I.V. infusion. Dose reduced in prior radiation or chemotherapy to 0.2 to 0.4 mg/kg. Dose based on ideal or actual body weight, whichever is less. *Neoplastic effusions—* **Adults:** 10 to 20 mg intracavitarily.	**Blood:** *nadir of leukopenia, thrombocytopenia, myelosuppression occurring by days 4 to 10, lasting 10 to 21 days;* mild anemia begins in 2 to 3 weeks, possibly lasting 7 weeks. **EENT:** tinnitus, *metallic taste,* immediately after dose; deafness in high doses. **GI:** *nausea, vomiting, and anorexia* begin within minutes, last 8 to 24 hours. **Metabolic:** hyperuricemia. **Local:** *thrombophlebitis, sloughing, severe irritation if drug extravasates or touches skin.* **Other:** *alopecia,* may precipitate herpes zoster.

♦ Available in U.S. and Canada. ♦♦ Available in Canada only. All other products (no symbol) available in U.S. only. Italicized side effects are common or life-threatening.

INTERACTIONS	NURSING CONSIDERATIONS
None significant.	• Use lower dose if renal function or bone marrow is impaired. Stop drug if WBC falls to 3,000/mm³ or platelets drop to 100,000/mm³. • Take temperature daily. Observe for signs of infection. • Monitor uric acid, CBC. • Discard refrigerated solution after 72 hours, room temperature solution after 8 hours. • Can cause false-positive cytology in all body secretions. • Avoid all I.M. injections when platelets are low. • Give I.V. infusion in 50 to 100 ml dextrose 5% in water over 30 minutes. May dilute further or slow infusion to decrease pain at infusion site. Make sure drug does not infiltrate. • For Hodgkin's disease, usually given with bleomycin, vinblastine, doxorubicin. • Anticoagulants should be used cautiously. Watch closely for signs of bleeding. • Administering antiemetics before giving dacarbazine may help decrease nausea. Nausea and vomiting usually subside after several doses.
None significant.	• Give 2 to 4 hours after meals. To avoid nausea, give antiemetic before administering. • May be useful in cancer involving CNS, since CSF level equals 30% to 50% of plasma level 1 hour after administration. • Monitor blood counts weekly. Don't give more often than every 6 weeks; bone marrow toxicity is cumulative and delayed. • Monitor uric acid, CBC. • Can cause false-positive cytology in all body secretions. • Avoid all I.M. injections when platelets are low. • For Hodgkin's disease, usually given with mechlorethamine. • Anticoagulants should be used cautiously. Watch closely for signs of bleeding. • Advise patient that drug can cause alopecia but hair will grow back.
None significant.	• Use cautiously in severe anemia, depressed neutrophil or platelet count, patients recently treated with radiation or chemotherapy. • Avoid contact with skin or mucous membranes. Wear gloves when preparing solution to prevent accidental skin contact. If contact occurs, wash with copious amounts of water. • Giving antiemetic before drug not always effective in reducing nausea. • Be sure I.V. doesn't infiltrate. If drug extravasates, apply cold compresses. • When given intracavitarily, turn patient from side to side every 15 minutes to 1 hour to distribute drug. • Monitor uric acid, CBC. • Severe herpes zoster may require stopping drug. • Very unstable solution. Prepare immediately before infusion. Use within 15 minutes. Discard unused solution. • To prevent hyperuricemia with resulting uric acid nephropathy, allopurinol may be given; keep patient well hydrated; alkalinize the urine. • Can cause false-positive cytology in all body secretions. • Avoid all I.M. injections when platelets are low. • One of the most effective drugs in treatment of Hodgkin's disease. • Has been used topically in treatment of mycosis fungoides. • Anticoagulants should be used cautiously. Watch closely for signs of bleeding.

NAME	INDICATIONS & DOSAGE	SIDE EFFECTS
melphalan Alkeran♦	*Multiple myeloma, malignant melanoma, testicular seminoma, reticulum cell sarcoma, osteogenic sarcoma, breast and ovarian cancer—* **Adults:** 6 mg P.O. daily for 2 to 3 weeks, then stop drug for up to 4 weeks or until WBC and platelets stop dropping and begin to rise again; resume with maintenance dose of 2 to 4 mg daily. Stop drug if WBC below 3,000/mm^3 or platelets below 100,000/mm^3. Alternate therapy: 0.15 mg/kg/day P.O. for 7 days, wait for WBC and platelets to recover, then resume with 0.05 mg/kg/day P.O.	**Blood:** *thrombocytopenia, leukopenia, agranulocytosis.* **GI:** anorexia, nausea, vomiting.
pipobroman Vercyte♦	*Polycythemia vera—* **Adults, and children over 15 years:** 1 mg/kg P.O. daily for 30 days; may increase to 1.5 to 3 mg/kg P.O. daily until hematocrit reduced to 50% to 55%, then 0.1 to 0.2 mg/kg daily maintenance. *Chronic myelocytic leukemia—* **Adults, and children over 15 years:** 1.5 to 2.5 mg/kg P.O. daily until WBC drops to 10,000/mm^3, then start maintenance 7 to 175 mg daily. Stop drug if WBC below 3,000/mm^3 or platelets below 150,000/mm^3.	**Blood:** *leukopenia and thrombocytopenia, delayed up to 4 weeks or longer.* **GI:** nausea, vomiting, cramping, diarrhea, anorexia. **Skin:** rash.
thiotepa Thiotepa♦	**Adults, and children over 12 years:** *Breast, lung, and ovarian cancer; Hodgkin's disease; lymphomas*—0.2 mg/kg I.V. daily for 5 days; then maintenance dose of 0.2 mg/kg I.V. q 1 to 3 weeks. *Bladder tumor*—60 mg in 60 ml water instilled in bladder once weekly for 4 weeks. *Neoplastic effusions*—10 to 15 mg intracavitarily, p.r.n. Stop drug or decrease dosage if WBC below 4,000/mm^3 or if platelets below 150,000/mm^3.	**Blood:** *leukopenia begins within 5 to 30 days; thrombocytopenia; neutropenia.* **GI:** nausea, vomiting, anorexia. **GU:** amenorrhea, decreased spermatogenesis. **Metabolic:** hyperuricemia. **Skin:** hives, rash. **Local:** intense pain at administration site. **Other:** headache, fever, tightness of throat, dizziness.

♦ Available in U.S. and Canada. ♦♦ Available in Canada only. All other products (no symbol) available in U.S. only. Italicized side effects are common or life-threatening.

INTERACTIONS	NURSING CONSIDERATIONS
None significant.	• Not recommended in severe leukopenia, thrombocytopenia, or anemia; chronic lymphocytic leukemia; or suppurative inflammation. • To reduce nausea, give antiemetic before administering. • Monitor uric acid, CBC. • Can cause false-positive cytology in all body secretions. • Avoid all I.M. injections when platelets are low. • May need dose reduction in renal impairment. • Drug of choice in multiple myeloma. • Anticoagulants should be used cautiously. Watch closely for signs of bleeding.
None significant.	• Use cautiously in bone marrow depression. • Do WBC and platelet count until desired response or toxicity occurs (platelets less than 150,000/mm^3 or WBC less than 3,000/mm^3). • Monitor CBC. • Anticoagulants should be used cautiously. Watch closely for signs of bleeding.
None significant.	• Use cautiously in bone marrow depression, chronic lymphocytic leukemia, renal or hepatic dysfunction. • Do WBC, RBC counts weekly for at least 3 weeks after last dose. Warn patient to report even mild infections. • GU side effects reversible in 6 to 8 months. • May require use of local anesthetic at injection site if intense pain occurs. • For bladder instillation: dehydrate patient 8 to 10 hours before therapy. Instill drug into bladder by catheter; ask patient to retain solution for 2 hours. Volume may be reduced to 30 ml if discomfort is too great with 60 ml. Reposition patient every 15 minutes for maximum area contact. • Toxicity delayed and prolonged because drug binds to tissues and stays in body several hours. • Monitor uric acid, CBC. • Refrigerate dry powder; protect from light. • Use only sterile water for injection to reconstitute. Refrigerated solution stable 5 days. • To prevent hyperuricemia with resulting uric acid nephropathy, allopurinol may be given; keep patient well hydrated; alkalinize the urine. • Can cause false-positive cytology in all body secretions.

(continued on following page)

NAME	INDICATIONS & DOSAGE	SIDE EFFECTS
thiotepa *(continued)*		
uracil mustard	*Chronic lymphocytic and myelocytic leukemia; Hodgkin's disease; non-Hodgkin's lymphomas of the histiocytic and lymphocytic types; reticulum cell sarcoma; lymphomas; mycosis fungoides; polycythemia vera; cancer of ovaries, cervix, and lungs—* **Adults:** 1 to 2 mg P.O. daily for 3 months or until desired response or toxicity; maintenance 1 mg daily for 3 out of 4 weeks until optimum response or relapse; or 3 to 5 mg P.O. for 7 days not to exceed total dose 0.5 mg/kg, then 1 mg daily until response, then 1 mg daily 3 out of 4 weeks.	**Blood:** bone marrow depression, delayed 2 to 4 weeks; *thrombocytopenia; leukopenia;* anemia. **CNS:** irritability, nervousness, mental cloudiness and depression. **GI:** *nausea, vomiting, diarrhea, epigastric distress,* abdominal pain, anorexia. **Metabolic:** hyperuricemia. **Skin:** pruritus, dermatitis, hyperpigmentation, alopecia.

♦ Available in U.S. and Canada. ♦♦ Available in Canada only. All other products (no symbol) available in U.S. only. Italicized side effects are common or life-threatening.

HOW NEOPLASTIC DISEASES RESPOND TO CHEMOTHERAPY WITH ALKYLATING AGENTS AND OTHER DRUGS

TYPE OF CANCER	USEFUL DRUGS	RESULTS EXPECTED
Prolonged survival or cure possible		
Burkitt's tumor	*cyclophosphamide*	50% cured
Testicular tumors (seminoma)	*cyclophosphamide* with radiotherapy	90% to 95% respond; 50% to 60% cured
Neuroblastoma	*cyclophosphamide,* doxorubicin, procarbazine, vincristine with surgery and/or with radiotherapy	Over 50% response (advanced stage); up to 80% long-term survival, depending on stage
Acute lymphoblastic leukemia	*carmustine,* daunorubicin, prednisone, vincristine, 6-mercaptopurine, methotrexate, L-asparaginase	90% remission; 70% survive beyond 5 years
Hodgkin's disease (stages IIB, IIIB, and IV)	*mechlorethamine,* vincristine, prednisone, doxorubicin, dacarbazine, procarbazine, vinblastine	70% respond; 40% survive beyond 5 years
Palliation and prolongation of life possible		
Breast carcinoma	*alkylating agents,* androgens, estrogens, 5-fluorouracil, vincristine, prednisone, methotrexate, doxorubicin	60% to 80% respond with probable prolongation of life

INTERACTIONS	NURSING CONSIDERATIONS
	• Avoid all I.M. injections when platelets are low. • Can be given by all parenteral routes, including direct injection into the tumor. • Anticoagulants should be used cautiously. Watch closely for signs of bleeding. • Discuss possible amenorrhea with female patients when drug therapy is initiated.
None significant.	• Not recommended in severe thrombocytopenia, aplastic anemia or leukopenia, acute leukemias. • Give at bedtime to reduce nausea. • Watch for signs of ecchymoses, easy bruising, petechiae. • Monitor uric acid. Do regular platelet count. Do CBC 1 to 2 times weekly for 4 weeks; then 4 weeks after stopping drug. • Don't give drug within 2 to 3 weeks after maximum bone marrow depression from past radiation or chemotherapy. • To prevent hyperuricemia and resulting uric acid nephropathy, allopurinol can be given; keep patient hydrated; alkalinize the urine. • Can cause false-positive cytology in all body secretions. • Avoid all I.M. injections when platelets are low. • Anticoagulants should be used cautiously. Watch closely for signs of bleeding.

TYPE OF CANCER	USEFUL DRUGS	RESULTS EXPECTED
Chronic lymphocytic leukemia and lymphosarcoma	*alkylating agents,* prednisone	50% respond with probable prolongation of life
Palliation possible but uncertain prolongation of life		
Chronic granulocytic leukemia	*alkylating agents,* 6-mercaptopurine, hydroxyurea	90% respond with good control during most of course
Multiple myeloma	*alkylating agents,* carmustine, prednisone, vincristine	60% respond
Ovary	*alkylating agents,* cisplatin	30% to 40% respond
Palliation possible but not usual		
Lung	*alkylating agents*	30% to 40% respond briefly
Head and neck	*alkylating agents,* cisplatin, methotrexate, bleomycin	20% to 30% respond briefly
Large bowel	*MeCCNU,** 5-fluorouracil, cytarabine, mitomycin C	30% to 50% respond
Cervix	*alkylating agents,* bleomycin	20% respond
Melanoma	*alkylating agents,* vinblastine, dacarbazine	20% respond

*An investigational alkylating agent (not listed in tables)

73 Antimetabolites

azathioprine
cytarabine
floxuridine
fluorouracil
hydroxyurea
mercaptopurine
methotrexate
methotrexate sodium
thioguanine

Antimetabolites, the first group of antineoplastics designed specifically as antitumor agents, function in one of two ways—as replacements for cellular components or as enzyme inhibitors. When they replace a necessary component in a cellular compound, the resulting cell product fails to function, blocking cell division. When antimetabolites inhibit a key enzyme reaction, they interfere with cellular metabolism.

Antimetabolites can be grouped as folic-acid antagonists (methotrexate and

HOW ANTIMETABOLITES AFFECT THE CELL CYCLE

Antimetabolites are cell-cycle specific antineoplastics. Like all antineoplastics, by interrupting protein synthesis they prevent cells—including cancer cells—from reproducing and surviving.

A cell's various proteins are manufactured at specific points during the cell cycle, which is divided into these distinct phases:

- **phase G_1:** the period immediately before DNA synthesis (at this time, the cell may also become dormant, a state designated G_0)
- **phase S:** DNA synthesis
- **phase G_2:** RNA synthesis
- **phase M:** mitosis (prophase, metaphase, anaphase, and telophase).

The duration of a cell's life cycle differs according to its tissue of origin, but on the average the process—excluding mitosis—takes 10 hours.

Antimetabolites act during the entire cell cycle but are most effective during phase S. They are divided into folic acid antagonists (which interfere with biosynthetic enzymes), and purine and pyrimidine antagonists (which take the place of normal components during both DNA and RNA synthesis). Antimetabolites destroy healthy cells as well as those that are diseased; their limited toxicity can be attributed to the different rates at which different cells grow. The degree of their toxicity is such, however, that they have the narrowest range of application of all antineoplastics.

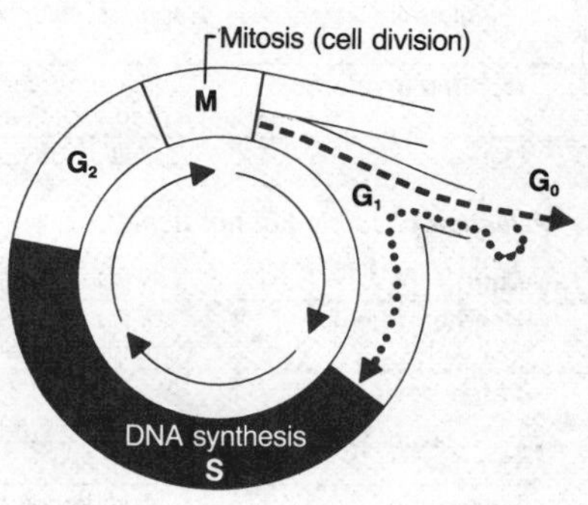

methotrexate sodium); purine antagonists (azathioprine, mercaptopurine, and thioguanine); and pyrimidine antagonists (cytarabine, floxuridine, and fluorouracil). Hydroxyurea also functions as an antimetabolite but cannot be assigned to any group.

Major uses

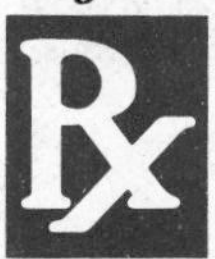

Antimetabolites, with the exception of azathioprine, are used to treat carcinomas (mostly of the breast and gastrointestinal tract), trophoblastic tumors such as choriocarcinomas and hydatidiform moles, medulloblastomas, and osteogenic sarcomas.

- Azathioprine produces immunosuppression in renal transplants and is also indicated in the treatment of severe, active rheumatoid arthritis when other measures aren't effective.

Mechanism of action

All the antimetabolites interfere with DNA synthesis, as follows:

- Azathioprine, mercaptopurine, and thioguanine inhibit purine synthesis.
- Cytarabine, floxuridine, and fluorouracil inhibit pyrimidine synthesis.
- Hydroxyurea inhibits ribonucleotide reductase.
- Methotrexate prevents reduction of folic acid to tetrahydrofolate by binding to dihydrofolate reductase.

Absorption, distribution, metabolism, and excretion

- Azathioprine, hydroxyurea, mercaptopurine, methotrexate, and thioguanine are well absorbed when given orally.
- Cytarabine, floxuridine, and fluorouracil are not absorbed after oral administration and must be given parenterally. However, fluorouracil can be administered orally in local treatment of some gastrointestinal carcinomas.
- All antimetabolites are distributed widely in body tissues and fluids, metabolized in the liver, and excreted in urine, largely as inactive metabolites.

Onset and duration

Therapeutic activity varies with the antimetabolite, disease, and patient response.

Combination products

None.

VITAMINS TO THE RESCUE IN HIGH-DOSE METHOTREXATE THERAPY

Your patient with cancer may be scheduled to receive a course of high-dose methotrexate therapy, followed by one or more doses of folinic acid (leucovorin calcium, citrovorum factor). In this follow-up procedure, known as *rescue therapy,* folinic acid selectively counteracts the toxic effects of large doses of methotrexate.

A folate antagonist, methotrexate inhibits the enyzme dihydrofolate reductase and thereby interferes with the important conversion of folic acid to tetrahydrofolate. This ultimately halts DNA synthesis, interrupting the cell life cycle at a crucial point before the divisional stage.

All cells are particularly vulnerable to chemotherapy during DNA synthesis. But cancer cells are more susceptible to destruction by methotrexate than are normal cells. This is due to different enzymatic processes that the cancer cells undergo.

To rescue remaining *normal cells* about to begin DNA synthesis, folinic acid is given. It bypasses the block created by methotrexate and delivers the metabolically active form of folic acid so normal cell reproduction can proceed.

Among the new targets of this aggressive treatment are cancers of the head and neck, squamous cell carcinoma of the lung, histiocytic lymphoma, and especially osteogenic sarcoma, a previously unresponsive tumor.

So, be sure your patient takes his folinic acid *on schedule*. It's an important part of his cancer therapy, not "just a vitamin."

NAME	INDICATIONS & DOSAGE	SIDE EFFECTS
azathioprine Imuran♦	*Immunosuppression in renal transplants—* **Adults and children:** initially, 3 to 5 mg/kg P.O. daily. Maintain at 1 to 2 mg/kg/day (dose varies considerably according to patient response). *Treatment of severe, refractory rheumatoid arthritis—* **Adults:** initially, 1 mg/kg taken as a single dose or as 2 doses. If patient response not satisfactory after 6 to 8 weeks, dosage may be increased by 0.5 mg/kg/day (up to a maximum of 2.5 mg/kg/day) at 4-week intervals.	**Blood:** *leukopenia, bone marrow depression,* anemia, pancytopeniathrombocytopenia. **GI:** nausea, vomiting, anorexia, pancreatitis, ascites, steatorrhea, mouth ulceration, esophagitis. **Hepatic:** hepatoxicity, jaundice. **Skin:** rash. **Other:** *immunosuppression (possibly profound),* arthralgia, muscle wasting, alopecia, pancreatitis.
cytarabine (ARA-C, cytosine arabinoside) Cytosar-U♦	*Acute myelocytic and other acute leukemias—* **Adults and children:** 2 to 3 mg/kg (100 mg/m²) I.V. or S.C. b.i.d. for 7 days; 2 to 3 mg/kg (100 mg/m²) daily for 7 days by 24-hour continuous infusion; or 10 to 30 mg/m² intrathecally, up to 3 times weekly. Maintenance 2 to 3 mg/kg I.V. or S.C. b.i.d. for 5 days.	**Blood:** WBC nadir 5 to 7 days after drug stopped; *leukopenia, anemia, thrombocytopenia,* reticulocytopenia; platelet nadir occurring on day 10; *megaloblastosis.* **GI:** *nausea, vomiting,* diarrhea, dysphagia; reddened area at juncture of lips, followed by sore mouth, oral ulcers in 5 to 10 days; high dose given via rapid I.V. may cause projectile vomiting. **Hepatic:** hepatotoxicity (usually mild and reversible). **Other:** flu-like syndrome.
floxuridine FUDR	*Brain, breast, head, neck, liver, gallbladder, and bile duct cancer—* **Adults:** 0.1 to 0.6 mg/kg daily by intra-arterial infusion (use pump for continuous, uniform rate); or 0.4 to 0.6 mg/kg daily into hepatic artery.	**Blood:** *leukopenia, anemia,* thrombocytopenia. **CNS:** cerebellar ataxia, vertigo, nystagmus, convulsions, depression, hemiplegia, hiccups, lethargy. **EENT:** blurred vision. **GI:** *stomatitis, cramps, nausea, vomiting, diarrhea, bleeding, enteritis.* **Skin:** *erythema,* dermatitis, pruritus, rash.

♦ Available in U.S. and Canada. ♦♦ Available in Canada only. All other products (no symbol) available in U.S. only. Italicized side effects are common or life-threatening.

INTERACTIONS	NURSING CONSIDERATIONS
Allopurinol: impaired inactivation of azathioprine. Decrease azathioprine dose to ¼ or ⅓ normal dose.	• Use cautiously in hepatic or renal dysfunction. • Watch for clay-colored stools, dark urine, pruritus, and yellow skin and sclera; and for increased alkaline phosphatase, bilirubin, SGOT, and SGPT. • In renal homotransplants, start drug 1 to 5 days before surgery. • Hemoglobin, WBC, platelet count should be done at least once a week; more often at beginning of treatment. Drug should be stopped immediately when WBC is less than 3,000/mm³ to prevent extension to irreversible bone marrow depression. • This is a potent immunosuppressive. Warn patient to report even mild infections (coryza, fever, sore throat, malaise). • Patient should avoid conception during therapy and up to 4 months after stopping therapy. • Warn patient that some thinning of hair is possible. • Avoid I.M. injections of any drugs in patients with severely depressed platelet counts (thrombocytopenia) to prevent bleeding. • When used to treat refractory rheumatoid arthritis, inform patient that drug may take up to 12 weeks to be effective.
None significant.	• Use cautiously in inadequate bone marrow reserve. Use cautiously in renal or hepatic disease and after other chemotherapy or radiation therapy. • Watch for signs of infection (leukoplakia, fever, sore throat). • Excellent mouth care can help prevent oral side effects. • Monitor intake/output carefully. Maintain high fluid intake and give allopurinol, if ordered, to avoid urate nephropathy in leukemia induction therapy. • Check uric acid, CBC with platelets, and hepatic function. • Use preservative-free normal saline solution for intrathecal use. • Optimum schedule is continuous infusion. • To reduce nausea, give antiemetic before administering. • Store dry powder in refrigerator; refrigerated, reconstituted solution stable 48 hours. Discard cloudy reconstituted solution. • Avoid I.M. injections of any drugs in patients with severely depressed platelet count (thrombocytopenia) to prevent bleeding. • Modify or discontinue therapy if polymorphonuclear granulocyte count is 1,000/mm³ or if platelet count is 50,000/mm³.
None significant.	• Use cautiously in poor nutritional state, bone marrow depression, or serious infection. Use cautiously following high-dose pelvic irradiation or use of alkylating agent, and in impaired hepatic or renal function. • Severe skin and GI side effects require stopping drug. Use of antacid eases but probably won't prevent GI distress. • Excellent mouth care can help prevent oral side effects. • Monitor intake/output, CBC, and renal and hepatic function. • Discontinue if WBC falls below 3,500/mm³ or if platelet count below 100,000/mm³. • Therapeutic effect may be delayed 1 to 6 weeks. Make sure patient is aware of time it may take for improvement to be noted. • Reconstitute with sterile water for injection. Dilute further in 5% dextrose in water or normal saline solution for actual infusion. • Always use infusion pump. • Avoid I.M. injections of any drugs in patients with thrombocytopenia to prevent bleeding. • Refrigerated solution stable no more than 2 weeks. • Observe arterial perfused area. Check line for bleeding, blockage, displacement, or leakage.

NAME	INDICATIONS & DOSAGE	SIDE EFFECTS
fluorouracil (5-fluorouracil) Adrucil, 5-FU	*Colon, rectal, breast, ovarian, cervical, bladder, liver, and pancreatic cancer—* **Adults:** 12.5 mg/kg I.V. daily for 3 to 5 days q 4 weeks; or 15 mg/kg weekly for 6 weeks. (Doses recommended based on lean body weight.) Maximum single recommended dose is 800 mg, although higher single doses (up to 1.5 g) have been used. The injectable form has been given orally but is not recommended.	**Blood:** *leukopenia, thrombocytopenia,* anemia. WBC nadir 9 to 14 days after first dose; platelet nadir in 7 to 14 days. **GI:** *stomatitis, GI ulcer may precede leukopenia, nausea, vomiting in 30% to 50% of patients; diarrhea.* **Skin:** *dermatitis,* hyperpigmentation (especially in Blacks), nail changes, pigmented palmar creases. **Other:** *alopecia in 5% to 20% of patients, weakness, malaise.*
hydroxyurea Hydrea	*Melanoma; resistant chronic myelocytic leukemia; recurrent, metastatic, or inoperable ovarian cancer—* **Adults:** 80 mg/kg P.O. as single dose q 3 days; or 20 to 30 mg/kg P.O. daily.	**Blood:** *leukopenia,* thrombocytopenia, anemia, *megaloblastosis; dose-limiting and dose-related bone marrow depression, with rapid recovery.* **CNS:** drowsiness. **GI:** *anorexia, nausea, vomiting, diarrhea,* stomatitis. **GU:** increased BUN, serum creatinine. **Metabolic:** hyperuricemia. **Skin:** rash, pruritus.
mercaptopurine Purinethol♦	*Acute lymphoblastic leukemia (in children), acute myeloblastic leukemia, chronic myelocytic leukemia—* **Adults:** 80 to 100 mg/m² P.O. daily as a single dose up to 5 mg/kg/day. **Children:** 70 mg/m² P.O. daily. Usual maintenance for adults and children: 1.5 to 2.5 mg/kg/day.	**Blood:** *decreased RBC; leukopenia, thrombocytopenia, bone marrow hypoplasia; all may persist several days after drug is stopped.* **GI:** *nausea, vomiting, and anorexia in 25% of patients;* painful oral ulcers. **Hepatic:** *jaundice, hepatic necrosis.* **Metabolic:** hyperuricemia.

♦ Available in U.S. and Canada. ♦♦ Available in Canada only. All other products (no symbol) available in U.S. only. Italicized side effects are common or life-threatening.

INTERACTIONS	NURSING CONSIDERATIONS
None significant.	• Use cautiously following major surgery; in poor nutritional state, serious infections, and bone marrow depression. Use cautiously following high-dose pelvic irradiation or use of alkylating agents, in impaired hepatic or renal function, or in widespread neoplastic infiltration of bone marrow. • Watch for stomatitis or diarrhea (signs of toxicity). May use topical oral anesthetic to soothe lesions. Discontinue if diarrhea occurs. • Give antiemetic before administering to reduce GI side effects. • Do WBC and platelet counts daily. Drug should be stopped when WBC is less than 3,500/mm^3. Watch for ecchymoses, petechiae, easy bruising, and anemia. Drug should be stopped if platelet count is less than 100,000/mm^3. • Skin and ocular side effects reversible when drug is stopped. Patient should use highly protective sun blockers to avoid inflammatory erythematous dermatitis. • Therapeutic concentrations don't reach cerebrospinal fluid. • Slowing infusion rate so it takes from 2 to 8 hours lessens toxicity but also lessens efficacy compared with rapid injection. • Monitor intake/output, CBC, and renal and hepatic functions. • Do not refrigerate fluorouracil. • Don't use cloudy solution. If crystals form, redissolve by warming. • Sometimes ordered as 5-FU. The number 5 is part of the drug name and should not be confused with dosage units. • Sometimes administered via hepatic arterial infusion in treatment of hepatic metastases. • Warn patient that alopecia may occur but is reversible. • To prevent bleeding, avoid I.M. injections of any drugs in patients with thrombocytopenia. • Fluorouracil toxicity is delayed for 1 to 3 weeks.
None significant.	• Use cautiously following other chemotherapy or radiation therapy. • Use with caution in renal dysfunction. Discontinue if WBC is less than 2,500/mm^3 or if platelet count is less than 100,000/mm^3. • If patient can't swallow capsule, he may empty contents into water and take immediately. • Monitor intake/output; keep patient hydrated. • Routinely measure BUN, uric acid, serum creatinine. • Drug crosses blood-brain barrier. • Auditory and visual hallucinations and blood toxicity increase when decreased renal function exists. • May exacerbate postirradiation erythema. • Avoid all I.M. injections when platelets are low.
Allopurinol: slowed inactivation of mercaptopurine. Decrease mercaptopurine to ¼ or ⅓ normal dose.	• Use cautiously following chemotherapy or radiation therapy, in depressed neutrophil or platelet count, and in impaired hepatic or renal function. • Observe for signs of bleeding and infection. • Hepatic dysfunction reversible when drug is stopped. Watch for jaundice, clay-colored stools, frothy dark urine. Drug should be stopped if hepatic tenderness occurs. • Do weekly blood counts; watch for precipitous fall. • Monitor intake/output. Push fluids (3 liters daily). • Sometimes ordered as 6-mercaptopurine or 6-MP. The number 6 is part of drug name and does not signify number of dosage units. • Warn patient that improvement may take 2 to 4 weeks or longer. • GI side effects less common in children than in adults. • Avoid all I.M. injections when platelets are low.

NAME	INDICATIONS & DOSAGE	SIDE EFFECTS
methotrexate **methotrexate sodium** Mexate	*Trophoblastic tumors (choriocarcinoma, hydatidiform mole)*— **Adults:** 15 to 30 mg P.O. or I.M. daily for 5 days. Repeat after 1 or more weeks, according to response or toxicity. *Acute lymphoblastic and lymphatic leukemia*— **Adults and children:** 3.3 mg/m² P.O., I.M., or I.V. daily for 4 to 6 weeks or until remission occurs; then 20 to 30 mg/m² P.O. or I.M. twice weekly. *Meningeal leukemia*— **Adults and children:** 0.2 to 0.5 mg/kg intrathecally q 2 to 5 days until cerebrospinal fluid is normal. Use only 20-, 50-, or 100-mg vials of powder with no preservatives, and dilute to concentration of 1 mg/ml using 0.9% NaCl injection *without* preservatives. Use only new vials of drug and diluent. Use immediately. *Burkitt's lymphoma* (Stage I or Stage II)— **Adults:** 10 to 25 mg P.O. daily for 4 to 8 days with 1-week rest intervals. *Burkitt's lymphoma* (Stage III)— **Adults:** up to 1 g/m²/day with cyclophosphamide and prednisolone. *Lymphosarcoma* (Stage III)— **Adults:** 0.625 to 2.5 mg/kg daily P.O., I.M., or I.V. *Mycosis fungoides*— **Adults:** 2.5 to 10 mg P.O. daily or 50 mg I.M. weekly; or 25 mg I.M. twice weekly. *Psoriasis*— **Adults:** 10 to 25 mg P.O., I.M., or I.V. as single weekly dose. To detect idiosyncratic reactions, 5 to 10 mg test dose recommended 1 week before methotrexate regimen.	**Blood:** WBC and platelet nadir occurring on day 7; anemia, *leukopenia, thrombocytopenia* (all dose-related). **CNS:** *arachnoiditis within hours of intrathecal use;* subacute neurotoxicity which may begin a few weeks later; necrotizing demyelinating leukoencephalopathy a few years later. **GI:** *stomatitis* (common); *diarrhea leading to hemorrhagic enteritis and intestinal perforation.* **GU:** *tubular necrosis.* **Hepatic:** hepatic dysfunction leading to cirrhosis or hepatic fibrosis. **Metabolic:** hyperuricemia. **Skin:** exposure to sun may aggravate psoriatic lesions, rash, photosensitivity. **Other:** alopecia; *pulmonary interstitial infiltrates;* long-term use in children may cause osteoporosis.
thioguanine Lanvis♦♦	*Acute leukemia, chronic granulocytic leukemia*— **Adults and children:** initially, 2 mg/kg/day P.O. (usually calculated to nearest 20 mg); then increased gradually to 3 mg/kg/day if no toxic effects occur.	**Blood:** *leukopenia,* anemia, *thrombocytopenia* (occurs slowly over 2 to 4 weeks). **GI:** nausea, vomiting, stomatitis, diarrhea, anorexia. **Hepatic:** hepatotoxicity, jaundice. **Metabolic:** hyperuricemia.

♦ Available in U.S. and Canada. ♦♦ Available in Canada only. All other products (no symbol) available in U.S. only. Italicized side effects are common or life-threatening.

INTERACTIONS	NURSING CONSIDERATIONS
Alcohol: increased hepatotoxicity; warn patient not to drink alcoholic beverages. *Probenecid, phenylbutazone, salicylates, sulfonamides:* increased methotrexate toxicity; don't use together if possible.	• Use cautiously in impaired hepatic or renal function, bone marrow depression, aplasia, leukopenia, thrombocytopenia, anemia. Use cautiously in infection, peptic ulcer, ulcerative colitis, and in very young, old, or debilitated patients. • Warn patient to avoid conception during and immediately after therapy because of possible abortion or congenital anomalies. • GI side effects may require stopping drug. • Rash, redness, or ulcerations in mouth or pulmonary side effects may signal serious complications. • Monitor uric acid. • Check thirst and urinary frequency. • Monitor intake/output daily. Force fluids (2 to 3 liters daily). • To alkalinize urine, the doctor may order $NaHCO_3$ tablets to prevent precipitation of drug, especially with high doses. Maintain urine pH at more than 6.5. The doctor may reduce dose if BUN 20 to 30 mg/100 ml or creatinine 1.2 to 2 mg/100 ml, or stop drug if BUN more than 30 mg/100 ml or creatinine more than 2 mg%. • Watch for increases in SGOT, SGPT, alkaline phosphatase; may signal hepatic dysfunction. • Watch for bleeding (especially GI) and infection. • Warn patient to use highly protective sun blocker when exposed to sunlight. • Take temperature daily, and watch for cough, dyspnea, cyanosis; corticosteroids may help reduce pulmonary side effects. • Leucovorin rescue: Leucovorin calcium (folinic acid) is given within 4 hours of administration of methotrexate and is usually continued 24 to 72 hours. Don't confuse with folic acid. This rescue technique is effective against systemic toxicity but does not interfere with the tumor cells' absorption of the methotrexate. • Avoid all I.M. injections in patients with thrombocytopenia.
None significant.	• Use cautiously in renal or hepatic dysfunction. • Stop drug if hepatotoxicity or hepatic tenderness occurs. Watch for jaundice; may reverse if drug stopped promptly. • Do CBC daily during induction, then weekly during maintenance therapy. • Monitor serum uric acid. • Sometimes ordered as 6-thioguanine. The number 6 is part of drug name and does not signify dosage units. • Avoid all I.M. injections when platelets are low.

74 Antibiotic antineoplastic agents

bleomycin sulfate
dactinomycin (actinomycin D)
daunorubicin hydrochloride
doxorubicin hydrochloride
mithramycin
mitomycin
procarbazine hydrochloride

Antibiotic antineoplastics are isolated from naturally occurring microorganisms that inhibit bacterial growth. But unlike the anti-infective drugs that they're related to, antibiotic antineoplastics can disrupt the functioning of both the host's cells and bacterial cells. Although procarbazine hydrochloride is not an antibiotic, it's included in this chapter because it acts in a similar manner.

Major uses

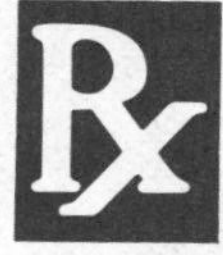

- Bleomycin, dactinomycin, doxorubicin, mitomycin, and procarbazine are used mainly to treat carcinomas, sarcomas, and lymphomas.
- Daunorubicin is used to treat acute leukemias.
- Mithramycin is used specifically to treat testicular carcinoma and hypercalcemia from various causes.

Mechanism of action

- Bleomycin inhibits deoxyribonucleic acid (DNA) synthesis and causes scission of DNA strands.
- Dactinomycin, daunorubicin, doxorubicin, and mithramycin interfere with DNA-dependent ribonucleic acid (RNA) synthesis by intercalation.
- Mithramycin also inhibits osteocytic activity, blocking calcium and phosphorus resorption from bone.
- Mitomycin acts like an alkylating agent, cross-linking strands of DNA. This causes an imbalance of cell growth, leading to cell death.
- Procarbazine inhibits DNA, RNA, and protein synthesis.

Absorption, distribution, metabolism, and excretion

- Procarbazine is well absorbed after oral administration. All the other drugs must be given parenterally.
- All are distributed to most body tissues and organs, especially the liver, spleen, kidneys, lungs, and heart.
- Mithramycin is the only drug that crosses the blood-brain barrier in significant amounts.
- The drugs are generally metabolized in the liver. Their inactive metabolites are eliminated in urine or through the bile in feces.

Onset and duration

Therapeutic activity varies with the drug, disease, and patient response.

Combination products

None.

ANTHRACYCLINE THERAPY: A PROGRESS REPORT

The presently available anthracyclines—doxorubicin and daunorubicin—effectively treat:

- acute leukemia
- Hodgkin's disease
- non-Hodgkin's lymphomas
- breast cancer
- sarcomas.

But, unfortunately, these drugs are corrosive when extravasated, and may present side effects such as:

- hematopoietic suppression
- nausea and vomiting
- alopecia
- and most important, *cardiomyopathy.*

Cardiomyopathy is the treatment-limiting toxicity associated with anthracycline therapy: The higher the total dose of anthracycline given, the greater the chance of toxicity. So the doctor has to choose between escalating the risk of cardiac toxicity and stopping this cancer therapy.

Recently, however, an effort has been made to seek out the ultimate anthracycline drug—one that works effectively with reduced side effects, particularly less cardiac toxicity. Although hundreds of anthracyclines have been developed, no currently approved anthracycline achieves the ideal. However, soon any one of the following investigational-use anthracyclines may be available for your patients:

DRUG	MAJOR USE	ADVANTAGES	ADVERSE REACTIONS	NURSING CONSIDERATIONS
aclacinomycin A	Acute leukemias	Less cardiac toxicity and mutagenicity than doxorubicin at equivalent dose levels	None reported	Greatest therapeutic potential of all the anthracyclines for your patient
carubicin	Soft-tissue sarcomas	Alopecia and extravasation problems are rare. No instances of cardiomyopathy.	Arrhythmias in 5% of patients	Well absorbed after oral or subcutaneous administration
zorubicin	Acute leukemias	Higher doses than daunorubicin possible without cardiac toxicity, but stronger therapeutic effect is questionable	Chills, fever, urticarial reactions	Use immediately after preparation

NAME	INDICATIONS & DOSAGE	SIDE EFFECTS
bleomycin sulfate Blenoxane♦	Dosage and indications may vary. Check patient's protocol with doctor. *Cervical, esophageal, head, neck, and testicular cancer—* **Adults:** 10 to 20 units/m² I.V., I.M., or S.C. 1 or 2 times weekly to total 300 to 400 units. *Hodgkin's disease*—10 to 20 units/m² I.V., I.M., or S.C. 1 or 2 times weekly. After 50% response, maintenance 1 unit I.M. or I.V. daily or 5 units I.M. or I.V. weekly. *Lymphomas*—first 2 doses should be 5 units or less, and patient should be monitored for any allergic reaction. If no reaction occurs, then follow above dosing schedule.	**CNS:** hyperesthesia of scalp and fingers, headache. **GI:** *stomatitis in 22% to 50% of patients, prolonged anorexia in 13% of patients, nausea, vomiting,* diarrhea. **Skin:** *erythema, vesiculation, and hardening and discoloration of palmar and plantar skin in 8% of patients;* desquamation of hands, feet, and pressure areas; *hyperpigmentation; acne.* **Other:** *alopecia,* swelling of interphalangeal joints, *pulmonary fibrosis in 10% of patients, pulmonary side effects (fine rales, fever, dyspnea), leukocytosis and nonproductive cough, allergic reaction (fever up to 106° F. [41.1° C.], with chills up to 5 hours after injection; anaphylaxis in 1% to 6% of patients).*
dactinomycin (actinomycin D) Cosmegen♦	Dosage and indications may vary. Check patient's protocol with doctor. *Melanomas, sarcomas, trophoblastic tumors in women, testicular cancer—* **Adults:** 500 mcg I.V. daily for 5 days; wait 2 to 4 weeks and repeat; or 2 mg I.V. single weekly dose for 3 weeks; wait for bone marrow recovery, then repeat in 3 to 4 weeks. *Wilms' tumor, rhabdomyosarcoma—* **Children:** 15 mcg/kg I.V. daily for 5 days. Maximum dose 500 mcg daily. Wait for marrow recovery.	**Blood:** anemia, *leukopenia, thrombocytopenia, pancytopenia.* **GI:** *anorexia, nausea, vomiting,* abdominal pain, diarrhea, *stomatitis.* **Skin:** *erythema;* desquamation; *hyperpigmentation of skin, especially in previously irradiated areas; acne-like eruptions (reversible).* **Local:** phlebitis, severe damage to soft tissue. **Other:** reversible alopecia.
daunorubicin hydrochloride Cerubidine♦	Dosage and indications may vary. Check patient's protocol. *Remission induction in acute nonlymphocytic leukemia (myelogenous, monocytic, erythroid) in adults—* **As a single agent:** 60 mg/m²/day I.V. on days 1, 2, 3 q 3 to 4 weeks. **In combination:** 45 mg/m²/day I.V. on days 1, 2, 3 of the first course and on days 1, 2 of subsequent courses with cytosine arabinoside infusions. *Note:* Dose should be reduced if hepatic function is impaired.	**Blood:** *bone marrow depression* (lowest blood counts 10 to 14 days after administration). **CV:** *cardiomyopathy (dose-related), EKG changes, arrhythmias,* pericarditis, myocarditis. **GI:** *nausea, vomiting, stomatitis, esophagitis,* anorexia, diarrhea. **Skin:** rash. **Local:** *severe cellulitis or tissue slough if drug extravasates.* **Other:** *generalized alopecia,* fever, chills.

♦ Available in U.S. and Canada. ♦♦ Available in Canada only. All other products (no symbol) available in U.S. only. Italicized side effects are common or life-threatening.

INTERACTIONS	NURSING CONSIDERATIONS
None significant.	• Use cautiously in renal or pulmonary impairment. • Drug concentrates in keratin of squamous epithelium. To prevent linear streaking, don't use adhesive dressings on skin. • Allergic reactions may be delayed for several hours, especially in lymphoma. • Monitor chest X-ray and listen to lungs. • Pulmonary function studies should be performed to establish baseline. Drug should be stopped if pulmonary function study shows a marked decline. • Pulmonary side effects common in patients over 70 years and in patients who receive a total dose of more than 400 mg. • Advise patient that alopecia may occur, but that it is usually reversible. • Refrigerated, reconstituted solution stable 4 weeks; at room temperature, stable 2 weeks. Solutions prepared in ampuls should be discarded if not used immediately. • Fatal pulmonary fibrosis occurs in 1% of patients, especially when cumulative dose exceeds 400 mg. • Bleomycin-induced fever is common and may be treated with antipyretics. • For treatment of anaphylaxis, see inside front cover.
None significant.	• Contraindicated in renal, hepatic, or bone marrow impairment; viral infection; or during chickenpox or herpes zoster infection. Use cautiously in metastatic testicular tumors, in combination with chlorambucil and methotrexate therapy. Extreme bone marrow and GI toxicity can occur with this combined therapy. • Stomatitis, diarrhea, leukopenia, thrombocytopenia may require stopping therapy. • Give antiemetic before administering to reduce nausea. • Monitor renal, hepatic functions. • Monitor CBCs daily and platelet counts every third day. • Observe for signs of bleeding. • Warn patient that alopecia may occur but is usually reversible. • Use only sterile water (without preservatives) as diluent for injection. • Administer through a running I.V. infusion. Avoid infiltration.
Heparin: don't mix. May form a precipitate.	• Use cautiously in myelosuppression, impaired cardiac function. • Stop drug immediately in signs of congestive heart failure or cardiomyopathy. Prevent by limiting cumulative dose to 550 mg/m²; 450 mg/m² when patient has been receiving radiation therapy that encompasses the heart or any other cardiotoxic agent. • Monitor EKG before treatment, monthly during therapy. • Note if resting pulse rate is high (a sign of cardiac side effects). • *Avoid extravasation;* inject into tubing of freely flowing I.V. *Never* give I.M. or subcutaneously. • Monitor CBC and hepatic function. • Warn patient urine may be red for 1 to 2 days and that it's a normal side effect, not hematuria. • Advise patient that alopecia may occur, but that it's usually reversible. • Don't use a scalp tourniquet or apply ice to prevent alopecia. May compromise effectiveness of drug. • Nausea and vomiting may be very severe and last 24 to 48 hours.

(continued on following page)

NAME	INDICATIONS & DOSAGE	SIDE EFFECTS
danunorubicin hydrochloride *(continued)*		
doxorubicin hydrochloride Adriamycin♦	Dosage and indications may vary. Check patient's protocol with doctor. *Bladder, breast, cervical, head, neck, liver, lung, ovarian, prostatic, stomach, testicular, and thyroid cancer; Hodgkin's disease; acute lymphoblastic and myeloblastic leukemia; Wilms' tumor; neuroblastomas; lymphomas; sarcomas—* **Adults:** 60 to 75 mg/m² I.V. as single dose q 3 weeks; or 30 mg/m² I.V. in single daily dose, days 1 to 3 of 4-week cycle. Maximum cumulative dose 550 mg/m².	**Blood:** *leukopenia, especially agranulocytosis, during days 10 to 15, with recovery by day 21; thrombocytopenia.* **CV:** *cardiac depression, seen in such EKG changes as sinus tachycardia, T-wave flattening, ST segment depression, voltage reduction; arrhythmias in 11% of patients; cardiomyopathy (sometimes with pulmonary edema) with mortality of 30% to 75%.* **GI:** *nausea, vomiting,* diarrhea, *stomatitis,* esophagitis. **GU:** red urine, enhancement of cyclophosphamide-induced bladder injury. **Skin:** *hyperpigmentation of skin, especially in previously irradiated areas.* **Local:** *severe cellulitis or tissue slough if drug extravasates.* **Other:** hyperpigmentation of nails and dermal creases, *complete alopecia within 3 to 4 weeks;* hair may regrow 2 to 5 months after drug is stopped.
mithramycin Mithracin	Dosage and indications may vary. Check patient's protocol with doctor. *Hypercalcemia—* **Adults:** 25 mcg/kg I.V. daily for 1 to 4 days. *Testicular cancer—* **Adults:** 25 to 30 mcg/kg I.V. daily for up to 8 to 10 days (based on ideal body weight or actual weight, whichever is less). I.V. infusions should be in 5% dextrose in water or 0.9% normal saline solution (1,000 ml over 4 to 6 hours).	**Blood:** *thrombocytopenia; bleeding syndrome, from epistaxis to generalized hemorrhage; facial flushing.* **GI:** *nausea, vomiting,* anorexia, diarrhea, stomatitis. **GU:** proteinuria; increased BUN, serum creatinine. **Metabolic:** *decreased serum calcium,* potassium, and phosphorus. **Skin:** periorbital pallor, usually the day before toxic symptoms occur. **Local:** extravasation causes irritation, cellulitis.

♦ Available in U.S. and Canada. ♦♦ Available in Canada only. All other products (no symbol) available in U.S. only. Italicized side effects are common or life-threatening.

INTERACTIONS	NURSING CONSIDERATIONS
	• Refrigerated, reconstituted solution stable for at least 36 hours; 24 hours at room temperature. Optimally, use within 8 hours of preparation. • Reddish color looks very similar to doxorubicin (Adriamycin). *Do not confuse the two drugs.*
None significant.	• Use cautiously in myelosuppression, impaired cardiac function. • Stop drug or slow rate of infusion if tachycardia develops. • Stop drug immediately in signs of congestive heart failure or cardiomyopathy. Prevent by limiting cumulative dose to 550 mg/m²; 450 mg/m² when patient is also receiving cyclophosphamide. • Monitor EKG before treatment, monthly during therapy. • Note if resting pulse is high: a signal of cardiac side effects. • *Avoid extravasation;* inject into tubing of freely flowing I.V. *Never* give I.M. or subcutaneously. • Monitor CBC and hepatic function. • Warn patient urine will be red for 1 to 2 days. • Dose should be reduced in hepatic dysfunction. • Warn patient that alopecia will occur. A scalp tourniquet or application of ice may decrease alopecia. However, *do not* use if treating leukemias or other neoplasms where tumor stem cells may be present in scalp. • Refrigerated, reconstituted solution stable 48 hours; at room temperature, stable 24 hours. • If cumulative dose exceeds 550 mg/m² body surface area, 30% of patients develop cardiac side effects, which begin 2 weeks to 6 months after stopping drug. • Decrease dose if serum bilirubin is increased: 50% dose when bilirubin is 1.2 to 3 mg/100 ml; 25% dose when bilirubin is greater than 3 mg/100 ml. • Esophagitis very common in patients who have also received radiation therapy. • Reddish color looks very similar to daunorubicin. *Do not confuse the two drugs.*
None significant.	• Contraindicated in thrombocytopenia and in coagulation and bleeding disorders. Use cautiously in renal, hepatic, or bone marrow impairment. • Slow infusion reduces nausea that develops with I.V. push. • Monitor LDH, SGOT, SGPT, alkaline phosphatase, BUN, creatinine, potassium, calcium, phosphorus. • Monitor platelet count and prothrombin time before and during therapy. • Observe for signs of bleeding. Facial flushing early indicator of bleeding. • Give antiemetic before administering to reduce nausea. • Avoid extravasation. If I.V. infiltrates, stop immediately; use ice packs. Restart I.V. • Avoid contact with skin or mucous membranes. • Therapeutic effect in hypercalcemia may not be seen for 24 to 48 hours; may last 3 to 15 days. • Precipitous drop in calcium possible. Monitor patient for tetany, carpopedal spasm, Chvostek's sign, muscle cramps; check serum calcium levels. • Store lyophilized powder in refrigerator. Remains stable after reconstitution for 24 hours; 48 hours in refrigerator.

NAME	INDICATIONS & DOSAGE	SIDE EFFECTS
mitomycin Mutamycin♦	Dosage and indications may vary. Check patient's protocol with doctor. *Breast, colon, head, neck, lung, pancreatic, and stomach cancer; malignant melanoma—* **Adults:** 2 mg/m² I.V. daily for 5 days. Stop drug for 2 days, then repeat dose for 5 more days; or 20 mg/m² as a single dose. Repeat cycle 6 to 8 weeks. Stop drug if WBC less than 4,000/mm³ or platelets less than 75,000/mm³.	**Blood:** *thrombocytopenia, leukopenia* (may be delayed up to 8 weeks). **CNS:** paresthesias. **GI:** nausea, vomiting, anorexia, stomatitis. **Local:** desquamation, induration, pruritus, *pain at site of injection.* Extravasation causes cellulitis, ulceration, sloughing. **Other:** *alopecia.*
procarbazine hydrochloride Matulane, Natulan♦♦	Dosage and indications may vary. Check patient's protocol with doctor. *Hodgkin's disease, lymphomas, brain and lung cancer—* **Adults:** 100 to 150 mg/m² P.O. for 10 days until WBC falls below 4,000/mm³ or platelets fall below 100,000/mm³. After bone marrow recovers, resume maintenance dose 50 to 100 mg P.O. daily. **Children:** 50 mg P.O. daily for first week, then 100 mg/m² until response or toxicity occurs. Maintenance dose is 50 mg P.O. daily after bone marrow recovery.	**Blood:** bleeding tendency, *leukopenia,* anemia. **CNS:** nervousness, depression, insomnia, nightmares, *hallucinations,* confusion. **EENT:** retinal hemorrhage, nystagmus, photophobia. **GI:** *nausea, vomiting, anorexia,* stomatitis, dry mouth, dysphagia, diarrhea, constipation. **Skin:** dermatitis. **Other:** alopecia, pleural effusion.

♦ Available in U.S. and Canada. ♦♦ Available in Canada only. All other products (no symbol) available in U.S. only. Italicized side effects are common or life-threatening.

INTERACTIONS	NURSING CONSIDERATIONS
None significant.	• Use cautiously when platelet count is less than 75,000/mm³, WBC is less than 4,000/mm³; in coagulation or bleeding disorders, serious infections, impaired renal function. • Continue CBC and blood studies at least 7 weeks after therapy is stopped. Observe for signs of bleeding. • Advise patient that alopecia may occur, but that it's usually reversible. • Reconstituted solution stable 1 week at room temperature, 2 weeks refrigerated.
Alcohol: disulfiram (Antabuse)-like reaction. Warn patient not to drink alcohol.	• Use cautiously in inadequate bone marrow reserve, leukopenia, thrombocytopenia, anemia, impaired hepatic or renal function. • Observe for signs of bleeding. • Warn patient that alopecia may occur. • Warn patient not to drink alcoholic beverages while taking this drug.

75 Antineoplastics altering hormone balance

dromostanolone propionate
megestrol acetate
mitotane
tamoxifen citrate
testolactone

For information on aminoglutethimide, see APPENDIX, *New Drugs*.

Synthetic sex hormones such as dromostanolone propionate, megestrol acetate, and testolactone counterbalance the tumor-stimulating effects of endogenous sex hormones. Tamoxifen citrate is not a synthetic hormone, but an estrogen antagonist. Mitotane, which is also not a hormone, is useful in managing cancer of the adrenal cortex.

These drugs are especially useful in treating cancer because they inhibit neoplastic growth in specific tissues without directly causing cytotoxicity.

Estrogens and androgens are also used as hormone manipulators in the treatment of cancer. (See Chapter 53, ANDROGENS AND ANABOLIC STEROIDS, and Chapter 55, ESTROGENS, for specific information.)

Major uses

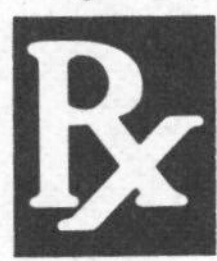

- Dromostanolone, tamoxifen, and testolactone are used as palliatives in postmenopausal metastatic breast cancer.
- Megestrol is a palliative in both breast and endometrial cancer.
- Mitotane is a palliative in inoperable adrenocortical carcinoma.

Mechanism of action

- Dromostanolone, megestrol, and testolactone change the tumor's hormonal environment and alter the neoplastic process.
- Mitotane selectively destroys adrenocortical tissue and hinders extra-adrenal metabolism of cortisol.
- Tamoxifen acts as an estrogen antagonist.

Absorption, distribution, metabolism, and excretion

Most of the drugs are well absorbed after oral administration and distributed widely in body tissues.

- Mitotane is partially absorbed when given orally (about 40%); dromostanolone must be given I.M.

All the drugs are metabolized in the liver and excreted in urine.

Onset and duration

Therapeutic activity varies with the drug, disease, and patient response.

Combination products

None.

HOW ESTROGEN ANTAGONISTS WORK

Estrogen antagonists, such as tamoxifen, bring about the death of estrogen-dependent tumors by preventing estrogen from nourishing tumor cells.

This occurs in two ways. First, through the process of competitive inhibition, tamoxifen binds with estrogen receptors in the cell cytoplasm, reducing the number of available receptors. Second, tamoxifen causes the estrogen that does enter the tumor cell nucleus to alter protein synthesis, thereby interfering with tumor cell division.

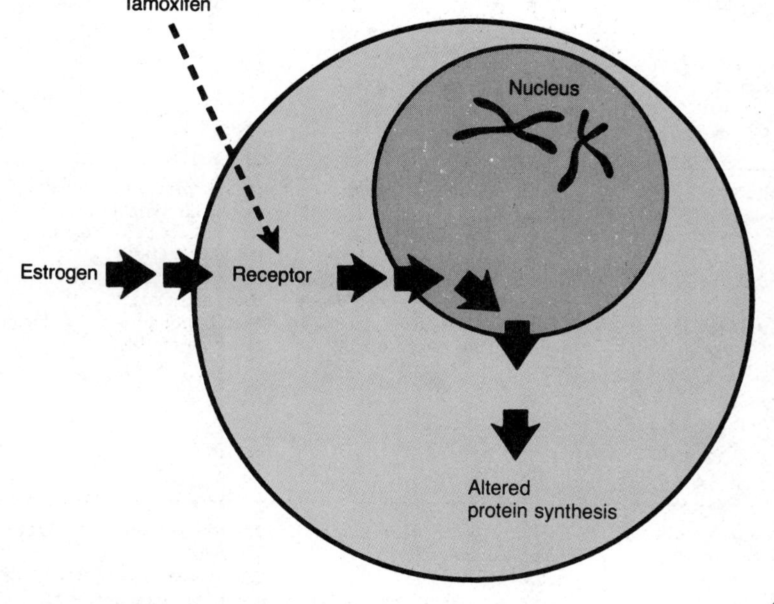

NAME	INDICATIONS & DOSAGE	SIDE EFFECTS
dromostanolone propionate Drolban	*Advanced, inoperable metastatic breast cancer, 1 to 5 years postmenopausal—* **Women:** 100 mg deep I.M. 3 times weekly.	**GU:** clitoral enlargement. **Metabolic:** hypercalcemia. **Skin:** acne. **Other:** *virilism (deepened voice, facial hair growth), which may be intense after long-term treatment;* edema, pain at injection site.
megestrol acetate Megace♦	*Breast cancer—* **Women:** 40 mg P.O. q.i.d. *Endometrial cancer—* **Women:** 40 to 320 mg P.O. daily in divided doses.	None reported.
mitotane Lysodren♦	*Inoperable adrenocortical cancer—* **Adults:** 9 to 10 g P.O. daily, divided t.i.d. to q.i.d. If severe side effects appear, reduce dose until maximum tolerated dose is achieved (varies from 2 to 16 g/day but is usually 8 to 10 g/day).	**CNS:** *depression, somnolence, vertigo;* brain damage and dysfunction in long-term, high-dose therapy. **GI:** *severe nausea, vomiting,* diarrhea, anorexia. **Metabolic:** adrenal insufficiency. **Skin:** dermatitis.
tamoxifen citrate Nolvadex♦	*Advanced premenopausal and postmenopausal breast cancer—* **Women:** 10 to 20 mg P.O. b.i.d.	**Blood:** transient fall in WBC or platelets. **GI:** nausea in 10% of patients, vomiting, anorexia. **GU:** vaginal discharge and bleeding. **Skin:** rash. **Other:** temporary bone or tumor pain, hot flashes in 7% of patients. Brief exacerbation of pain from osseous metastases.
testolactone Teslac♦	*Advanced postmenopausal breast cancer—* **Women:** 100 mg deep I.M. 3 times weekly; or 250 mg P.O. q.i.d.	**Local:** pain, inflammation at injection site. **Metabolic:** hypercalcemia.

♦ Available in U.S. and Canada. ♦♦ Available in Canada only. All other products (no symbol) available in U.S. only. Italicized side effects are common or life-threatening.

INTERACTIONS	NURSING CONSIDERATIONS
None significant.	• Contraindicated by any route other than I.M.; in male breast cancer and premenopausal women. Use cautiously in hepatic disease, cardiac decompensation, nephritis, nephrosis, and prostatic cancer. • If severe hypercalcemia develops or disease accelerates, drug should be stopped. • Therapeutic effect may be delayed 8 to 12 weeks. Reassure patient that results are not immediate. • Do not store in refrigerator; drug precipitates at cold temperatures. • Explain possible virilizing effects, skin and libido changes to female patients to prevent undue alarm.
None significant.	• Use cautiously in patients with history of thrombophlebitis. • Adequate trial is 2 months. Reassure patient that therapeutic response isn't immediate.
None significant.	• Use cautiously in hepatic disease. • Drug should be stopped if shock or trauma occurs. Use of corticosteroids may avoid acute adrenocorticoid insufficiency. • Assess and record behavioral and neurologic signs for baseline data daily throughout therapy. • Give antiemetic before administering to reduce nausea. • Dosage may be reduced if GI or skin side effects are severe. • Obese patients may need higher dosage and may have longer-lasting side effects, since drug distributes mostly to body fat. • Warn ambulatory patient of CNS side effects; advise him to avoid hazardous tasks requiring mental alertness or physical coordination. • Monitor effectiveness by reduction in pain, weakness, anorexia. • Adequate trial is at least 3 months, but therapy can continue if clinical benefits are observed.
None significant.	• Use cautiously in preexisting leukopenia, thrombocytopenia. • Use analgesic to relieve pain. • Monitor WBC and platelet counts. • Acts as an "antiestrogen." Best results in patients with positive estrogen receptors. • Side effects are usually minor and are well tolerated. • Reassure patient that acute exacerbation of bone pain during tamoxifen therapy usually indicates drug will produce good response.
None significant.	• Contraindicated in male breast cancer and not recommended in premenopausal females. • Adequate trial is 3 months. Reassure patient that therapeutic response isn't immediate. • Monitor fluids and electrolytes, especially calcium levels. • Immobilized patients are prone to hypercalcemia. Exercise may prevent it. Force fluids to aid calcium excretion. • Shake vial vigorously before drawing up injection. Do not refrigerate. • Use 1½" needle and inject into upper outer quadrant of gluteal region. Rotate injection sites. • No advantage over testosterone, except less virilization. • Higher than recommended doses do not increase incidence of remission.

76 Vinca alkaloids, podophyllin derivatives, and asparaginase

asparaginase (L-asparaginase)
etoposide (VP-16)
vinblastine sulfate
vincristine sulfate
vindesine sulfate
VM-26 (teniposide)

Vinblastine, vincristine, and vindesine are used as palliative treatment of various malignant neoplastic conditions. Closely related derivatives of the periwinkle plant, they are referred to as vinca alkaloids.

The podophyllin derivatives etoposide (VP-16) and VM-26 (teniposide) are used for the same purpose as the vinca alkaloids.

Asparaginase, derived from *Escherichia coli* and a number of other sources, is usually given in combination with other antineoplastic drugs.

Major uses

℞ All the drugs furnish supplemental or adjunctive therapy for acute lymphocytic leukemia.

• Podophyllin derivatives and vinca alkaloids are used as palliative therapy for lymphomas, leukemias, sarcomas, and some carcinomas.

Mechanism of action

• Asparaginase destroys the amino acid asparagine, which is needed for protein synthesis in acute lymphocytic leukemia. This leads to death of the leukemic cell.

• Podophyllin derivatives and vinca alkaloids all arrest metaphase in mitosis, blocking cell division.

BACKGROUND ON VINCA ALKALOIDS

The vinca alkaloids, commonly used in cancer treatment, are derived from the periwinkle *(Vinca rosea)*, a species of myrtle. The beneficial properties of the periwinkle have been described in folklore.

In 1949, an alleged activity as an oral hypoglycemic agent prompted research on crude extracts from the plant. Working with periwinkle extracts, in 1958, Noble and co-workers were unable to back up the claims for hypoglycemic activity in laboratory animals. They did, however, see granulocytopenia and bone marrow suppression in rats—effects that led to the extraction and purification of an active alkaloid, originally termed vincaleukoblastine. Other investigations by Johnson and associates supplemented this work.

A frequent side effect with vinca alkaloid usage is peripheral neuropathy, especially prevalent in fingers and hands. This side effect generally subsides several weeks after drug treatment is discontinued.

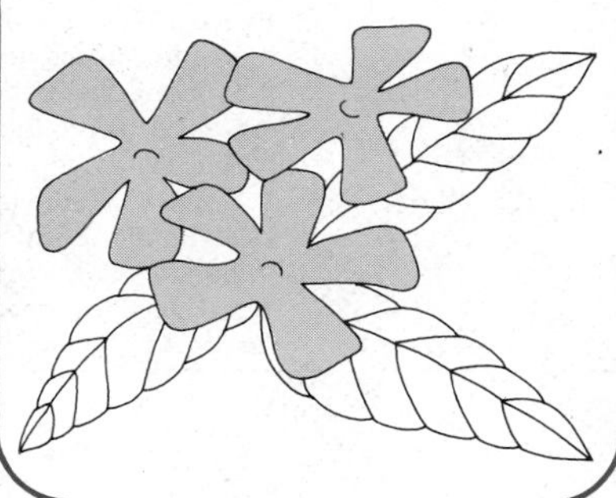

Absorption, distribution, metabolism, and excretion

- Although all the drugs are rapidly cleared from the blood and distributed in body tissues, they penetrate the blood-brain barrier poorly.
- Asparaginase is well absorbed after I.M. injection; it can also be administered I.V.

Its metabolism and route of excretion are unknown. Only trace amounts are excreted in urine.

- Podophyllin derivatives and vinca alkaloids are given I.V. only. They are extensively metabolized in the liver and eliminated both in urine and—through the bile—in feces.

Onset and duration

Therapeutic activity varies with the drug, disease, and patient response.

Combination products

None.

PRECAUTIONS

A DOUBLE-CHECK PAYS... AND SO DOES CAREFUL MONITORING

Naturally, you know to check the drug label to make sure it's what the doctor ordered; you'd do that with any medication. But with vinca alkaloids, you'd be wise to double-check or have another nurse double-check for you, since these drugs have similar names. Check the doctor's order sheet—not just a medication card—and be sure to check the dose too. Fatal mistakes can occur.

If the drug is to be administered I.V., also check the method: Some are given I.V. push; some are mixed with a specific amount of solution; some are administered only into an already established free-flowing I.V. infusion; and some are delivered by I.V. drip at a specified rate.

Monitor I.V. infusion carefully, since too rapid an infusion may produce severe toxic effects. *Some drugs—particularly vinblastine—cause severe local tissue damage if extravasation occurs.* If you see signs of this damage, stop the infusion and notify the doctor immediately; he may order treatment to help lessen local tissue damage.

NAME	INDICATIONS & DOSAGE	SIDE EFFECTS
asparaginase (or L-asparaginase) Elspar	*Acute lymphocytic leukemia (when used along with other drugs)*— **Adults and children:** 1,000 international units (IU)/kg I.V. daily for 10 days, injected over 30 minutes or by slow I.V. push; or 6,000 IU/m² I.M. at intervals specified in protocol. Sole induction agent—200 IU/kg I.V. daily for 28 days.	**Blood:** *hypofibrinogenemia* and depression of other clotting factors, thrombocytopenia, *leukopenia,* depression of serum albumin. **GI:** *vomiting (may last up to 24 hours), anorexia, nausea,* cramps, weight loss. **GU:** *azotemia,* renal failure, uric acid nephropathy, glycosuria, polyuria. **Hepatic:** elevated SGOT, SGPT; *hepatotoxicity.* **Metabolic:** elevated alkaline phosphatase and bilirubin (direct and indirect); increase or decrease in total lipids; *hyperglycemia; increased blood ammonia.* **Skin:** *rash, urticaria.* **Other:** *hemorrhagic pancreatitis, anaphylaxis (relatively common).*
etoposide (VP-16)	*Small cell carcinoma of the lung, acute nonlymphocytic leukemia, lymphosarcoma, Hodgkin's disease, testicular carcinoma*— **Adults:** 45 to 75 mg/m²/day I.V. for 3 to 5 days repeated q 3 to 5 weeks; or 200 to 250 mg/m² I.V. weekly; or 125 to 140 mg/m²/day I.V. 3 times a week q 5 weeks.	**Blood:** *myelosuppression (dose-limiting), leukopenia,* thrombocytopenia. **CV:** hypotension from rapid infusion. **GI:** nausea and vomiting. **Local:** infrequent phlebitis. **Other:** occasional headache and fever, *alopecia, anaphylaxis* (rare).
vinblastine sulfate (VLB) Velban, Velbe♦♦	*Breast or testicular cancer, generalized Hodgkin's disease, choriocarcinoma, lymphosarcoma,*	**Blood:** *leukopenia* (nadir days 4 to 10 and lasts another 7 to 14 days), *thrombocytopenia.*

♦ Available in U.S. and Canada. ♦♦ Available in Canada only. All other products (no symbol) available in U.S. only. Italicized side effects are common or life-threatening.

INTERACTIONS	NURSING CONSIDERATIONS
None significant.	• Contraindicated in pancreatitis, previous hypersensitivity unless desensitized. Use cautiously in preexisting hepatic dysfunction. • Should be administered in hospital setting with close supervision. • Don't use as sole agent to induce remission unless combination therapy is inappropriate. Not recommended for maintenance therapy. • Risk of hypersensitivity increases with repeated doses. Patient may be desensitized, but this doesn't rule out risk of allergic reactions. Routine administration of 2-unit I.V. test dose may identify high-risk patients. • Intravenous administration of asparaginase with or immediately before vincristine or prednisone may increase toxicity reactions. • Give I.V. injection over 30-minute period through a running infusion of sodium chloride injection or 5% dextrose injection. • For I.M. injection, limit dose at single injection site to 2 ml. • Due to vomiting, patient may need parenteral fluids for 24 hours or until oral fluids are tolerated. • Monitor blood count and bone marrow levels. Bone marrow regeneration may take 5 to 6 weeks. • Obtain frequent serum amylase determinations to check pancreatic status. If elevated, asparaginase should be discontinued. • Watch for uric acid nephropathy. Prevent occurrence by increasing fluid intake, alkalinization of urine. Allopurinol may be ordered. • Watch for signs of bleeding, such as petechiae and melena. • Monitor blood sugar and test urine for sugar before and during therapy. Watch for signs of hyperglycemia such as glycosuria, polyuria. • Reconstitute with 2 to 5 ml sterile water for injection or sodium chloride injection. • Don't shake vial. May cause loss of potency. Don't use cloudy solutions. • Refrigerate unopened dry powder. Reconstituted solution stable 6 hours at room temperature, 24 hours refrigerated. • Keep epinephrine, diphenhydramine, and I.V. corticosteroids available for treatment of anaphylaxis. • For treatment of anaphylaxis, see inside front cover.
None significant.	• Intraperitoneal, intrapleural, and intrathecal administration of this drug is contraindicated. • Give drug by slow I.V. infusion (over at least 30 minutes) to prevent severe hypotension. • Patients receiving drug over less than 2 hours should be in the recumbent position. • Blood pressure should be monitored before infusion and at 30-minute intervals during infusion. If systolic blood pressure falls below 90 mm Hg, infusion should be stopped and doctor notified. • Do *not* dilute in 5% dextrose in water due to physical incompatibility (precipitate will form). • Drug must be diluted to a concentration of 1 mg/ml or less with normal saline solution before giving. Discard cloudy solutions. • Solutions containing 1 mg/ml are stable for 30 minutes; 0.4 mg/ml, stable 3 hours; 0.2 mg/ml, stable 6 hours. • Have diphenhydramine, hydrocortisone, epinephrine, and airway available in case of an anaphylactic reaction. • Monitor CBC. Observe patient for signs of bone marrow depression. • An investigational drug. • For treatment of anaphylaxis, see inside front cover.
None significant.	• Contraindicated in severe leukopenia, bacterial infection. Use cautiously in jaundice or hepatic dysfunction. • Give antiemetic before administering to reduce nausea.

(continued on following page)

NAME	INDICATIONS & DOSAGE	SIDE EFFECTS
vinblastine sulfate *(continued)*	*neuroblastoma, mycosis fungoides, histiocytosis*— **Adults and children:** 0.1 mg/kg or 3.7 mg/m² I.V. weekly or q 2 weeks. May be increased to maximum dose (adults) of 0.5 mg/kg or 18.5 mg/m² I.V. weekly according to response. Dose should not be repeated if WBC less than 4,000/mm³.	**CNS:** depression, *paresthesias, peripheral neuropathy and neuritis, numbness, loss of deep tendon reflexes, muscle pain and weakness.* **EENT:** pharyngitis. **GI:** *nausea, vomiting, stomatitis,* ulcer and bleeding, *constipation, ileus, anorexia, weight loss,* abdominal pain. **GU:** oligospermia, aspermia, urinary retention. **Skin:** dermatitis, vesiculation. **Local:** *irritation, phlebitis,* cellulitis, necrosis if I.V. extravasates. **Other:** reversible alopecia in 5% to 10% of patients; *pain in tumor site,* low fever.
vincristine sulfate Oncovin♦	*Acute lymphoblastic and other leukemias, Hodgkin's disease, lymphosarcoma, reticulum cell sarcoma, neuroblastoma, rhabdomyosarcoma, Wilms' tumor, osteogenic and other sarcomas, lung and breast cancer*— **Adults:** 1 to 2 mg/m² I.V. weekly. **Children:** 1.5 to 2 mg/m² I.V. weekly. Maximum single dose (adults and children) is 2 mg.	**Blood:** rapidly reversible mild anemia and leukopenia. **CNS:** *peripheral neuropathy,* sensory loss, *deep tendon reflex loss, paresthesias, wrist and foot drop,* ataxia, cranial nerve palsies (headache, *jaw pain,* hoarseness, vocal cord paralysis, visual disturbances), *muscle weakness and cramps,* depression, agitation, insomnia; neurotoxicities may be permanent. **EENT:** diplopia, optic and extraocular neuropathy, ptosis. **GI:** *constipation, cramps,* ileus that mimics surgical abdomen, *nausea, vomiting,* anorexia, *stomatitis,* weight loss, dysphagia. **GU:** urinary retention. **Local:** *phlebitis,* cellulitis. **Other:** *reversible alopecia (up to 71% of patients).*
vindesine sulfate DAVA, Eldesine	*Acute lymphoblastic leukemia, breast cancer, malignant melanoma, lymphosarcoma, non-small cell lung carcinoma*— **Adults:** 3 to 4 mg/m² I.V. q 7 to 14 days, or continuous I.V. infusion 1.2 to 1.5 mg/m²/day for 5 days every 3 weeks.	**Blood:** *leukopenia, thrombocytopenia.* **CNS:** *paresthesias, decreased deep tendon reflex, muscle weakness.* **GI:** *constipation, abdominal cramping,* nausea, vomiting. **Local:** *phlebitis,* necrosis on extravasation. **Other:** *alopecia,* jaw pain, fever with continuous infusions.

INTERACTIONS	NURSING CONSIDERATIONS
	• Drug should be stopped if stomatitis occurs. • Give laxatives as needed. May use stool softeners prophylactically. • Don't repeat dose more frequently than every 7 days or severe leukopenia will develop. • Less neurotoxic than vincristine. • Should be injected directly into vein or tubing of running I.V. over 1 minute. May also be given in 50 ml dextrose in water or normal saline solution and infused over 15 minutes. If extravasation occurs, stop infusion. Apply ice packs on and off every 2 hours for 24 hours. • Warn patient that alopecia may occur but is usually reversible. • Adequate trial 12 weeks; reassure patient that therapeutic response isn't immediate. • Reconstitute 10-mg vial with 10 ml of sodium chloride injection or sterile water. This yields 1 mg/ml. • Refrigerate reconstituted solution. Discard after 30 days. • Don't confuse vinblastine with vincristine or the investigational agent vindesine.
None significant.	• Use cautiously in jaundice or hepatic dysfunction, neuromuscular disease, infection, or with other neurotoxic drugs. • Because of neurotoxicity, don't give drug more than once a week. Children more resistant to neurotoxicity than adults. • Should be given directly into vein or tubing of running I.V. slowly over 1 minute. May also be given in 50 ml dextrose in water or normal saline solution and infused over 15 minutes. If drug infiltrates, apply ice packs on and off every 2 hours for 24 hours. • Check for depression of Achilles tendon reflex, numbness, tingling, foot or wrist drop, difficulty in walking, ataxia, slapping gait. Also check ability to walk on heels. Support patient when walking. • Monitor bowel function. Give stool softener, laxative, or water before dosing. Constipation may be an early sign of neurotoxicity. • Reconstitute with sodium chloride injection, normal saline solution, or sterile water. • Refrigerate reconstituted solution. Discard after 14 days. • Warn patient that alopecia may occur but is usually reversible. • Be extremely careful about doses. Don't confuse vincristine with vinblastine or the investigational agent vindesine.
None significant.	• Do not give as a continuous infusion unless patient has a central I.V. line. • To prevent paralytic ileus, encourage patient to force fluids, increase ambulation, and use stool softeners. • Instruct patient to report any signs of neurotoxicity: numbness and tingling of extremities, jaw pain, constipation (may be early signs of neurotoxicity). • Assess for depression of Achilles tendon reflex, foot or wrist drop, slapping gait (late signs of neurotoxicity). • Neuropathy may be assessed by recording patient signatures before each course of therapy and observing for deterioration of handwriting. • Monitor CBC. • Avoid extravasation. Drug is a painful vesicant. Give 10 ml normal saline solution flush before drug to test vein patency, and 10 ml normal saline solution flush to remove any remaining drug from tubing after drug is given.

(continued on following page)

NAME	INDICATIONS & DOSAGE	SIDE EFFECTS
vindesine sulfate *(continued)*		
VM-26 (teniposide)	*Hodgkin's and non-Hodgkin's lymphomas, acute lymphocytic leukemia, bladder carcinoma*— **Adults:** 50 to 100 mg/m² I.V. once or twice weekly for 4 to 6 weeks, or 40 to 50 mg/m²/day I.V. for 5 days repeated every 3 to 4 weeks.	**Blood:** *myelosuppression (dose-limiting), leukopenia,* some thrombocytopenia. **CV:** hypotension from rapid infusion. **GI:** nausea and vomiting. **Local:** *phlebitis,* extravasation. **Other:** alopecia (rare), *anaphylaxis* (rare).

♦ Available in U.S. and Canada. ♦♦ Available in Canada only. All other products (no symbol) available in U.S. only. Italicized side effects are common or life-threatening.

INTERACTIONS	NURSING CONSIDERATIONS
	• When reconstituted with the 10 ml diluent provided or normal saline solution, the drug is stable for 2 weeks under refrigeration. • Do not mix vindesine with other drugs; compatibility with other drugs has not yet been determined. • An investigational drug.
None significant.	• May be diluted for infusion in either 5% dextrose in water or normal saline solution, but cloudy solutions should be discarded. • Infuse over 45 to 90 minutes to prevent hypotension. • Solutions containing 0.5 to 2 mg/ml are stable for 4 hours. Solutions containing 0.1 to 0.2 mg/ml are stable for 6 hours. • Blood pressure should be monitored before infusion and at 30-minute intervals during infusion. If systolic blood pressure falls below 90 mm Hg, infusion should be stopped and doctor notified. • Have diphenhydramine, hydrocortisone, epinephrine, and airway available in case of an anaphylactic reaction. • Monitor CBC. Observe patient for signs of bone marrow depression. • Avoid extravasation. • Drug may be given by local bladder instillation as a treatment for bladder cancer. • An investigational drug. • For treatment of anaphylaxis, see inside front cover.

DRUG ALERT

WATCH FOR VINCRISTINE NEUROTOXICITY

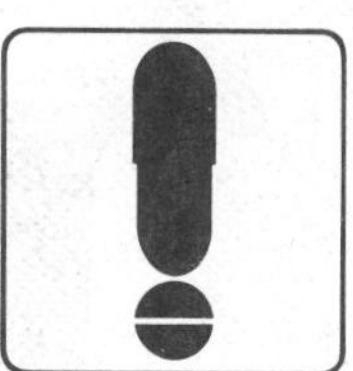

Vincristine causes neural damage, so have the patient on this drug report early symptoms of neural drug toxicity, such as constipation, tingling, numbness and tremors in his extremities.

A later effect of neurotoxicity is loss of deep tendon reflexes. Check the patient's reflexes regularly, especially the Achilles tendon. By the time the patient has difficulty heel-walking or rising from chairs, the damage is severe.

Although the drug may be discontinued, side effects can persist up to 2 years. Some effects may be permanent.

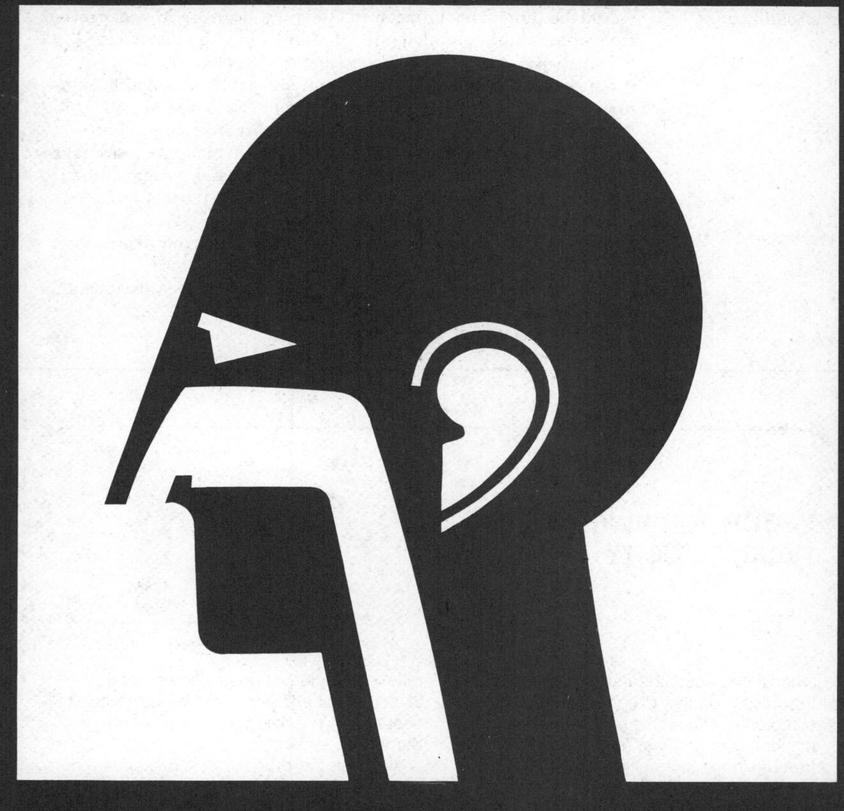

XII Eye, Ear, Nose, and Throat Drugs

Ophthalmic anti-infectives

bacitracin
benzalkonium chloride
boric acid
chloramphenicol
chlortetracycline hydrochloride
erythromycin
gentamicin sulfate
idoxuridine (IDU)
natamycin
neomycin sulfate
polymyxin B sulfate
silver nitrate 1%
sulfacetamide sodium
tetracycline hydrochloride
trifluridine
vidarabine

For information on tobramycin ophthalmic, see APPENDIX, *New Drugs.*

Ophthalmic anti-infectives have antibacterial, antiviral, or antifungal activity. Most are antibiotics, but others, such as boric acid and benzalkonium chloride, are not. Although sulfacetamide sodium belongs to this group, other antibiotics have largely replaced it, except for use in minor infections. Idoxuridine, trifluridine, and vidarabine are specific antiviral agents.

These agents are available as solutions, suspensions, or ointments.

Major uses

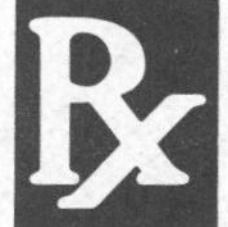

• Bacitracin, chloramphenicol, chlortetracycline, erythromycin, gentamicin, neomycin, polymyxin B, sulfacetamide, and tetracycline are used to treat surface infections of the conjunctiva or cornea caused by such microorganisms as *Chlamydia trachomatis, Pseudomonas,* and *Staphylococcus.*

• Benzalkonium chloride is a weak bactericide used as a wetting solution and a preservative; it also facilitates transcorneal penetration of other ophthalmic drugs.

• Boric acid is a bacteriostatic and fungistatic irrigating solution.

• Idoxuridine, trifluridine, and vidarabine are used to treat acute keratoconjunctivitis or recurrent epithelial keratitis caused by herpes simplex types I and II.

• Natamycin is used to treat ophthalmic fungal infections.

• Silver nitrate is used to prevent gonorrheal ophthalmia neonatorum.

Mechanism of action

• Bacitracin, chloramphenicol, erythromycin, gentamicin, neomycin, polymyxin B, and the tetracyclines inhibit protein synthesis in susceptible microorganisms.

• Benzalkonium chloride increases corneal permeability, enabling greater penetration of other drugs.

• Boric acid's mechanism of action is unknown.

• Idoxuridine, trifluridine, and vidarabine interfere with DNA synthesis.

• Natamycin increases fungal cell-membrane permeability.

• Silver nitrate causes protein denaturation, which prevents gonorrheal ophthalmia neonatorum.

• Sulfacetamide prevents uptake of

para-aminobenzoic acid, a metabolite of bacterial folic-acid synthesis.

Absorption, distribution, metabolism, and excretion

Bacitracin, chloramphenicol, and neomycin penetrate the cornea and conjunctiva, and are excreted by the nasolacrimal system.

- Benzalkonium chloride and silver nitrate do not penetrate intraocularly.
- Boric acid and idoxuridine are poorly absorbed topically.
- Chloramphenicol penetrates the aqueous humor; both chloramphenicol and gentamicin are excreted through the nasolacrimal system.
- Erythromycin, gentamicin, polymyxin B, and the tetracyclines penetrate poorly through an intact cornea but well through corneal abrasions.
- Natamycin does not reach measurable levels in deeper corneal layers unless there's a defect in the epithelium.
- Sulfacetamide's intraocular penetration varies.
- Trifluridine and vidarabine are found in trace amounts in the aqueous humor after topical application to a cornea with an epithelial defect or inflammation, but neither drug is significantly absorbed systemically.

Onset and duration

As a rule, ophthalmic anti-infectives are administered often—sometimes as frequently as every 2 hours. Onset and duration vary according to the condition and patient response.

Combination products

BLEPHAMIDE LIQUIFILM SUSPENSION: sodium sulfacetamide 10%, prednisolone acetate 0.2%, and phenylephrine hydrochloride 0.12%.

BPN OPHTHALMIC OINTMENT: bacitracin 500 units, polymyxin B sulfate 5,000 units, and neomycin sulfate 5 mg per g.

CETAPRED OINTMENT♦: sodium sulfacetamide 10% and prednisolone acetate 0.25%.

CHLOROMYCETIN HYDROCORTISONE OPHTHALMIC♦: chloramphenicol 1.25% and hydrocortisone acetate 2.5%.

CHLOROMYXIN OPHTHALMIC♦: chloramphenicol 10 mg and polymyxin B sulfate 5,000 units.

CHLOROPTIC-P S.O.P.: chloramphenicol 1% and prednisolone alcohol 0.5%.

CORTISPORIN OPHTHALMIC OINTMENT♦: polymyxin B sulfate 5,000 units, bacitracin zinc 400 units, neomycin sulfate 0.5%, and hydrocortisone 1%.

CORTISPORIN OPHTHALMIC SUSPENSION♦: polymyxin B sulfate 10,000 units, neomycin sulfate 0.5%, and hydrocortisone 1%.

ISOPTO CETAPRED SUSPENSION♦: sulfacetamide 10% and prednisolone acetate 0.25%.

MAXITROL OPHTHALMIC OINTMENT/SUSPENSION♦: dexamethasone 0.1%, neomycin sulfate 3.5 mg, and polymyxin B sulfate 6,000 units.

METIMYD OPHTHALMIC OINTMENT/SUSPENSION: sodium sulfacetamide 10% and prednisolone acetate 0.5%.

MYCITRACIN OPHTHALMIC: polymyxin B sulfate 5,000 units, neomycin sulfate 5 mg, and bacitracin 500 units.

NEO-CORTEF OPHTHALMIC♦: hydrocortisone 0.5% or 1.5% and neomycin sulfate 0.5%.

NEODECADRON OPHTHALMIC OINTMENT: dexamethasone phosphate 0.5% and neomycin sulfate 0.5%.

NEO-MEDROL OINTMENT: methylprednisolone 0.1% and neomycin sulfate 0.5%.

NEOSPORIN OPHTHALMIC OINTMENT♦: polymyxin B sulfate 5,000 units, neomycin sulfate 5 mg, and bacitracin zinc 100 units per g.

POLYSPORIN OPHTHALMIC OINTMENT: neomycin sulfate 5 mg, polymyxin B sulfate 10,000 units, and bacitracin zinc 500 units.

VASOCIDIN OINTMENT: sodium sulfacetamide 10%, prednisolone acetate 0.2%, and phenylephrine HCl 0.125%.

VASOCIDIN SOLUTION♦: sodium sulfacetamide 10%, prednisolone phosphate 0.2%, and phenylephrine HCl 0.125%.

VASOSULF SOLUTION♦: sodium sulfacetamide 15% and phenylephrine HCl 0.125%.

NAME	INDICATIONS & DOSAGE	SIDE EFFECTS
bacitracin Baciguent Ophthalmic Ointment♦	*Ocular infections*— **Adults and children:** apply small amount into conjunctival sac several times a day or p.r.n. until favorable response is observed.	**Eye:** slowed corneal wound healing, temporary visual haze. **Other:** overgrowth of nonsusceptible organisms.
benzalkonium chloride Spensomide, Zephiran♦	*To increase transcorneal penetration of drugs*— **Adults and children:** 1:5,000 to 1:2,000 concentration used in some irrigating solutions for its antiseptic as well as its surface-active qualities. *To sterilize ophthalmic solutions:* use 1:5,000 concentration. An ingredient in germicidal cleaning solutions for contact lens.	**Eye:** toxic to abraded cornea and to endothelial cells of cornea if introduced into anterior chamber.
boric acid Blinx, Collyrium, Neo-Flo	*For irrigation following tonometry, gonioscopy, foreign body removal, or use of fluorescein; used to soothe and cleanse the eye; used in conjunction with contact lens*— **Adults:** irrigate eye with 2% solution or apply 5% or 10% ointment, p.r.n.	Note: toxic if absorbed from abraded skin areas, granulating wounds, or ingestion.
chloramphenicol Antibiopto, Chloromycetin Ophthalmic♦, Chloroptic Ophthalmic♦, Chloroptic S.O.P.,	*Surface bacterial infection involving conjunctiva or cornea*— **Adults and children:** instill 2 drops of solution in eye q 1 hour until condition improves, or instill q.i.d., depending on severity of infection. Apply	Note: systemic adverse reactions have not been reported with short-term topical use. **Blood:** *bone marrow hypoplasia with prolonged use.* **Eye:** optic atrophy in children, stinging or burning of eye after

♦ Available in U.S. and Canada. ♦♦ Available in Canada only. All other products (no symbol) available in U.S. only. Italicized side effects are common or life-threatening.

INTERACTIONS	NURSING CONSIDERATIONS
Heavy metals (silver nitrate): inactivate bacitracin. Don't use together.	• Use cautiously in patients with hereditary predisposition to antibiotic hypersensitivity. • Warn patient to avoid sharing washcloths and towels with family members. • Always wash hands before and after applying ointment. • Cleanse eye area of excessive exudate before application. • Tell patient to watch for signs of sensitivity, such as itching lids or constant burning. Patient who develops such signs should stop drug and notify doctor immediately. • Show patient how to apply. Stress importance of compliance with recommended therapy. • Warn patient not to touch tip of tube to any part of eye or surrounding tissue. • Solution not commercially available but may be prepared by pharmacy. May be stored up to 3 weeks in refrigerator. • Bactericidal or bacteriostatic, depending on concentration and infection. • Store in tightly closed, light-resistant container. • Tell patient not to share eye medications with family members. If a family member develops the same symptoms, instruct him to contact the doctor.
Fluorescein: destroys benzalkonium chloride antibacterial activity. May cause corneal staining. Don't use together. *Sulfonamides (ophthalmic):* incompatible. Don't apply at same time.	• Never prepare a straight benzalkonium chloride solution for use in eye. • Warn patient to avoid sharing washcloths and towels with family members. • Don't use concentrations greater than 1:5,000 in the eye; may be irritating. • Tell patient to watch for signs of sensitivity, such as itching lids or constant burning. If he develops such signs, patient should stop drug and notify doctor immediately. • Warn patient not to touch applicator to eye or surrounding tissue. • Always wash hands before and after applying drug. • Cleanse eye area of excessive exudate before application. • Present in most combination topical eye preparations commercially available. • Tell patient not to share eye medications with family members. If a family member develops the same symptoms, instruct him to contact the doctor.
Polyvinyl alcohol (Liquifilm): may form insoluble complex. Check with pharmacy on contents in eye drugs and contact lens wetting solutions.	• Contraindicated in eye abrasions. • Don't apply to abraded cornea or skin. • Lethal dose is 5 to 6 g in infants and 15 to 20 g in adults. • Always wash hands before and after instilling solution or ointment. • Not for use with soft contact lenses. • Weak bacteriostatic, fungistatic agent. • Tell patient not to share eye medications with family members. If a family member develops the same symptoms, instruct him to contact the doctor.
None significant.	• Not for long-term use. Notify doctor if no improvement in 3 days. • If patient has more than a superficial infection, systemic therapy should also be used. • Bacteriostatic. • One of the safest topical ocular antibiotics, especially for endophthalmitis. • Warn patient to avoid sharing washcloths and towels with family

(continued on following page)

NAME	INDICATIONS & DOSAGE	SIDE EFFECTS
chloramphenicol *(continued)* Econochlor Ophthalmic, Fenicol♦♦, Isopto Fenicol♦♦, Nova-Phenicol♦♦, Ophthoclor Ophthalmic, Pentamycetin♦♦	small amount of ointment to lower conjunctival sac at bedtime as supplement to drops. May use ointment alone by applying a small amount of ointment to lower conjunctival sac q 3 to 6 hours or more often, if necessary. Continue until condition improves.	instillation. **Other:** overgrowth of nonsusceptible organisms; hypersensitivity, including itching and burning eye, dermatitis, angioedema.
chlortetracycline hydrochloride Aureomycin Ophthalmic	*Superficial ocular infection—* **Adults and children:** apply 1% ointment to eye q 2 hours or more, p.r.n.	**Eye:** itching and burning. **Other:** overgrowth of nonsusceptible organisms with long-term use, dermatitis.
erythromycin Ilotycin Ophthalmic♦	*Acute and chronic conjunctivitis, other eye infections—* **Adults and children:** apply 0.5% ointment 1 or more times daily, depending upon severity of infection.	**Eye:** slowed corneal wound healing. **Other:** overgrowth of nonsusceptible organisms with long-term use; hypersensitivity, including itchy and burning eye, urticaria, dermatitis, angioedema.

♦ Available in U.S. and Canada. ♦♦ Available in Canada only. All other products (no symbol) available in U.S. only. Italicized side effects are common or life-threatening.

INTERACTIONS	NURSING CONSIDERATIONS
	members. • Always wash hands before and after applying ointment or solution. • Cleanse eye area of excessive exudate before application. • Tell patient to watch for signs of sensitivity, such as itching lids or constant burning. Patient who develops such signs should stop drug and notify doctor immediately. • Show patient how to instill. Stress importance of compliance with recommended therapy. • Warn patient not to touch tip of applicator to eye or surrounding tissue. • If chloramphenicol drops are to be given q 1 hour, then tapered, follow order closely to ensure adequate anterior chamber levels. • Store in tightly closed, light-resistant container. • Tell patient not to share eye medications with family members. If a family member develops the same symptoms, instruct him to contact the doctor.
None significant.	• Contraindicated in tetracycline hypersensitivity. • *Pseudomonas, Proteus,* and *Staphylococcus* resistant to drug. Used mainly for trachoma in conjunction with oral therapy. Trachoma treatment may continue 2 months or more. Trachoma may cause blindness if untreated or if treated improperly. • Warn patient to avoid sharing washcloths and towels with family members. • Always wash hands before and after applying ointment. • Cleanse eye area of excessive exudate before application. • Tell patient to watch for signs of sensitivity, such as itching lids or constant burning. Patient who develops such signs should stop drug and notify doctor immediately. • Show patient how to instill. Stress importance of compliance with recommended therapy. • Warn patient not to touch tip of tube to eye or surrounding tissue. • Bacteriostatic. • Store in tightly closed, light-resistant container. • Tell patient not to share eye medications with family members. If a family member develops the same symptoms, instruct him to contact the doctor.
None significant.	• Bacteriostatic but may be bactericidal in high concentrations or against highly susceptible organisms. • Has a limited antibacterial spectrum. Use only when sensitivity studies show it is effective against infecting organisms. Don't use in infections of unknown etiology. • Warn patient to avoid sharing washcloths and towels with family members. • Always wash hands before and after applying ointment. • Cleanse eye area of excessive exudate before application. • Tell patient to watch for signs of sensitivity, such as itching lids or constant burning. Patient who develops such signs should stop drug and notify doctor immediately. • Show patient how to apply. Stress importance of compliance with recommended therapy. • Warn patient not to touch tube to eye or surrounding tissue. • Store at room temperature in tightly closed, light-resistant container. • Tell patient not to share eye medications with family members. If a family member develops the same symptoms, instruct him to contact the doctor.

NAME	INDICATIONS & DOSAGE	SIDE EFFECTS
gentamicin sulfate Garamycin Ophthalmic♦, Genoptic	*External ocular infections (conjunctivitis, keratoconjunctivitis, corneal ulcers, blepharitis, blepharoconjunctivitis, meibomianitis, and dacryocystitis) due to susceptible organisms, especially* Pseudomonas aeruginosa, Proteus *sp,* Klebsiella pneumoniae, Escherichia coli— **Adults and children:** instill 1 to 2 drops in eye q 4 hours. In severe infections, may use up to 2 drops q 1 hour. Apply ointment to lower conjunctival sac b.i.d. to t.i.d.	Note: systemic absorption from excessive use may cause systemic toxicities. **Eye:** burning or stinging with ointment, transient irritation from solution. **Other:** hypersensitivity, overgrowth of nonsusceptible organisms with long-term use.
idoxuridine (IDU) Dendrid, Herplex, Stoxil♦	*Herpes simplex keratitis*— **Adults and children:** instill 1 drop of solution into conjunctival sac q 1 hour during day and q 2 hours at night, or apply ointment to conjunctival sac q 4 hours or 5 times daily, with last dose at bedtime. A response should be seen in 7 days; if not, discontinue and begin alternate therapy. Therapy should not be continued longer than 21 days.	**Eye:** temporary visual haze; irritation, pain, burning, or inflammation of eye; mild edema of eyelid or cornea; photosensitivity; small punctate defects in corneal epithelium; slowed corneal wound healing with ointment. **Other:** hypersensitivity.
natamycin Natacyn	*Treatment of fungal keratitis*— **Adults:** initial dosage 1 drop instilled in conjunctival sac q 1 to 2 hours. After 3 to 4 days, reduce dosage to 1 drop 6 to 8 times daily.	**Eye:** ocular edema, hyperemia.

♦ Available in U.S. and Canada. ♦♦ Available in Canada only. All other products (no symbol) available in U.S. only. Italicized side effects are common or life-threatening.

INTERACTIONS	NURSING CONSIDERATIONS
None significant.	• Contraindicated in aminoglycoside hypersensitivity. Use cautiously in impaired renal function. • Have culture taken before giving drug. • Stress importance of following recommended therapy. *Pseudomonas* infections can cause complete vision loss within 24 hours if infection is not controlled. • Warn patient to avoid sharing washcloths and towels with family members. • Always wash hands before and after applying ointment or solution. • Cleanse eye area of excessive exudate before application. • Tell patient to watch for signs of sensitivity, such as itching lids or constant burning. Patient who develops such signs should stop drug and notify doctor immediately. • Show patient how to instill. • Warn patient not to touch tip of tube or dropper to eye or surrounding tissue. • Store away from heat. • Tell patient not to share eye medications with family members. If a family member develops the same symptoms, instruct him to contact the doctor.
None significant.	• Contraindicated in deep ulceration. • Not for long-term use. • Idoxuridine should not be mixed with other medications. • Don't use old solution; causes ocular burning and has no antiviral activity. • Warn patient to avoid sharing washcloths and towels with family members. • Always wash hands before and after applying ointment or solution. • Cleanse eye area of excessive exudate before application. • Tell patient to watch for signs of sensitivity, such as itching lids or constant burning. Patient who develops such signs should stop drug and notify doctor immediately. • Show patient how to apply. Stress importance of compliance with recommended therapy. • Warn patient not to touch tip of tube or dropper to eye or surrounding tissue. • Refrigerate idoxuridine 0.1% solution. Store in tightly closed, light-resistant container. • Tell patient not to share eye medications with family members. If a family member develops the same symptoms, instruct him to contact the doctor.
None significant.	• Only antifungal available as ophthalmic preparation. • Treatment of choice for fungal keratitis. May also be used to treat fungal blepharitis and conjunctivitis. • Therapy should be continued for 14 to 21 days, or until active disease subsides. • Reduce dosage gradually at 4- to 7-day intervals to assure that organism has been eliminated. • If infection does not improve with 7 to 10 days of therapy, clinical and laboratory reevaluation is recommended. • Warn patient to avoid sharing washcloths and towels with family members. • Always wash hands before and after applying. • Cleanse eye area of excessive exudate before application. • Show patient how to apply. Stress importance of compliance with recommended therapy.

(continued on following page)

NAME	INDICATIONS & DOSAGE	SIDE EFFECTS
natamycin *(continued)*		
neomycin sulfate Myciguent Ophthalmic	*Used alone or in combination with other antibiotics in treating superficial ocular infections involving conjunctiva or cornea—* **Adults and children:** apply ointment to lower conjunctival sac daily to t.i.d.	**Other:** hypersensitivity reactions (itching and burning eye, erythema, dermatitis, urticaria); after long-term use, overgrowth of nonsusceptible organisms.
polymyxin B sulfate Aerosporin♦	*Used alone or in combination with other agents for treating corneal ulcers resulting from* Pseudomonas *infection or other gram-negative organism infections—* **Adults and children:** instill 1 to 3 drops of 0.1% to 0.25% (10,000 to 25,000 units per ml) q 1 hour. Increase interval according to patient response; or up to 10,000 units subconjunctivally daily by doctor.	**Eye:** eye irritation, conjunctivitis. **Other:** overgrowth of nonsusceptible organisms, hypersensitivity (local burning, itching).
silver nitrate 1%	*Prevention of gonorrheal ophthalmia neonatorum—* **Neonates:** cleanse lids thoroughly; instill 1 drop of 1% solution into each eye.	**Eye:** periorbital edema, temporary staining of lids and surrounding tissue, conjunctivitis (with concentrations greater than 1%).

INTERACTIONS	NURSING CONSIDERATIONS
	• Warn patient not to touch tip of dropper to eye or surrounding tissue. • Tell patient not to share eye medications with family members. If a family member develops the same symptoms, instruct him to contact the doctor.
None significant.	• Contraindicated in aminoglycoside hypersensitivity. • Effective against gram-positive and gram-negative organisms. • Warn patient to avoid sharing washcloths and towels with family members. • Always wash hands before and after applying ointment. • Cleanse eye area of excessive exudate before application. • Tell patient to watch for signs of sensitivity, such as itching lids or constant burning. Patient who develops such signs should stop drug and notify doctor immediately. • Show patient how to apply. Stress importance of compliance with recommended therapy. • Warn patient not to touch tip of tube to eye or surrounding tissue. • Bactericidal. • Tell patient not to share eye medications with family members. If a family member develops the same symptoms, instruct him to contact the doctor.
None significant.	• One of the most effective antibiotics against gram-negative organisms, especially *Pseudomonas*. • Often used in combination with neomycin sulfate. • Warn patient to avoid sharing washcloths and towels with family members. • Always wash hands before and after instilling solution. • Cleanse eye area of excessive exudate before application. • Tell patient to watch for signs of sensitivity, such as itching lids and lashes or constant burning. Patient who develops such signs should stop drug and notify doctor immediately. • Show patient how to instill. Stress importance of compliance with recommended therapy. • Warn patient not to touch tip of dropper to eye or surrounding tissue. • Bactericidal. • Not commercially available. Polymyxin B sulfate powder must be reconstituted with sterile water for injection or normal saline solution. Refrigerated solutions stable for 6 months. • Reconstitute carefully to ensure correct drug concentration in solution. • Tell patient not to share eye medications with family members. If a family member develops the same symptoms, instruct him to contact the doctor.
Bacitracin: inactivates silver nitrate. Don't use together.	• Legally required for neonates in most states. • Don't use repeatedly. • If 2% solution is accidentally used in eye, prompt irrigation with isotonic sodium chloride is advised to prevent eye irritation. • May delay instillation slightly to allow neonate to bond with mother. • Always wash hands before instilling solution. • Store wax ampuls away from light and heat. • Bacteriostatic, germicidal, and astringent. • Don't irrigate eyes after instillation.

NAME	INDICATIONS & DOSAGE	SIDE EFFECTS
sulfacetamide sodium 10% Bleph-10 Liquifilm Ophthalmic♦, Cetamide Ophthalmic♦, 10% Sodium Sulamyd Ophthalmic, Sulf-10 Ophthalmic♦ **sulfacetamide sodium 15%** Isopto Cetamide Ophthalmic♦, Sulfacel-15 Ophthalmic **sulfacetamide sodium 30%** Sodium Sulamyd 30% Ophthalmic♦	*Inclusion conjunctivitis, corneal ulcers, trachoma, prophylaxis to ocular infection*— **Adults and children:** instill 1 to 2 drops of 10% solution into lower conjunctival sac q 2 to 3 hours during day, less often at night; or instill 1 to 2 drops of 15% solution into lower conjunctival sac q 1 to 2 hours initially, increasing interval as condition responds; or instill 1 drop of 30% solution into lower conjunctival sac q 2 hours. Instill ½ to 1 inch of 10% ointment into conjunctival sac q.i.d. and at bedtime. May use ointment at night along with drops during the day.	**Eye:** slowed corneal wound healing (ointment), pain on instilling eye drop. **Other:** hypersensitivity (including itching or burning), overgrowth of nonsusceptible organisms.
tetracycline hydrochloride Achromycin Ophthalmic♦	**Adults and children:** *Superficial ocular infections and inclusion conjunctivitis*— instill 1 to 2 drops in eye b.i.d., q.i.d., or more often, depending on severity of infection. *Trachoma*—instill 2 drops in each eye b.i.d., t.i.d., or q.i.d. Continue for 1 to 2 months or longer, or use 1% ointment t.i.d. to q.i.d. for 30 days.	**Eye:** itching. **Other:** hypersensitivity (eye itching and dermatitis), overgrowth of nonsusceptible organisms with long-term use.
trifluridine Viroptic Ophthalmic Solution 1%	*Primary keratoconjunctivitis and recurrent epithelial keratitis due to herpes simplex virus, types 1 and 2*— **Adults** 1 drop of solution q 2 hours while patient is awake, to a maximum of 9 drops daily until re-epithelialization of the corneal ulcer occurs; then 1 drop q 4 hours (minimum	**Eye:** stinging upon instillation, edema of eyelids.

♦ Available in U.S. and Canada. ♦♦ Available in Canada only. All other products (no symbol) available in U.S. only. Italicized side effects are common or life-threatening.

INTERACTIONS	NURSING CONSIDERATIONS
Local anesthetics (procaine, tetracaine), p-aminobenzoic acid derivatives: decreased sulfacetamide sodium action. Wait ½ to 1 hour after instilling anesthetic or *p*-aminobenzoic acid derivative before instilling sulfacetamide.	• Contraindicated in sulfonamide hypersensitivity. • Often used with systemic tetracycline in treating trachoma and inclusion conjunctivitis. • Replaced by antibiotics in treating major ocular infections; still used in minor ocular infections. • Purulent exudate interferes with sulfacetamide action. Remove as much exudate as possible from lids before instilling sulfacetamide. • Incompatible with silver preparations. • Warn patient eye drop is painful. • Warn patient to avoid sharing washcloths and towels with family members. • Always wash hands before and after applying ointment or solution. • Tell patient to watch for signs of sensitivity, such as itching lids or constant burning. Patient who develops such signs should stop drug and notify doctor immediately. • Show patient how to instill. Stress importance of compliance with recommended therapy. • Warn patient not to touch tip of tube or dropper to eye or surrounding tissue. • Store in tightly closed, light-resistant container away from heat. • Don't use discolored (dark brown) solution. • Tell patient not to share eye medications with family members. If a family member develops the same symptoms, instruct him to contact the doctor.
None significant.	• Tell patient or family that trachoma therapy should continue for 1 to 2 months or longer. Trachoma may cause blindness if left untreated or if not treated properly. • Tell patient that gnats and flies are vectors of the trachoma organism. Warn patient with trachoma not to let them settle around eye area. Also explain that infection is spread by direct contact, so handwashing is essential to prevent spread. • Warn patient to avoid sharing washcloths and towels with family members. • Always wash hands before and after applying solution. • Cleanse eye area of excessive exudate before application. • Tell patient to watch for signs of sensitivity, such as itching lids or constant burning. Patient who develops such signs should stop drug and notify doctor immediately. • Show patient how to instill. Stress importance of compliance with recommended therapy. • Warn patient not to touch tip of dropper to eye or surrounding tissue. • Store in tightly closed, light-resistant container. • Tell patient not to share eye medications with family members. If a family member develops the same symptoms, instruct him to contact the doctor.
None significant.	• Should be prescribed only for those patients with clinical diagnosis of herpetic keratitis. • Consider another form of therapy if improvement doesn't occur after 7 days' treatment or complete re-epithelialization after 14 days' treatment. Trifluridine shouldn't be used more than 21 days continuously due to potential ocular toxicity. • Reassure patient that mild local irritation of the conjunctiva and cornea that occurs when solution is instilled is usually temporary. • Drug should be refrigerated. • More effective drug than vidarabine with fewer side effects.

(continued on following page)

NAME	INDICATIONS & DOSAGE	SIDE EFFECTS
trifluridine *(continued)*	5 drops daily) for an additional 7 days.	
vidarabine Vira-A Ophthalmic♦	*Acute keratoconjunctivitis, superficial keratitis, and recurrent epithelial keratitis resulting from herpes simplex types 1 and 2—* **Adults and children:** instill ½ inch ointment into lower conjunctival sac 5 times daily at 3-hour intervals.	**Eye:** temporary visual burning, itching, mild irritation of eye, lacrimation, foreign body sensation, conjunctival injection, superficial punctate keratitis, eye pain, photosensitivity. **Other:** hypersensitivity.

INTERACTIONS	NURSING CONSIDERATIONS
	• Warn patient to avoid sharing washcloths and towels with family members. • Wash hands before and after administration. • Warn patient not to touch tip of dropper to eye or surrounding tissue. • Tell patient not to share eye medications with family members. If a family member develops the same symptoms, instruct him to contact the doctor.
None significant.	• Not for long-term use. • A relatively new alternative in treating herpes simplex ocular infections. • Warn patient not to exceed recommended frequency or duration of dosage. • Not effective against RNA virus or adenoviral ocular infections, or against bacterial, fungal, or chlamydial infections. • Warn patient to avoid sharing washcloths and towels with family members. • Always wash hands before and after applying ointment. • Tell patient to watch for signs of sensitivity, such as itching lids or constant burning. Patient who develops such signs should stop drug and notify doctor immediately. • Show patient how to instill. • Warn patient not to touch tip of tube to eye or surrounding tissue. • Available in 3% ointment. • Store in tightly closed, light-resistant container. • Tell patient not to share eye medications with family members. If a family member develops the same symptoms, instruct him to contact the doctor.

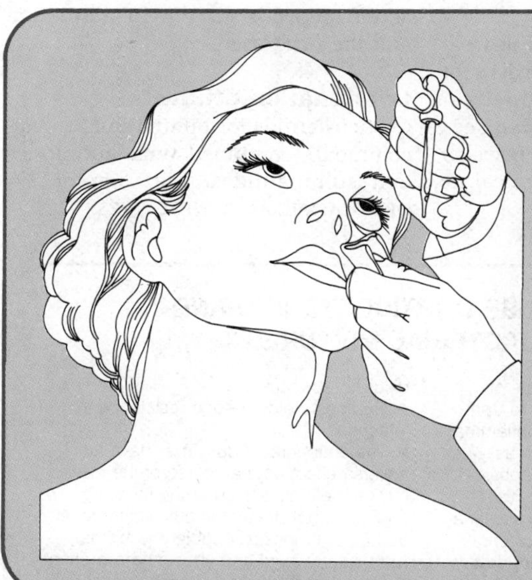

INSTILLING EYE DROPS

Before you instill any eye medication:

- Wash your hands.
- Position your patient's head back and to the side (with the unaffected eye up), with eyes open and looking up.
- Pull down the lower eyelid. Instill the drops in the conjunctival sac. Be careful and gentle, especially when the patient's eyes are irritated.

78 Ophthalmic anti-inflammatory agents

dexamethasone
dexamethasone sodium phosphate
fluorometholone
hydrocortisone
hydrocortisone acetate
medrysone
prednisolone acetate
prednisolone sodium phosphate

These potent corticosteroids are used topically in the eye to treat inflammatory ophthalmic conditions. Their use should be supervised.

Major uses

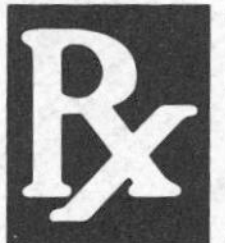

The drugs are used to treat inflammatory disorders of the eyelids, conjunctiva, cornea, and anterior segment of the globe. They also treat corneal injury from chemical or thermal burns.

Mechanism of action

The drugs decrease the infiltration of leukocytes at the site of inflammation.

Absorption, distribution, metabolism, and excretion

Absorption through the intact corneal membrane is minimal. The drugs available as suspensions are generally absorbed to a greater extent than are the solutions.

Onset and duration

Onset and duration vary. Therapeutic action depends on the inflammation and the drug used.

Combination products

Corticosteroids for ophthalmic use are commonly combined with antibiotics and sulfonamides. See Chapter 77, OPHTHALMIC ANTI-INFECTIVES.

WHEN TO USE CORTICOSTEROID AND ANTIBACTERIAL MIXTURES

Ophthalmologists use combinations of corticosteroids and antibacterials to treat conditions that require both anti-inflammatory and anti-infective action, such as marginal keratitis secondary to staphylococcal infection, blepharoconjunctivitis, allergic conjunctivitis with chronic bacterial conjunctivitis, phlyctenular keratoconjunctivitis, and selected cases of postoperative inflammation.

These mixtures are not used to treat routine ocular infections or inflammatory disorders because:

- Corticosteroids reduce resistance to infection.
- The antibacterial drug may have an adverse effect on the course of the disease if it's not effective against the invading organism, not present in sufficient concentration, or if nonsusceptible organisms (particularly fungi and viruses) are present.
- Hypersensitivity to the antibacterial may develop but go unnoticed because corticosteroids can mask an allergic response.

PATIENT-TEACHING AID

HOW TO USE EYE DROPS AND EYE OINTMENT

Dear Patient:

To relieve your eye infection or irritation, the doctor has prescribed either eye drops or eye ointment. Here's how to use them.

To instill eye drops

- First, wash your hands thoroughly.
- Hold the bottle to the light and examine it. If the medication is discolored or contains sediment, discard it and have the prescription refilled. If it looks OK, warm the medication to room temperature by holding the bottle between your palms for 2 minutes.
- Next, moisten a cotton ball or tissue with water, and clean all secretions from around your eyes. Use a fresh cotton ball or tissue for each eye, so you don't spread infection.
- Stand or sit before a mirror. Squeeze the bulb of the eyedropper to fill the dropper with medication.
- Tilt your head back slightly and toward the eye you're treating. Pull down your lower eyelid. (Don't pull your upper eyelid, or you'll put unnecessary pressure on your eye.)
- Position the dropper over the area between your lower lid and the white of your eye. Steady your hand by resting two fingers against your cheek or nose.

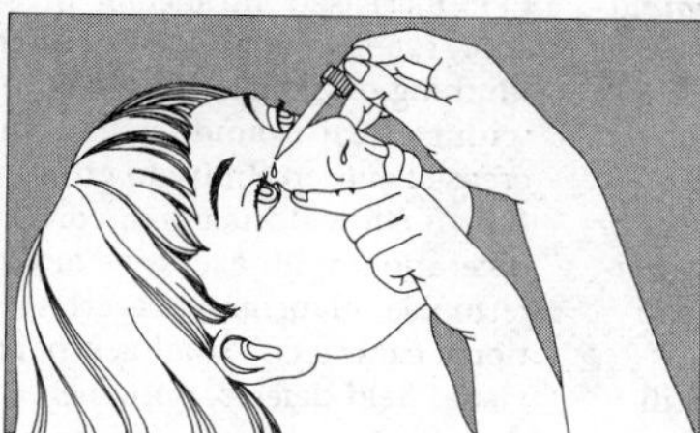

- Look away from the dropper. Then, squeeze the prescribed number of drops into the sac of the lower lid of your eye. (See illustration.) Take care not to drop the medication directly onto your eyeball or touch the dropper to your eye or eyelashes. Wipe away excess medication with a clean tissue.
- Recap the medication. Store the bottle away from light and extreme heat.

To instill eye ointment

- First, cleanse your eyelids and lashes with an irrigating solution.
- Then, remove the cap from the tube, taking care not to contaminate the applicator end by letting it touch anything.

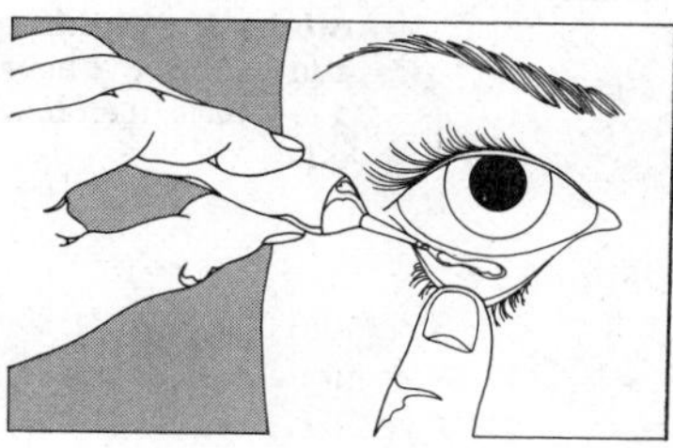

- Squeeze a small ribbon of medication along the inside of your lower eyelid. (See illustration.)
- Keep your eyelids closed for 1 to 2 minutes after application to allow the medication to spread and be absorbed.

You may experience blurred vision for a few minutes after the ointment is applied. This is normal.

A final caution

Never put any medication in your eyes unless the label reads FOR OPHTHALMIC USE or FOR USE IN THE EYES. Call your doctor immediately if you notice such side effects as decreased visual acuity, persistent blurred vision, or unusual redness or irritation when using medication.

NAME	INDICATIONS & DOSAGE	SIDE EFFECTS
dexamethasone Maxidex Ophthalmic Suspension♦ **dexamethasone sodium phosphate** Decadron Phosphate Ophthalmic♦, Maxidex Ophthalmic♦, Novadex♦♦, Opto-Methasone♦♦	*Uveitis; iridocyclitis; inflammatory condition of eyelids, conjunctiva, cornea, anterior segment of globe; corneal injury from chemical or thermal burns, or penetration of foreign bodies; allergic conjunctivitis—* **Adults and children:** instill 1 to 2 drops into conjunctival sac. In severe disease, drops may be used hourly, tapering to discontinuation as condition improves. In mild conditions, drops may be used up to 4 to 6 times daily. Treatment may extend from a few days to several weeks.	**Eye:** increased intraocular pressure, especially in elderly patients; thinning of cornea, interference with corneal wound healing, increased susceptibility to viral or fungal corneal infection, corneal ulceration; with excessive or long-term use, glaucoma exacerbations, cataracts, defects in visual acuity and visual field, optic nerve damage. **Other:** systemic effects and adrenal suppression with excessive or long-term use.
fluorometholone FML Liquifilm Ophthalmic♦	*Inflammatory and allergic conditions of cornea, conjunctiva, sclera, anterior uvea—* **Adults and children:** instill 1 to 2 drops q 1 hour for first 1 to 2 days, then b.i.d., t.i.d., or q.i.d.	**Eye:** increased intraocular pressure, especially in elderly patients; thinning of cornea, interference with corneal wound healing, corneal ulceration, increased susceptibility to viral or fungal corneal infections; with excessive or long-term use, glaucoma exacerbations, cataracts, decreased visual acuity, diminished visual field; optic nerve damage. **Other:** systemic effects and adrenal suppression in excessive or long-term use.
hydrocortisone Optef **hydrocortisone acetate** Cortamed♦♦, Hydrocortone♦	*Uveitis, iridocyclitis, inflammatory condition of eyelids, conjunctiva, cornea, anterior segment of globe; to prevent corneal scarring in visual axis; corneal injury from chemical or thermal burns, or penetration of foreign bodies; allergic conjunctivitis—* **Adults and children:** instill 1 to 3 drops into conjunctival sac q 1 hour during the day and q 2 hours during the night in acute situations. May be decreased to 1 drop t.i.d. or q.i.d.; or instill ointment t.i.d. to q.i.d. initially. May decrease to daily or b.i.d.	**Eye:** increased intraocular pressure, especially in elderly patients; thinning of cornea, interference with corneal wound healing, increased susceptibility to viral or fungal corneal infection, corneal ulceration; with excessive or long-term use, glaucoma exacerbations, cataracts, visual acuity and visual field defects, optic nerve damage. **Other:** systemic effects and adrenal suppression with excessive or long-term use.

♦ Available in U.S. and Canada. ♦♦ Available in Canada only. All other products (no symbol) available in U.S. only. Italicized side effects are common or life-threatening.

INTERACTIONS	NURSING CONSIDERATIONS
None significant.	• Contraindicated in acute superficial herpes simplex (dendritic keratitis), vaccinia, varicella, or other fungal or viral diseases of cornea and conjunctiva; presence of active diabetes; ocular tuberculosis, or any acute, purulent, untreated infection of the eye. Use cautiously in corneal abrasions, since these may be infected (especially with herpes); patients with glaucoma (any form), due to possibility of increasing intraocular pressure (miotic medication drug regimen may need to be increased to compensate). • Viral and fungal infections of the cornea may be exacerbated by the application of steroids. • Warn patient to call doctor immediately and to stop drug if visual acuity changes or visual field diminishes. • Not for long-term use. • May use eye pad with ointment for increased effect. • Watch for corneal ulceration; may require stopping drug. • Dexamethasone has greater anti-inflammatory effect than dexamethasone sodium phosphate. • Warn patient not to use leftover medication for a new eye infection; can cause serious problems. • Tell patient never to share eye medications. If a family member develops similar symptoms, instruct him to contact the doctor.
None significant.	• Contraindicated in vaccinia, varicella, acute superficial herpes simplex (dendritic keratitis), or other fungal or viral eye diseases; ocular tuberculosis; or any acute, purulent, untreated eye infection. Use cautiously in corneal abrasions since they are commonly contaminated (especially with herpes). • Not for long-term use. • Less likely to cause increased intraocular pressure with long-term use than other ophthalmic anti-inflammatory drugs (except medrysone). • Store in tightly covered, light-resistant container. • Warn patient to call doctor immediately and to stop drug if visual acuity decreases or visual field diminishes. • Shake well before using. • Warn patient not to use leftover medication for a new eye infection; can cause serious problems. • Tell patient never to share eye medications. If a family member develops similar symptoms, instruct him to contact the doctor.
None significant.	• Contraindicated in acute superficial herpes simplex (dendritic keratitis), vaccinia, varicella, or other fungal or viral diseases of cornea and conjunctiva; presence of active diabetes; ocular tuberculosis; or any acute, purulent, untreated eye infection. Use cautiously in corneal abrasions since they are commonly contaminated (especially with herpes). • Viral and fungal infections of the cornea may be exacerbated by the application of steroids. • Keep in mind possibility of increasing intraocular pressure. • Warn patient to call doctor immediately and to stop drug if visual acuity changes or visual field diminishes. • Not for long-term use. • May use eye pad with ointment for increased effect. • Watch for corneal ulceration; may require stopping drug. • Warn patient not to use leftover medication for a new eye infection; can cause serious problems. • Tell patient never to share eye medications. If a family member develops similar symptoms, instruct him to contact the doctor.

NAME	INDICATIONS & DOSAGE	SIDE EFFECTS
medrysone HMS Liquifilm Ophthalmic♦	*Allergic conjunctivitis, spring conjunctivitis, episcleritis, ophthalmic epinephrine sensitivity reaction—* **Adults and children:** instill 1 drop in conjunctival sac b.i.d. to q.i.d. May use q 1 hour during first 1 to 2 days if needed.	**Eye:** thinning of cornea, interference with corneal wound healing, increased susceptibility to viral or fungal corneal infection, corneal ulceration; with excessive or long-term use, glaucoma exacerbations, cataracts, visual acuity and visual field defects, optic nerve damage. **Other:** systemic effects and adrenal suppression with excessive or long-term use.
prednisolone acetate (suspensions) Econopred Ophthalmic, Econopred Plus Ophthalmic, Pred-Forte♦, Pred Mild Ophthalmic♦, Prednicon♦♦, Predulose Ophthalmic **prednisolone sodium phosphate (solutions)** Hydeltrasol Ophthalmic, Inflamase Forte♦, Inflamase Ophthalmic♦, Metreton Ophthalmic, Nova-Pred Forte♦♦	*Inflammation of palpebral and bulbar conjunctiva, cornea, and anterior segment of globe—* **Adults and children:** instill 2 drops in eye. In severe conditions, may be used hourly, tapering to discontinuation as inflammation subsides. In mild conditions, may be used up to 4 to 6 times daily.	**Eye:** increased intraocular pressure, especially in elderly patients; thinning of cornea, interference with corneal wound healing, increased susceptibility to viral or fungal corneal infection, corneal ulceration; with excessive or long-term use, glaucoma exacerbations, cataracts, visual acuity and visual field defects, optic nerve damage. **Other:** systemic effects and adrenal suppression with excessive or long-term use.

♦ Available in U.S. and Canada. ♦♦ Available in Canada only. All other products (no symbol) available in U.S. only. Italicized side effects are common or life-threatening.

INTERACTIONS	NURSING CONSIDERATIONS
None significant.	• Contraindicated in vaccinia, varicella, acute superficial herpes simplex (dendritic keratitis), viral diseases of conjunctiva and cornea, ocular tuberculosis, fungal or viral eye diseases, iritis, uveitis, or any acute, purulent, untreated eye infection. Use cautiously in corneal abrasions since they are commonly contaminated (especially with herpes). • Shake well before using. Don't freeze. • Warn patient not to use leftover medication for a new eye infection; can cause serious problems. • Tell patient never to share eye medications. If a family member develops similar symptoms, instruct him to contact the doctor.
None significant.	• Contraindicated in acute, untreated, purulent ocular infections, acute superficial herpes simplex (dendritic keratitis), vaccinia, varicella, or other viral or fungal eye diseases, ocular tuberculosis. Use cautiously in corneal abrasions since they are commonly contaminated (especially with herpes). • Tell patient on long-term therapy to have frequent tonometric examinations. • Shake suspensions before using, and store in tightly covered container. • Don't stop therapy prematurely. • Warn patient not to use leftover medication for a new eye infection; can cause serious problems. • Tell patient never to share eye medications. If a family member develops similar symptoms, instruct him to contact the doctor.

79 Miotics

acetylcholine chloride
carbachol
demecarium bromide
echothiophate iodide
isoflurophate
physostigmine salicylate
pilocarpine hydrochloride
pilocarpine nitrate

Miotics are topical drugs that cause pupillary constriction (miosis). They're used in chronic ophthalmic conditions and in surgical procedures for ocular disorders.

Major uses

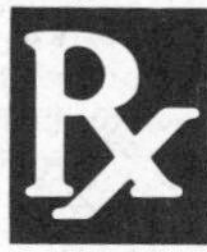

Miotics are used to treat open-angle and narrow-angle glaucoma. They are also therapeutic in iridectomy, anterior segment surgery, and other ocular surgery. When used with mydriatics, they prevent adhesions after ocular surgery.

Mechanism of action

• Acetylcholine chloride, carbachol, and pilocarpine hydrochloride (cholinergic drugs) cause contraction of the

RECOGNIZING HIGH-RISK GLAUCOMA PATIENTS

Do you know when your patient has glaucoma? You won't know for certain until he's been tested. But you can help detect vulnerable patients. Increasing intraocular pressure may be the first sign of glaucoma, so early tonometry screening is essential. Vulnerable persons who should be screened at least every 2 years are:

• *everyone between ages 55 and 65.*

• *those with diabetes.* Primary open-angle glaucoma occurs approximately three times more frequently in such persons; and visual field loss appears to develop at lower pressures. Therefore, urge your patients with diabetes to have an ophthalmologic examination regularly.

• *blacks.* Reportedly, the black population has eight times more glaucoma-related blindness than the white population. No physiological cause is known, but some attribute the increased incidence to poor preventive care.

• *hypertensive patients with primary open-angle glaucoma.* In these patients, lowering of blood pressure may reduce the blood flow to the optic nerve, making it more vulnerable to damage.

• *patients with family histories of glaucoma.* The genetic factor is so strongly indicated (about one third of patients with chronic open-angle glaucoma have relatives with the disease) that any patient with glaucoma in the family within two generations should be regularly screened from age 25 on.

• *large-eyed children.* If a child has frequent tearing, photophobia (light sensitivity), or blepharospasm (continual blinking), and seems to have exceptionally large corneas (normal corneal diameter is approximately 11.5 mm), these could be indications of congenital glaucoma. (However, this is a rare variation of the disease.)

• *patients who've suffered eye injuries.* Be especially alert for signs of glaucoma in patients who've had eye injuries caused by the blow of a tennis ball, a fist, or blunt instruments.

THERAPEUTIC ACTIVITY OF MIOTICS

DRUG	ONSET	DURATION	ADVANTAGES OR DISADVANTAGES
acetylcholine	10 to 15 sec	15 min	Best for surgery
carbachol	10 to 20 min	4 to 8 hr	Stronger than pilocarpine but doesn't penetrate as well
demecarium	15 to 30 min	12 to 48 hr	May cause prolonged and serious systemic side effects, but a more stable compound than echothiophate
echothiophate	15 to 30 min	1 to 2 wk	May cause prolonged and serious systemic side effects; very unstable
isoflurophate	5 to 10 min	2 to 4 wk	Very unstable
physostigmine	10 to 30 min	24 to 48 hr	Commonly causes headache
pilocarpine	15 min	4 to 8 hr	Tolerance develops; usually strength must be increased

sphincter muscles of the iris, resulting in miosis. They also produce ciliary spasm, deepening of the anterior chamber, and vasodilation of conjunctival vessels of the outflow tract.

• Demecarium bromide, echothiophate iodide, isoflurophate, and physostigmine salicylate (anticholinesterase drugs) inhibit the enzymatic destruction of acetylcholine by inactivating cholinesterase. This leaves acetylcholine free to act on the effector cells of the iridic sphincter and ciliary muscles, causing pupillary constriction and accommodation spasm.

Absorption, distribution, metabolism, and excretion

Although some systemic absorption is possible with all agents except acetylcholine, systemic side effects are unusual. Among all the drugs, demecarium and echothiophate are most likely to produce systemic side effects when used excessively. Drug-related symptoms of significant absorption include hypersalivation, nausea, vomiting, and bronchospasm.

Onset and duration

The accompanying chart summarizes the therapeutic activity of the miotics.

Combination products

E-CARPINE♦: epinephrine bitartrate 0.5% and pilocarpine HCl 1%, 2%, 3%, 4%, or 6%.

E-PILO♦: epinephrine bitartrate 1%; pilocarpine HCl 1%, 2%, 3%, 4%, or 6%.

ISOPTO P-ES: pilocarpine HCl 2% and physostigmine salicylate 0.125%.

P_1E_1, P_2E_1, P_3E_1, P_4E_1, P_6E_1: epinephrine bitartrate 1% and pilocarpine HCl 1%, 2%, 3%, 4%, or 6%.

NAME	INDICATIONS & DOSAGE	SIDE EFFECTS
acetylcholine chloride Miochol♦	*Anterior segment surgery—* **Adults and children:** doctor instills 0.5 to 2 ml of 1% solution gently in anterior chamber of eye.	None reported with 1% concentration. Iris atrophy possible with higher concentrations.
carbachol (intraocular) Miostat **carbachol (topical)** Carbacel, Isopto Carbachol♦	*Ocular surgery (to produce pupillary miosis)—* **Adults:** doctor should gently instill 0.5 ml into the anterior chamber for production of satisfactory miosis. It may be instilled before or after securing sutures. *Open-angle or narrow-angle glaucoma—* **Adults:** instill 1 drop into eye daily, b.i.d., t.i.d., or q.i.d. Ointment form also available with b.i.d. dosage.	**CNS:** headache. **Eye:** accommodative spasm, blurred vision, conjunctival vasodilation, eye and brow pain. **GI:** abdominal cramps, diarrhea. **Other:** sweating, flushing, asthma.
demecarium bromide Humorsol	*Glaucoma, postiridectomy—* **Adults:** instill 1 drop 0.125% or 0.25% solution in eyes twice weekly up to b.i.d., depending on intraocular pressure. *Accommodative esotropia—* **Children:** instill 1 drop 0.125% solution in each eye daily for 2 to 3 weeks, taper to 1 drop q 2 days for 3 to 4 weeks, then 1 drop twice weekly. Therapy should be discontinued after 4 months if control of condition still requires every other day therapy or if patient shows no response.	**CNS:** headache. **CV:** hypotension, bradycardia. **Eye:** iris cysts (reversible with discontinuation), lens opacity, ciliary or accommodative spasm, blurred vision, eye or brow pain, photosensitivity, eyelid twitching, congestive iritis, iridocyclitis, conjunctival and intraocular hyperemia, ocular pain, photophobia, acute attack of narrow-angle glaucoma. **GI:** nausea, vomiting, abdominal pain, diarrhea, excessive salivation. **GU:** frequent urination. **Skin:** contact dermatitis. **Other:** flushing, bronchial constriction.

INTERACTIONS	NURSING CONSIDERATIONS
None significant.	• Shake vial gently until clear solution is obtained. • Reconstitute immediately before using. • Discard any unused solution. • Complete miosis occurs within seconds. • Don't gas-sterilize vial. Ethylene oxide may produce formic acid.
None significant.	• Contraindicated in acute iritis, corneal abrasion. Use cautiously in acute heart failure, bronchial asthma, peptic ulcer, hyperthyroidism, GI spasm, urinary tract obstruction, parkinsonism. • A cholinergic agent. • Used in glaucoma, especially when patient is resistant or allergic to pilocarpine HCl or nitrate. • Show patient how to instill. Warn him not to exceed recommended dosage. • For single-dose intraocular use only. Premixed; discard unused portions. • Warn patient not to touch tip of dropper to eye or surrounding tissue. • Tell glaucoma patient that long-term use may be necessary. Stress compliance. Tell him to remain under medical supervision for periodic tonometric readings. • In case of toxicity, atropine should be given parenterally. • Caution patient not to drive for 1 or 2 hours after administration. • Reassure patient that blurred vision usually diminishes with prolonged use.
Systemic anticholinesterase for myasthenia gravis: additive effects. Monitor patient for signs of toxicity. *Echothiophate iodide:* decreased duration of miosis if demecarium bromide is given first. Give echothiophate iodide first. *Organophosphate insecticides:* additive effects. Warn patient exposed to insecticides of this danger. *Pilocarpine:* interferes with miosis. Do not use together. *Succinylcholine:* respiratory or cardiovascular collapse. Don't use together.	• Contraindicated in active uveal inflammation, narrow-angle glaucoma, secondary glaucoma resulting from iridocyclitis, ocular hypertension, vasomotor instability, bronchial asthma, spastic GI conditions, peptic ulcer, severe bradycardia, hypotension, recent myocardial infarction, epilepsy, parkinsonism, history of retinal detachment. Use cautiously in patients with myasthenia gravis receiving systemic anticholinesterase therapy; in patients exposed to organophosphate insecticides. • Systemic absorption may be minimized by compressing inner canthus of eye for 1 to 2 minutes after instilling drops. • Dangerous drug capable of producing cumulative systemic side effects. Closely follow prescribed concentration and dosage schedule and monitor patient carefully. • Atropine sulfate given subcutaneously or I.V., and pralidoxine chloride are antidotes of choice. • Tell patient to stop drug and report immediately if excessive salivation, diaphoresis, urinary incontinence, diarrhea, or muscle weakness occurs. • Instruct patient to use at bedtime since drug blurs vision. • Warn patient not to exceed recommended dosage. • Show patient how to instill. Warn him not to touch tip of dropper to eye or surrounding tissue. Store in tightly closed container. • Stop drug at least 2 weeks preoperatively. • If solution contacts skin, wash promptly with large amount of water. • Wash hands immediately before and after administering. • Monitor patient for lenticular opacities every 6 months. • Treat any extraocular pressure changes with rapid instillation of 1% to 2% epinephrine at 5-minute intervals. • Antidote for atropine for glaucoma patients, and used to control preoperative and postoperative intraocular pressure of glaucoma. • An extremely potent, long-lasting anticholinesterase drug. • Reassure patient that blurred vision usually diminishes with prolonged use.

NAME	INDICATIONS & DOSAGE	SIDE EFFECTS
echothiophate iodide Echodide, Phospholine Iodide♦	*Open-angle glaucoma, conditions obstructing aqueous outflow, accommodative esotropia—* **Adults and children:** instill 1 drop 0.03% to 0.125% solution into conjunctival sac daily. Maximum 1 drop b.i.d. Use lowest possible dosage to continuously control intraocular pressure.	**CNS:** fatigue, muscle weakness, paresthesias, headache. **CV:** bradycardia, hypotension. **Eye:** ciliary or accommodative spasm, ciliary or conjunctival injection, nonreversible cataract formation (time- and dose-related), reversible iris cysts, pupillary block, blurred or dimmed vision, eye or brow pain, lid twitching, hyperemia, photosensitivity, lens opacities, lacrimation, retinal detachment. **GI:** diarrhea, nausea, vomiting, abdominal pain, intestinal cramps, salivation. **GU:** frequent urination. **Other:** flushing, sweating, bronchial constriction.
isoflurophate Floropryl	*Glaucoma—* **Adults and children:** instill ¼" strip 0.025% ointment in conjunctival sac q 8 to 72 hours. *Esotropia uncomplicated by amblyopia or anisometropia—* **Adults and children:** ¼" of ointment every night for 2 weeks.	**CNS:** headache, muscle weakness. **Eye:** moderate conjunctival hyperemia, eye pain, ciliary spasm causing discomfort, iris cysts, cataract formation, retinal detachment, paradoxical increase in intraocular pressure; precipitates attacks of acute narrow-angle glaucoma. **GI:** diarrhea, salivation. **Other:** sweating, bronchial constriction.

♦ Available in U.S. and Canada. ♦♦ Available in Canada only. All other products (no symbol) available in U.S. only. Italicized side effects are common or life-threatening.

INTERACTIONS	NURSING CONSIDERATIONS
Organophosphate insecticides (parathion, malathion): may have an additive effect that could cause systemic effects. Warn patient exposed to insecticides of this danger. *Succinylcholine:* respiratory and cardiovascular collapse. Don't use together. *Systemic anticholinesterase for myasthenia gravis:* effects may be additive. Monitor patient for signs of toxicity.	• Contraindicated in narrow-angle glaucoma, epilepsy, vasomotor instability, parkinsonism, iodide hypersensitivity, active uveal inflammation, ocular hypertension with intraocular inflammatory processes, bronchial asthma, spastic GI conditions, urinary tract obstruction, peptic ulcer, severe bradycardia or hypotension, vascular hypertension, myocardial infarction, history of retinal detachment. Use cautiously in patients routinely exposed to organophosphate insecticides. May cause nausea, vomiting, and diarrhea, progressing to muscle weakness and respiratory difficulty. Use cautiously in patients with myasthenia gravis receiving anticholinesterase therapy. • Toxicity is cumulative. Toxic systemic symptoms don't appear for weeks or months after initiating therapy. • Reconstitute powder carefully to avoid contamination. Use only diluent provided. Discard refrigerated, reconstituted solution after 6 months; solution at room temperature after 1 month. • Warn patient that transient brow pain or dimmed or blurred vision is common at first but usually disappears within 5 to 10 days. • Systemic absorption may be minimized by compressing inner canthus of eye for 1 to 2 minutes after instilling drops. • Instill at bedtime since drug causes transient blurred vision. • Tell patient to remain under constant medical supervision. Warn him not to exceed recommended dosage. • Report salivation, diarrhea, profuse sweating, urinary incontinence, or muscle weakness. • Stop drug at least 2 weeks preoperatively. • Atropine sulfate (subcutaneous, I.M., or I.V.) is antidote of choice. • A potent, long-acting, irreversible anticholinesterase. • Show patient how to instill. Warn him not to touch tip of dropper to eye or surrounding tissue. • Wash hands before and after administering medication.
Demecarium, physostigmine: competitive action. Decreased duration of miosis if isoflurophate given second. Give isoflurophate first. *Pilocarpine:* interferes with miosis. Use cautiously for ciliary spasm. *Succinylcholine:* respiratory or cardiovascular collapse. Don't use together. *Systemic anticholinesterase for myasthenia gravis:* additive effects. Monitor patient for signs of toxicity.	• Contraindicated in hypersensitivity to organophosphate compounds, peanut oil, and polyethylene mineral oil; in patients with uveal inflammation, narrow-angle glaucoma, ocular hypertension, bronchial asthma, peptic ulcer, severe bradycardia, hypotension, recent MI, epilepsy, parkinsonism, or history of retinal detachment. Use cautiously in patients exposed to organophosphate insecticides; patients with myasthenia gravis receiving concurrent anticholinesterase drugs. • Tell patient with glaucoma to use at bedtime if possible because of blurred vision and ciliary spasm. • Show patient how to instill. Warn him not to touch tip of tube to eye, surrounding tissues, or moist surface. • Warn patient that close, constant medical supervision is vital and that he should not exceed prescribed dosage. • Treat paradoxical pressure changes with rapid instillation of 1% to 2% epinephrine at 5-minute intervals. • Instruct patient to stop therapy at once and notify doctor if he experiences excessive salivation, diarrhea, sweating, muscle weakness. • Systemic absorption may be minimized by compressing inner canthus of eye for 1 to 2 minutes after instilling drops. • Unstable and inactivated in the presence of water. • Store in refrigerator in a tightly closed container. • Rapidly absorbed through skin. • A potent parasympathomimetic, or anticholinesterase, drug. • Wash hands before and after administering medication.

NAME	INDICATIONS & DOSAGE	SIDE EFFECTS
physostigmine salicylate Eserine Salicylate, Isopto Eserine	*Atropine mydriasis, acute narrow-angle glaucoma*— **Adults and children:** instill ¼" 0.25% ophthalmic ointment in conjunctival sac, or instill 1 to 2 drops 0.25% to 0.5% solution in conjunctival sac t.i.d. Repeat p.r.n. to obtain miosis.	**CNS:** *headache.* **Eye:** twitching of eyelids, conjunctival irritation, reversible depigmentation of lid skin in Blacks allergic to ointment, eye and brow pain, marked miosis, lacrimation, dimmed or blurred vision, follicular cysts. **Skin:** allergic dermatitis.
pilocarpine hydrochloride Adsorbocarpine♦, Almocarpine, Isopto Carpine♦, Miocarpine♦♦, Nova-Carpine♦♦, Ocusert Pilo♦, Opto-Pilo♦♦, Pilocar, Pilocel, Pilomiotin **pilocarpine nitrate** P.V. Carpine Liquifilm♦	*Chronic open-angle glaucoma, before emergency surgery in acute narrow-angle glaucoma*— **Adults and children:** instill 1 to 2 drops in eye daily b.i.d., t.i.d., q.i.d., or as directed by doctor.	**Eye:** suborbital headache, *myopia,* ciliary spasm, *blurred vision,* conjunctival irritation, lacrimation, changes in visual field, *brow pain.* **GI:** nausea, vomiting, abdominal cramps, diarrhea, salivation. **Other:** bronchiolar spasm, pulmonary edema, hypersensitivity.

♦ Available in U.S. and Canada. ♦♦ Available in Canada only. All other products (no symbol) available in U.S. only. Italicized side effects are common or life-threatening.

INTERACTIONS	NURSING CONSIDERATIONS
Isoflurophate: decreased miosis if isoflurophate given second. Give isoflurophate first. *Organophosphate insecticides:* additive effect. Warn patient exposed to insecticides of this danger. *Pilocarpine:* prolonged miosis. May be used together therapeutically. *Succinylcholine:* additive effect. Don't use together.	• Contraindicated in inflammatory diseases of iris or ciliary body, asthma, diabetes mellitus, gangrene, cardiovascular disease, mechanical obstruction of intestinal or urogenital tract, vagotonia, secondary glaucoma. Use cautiously in bradycardia, epilepsy, parkinsonism, and in patients exposed to organophosphate insecticides. • Glaucoma therapy is long-term. Stress patient compliance. Warn not to exceed dosage. • Lid twitching, temporarily blurred vision, and difficulty in seeing in the dark are common side effects. • Irritating to eye. Watch for signs of conjunctivitis or allergic reactions. • Show patient how to instill. Warn him not to touch dropper or tip of tube to eye or surrounding tissue. • Systemic absorption may be minimized by compressing inner canthus of eye for 1 to 2 minutes after instilling drops. • Discard discolored (rusty or pink) solution or ointment. Aqueous solutions oxidize on exposure to light or air. • Anticholinesterase. • Used in ocular myasthenia gravis. • May be used alternately with atropine as a miotic to break adhesions between the iris and lens. • Wash hands before and after administering medication.
Carbachol: additive effect. Do not use together. *Phenylephrine HCl:* decreased dilation by phenylephrine HCl. Don't use together.	• Contraindicated in acute iritis, acute inflammatory disease of anterior segment of eye, secondary glaucoma. Use cautiously in bronchial asthma, hypertension. • Warn patient that vision will be temporarily blurred. • Transient brow pain and myopia are common at first; usually disappear in 10 to 14 days. • Warn patient not to exceed recommended dosage. • Show patient how to instill. Warn him not to touch dropper to eye or surrounding tissue. • Glaucoma therapy is necessarily prolonged. Stress compliance. Warn that glaucoma can cause blindness. • Most widely used drug in initial treatment of chronic open-angle glaucoma. • Systemic absorption may be minimized by compressing inner canthus of eye for 1 to 2 minutes after instilling drops. • Also used to counteract effects of mydriatics and cycloplegics after surgery or ophthalmoscopic examination. • May be used alternately with atropine to break adhesions between iris and lens. • In acute narrow-angle glaucoma before surgery, may be used alone or with physostigmine or mannitol, urea, or glycerol. • Wash hands before and after administration.

80 Mydriatics

atropine sulfate
cyclopentolate hydrochloride
epinephrine bitartrate
epinephrine hydrochloride
epinephryl borate
homatropine hydrobromide
hydroxyamphetamine hydrobromide
phenylephrine hydrochloride
scopolamine hydrobromide
tropicamide

Both anticholinergics (atropine, cyclopentolate, homatropine, scopolamine, and tropicamide) and adrenergics (epinephrine, epinephryl borate, hydroxyamphetamine, and phenylephrine) produce mydriasis (pupillary dilation) when applied topically to the eye. In addition, the anticholinergics produce cycloplegia (paralysis of accommodation).

Major uses

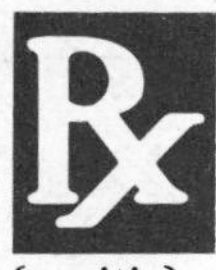

- Atropine, homatropine, and scopolamine are used in acute inflammation of the iris (iritis), or of the iris, ciliary body, and choroid (uveitis).
- Cyclopentolate, hydroxyamphetamine, phenylephrine, and tropicamide are used in diagnostic procedures.
- The epinephrine salts are used with or without miotics to lower intraocular pressure in open-angle glaucoma.

Mechanism of action

- Anticholinergics block acetylcholine, leaving the pupil under the unopposed influence of its sympathetic or adrenergic nerve supply. This causes the pupil to dilate. Relaxation of the ciliary muscle allows the lens to flatten.
- Adrenergics dilate the pupil by contracting the dilator muscle of the pupil.

Absorption, distribution, metabolism, and excretion

- Anticholinergics can be systemically absorbed, causing side effects, particularly in children and elderly persons. (For more information on absorption of anticholinergics, see Chapter 38, CHOLINERGIC BLOCKERS.) Side effects such as dry mouth and tachycardia are most common after instillation of atropine, scopolamine, and cyclopentolate.
- Penetration by adrenergics is heightened during surgical procedures and in the traumatized eye. (For greater detail, see Chapter 39, ADRENERGICS.)
- Adrenergics are systemically absorbed less often than anticholinergics. Repeated instillation of phenylephrine (10% solution) may exacerbate hypertension.

Onset and duration

- Atropine produces mydriasis in 30 to 40 minutes; dilation can last 12 to 14 days before complete recovery. The drug causes cycloplegia within a few hours; this effect lasts 2 weeks or more before complete recovery.
- Cyclopentolate produces mydriasis in 15 to 30 minutes that lasts up to 24 hours. Cyclopentolate produces cy-

MYDRIATICS FACILITATE EYE EXAMINATION

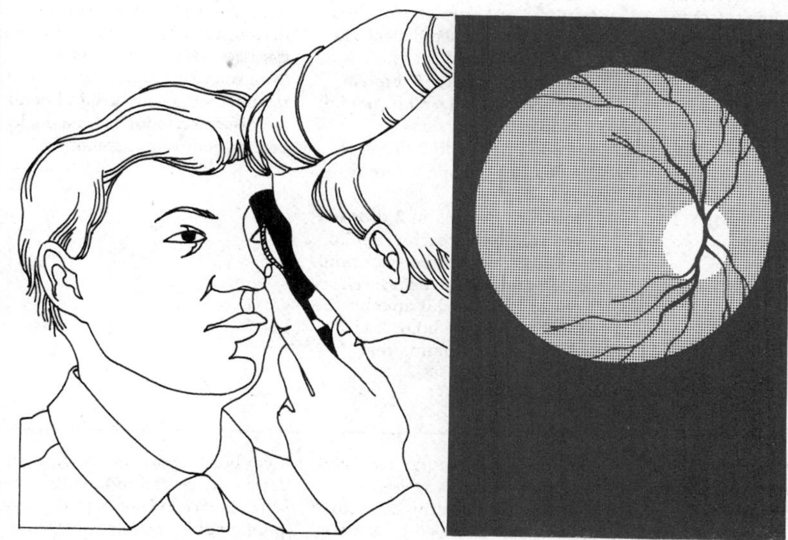

Mydriatics and cycloplegics are used to dilate the pupil and paralyze the muscles of accommodation so that the eyegrounds can be visualized during ophthalmic examination.

cloplegia in 15 to 45 minutes that lasts up to 24 hours

- Epinephrine produces mydriasis within minutes after instillation; dilation lasts several hours. Epinephrine lowers intraocular pressure for variable lengths of time. The maximal interval is 4 to 8 hours; recovery occurs in 12 to 24 or more hours. (Epinephrine also causes, in 5 minutes, vasoconstriction that lasts 1 hour.)
- Homatropine hydrobromide has a shorter duration than atropine. Cycloplegia begins in 30 to 90 minutes, and recovery takes 10 to 48 hours. Maximal cycloplegia occurs within 1 hour; recovery is in 1 to 3 days.
- Hydroxyamphetamine produces maximal dilation within 40 minutes after instillation. The dilation continues for several hours. Cycloplegia begins in 30 to 60 minutes; recovery takes 20 hours for adults and several days for children.
- Phenylephrine (2.5% solution) produces dilation within minutes after instillation. Maximal dilation occurs in 15 to 60 minutes and lasts up to 3 hours.
- Scopolamine produces maximal dilation within 40 minutes after instillation; recovery occurs in 3 to 7 days. Cycloplegia, which begins in 10 to 30 minutes, reaches a maximum within 30 to 45 minutes. Complete recovery may take several days.
- Tropicamide produces maximal dilation in 20 to 25 minutes after application, and cycloplegia that lasts about 20 minutes. Recovery is complete in about 6 hours.

Combination products

CYCLOMYDRIL: cyclopentolate HCl 0.2% and phenylephrine HCl 1%.

MYDRAPRED: prednisolone acetate 0.25% and atropine sulfate 1%.

MUROCOLL-2: scopolamine HBr 0.3% and phenylephrine HCl 10%.

NAME	INDICATIONS & DOSAGE	SIDE EFFECTS
atropine sulfate Atropisol, BufOpto Atropine, Isopto Atropine♦, Opto-Tropinal♦♦	*Acute iris inflammation (iritis)*— **Adults:** 1 to 2 drops of 1% solution or small amount of ointment 2 to 3 times daily, b.i.d., or t.i.d. **Children:** instill 1 to 2 drops of 0.5% solution daily, b.i.d., or t.i.d. *Cycloplegic refraction*— **Adults:** instill 1 to 2 drops of 1% solution 1 hour before refracting. **Children:** instill 1 to 2 drops of 0.5% solution to each eye b.i.d. for 1 to 3 days before eye examination and 1 hour before refraction, or instill small amount ointment daily or b.i.d. 2 to 3 days before examination.	**Eye:** increased intraocular pressure, ocular congestion in long-term use, conjunctivitis, contact dermatitis, edema, *blurred vision,* eye dryness, *photophobia.* **Systemic:** flushing, dry skin and mouth, fever, tachycardia, abdominal distention in infants, ataxia, irritability, confusion, somnolence.
cyclopentolate hydrochloride Cyclogyl♦, Mydplegic♦♦, Nova-Cyclo♦♦, Opto-Pentolate♦♦	*Diagnostic procedures requiring mydriasis and cycloplegia*— **Adults:** instill 1 drop 1% solution in eye, followed by 1 more drop in 5 minutes. Use 2% solution in heavily pigmented irises. **Children:** instill 1 drop of 0.5%, 1%, or 2% solution in each eye, followed in 5 minutes with 1 drop 0.5% or 1% solution, if necessary. Not recommended for children under 6 years.	**Eye:** burning sensation on instillation, increased intraocular pressure, blurred vision, eye dryness, *photophobia,* ocular congestion, contact dermatitis, conjunctivitis. **Systemic:** flushing, tachycardia, urinary retention, dry skin, fever, ataxia, irritability, confusion, somnolence, convulsions.
epinephrine bitartrate E1, E2, Epitrate♦, Lyophrin, Murocoll, Mytrate **epinephrine hydrochloride** Epifrin♦, Glaucon♦ **epinephryl borate** Epinal♦, Eppy/N♦	**Adults and children:** *Intraocular injection*—0.1 to 0.2 ml of 0.01% or 0.1% epinephrine HCl by doctor. *Open-angle glaucoma*—instill 1 to 2 drops of 1% or 2% bitartrate solution in eye with frequency determined by tonometric readings (once q 2 to 4 days up to q.i.d.), or instill 1 drop 0.5%, 1%, or 2% HCl solution (or 0.25%, 0.5%, or 1% epinephryl borate solution) in eye b.i.d. *During surgery*—1 or more drops of 0.1% epinephrine HCl up to 3 times.	**Eye:** corneal or conjunctival pigmentation or corneal edema in long-term use; follicular hypertrophy; chemosis; conjunctivitis; iritis; hyperemic conjunctiva; maculopapular rash; severe stinging, burning, and tearing upon instillation; brow pain. **Systemic:** palpitations, tachycardia.

♦ Available in U.S. and Canada. ♦♦ Available in Canada only. All other products (no symbol) available in U.S. only. Italicized side effects are common or life-threatening.

INTERACTIONS	NURSING CONSIDERATIONS
None significant.	• Contraindicated in primary glaucoma (shallow anterior chamber or narrow-angle), increased intraocular pressure. Use cautiously in infants, children, elderly or debilitated patients. • Warn patient vision will be temporarily blurred. Dark glasses ease discomfort of photophobia. • Not for internal use. Treat drops and ointment as poison. Keep physostigmine available as antidote for poisoning. Signs of poisoning are disorientation and confusion. • Don't touch dropper or tip of tube to eye or surrounding tissue. • Watch for signs of glaucoma: increased intraocular pressure, ocular pain, headache, progressive blurring of vision. • Most potent mydriatic and cycloplegic available; long duration of action. • Warn patient not to operate machinery or drive a car until the temporary visual impairment caused by this drug wears off. • Warn patient not to exceed recommended dosage. • Systemic absorption may be minimized by compressing inner canthus of eye for 1 to 2 minutes after instilling drops. • Show patient how to instill. Wash hands before and after administration. • For toxicity (if ingested), see APPENDIX, *Drug Toxicities*.
None significant.	• Contraindicated in narrow-angle glaucoma. Use cautiously in elderly patients. • Systemic absorption may be minimized by compressing inner canthus of eye for 1 to 2 minutes after instilling drops. • Close container after each use to avoid contamination. • Wash hands before and after administration. • Potent drug with mydriatic and cycloplegic effect; superior to homatropine hydrobromide and has shorter duration of action. • Instruct patient to wear dark glasses to ease discomfort of photophobia. • Warn patient drug will burn when instilled. • Warn patient not to operate machinery or drive until the temporary visual impairment caused by this drug has worn off.
Cyclopropane or halogenated hydrocarbons: arrhythmias, tachycardia. Use together cautiously, if at all. *Tricyclic antidepressants, antihistamines:* potentiated cardiac effects of epinephrine. Use together cautiously.	• Contraindicated in shallow anterior chamber or narrow-angle glaucoma. • Use cautiously in diabetes mellitus, hypertension, Parkinson's disease, hyperthyroidism, aphakia (eye without lens), cardiac disease, or cerebral arteriosclerosis; in elderly patients or pregnant women. • May stain soft contact lenses. • Use with pilocarpine: additive effect in lowering intraocular pressure. • Monitor blood pressure and other systemic effects. • Protect from light and heat. • Don't use darkened solution. • Also used during surgery to control local bleeding, or injected into the anterior chamber to produce rapid mydriasis during cataract removal. • Warn patient not to touch dropper to eye or surrounding tissue. • Wash hands before and after administration.

NAME	INDICATIONS & DOSAGE	SIDE EFFECTS
homatropine hydrobromide Homatrocel Ophthalmic, Isopto Homatropine♦	**Adults and children:** *Cycloplegic refraction*—instill 1 to 2 drops 2% or 5% solution in eye; repeat in 5 to 10 minutes. *Uveitis*—instill 1 to 2 drops 2% or 5% solution in eye up to every 3 to 4 hours.	**Eye:** eye irritation, *blurred vision, photophobia.* **Systemic:** flushing, dry skin and mouth, fever, tachycardia, ataxia, irritability, confusion, somnolence.
hydroxy-amphetamine hydrobromide Paredrine	*Diagnosis of Horner's syndrome*— **Adults, and children over 12 years:** instill 1 to 2 drops 1% solution into conjunctival sac.	**Eye:** increased intraocular pressure, blurred vision, *photophobia.*
phenylephrine hydrochloride Mydfrin, Neo-Synephrine♦	**Adults and children:** *Mydriasis (without cycloplegia)*—instill 1 drop 2.5% or 10% solution in eye before examination. *Posterior synechia (adhesion of iris)*—instill 1 drop 10% solution in eye. Do not use 10% concentration in infants; use cautiously in elderly patients.	**Eye:** transient burning or stinging on instillation, blurred vision, reactive hyperemia, allergic conjunctivitis, iris floaters, narrow-angle glaucoma, rebound miosis, allergic conjunctivitis, dermatitis. **CNS:** headache, brow pain. **CV:** *hypertension,* tachycardia, palpitations, premature ventricular contractions. **Other:** pallor, trembling, sweating.

♦ Available in U.S. and Canada. ♦♦ Available in Canada only. All other products (no symbol) available in U.S. only. Italicized side effects are common or life-threatening.

INTERACTIONS	NURSING CONSIDERATIONS
None significant.	• Contraindicated in primary glaucoma (shallow anterior chamber or narrow-angle). Use cautiously in infants, elderly or debilitated patients, or patients with hypertension, cardiac disease, or increased intraocular pressure. • Warn patient vision will be temporarily blurred after instillation. Tell him not to drive a car or operate machinery until this wears off. Dark glasses should be worn to decrease photophobia. • Long-term frequent use may produce symptoms of atropine SO_4 poisoning, such as severe dryness of mouth, tachycardia. • Not for internal use. Treat as poison. Keep physostigmine available as antidote for poisoning. • Systemic absorption may be minimized by compressing inner canthus of eye for 1 to 2 minutes after instilling drops. • Show patient how to instill. • Warn patient not to touch dropper tip to eye or surrounding tissue. • Wash hands before and after administration. • Similar to atropine SO_4 but weaker, with a shorter duration of action. • For toxicity (if ingested), see APPENDIX, *Drug Toxicities.*
None significant.	• Contraindicated in narrow-angle glaucoma. Use cautiously in hypertension, hyperthyroidism, diabetes mellitus, increased intraocular pressure. • Instruct patient to wear dark glasses to ease discomfort of photophobia. • May cause blurred vision. Warn patient not to drive car or operate machinery until this effect wears off. • Store in tightly closed container. Do not use discolored solution. • Wash hands before and after administration. • If ingested, toxic symptoms include arrhythmias, headache, nausea, vomiting. Contact doctor immediately.
Guanethidine: increased mydriatic and pressor effects of phenylephrine HCl. Use together cautiously. *Levodopa (systemic):* reduced mydriatic effect of phenylephrine HCl. Use together cautiously. *MAO inhibitors:* may cause arrhythmias due to increased pressor effect. Use together cautiously. *Tricyclic antidepressants:* potentiated cardiac effects of epinephrine. Use together cautiously.	• Contraindicated in narrow-angle glaucoma, soft contact lens use. Use cautiously in marked hypertension, cardiac disorders, and in children of low body weight. • Should be avoided in patients with idiopathic orthostatic hypotension. May produce high blood pressure response. • Protect from light and heat. • Warn patient not to exceed recommended dosage. Systemic effects can result. Monitor blood pressure and pulse rate. • Warn patient not to touch dropper tip to eye or surrounding tissue. • Systemic absorption can be minimized by compressing inner canthus of eye for 1 to 2 minutes after instilling drops. • Potential for systemic side effects less severe with 2.5% solution. • Show patient how to instill. • Wash hands before and after administration. • May cause blurred vision. Warn patient not to drive car or operate machinery until this effect wears off.

NAME	INDICATIONS & DOSAGE	SIDE EFFECTS
scopolamine hydrobromide Isopto Hyoscine	*Cycloplegic refraction*— **Adults:** instill 1 to 2 drops 0.5% to 1% solution in eye 1 hour before refraction. **Children:** instill 1 drop 0.2% or 0.25% solution or ointment b.i.d. for 2 days before refraction. *Iritis*— **Adults:** 1 to 2 drops of 0.1% solution daily, b.i.d., or t.i.d.	**Eye:** ocular congestion with prolonged use, conjunctivitis, *blurred vision,* eye dryness, increased intraocular pressure, *photophobia,* contact dermatitis. **Systemic:** flushing, fever, dry skin and mouth, tachycardia, hallucinations, ataxia, irritability, confusion, delirium, somnolence.
tropicamide Mydriacyl♦	**Adults and children:** *Cycloplegic refractions*—instill 1 to 2 drops of 1% solution in each eye; repeat in 5 minutes. Additional drop may be instilled in 20 to 30 minutes. *Fundus examinations*—instill 1 to 2 drops 0.5% solution in each eye 15 to 20 minutes before examination.	**EENT:** *transient stinging on instillation,* increased intraocular pressure (less than with other mydriatic agents because of shorter duration of action), *blurred vision, photophobia,* dry mouth and throat.

♦ Available in U.S. and Canada. ♦♦ Available in Canada only. All other products (no symbol) available in U.S. only. Italicized side effects are common or life-threatening.

INTERACTIONS	NURSING CONSIDERATIONS
None significant.	• Contraindicated in primary glaucoma (shallow anterior chamber or narrow-angle). Use cautiously in cardiac disease, increased intraocular pressure, and in patients over 40 years. • Observe patient closely for systemic effects (disorientation, delirium). • Warn patient vision will be temporarily blurred; tell him not to drive car or operate machinery until this effect wears off. • Instruct patient to wear dark glasses to ease discomfort of photophobia. • Not for internal use. • May be used when patient is sensitive to atropine. Faster acting and has shorter duration of action and fewer side effects. • Show patient how to instill. Warn him not to touch dropper tip to eye or surrounding tissue. Wash hands before and after administration. • Systemic absorption may be minimized by compressing inner canthus of eye for 1 to 2 minutes after instilling drops. • For toxicity (if ingested), see APPENDIX, *Toxicities*.
None significant.	• Contraindicated in narrow-angle and shallow anterior chamber glaucoma. Use cautiously in elderly patients. • Shortest acting cycloplegic, but mydriatic effect greater than cycloplegic effect. • Causes transient stinging; vision temporarily blurred. Warn patient not to drive car or operate machinery until this effect wears off. • Instruct patient to wear dark glasses if photosensitivity occurs (lasts about 2 hours). • Store at room temperature in tightly closed container.

HOW PUPILS DILATE

The pupil helps control the amount of light that strikes the retina. Pupillary dilation (mydriasis) occurs when the dilator muscle fibers of the iris contract. (See illustration.) In normal indoor lighting, pupil dilation ranges from 3 to 6 mm in diameter. However, pupil size can range from a diameter of 2 mm to about 8 mm.

Although the tiny muscle fibers aren't visible to the naked eye, you can readily observe the action they produce. Pupillary dilation may indicate brain activity, emotional states, and interest levels. For example:

- Brain death has occurred when the pupil dilates to about 6 mm and does not contract when light is shown on the eye.
- Unequally dilated pupils may indicate increased intracranial pressure.
- Pupil dilation occurs in fight-or-flight reactions.
- Even advertisers have observed pupil dilation to measure viewer interest in their advertisements. The greater the pupil dilation, the greater the viewer's interest.

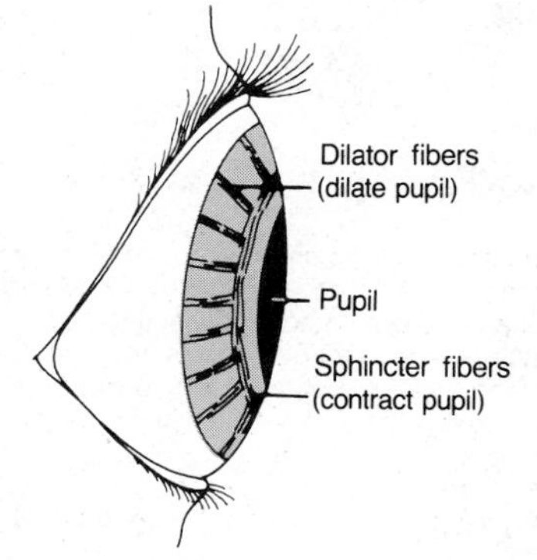

Ophthalmic vasoconstrictors

naphazoline hydrochloride
phenylephrine hydrochloride
tetrahydrozoline hydrochloride
zinc sulfate

Ophthalmic vasoconstrictors relieve the itching and redness of ocular irritations and inflammations. They are available as eye drops, without a prescription.

Major uses

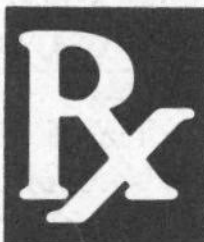

Ophthalmic vasoconstrictors furnish symptomatic relief of ocular congestion, irritation, and itching due to allergic conditions.

Mechanism of action

• Naphazoline, phenylephrine, and tetrahydrozoline produce vasocon-

PATIENT-TEACHING AID

WHEN YOU HAVE RED EYES

Dear Patient:

Irritated red eyes are a symptom of many serious eye diseases. How do you decide when to see a doctor and when to self-medicate with an over-the-counter (OTC) preparation? Consult a doctor if you notice any of the following symptoms:

• your vision is impaired
• your eye is painful
• your eye hurts when exposed to bright light
• your eyelids stick together
• there is any discharge of pus from your eyes
• the redness does not subside after using OTC decongestant eye drops for 2 days
• you suspect you have a foreign body in your eye.

Note: OTC decongestant eye drops should not be used by persons with *narrow-angle* glaucoma or an injured cornea. These preparations make the pupils dilate, which can precipitate a severe glaucoma attack. These attacks can cause blindness. Although the label carries the warning "Do not use in cases of glaucoma," OTC decongestant eye drops can be used by persons with *open-angle* glaucoma.

MATCHING SYMPTOMS WITH CAUSES OF CONJUNCTIVITIS

SYMPTOM	VIRAL	BACTERIAL Purulent	BACTERIAL Nonpurulent	FUNGAL AND PARASITIC	ALLERGIC
Discharge	Minimum	Copious	Minimum	Minimum	Minimum
Tearing	Copious	Moderate	Moderate	Minimum	Moderate
Itching	Minimum	Minimum	None	None	Marked
Localized conjunctival lesions	None	None	Common	Common	None
Preauricular nodes	Common	Uncommon	Common	Common	None
Associated sore throat and fever	Occasionally	Uncommon	None	None	None

Reproduced with permission from Vaughan, D., Asbury, T.: *General Ophthalmology,* 9th ed. Copyright 1980 by Lange Medical Publications, Los Altos, California.

striction by local adrenergic action on the blood vessels of the conjunctiva.
- Zinc sulfate produces astringent action on the conjunctiva.

Absorption, distribution, metabolism, and excretion
- Naphazoline, phenylephrine, and tetrahydrozoline are variably absorbed. The drugs may, however, be absorbed in high enough concentrations to cause systemic side effects, such as transient stinging and irritation, especially in young children.
- Zinc sulfate is not absorbed and has a local effect only.

Onset and duration
- Naphazoline, tetrahydrozoline, and zinc sulfate begin to act within 5 minutes after instillation. Naphazoline acts for as long as 3 to 4 hours; tetrahydrozoline and zinc sulfate are shorter-acting.
- Phenylephrine begins to act within 5 minutes after application; its effect continues for up to 3 hours.

Combination products
ALBALON-A♦: naphazoline hydrochloride 0.05% and antazoline phosphate 0.5%.
BLEPHAMIDE♦: phenylephrine hydrochloride 0.12%, sulfacetamide sodium 10%, and prednisolone acetate 0.2%.
M-Z: phenylephrine hydrochloride 0.12%, zinc sulfate 0.25%, and piperocaine hydrochloride 0.75%.
NEOZIN OPHTH: phenylephrine hydrochloride 0.125% and zinc sulfate 0.25%.
PHENYLZIN DROPS: zinc sulfate 0.25% and phenylephrine hydrochloride 0.12%.
PREFRIN-A♦: phenylephrine hydrochloride 0.12%, pyrilamine maleate 0.1%, and antipyrine 0.1%.
PREFIN-Z: phenylephrine hydrochloride 0.12% and zinc sulfate 0.24%.
VASOCIDIN♦: phenylephrine hydrochloride 0.125%, sodium sulfacetamide 10%, and prednisolone sodium phosphate 0.2%.
VASOCON-A♦: naphazoline hydrochloride 0.05% and antazoline phosphate 0.5%.

NAME	INDICATIONS & DOSAGE	SIDE EFFECTS
naphazoline hydrochloride 0.012%, 0.1%, 0.02% Albalon Liquifilm Ophthalmic♦, Clear Eyes, Naphcon, Naphcon Forte Ophthalmic♦, Opto-Zoline♦♦, Vasoclear, Vasocon Regular Ophthalmic♦	*Ocular congestion, irritation, itching—* **Adults:** instill 1 to 2 drops in eye q 3 to 4 hours.	**Eye:** transient stinging, pupillary dilation, increased intraocular pressure, irritation.
phenylephrine hydrochloride Isopto Frin, Prefrin, Tear-Efrin	*Decongestant, minor eye irritations—* **Adults and children:** 2 drops of 0.12% or 0.25% in affected eye. May repeat in 3 to 4 hours, p.r.n.	**CNS:** headache. **Eye:** transient stinging, iris floaters, narrow-angle glaucoma, blurred vision, reactive hyperemia, brow pain.
tetrahydrozoline hydrochloride Clear & Bright, Murine 2, Soothe, Tetrasine, Visine	*Ocular congestion, irritation, and allergic conditions—* **Adults, and children over 2 years:** instill 1 to 2 drops in eye b.i.d. or t.i.d., or as directed by doctor.	**Eye:** transient stinging, pupillary dilation, increased intraocular pressure, irritation, iris floaters in elderly. **Systemic:** drowsiness, CNS depression, cardiac irregularities, headache, dizziness, tremors, insomnia.
zinc sulfate Bufopto Zinc Sulfate, Eye-Sed Ophthalmic, Op-Thal-Zin	*Ocular congestion, irritation—* **Adults and children:** solution 0.2%—instill 1 to 2 drops in eye b.i.d. or t.i.d.	**Eye:** irritation.

INTERACTIONS	NURSING CONSIDERATIONS
MAO inhibitors: hypertensive crisis if naphazoline HCl is systemically absorbed. Use together cautiously.	• Contraindicated in narrow-angle glaucoma, hypersensitivity to any ingredients. Use cautiously in patients with hyperthyroidism, cardiac disease, hypertension, and diabetes mellitus, and in elderly patients. • Can produce marked sedation and coma if ingested by child. • Advise patient that photophobia may follow pupil dilation if he is sensitive to drug. Tell patient to report this to the doctor if it occurs. • Warn patient not to exceed recommended dosage. Rebound congestion and rhinitis may occur with frequent or prolonged use. • Notify doctor if blurred vision, pain, or lid edema develops. • Store in tightly closed container. • Most effective and widely used ocular decongestant. • Show patient how to instill. Do not touch tip of dropper to eye or surrounding tissues.
MAO inhibitors: may cause hypertensive crisis. Don't use together.	• Contraindicated in narrow-angle glaucoma, in patients taking tricyclic antidepressants or MAO inhibitors, and in hypersensitivity to any ingredient. • May exacerbate hypertension in hypertensive patients. • Do not use butacaine drops as local anesthetic, since phenylephrine and butacaine are incompatible. • Do not exceed prescribed dose. • Monitor blood pressure and pulse rate; watch for overdosage. • Do not use if solution is dark brown or contains precipitate. • Keep container tightly sealed and away from light. • Do not touch tip of dropper to eye or surrounding tissues. • Show patient how to instill. • Caution patient not to share eye medications with others.
MAO inhibitors: hypertensive crisis if tetrahydrozoline HCl is systemically absorbed. Don't use together.	• Contraindicated in patients receiving MAO inhibitors, and in those with hypersensitivity to any ingredients or narrow-angle glaucoma. Use cautiously in patients with hyperthyroidism, heart disease, hypertension, and diabetes mellitus, and in elderly patients. • Do not exceed recommended dosage. Rebound congestion and rhinitis may occur with frequent or prolonged use. • Warn patient to stop drug and notify doctor if relief is not obtained within 48 hours, or if redness or irritation persists or increases. • Available without prescription. • Available in 0.05% concentration; less effective than naphazoline hydrochloride 0.1%. • Warn patient not to touch dropper tip to eye or surrounding tissues. • Show patient how to instill. • Caution patient not to share eye medications with others.
None significant.	• Use cautiously in patients with a shallow anterior chamber, predisposition to narrow-angle glaucoma. • A decongestant astringent. • Store in tightly closed container. • Warn patient not to touch dropper tip to eye or surrounding tissues. • Show patient how to instill drops. • Caution patient not to share eye medications with others.

Topical ophthalmic anesthetics

cocaine hydrochloride
proparacaine hydrochloride
tetracaine hydrochloride

Topical ophthalmic anesthetics are used for various diagnostic and minor surgical procedures. They are not for self-medication and should be used only under a doctor's supervision.

Major uses

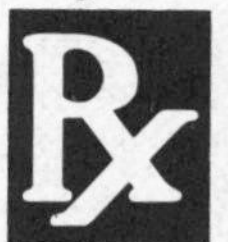

The drugs supply anesthesia in tonometric and gonioscopic procedures, suture removal from the cornea, and extraction of a foreign object from the cornea. They are also used as part of emergency management before flushing chemicals from the eye.

- Cocaine hydrochloride is also used to diagnose Horner's syndrome.

Mechanism of action

Topical ophthalmic anesthetics produce anesthesia by preventing initiation and transmission of impulses at the nerve-cell membrane.

- Cocaine hydrochloride also has an adrenergic action that produces mydriasis and constriction of conjunctival vessels.

Absorption, distribution, metabolism, and excretion

- Proparacaine and tetracaine are not absorbed systemically.
- Cocaine hydrochloride is absorbed systemically, metabolized in the liver, and excreted in urine.

Onset and duration

- Cocaine hydrochloride begins to act within 30 seconds; proparacaine, within 20 seconds; and tetracaine hydrochloride, within 1 minute after administration.
- Proparacaine provides anesthesia up to 15 minutes; tetracaine, up to 20 minutes.
- Cocaine hydrochloride provides complete anesthesia for 10 minutes, moderate anesthesia for another 5 to 10 minutes, and minimal anesthesia for as long as 2 hours.

Combination products

None.

HOW TO PROTECT THE ANESTHETIZED EYE

After applying topical ophthalmic anesthetics, the doctor may order an eye patch, to protect the patient's eye from dust, smoke, or other irritants. Here's how to apply it:

1. First, wash your hands. Ask the patient to close both eyes. Then, use as many sterile gauze pads as you need to fill the patient's orbital space. Next, grasp the sterile eye patch in the center and place it over the gauze pads, as shown here.

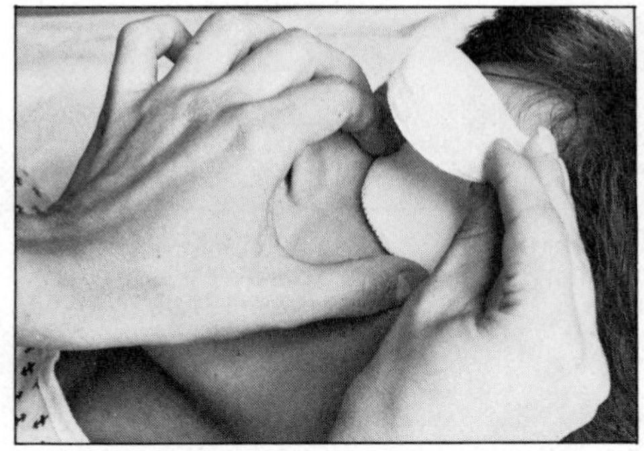

2. Secure the patch with two parallel strips of nonallergenic tape, preferably plastic. Work from the patient's mid-forehead to the cheekbone, as the nurse is doing here.

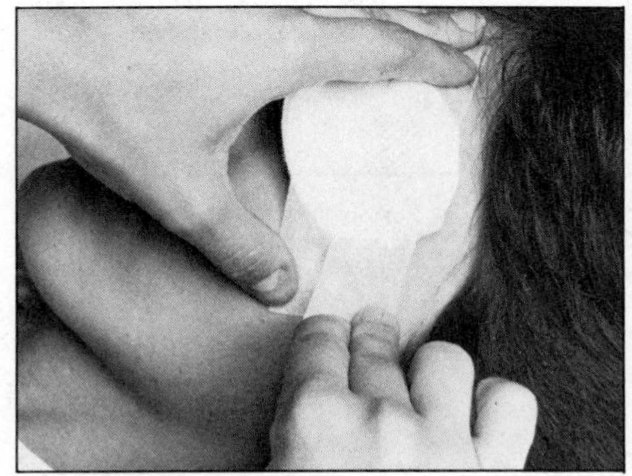

3. For added protection, the doctor may order an eyeshield (or eyecone). The eyeshield rests on the bony prominences of the brow, cheek, and nose without touching the underlying dressing. Tape the shield (or cone) in place, as shown here.

When it's time to instill the next dose of medication, remove the patch by loosening the tape from the forehead down. If you notice any drainage on the gauze or the patch, document your findings on the patient's chart.

Replace the gauze pads and patch (if soiled) each time you instill medication.

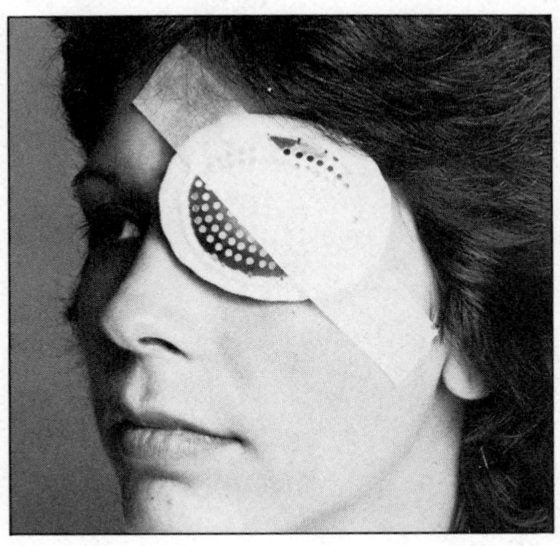

NAME	INDICATIONS & DOSAGE	SIDE EFFECTS
cocaine hydrochloride	*Diagnosis of Horner's syndrome, topical anesthesia for minor surgery or examinations*— **Adults and children:** instill 1 to 2 drops 4% solution in eye just before procedure or examination.	**Eye:** *blurring,* corneal ulceration or scarring in excessive or long-term use. Varying effects on intraocular pressure. **Systemic:** excitation; nervousness; rapid, shallow respirations; emesis; chills; fever; tachycardia; hypertension; euphoria; anxiety; delirium; convulsions; respiratory and circulatory failure.
proparacaine hydrochloride Alcaine♦, Ophthaine♦, Ophthetic♦	**Adults and children:** *Anesthesia for tonometry, gonioscopy; suture removal from cornea, removal of corneal foreign bodies*—instill 1 to 2 drops 0.5% solution in eye just before procedure. *Anesthesia for cataract extraction, glaucoma surgery*—instill 1 drop 0.5% solution in eye every 5 to 10 minutes for 5 to 7 doses.	**Eye:** occasional conjunctival redness, transient pain. **Other:** hypersensitivity.
tetracaine hydrochloride Anacel, Pontocaine♦	*Anesthesia for tonometry, gonioscopy; removal of corneal foreign bodies, suture removal from cornea; other diagnostic and minor surgical procedures*— **Adults and children:** instill 1 to 2 drops 0.5% solution in eye just before procedure.	**Eye:** transient stinging in eye 30 seconds after initial instillation, epithelial damage in excessive or long-term use. **Other:** sensitization in repeated use (allergic skin rash, urticaria).

♦ Available in U.S. and Canada. ♦♦ Available in Canada only. All other products (no symbol) available in U.S. only. Italicized side effects are common or life-threatening.

INTERACTIONS	NURSING CONSIDERATIONS
Epinephrine (topical): increased epinephrine effect. Use together cautiously.	• Use cautiously and sparingly in patients with known allergies, cardiac disease, hyperthyroidism, or open lesions. • Patient should be given short-acting barbiturate before administering to avoid CNS stimulation. • Solutions not commercially available; must be prepared specially by pharmacist. Rarely used. • Monitor heart rate after instillation; observe for systemic effects. • Warn patient that vision will be blurred for several hours. • Warn patient not to rub eye for at least 20 minutes after instillation. • Protective eyepatch recommended following procedure. • Solution should be pink. Return discolored solution to pharmacy. • Doesn't require refrigeration.
None significant.	• Use cautiously in cardiac diseases and hyperthyroidism. • *Not* for long-term use; may delay wound healing. • Warn patient not to rub or touch eye while cornea is anesthetized, since this may cause corneal abrasion and greater discomfort when anesthesia wears off. • Protective eyepatch recommended following procedure. • Warn patient corneal pain is relieved only temporarily in abrasion. • Systemic reactions unlikely when used in recommended doses. • Topical ophthalmic anesthetic of choice in diagnostic and minor surgical procedures. • Don't use discolored solution. • Store in tightly closed container. • Ophthaine brand packaged in bottle that looks similar in size and shape to Hemoccult. When taking bottle from shelf, check label carefully.
Sulfonamides: interference with sulfonamide antibacterial activity. Wait ½ hour after anesthesia before instilling sulfonamide.	• Systemic absorption unlikely in recommended doses. • Avoid repeated use. • Does not dilate the pupil, paralyze accommodation, or increase intraocular pressure. • Protective eyepatch recommended following procedure. • Don't use discolored solution. Keep container tightly closed.

83 Artificial tears

artificial tears
eye irrigation solutions

Artificial tears and external eye irrigation solutions are applied topically to relieve eyes that are deficient in or completely devoid of tear production. Among the components that make up these drugs are salts that are isotonic with tears, buffering agents for pH adjustment, viscosity agents to promote length of contact time with the eye, and preservatives to maintain solution integrity. Many of the drugs are available over the counter and without a prescription. The patient may have to try several of the commerically available products before he finds one that suits him.

Major uses

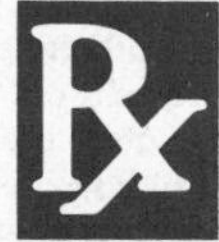

• Artificial tears are instilled in the eye to lubricate, remove debris, and protect against infection when tear production is insufficient.

• External eye irrigation solutions are sterile isotonic preparations used to irrigate the eyes after tonometry, gonioscopy, fluorescein dye examination, foreign-body removal, and other pro-

NURSING TIP

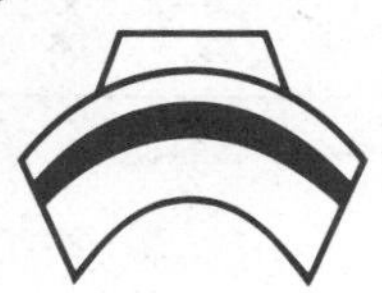

HOW TO IRRIGATE YOUR PATIENT'S EYE

Be sure to wash your hands before instilling eye irrigation. Then:

• Have the patient sit or lie with head tilted toward the affected side. Irrigating solution will flow from the inner canthus of the affected eye toward the outer canthus.

• Place a curved basin at the cheek on the side of the affected eye, to catch irrigating solution.

• Use gentle force to remove secretions as you direct the flow from the inner to the outer canthus. Do not touch any part of the eye with the irrigating tip.

• After irrigation, have the patient close her eyes and wipe excess solution from the lids and lashes.

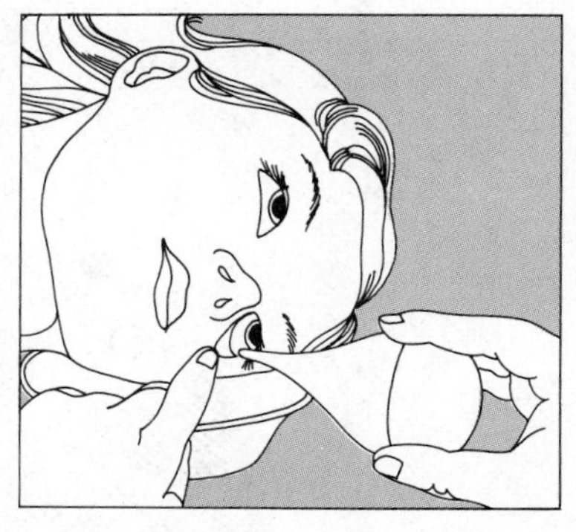

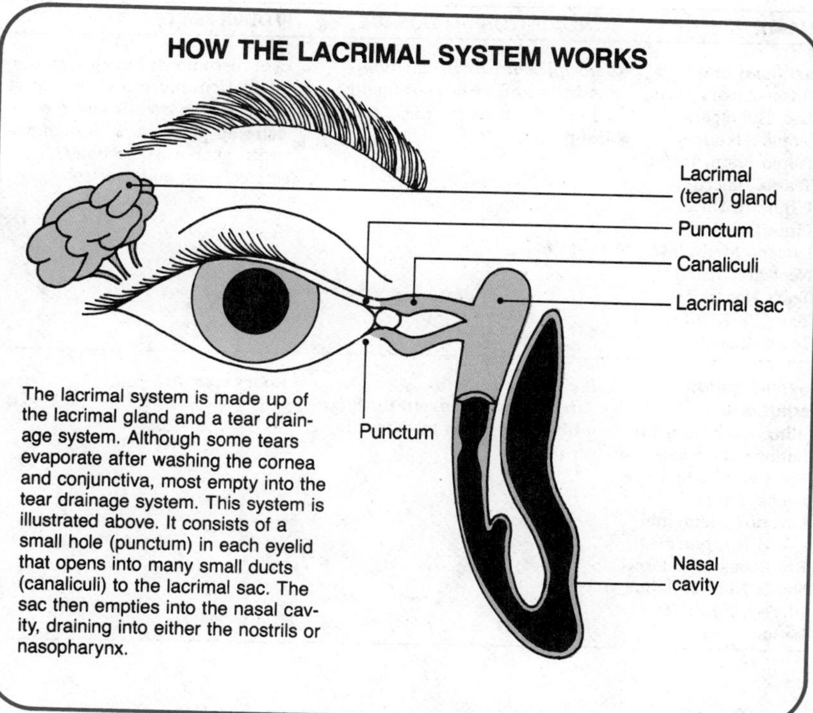

cedures. They also soothe minor eye irritation and are used in large quantities for caustic chemical injury.

HOW THE LACRIMAL SYSTEM WORKS
Lacrimal (tear) gland
Punctum
Canaliculi
Lacrimal sac
Punctum
Nasal cavity
The lacrimal system is made up of the lacrimal gland and a tear drainage system. Although some tears evaporate after washing the cornea and conjunctiva, most empty into the tear drainage system. This system is illustrated above. It consists of a small hole (punctum) in each eyelid that opens into many small ducts (canaliculi) to the lacrimal sac. The sac then empties into the nasal cavity, draining into either the nostrils or nasopharynx.

Mechanism of action

- Artificial tears augment insufficient tear production.
- External irrigation solutions clean the eye.

Absorption, distribution, metabolism, and excretion

The drugs are not systemically absorbed.

Onset and duration

The higher the viscosity of the artificial tear products, the longer the action. Duration of some artificial tear products are:

- Adsorbotear: 90 minutes or more
- Isopto Tears: 60 minutes
- Liquifilm Tears: 60 minutes
- Lyteers: 45 minutes
- Tearisol: 40 minutes or more
- Tears Naturale: 90 minutes or more.

Combination products

None.

NAME	INDICATIONS & DOSAGE	SIDE EFFECTS
artificial tears Adsorbotear♦, Bro-Lac, Hypotears, Isopto Alkaline, Isopto Plain, Isopto Tears♦, Lacril♦, Liquifilm Forte, Liquifilm Tears, Lyteers, Methulose, Neotears, Tearisol, Tears Naturale♦, Tears Plus, Ultra Tears, Visculose	*Insufficient tear production*— **Adults and children:** instill 1 to 2 drops in eye t.i.d., q.i.d., or p.r.n.	**Eye:** discomfort; burning, pain on instillation; blurred vision; crust formation on eyelids and eyelashes in products with high viscosity, such as Adsorbotear, Isopto Tears, and Tearisol.
eye irrigation solutions Blinx, Collyrium Eye Lotion♦, Dacriose, EyeStream, I-Lite Eye Drops, Lauro, Lavoptik Medicinal Eye Wash, Murine Eye Drops, Neo-Flow, Sterile Normal Saline (0.9%), Zoptic Eye Lotion	*Eye irrigation*— **Adults and children:** flush eye with 1 to 2 drops t.i.d., q.i.d., or p.r.n.	None reported.

♦ Available in U.S. and Canada. ♦♦ Available in Canada only. All other products (no symbol) available in U.S. only. Italicized side effects are common or life-threatening.

INTERACTIONS	NURSING CONSIDERATIONS
Borate external irrigation solutions: may form gummy deposits on the lid when used with artificial tear products containing polyvinyl alcohol (Liquifilm Forte, Liquifilm Tears). Keep patient's eyelids clean.	• Contraindicated in hypersensitivity to active product or preservatives. • Show patient how to instill. • Warn patient not to touch tip of container to eye, surrounding tissue, or other surface, to avoid contamination of solution. • Instruct patient that product should be used by one person only.
Products containing polyvinyl alcohol: may form gel and gummy deposits on the eye. Keep eyelids clean.	• Contraindicated in hypersensitivity to active ingredient or preservatives. • Don't touch tip of container to eye, surrounding tissue, or other surface, to avoid contamination. • Check date of expiration to make sure solution is potent. • Store in tightly closed, light-resistant container. • Show patient how to instill. • Should be used by one person only. • When irrigating, have patient turn his head to side and irrigate from inner to outer canthus. Have tissues handy.

NURSING TIP

TREATING A CHEMICAL EYE INJURY

When a patient has a chemical eye injury like the one illustrated here, what should you do until the doctor arrives? The general rule is to irrigate your patient's eye for at least 20 minutes with an irrigant solution, normal saline solution, or even tap water if you're at home. Irrigating the eye immediately can minimize further injury to delicate eye tissues. Irrigation can continue for up to an hour depending on the chemical involved. Don't worry about irrigating too much because, as one authority notes, "the proper method of irrigation is overirrigation."

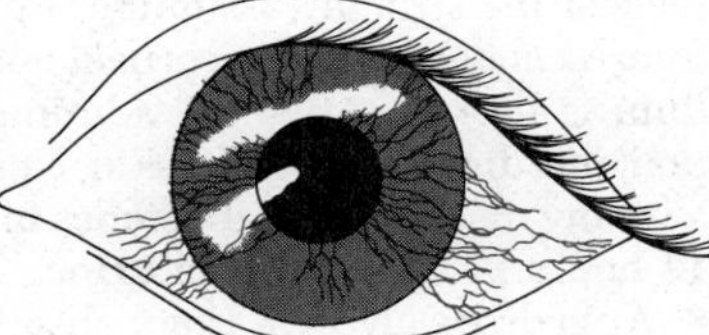

If you suspect an alkaline injury, the doctor will probably want you to check the pH during irrigation until neutral pH (7.0) is achieved. To do so, touch pH paper to the inner surface of the upper lid.

When the doctor arrives, depending on the severity of the injury, he may tell you to:

- dilate the pupil with 0.3% scopolamine drops to reduce pain caused by iris spasm
- instill an antibiotic eye drop
- administer a systemic analgesic.

If the injury involves the cornea, the doctor may:

- administer local corticosteroids
- apply a continuous-wear soft contact lens to encourage the growth of an epithelium over the injured area
- perform a corneal transplant if the cornea does not clear after healing has occurred.

Adapted with permission from "The Ailing Eye: Treat, Consult, Refer?" *Patient Care*, April 15, 1980.

Miscellaneous ophthalmics

alpha-chymotrypsin
dipivefrin
fluorescein sodium
glycerin, anhydrous
sodium chloride, hypertonic
timolol maleate

For information on isosorbide solution, see APPENDIX, *New Drugs*.

These drugs are used for various purposes in medical, surgical, and diagnostic procedures.

Major uses

- Alpha-chymotrypsin is a fast-acting proteolytic enzyme that aids cataract extraction.
- Dipivefrin reduces intraocular pressure in chronic open-angle glaucoma.
- Fluorescein is a dye used for various diagnostic procedures.
- Anhydrous glycerin temporarily restores transparency when the cornea is too edematous to permit diagnosis in ophthalmoscopy or gonioscopy.
- Hypertonic sodium chloride reduces edema after surgery and in trauma, bullous keratopathy, and corneal edema associated with excessive use of contact lenses.
- Timolol lowers intraocular pressure in open-angle glaucoma, ocular hypertension, aphakic glaucoma, and secondary glaucoma.

Mechanism of action

- Alpha-chymotrypsin dissolves filaments or zonules holding the lens.
- Dipivefrin is a prodrug of epinephrine (in the eye, dipivefrin is converted to epinephrine). The liberated epinephrine appears to decrease aqueous production and increase aqueous outflow.
- Fluorescein produces an intense green fluorescence in alkaline solution (pH 5.0 or less) or a bright yellow if viewed under cobalt blue illumination.
- Glycerin and sodium chloride remove excess fluid from the cornea.
- Timolol, classified as a beta blocker, reduces aqueous formation and possibly increases aqueous outflow. It has little or no effect on pupil size.

Absorption, distribution, metabolism, and excretion

- Alpha-chymotrypsin is not absorbed and must be instilled into the posterior chamber. It is removed by irrigation with saline solution.
- Dipivefrin and hypertonic sodium chloride are not absorbed when recommended dosages are used.
- Fluorescein doesn't penetrate an intact corneal epithelium but is distributed to the stroma (assuming a green fluorescence) when the corneal epithelium is broken. After I.V. administration, it is distributed to the skin, causing a yellow discoloration that fades in 6 to 12 hours. It is excreted in urine.
- Anhydrous glycerin is not absorbed.
- Timolol is absorbed systemically in varying amounts. The beta blockade may cause systemic side effects such as

HOW TO USE FLUORESCEIN STAIN

Moisten a fluorescein paper strip or prepare fluorescein solution, and instill the dye in the inferior conjunctival cul-de-sac (illustration 1). The dye will distribute itself over the cornea in the tear film.

When surface irregularities are present, fluorescein-stained tears pool in the corneal depressions (illustration 2) and fluoresce bright yellow-green in cobalt blue or ultraviolet light.

Such depressions may be minor surface irregularities of the healthy cornea (illustration 3). If so, irrigation of the corneal surface washes pooled fluorescein out of these depressions.

If the depression is caused by an abrasion that has scraped away the corneal epithelium and exposed the underlying stromal connective tissue (illustration 4), fluorescein stains the underlying tissue. In this case, the fluorescein stain remains after irrigation, indicating injury.

Note: Remove soft contact lenses before applying fluorescein, as dye may permanently stain the lenses. Rinse the eye thoroughly after examination, to prevent chemical conjunctivitis from fluorescein residue.

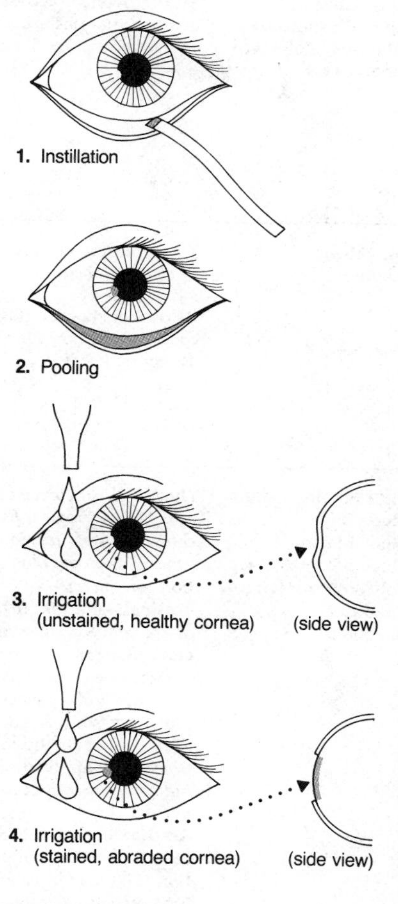

Adapted with permission from George O. Waring III, "The Eye at First Sight," *Emergency Medicine,* November 15, 1979.

bradycardia and bronchospasm.

Onset and duration

- Alpha-chymotrypsin and anhydrous glycerin begin to act within 1 to 2 minutes after administration. Both drugs have a short duration of action (only minutes).
- Dipivefrin and timolol begin to work within 30 minutes after administration. Maximal effect occurs in 1 hour. Therapeutic action lasts up to 24 hours.
- Fluorescein begins to act immediately after instillation, and its duration is about 30 minutes. After I.V. administration, fluorescein dye appears in the retinal vessels after 13 seconds and remains 20 seconds.
- Hypertonic sodium chloride's effect lasts up to 4 hours.

Combination products

FLURESS: sodium fluorescein 0.25% and benoxinate HCl 0.4%.

NAME	INDICATIONS & DOSAGE	SIDE EFFECTS
alpha-chymotrypsin Alpha Chymar, Alpha Chymolean♦♦, Catarase♦, Zolyse♦, Zonulyn♦♦	*Zonulysis in cataract surgery—* **Adults over 20 years:** 1 to 2 ml instilled into posterior chamber under the iris, by doctor.	**Eye:** transient increase in intraocular pressure (dose-related), moderate uveitis, corneal edema and striation.
dipivefrin Propine	*To reduce intraocular pressure in chronic open-angle glaucoma—* **Adults:** for initial glaucoma therapy, 1 drop in eye q 12 hours.	**Eye:** burning, stinging. **CV:** tachycardia, hypertension.
fluorescein sodium Fluorescite, Fluor-I-Strip, Fluor-I-Strip-A.T.♦, Ful-Glo Strips♦, Funduscein Injections	*Diagnostic in corneal abrasions and foreign bodies; fitting hard contact lenses; lacrimal patency; fundus photography; applanation tonometry—* **Topical:** Solution: instill 1 drop of 2% solution followed by irrigation, or moisten strip with sterile water. Touch conjunctiva or fornix with moistened tip. Flush eye with irrigating solution. Patient should blink several times after application. *Indicated in retinal angiography—* **Adults:** 5 ml of 10% solution (500 mg) or 3 ml of 25% solution (750 mg) injected rapidly into antecubital vein, by doctor. **Children:** 0.077 ml of 10% solution (7.7 mg/kg body weight) or 0.044 ml of 25% solution (11 mg/kg body weight) injected rapidly into antecubital vein, by doctor.	Topical use: **Eye:** stinging, burning. Intravenous use: **CNS:** headache persisting for 24 to 36 hours. **GI:** nausea, vomiting. **GU:** bright yellow urine (persists for 24 to 36 hours). **Skin:** yellow skin discoloration (fades in 6 to 12 hours). **Local:** extravasation at injection site, thrombophlebitis. **Other:** hypersensitivity, including urticaria and *anaphylaxis.*
glycerin, anhydrous Ophthalgan	*Corneal edema before ophthalmoscopy or gonioscopy in acute glaucoma and bullous keratitis—* **Adults and children:** instill 1 to 2 drops glycerin, anhydrous after instilling a local anesthetic.	**Eye:** pain if instilled without topical anesthetic.

♦ Available in U.S. and Canada. ♦♦ Available in Canada only. All other products (no symbol) available in U.S. only. Italicized side effects are common or life-threatening.

INTERACTIONS	NURSING CONSIDERATIONS
Alcohol, surgical detergent: inactivated alpha-chymotrypsin. Rinse off all alcohol or detergents from surgical instruments and syringe with saline solution.	• Contraindicated in high vitreous pressure with gaping incisional wound; congenital cataract. • Solutions very unstable. Use only freshly reconstituted solution. Don't use if it is cloudy or has precipitated. Discard unused portions, including diluent, except for Zonulyn. Retains potency 1 week at room temperature, or for 1 month when refrigerated. • Remove drug by irrigating with intraocular balanced saline solution. • Don't autoclave powder or reconstituted solution; excess heat will inactivate the enzyme. • Delayed healing of incision has been reported but not confirmed.
None significant.	• Contraindicated in narrow-angle glaucoma. • Use cautiously in patients with aphakia. • Dipivefrin is a prodrug of epinephrine: converted to epinephrine when it enters the eye. • May have fewer side effects than conventional epinephrine therapy. • Often used concomitantly with other antiglaucoma drugs. • Available as a 0.1% solution in 5-, 10-, and 15-ml dropper bottles. • Teach patient how to instill. • Wash hands before and after administration. • Don't touch dropper to eye or surrounding tissue.
None significant.	• Use with caution in patients with history of allergy or bronchial asthma. • Use topical anesthetic before instilling to partially relieve burning and irritation. • Always use sterile technique. Easily contaminated by *Pseudomonas.* • Yellow skin discoloration may persist 6 to 12 hours. • Warn patient urine will be bright yellow after I.V. injection. • Routine urinalysis will be abnormal within 1 hour after I.V. injection. • A water-soluble dye. • Don't freeze; store below 80° F. (26.7° C.). • Defects appear green under normal light, or bright yellow under cobalt blue illumination. Foreign bodies are surrounded by a green ring. Similar lesions of the conjunctiva are delineated in orange-yellow. • Always keep an emergency tray with antihistamine, epinephrine, and oxygen available when giving parenterally. • For symptoms and treatment of anaphylaxis, see inside front cover.
None significant.	• Use topical tetracaine HCl or proparacaine HCl before instilling to prevent discomfort. • Don't touch tip of dropper to eye, surrounding tissues, or tear-film; glycerin will absorb moisture. • Used to temporarily restore corneal transparency when cornea is too edematous to permit diagnosis. • Store in tightly closed container.

NAME	INDICATIONS & DOSAGE	SIDE EFFECTS
sodium chloride, hypertonic Adsorbonac Ophthalmic Solution, Hypersal Ophthalmic Solution, Methylcellulose Ophthalmic Solution, Muro Ointment, Murocoll, Sodium Chloride Ointment 5%	*Corneal edema (postoperative) after cataract extraction or corneal transplantation; also in trauma or bullous keratopathy—* **Adults and children:** instill 1 to 2 drops q 3 to 4 hours, or apply ointment at bedtime.	**Eye:** slight stinging. **Other:** hypersensitivity.
timolol maleate Timoptic Solution	*Chronic open-angle glaucoma, secondary glaucoma, aphakic glaucoma, ocular hypertension—* **Adults:** initially, instill 1 drop 0.25% solution in each eye b.i.d.; reduce to 1 drop daily for maintenance. If patient doesn't respond, instill 1 drop 0.5% solution in each eye b.i.d. If intraocular pressure is controlled, dosage may be reduced to 1 drop in each eye daily.	**Eye:** minor irritation. Long-term use may decrease corneal sensitivity. **CV:** bradycardia, syncope. **Other:** apnea in infants, *respiratory distress (evidence of beta blockade and systemic absorption).*

◆ Available in U.S. and Canada. ◆◆ Available in Canada only. All other products (no symbol) available in U.S. only. Italicized side effects are common or life-threatening.

INTERACTIONS	NURSING CONSIDERATIONS
None significant.	• An osmotic agent used to reduce corneal edema when repeated instillation is indicated. • May use few drops of sterile irrigation solution inside bottle cap to prevent caking on dropper bottle tip. • Store in tightly closed container. • Don't touch tip of dropper or tube to eye or surrounding tissue. • Show patient how to instill.
Propranolol HCl, metoprolol tartrate, other oral beta-adrenergic blocking agents: increased ocular and systemic effect. Use together cautiously. *MAO inhibitors, other adrenergic-augmenting psychotropic drugs:* hazardous increased effect. Use together cautiously.	• Contraindicated in bronchial asthma, and severe chronic obstructive pulmonary disease. Use cautiously in sinus bradycardia, second- and third-degree heart block, cardiogenic shock, right ventricular failure resulting from pulmonary hypertension, congestive heart failure, severe cardiac disease, and in infants with congenital glaucoma. • Warn patient not to touch dropper to eye or surrounding tissue. • Beta-adrenergic blocking agent in ophthalmic solution. • Can be used safely in patient with glaucoma who wears conventional (PMMA) hard contact lenses. • Show patient how to instill. Teach patient to lightly press lacrimal sac with finger after drug administration to decrease chance of systemic absorption.

DRUG ALERT

NEW CAUTIONS FOR USING TIMOLOL

Timolol maleate (Timoptic) now carries additional warnings concerning ocular irritations, hypersensitivity reactions, visual disturbances, and precipitation or aggravation of certain cardiovascular and pulmonary disorders.

This beta blocker is absorbed into the systemic circulation and can cause bradycardia, hypotension, syncope, and bronchospasm (mostly in patients with preexisting bronchospastic disease).

FDA reports associate the use of timolol eye drops not only with precipitation and aggravation of bronchospasm, but also with one fatality, that of a patient with status asthmaticus.

85 Otics

acetic acid
benzocaine
boric acid
carbamide peroxide
chloramphenicol
colistin B sulfate
dexamethasone sodium phosphate
hydrocortisone
hydrocortisone acetate
methylprednisolone disodium phosphate
neomycin sulfate
oxytetracycline hydrochloride
polymyxin B sulfate
triethanolamine polypeptide oleate-condensate

Most otics act locally; many are combinations of two or more drugs.

Major uses

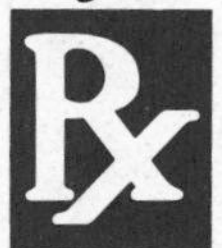

The otics are used to treat infection, inflammation, and pain of internal or external ear disorders (swimmer's ear, perforation, and otitis media) and are therapeutic adjuncts in surgical procedures (myringotomy and fenestration).

- Carbamide peroxide and triethanolamine also soften impacted cerumen.

Mechanism of action

- Anti-infectives (acetic acid, boric acid, chloramphenicol, colistin B, neomycin, oxytetracycline, and polymyxin B) inhibit or destroy bacteria present in the ear canal.
- Corticosteroids (dexamethasone, hydrocortisone, and methylprednisolone) control inflammation, edema, and pruritus.
- The local anesthetic benzocaine produces analgesic effects.
- Ceruminolytics (carbamide peroxide and triethanolamine) emulsify and disperse accumulated cerumen.

Absorption, distribution, metabolism, and excretion

Long-term use of corticosteroids and certain antibiotics (for example, neomycin) may result in some systemic absorption. The other drugs aren't significantly absorbed systemically.

Onset and duration

- Most otics begin to act within 1 hour, but full therapeutic effect may not be seen for 2 or 3 days.
- The short action of benzocaine requires repeated doses every 2 hours.

Combination products

ADRENOMYXIN♦♦: Each ml contains neomycin SO_4 5 mg, polymyxin B SO_4 10,000 units, and hydrocortisone 10 mg.
COLY-MYCIN S OTIC: Each ml contains neomycin SO_4 5 mg, colistin SO_4 3 mg, hydrocortisone acetate 10 mg, and thonzonium bromide 0.5%.
CORTISPORIN OTIC♦: Each ml contains neomycin SO_4 5 mg, polymyxin B SO_4 10,000 units, and hydrocortisone 1%.
LIDOSPORIN OTIC♦: Each ml contains polymyxin B SO_4 10,000 units and lidocaine HCl 50 mg.
NEO-CORT-DOME OTIC : Each ml con-

tains neomycin SO_4 5 mg, acetic acid 2%, and hydrocortisone 1%.
NEOCORTEF♦♦: Each ml contains neomycin SO_4 5 mg and hydrocortisone acetate 5 mg.
PENTAMYCETIN HC♦♦: Each ml contains chloramphenicol 2 mg and hydrocortisone acetate 10 mg.

PATIENT-TEACHING AID

HOME CARE: USING EAR DROPS CORRECTLY

Dear Patient:

Here's how to administer ear drops safely to yourself or to a child. The general directions apply to both procedures.

General directions

- Wash your hands thoroughly.
- Check the drops for discoloration and sediment. If the drops are in a clear bottle, hold the bottle to the light. If they're in a dark bottle, shake the bottle well, draw some medication into the dropper, and hold the dropper to the light. If the drops are discolored or contain sediment, have the prescription refilled.
- Warm the drops by rolling the bottle between your palms for 2 minutes.
- After instilling the drops, recap the bottle and store it in a cool, dark place.

Giving drops to yourself

- Shake the bottle, if directed, and open it. Fill the dropper and place the bottle within reach.
- Lie on your side so that the ear to be treated is facing up. Then, gently pull the top of your ear up and back to straighten the ear canal.
- Position the dropper above, but not touching the ear, and release the prescribed number of drops.
- To retain the drops in the ear, remain on your side for 10 minutes. If desired, plug the ear with cotton moistened with the ear drops. Don't use dry cotton, because it will absorb the drops.
- If directed, repeat the procedure for the other ear.

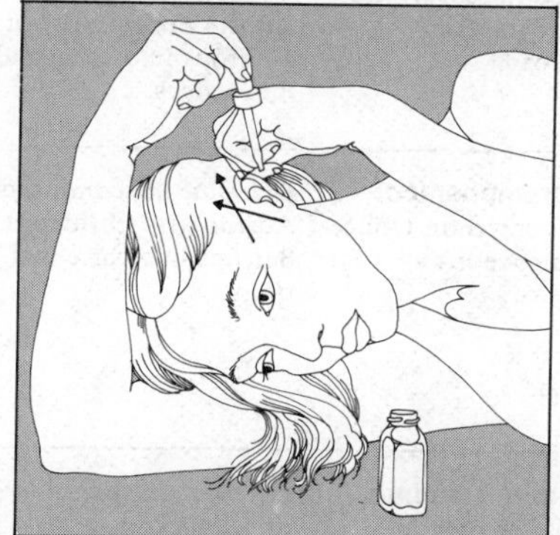

Giving drops to a child

- Lay the child on his side so that the ear to be treated is facing up.
- Gently pull the ear down and back, then slowly release the prescribed number of drops. (Note the difference in the direction the ear is moved for a child. This is due to the immaturity of the child's ear cartilage.)
- If the child has any pain after you've given the drops, notify the doctor.

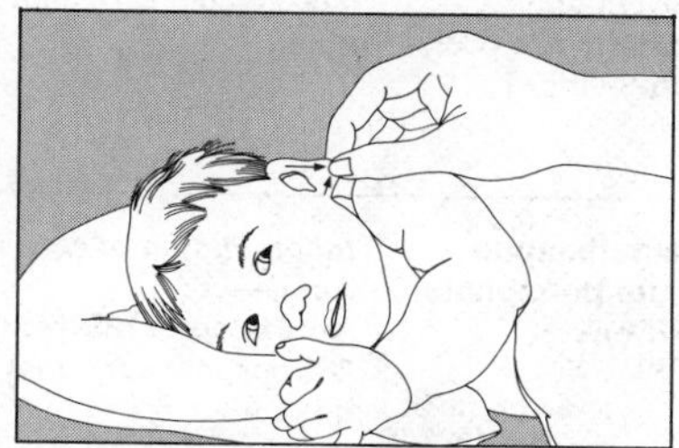

NAME	INDICATIONS & DOSAGE	SIDE EFFECTS
acetic acid Domeboro Otic♦, VoSol Otic♦	*External ear canal infection—* **Adults and children:** 4 to 6 drops into ear canal t.i.d. or q.i.d., or insert saturated wick for first 24 hours, then continue with instillations. *Prophylaxis of swimmer's ear—* **Adults and children:** 2 drops in each ear b.i.d.	**Ear:** irritation or itching. **Skin:** urticaria. **Other:** overgrowth of nonsusceptible organisms.
benzocaine Americaine-Otic, Auralgan♦, Aurasol, Eardro, Myringacaine, Tympagesic	*Cerumen removal—* **Adults and children:** fill ear canal t.i.d. for 2 days. *Pain from otitis media—* **Adults and children:** fill ear canal with solution and plug with cotton. May repeat q 1 to 2 hours, p.r.n.	**Ear:** irritation or itching. **Skin:** urticaria. **Other:** edema.
boric acid Ear-Dry, Swim-Ear, Swim 'n Clear	*External ear canal infection—* **Adults and children:** fill ear canal with solution and plug with cotton. Repeat t.i.d. or q.i.d.	**Ear:** irritation or itching. **Skin:** urticaria. **Other:** overgrowth of nonsusceptible organisms.
carbamide peroxide Benadyne Ear, Debrox♦	*Impacted cerumen—* **Adults and children:** 5 to 10 drops into ear canal b.i.d. for 3 to 4 days.	None reported.
chloramphenicol Chloromycetin Otic♦, Sopamycetin♦♦	*External ear canal infection—* **Adults and children:** 2 to 3 drops into ear canal t.i.d. or q.i.d.	**Ear:** itching or burning. **Local:** pruritus, burning, urticaria, vesicular or maculopapular dermatitis. **Systemic:** sore throat, angioedema. **Other:** overgrowth of nonsusceptible organisms.
colistin B sulfate available only in combination with neomycin and hydrocortisone (Coly-Mycin-S-Otic♦)	*External ear canal infection and otitis media—* **Adults and children:** 3 to 5 drops into ear canal t.i.d. or q.i.d.	**Ear:** ototoxicity in patient with a perforated eardrum and in patient undergoing tympanoplasty; irritation, itching. **Other:** overgrowth of nonsusceptible organisms.
dexamethasone sodium phosphate Decadron♦	*Inflammation of external ear canal—* **Adults and children:** 1 to 2 drops into ear canal t.i.d. or q.i.d.	**Systemic:** adrenal suppression with long-term use. **Other:** masking or exacerbation of underlying infection.

♦ Available in U.S. and Canada. ♦♦ Available in Canada only. All other products (no symbol) available in U.S. only. Italicized side effects are common or life-threatening.

INTERACTIONS	NURSING CONSIDERATIONS
None significant.	• Use cautiously in perforated eardrum. • Has anti-infective, anti-inflammatory, and antipruritic effects. • *Pseudomonas aeruginosa* particularly sensitive to drug. • Reculture persistent drainage.
None significant.	• Contraindicated in perforated eardrum. • Local anesthetic effect only. • Use with antibiotic to treat underlying cause of pain, because use alone may mask more serious condition. • Tell patient to call doctor if pain lasts longer than 48 hours. • Avoid touching ear with dropper. Do not rinse dropper. • Irrigate ear gently to remove impacted cerumen. • Keep container tightly closed and away from moisture.
None significant.	• Contraindicated in perforated eardrum or excoriated membranes in ear. • Watch for signs of superinfection (continual pain, inflammation, fever). • Weak bacteriostatic action; also fungistatic agent. • If cotton plug used, always moisten with medication. • Avoid touching ear with dropper.
None significant.	• Contraindicated in perforated eardrum. • Tell patient to call doctor if redness, pain, or swelling persists. • Ceruminolytic agent. • Irrigation of ear may be necessary to aid in removal of cerumen. • Tip of dropper should not touch ear or ear canal.
None significant.	• Avoid prolonged use. • Obtain history of use and reaction to drug. • Watch for signs of superinfection (continued pain, inflammation, fever). • Reculture persistent drainage. • Watch for signs of sore throat (early sign of toxicity). • Bacteriostatic agent. • Avoid touching ear with dropper.
None significant.	• Watch for signs of superinfection (continued pain, inflammation, fever). • Reculture persistent drainage. • Observe for signs of hearing loss. • Bactericidal agent. • Avoid prolonged use. • Shake well before using. • Avoid touching ear with dropper.
None significant.	• Contraindicated in perforated eardrum, fungal infections, herpes or other viral infections. • Use with antibiotic to treat inflammation caused by infection. • Use alone in allergic otitis externa. • Anti-inflammatory agent. • Avoid touching ear with dropper.

NAME	INDICATIONS & DOSAGE	SIDE EFFECTS
hydrocortisone **hydrocortisone acetate** Cortamed♦♦, Otall	*Inflammation of external ear canal—* **Adults and children:** 3 to 5 drops into ear canal t.i.d. or q.i.d. Available in 0.25%, 0.5%, and 1% concentrations.	**Systemic:** adrenal suppression with long-term use. **Other:** may mask or exacerbate underlying infection.
methylprednisolone disodium phosphate Medrol♦♦	*Inflammation of external ear canal—* **Adults and children:** 2 to 3 drops into ear canal t.i.d. or q.i.d.	**Systemic:** adrenal suppression with long-term use. **Other:** may mask or exacerbate underlying infection.
neomycin sulfate Otobiotic	*External ear canal infection—* **Adults and children:** 2 to 5 drops into ear canal t.i.d. or q.i.d.	**Ear:** ototoxicity (in patients undergoing tympanoplasty). **Local:** burning, erythema, vesicular dermatitis, urticaria. **Other:** overgrowth of nonsusceptible organisms.
oxytetracycline hydrochloride available only in combination with polymyxin B sulfate (Terramycin) or polymyxin B sulfate and hydrocortisone (Terra-Cortril♦♦)	*External ear canal infection—* **Adults and children:** instill ½ inch of ointment into external ear canal t.i.d. or q.i.d.	**Ear:** irritation, itching, urticaria. **Other:** overgrowth of nonsusceptible organisms.
polymyxin B sulfate Aerosporin♦	*Acute and chronic otitis externa, otitis media if tympanic membrane perforated; otomycosis—* **Adults and children:** 3 to 4 drops t.i.d. or q.i.d.	**Ear:** irritation, itching, urticaria. **Other:** overgrowth of nonsusceptible organisms.
triethanolamine polypeptide oleate-condensate Cerumenex♦	*Impacted cerumen—* **Adults and children:** fill ear canal with solution and insert cotton plug. After 15 to 30 minutes, flush ear with warm water.	**Ear:** erythema, pruritus. **Skin:** severe eczema.

♦ Available in U.S. and Canada. ♦♦ Available in Canada only. All other products (no symbol) available in U.S. only. Italicized side effects are common or life-threatening.

INTERACTIONS	NURSING CONSIDERATIONS
None reported.	• Contraindicated in perforated eardrum, fungal infections, herpes or other viral infections. • Use with antibiotic to treat inflammation caused by infection. • Use alone in allergic otitis externa. • Anti-inflammatory agent. • Avoid touching ear with dropper.
None significant.	• Contraindicated in perforated eardrum, fungal infection, herpes or other viral infections. • Use with antibiotic to treat inflammation caused by infection. • Use alone to treat seborrheic, contact, or uninfected eczematoid dermatitis. • Anti-inflammatory agent. • Avoid touching ear with dropper.
None significant.	• Contraindicated in perforated eardrum. • Obtain history of use and reaction to neomycin. • Observe for signs of hearing loss. • Watch for signs of superinfection (continued pain, inflammation, fever). • Reculture persistent drainage. • Bactericidal agent. • Best used in combination with other antibiotics. • Avoid touching ear with dropper.
None significant.	• Obtain history of reaction to tetracyclines. • Watch for signs of superinfection (continued pain, inflammation, fever). • Reculture persistent drainage. • Bacteriostatic agent.
None significant.	• Watch for signs of superinfection (continued pain, inflammation, fever). • Reculture persistent drainage. • Bactericidal agent. • Best used in combination with other antibiotics. • Keep container tightly closed and away from moisture. • Avoid touching ear with dropper.
None significant.	• Contraindicated in perforated eardrum, otitis media, and allergies. Do patch test by placing 1 drop of drug on inner forearm; cover with small bandage. Read in 24 hours. If any reaction (redness, swelling) occurs, don't use drug. • Tell patient not to use drops more often than prescribed. Flush ear gently with warm water, using soft rubber bulb ear syringe, within 30 minutes after instillation. • Ceruminolytic agent. • Moisten cotton plug with medication before insertion. • Keep container tightly closed and away from moisture. • Avoid touching ear with dropper.

86 Oral and nasal agents

benzocaine
carbamide peroxide
cocaine hydrochloride
dexamethasone sodium phosphate
ephedrine sulfate
epinephrine hydrochloride
lidocaine hydrochloride
naphazoline hydrochloride
oxymetazoline hydrochloride
phenylephrine hydrochloride
piperocaine hydrochloride
tetrahydrozoline hydrochloride
triamcinolone acetonide
xylometazoline hydrochloride

For information on beclomethasone dipropionate and flunisolide, see APPENDIX, *New Drugs*.

Oral and nasal agents are used alone or with other drugs to treat conditions affecting the nose and mouth. Many over-the-counter preparations are combinations of these drugs. Combinations for nasal use may also contain antihistamines.

Major uses

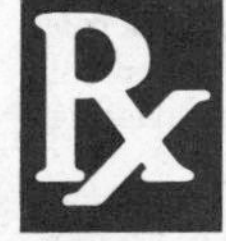

• Carbamide peroxide cleans and debrides, provides antimicrobial activity, and is a therapeutic adjunct in oral inflammations.

• Corticosteroids (dexamethasone and triamcinolone) reduce inflammation in allergic or inflammatory conditions and in nasal polyps. They're also used to treat stomatitis and traumatic oral lesions.

• Local anesthetics (benzocaine, cocaine hydrochloride, lidocaine, and piperocaine) produce anesthesia for rhinolaryngologic examination, laryngoscopic or bronchoscopic surgical procedures, and endotracheal intubation. They also relieve the pain of dental extractions.

• Sympathomimetic vasoconstrictors, (ephedrine, epinephrine, naphazoline, oxymetazoline, phenylephrine, tetrahydrozoline, and xylometazoline) relieve nasal congestion of the common cold, sinusitis, allergy, or chronic or vasomotor rhinitis.

Epinephrine also controls local superficial bleeding.

Mechanism of action

• Carbamide peroxide serves as a source of hydrogen peroxide to produce nascent oxygen, which aids in cleaning and debriding.

• Corticosteroids reduce inflammation and help heal oral ulcers and lesions by interfering with the protein synthesis of various enzymes.

• Local anesthetics block nerve conduction through sensory nerve fibers.

• Sympathomimetic agents produce local vasoconstriction of dilated arterioles to reduce blood flow and nasal congestion.

Absorption, distribution, metabolism, and excretion

Oral and nasal agents are minimally absorbed when used in recommended dosages.

Onset and duration

Onset and duration of action vary with

POSITIONING A PATIENT TO TREAT SINUSES

Proetz position

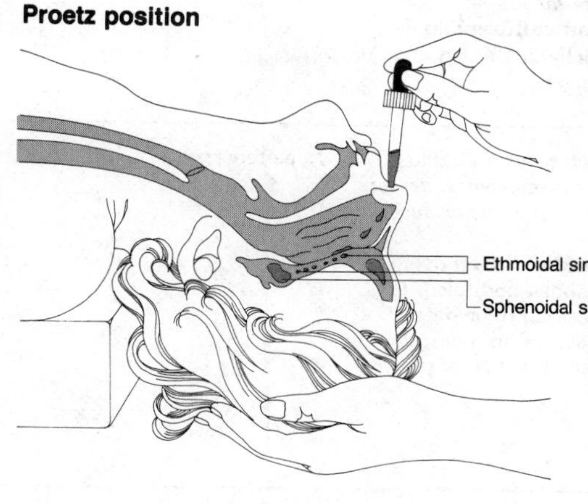

To instill medication in both the ethmoidal and the sphenoidal sinuses, place your patient on his back, with shoulders elevated and head tilted back. This is the Proetz position.

Parkinson position

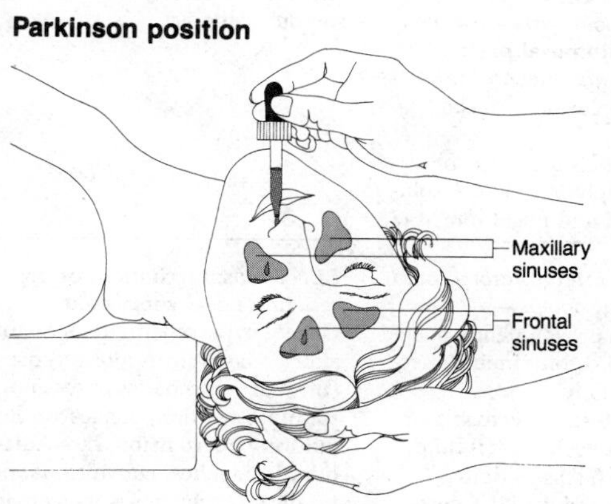

Use the Parkinson position to treat the maxillary and the frontal sinuses, located on each side of the face. As you can see here, this position is like the Proetz position, except the patient's head is tilted to one side instead of straight back.

Important: No matter which position you use, take care not to contaminate the dropper by touching the nostrils.

the drug, patient response, and conditions being treated. In general, oral and nasal drugs begin to act quickly due to their easy penetration into mucous membranes. The duration of action of local anesthetics depends on the amount of time the drug is in contact with nerve tissue.

Combination products

CHLOROHIST NASAL SPRAY: phenylephrine hydrochloride 0.25%, methapyriline hydrochloride 0.15%, and benzalkonium chloride 0.02%.

4-WAY NASAL SPRAY: phenylephrine hydrochloride 0.5%, naphazoline hydrochloride 0.05%, and pyrilamine maleate 0.2%.

NEO-VADRIN NASAL DECONGESTANT DROPS: phenylephrine hydrochloride 0.15% and phenylpropanolamine hydrochloride 0.4%, with chlorobutanol 0.15% and benzalkonium chloride 0.005%.

NTZ NASAL DROPS: phenylephrine hydrochloride 0.5% and thenyldiamine hydrochloride 0.1%, with benzalkonium chloride 1:5,000.

NAME	INDICATIONS & DOSAGE	SIDE EFFECTS
benzocaine Colrex, Dentition Syrup♦♦, Orabase with Benzocaine, Oracin, Ora-Jel, Spec-T Anesthetic, Trocaine, Tyzomint	*Pain from toothache, cold sore, canker sore, oral irritation, minor sore throat—* **Adults and children:** apply syrup or jelly to affected area, or suck lozenges.	**Skin:** hypersensitivity. **Other:** possible tolerance.
carbamide peroxide Cank-aid, Clear Drops, Gly-Oxide♦, Proxigel	*Canker sores, herpetic and other lesions, gingivitis, denture irritation, traumatic or surgical wounds—* **Adults, and children over 3 years:** apply, undiluted, to oral mucosa q.i.d. or p.r.n., leave for several minutes, then expectorate. Don't rinse out mouth.	None reported.
cocaine hydrochloride Controlled Substance Schedule II	**Adults and children:** *Acute rhinosinusitis*—use 1% solution with nasal pack. *Diagnostic nasal examination*—apply 4% solution to nasal mucosa. *Local anesthesia of nose or throat*—apply 5% to 10% solution to oral and nasal mucosa.	**CNS:** nervousness, excitation, vasomotor collapse.
dexamethasone sodium phosphate Decadron Phosphate♦, Decadron Phosphate Respihaler, Turbinaire	*Allergic or inflammatory conditions, nasal polyps—* **Adults:** 2 sprays in each nostril b.i.d. or t.i.d. Maximum 12 sprays daily. **Children 6 to 12 years:** 1 or 2 sprays in each nostril b.i.d. Maximum 8 sprays daily. Each spray delivers 0.1 mg dexamethasone sodium phosphate equal to 0.084 mg dexamethasone.	**EENT:** nasal irritation, dryness, rebound nasal congestion. **Other:** hypersensitivity, systemic side effects with prolonged use (pituitary-adrenal suppression, sodium retention, congestive heart failure, hypertension, hypokalemia, headaches, convulsions, peptic ulcer, ecchymoses, petechiae, masking of secondary infection).
ephedrine sulfate Ephedsol-1%, I-Sedrin Plain, Isofedrol, Nasdro	*Nasal congestion—* **Adults and children:** apply 3 to 4 drops 0.5% to 3% solution to nasal mucosa. Use no more frequently than q 4 hours.	**CNS:** nervousness, excitation. **CV:** *tachycardia.* **EENT:** rebound nasal congestion with long-term or excessive use. **Local:** mucosal irritation.
epinephrine hydrochloride Adrenalin Chloride	*Nasal congestion, local superficial bleeding—* **Adults and children:** apply	**CNS:** nervousness, excitation. **CV:** *tachycardia.* **EENT:** rebound nasal congestion,

♦ Available in U.S. and Canada. ♦♦ Available in Canada only. All other products (no symbol) available in U.S. only. Italicized side effects are common or life-threatening.

INTERACTIONS	NURSING CONSIDERATIONS
None significant.	• Contraindicated in infants under 1 year. Use cautiously in children under 6 years and in severe oral trauma or sepsis. • Not intended for use in the presence of infection. • Obtain history of reactions to local anesthetics. • Watch for allergic reactions, such as reddening or swelling. If condition persists, drug should be stopped and doctor notified. • Show patient how to apply.
None significant.	• Use only as adjunct to regular professional care. • Don't dilute. Gently massage affected area with medication. Show patient how to apply. Tell him not to drink or rinse his mouth for 5 minutes after use. • Warn patient that drug foams in mouth when mixed with saliva. • Use after meals and at bedtime for best results. • If severe or persistent inflammation continues, patient should notify doctor or dentist. • Provides chemomechanical cleansing, debriding action, and has nonselective microbial activity. • An oxygenating agent. • Store in cool place. • Only one person should use dropper bottle or tube.
None significant.	• Store under lock and key with other controlled drugs. • Patient should be given a short-acting barbiturate before giving cocaine HCl to prevent excess CNS stimulation or vasomotor collapse. • Nasal surgery performed with cocaine HCl anesthetic may cause a delayed capillary hemorrhage resulting from capillary dilation. Watch for postoperative nasal bleeding when effect of cocaine wears off. • Obtain history of reactions to local anesthetics.
None significant.	• Contraindicated in cutaneous tuberculosis, fungal and herpetic lesions. Use cautiously in diabetes mellitus, peptic ulcer, tuberculosis, as systemic absorption can activate disease. • Mothers should not breast-feed, as systemic absorption can occur. • Control underlying bacterial infection with anti-infectives. • Irritation or sensitivity may require stopping drug. • Don't break, incinerate, or store in extreme heat; contents under pressure. • Gradually reduce dose as nasal condition improves. • Fluid retention can occur as a result of systemic absorption. • Show patient how to apply. Only one person should use nasal spray. • Hypertension and hypokalemia can occur with systemic absorption. Monitor blood pressure, serum potassium frequently. • Should not be used for prolonged periods.
MAO inhibitors: hypertensive crisis if ephedrine is absorbed. Don't use together.	• Use cautiously in hyperthyroidism, coronary artery disease, hypertension, or diabetes mellitus, as systemic absorption can occur. • Tell patient not to exceed recommended dose. Use only when needed. • Show patient how to apply. Only one person should use dropper bottle or nasal spray.
None significant.	• Use cautiously in hyperthyroidism, coronary artery disease, hypertension, or diabetes mellitus, as systemic absorption can occur. • Tell patient not to exceed recommended dose.

(continued on following page)

NAME	INDICATIONS & DOSAGE	SIDE EFFECTS
epinephrine hydrochloride *(continued)*	0.1% solution to oral or nasal mucosa.	slight sting upon application.
lidocaine hydrochloride Xylocaine♦, Xylocaine Viscous♦	*Local anesthesia, pain from dental extractions, stomatitis—* **Adults and children:** apply 2% to 5% solution, ointment, or 15 ml of Xylocaine Viscous q 3 to 4 hours to oral or nasal mucosa.	**EENT:** interference with pharyngeal stage of swallowing. **Other:** hypersensitivity (CNS symptoms are excitatory or depressant; CV symptoms are depressant); systemic absorption when used repeatedly.
naphazoline hydrochloride Privine♦	*Nasal congestion—* **Adults:** apply 2 drops or sprays of 0.05% to 0.1% solution to nasal mucosa q 3 to 4 hours. **Children 6 to 12 years:** 1 to 2 drops or sprays of 0.05% solution. Repeat q 3 to 6 hours, p.r.n. Use no longer than 3 to 5 days.	**EENT:** rebound nasal congestion with excessive or long-term use, sneezing, stinging, dryness of mucosa. **Other:** systemic side effects in children after excessive or long-term use; marked sedation.
oxymetazoline hydrochloride Afrin, Duration, Nafrine♦♦, St. Joseph's Decongestant for Children	*Nasal congestion—* **Adults, and children over 6 years:** apply 2 to 4 drops or sprays 0.05% solution to nasal mucosa b.i.d. **Children 2 to 5 years:** apply 2 to 3 drops 0.025% solution to nasal mucosa b.i.d. Use no longer than 3 to 5 days. Dosage for younger children has not been established.	**CNS:** headache, drowsiness, dizziness, insomnia. **CV:** palpitations. **EENT:** rebound nasal congestion or irritation with excessive or long-term use, dryness of nose and throat, increased nasal discharge, stinging, sneezing. **Other:** systemic side effects in children with excessive or long-term use; possible sedation.
phenylephrine hydrochloride Alconefrin, Coricidin Nasal Mist, Coryzine, Ephrine, Isophrin, Neo-Synephrine♦, Pyracort-D, Rhinall, Sinarest Nasal Spray, Sinophen Intranasal, SuperAnahist Nasal Spray, Synasal, Vacon	*Nasal congestion—* **Adults:** 2 to 3 drops or sprays 0.25% to 1% solution; apply jelly or spray to nasal mucosa. **Children 6 to 12 years:** apply 2 to 3 drops or sprays of 0.25% solution. **Children under 6 years:** apply 2 to 3 drops or sprays 0.125% solution. Drops, spray, or jelly can be given q 4 hours, p.r.n.	**CNS:** headache, tremors, dizziness, nervousness. **CV:** *palpitations, tachycardia,* premature ventricular contractions, hypertension, pallor. **EENT:** transient burning, stinging; dryness of nasal mucosa; rebound nasal congestion may occur with continued use. **GI:** nausea.
piperocaine hydrochloride Metycaine HCl	*Anesthetic in dental procedures—* **Adults and children:** apply 5% to 10% solution as a spray or 1% to 2% solution by infiltration to oral or nasal mucosa. *Local anesthetic in rhinolaryngologic examinations—*	**EENT:** interference with pharyngeal stage of swallowing. **Other:** hypersensitivity.

♦ Available in U.S. and Canada. ♦♦ Available in Canada only. All other products (no symbol) available in U.S. only. Italicized side effects are common or life-threatening.

INTERACTIONS	NURSING CONSIDERATIONS
	• Use only when needed. • Show patient how to apply. Only one person should use dropper bottle or nasal spray.
None significant.	• Use cautiously in cardiac disease, hyperthyroidism, or severe oral or nasal trauma or sepsis, as systemic absorption can occur. • Chronic, prolonged use for oropharynx anesthesia can lead to systemic absorption and toxicity. • Instruct patient how to use. Xylocaine Viscous should be swished around in mouth and can be swallowed. Warn patient to eat or drink cautiously within 60 minutes after oral application, to avoid food aspiration. • Obtain history of reactions to local anesthetics. • Taste can be improved by adding a drop of oil of peppermint.
None significant.	• Contraindicated in glaucoma. Use cautiously in hyperthyroidism, heart disease, hypertension, or diabetes mellitus, as systemic absorption can occur. • Warn patient not to exceed recommended dosage. • Tell patient to notify doctor if nasal congestion persists after 5 days. • Show patient how to apply. Hold container upright. Only one person should use dropper bottle or nasal spray. • Do not shake container.
None significant.	• Use cautiously in hyperthyroidism, cardiac disease, hypertension, or diabetes mellitus, as systemic absorption can occur. • Tell patient not to exceed recommended dose. Use only when needed. • Show patient how to apply. Have patient bend head forward and sniff spray briskly. Only one person should use dropper bottle or nasal spray.
None significant.	• Contraindicated in narrow-angle glaucoma. Use cautiously in hyperthyroidism, hypertension, diabetes mellitus, or ischemic cardiac disease, as systemic absorption may occur. • Tell patient not to exceed recommended dose. Use only when needed. • Show patient how to apply: keep head erect to minimize swallowing of medication. Only one person should use dropper bottle or nasal spray.
None significant.	• Use cautiously in cardiac disease, hyperthyroidism, severe trauma, or sepsis of oral or nasal mucosa, as systemic absorption can occur. • Obtain history of reaction to topical anesthetics. • Warn patient not to eat or drink for 60 minutes after oral application, to prevent possible food aspiration.

(continued on following page)

NAME	INDICATIONS & DOSAGE	SIDE EFFECTS
piperocaine hydrochloride *(continued)*	**Adults and children:** apply 2% solution as a spray to oral or nasal mucosa.	
tetrahydrozoline hydrochloride Tyzine HCl, Tyzine Pediatric	*Nasal congestion—* **Adults, and children over 6 years:** apply 2 to 4 drops 0.1% solution or spray to nasal mucosa q 4 to 6 hours, p.r.n. **Children 2 to 6 years:** apply 2 to 3 drops 0.05% solution to nasal mucosa q 4 to 6 hours, p.r.n.	**EENT:** transient burning, stinging; sneezing, rebound nasal congestion in excessive or long-term use.
triamcinolone acetonide Kenalog in Orabase	*Stomatitis; erosive lichen planus; traumatic oral lesions, including sore denture spots—* **Adults and children:** press ¼ inch of 0.1% emollient dental paste onto affected area until thin film develops. Repeat b.i.d. or t.i.d. Don't rub in or protection of film will be lost.	**Systemic:** with prolonged use, adrenal insufficiency, altered glucose metabolism, peptic ulcer activation.
xylometazoline hydrochloride 4-Way Long Acting, Neo-Synephrine II, Otrivin♦, Sine-Off Nasal Spray, Sinex-L.A.	*Nasal congestion—* **Adults, and children over 12 years:** apply 2 to 3 drops or 2 sprays of 0.1% solution to nasal mucosa q 8 to 10 hours. **Children under 12 years:** apply 2 to 3 drops or 1 spray of 0.05% solution to nasal mucosa q 8 to 10 hours.	**EENT:** rebound nasal congestion or irritation with excessive or long-term use; transient burning, stinging; dryness or ulceration of nasal mucosa; sneezing.

INTERACTIONS	NURSING CONSIDERATIONS
None significant.	• Contraindicated in glaucoma. Use cautiously in hyperthyroidism, hypertension, diabetes mellitus. • Don't use 0.1% solution in children under 6 years. • Tell patient not to exceed recommended dose. Use only as needed. • Show patient how to apply. Only one person should use dropper or nasal spray.
None significant.	• Contraindicated in oral herpetic or viral lesions. Use cautiously in diabetes mellitus, peptic ulcer, or tuberculosis, as systemic absorption can occur. • Apply after meals and at bedtime for best results.
None significant.	• Contraindicated in narrow-angle glaucoma. Use cautiously in hyperthyroidism, cardiac disease, hypertension, diabetes mellitus, and advanced arteriosclerosis, as systemic absorption can occur. • Tell patient not to exceed recommended dose. • Show patient how to apply. Only one person should use dropper bottle or nasal spray.

NASAL SPRAYS CAN BE ADDICTIVE

Although nasal sprays don't cause addiction in the usual sense—a craving for a particular substance—they do cause a physical dependency called the rebound phenomenon.

Rebound phenomenon occurs when a patient uses a nasal spray for initial relief and then continues to use the spray more heavily each time he becomes congested. After the nasal blood vessels constrict many times—in response to each dose of the spray—they become tired, so they relax, engorge, and become more congested.

According to the directions for using most nasal sprays, short-term use (2 or 3 days) doesn't lead to "addiction." But if long-term use of a nasal spray is required, the patient should consult an eye, ear, nose, and throat specialist. Continuous nasal congestion may be a sign of an underlying allergy, infection, or some structural defect that can be corrected in other, less dangerous ways.

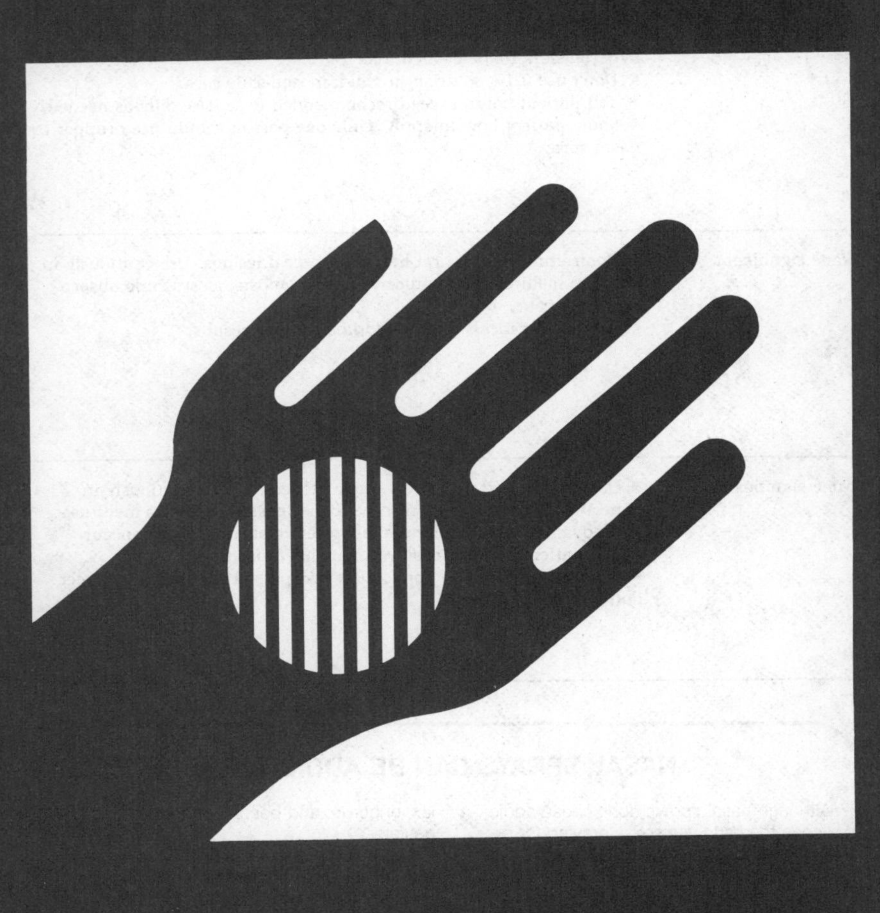

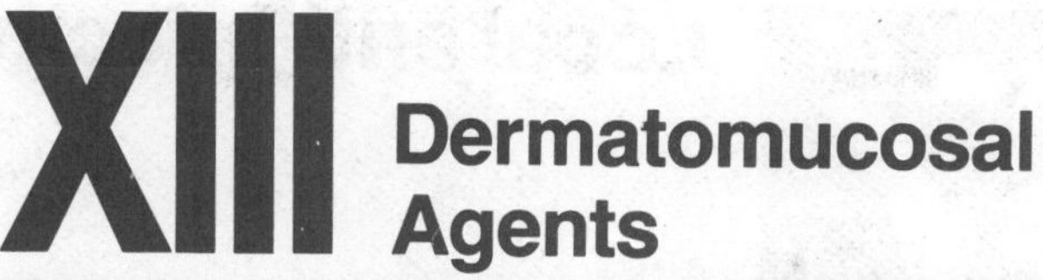

XIII Dermatomucosal Agents

87 Local anti-infectives

amphotericin B
bacitracin
carbol-fuchsin solution
chloramphenicol
chlortetracycline hydrochloride
clotrimazole
erythromycin
gentamicin sulfate
gentian violet (methylrosaniline chloride)
haloprogin
iodochlorhydroxyquin
mafenide acetate
miconazole nitrate 2%
neomycin sulfate
nitrofurazone
nystatin
silver sulfadiazine
tetracycline hydrochloride
tolnaftate
undecylenic acid (zinc undecylenate)

For information on meclocycline sulfosalicylate, see APPENDIX, *New Drugs*.

Local anti-infective drugs are widely used in treatment of local bacterial and fungal infections. Bacteriostatic and fungistatic drugs suppress growth of microorganisms; bactericidal antibiotics and fungicidal agents destroy them. *Bacteriostatic* antibiotics include chloramphenicol, chlortetracycline, erythromycin, mafenide, nitrofurazone, and tetracycline. *Bactericidal* antibiotics include bacitracin, gentamicin, and neomycin.

The effectiveness of the antifungal agents depends on concentration: most of them are fungistatic at low concentrations or against some organisms, but fungicidal at higher concentrations or against other organisms. *Fungistatic* drugs include iodochlorhydroxyquin, nystatin, tolnaftate, and undecylenic acid. The agents that are generally considered *fungicidal* are amphotericin B, carbol-fuchsin, clotrimazole, gentian violet, haloprogin, miconazole, and silver sulfadiazine.

Major uses

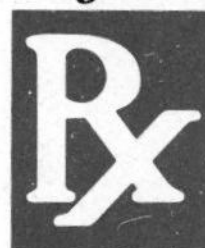

- Antibiotics are used to treat bacterial infections that are due to susceptible organisms and responsive to local therapy.
- Antifungal agents are used topically to treat fungal infections.

Mechanism of action

- Amphotericin B and nystatin act mainly by altering the permeability of the cell membrane; the other antifungals act primarily by removing diseased tissue (softening and dissolving the horny layer of the epidermis).
- Bacitracin acts by inhibiting cell-wall synthesis; the other antibiotics act primarily by disrupting protein synthesis of bacterial ribosomes.

Absorption, distribution, metabolism, and excretion

Most topical anti-infectives, in the absence of inflammation, undergo minimal systemic absorption; however, absorption increases when they're ap-

NEW THREE-DAY CLOTRIMAZOLE REGIMEN FOR VULVOVAGINAL CANDIDIASIS

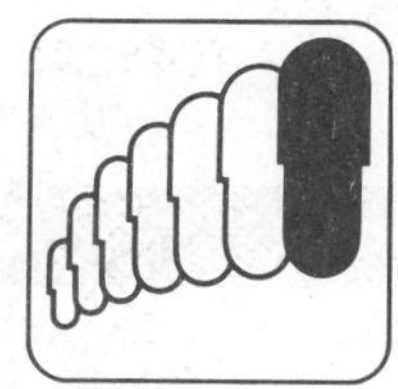

Studies show that a new 3-day regimen of clotrimazole vaginal tablets is just as effective as the standard 7-day regimen for treating vulvovaginal candidiasis in nonpregnant women. The incidence of side effects is comparable with both regimens. But because compliance has been a problem with the 7-day regimen, the shortened dosage schedule represents a significant therapeutic advance.

In the new regimen, two clotrimazole tablets are inserted intravaginally once daily for 3 consecutive days. The 3-day course has *not* proven effective in pregnant women, however. So the 7-day regimen should be used during pregnancy.

Adapted with permission from "Three-day Clotrimazole Regimen Effective in Vulvovaginal Candidiasis," *Drug Therapy,* December 1980.

plied to large areas of denuded or inflamed skin. Applied externally, anti-infectives generally penetrate quickly and easily into the skin.

- Gentamicin and neomycin are systemically absorbed to a greater extent than the other anti-infectives, and special caution is needed with their use. Gentamicin cream may be absorbed more readily than the ointment, with up to 2% to 5% of the drug appearing in urine. Loss of hearing has been reported in persons with normal renal function after topical application of large amounts of neomycin. Large amounts of gentamicin may also cause hearing loss.

Onset and duration

- Onset of local anti-infectives is rapid—usually within minutes. The antifungal agents that remove diseased tissue have a more prolonged onset of action than other antifungals. Therapeutic benefit may not appear for 1 to 3 weeks.
- Duration of action of local anti-infectives is limited because they're often inactivated by components of blood, pus, and exudates. They should generally be applied often (three to six times a day) after the skin is cleansed of adherent crusts and debris.

Combination products

AUREOCORT OINTMENT♦♦: triamcinolone acetonide 0.1% and chlortetracycline HCl 3% per 15-g tube.

BACIMYCIN OINTMENT: zinc bacitracin 500 units and neomycin sulfate 5 mg per g.

BACIMIN OINTMENT: polymyxin B sulfate 5,000 units, neomycin sulfate 5 mg, and bacitracin 400 units per g.

BIOTRES OINTMENT: polymyxin B sulfate 10,000 units and zinc bacitracin 500 units per g.

CORDRAN-N CREAM, OINTMENT: flurandrenolide 0.05% and neomycin sulfate 0.5%.

CORTISPORIN CREAM: hydrocortisone acetate 0.5%, neomycin sulfate 0.5%, gramicidin 0.25 mg, and polymyxin B sulfate 10,000 per g.

CORTISPORIN OINTMENT♦: hydrocortisone 1%, neomycin sulfate 0.5%, bacitracin zinc 400 units and polymyxin B sulfate 5,000 units per g.

MYCITRACIN OINTMENT: polymyxin B sulfate 5,000 units, bacitracin 500 units, and neomycin sulfate 5 mg/g.

MYCOLOG CREAM, OINTMENT: triamcinolone acetonide 0.1%, gramicidin 0.25 mg, nystatin 100,000 units, and

TOPICAL THERAPY: MATCHING THE VEHICLE TO THE CONDITION

ACUTE	CLINICAL SIGNS	TYPE OF VEHICLE
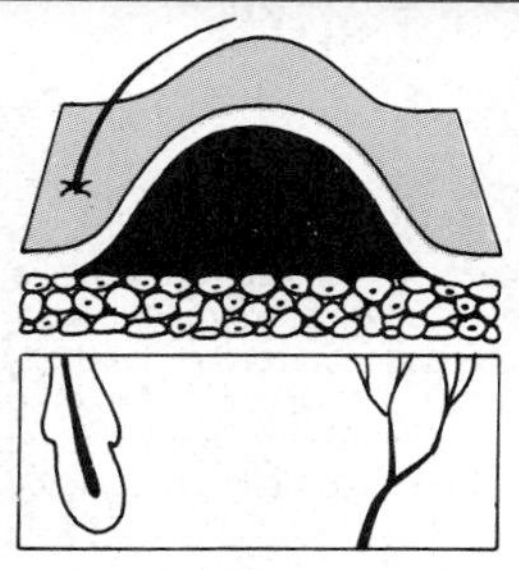	Inflammation is marked. The lesion is erythematous, edematous, and vesicular. To the patient, these often-weepy lesions feel tender, itchy, and hot or burning.	*Apply a wet compress* as often as possible, changing it before it dries. Leave the compress uncovered so as not to impede evaporation, which soothes, cools, and also helps heal through its antipruritic, anti-inflammatory action.

SUBACUTE	CLINICAL SIGNS	TYPE OF VEHICLE
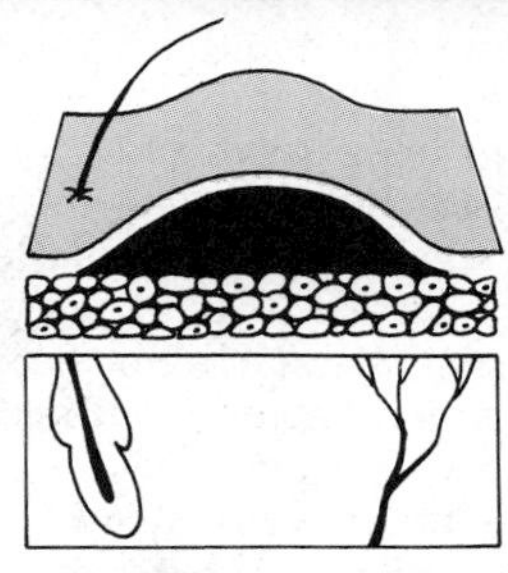	Inflammation is present but is often restricted to the areas immediately surrounding the lesions. Total appearance suggests a drying-out process.	*Apply lotions or creams,* which are protective and lubricating yet not occlusive enough to stop the still-needed evaporation.

CHRONIC	CLINICAL SIGNS	TYPE OF VEHICLE
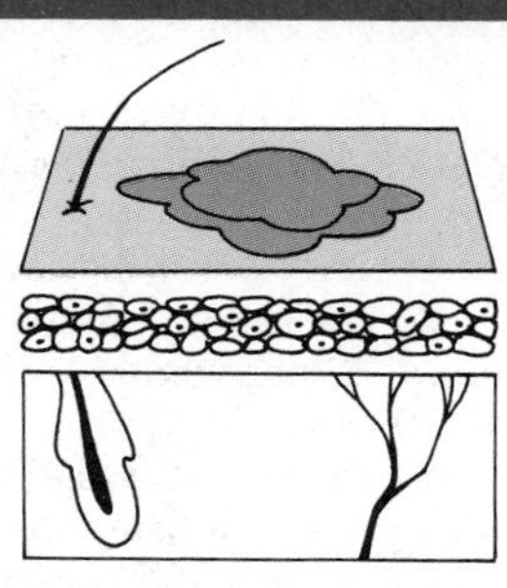	Limited inflammation may still be present. Chronic lesions may assume a scaly, lichenified appearance.	*Apply ointments,* which are occlusive and lubricating, and help the skin to retain moisture and natural skin emollients. At this stage, active medications can be continued in the ointments.

neomycin sulfate 0.25%.

NEO-CORTEF LOTION: hydrocortisone acetate 1% and neomycin sulfate 0.5%.

NEO-CORTEF OINTMENT♦: hydrocortisone acetate 0.5% together with neomycin sulfate 0.5%.

NEODECADRON CREAM: dexamethasone phosphate 0.1% and neomycin sulfate 0.5%.

NEO-DELTA-CORTEF OINTMENT: prednisolone acetate 0.5% and neomycin sulfate 0.5%.

NEO-POLYCON OINTMENT: polymyxin B sulfate 5,000 units, neomycin sulfate 5 mg, and zinc bacitracin 400 units/g.

POLYSPORIN CREAM♦♦: polymyxin B sulfate 10,000 units and gramicidin 0.25 mg per g.

POLYSPORIN OINTMENT♦: polymyxin B sulfate 10,000 units and zinc bacitracin 500 units per g.

SOFRAMYCIN OINTMENT♦♦: framycetin sulfate 15 mg, gramicidin 50 mcg, and anhydrous lanolin 10% per g.

SPECTROCIN OINTMENT: neomycin sulfate 3.6 mg and gramicidin 0.25 mg per g.

STERISPRAY♦♦: neomycin sulfate 500 mg, polymyxin B sulfate 165,000 units, and zinc bacitracin 10,000 units per 110-g container.

TERRAMYCIN WITH POLYMYXIN B SULFATE OINTMENT♦, POWDER: oxytetracycline HCl 30 mg and polymyxin B sulfate 10,000 units per g.

TRICILONE NNG CREAM: triamcinolone acetonide 0.1%, nystatin 100,000 units, neomycin sulfate 0.25%, and gramicidin 0.25 mg per g.

VALISONE-G CREAM♦♦, OINTMENT♦♦: bethamethasone valerate NF 1.22 mg and gentamicin sulfate 1.67 mg/g.

Combination products (antifungal combinations)

CORTIN CREAM: iodochlorhydroxyquin 3% and hydrocortisone 0.5% or 1%.

DRENIFORM CREAM♦♦: iodochlorhydroxyquin 3% and flurandrenolide 0.0125% per 20-g tube.

HYSONE OINTMENT: iodochlorhydroxyquin 3% and hydrocortisone 1%.

IODOCORT CREAM♦: iodochlorhydroxyquin 3% and hydrocortisone 1%.

KOMED LOTION: sodium thiosulfate 8%, salicylic acid 2%, and isopropyl alcohol 25% per g.

LOCACORTEN-VIOFORM CREAM♦♦, OINTMENT♦♦: iodochlorhydroxyquin 3% and flumethasone pivalate 0.02% per g.

MYCOLOG CREAM, OINTMENT: gramicidin 0.25 mg, neomycin sulfate 0.25%, triamcinolone acetonide 0.1%, and nystatin 100,000 units per g.

NEO-POLYCIN HC OINTMENT♦♦: neomycin sulfate 3.5 mg, polymyxin B sulfate 5,000 units, zinc bacitracin 400 units, and hydrocortisone acetate 10 mg per g.

NEOSPORIN CREAM♦♦: polymyxin B sulfate 10,000 units, neomycin sulfate 5 mg, and gramicidin 0.25 mg per g.

NEOSPORIN OINTMENT♦: polymyxin B sulfate 5,000 units, zinc bacitracin 400 units, neomycin sulfate 5 mg/g.

NEOSPORIN-G CREAM: polymyxin B sulfate 10,000 units, neomycin sulfate 5 mg, and gramicidin 0.25 mg per g.

NEO-SYNALAR CREAM♦: fluocinolone acetonide 0.025% and neomycin sulfate 0.5%.

NYSTAFORM OINTMENT♦: nystatin 100,000 units per g and iodochlorhydroxyquin 1%.

NYSTAFORM-HC CREME♦♦, LOTION♦♦, OINTMENT♦: nystatin 100,000 units per g, iodochlorhydroxyquin 3% and hydrocortisone alcohol, 5% or 1%.

P.B.N. OINTMENT: polymyxin B sulfate 5,000 units, neomycin sulfate 5 mg, and bacitracin 400 units per g.

RACET CREAM: iodochlorhydroxyquin 3% and hydrocortisone 0.5%.

TINVER LOTION♦: sodium thiosulfate 25%, salicylic acid 1%, and isopropyl alcohol 10%.

VIOFORM-HYDROCORTISONE CREAM♦, LOTION, OINTMENT♦: iodochlorhydroxyquin 3% and hydrocortisone 1%.

VIOFORM-HYDROCORTISONE MILD CREAM♦, OINTMENT♦: iodochlorhydroxyquin 3% and hydrocortisone 0.5%.

WHITFIELD'S OINTMENT: benzoic acid 12% and salicylic acid 6%.

NAME	INDICATIONS & DOSAGE	SIDE EFFECTS
amphotericin B Fungizone Cream, Lotion, Ointment (3% amphotericin B)	*Cutaneous or mucocutaneous candidal infections—* **Adults and children:** apply liberally b.i.d., t.i.d., or q.i.d. for 1 to 3 weeks; up to several months for interdigital lesions, paronychias, and onychomycosis (where relapses are frequent).	**Skin:** possible drying, contact sensitivity, erythema, burning, pruritus.
bacitracin Baciguent♦, Bacitin♦♦	*Topical infections, impetigo, abrasions, cuts, minor wounds, seborrheic dermatitis, acne, contact dermatitis, psoriasis—* **Adults and children:** apply thin film b.i.d. or t.i.d. or more often, depending on severity of condition.	**Skin:** rashes and other allergic reactions; itching, burning, swelling of lips or face. **Other:** *possible systemic side effects when used over large areas for prolonged periods: potentially nephrotoxic and ototoxic;* tightness in chest, hypotension.
carbol-fuchsin solution Carfusin, Castaderm, Castellani's Paint	*Tinea, dermatophytosis, skin infections—* **Adults and children:** apply liberally 1 or 2 times daily.	**Blood:** possibility of bone marrow hypoplasia with use over long periods or at frequent intervals. **Skin:** *contact dermatitis.*
chloramphenicol Chloromycetin♦ (1% chloramphenicol)	*Superficial skin infections caused by susceptible bacteria—* **Adults and children:** after thorough cleansing, apply t.i.d. or q.i.d.	**Skin:** possible contact sensitivity; itching, burning, urticaria, angioneurotic edema in patients hypersensitive to any of the components.
chlortetracycline hydrochloride Aureomycin 3%♦	*Superficial infections of the skin caused by susceptible bacteria—* **Adults and children:** rub into affected area b.i.d. or t.i.d.	**Skin:** *rashes, dermatitis.*
clotrimazole Canesten♦♦, Gyne-Lotrimin, Lotrimin (1% clotrimazole)	*Superficial fungal infections (tinea pedis, tinea cruris, tinea versicolor, candidiasis, and tinea corporis)—* **Adults and children:** apply thinly and massage into affected and surrounding area, morning and evening, 1 to 8 weeks. *Candidal vulvovaginitis—* **Adults:** insert 1 applicatorful or 1 tablet intravaginally daily for	**GU:** *with vaginal use: mild vaginal burning, irritation.* **Skin:** blistering, *erythema,* edema, pruritus, burning, stinging, peeling, urticaria, skin fissures, general irritation.

♦ Available in U.S. and Canada. ♦♦ Available in Canada only. All other products (no symbol) available in U.S. only. Italicized side effects are common or life-threatening.

INTERACTIONS	NURSING CONSIDERATIONS
None significant.	• Cream or lotion preferred for areas such as folds of groin, armpit, and neck creases. • Cream discolors skin slightly when rubbed in; lotion or ointment doesn't. Lotion may stain nail lesions. • Watch for and report signs of local irritation. • Avoid occlusive dressings and ointments. • Store at room temperature; avoid freezing. • Well tolerated, even by infants, for long periods. • Tell patient to continue using medication for full time prescribed even though condition has improved.
None significant.	• Contraindicated in hypersensitivity to any of the components and for application in the external ear canal if the eardrum is perforated. • If used on burns that cover more than 20% of body surface, and especially if patient suffers impaired renal function, apply only once daily. • If no improvement or if condition worsens, stop using and notify doctor. • Prolonged use may result in overgrowth of nonsusceptible organisms. • Avoid excess application.
None significant.	• Do not use on large areas or on eroded skin. • Do not continue use after 1 week if no improvement shown; consult doctor. Toxicities develop in long-term use. • Poisonous; warn against swallowing. • Clean and dry skin thoroughly before applying. • Instruct patient to continue using for full treatment period prescribed, even if condition has improved. • Will stain clothing.
None significant.	• Contraindicated in hypersensitivity to any of the components. • If no improvement or if condition worsens, stop using and report to doctor. • Prolonged use may result in overgrowth of nonsusceptible organisms. • For all but very superficial infections, topical use of this drug should be supplemented by appropriate systemic medication. • Discontinue if signs of hypersensitivity develop. • Tell patient to continue using for full treatment period prescribed, even if condition has improved.
None significant.	• Contraindicated in hypersensitivity to any of the components. • Prolonged use may result in overgrowth of nonsusceptible organisms. • If no improvement or if condition worsens, stop using and report to doctor.
None significant.	• Contraindicated in hypersensitivity to any of the components. • Not for ophthalmic use. • Watch for and report irritation or sensitivity. Discontinue use. • Improvement usually within a week; if none in 4 weeks, diagnosis should be reviewed. • Shortened dosage schedule with tablets may be used when compliance is a problem. • Do not use occlusive dressings.

(continued on following page)

NAME	INDICATIONS & DOSAGE	SIDE EFFECTS
clotrimazole *(continued)*	7 to 14 days at bedtime. Alternatively, insert 2 tablets once daily for 3 consecutive days.	
erythromycin Erythrocin♦♦, Ilotycin♦	*Superficial skin infections due to susceptible organisms—* **Adults and children:** clean affected area; apply t.i.d. or q.i.d.	**Skin:** sensitivity reactions.
gentamicin sulfate Garamycin♦	*Primary and secondary bacterial infections, superficial burns, skin ulcers, infected insect bites and stings, infected lacerations and abrasions, wounds from minor surgery—* **Adults, and children over 1 year:** rub in small amount gently t.i.d. or q.i.d., with or without gauze dressing.	**Skin:** small percentage of minor skin irritation; possible photosensitivity.
gentian violet (methylrosaniline chloride) Bismuth Violet solution (1% and 2%), Crystal Violet	*Superficial infections of skin; lesions, except ulcerative lesions of face, particularly* Candida albicans— **Adults and children:** apply with swab b.i.d. or t.i.d. Keep affected area clean, dry, and exposed to air to prevent spread of infection.	**Skin:** *permanent discoloration if applied to granulation tissue;* ulceration of mucous membranes.
haloprogin Halotex♦	*Superficial fungal infections (tinea pedis, tinea cruris, tinea corporis, tinea manuum, and tinea versicolor)—* **Adults and children:** apply liberally b.i.d. for 2 to 3 weeks.	**Skin:** burning sensation, irritation, vesicle formation, increased maceration, *pruritus or exacerbation of preexisting lesions.*
iodochlorhydroxyquin Gentleline, Quinoform, Torofor, Vioform	*Inflamed skin conditions, including eczema, athlete's foot, other fungal infections; cutaneous or mucocutaneous mycotic infections caused by* Candida *species* (Monilia)— **Adults and children:** apply a thin layer b.i.d., t.i.d., q.i.d., or as directed. Continue for 1 week after clinical cure.	**Skin:** *possible burning, itching, acneiform eruptions.* **Systemic:** electrolyte imbalance, adrenal suppression.
mafenide acetate Sulfamylon♦	*Adjunctive treatment of second- and third-degree burns—* **Adults and children:** apply $^1/_{16}$ inch daily or b.i.d. to cleansed, debrided wounds.	**Blood:** eosinophilia. **Skin:** pain, *burning sensation,* rash, itching, swelling, hives, blisters, erythema. **Other:** facial edema.

♦ Available in U.S. and Canada. ♦♦ Available in Canada only. All other products (no symbol) available in U.S. only. Italicized side effects are common or life-threatening.

INTERACTIONS	NURSING CONSIDERATIONS
None significant.	• Prolonged use may result in overgrowth of nonsusceptible organisms. • If no improvement or if condition worsens, stop using and tell doctor. • Usually a bacteriostatic agent, but in high concentrations or against highly susceptible organisms, may be bactericidal.
None significant.	• Contraindicated in hypersensitivity to any of the components. • If no improvement or if condition worsens, stop using and report to doctor. • Avoid use on large skin lesions or over a wide area because of possible systemic toxic effects. • Prolonged use may result in overgrowth of nonsusceptible organisms. • May clear bacterial infections that have not responded to other antibacterial agents. • Useful for treating patients who are sensitive to neomycin. • Useful for infected skin cysts, preceded by incision and draining. • Store in cool place. • Remove crusts before application of gentamicin in impetigo contagiosa.
None significant.	• Contraindicated in hypersensitivity to any of the components. • Do not use on ulcerative lesions of the face. • Apply carefully to avoid undue staining. Will stain skin and clothing. • When used in infant with oral candidiasis, turn infant face down after application to minimize amount swallowed. • Do not use occlusive dressings.
None significant.	• Contraindicated in hypersensitivity to any of the components. • Diagnosis should be reconsidered if no improvement in 4 weeks. • Tell patient to continue using for full treatment period prescribed, even if condition has improved.
Systemic corticosteroids: possible increased absorption. Use together cautiously.	• Contraindicated in hypersensitivity to iodine or iodine-containing preparations. Contraindicated in tuberculosis, vaccinia, and varicella. • Note all side effects and precautions of each component in the combination antifungals. • Presence in urine may cause false-positive result for phenylketonuria (PKU) or inaccurate thyroid function tests. Discontinue at least 1 month before thyroid function tests. • Drug will stain fabric and hair.
None significant.	• Use with caution in acute renal failure and in known hypersensitivity to mafenide. • Closely monitor acid-base balance, especially in the presence of pulmonary and renal dysfunction. • If acidosis occurs, discontinue use for 24 to 48 hours. • Causes pain at application site. Check for pain and burning; if they occur, notify doctor. Severe and prolonged pain may indicate allergy.

(continued on following page)

NAME	INDICATIONS & DOSAGE	SIDE EFFECTS
mafenide acetate *(continued)*		
miconazole nitrate 2% Micatin	*Tinea pedis, tinea cruris, tinea corporis, cutaneous candidiasis (moniliasis), infections from common dermatophytes—* **Adults and children:** apply sparingly b.i.d. for 2 to 4 weeks.	**Skin:** isolated reports of irritation, burning, maceration.
neomycin sulfate Herisan Antibiotic♦♦, Mycifradin♦♦, Myciguent♦, Neocin♦♦	*Topical bacterial infections, burns, wounds, skin grafts, following surgical procedure, lesions, pruritus, trophic ulcerations, edema—* **Adults and children:** rub in small quantity gently b.i.d., t.i.d., or as directed.	**Skin:** *rashes.* **Other:** *possible nephrotoxicity, ototoxicity, and neuromuscular blockade; possible systemic absorption when used on extensive areas of the body.*
nitrofurazone Furacin♦, Furazyme	*Adjunctive treatment of second- and third-degree burns (especially when resistance to other antibiotics and sulfonamides occurs); skin grafting—* **Adults and children:** apply directly to lesion daily or every few days, depending on severity of burn.	**GU:** possible renal toxicity. **Skin:** *erythema, pruritus,* burning, edema, severe reactions (vesiculation, denudation, ulceration).
nystatin Candex, Mycostatin♦, Nadostine♦♦, Nilstat	*Infant eczema, pruritus ani and vulvae, superficial bacterial infections, localized forms of candidiasis—* **Adults and children:** apply and rub into area b.i.d. for 2 weeks.	**Skin:** occasional contact dermatitis from preservatives present in some formulations. **Systemic:** possible nephrotoxicity or ototoxicity with prolonged or frequent use.

INTERACTIONS	NURSING CONSIDERATIONS
	If other allergic reactions occur, treatment may have to be temporarily discontinued. • Cleanse area before applying. Mafenide washes off with water. • Accidental ingestion may cause diarrhea. • Keep burn areas medicated at all times. • Bathe patient daily, if possible. • Safety of use during pregnancy has not yet been established. • For burns, using reverse isolation technique with sterile gloves and instruments to apply cream prevents further wound contamination.
None significant.	• For external use only. Keep out of eyes. • Discontinue if sensitivity or chemical irritation occurs. • Tell patient to continue using for full treatment period prescribed, even if condition has improved. • Do not use occlusive dressings.
None significant.	• Contraindicated in hypersensitivity to any of the components, atopy, vaccinia, varicella, fungal or viral lesions. • If no improvement or if condition worsens, stop drug; call doctor. • If used on more than 20% of the body surface and on patient with impaired renal function, apply only once daily. • Prolonged use may result in overgrowth of nonsusceptible organisms. • In those combination products that contain corticosteroids, use of occlusive dressings increases corticosteroid absorption and the likelihood of systemic effects. • Particularly well absorbed on denuded or abraded areas. • Watch for signs of hypersensitivity and contact dermatitis. • Evaluate patient for signs of ototoxicity.
None significant.	• Contraindicated in previous hypersensitivity to drug. • Use cautiously in patients with known or suspected renal impairment. The polyethylene glycols present in the base can be absorbed through denuded skin and may cause kidney damage. • If irritation, sensitization, or infection occurs, discontinue use. • With wet dressing, protect skin around wound with zinc oxide. • Cleanse wound as indicated by doctor at each dressing change. • Remove adherent dressings by flushing with solution of nitrofurazone and sterile wsterile normal saline solution. • Solution should be stored inlight-resistant containers (brown bottles). Avoid expsolution at all times to direct light, prolonged heat, and alkaline materials. • Drug may discolor in light but is still potent and usable. • Discard cloudy solutions if warming to 55° to 60° C. (131° to 140° F.) does not restore clarity. • Use reverse isolation and/or sterile application technique to prevent further wound contamination.
None significant.	• Contraindicated in viral diseases of the skin (vaccinia and varicella), fungal lesions (except candidiasis), and markedly impaired circulation. • Generally well tolerated by all age-groups, including debilitated infants. • Preparation does not stain skin or mucous membranes. • Cream recommended for intertriginous areas, powder for very moist areas, ointment for dry areas. • Tell patient to continue using for full treatment period prescribed, even if condition has improved. • Do not use occlusive dressings.

NAME	INDICATIONS & DOSAGE	SIDE EFFECTS
silver sulfadiazine Flamazine♦♦, Silvadene	*Prevention and treatment of wound infection for second- and third-degree burns—* **Adults and children:** apply $^1/_{16}$ inch thickness of ointment to cleansed and debrided burn wound, then apply daily or b.i.d.	**Blood:** *neutropenia (in 3% to 5%).* **Skin:** pain, burning, rashes, itching. **Other:** fungal infections.
tetracycline hydrochloride Achromycin♦, Topicycline	*Superficial skin infections caused by susceptible bacteria, acne—* **Adults and children:** rub into cleansed affected area b.i.d. or t.i.d. *Acne—* **Adults:** apply Topicycline generously to affected areas b.i.d. until skin is thoroughly wet.	**Skin:** dermatitis with Achromycin; with Topicycline, temporary stinging or burning on application, slight yellowing of treated skin, especially in patients with light complexions; severe dermatitis; treated skin areas fluoresce under ultraviolet light.
tolnaftate Aftate, Tinactin♦	*Superficial fungal infections of the skin, infections due to common pathogenic fungi, tinea pedis, tinea cruris, tinea corporis, tinea manuum, tinea versicolor—* **Adults and children:** ¼- to ½-inch ribbon of cream or 1 or 3 drops of lotion to cover area of one hand; same amount of cream or 2 to 3 drops of lotion to cover the toes and interdigital webs of one foot. Apply and massage gently into skin b.i.d. for 2 or 3 weeks, up to 6 weeks.	None significant.
undecylenic acid (zinc undecylenate) Desenex, Ting, Unde-Jen	*Athlete's foot and ringworm of the body exclusive of nails and hairy areas—* **Adults and children:** clean thoroughly. Apply ointment liberally at night and powder during the day. Use regularly to prevent fungal infections.	**Skin:** possible irritation in hypersensitive person.

♦ Available in U.S. and Canada. ♦♦ Available in Canada only. All other products (no symbol) available in U.S. only. Italicized side effects are common or life-threatening.

INTERACTIONS	NURSING CONSIDERATIONS
Topical proteolytic enzymes: inactivity of enzymes when used together. Do not use together.	• Contraindicated in premature and newborn infants during first month of life. (Drug may increase possibility of kernicterus.) Use with caution in hypersensitivity to drug or sulfonamides. • Inspect patient's skin daily, and note any changes. Notify doctor if burning or excessive pain develops. • Use only on affected areas. Keep medicated at all times. • For patients with extensive burns, monitor serum sulfa concentrations and renal function, and check urine for sulfa crystals. • Bathe patient daily, if possible. • Discard darkened cream. • Should be discontinued if infection is suspected. • Reverse isolation and/or sterile application technique recommended to prevent wound contamination.
None significant.	• Contraindicated in hypersensitivity to any of the components. • If no improvement or if condition worsens, stop using and notify doctor. • Prolonged use may result in overgrowth of nonsusceptible organisms. • Patient may continue normal use of cosmetics. • Store at room temperature, away from excessive heat. • Medication to be used by one person only. Tell patient not to share with family members. • Apply in morning and evening. Warn that drug should be used within 2 months. • Explain that floating plug in bottle of Topicycline—an inert and harmless result of proper reconstitution of the preparation—shouldn't be removed. • Serum levels of topical tetracycline HCl are much lower than those for orally administered drug, so systemic effects are unlikely. • To control flow rate of solution, increase or decrease pressure of the applicator against the skin.
None significant.	• Discontinue if condition worsens. Check with doctor. • Odorless, greaseless. Won't stain or discolor skin, hair, nails, or clothing. • Only a small quantity of cream or lotion is needed; area should not be wet with solution when application is completed. • Commonly available product used to treat athlete's foot (tinea pedis). • Tell patient to continue using for full treatment period prescribed, even if condition has improved.
None significant.	• Consult doctor before using on person with peripheral neuropathy and peripheral vascular diseases or diabetes. • Tell patient to continue using for full treatment period prescribed, even if condition has improved.

Scabicides and pediculicides

benzyl benzoate lotion
copper oleate solution
(with tetrahydronaphthalene)
crotamiton
gamma benzene hexachloride
(or lindane)
pyrethrins
sulfa (6%) in petrolatum

Scabicides and pediculicides destroy the most common parasitic arthropods that infest man.

Persistent itching after adequate therapy indicates either continued infestation, slow-resolving hypersensitivity, or irritation from the drug. Laundering or dry cleaning all contaminated linens and clothing is essential to eradicate infestations. Commercial sprays can be used to decontaminate furniture or rugs that may harbor the parasites.

Major uses

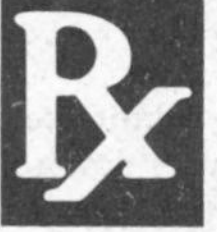

These drugs eradicate parasitic arthropod infestations such as scabies and pediculosis. They're used against *Sarcoptes scabiei* (scabies), *Pediculus humanus* var.

SHAMPOOING OUT SCABIES AND PEDICULOSIS

To wash the hair of a bedridden patient with scabies or pediculosis, follow these steps:

- Wear gloves and a paper gown over your uniform.
- Thoroughly pad the patient's back and neck for comfort.
- Arrange pillows on a slight incline to let water drain away from the patient's head.
- Make a water-draining trough from a bath blanket, towels, or sheets rolled into a log. Shape the log into a U inside a large plastic bag, such as those used for contaminated waste. Arrange the bag under the patient's head, with the bag's open end extending over the edge of the bed and into a bucket on the floor.
- Produce a good lather in the hair. Rinse two or three times.
- Dry immediately.
- Inspect the patient's scalp for scabies, pediculosis, or other abnormalities. Note observations.
- When finished, change bed linens. Discard all towels and linens, gown and gloves in separate, labeled containers. Wash your hands. When caring for those with scabies or pediculosis, pay extra attention to isolation and aseptic procedures.

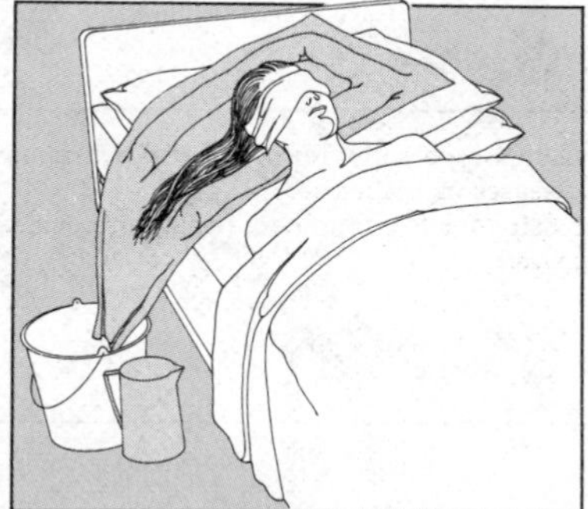

capitis (head louse), *Pediculus humanus* var. *corporis* (body louse), and *Phthirus pubis* (crab louse). One application is usually enough to kill adult forms, but repeated applications are necessary to destroy nits.

Mechanism of action

Gamma benzene hexachloride appears to inhibit neuronal-membrane function in arthropods.

The mechanism of action of the other agents is unknown.

Absorption, distribution, metabolism, and excretion

Gamma benzene hexachloride is absorbed through intact skin when applied topically. Absorption through skin is usually greatest when drug is applied to face, scalp, neck, axillae, scrotum, or damaged skin. No information is available on systemic absorption of the other drugs.

Gamma benzene hexachloride is stored in body fat, metabolized in the liver, and eliminated in urine and feces.

Onset and duration

Onset of all the drugs is immediate. Duration of action is limited. The drug must be reapplied, if necessary, according to product information.

Combination products

None.

PARENT-TEACHING AID

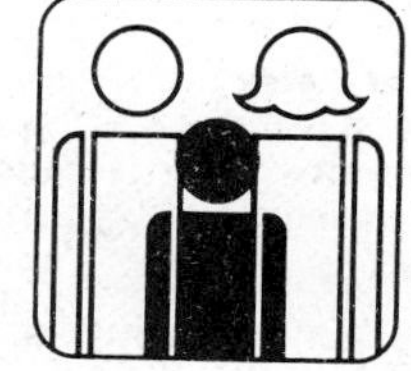

HOW TO GET RID OF HEAD LICE

Dear Parent:

Having head lice is not a disgrace: anyone can get them. They don't necessarily result from poor grooming or bad health habits, but instead can be spread by close contact with those who have lice in schools, locker rooms, buses, and other public places, or by sharing clothing or hairbrushes. Here's how you can relieve your child's itching and help eliminate the lice:

1. Wash your child's hair for 4 minutes with a lindane-medicated shampoo (Kwell), Cuprex shampoo, or pyrinate shampoo. This will destroy lice and nits (lice eggs), but nits will remain attached to hair shafts.
2. Remove nits from hair with a brush or fine-toothed comb dipped in vinegar.
3. Repeat steps #1 and #2 on 2 consecutive days or at weekly intervals.
4. Wash or dry clean all your child's clothing, because nits can survive away from the body for up to 30 days.
5. Spray upholstered furniture and rugs with a pyrethrum spray (R&C). Animals don't become infested, so don't worry about treating family pets.
6. Examine your child's head regularly for recurrent infestation. You can detect head lice and nits with the naked eye. Usually you won't find many adult lice moving through your child's hair. Instead, you'll find nits attached to the hair shafts. Be careful not to mistake hair casts (normal root sheaths that encircle the hair shaft), hair-spray globules, or severe scalp scaling (from psoriasis or seborrhea) for head lice. If you have any questions, consult your child's doctor.

NAME	INDICATIONS & DOSAGE	SIDE EFFECTS
benzyl benzoate lotion Scabanca♦♦	*Parasitic infestation (scabies,* Phthirus pubis)— **Adults and children:** first, scrub entire body with soap and water. Then apply the 25% lotion undiluted over entire body, except the face, while still damp. Be sure to apply around nails. Let dry. Apply second coat on the most involved areas. Bathe after 24 to 48 hours. Adults require 30 ml. Children require 20 ml. *Pediculosis capitis—* **Adults and children:** apply to scalp and leave on overnight; shampoo out in morning. Repeat next night if necessary.	**Skin:** *irritation, itching; contact dermatitis with repeated applications.*
copper oleate solution (with tetrahydronaphthalene) Cuprex	*Parasitic infestation (pediculoses capitis and pubis)—* **Adults and children:** first, scrub entire body with soap and water. Apply gently and sparingly 3 to 4 tablespoonfuls onto affected areas; after 15 minutes wash off with soap and water.	**Skin:** *irritation with repeated use, or if used on raw or inflamed skin.*
crotamiton Eurax♦	*Parasitic infestation (scabies)—* **Adults and children:** scrub entire body with soap and water. Then, apply a thin layer of cream over entire body, from chin down, with special attention to folds, creases, interdigital spaces, genital area. Apply second coat within 24 hours. Wait 48 hours, then wash off. *General itching*—apply locally b.i.d. or t.i.d.	**Skin:** *irritation with repeated use.*

♦ Available in U.S. and Canada. ♦♦ Available in Canada only. All other products (no symbol) available in U.S. only. Italicized side effects are common or life-threatening.

INTERACTIONS	NURSING CONSIDERATIONS
None significant.	• Contraindicated when skin is raw or inflamed. Notify doctor immediately if skin irritation or hypersensitivity develops; tell patient to discontinue drug and to wash it off skin. • Do not apply to face, eyes, mucous membranes, or urethral meatus. If accidental contact with eyes does occur, flush with water and notify doctor. • Instruct patient to change and sterilize (boil, launder, dry clean, or apply very hot iron) all clothing and bed linen after drug is washed off. • Itching may continue for several weeks; this does not indicate that therapy is ineffective. To prevent acarophobia, reassure patient that itching will cease. • Tendency to overuse this drug. Estimate amount needed. • Topical corticosteroids may be needed if dermatitis develops from scratching. • Question other family members about possible infestation. • After application, use a fine comb dipped in white vinegar on hair to remove nits. • Instruct patient to reapply if washed off (hands, for example) during treatment time. • Hospitalized patients should be placed in isolation with linen handling precautions until treatment is completed.
None significant.	• Contraindicated when skin is raw or inflamed, or when there is a severe infection. Notify doctor immediately if skin irritation or hypersensitivity develops; tell patient to discontinue drug and to wash it off skin. • Do not apply more than twice within 48 hours. • Do not apply to face, eyes, mucous membranes, or urethral meatus. If accidental contact with eyes does occur, flush with water and notify doctor. • Instruct patient to change and sterilize (boil, launder, dry clean, or apply very hot iron) all clothing and bed linen after application. • After application, use a fine comb dipped in white vinegar on hair to remove nits. • Question other family members about possible infestation. • Tendency for overuse of pediculicides. Estimate amount needed. • Hospitalized patients should be placed in isolation with linen handling precautions until treatment is completed.
None significant.	• Contraindicated when skin is raw or inflamed. Notify doctor immediately if skin irritation or hypersensitivity develops; tell patient to discontinue drug and to wash it off skin. • Do not apply to face, eyes, mucous membranes, or urethral meatus. If accidental contact with eyes does occur, flush with water and notify doctor. • Instruct patient to change and sterilize (boil, launder, dry clean, or apply very hot iron) all clothing and bed linen after drug is washed off. • Topical corticosteroids may be needed if dermatitis develops from scratching. • Tendency to overuse scabicides. Estimate amount needed. • Question other family members about possible infestation. • Instruct patient to reapply if washed off (hands, for example) during treatment time. • Hospitalized patients should be placed in isolation with special linen handling precautions until treatment is completed.

NAME	INDICATIONS & DOSAGE	SIDE EFFECTS
gamma benzene hexachloride (or lindane) Gamene, GBH♦♦, Kwell, Kwellada♦♦	*Parasitic infestation (scabies, pediculosis)—* **Adults and children:** scrub entire body with soap and water. Cream or lotion—apply thin layer over entire skin surface (with special attention to folds, creases, interdigital spaces, genital area) for scabies, or to hairy areas for pediculosis. After 8 to 12 hours, wash off drug. If second application needed for scabies, wait 1 week before repeating. For pediculosis, may be repeated after 7 days but never more than twice in a week. Shampoo—apply 30 to 60 ml onto affected area and work into lather for 4 to 5 minutes. Rinse thoroughly and rub with dry towel.	**Skin:** *irritation with repeated use.*
pyrethrins Rid, A-200 Pyrinate, Pyrin-Aid, Pyrinyl, Barc, TISIT, Triple X (See chapter 88 for information about other pediculicides.)	*Treatment of infestations of head, body, and pubic (crab) lice and their eggs—* **Adults and children:** apply to hair, scalp, or other infested area until entirely wet. Allow to remain for 10 minutes, but no longer. Wash thoroughly with warm water and soap, or shampoo. Remove dead lice and eggs with fine-toothed comb. Treatment may be repeated, if necessary, but don't exceed 2 applications within 24 hours.	**Skin:** *irritation with repeated use.*
sulfa (6%) in petrolatum	*Parasitic infestation (scabies)—* **Adults and children (preferred treatment for infants and pregnant women):** after taking a soapy bath, patient should apply drug nightly for 2 to 3 nights consecutively. He should take soapy bath 24 hours after last application.	**Skin:** *may produce dermatitis if applied continually for several days.*

♦ Available in U.S. and Canada. ♦♦ Available in Canada only. All other products (no symbol) available in U.S. only. Italicized side effects are common or life-threatening.

INTERACTIONS	NURSING CONSIDERATIONS
None significant.	• Contraindicated when skin is raw or inflamed. Notify doctor immediately if skin irritation or hypersensitivity develops; tell patient to discontinue drug and to wash it off skin. Use cautiously in infants and small children. • Do not apply to open areas or acutely inflamed skin, or to face, eyes, mucous membranes, or urethral meatus. If accidental contact with eyes does occur, flush with water and notify doctor. • Warn parents not to let infants or children suck their fingers after drug application. • Discourage repeated use, which can lead to skin irritation and possible systemic toxicity. • Warn patient itching may continue several weeks, especially in scabies. • Topical corticosteroids may be needed if dermatitis develops from scratching. • Instruct patient to change and sterilize (boil, launder, dry clean, or apply very hot iron) all clothing and bed linen after drug is washed off. • After application, use a fine comb dipped in white vinegar on hair to remove nits. • Gamma benzene hexachloride shampoo can be used to clean comb or brushes; wash them thoroughly afterward. Warn patient not to use gamma benzene hexachloride as routine shampoo. • Question other family members about possible infestation. • Tendency for overuse. Estimate amount needed. • Instruct patient to reapply if washed off (hands, for example) during treatment time. • Hospitalized patients should be placed in isolation with special linen handling precautions until treatment is completed.
None significant.	• Contraindicated when skin is raw or inflamed. Notify doctor immediately if skin irritation develops; tell patient to discontinue drug and to wash it off skin. Use cautiously in infants and small children. • Do not apply to open areas or acutely inflamed skin, or to face, eyes, mucous membranes, or urethral meatus. After accidental contact with eyes, flush with water and notify doctor. • Warn parents not to let infants or children suck their fingers after drug application. • Discourage repeated use, which can lead to skin irritation and possible systemic toxicity. • Topical corticosteroids may be needed if dermatitis develops from scratching. • Instruct patient to change and sterilize (boil, launder, dry clean, or apply very hot iron) all clothing and bed linen after drug is washed off. • Products containing pyrethrins are available without prescription. Some authorities consider pyrethrins and gamma benzene hexachloride (Kwell) equally effective for lice infestation.
None significant.	• Instruct patient to change and sterilize (boil, launder, dry clean, or apply very hot iron) all clothing and bed linen after drug is washed off. • Warn patient product has an odor, is messy, and stains clothing. • Question other members of family about possible infestation. • Tendency to overuse scabicides. Estimate amount needed. • Hospitalized patients should be placed in isolation with special linen handling precautions until treatment is completed.

Topical corticosteroids

amcinonide
betamethasone
betamethasone benzoate
betamethasone dipropionate
betamethasone valerate
desonide
desoximetasone
dexamethasone
dexamethasone sodium phosphate
diflorasone diacetate
flumethasone pivalate
fluocinolone acetonide
fluocinonide
fluorometholone
flurandrenolide
halcinonide
hydrocortisone
hydrocortisone acetate
hydrocortisone valerate
methylprednisolone acetate
prednisolone
triamcinolone acetonide

For information on clocortolone pivalate, see APPENDIX, *New Drugs*.

Topical corticosteroids reduce inflammation, constrict blood vessels, and occasionally relieve itching. Their potency depends on the drug, the method of application, and the degree of penetration. The base or vehicle of the drug may also affect its release and therefore its potency. Ointments furnish most complete penetration of the skin by the drug; gels, creams, and lotions are less penetrating, in descending order. Topical corticosteroids reduce inflammation without curing the underlying disease; use them with caution.

After the drug is applied to the affected site, it may be covered by an occlusive dressing. The dressing facilitates the drug's absorption through the skin. Tape is used to hold the dressing in place. It protects the adjacent unaffected skin from abrasion, rubbing, discoloration, and chemical irritation. It also acts as a mechanical splint for fissured skin and prevents medication from being removed by washing or rubbing against clothing.

Major uses

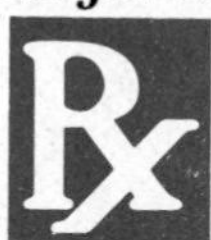

Topical corticosteroids are used to treat acute and chronic inflammatory dermatoses; psoriasis; atopic and infantile eczemas; pruritus ani and vulvae; neurodermatitis, and contact, seborrheic, and exfoliative dermatitis.

Occlusive dressings are used in the medical management of psoriasis or such resistant conditions as localized neurodermatitis or lichen planus.

Creams are useful for wet lesions; *lotions,* for areas subject to chafing (axillae, feet, or groin); and *ointments,* for dry, scaly lesions.

Mechanism of action

Exactly how these drugs work is unknown. Some investigators believe that corticosteroids attach to tissue receptors, decreasing membrane permeability and inhibiting release of toxins. They may also control the rate of protein synthesis. Their actions on the in-

RELATIVE POTENCY OF TOPICAL CORTICOSTEROIDS

DRUG	CONCENTRATION(%)	VEHICLE
Most potent:		
fluocinonide*	0.05	C, G, O, S
halcinonide*	0.1	C, O
diflorasone diacetate*	0.05	C, O
desoximetasone*	0.25	C
fluocinolone*	0.2	C
triamcinolone acetonide*	0.5	C, O
betamethasone dipropionate*	0.05	C, L, O
Moderately potent:		
betamethasone benzoate*	0.025	C, G, L
halcinonide*	0.025	C, O
triamcinolone acetonide*	0.1	C, L, O
flurandrenolide*	0.05	C, L, O
amcinonide*	0.1	C
fluocinolone acetonide*	0.025	C, O
desonide	0.05	C, O
betamethasone valerate*	0.1	C, L, O
Mildly potent:		
flumethasone pivalate*	0.03	C
triamcinolone acetonide*	0.025	C, O
fluorometholone*	0.025	C
flurandrenolide*	0.025	C, O
betamethasone valerate*	0.01	C
hydrocortisone valerate	0.2	C
fluocinolone acetonide*	0.01	C, S
Least potent:		
betamethasone*	0.2	C
betamethasone*	0.1	C
prednisolone	0.5	C
methylprednisolone acetate	1.0	O
dexamethasone*	0.1	C
dexamethasone*	0.04	C
methylprednisolone acetate	0.25	O
hydrocortisone	2.5	C, O
hydrocortisone	1.0	C, L, O
hydrocortisone	0.5	C, L, O
hydrocortisone	0.25	C, L

KEY: C = cream; G = gel; L = lotion; O = ointment; S = solution

Note: Within each group, the more potent precedes the less potent drug. Potency is, at best, an approximation based on vasoconstrictor assays, double-blind studies, and general clinical observations. Hence, no *significant* difference exists among drugs within any given group.

*Compounds with fluoro substituents

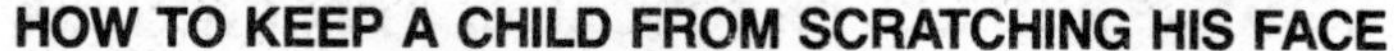

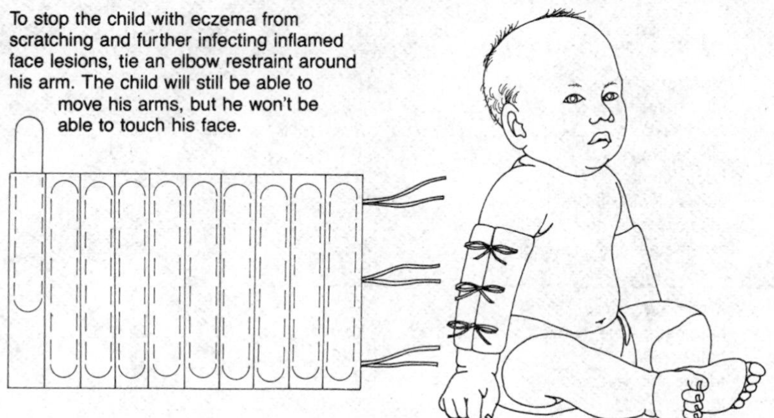

To stop the child with eczema from scratching and further infecting inflamed face lesions, tie an elbow restraint around his arm. The child will still be able to move his arms, but he won't be able to touch his face.

Because children find restraints so distressing, avoid using them whenever possible. Fortunately, antipruritic medications and lotions usually relieve itching sufficiently. When they don't, first try mild restraint, such as mittens made of stockinette or an undershirt. Mitten restraints are especially effective if the child's skin lesions are on the forearm, ruling out the cuff restraint (shown above).

flammatory process include inhibition of edema, fibrin deposition, capillary dilation, migration of leukocytes into the inflamed area, and phagocytic activity. They may also moderate later inflammatory developments such as capillary and fibroblast proliferation and deposition of collagen.

Cortiscosteroid-induced vasoconstriction decreases extravasation of blood, swelling, and itching. The drugs also act as antimitotics, reducing cell multiplication in psoriasis.

Absorption, distribution, metabolism, and excretion

• Corticosteroids are absorbed through the skin, and absorption varies markedly with the area of the body on which the drugs are applied. If the skin is well hydrated, absorption will be increased four to five times. Inflamed or damaged skin also allows increased penetration. Occlusive dressings increase absorption significantly (up to a hundred times). They retain insensible perspiration, causing hydration of the stratum corneum.

Absorption of these drugs in dressings that occlude extensive areas of skin can lead to adrenal suppression. Adrenal suppression may develop even in the absence of occlusion, if drug use is prolonged.

• These drugs enter the circulation and are metabolized primarily in the liver. The metabolites are excreted in urine. (For greater detail, see Chapter 52, CORTICOSTEROIDS.)

Onset and duration

Topical corticosteroids begin to act within 30 minutes after application. Because their action lasts only 4 to 6 hours, apply 2 to 4 times daily.

Combination products

Corticosteroids are commonly combined with antibiotics, antifungals, and sulfonamides. (See also Chapter 17, SULFONAMIDES, and Chapter 74, ANTIBIOTIC ANTINEOPLASTIC AGENTS.)

HOW TO APPLY OCCLUSIVE DRESSINGS

To create an occlusive dressing, put a plastic bag over the treated area. Seal the open ends with tape. Try to minimize the size of air pockets under the plastic since these may influence moisture retention and reduce the amount of medication in contact with the lesion.

The illustration below shows how an occlusive dressing would look on a foot.

Note: When there is no toe involvement, the tip of the plastic bag should be cut off and the edges sealed with tape.

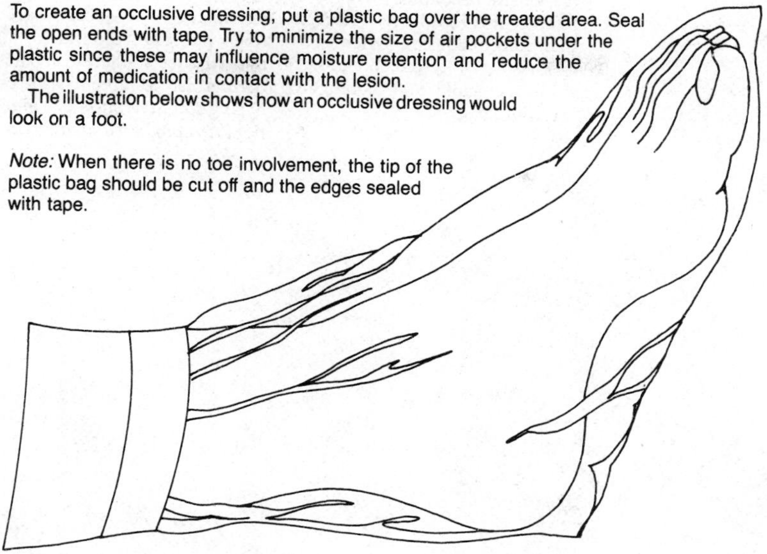

NAME	INDICATIONS & DOSAGE	SIDE EFFECTS
amcinonide Cyclocort♦	*Inflammation of corticosteroid-responsive dermatoses*— **Adults and children:** apply a light film to affected areas 2 or 3 times daily. Cream should be rubbed in gently and thoroughly until it disappears.	**Skin:** burning, itching, irritation, dryness, folliculitis, hypopigmentation, striae, acneiform eruptions, perioral dermatitis, hypertrichosis, allergic contact dermatitis. *With occlusive dressings: secondary infection, maceration, atrophy, striae, miliaria.*
betamethasone Celestone♦	*Inflammation of corticosteroid-responsive dermatoses*— **Adults and children:** clean area; apply cream sparingly b.i.d. or t.i.d. Massage gently until it disappears. Apply thick layer with occlusive dressing to manage deep-seated dermatoses, such as neurodermatitis.	**Skin:** burning, itching, irritation, dryness, folliculitis, hypopigmentation, acneiform eruptions, hypertrichosis, allergic contact dermatitis. *With occlusive dressings: secondary infection, maceration, skin atrophy, striae, miliaria.*

♦ Available in U.S. and Canada. ♦♦ Available in Canada only. All other products (no symbol) available in U.S. only. Italicized side effects are common or life-threatening.

INTERACTIONS	NURSING CONSIDERATIONS
None significant.	• Use cautiously in viral diseases of skin, such as varicella, vaccinia, herpes simplex; fungal infections; skin tuberculosis; impaired circulation. • Avoid application in or near eyes. Do not use on face, armpits, groin, or under breasts unless specifically ordered. • Due to alcohol content of vehicle, gel preparations may cause mild, transient stinging without irritation if used on or near excoriated skin. • Systemic absorption especially likely with occlusive dressings, prolonged treatment, or extensive body-surface treatment. • Stop drug and notify doctor if patient develops signs of systemic absorption, skin irritation or ulceration, signs of hypersensitivity, infection. (If antifungals or antibiotics are being used with corticosteroids and infection does not respond immediately, corticosteroids should be stopped until infection is controlled.) • Before applying, gently wash skin. To prevent damage to skin, rub in medication gently, leaving a thin coat. When treating hairy sites, part hair and apply directly to lesion. Apply lotions to scalp immediately after shampoo, while scalp is still damp. • Occlusive dressing: apply cream heavily, then cover with a thin, pliable, nonflammable plastic film; seal to adjacent normal skin with hypoallergenic tape. Minimize adverse reactions by using occlusive dressing intermittently. • For patient with eczematous dermatitis who may develop irritation with adhesive material, hold dressing in place with gauze, elastic bandages, stockings, or stockinette. • Notify doctor and remove occlusive dressing if body temperature rises. • Occlusive dressings are generally not used in presence of infections or with weeping or exudative lesions. • Change dressings as ordered by doctor. Inspect skin for infection, striae, and atrophy. Discontinue drug and notify doctor if these occur. • Treatment should be continued for a few days after clearing of lesions to prevent recurrence. • Instruct patient to report signs of drug sensitivity.
None significant.	• Use cautiously in viral diseases of skin, such as vaccinia, varicella, herpes simplex; fungal infections; skin tuberculosis; impaired circulation. • Avoid application in or near eyes. • Systemic absorption especially likely with occlusive dressings, prolonged treatment, or extensive body-surface treatment. • Stop drug and notify doctor if patient develops signs of systemic absorption, skin irritation or ulceration, hypersensitivity, infection. (If antifungals or antibacterials are being used with corticosteroids and infection does not respond immediately, corticosteroids should be stopped until infection is controlled.) • Before applying, gently wash skin. To prevent damage to skin, rub medication in gently, leaving a thin coat. • Occlusive dressing: apply cream heavily, then cover with a thin, pliable, nonflammable plastic film; seal to adjacent normal skin with hypoallergenic tape. Minimize adverse reactions by using occlusive dressing intermittently. • For patient with eczematous dermatitis who may develop irritation with adhesive material, hold dressing in place with gauze, elastic bandages, stockings, or stockinette. • Notify doctor and remove occlusive dressing if body temperature rises.

(continued on following page)

NAME	INDICATIONS & DOSAGE	SIDE EFFECTS
betamethasone *(continued)*		
betamethasone benzoate Beben♦, Benisone, Uticort	*Inflammation of corticosteroid-responsive dermatoses—* **Adults and children:** clean area; apply cream, lotion, or gel sparingly daily to q.i.d.	**Skin:** burning, itching, irritation, dryness, folliculitis, hypopigmentation, striae, acneiform eruptions, perioral dermatitis, hypertrichosis, allergic contact dermatitis. *With occlusive dressings: secondary infection, maceration, atrophy, striae, miliaria.*
betamethasone dipropionate Diprosone♦	*Inflammation of corticosteroid-responsive dermatoses—* **Adults and children:** clean area; apply cream, lotion, or ointment sparingly b.i.d. Aerosol: Direct spray onto affected area from a distance of 6 inches for only 3 seconds t.i.d.	**Skin:** burning, itching, irritation, dryness, folliculitis, hypopigmentation, perioral dermatitis, allergic contact dermatitis, hypertrichosis, acneiform eruptions. *With occlusive dressings: maceration of skin, secondary infection, atrophy, striae, miliaria.*

♦ Available in U.S. and Canada. ♦♦ Available in Canada only. All other products (no symbol) available in U.S. only. Italicized side effects are common or life-threatening.

INTERACTIONS	NURSING CONSIDERATIONS
	• Occlusive dressings are generally not used in presence of infection or with weeping or exudative lesions. • Change dressing as ordered by doctor. Inspect skin for infection, striae, and atrophy. Discontinue drug and notify doctor if these occur. • Treatment should be continued for a few days after clearing of lesions to prevent recurrence. • Instruct patient to report signs of drug sensitivity.
None significant.	• Use cautiously in viral diseases of skin, such as varicella, vaccinia, herpes simplex; fungal infections; skin tuberculosis; impaired circulation. • Avoid application in or near eyes. • Due to alcohol content of vehicle, gel preparations may cause mild, transient stinging without irritation if used on or near excoriated skin. • Systemic absorption especially likely with occlusive dressings, prolonged treatment, or extensive body-surface treatment. • Stop drug and notify doctor if patient develops signs of systemic absorption, skin irritation or ulceration, signs of hypersensitivity, infection. (If antifungals or antibiotics are being used with corticosteroids and infection does not respond immediately, corticosteroids should be stopped until infection is controlled.) • Before applying, gently wash skin. To prevent damage to skin, rub in medication gently, leaving a thin coat. When treating hairy sites, part hair and apply directly to lesion. • Occlusive dressing: apply cream heavily, then cover with a thin, pliable, nonflammable plastic film; seal to adjacent normal skin with hypoallergenic tape. Minimize adverse reactions by using occlusive dressing intermittently. • For patient with eczematous dermatitis who may develop irritation with adhesive material, hold dressing in place with gauze, elastic bandages, stockings, or stockinette. • Notify doctor and remove occlusive dressing if body temperature rises. • Occlusive dressings are generally not used in presence of infections or with weeping or exudative lesions. • Change dressings as ordered by doctor. Inspect skin for infection, striae, and atrophy. Discontinue drug and notify doctor if these occur. • Treatment should be continued for a few days after clearing of lesions to prevent recurrence. • Instruct patient to report signs of drug sensitivity.
None significant.	• Use cautiously in viral diseases of skin, such as varicella, vaccinia, herpes simplex; fungal infections; skin tuberculosis; impaired circulation. • Avoid application in or near eyes. • Systemic absorption especially likely with occlusive dressings, prolonged treatment, or extensive body-surface treatment. • Stop drug and notify doctor if patient develops signs of systemic absorption, skin irritation or ulceration, hypersensitivity, infection. (If antifungals or antibiotics are being used with corticosteroids and infection does not respond immediately, corticosteroids should be stopped until infection is controlled.) • Before applying, gently wash skin. To prevent damage to skin, rub in medication gently, leaving a thin coat. When treating hairy sites, part hair and apply directly to lesion. • Aerosol preparation contains alcohol and may produce irritation or burning in open lesions. When using about the face, cover patient's

(continued on following page)

NAME	INDICATIONS & DOSAGE	SIDE EFFECTS
betamethasone dipropionate *(continued)*		
betamethasone valerate Betnovate♦♦, Betnovate 1/2♦♦, Celestoderm-V♦♦, Celestoderm-V/2♦♦, Valisone	*Inflammation of corticosteroid-responsive dermatoses—* **Adults and children:** clean area; apply cream, lotion, ointment, or aerosol sparingly daily to q.i.d. Aerosol: shake can well. Direct spray onto affected area from a distance of 6 inches. Apply for only 3 seconds t.i.d. to q.i.d. Betnovate 1/2 and Celestoderm V/2 contain less betamethasone.	**Skin:** burning, itching, irritation, dryness, folliculitis, hypopigmentation, hypertrichosis, acneiform eruptions, perioral dermatitis, allergic contact dermatitis. *With occlusive dressings: maceration of skin, secondary infection, atrophy, striae, miliaria.*
desonide Tridesilon♦	*Adjunctive therapy for inflammation in acute and chronic corticosteroid-responsive dermatoses—* **Adults and children:** clean area; apply cream, lotion, or gel sparingly b.i.d. to t.i.d.	**Skin:** burning, itching, irritation, dryness, folliculitis, hypopigmentation, perioral dermatitis, allergic contact dermatitis, hypertrichosis, acneiform eruptions. *With occlusive dressings: maceration of skin, secondary infection, atrophy, striae, miliaria.*

INTERACTIONS	NURSING CONSIDERATIONS
	eyes and warn against inhalation of spray. To avoid freezing tissues, do not spray longer than 3 seconds or closer than 6 inches. • For patient with eczematous dermatitis who may develop irritation with adhesive material, hold dressing in place with gauze, elastic bandages, stockings, or stockinette. • Occlusive dressings are generally not used in presence of infection or with weeping or exudative lesions. • Change dressing as ordered by doctor. Inspect skin for infection, striae, and atrophy. Discontinue drug and notify doctor if these occur. • Instruct patient to report signs of drug sensitivity.
None significant.	• Use cautiously in viral diseases of skin, such as varicella, vaccinia, herpes simplex; fungal infections; skin tuberculosis; impaired circulation. • Avoid application in or near eyes. • Systemic absorption especially likely with occlusive dressings, prolonged treatment, or extensive body-surface treatment. • Stop drug and notify doctor if patient develops signs of systemic absorption, skin irritation or ulceration, hypersensitivity, infection. (If antifungals or antibiotics are being used with corticosteroids and infection does not respond immediately, corticosteroids should be stopped until infection is controlled.) • Before applying, gently wash skin. To prevent damage to skin, rub in medication gently, leaving a thin coat. When treating hairy sites, part hair and apply directly to lesions. • Aerosol preparation contains alcohol and may produce irritation or burning in open lesions. When using about the face, cover patient's eyes and warn against inhalation of the spray. To avoid freezing tissues, do not spray longer than 3 seconds or closer than 6 inches. • Occlusive dressing: apply cream or ointment heavily, then cover with a thin, pliable, nonflammable plastic film; seal to adjacent normal skin with hypoallergenic tape. Minimize adverse reactions by using occlusive dressing intermittently. • For patient with eczematous dermatitis who may develop irritation with adhesive material, hold dressing in place with gauze, elastic bandages, stockings, or stockinette. • Notify doctor and remove occlusive dressing if body temperature rises. • Occlusive dressings are generally not used in presence of infection or with weeping or exudative lesions. • Change dressing as ordered by doctor. Inspect skin for infection, striae, and atrophy. Discontinue drug and notify doctor if these occur. • Treatment should be continued for a few days after clearing of lesions to prevent recurrence. • Instruct patient to report signs of drug sensitivity.
None significant.	• Use cautiously in viral diseases of skin, such as varicella, vaccinia, herpes simplex; fungal infections; skin tuberculosis; impaired circulation. • Avoid application in or near eyes. • Systemic absorption especially likely with occlusive dressings, prolonged treatment, or extensive body-surface treatment. • Stop drug and notify doctor if patient develops signs of systemic absorption, skin irritation or ulceration, hypersensitivity, infection. (If antifungals or antibiotics are being used with corticosteroids and infection does not respond immediately, corticosteroids should be stopped until infection is controlled.)

(continued on following page)

NAME	INDICATIONS & DOSAGE	SIDE EFFECTS
desonide *(continued)*		
desoximetasone Topicort♦	*Inflammation of corticosteroid-responsive dermatoses*— **Adults and children:** clean area; apply cream sparingly b.i.d.	**Skin:** burning, itching, irritation, dryness, folliculitis, hypopigmentation, hypertrichosis, acneiform eruptions, perioral dermatitis, allergic contact dermatitis. *With occlusive dressings: maceration of skin, secondary infection, atrophy, striae, miliaria.*
dexamethasone Aeroseb-Dex, Decaderm, Decaspray, Hexadrol♦	*Inflammation of corticosteroid-responsive dermatoses*— **Adults and children:** clean area; apply cream, gel, or aerosol sparingly b.i.d. to q.i.d. Aerosol use on scalp: shake can well and apply to dry scalp after	**Skin:** burning, itching, irritation, dryness, folliculitis, hypopigmentation, hypertrichosis, acneiform eruptions, perioral dermatitis, allergic contact dermatitis. *With occlusive dressings: maceration of skin, secondary infection,*

♦ Available in U.S. and Canada. ♦♦ Available in Canada only. All other products (no symbol) available in U.S. only. Italicized side effects are common or life-threatening.

INTERACTIONS	NURSING CONSIDERATIONS
	• Before applying, gently wash skin. To prevent damage to skin, rub in medication gently, leaving a thin coat. When treating hairy sites, part hair and apply directly to lesion. • Occlusive dressing: apply cream or ointment heavily, then cover with a thin, pliable, nonflammable plastic film; seal to adjacent normal skin with hypoallergenic tape. Minimize adverse reactions by using occlusive dressing intermittently. • For patient with eczematous dermatitis who may develop irritation with adhesive material, hold dressing in place with gauze, elastic bandages, stockings, or stockinette. • Notify doctor and remove occlusive dressing if body temperature rises. • Occlusive dressings are generally not used in presence of infection or with weeping or exudative lesions. • Change dressing as ordered by doctor. Inspect skin for infection, striae, and atrophy. Discontinue drug and notify doctor if these occur. • Treatment should be continued for a few days after clearing of lesions to prevent recurrence. • Instruct patient to report signs of drug sensitivity.
None significant.	• Use cautiously in viral diseases of skin, such as varicella, vaccinia, herpes simplex; fungal infections; skin tuberculosis; impaired circulation. • Avoid application in or near eyes. • Systemic absorption especially likely with occlusive dressings, prolonged treatment, or extensive body-surface treatment. • Stop drug and notify doctor if patient develops signs of systemic absorption, skin irritation or ulceration, hypersensitivity, infection. (If antifungals or antibiotics are being used with corticosteroids and infection does not respond immediately, corticosteroids should be stopped until infection is controlled.) • Before applying, gently wash skin. To prevent damage to skin, rub in medication gently, leaving a thin coat. When treating hairy sites, part hair and apply directly to lesions. • Occlusive dressing: apply cream heavily, then cover with a thin, pliable, nonflammable plastic film; seal to adjacent normal skin with hypoallergenic tape. To minimize adverse reactions, use occlusive dressing intermittently. • For patient with eczematous dermatitis who may develop irritation with adhesive material, hold dressing in place with gauze, elastic bandages, stockings, or stockinette. • Notify doctor and remove occlusive dressing if body temperature rises. • Occlusive dressings are generally not used in presence of infection or with weeping or exudative lesions. • Change dressing as ordered by doctor. Inspect skin for infection, striae, and atrophy. Discontinue drug and notify doctor if these occur. • Treatment should be continued for a few days after clearing of lesions to prevent recurrence. • Instruct patient to report signs of drug sensitivity.
None significant.	• Use cautiously in viral diseases of skin, such as varicella, vaccinia, herpes simplex; fungal infections; skin tuberculosis; impaired circulation. • Avoid application in or near eyes. • Systemic absorption especially likely with occlusive dressings, prolonged treatment, or extensive body-surface treatment. • Stop drug and notify doctor if patient develops signs of systemic

(continued on following page)

NAME	INDICATIONS & DOSAGE	SIDE EFFECTS
dexamethasone *(continued)*	shampooing. Hold can upright. Slide applicator tube under hair so that it touches scalp. Spray while moving tube to all affected areas, keeping tube under hair and in contact with scalp throughout spraying, which should take about 2 seconds. Inadequately covered areas may be spot sprayed. Slide applicator tube through hair to touch scalp, press and immediately release spray button. Don't massage medication into scalp or spray forehead or eyes.	*atrophy, striae, miliaria.*
dexamethasone sodium phosphate Decadron Phosphate♦	*Inflammation of corticosteroid-responsive dermatoses*— **Adults and children:** clean area; apply cream sparingly b.i.d. to t.i.d.	**Skin:** burning, itching, irritation, dryness, folliculitis, hypopigmentation, hypertrichosis, acneiform eruptions, perioral dermatitis, allergic contact dermatitis. *With occlusive dressings: maceration of skin, secondary infection, atrophy, striae, miliaria.*

INTERACTIONS	NURSING CONSIDERATIONS
	absorption, skin irritation or ulceration, signs of hypersensitivity, infection. (If antifungals or antibiotics are being used with corticosteroids and infection does not respond immediately, corticosteroids should be stopped until infection is controlled.) • Before applying, gently wash skin. To prevent damage to skin, rub in medication gently, leaving a thin coat. When treating hairy sites, part hair and apply directly to lesions. • Occlusive dressing: apply cream heavily and cover with a thin, pliable, nonflammable plastic film; seal to adjacent normal skin with hypoallergenic tape. To minimize adverse reactions, use occlusive dressing intermittently. • For patient with eczematous dermatitis who may develop irritation with adhesive material, hold dressing in place with gauze, elastic bandages, stockings, or stockinette. • Notify doctor and remove occlusive dressing if body temperature rises. • Change dressing as ordered by doctor. Inspect skin for infection, striae, and atrophy. Discontinue drug and notify doctor if these occur. • Occlusive dressings are generally not used in presence of infection or with weeping or exudative lesions. • Aerosol preparation contains alcohol and may produce irritation or burning in open lesions. When using about the face, cover patient's eyes and warn against inhalation of the spray. To avoid freezing tissues, do not spray longer than 3 seconds or closer than 6 inches. • Treatments should be continued for a few days after clearing of lesions to prevent recurrence. • Instruct patient to report signs of drug sensitivity.
None significant.	• Use cautiously in viral diseases of skin, such as varicella, vaccinia, herpes simplex; fungal infections; skin tuberculosis; impaired circulation. • Avoid application in or near eyes. • Systemic absorption especially likely with occlusive dressings, prolonged treatment, or extensive body-surface treatment. • Stop drug and notify doctor if patient develops signs of systemic absorption, skin irritation or ulceration, hypersensitivity, infection. (If antifungals or antibiotics are being used along with corticosteroids and infection does not respond immediately, corticosteroids should be stopped until infection is controlled.) • Before applying, gently wash skin. To prevent damage to skin, rub in medication gently, leaving a thin coat. When treating hairy sites, part hair and apply directly to lesions. • Occlusive dressing: apply cream heavily, then cover with a thin, pliable, nonflammable plastic film; seal to adjacent normal skin with hypoallergenic tape. To minimize adverse reactions, use occlusive dressing intermittently. Occlusive dressings are generally not used in presence of infection or with weeping or exudative lesions. • For patient with eczematous dermatitis who may develop irritation with adhesive material, hold dressing in place with gauze, elastic bandages, stockings, or stockinette. • Notify doctor and remove occlusive dressing if body temperature rises. • Change dressing as ordered by doctor. Inspect skin for infection, striae, and atrophy. Discontinue drug and notify doctor if these occur. • Treatment should be continued for a few days after clearing of lesions to prevent recurrence. • Instruct patient to report signs of drug sensitivity.

NAME	INDICATIONS & DOSAGE	SIDE EFFECTS
diflorasone diacetate Florone, Maxiflor	*Inflammation of corticosteroid-responsive dermatoses*— **Adults and children:** clean area; apply ointment daily to t.i.d.; apply cream b.i.d. to q.i.d. Apply sparingly in a thin film.	**Skin:** burning, itching, irritation, dryness, folliculitis, hypopigmentation, perioral dermatitis, hypertrichosis, acneiform eruptions. *With occlusive dressings: maceration, secondary infection, atrophy, striae, miliaria.*
flumethasone pivalate Locacorten♦♦, Locorten	*Inflammation of corticosteroid-responsive dermatoses*— **Adults and children:** clean area; apply cream sparingly t.i.d. to q.i.d.	**Skin:** burning, itching, irritation, dryness, folliculitis, hypopigmentation, hypertrichosis, acneiform eruptions, perioral dermatitis, allergic contact dermatitis. *With occlusive dressings: maceration of skin, secondary infection, atrophy, striae, miliaria.*

INTERACTIONS	NURSING CONSIDERATIONS
None significant.	• Use cautiously in viral diseases of skin, such as varicella, vaccinia, herpes simplex; fungal infections; skin tuberculosis; impaired circulation. • Avoid application in or near eyes. • Systemic absorption especially likely with occlusive dressings, prolonged treatment, or extensive body-surface treatment. • Stop drug and notify doctor if patient develops signs of systemic absorption, skin irritation or ulceration, hypersensitivity, infection. (If antifungals or antibiotics are being used concomitantly, corticosteroids should be stopped until infection is controlled.) • Before applying, gently wash skin. To prevent damage to skin, rub in medication gently, leaving a thin coat. When treating hairy sites, part hair and apply directly to lesion. • Occlusive dressing: apply cream or ointment heavily, then cover with a thin, pliable, nonflammable plastic film; seal to adjacent normal skin with hypoallergenic tape. Minimize adverse reactions by using occlusive dressing intermittently. Occlusive dressings are generally not used in presence of infection or with weeping or exudative lesions. • For patient with eczematous dermatitis who may develop irritation with adhesive material, hold dressing in place with gauze, elastic bandages, stockings, or stockinette. • Notify doctor and remove occlusive dressing if body temperature rises. • Change dressing as ordered by doctor. Inspect skin for infection, striae, and atrophy. Discontinue drug and notify doctor if these occur. • Instruct patient to report signs of drug sensitivity. • Diflorasone is often effective with once-daily application.
None significant.	• Use cautiously in viral diseases of skin, such as varicella, vaccinia, and herpes simplex; fungal infections; skin tuberculosis; and impaired circulation. • Avoid application in or near eyes. • Systemic absorption especially likely with occlusive dressings, prolonged treatment, or extensive body-surface treatment. • Stop drug and notify doctor if patient develops signs of systemic absorption, skin irritation or ulceration, hypersensitivity, infection. (If antifungals or antibiotics are being used along with corticosteroids and infection does not respond immediately, corticosteroids should be stopped until infection is controlled.) • Before applying, gently wash skin. To prevent damage to skin, rub in medication gently, leaving a thin coat. When treating hairy sites, part hair and apply directly to lesion. • Occlusive dressing: apply cream or ointment heavily, then cover with a thin, pliable, nonflammable plastic film; seal to adjacent normal skin with hypoallergenic tape. To minimize adverse reactions, use occlusive dressing intermittently. Occlusive dressings are generally not used in presence of infection or with weeping or exudative lesions. • For patient with eczematous dermatitis who may develop irritation with adhesive material, hold dressing in place with gauze, elastic bandages, stockings, or stockinette. • Notify doctor and remove occlusive dressing if body temperature rises. • Change dressing as ordered by doctor. Inspect skin for infection, striae, and atrophy. Discontinue drug and notify doctor if these occur. • Treatment should be continued for a few days after clearing of lesions to prevent recurrence. • Instruct patient to report signs of drug sensitivity.

NAME	INDICATIONS & DOSAGE	SIDE EFFECTS
fluocinolone acetonide Fluonid, Synalar♦, Synalar-HP♦, Synamol♦, Synemol	*Inflammation of corticosteroid-responsive dermatoses*— **Adults, and children over 2 years:** clean area; apply cream, ointment, or solution sparingly b.i.d. to q.i.d. Treat multiple or extensive lesions sequentially, applying to only small areas at any one time.	**Skin:** burning, itching, irritation, dryness, folliculitis, hypopigmentation, hypertrichosis, acneiform eruptions, perioral dermatitis, allergic contact dermatitis. *With occlusive dressings: maceration of skin, secondary infection, atrophy, striae, miliaria.*
fluocinonide Lidemol♦♦, Lidex♦, Lidex-E, Topsyn♦	*Inflammation of corticosteroid-responsive dermatoses*— **Adults and children:** clean area; apply cream, ointment, or gel sparingly t.i.d. to q.i.d.	**Skin:** burning, itching, irritation, dryness, folliculitis, hypopigmentation, hypertrichosis, acneiform eruptions, perioral dermatitis, allergic contact dermatitis. *With occlusive dressings: maceration of skin, secondary infection, atrophy, striae, miliaria.*

♦ Available in U.S. and Canada. ♦♦ Available in Canada only. All other products (no symbol) available in U.S. only. Italicized side effects are common or life-threatening.

INTERACTIONS	NURSING CONSIDERATIONS
None significant.	• Use cautiously in viral diseases of skin, such as varicella, vaccinia, herpes simplex; fungal infections; skin tuberculosis; impaired circulation. • Avoid application in or near eyes. • Systemic absorption especially likely with occlusive dressings, prolonged treatment, or extensive body-surface treatment. • Stop drug and notify doctor if patient develops signs of systemic absorption, skin irritation or ulceration, hypersensitivity, infection. (If antifungals or antibiotics are being used with corticosteroids and infection does not respond immediately, corticosteroids should be stopped until infection is controlled.) • Before applying, gently wash skin. To prevent damage to skin, rub in medication gently, leaving a thin coat. When treating hairy sites, part hair and apply directly to lesion. • Occlusive dressing: apply gently and sparingly to the lesion until cream disappears. Then reapply, leaving a thin coat. Cover with a thin, pliable, nonflammable plastic film; seal to adjacent normal skin with hypoallergenic tape. To minimize adverse reactions, use occlusive dressing intermittently. Occlusive dressings are generally not used in presence of infection or with weeping or exudative lesions. • For patient with eczematous dermatitis who may develop irritation with adhesive material, hold dressing in place with gauze, elastic bandages, stockings, or stockinette. • Notify doctor and remove occlusive dressing if body temperature rises. • Change dressing as ordered by doctor. Inspect skin for infection, striae, and atrophy. Discontinue drug and notify doctor if these occur. • Instruct patient to report signs of drug sensitivity. • Fluonid solution on dry lesions may increase dryness, scaling, or itching; on denuded or fissured areas, may produce burning or stinging. If burning or stinging persists and dermatitis has not improved, solution should be discontinued.
None significant.	• Use cautiously in viral diseases of skin, such as varicella, vaccinia, and herpes simplex; untreated purulent bacterial skin infections; fungal infections; skin tuberculosis; impaired circulation. • Avoid application in or near eyes. • Systemic absorption especially likely with occlusive dressings, prolonged treatment, or extensive body-surface treatment. • Stop drug and notify doctor if patient develops signs of systemic absorption, skin irritation or ulceration, hypersensitivity, infection. (If antifungals or antibiotics are being used with corticosteroids and infection does not respond immediately, corticosteroids should be stopped until infection is controlled.) • Before applying, gently wash skin. To prevent damage to skin, rub in medication gently, leaving a thin coat. When treating hairy sites, part hair and apply directly to lesion. • Occlusive dressing: apply cream or ointment heavily, then cover with a thin, pliable, nonflammable plastic film; seal to adjacent normal skin with hypoallergenic tape. To minimize adverse reactions, use occlusive dressing intermittently. Occlusive dressings are generally not used in presence of infection or with weeping or exudative lesions. • For patient with eczematous dermatitis who may develop irritation with adhesive material, hold dressing in place with gauze, elastic bandages, stockings, or stockinette. • Notify doctor and remove occlusive dressing if body temperature rises.

(continued on following page)

NAME	INDICATIONS & DOSAGE	SIDE EFFECTS
fluocinonide *(continued)*		
fluorometholone Oxylone	*Inflammation of corticosteroid-responsive dermatoses*— **Adults and children:** clean area; apply cream sparingly daily to t.i.d.	**Skin:** burning, itching, irritation, dryness, folliculitis, hypopigmentation, hypertrichosis, acneiform eruptions, perioral dermatitis, allergic contact dermatitis. *With occlusive dressings: maceration of skin, secondary infection, atrophy, striae, miliaria.*
flurandrenolide Cordran, Cordran SP, Cordran Tape, Drenison♦♦, Drenison ¼♦♦, Drenison Tape♦♦	*Inflammation of corticosteroid-responsive dermatoses*— **Adults and children:** clean area; apply cream, lotion, or ointment sparingly b.i.d. or t.i.d. Apply tape q 12 to 24 hours. Before applying tape, cleanse skin carefully, removing scales, crust, and dried exudates. Allow skin to dry for 1 hour before applying new tape. Shave or clip hair to allow good contact with skin and comfortable removal. If tape ends loosen prematurely, trim off and replace with fresh tape. Lowest incidence of adverse reactions if tape is replaced q 12 hours, but may be left in place for 24 hours if well tolerated and adheres satisfactorily. Drenison ¼: for maintenance	**Skin:** burning, itching, irritation, dryness, folliculitis, hypopigmentation, hypertrichosis, acneiform eruptions, allergic contact dermatitis. *With occlusive dressings: maceration of skin, secondary infection, atrophy, striae, miliaria.* With tape: purpura, stripping of epidermis, furunculosis.

♦ Available in U.S. and Canada. ♦♦ Available in Canada only. All other products (no symbol) available in U.S. only. Italicized side effects are common or life-threatening.

INTERACTIONS	NURSING CONSIDERATIONS
	• Change dressing as ordered by doctor. Inspect skin for infection, striae, and atrophy. Discontinue drug and notify doctor if these occur. • Treatment should be continued for a few days after clearing of lesions to prevent recurrence. • Instruct patient to report signs of drug sensitivity.
None significant.	• Use cautiously in viral diseases of skin, such as varicella, vaccinia, herpes simplex; fungal infections; skin tuberculosis; impaired circulation. • Avoid application in or near eyes. • Systemic absorption especially likely with occlusive dressings, prolonged treatment, or extensive body-surface treatment. • Stop drug and notify doctor if patient develops signs of systemic absorption, skin irritation or ulceration, hypersensitivity, infection. (If antifungals or antibiotics are being used with corticosteroids and infection does not respond immediately, corticosteroids should be stopped until infection is controlled.) • Before applying, gently wash skin. To prevent damage to skin, rub in medication gently, leaving a thin coat. When treating hairy sites, part hair and apply directly to lesion. • Occlusive dressing: apply cream heavily, then cover with a thin, pliable, nonflammable plastic film; seal to adjacent normal skin with hypoallergenic tape. To minimize adverse reactions, use occlusive dressing intermittently. Occlusive dressings are generally not used in presence of infection or with weeping or exudative lesions. • For patient with eczematous dermatitis who may develop irritation with adhesive material, hold dressing in place with gauze, elastic bandages, stockings, or stockinette. • Notify doctor and remove occlusive dressing if body temperature rises. • Change dressing as ordered by doctor. Inspect skin for infection, striae, and atrophy. Discontinue drug and notify doctor if these occur. • Treatment should be continued for a few days after clearing of lesions to prevent recurrence. • Instruct patient to report signs of drug sensitivity.
None significant.	• Use cautiously in viral diseases of skin, such as varicella, vaccinia, herpes simplex; fungal infections; skin tuberculosis; impaired circulation. • Tape not advised for exudative lesions or those in intertriginous areas. • Avoid application in or near eyes. • Systemic absorption especially likely with occlusive dressings, prolonged treatment, or extensive body-surface treatment. • Stop drug and notify doctor if patient develops signs of systemic absorption, skin irritation or ulceration, hypersensitivity, infection. (If antifungals or antibiotics are being used with corticosteroids and infection does not respond immediately, corticosteroids should be stopped until infection is controlled.) • Before applying, gently wash skin. To prevent damage to skin, rub in medication gently, leaving a thin coat. When treating hairy sites, part hair and apply directly to lesion. • Occlusive dressing: apply cream heavily, then cover with a thin, pliable, nonflammable plastic film; seal to adjacent normal skin with hypoallergenic tape. To minimize adverse reactions, use occlusive dressing intermittently. Occlusive dressings are generally not used in presence of infection or with weeping or exudative lesions. • For patient with eczematous dermatitis who may develop irritation

(continued on following page)

NAME	INDICATIONS & DOSAGE	SIDE EFFECTS
flurandrenolide *(continued)*	therapy of widespread or chronic lesions.	
halcinonide Halciderm, Halog♦	*Inflammation of acute and chronic corticosteroid-responsive dermatoses—* **Adults and children:** clean area; apply cream, ointment, or solution sparingly b.i.d. to t.i.d.	**Skin:** burning, itching, irritation, dryness, folliculitis, hypopigmentation, hypertrichosis, acneiform eruptions, allergic contact dermatitis. *With occlusive dressings: maceration of skin, secondary infection, atrophy, striae, miliaria.*
hydrocortisone Acticort, Aeroseb-HC♦, Alphaderm, Carmol-HC, Cetacort, Cortaid, Cort-Dome♦, Corticreme♦♦, Cortinal, Cortril♦, Cotacort, Cremesone, Delacort, Dermacort,	*Inflammation of corticosteroid-responsive dermatoses; adjunctive typical management of seborrheic dermatitis of scalp; may be safely used on face, groin, armpits, and under breasts—* **Adults and children:** clean area; apply cream, lotion, ointment, or aerosol sparingly daily	**Skin:** burning, itching, irritation, dryness, folliculitis, hypopigmentation, hypertrichosis, acneiform eruptions, allergic contact dermatitis. *With occlusive dressings: maceration of skin, secondary infection, atrophy, striae, miliaria.*

♦ Available in U.S. and Canada. ♦♦ Available in Canada only. All other products (no symbol) available in U.S. only. Italicized side effects are common or life-threatening.

INTERACTIONS	NURSING CONSIDERATIONS
	with adhesive material, hold dressing in place with gauze, elastic bandages, stockings, or stockinette. • Notify doctor and remove occlusive dressing if body temperature rises. • Change dressing as ordered by doctor. Inspect skin for infection, striae, and atrophy. Discontinue drug and notify doctor if these occur. • Treatment should be continued for a few days after clearing of lesions to prevent recurrence. • Instruct patient to report signs of drug sensitivity.
None significant.	• Use cautiously in viral diseases of skin, such as varicella, vaccinia, herpes simplex; fungal infections; skin tuberculosis; impaired circulation. • Avoid application in or near eyes. • Systemic absorption especially likely with occlusive dressings, prolonged treatment, or extensive body-surface treatment. • Stop drug and notify doctor if patient develops signs of systemic absorption, skin irritation or ulceration, hypersensitivity, infection. (If antifungals or antibiotics are being used with corticosteroids and infection does not respond immediately, corticosteroids should be stopped until infection is controlled.) • Before applying, gently wash skin. To prevent damage to skin, rub in medication gently, leaving a thin coat. When treating hairy sites, part hair and apply directly to lesion. • Occlusive dressing with cream: gently rub small amount into lesion until it disappears. Reapply, leaving a thin coating on lesion, and cover with occlusive dressing. With ointment: apply to lesion and cover with occlusive dressing. Cover with a thin, pliable, nonflammable plastic film; seal to adjacent normal skin with hypoallergenic tape. To minimize adverse reactions, use occlusive dressing intermittently; or with extensive lesions, occlude one part of the body at a time. • Good results have been obtained by applying occlusive dressings in the evening and removing them in the morning (i.e., 12-hour occlusion). Medication should then be reapplied in the morning, without using the occlusive dressings during the day. • For patient with eczematous dermatitis who may develop irritation with adhesive material, hold dressing in place with gauze, elastic bandages, stockings, or stockinette. • Notify doctor and remove occlusive dressing if body temperature rises. • Occlusive dressings are generally not used in presence of infection or with weeping or exudative lesions. • Change dressing as ordered by doctor. Inspect skin for infection, striae, and atrophy. Discontinue drug and notify doctor if these occur. • Treatment should be continued for a few days after clearing of lesions to prevent recurrence. • Instruct patient to report signs of drug sensitivity.
None significant.	• Use cautiously in viral diseases of skin, such as varicella, vaccinia, herpes simplex; fungal infections; skin tuberculosis; impaired circulation. • Avoid application in or near eyes. • Systemic absorption especially likely with occlusive dressings, prolonged treatment, or extensive body-surface treatment. • Stop drug and notify doctor if patient develops signs of systemic absorption, skin irritation or ulceration, hypersensitivity, infection. (If antifungals or antibiotics are being used with corticosteroids and

(continued on following page)

NAME	INDICATIONS & DOSAGE	SIDE EFFECTS
hydrocortisone *(continued)* Dermolate, Durel-Cort, Ecosone, Eldecort, Emo-Cort◆◆, HC Cream, Heb-Cort, HI-COR-2.5, Hycort, Hycortole, Hydrocortex, Hydro-Cortilean◆◆, Hytone, Ivocort, Manticor◆◆, Maso-Cort, Microcort◆, Nutracort◆, Penetrate, Proctocort, Rectocort◆◆, Relecort, Rhus Tox HC, Rocort, Tarcortin, Ulcort, Unicort	to q.i.d. Aerosol: shake can well. Direct spray onto affected area from a distance of 6 inches. Apply for only 3 seconds (to avoid freezing tissues). Apply to dry scalp after shampooing; no need to massage or rub medication into scalp after spraying. Apply daily until acute phase is controlled, then reduce dosage to 1 to 3 times a week as needed to maintain control.	
hydrocortisone acetate Cortifoam, Cortiprel, Cortef Acetate, Epifoam, Hydrocortisone Acetate, Hydrocortone Acetate, My-Cort Lotion **hydrocortisone valerate** Westcort Cream	*Inflammation of corticosteroid-responsive dermatoses*— **Adults and children:** clean area; apply lotion, cream, ointment, or foam (acetate) sparingly daily to q.i.d. Massage gently (valerate) 2 to 3 times daily p.r.n.	**Skin:** burning, itching, irritation, dryness, folliculitis, hypopigmentation, hypertrichosis, acneiform eruptions, perioral dermatitis, allergic contact dermatitis. *With occlusive dressings: maceration of skin, secondary infection, atrophy, striae, miliaria.*

◆ Available in U.S. and Canada. ◆◆ Available in Canada only. All other products (no symbol) available in U.S. only. Italicized side effects are common or life-threatening.

INTERACTIONS	**NURSING CONSIDERATIONS**
	infection does not respond immediately, corticosteroids should be stopped until infection is controlled.) • Before applying, gently wash skin. To prevent damage to skin, rub in medication gently, leaving a thin coat. When treating hairy sites, part hair and apply directly to lesions. • Occlusive dressing: apply cream heavily, then cover with a thin, pliable, nonflammable plastic film; seal to adjacent normal skin with hypoallergenic tape. To minimize adverse reactions, use occlusive dressing intermittently. Occlusive dressings are generally not used in presence of infection or with weeping or exudative lesions. • For patient with eczematous dermatitis who may develop irritation with adhesive material, it may be helpful to hold dressing in place with gauze, elastic bandages, stockings, or stockinette. • Notify doctor and remove occlusive dressing if body temperature rises. • Aerosol preparation contains alcohol and may produce irritation or burning in open lesions. When using about the face, cover patient's eyes and warn against inhalation of the spray. To avoid freezing tissues, do not spray longer than 3 seconds or closer than 6 inches. • Change dressing as ordered by doctor. Inspect skin for infection, striae, and atrophy. Discontinue drug and notify doctor if these occur. • Treatment should be continued for a few days following clearing of lesions to prevent recurrence. • Instruct patient to report signs of drug sensitivity. • The 0.5% strength is available without prescription.
None significant.	• Use cautiously in viral diseases of skin, such as varicella, vaccinia, herpes simplex; fungal infections; skin tuberculosis; impaired circulation. • Avoid application in or near eyes. • Systemic absorption especially likely with occlusive dressings, prolonged treatment, or extensive body-surface treatment. • Stop drug and notify doctor if patient develops signs of systemic absorption, skin irritation or ulceration, hypersensitivity, infection. (If antifungals or antibiotics are being used with corticosteroids and infection does not respond immediately, corticosteroids should be stopped until infection is controlled.) • Before applying, gently wash skin. To prevent damage to skin, rub in medication gently, leaving a thin coat. When treating hairy sites, part hair and apply directly to lesion. • Occlusive dressing: apply cream or ointment heavily, then cover with a thin, pliable, nonflammable plastic film; seal to adjacent normal skin with hypoallergenic tape. To minimize adverse reactions, use occlusive dressings intermittently. Occlusive dressings are generally not used in presence of infection or with exudative lesions. • For patient with eczematous dermatitis who may develop irritation with adhesive material, hold dressing in place with gauze, elastic bandages, stockings, or stockinette. • Notify doctor and remove occlusive dressing if body temperature rises. • Lotions and foams are not used with occlusive dressings. • Change dressing as ordered by doctor. Inspect skin for infection, striae, and atrophy. Discontinue drug and notify doctor if these occur. • Treatment should be continued for a few days after clearing of lesions to prevent recurrence. • Instruct patient to report signs of drug sensitivity. • The 0.5% strength of hydrocortisone acetate is available without prescription.

NAME	INDICATIONS & DOSAGE	SIDE EFFECTS
methylprednisolone acetate Medrol Acetate♦	*Inflammation of corticosteroid-responsive dermatoses*— **Adults and children:** clean area; apply ointment daily to t.i.d.	**Skin:** burning, itching, irritation, dryness, folliculitis, hypopigmentation, hypertrichosis, acneiform eruptions, allergic contact dermatitis. *With occlusive dressings: maceration of skin, secondary infection, atrophy, striae, miliaria.*
prednisolone Meti-Derm	*Inflammation of corticosteroid-responsive dermatoses*— **Adults and children:** clean area; apply cream t.i.d. or q.i.d.	**Skin:** burning, itching, irritation, dryness, folliculitis, hypopigmentation, hypertrichosis, acneiform eruptions, perioral dermatitis, allergic contact dermatitis. *With occlusive dressings: maceration of skin, secondary infection, atrophy, striae, miliaria.*

♦ Available in U.S. and Canada. ♦♦ Available in Canada only. All other products (no symbol) available in U.S. only. Italicized side effects are common or life-threatening.

INTERACTIONS	NURSING CONSIDERATIONS
None significant.	• Use cautiously in viral diseases of skin, such as varicella, vaccinia, herpes simplex; fungal infections; skin tuberculosis; impaired circulation. • Avoid application in or near eyes. • Systemic absorption especially likely with occlusive dressings, prolonged treatment, or extensive body-surface treatment. • Stop drug and notify doctor if patient develops signs of systemic absorption, skin irritation or ulceration, hypersensitivity, infection. (If antifungals or antibiotics agents are being used with corticosteroids and infection does not respond immediately, corticosteroids should be stopped until infection is controlled.) • Before applying, gently wash skin. To prevent damage to skin, rub in medication gently, leaving a thin coat. When treating hairy sites, part hair and apply directly to lesion. • Occlusive dressing: apply ointment heavily, then cover with a thin, pliable, nonflammable plastic film; seal to adjacent normal skin with hypoallergenic tape. To minimize adverse effects, use occlusive dressing intermittently. Occlusive dressings are generally not used in presence of infection or with weeping or exudative lesions. • For patient with eczematous dermatitis who may develop irritation with adhesive material, hold dressing in place with gauze, elastic bandages, stockings, or stockinette. • Notify doctor and remove occlusive dressing if body temperature rises. • Change dressing as ordered by doctor. Inspect skin for infection, striae, and atrophy. Discontinue drug and notify doctor if these occur. • Treatment should be continued for a few days after clearing of lesions to prevent recurrence. • Instruct patient to report signs of drug sensitivity.
None significant.	• Use cautiously in viral diseases of skin, such as varicella or vaccinia; fungal infections; skin tuberculosis; impaired circulation. • Avoid application in or near eyes. • Systemic absorption especially likely with occlusive dressings, prolonged treatment, or extensive body-surface treatment. • Stop drug and notify doctor if patient develops signs of systemic absorption, skin irritation or ulceration, hypersensitivity, infection. (If antifungals or antibiotics are being used with corticosteroids and infection does not respond immediately, corticosteroids should be stopped until infection is controlled.) • Before applying, gently wash skin. To prevent damage to skin, rub in medication gently, leaving a thin coat. When treating hairy sites, part hair and apply directly to lesions. • Occlusive dressing: apply cream heavily and cover with a thin, pliable, nonflammable plastic film; seal to adjacent normal skin with hypoallergenic tape. To minimize adverse reactions, use occlusive dressing intermittently. Occlusive dressings are generally not used in presence of infection or with weeping or exudative lesions. • For patient with eczematous dermatitis who may develop irritation with adhesive material, hold dressing in place with gauze, elastic bandages, stockings, or stockinette. • Notify doctor and remove occlusive dressing if body temperature rises. • Change dressing as ordered by doctor. Inspect skin for infection, striae, and atrophy. Discontinue drug and notify doctor if these occur. • Treatment should be continued for a few days after clearing of lesions to prevent recurrence. • Instruct patient to report signs of drug sensitivity.

NAME	INDICATIONS & DOSAGE	SIDE EFFECTS
triamcinolone acetonide Aristocort♦, Aristocort A, Kenalog♦, Triamalone♦♦	*Inflammation of corticosteroid-responsive dermatoses*— **Adults and children:** clean area; apply cream, ointment, lotion, foam, or aerosol sparingly b.i.d. to q.i.d. Aerosol: shake can well. Direct spray onto affected area from a distance of approximately 6 inches and apply for only 3 seconds.	**Skin:** burning, itching, irritation, dryness, folliculitis, hypopigmentation, hypertrichosis, acneiform eruptions, perioral dermatitis, allergic contact dermatitis. *With occlusive dressings: maceration of skin, secondary infection, atrophy, striae, miliaria.*

♦ Available in U.S. and Canada. ♦♦ Available in Canada only. All other products (no symbol) available in U.S. only. Italicized side effects are common or life-threatening.

DRUG ALERT

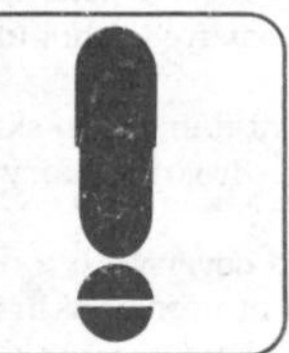

BE CAREFUL: TOPICAL STEROIDS CAN BE ABSORBED

If improperly used, topical steroids can be absorbed from local application sites, and if doses are large enough, these drugs may eventually produce adverse systemic effects.

They can be absorbed systemically when administered by these routes:

- ophthalmic
- inhalation (for asthma)
- intranasal (for nasal polyps)
- intrasynovial (for bursitis)
- rectal (for ulcerative colitis)

INTERACTIONS	NURSING CONSIDERATIONS
None significant.	• Use cautiously in viral diseases of skin, such as varicella, vaccinia, herpes simplex; fungal infections; skin tuberculosis; impaired circulation. • Avoid application in or near eyes. • Systemic absorption especially likely with occlusive dressings, prolonged treatment, or extensive body-surface treatment. • Stop drug and notify doctor if patient develops signs of systemic absorption, skin irritation or ulceration, hypersensitivity, infection. (If antifungals or antibiotics are being used with corticosteroids and infection does not respond immediately, corticosteroids should be stopped until infection is controlled.) • Before applying, gently wash skin. To prevent damage to skin, rub in medication gently, leaving a thin coat. When treating hairy sites, part hair and apply directly to lesion. • Aerosol preparation contains alcohol and may produce irritation or burning in open lesions. When using about the face, cover patient's eyes and warn against inhalation of the spray. To avoid freezing tissues, do not spray longer than 3 seconds or closer than 6 inches. • Occlusive dressing: apply cream or ointment heavily, then cover with a thin, pliable, nonflammable plastic film; seal to adjacent normal skin with hypoallergenic tape. To minimize adverse reactions, use occlusive dressing intermittently. Occlusive dressings are generally not used in presence of infection or with exudative lesions. • For patient with eczematous dermatitis who may develop irritation with adhesive material, hold dressing in place with gauze, elastic bandages, stockings, or stockinette. • Notify doctor and remove occlusive dressing if body temperature rises. • Change dressing as ordered by doctor. Inspect skin for infection, striae, and atrophy. Discontinue drug and notify doctor if these occur. • Treatment should be continued for a few days after clearing of lesions to prevent recurrence. • Instruct patient to report signs of drug sensitivity.

- intralesional injection (for psoriasis)
- topical (for allergic dermatoses).

Topical steroid absorption may vary at different sites of the body. Hydrocortisone is absorbed **0.14** times as well through the plantar foot arch as it is through the forearm; **0.83** times as well through the palms; **1.7** times as well through the back; **3.5** times as well through the scalp; **6** times as well through the forehead; **13** times as well through the cheeks at the jaw angle; and **42** times as well through scrotal skin.

Although the FDA has approved nonprescription use of hydrocortisone and hydrocortisone acetate as antipruritics in concentrations up to 0.5%, make sure they're *not* used:

- **in children under age 2.** Absorption of these products may cause growth retardation, weight gain, and hypertension.
- **in the eyes.** Activation of viral eye infections, ocular hypertension, glaucoma, and cataract formation may result from unsupervised ophthalmic use.
- **as self-medication therapy for longer than 7 days,** especially in large doses, since systemic absorption occurs even in adults.

Important: Advise patients who use over-the-counter corticosteroid preparations to follow package directions carefully.

Antipruritics and topical anesthetics

benzocaine
camphor
dibucaine hydrochloride
dimethisoquin hydrochloride
diperodon monohydrate
dyclonine hydrochloride
ethyl chloride
lidocaine
lidocaine hydrochloride
menthol
phenol
pramoxine hydrochloride
tars
tetracaine
tetracaine hydrochloride

These topical drugs are used to produce local anesthesia and relieve discomfort and pruritus. Since they do not penetrate the stratum corneum, their effectiveness on intact skin is limited. But since mucosal surfaces lack a stratum corneum, topical anesthetics can be both effective and useful, as in some oral or anogenital disorders. Because these agents can cause sensitization, leading to contact dermatitis, their use should not be prolonged.

Hypersensitivity is most prevalent in reaction to local anesthetics of the ester type (tetracaine) and commonly develops when chemically related drugs are used. Drugs of the amide type (dibucaine and lidocaine) can usually be given to a patient who is allergic to ester-type drugs because incidence of hypersensitivity is much lower. As an alternative, a compound of a completely different class—such as benzocaine, dyclonine hydrochloride, or pramoxine hydrochloride—might be used.

Major uses

Rx

• Antipruritics relieve skin discomfort caused by minor burns, cuts, diaper rash, fungal infections, sunburn, hemorrhoids, insect bites, hives, eczema, skin ulcers, and pruritus ani and vulvae.

• Topical anesthetics anesthetize mucous membranes, as in the rectum, and are commonly used before endoscopic procedures.

Mechanism of action

• The general effect of all these drugs is to block conduction of impulses at the sensory nerve endings by interfering with the cell membrane's permeability to ions.

• Ethyl chloride produces local anesthesia by producing the sensation of cold.

• The specific mechanism of action of the other drugs is largely unknown. Menthol and phenol are general protoplasmic poisons.

Absorption, distribution, metabolism, and excretion

• These agents may be absorbed through mucous membranes and abraded skin, but are poorly absorbed when applied to intact skin.

• Esters such as tetracaine are metabolized extensively in the blood and to a lesser extent in the liver. They are excreted in urine.

- Amides such as dibucaine and lidocaine are metabolized mostly in the liver and excreted in urine.
- The remaining agents follow various routes of metabolism and are excreted in urine.

Onset and duration

Onset is rapid (within minutes). Duration varies according to the specific drug.

- Benzocaine and pramoxine hydrochloride have a prolonged duration of 2 to 4 hours.
- Dibucaine is one of the most potent and longest-acting of the topical anesthetics, with a duration of 3 hours.
- Dimethisoquin's action lasts 2 to 4 hours.
- Dyclonine is effective for ½ to 1 hour.
- The other drugs have a duration of action from 1 to 3 hours.

Combination products

BALNETAR♦: water-dispersible emollient tar 2.5% in lanolin fraction, mineral oil, and nonionic emulsifiers.

CARMOL HC: urea 10% and hydrocortisone acetate 1%.

CETACAINE LIQUID: benzocaine 14%, tetracaine HCl 2%, benzalkonium chloride 0.5%, butyl aminobenzoate 2%, and cetyl dimethyl ethyl ammonium bromide in a bland water-soluble base.

CETACAINE OINTMENT: benzocaine 14%, tetracaine HCl 2%, butyl aminobenzoate 2%, benzalkonium chloride 0.5%, and cetyl dimethyl ethyl ammonium bromide in a bland water-soluble base.

CHIGGER-TOX LIQUID: benzocaine 2.1% and benzyl benzoate in an isopropanol base.

COR-TAR-QUIN♦: coal tar solution USP 2%, diiodohydroxyquin 1% with hydrocortisone 0.25%, 0.5%, or 1% in an acid-mantle vehicle.

CUTAR BATH OIL EMULSION: coal tar solution 7.5% in liquid petrolatum isopropyl myristate, acetylated lanolin, lanolin alcohols extract, and water.

DERMA MEDICONE OINTMENT: benzocaine 2%, zinc oxide 13.7%, oxyquinoline sulfate 1.05%, ichthammol 1%, and menthol 0.48% in petrolatum and lanolin base.

DERMOPLAST SPRAY: benzocaine 20% and menthol 0.5%.

ESTAR GEL♦: coal tar 5% and alcohol 29%.

LAVATAR♦: tar distillate 33.3% in water-miscible emulsion base.

MEDICONE DRESSING (CREAM): benzocaine 0.5%, 8-hydroxyquinoline sulfate 0.05%, cod liver oil 12.5%, zinc oxide 12.5%, and menthol 0.18% with petrolatum, lanolin, talcum, and paraffin.

POLYTAR BATH: polytar 25% (juniper, pine, and coal tars, vegetable oil and solubilized crude coal tar) in water-miscible emulsion base.

PRAGMATAR OINTMENT♦: cetyl alcohol-coal tar distillate 4%, precipitated sulfur 3%, and salicylic acid 3% in an oil-in-water emulsion base.

SEBUTONE♦: tar (equivalent to 0.5% coal tar) in surface-active soapless cleansers and wetting agents, sulfur 2%, and salicylic acid 2%.

TAR DOAK LOTION♦: tar distillate 5% and nonionic emulsifiers.

VANSEB-T♦: coal tar solution USP 5% salicylic acid 1%, sulfur 2% in perfumed base.

ZETAR EMULSION♦: 30% colloidal whole coal tar in polysorbates.

ZETAR SHAMPOO♦: whole coal tar 1% and parachlorometaxylenol 0.5% in foam shampoo base.

APPLYING TOPICAL ANESTHETICS

Take care when applying the topical anesthetics dyclonine hydrochloride (Dyclone) and ethyl chloride (Ethyl Chloride Spray.) If you get any of these preparations on your fingers, you'll experience temporary numbness, which may last up to 45 minutes.

NAME	INDICATIONS & DOSAGE	SIDE EFFECTS
benzocaine Aerocaine, Americaine, Anbesol, Ben-Caine B.B., Benzocol, Col-Vi-Nol, Dermoplast, Hurricaine, Morusan, Rhulicream, Rhulihist, Solarcaine, Urolocaine	*Local anesthetic for pruritic dermatoses, localized idiopathic pruritus, and sunburn—* **Adults and children:** apply locally 2 or 3 times a day. *Hemorrhoids or rectal irritation—* **Adults and children:** apply ointment 2 or 3 times a day. Suppository: insert well into rectum morning, evening, and after each bowel movement.	**Blood:** methemoglobinemia (infants). **Local:** sensitization rash.
camphor	*Mild antipruritic and local anesthetic; counterirritant for use in sprains and rheumatic conditions—* **Adults and children:** apply a 1% to 3% lotion or ointment of camphor, as needed.	**Local:** sensitization, rash.
dibucaine hydrochloride D-Caine, Dulzit, Nupercainal Cream♦, Nupercainal Ointment♦, Nupercainal Suppositories, Nuporals (Troches)	*Abrasions, sunburn, minor burns, hemorrhoids, and other painful skin conditions—* **Adults and children:** 0.5% to 1% lotion or ointment applied locally several times a day. Suppositories: insert rectally morning, evening, and after every bowel movement. Also used as a local anesthetic for mouth and throat.	**Local:** *hypersensitivity.*
dimethisoquin hydrochloride Quotane Cream♦♦, Quotane Ointment	*Surface pain and itching—* **Adults and children:** 0.5% ointment or lotion applied topically up to 4 times daily or as directed.	**Skin:** *sensitization and contact dermatitis can develop but incidence is low.*
diperodon monohydrate Diothane Ointment♦, Proctodon	*Pain caused by minor burns and cuts (cream); pain caused by anorectal disorders (ointment)—* **Adults and children:** apply 3 to 4 times a day.	**Skin:** rash, irritation, and other allergic manifestations.
dyclonine hydrochloride Dyclone	*To relieve surface pain and itching caused by minor burns or trauma, surgical wounds, pruritus ani or vulvae, insect bites, and pruritic dermatoses. Also, to anesthetize mucous membranes before endoscopic procedures—* **Adults and children:** 0.5% solution or 1% ointment applied 3 or 4 times daily. *Urethral dilation or*	**Local:** *irritation at site of application may occur.*

♦ Available in U.S. and Canada. ♦♦ Available in Canada only. All other products (no symbol) available in U.S. only. Italicized side effects are common or life-threatening.

INTERACTIONS	NURSING CONSIDERATIONS
None significant.	• Contraindicated in hypersensitivity to procaine or other para-aminobenzoic acid (PABA) derivatives (often used in topical sun-blocking agents). • Discontinue if rash develops. • Avoid contact with eyes. • If spray preparation used, hold can 6 to 12 inches from affected area and spray liberally. Avoid inhalation. • If using rectally, cleanse and thoroughly dry rectal area before applying.
None significant.	• Extremely toxic if taken orally. • Avoid contact with eyes. • Do not apply to broken skin or mucous membranes. • Discontinue use if rash develops.
None significant.	• Avoid contact with eyes. • Before applying cream or ointment rectally or inserting suppository, cleanse and thoroughly dry rectal area. • Discontinue use if rash develops.
None significant.	• Useful in patients sensitive to ester- or amide-type agents. • Don't apply to extensive areas. • Avoid contact with eyes. • Avoid prolonged use for patients with chronic conditions. • Discontinue use if rash develops.
None significant.	• Before applying cream or ointment rectally, cleanse and thoroughly dry rectal area. • Discontinue use if rash develops.
None significant.	• Avoid prolonged use in patients with chronic conditions. • May be useful in patients hypersensitive to other local anesthetics because it is a ketone. • Contraindicated in cystoscopic examinations following an intravenous pyelogram. Iodine-containing contrast material will cause precipitate to form with dyclonine. • Can be combined with diphenhydramine elixir to provide an effective treatment for stomatitis. • Avoid accidental contact with drug; it produces temporary numbness.

(continued on following page)

NAME	INDICATIONS & DOSAGE	SIDE EFFECTS
dyclonine hydrochloride *(continued)*	*cystourethroscopy—* **Adults:** 10 ml of 0.5% solution may be instilled into the urethra.	
ethyl chloride Ethyl Chloride Spray	*For irritation—* **Adults and children:** hold container about 24 inches from skin and spray rhythmically to cover area evenly once or twice. Application may be repeated. *As a local anesthetic in minor operative procedures; relieves pain caused by insect stings and burns, and irritation caused by myofascial and visceral pain syndromes—* **Adults and children:** dosage varies with different procedures. Use smallest dosage needed to produce desired effect. For local anesthesia, hold container about 12 inches from area to produce a fine spray. **Infants:** hold a cotton ball saturated with ethyl chloride to injection site, and make injection when site dries.	**Skin:** sensitization; *frostbite and tissue necrosis may occur with prolonged spraying.* **Other:** excessive cooling may increase pain and muscle spasms.
lidocaine **lidocaine hydrochloride** Lida-Mantle Cream, Stanacaine, Xylocaine Jelly (2%), Xylocaine Ointment (2.5%)♦, Xylocaine Ointment (5%)♦, Xylocaine Solution (4%)♦, Xylocaine Viscous Solution (2%)	*Local anesthesia of skin or mucous membranes—* **Adults and children:** apply liberally. *In procedures involving the male or female urethra—* **Adults:** instill about 15 ml (male) or 3 to 5 ml (female) into urethra. *Pain, burning, or itching caused by burns, sunburn, or skin irritation—* **Adults and children:** apply liberally.	**Local:** rash, *hypersensitivity.*
menthol	*As an antipruritic—* **Adults and children:** apply 0.25% to 2% lotion or ointment, as needed. Often added with phenol to an ointment.	None reported.
phenol	*As an antipruritic—* **Adults, and children over 6 months:** apply 0.5% to 2% preparations locally several times a day.	None at recommended strengths.

♦ Available in U.S. and Canada. ♦♦ Available in Canada only. All other products (no symbol) available in U.S. only. Italicized side effects are common or life-threatening.

INTERACTIONS	NURSING CONSIDERATIONS
None significant.	• Do not apply to broken skin or mucous membranes. • Protect skin adjacent to treated area with petrolatum to avoid tissue sloughing. • Avoid use near eyes. • Avoid inhalation when spraying. • Highly flammable; do not use in areas where open flames or sparks are possible. • Avoid accidental contact with drug; it produces temporary numbness.
None significant.	• Use with caution on severely traumatized mucosa or where sepsis is present or for anesthesia of oropharyngeal mucosa, since gag reflex may be suppressed by lidocaine and aspiration may occur. • The 4% solution can be sprayed or poured onto abrasions to facilitate cleansing and removal of foreign substances (gravel, glass, etc.). • Discontinue use if rash develops. • Apply Xylocaine Ointment carefully to prevent contact with skin; it produces numbness.
None significant.	• Relieves itching by substituting a cooling effect. • Avoid contact with eyes. • Discontinue use if rash develops.
None significant.	• Avoid accidental contact with normal skin. If contact occurs, remove phenol with alcohol or vegetable oil. • Tissue necrosis possible with higher than usual concentration or extensive use. • Avoid contact with eyes. • Do not use under occlusive dressings, bandages, or diapers.

NAME	INDICATIONS & DOSAGE	SIDE EFFECTS
pramoxine hydrochloride Proctofoam, Tronothane♦	*Pain and itching caused by dermatoses, minor burns, surgical wounds, insect bites, and hemorrhoids—* **Adults and children:** apply every 3 to 4 hours.	**Local:** stinging or burning, sensitization.
tars	*As an antipruritic—* **Adults and children:** apply preparations 2 or 3 times daily.	**Skin:** irritation, folliculitis, erythema, photosensitivity.
tetracaine **tetracaine hydrochloride** Pontocaine♦	*For relief of pain in hemorrhoids, minor burns, ulcers, sunburn, and poison ivy—* **Adults and children:** apply 5% ointment or 1% cream—no more than 1 oz for adults or ¼ oz for children in 24 hours.	**Local:** *sensitization.*

♦ Available in U.S. and Canada. ♦♦ Available in Canada only. All other products (no symbol) available in U.S. only. Italicized side effects are common or life-threatening.

INTERACTIONS	NURSING CONSIDERATIONS
None significant.	• Can be safely used in those allergic to other local anesthetics. • May be applied with gauze or sprayed directly on skin. Avoid contact with eyes. • Cleanse and thoroughly dry rectal area before applying ointment or cream, or inserting suppository.
None significant.	• Use caution in applying tar preparations to patients with exacerbation of psoriasis. Excessive use may precipitate total body exfoliation. • Never use under occlusive dressings. • Avoid excessive exposure to sunlight. May produce photosensitization. • Darkens color of blond hair when applied to scalp. • May stain skin and clothing. Use mineral oil to remove from skin, especially if 1% to 5% crude coal tar is used.
None significant.	• Contraindicated in hypersensitivity to procaine or other para-aminobenzoic acid (PABA) derivatives (often used in topical sun-blocking agents). • Before applying cream or ointment rectally, cleanse and thoroughly dry rectal area.

NURSING TIP

RELIEVING SUNBURN PAIN

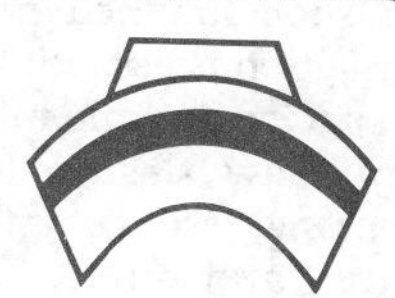

As you know, sunburn results from overexposure to the sun's ultraviolet rays. Unless the burn is severe, it's a benign, self-limiting condition that necessitates no treatment other than application of cool compresses, cool tap water, or local anesthetic preparations to relieve pain.

Among the most popular over-the-counter sunburn pain remedies are preparations containing the -caine derivatives benzocaine, dibucaine, lidocaine, and tetracaine. These products provide local anesthesia by blocking conduction of nerve impulses at sensory nerve endings.

These local anesthetics are available in ointments, creams, solutions, and aerosols. You can help your patient choose an appropriate product by keeping in mind the following considerations:

• Ointments are the least desirable form of local anesthetic because the greasy base may facilitate microbial infection of burns. Also, ointments must be removed before a doctor can examine and treat the sunburn, should this become necessary.

• Creams, solutions, and aerosols are easier to remove than ointments. They also have a cooling effect that may aid in relieving pain.

• Sprays and aerosols are easiest for the patient to use; however, he must be careful to avoid inhaling the fumes or getting the preparation in his eyes, nose, or mouth.

91 Astringents

acetic acid lotion
aluminum acetate
aluminum sulfate
hamamelis water
tannic acid

Externally applied, astringents are toners, tonics, and comforting agents.

Astringents applied locally cause precipitation of proteins. These drugs have such low cell penetrability that their action is essentially limited to the cell surface and the interstitial spaces. They draw tissues together, cause blanching, reduce inflammation and oozing, and have a soothing effect. Most of them also have antiseptic action (see Chapter 92, ANTISEPTICS AND DISINFECTANTS).

Because most astringents are irritating or caustic in moderate to high concentrations, pay strict attention to appropriate concentrations. Long-term use of these agents may result in excessively dry skin.

Major uses

Astringents are used to:

- arrest hemorrhage by coagulating blood (styptic action
- reduce inflammation of mucous membranes, as in trench mouth, gingivitis, and minor external hemorrhoidal and outer vaginal discomfort
- promote healing and toughen the skin
- treat poison ivy, poison oak, sunburn, heat rash, and minor burns
- treat acute inflammations attended by exudation, oozing, and crusting (in solutions for wet dressings)
- decrease sweating (as an ingredient in many antiperspirants).

Mechanism of action

Astringents precipitate protein, causing tissue to contract. The cement substance of the capillary endothelium is hardened so that transcapillary movement of plasma protein is inhibited. Local edema, inflammation, and exudation are thereby reduced.

Mucus or other secretions may also

NURSING TIP

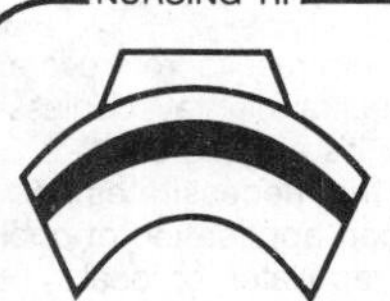

HOW TO APPLY TANNIC ACID

When treating burns, follow these procedures:

- First, flush the burned areas with water or saline solution.
- Next, apply a thick layer of tannic acid to gauze dressings. Place the dressings on burned areas.
- Later, soak loose adherent gauze with normal or slightly hypertonic saline solution.
- A dark eschar will probably form. Leave it until it loosens and peels off on its own. You may, however, trim or cut away the edges, if hospital policy permits.

be reduced so that the affected area becomes drier.

Absorption, distribution, metabolism and excretion

• Astringents penetrate the cell so poorly that their action is confined to the cell surface. Hence, absorption is minimal unless the drugs are applied to large areas of denuded skin.

Tannic acid, when used over large areas of burned tissue, may be absorbed and cause significant hepatic damage. It also causes necrosis of viable tissue in the burned area.

• Distribution of the drugs is generally confined to the area of application.

Onset and duration

Astringents begin to act almost immediately. Their duration of action is limited, and repeated applications may be required for optimal effects.

Combination products

ASTRINGENTS WITH ANESTHETICS, for example, Nupercainal Suppositories.

ASTRINGENTS WITH ANTIPRURITIC/ANTIHISTAMINE, for example, Caladryl, Ziradryl.

ASTRINGENTS WITH ANTIPRURITIC/ANTIHISTAMINE AND ANESTHETIC, for example, Rhulicream, Rhulihist, Rhulispray.

ASTRINGENTS WITH ANTISEPTICS, for example, Tucks Pads, Tanac, Lavoris.

ASTRINGENTS WITH ANTISEPTICS AND ANESTHETICS, for example, Rectal Medicone Suppositories and Unguent, Tanicaine Suppositories and Ointment, Wyanoid Ointment, Pazo Hemorrhoid Suppositories and Ointment.

ASTRINGENTS WITH DEODORANTS, for example, antiperspirant/deodorants.

DRUG ERROR

BEWARE OF TELEPHONE ORDERS

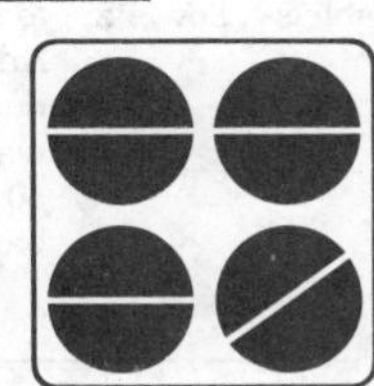

A nurse took a telephone order from a doctor to irrigate a patient's bladder with sterile Neosporin G.U. Irrigant, an antibiotic solution manufactured by the Burroughs-Wellcome Co. When referring to the irrigant, however, the doctor incorrectly called it *Burrough's* solution.

The nurse assumed the doctor meant *Burow's* solution, a topical astringent. So she wrote on the patient's chart: Irrigate bladder b.i.d. via catheter, with Burow's solution.

The doctor found the error when he countersigned the order. By this time, the patient had received several irrigations with Burow's solution. Fortunately, the patient suffered no ill effects from irrigation with the nonsterile astringent, but he hadn't received the intended antibiotic's benefits either.

To prevent this kind of error from happening to you:

• Always question the doctor when you're not familiar with a drug's name.
• When you check with the pharmacist, tell him exactly why the drug's being prescribed.
• Work toward establishing a policy that doctors countersign telephone orders within 24 hours.
• Limit telephone orders to emergencies whenever practical.

NAME	INDICATIONS & DOSAGE	SIDE EFFECTS
acetic acid lotion (0.1% glacial acetic acid in alcohol)	*Superficial fungal or bacterial infection to toughen skin and prevent bedsores—* **Adults and children:** apply and work into area, p.r.n.	**Skin:** burning and irritation of denuded skin and mucous membranes.
aluminum acetate (modified Burow's solution) Acid Mantle Creme and Lotion♦, Burosol, Burowets, Burow's Emulsion, Burow's Lotion, Burow's Ointment	*Mild skin irritation from exposure to soaps, detergents, chemicals, diaper rash, acne, scaly skin, eczema—* **Adults and children:** apply p.r.n. *Relieve inflammation of poison ivy, insect bites, athlete's foot—* **Adults and children:** apply as wet dressing, p.r.n. *Ulcerative skin conditions—* **Adults and children:** apply ointment, p.r.n.	**Skin:** irritation; extension of inflammation possible.
aluminum sulfate Bluboro Powder, Domeboro Powder♦ and Tablets♦, Soy-Sitz Powder	*Skin inflammation, insect bites, poison ivy or other contact dermatoses, swelling, athlete's foot—* **Adults and children:** mix powder with 1 pint of lukewarm tap water and apply for 15 to 30 minutes every 4 to 8 hours; bandage loosely.	**Skin:** irritation; extension of inflammation possible.
hamamelis water (witch hazel) Hazel-Balm, Mediconet (wipes), Tucks (Cream, Ointment, Pads)	*Anal discomfort, itching, burning, minor external hemorrhoidal or outer vaginal discomfort, diaper rash—* **Adults and children:** apply t.i.d. or q.i.d.	**Skin:** hypersensitivity.
tannic acid Amertan Jelly, Dalidyne Lotion, Tanac	*Denture irritation; teething irritation; trench mouth; gingivitis; throat irritation; herpes simplex; oral cavity lesions; adjunctive treatment of second- and third-degree thermal, chemical, or electrical burns—* **Adults:** apply with cotton applicator. As gargle or mouthwash, ½ teaspoon of solution in ½ glass of warm water, p.r.n. *Cold sores, throat irritation, oral cavity lesions, some second- and third-degree burns—* **Children:** apply with cotton applicator.	**Local:** stinging. **Other:** large amounts in burn treatment can cause hepatic damage.

♦ Available in U.S. and Canada. ♦♦ Available in Canada only. All other products (no symbol) available in U.S. only. Italicized side effects are common or life-threatening.

INTERACTIONS	NURSING CONSIDERATIONS
Heavy metals: causes precipitation of the metal acetate.	• Contraindicated under occlusive dressings. • Never confuse acetic acid solutions with *glacial* acetic acid solutions. Glacial form is a concentrate. • Keep away from eyes and mucous membranes. • Always apply to freshly cleansed area, free of other medications. • Especially good for treating topical infection due to *Pseudomonas aeruginosa.*
None significant.	• Contraindicated under occlusive dressings. • Keep away from eyes and mucous membranes. • Always apply to freshly cleansed area, free of other medications. • May be used in place of boric acid ointment. • Powder must be diluted in water to prescribed concentration. • Discontinue if irritation develops. • Clear solution may be stored at room temperature for up to 7 days.
None significant.	• Contraindicated under occlusive dressings; use open wet dressings only. • When solution is prepared, immediately decant clear portion. Discard precipitate. Use only clear solution, *not* precipitate, for soaks. Never strain or filter solutions. Decanted portion may be stored at room temperature for up to 7 days. • In general, no more than a third of the body should be treated at any one time, since excessive wet dressings may cause chilling and hypothermia. • Keep away from eyes and mucous membranes. • Discontinue if irritation develops.
None significant.	• Discontinue if irritation or itching does not improve. • Use pads or wipes after toilet tissue to help prevent pruritus ani, vulvae. • Cream can be used by breast-feeding mother for nipple care, but wash area clean before breast-feeding baby. • Some products contain potential allergic sensitizers. Observe for allergic reactions.
Organic salts of heavy metals: will precipitate tannate salt of heavy metal. Do not apply.	• Incompatible with organic salts of heavy metals. Apply only to surfaces free of other medication. • Produces a firm eschar on burned area that helps protect burned tissue from infection and loss of body fluids, and comforts patient. • Apply only after proper debridement of burn. • Use only freshly prepared aqueous solutions, as they are unstable. • Light and air cause solution to darken, which reduces potency. • Avoid extensive application and prolonged use on denuded tissue to decrease possibility of systemic toxicity from absorption. • Slight stinging on application soon subsides.

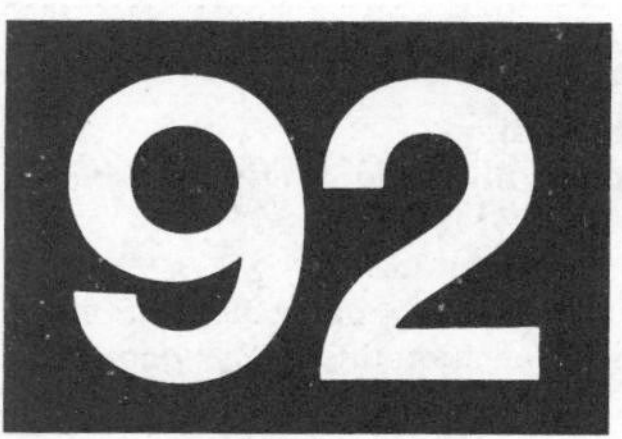

Antiseptics and disinfectants

alcohol, ethyl
alcohol, isopropyl
benzalkonium chloride
boric acid
chlorhexidine gluconate
formaldehyde
glutaraldehyde
hexachlorophene
hydrogen peroxide
iodine
merbromin
nitromersol
oxychlorosene calcium
oxychlorosene sodium
phenylmercuric nitrate
poloxamer iodine
potassium permanganate
povidone-iodine
silver protein, mild
sodium hypochlorite
thimerosal

Antiseptics inhibit growth of microorganisms; disinfectants destroy them. Antiseptics are used mainly on living tissue, whereas disinfectants are generally applied to inanimate objects. The effectiveness of these drugs depends on their mechanism of action, concentration, the number of microorganisms, the length of time the microorganisms are in contact with the drug, and the temperature and amount of organic matter present.

The antiseptics are boric acid, hexachlorophene, merbromin, oxychlorosene, and potassium permanganate. The rest of the drugs listed in this chapter are disinfectants.

WHAT TO LOOK FOR IN A GOOD ANTISEPTIC OR DISINFECTANT

The ideal antiseptic should:

- be lethal to microorganisms, rather than just inhibit their growth
- have a wide antimicrobial spectrum (although a limited spectrum may be useful in some situations)
- have a low surface tension (if used for topical application)
- retain its activity even in the presence of body fluids, including the exudates in infection
- have a rapid germicidal onset of action
- have a sustained duration of action
- have a wide therapeutic index (effective but nontoxic)
- have a low incidence of hypersensitivity reactions.

The ideal disinfectant should:

- have high germicidal efficacy
- have a wide antimicrobial spectrum
- be rapidly lethal
- be able to penetrate into crevices and cavities
- be germicidal in the presence of blood, sputum, and fecal material
- be compatible with soaps and other chemical substances
- be chemically stable
- be noncorrosive to surgical instruments
- have a pleasant odor and color
- be inexpensive.

HOW TO WASH YOUR HANDS PROPERLY

Proper handwashing is the key to medical asepsis. Before administering medications, remove your rings and watch, then wash your hands.

- Using warm running water, lather well for 30 to 60 seconds; be sure to clean your fingernails and interdigital spaces well.
- Rinse your hands; dry with a paper towel.
- Turn faucet off with a clean, dry paper towel.

Note: Don't lean against sink or splash water.

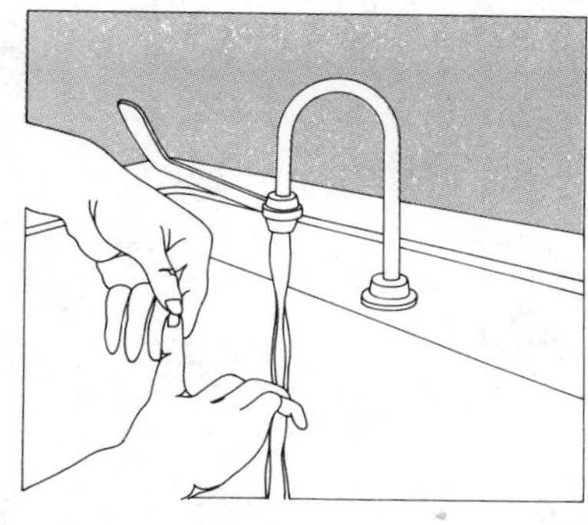

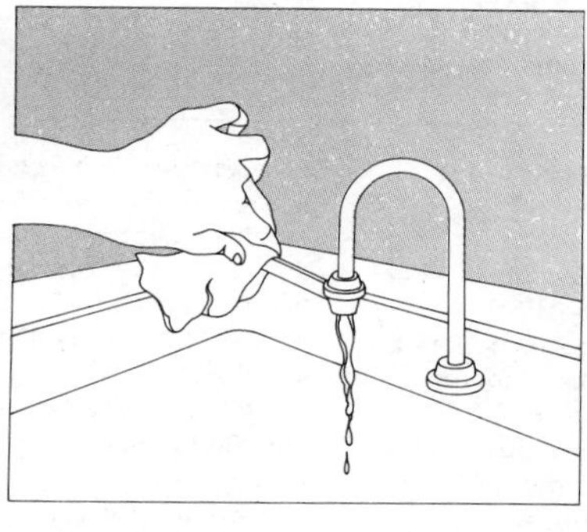

Major uses

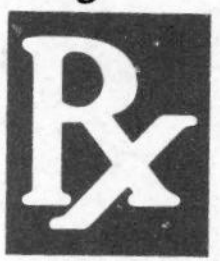

These drugs are used to control and prevent infection: antiseptics immobilize and disinfectants destroy pathogens.

- Povidone-iodine, a disinfectant, is especially useful as a preoperative skin disinfectant.

Mechanism of action

These drugs denature protein in microorganisms, changing their chemical structure. They lower surface tension, increasing cell permeability and causing lysis of the cell's contents, and also interfere with cellular metabolic processes.

Absorption, distribution, metabolism, and excretion

Not applicable.

Onset and duration

Onset of all these drugs except alcohol and hexachlorophene is immediate.

- Alcohol, to be effective in reducing bacterial count to 5% of normal, must be left on the skin for at least 2 minutes.
- Hexachlorophene is a chlorinated phenol used as a bacteriostatic cleansing agent. Its antibacterial action develops only after repeated daily application. The residual phenol retained on the skin greatly reduces bacterial flora.

Combination products

B.F.I. POWDER: bismuth-formic-iodide, zinc phenosulfonate, amol, potassium alum, bismuth subgallate, boric acid, menthol, eucalyptol, and thymol.

MERCRESIN: secondary-amyltricresols 0.1%, orthohydroxyphenylmercuric chloride 0.1%, acetone 10%, and alcohol 50%.

OBTUNDIA: camphor and metacresol in lanolin-petroleum base.

OBTUNDIA CALAMINE: camphor, metacresol, zinc oxide, and calamine.

S.T. 37: hexylresorcinol 0.1% in glycerin aqueous solution.

ZEASORB POWDER: parachlorometaxylenol 0.5%, aluminum dihydroxy allantoinate 0.2%, and microporous cellulose 45%.

NAME	INDICATIONS & DOSAGE	SIDE EFFECTS
alcohol, ethyl Alcohol, Ethanol	*To disinfect skin, instruments, and ampuls*—disinfect as needed.	**Skin:** dryness.
alcohol, isopropyl isopropyl alcohol 99%, isopropyl rubbing alcohol 70%, isopropyl aqueous alcohol 75%	*To disinfect skin, instruments, and ampuls*— disinfect as needed.	**Skin:** dryness.
benzalkonium chloride Benasept, Benzachlor-50♦♦, Benz-All, Drapolex♦♦, Ionax Foam♦♦, Ionax Scrub♦♦, Sabol♦♦, Spensomide, Zalkon, Zalkonium Chloride, Zephiran	*Preoperative disinfection of unbroken skin*—apply 1:750 to 1:1,000 tincture or spray. *Disinfection of mucous membranes and denuded skin*—apply 1:10,000 to 1:5,000 aqueous solution. *Irrigation of vagina*—instill 1:5,000 to 1:2,000 aqueous solution. *Irrigation of bladder or urethra*—instill 1:20,000 to 1:5,000 aqueous solution. *Irrigation of deep infected wounds*—instill 1:20,000 to 1:3,000 aqueous solution. *Preservation of metal instruments, thermometers, and rubber articles*—wipe or soak objects in 1:5,000 to 1:750 solution. *Disinfection of operating room equipment*—wipe with 1:5,000 solution.	**Skin:** hypersensitivity.
boric acid Bluboro, boric acid solution 5%, Borofax♦, Ting	*Skin conditions (athlete's foot) as a compress, powder, or ointment (2% to 5%)*— **Adults and children:** apply as directed.	Signs of systemic absorption: **CNS:** delirium, convulsions, restlessness, headache. **CV:** *circulatory collapse*, tachycardia. **GI:** irritation, nausea, vomiting, diarrhea. **GU:** renal damage. **Other:** hypothermia.
chlorhexidine gluconate Hibiclens Liquid, Hibitane	*Surgical hand scrub, hand wash, skin wound cleanser*—use p.r.n.	**EENT:** irritating to eyes. Causes deafness if instilled into middle ear through perforated eardrum.
formaldehyde Formalin (37% solution of formaldehyde)	*Cold sterilization of equipment*—disinfect as needed. *Tissue preservative*—cover tissue.	**EENT:** fumes cause eye, nose, and throat irritation. **Skin:** irritation. **Other:** pungent odor.

♦ Available in U.S. and Canada. ♦♦ Available in Canada only. All other products (no symbol) available in U.S. only. Italicized side effects are common or life-threatening.

INTERACTIONS	NURSING CONSIDERATIONS
None significant.	• Effective as fat solvent germicidal; ineffective against spore-forming organisms, tubercle bacilli, viruses. • Alcohol used as 70% solution known commonly as "rubbing alcohol." • Don't use on skin before insulin administration. May affect potency of insulin.
None significant.	• Isopropyl alcohol is slightly more effective than ethyl alcohol as an antibacterial agent, but it also tends to cause more dryness. • 75% solution for disinfection and storage of thermometers. • Not effective against spore-forming organisms, tubercle bacilli, or viruses. • Combined with formaldehyde, makes effective germicide.
Soaps: inactivate benzalkonium chloride. Remove soap traces with alcohol.	• Germicidal for some nonspore-forming organisms and fungi. No effect on tubercle bacilli. Limited viricidal use. • Used as preservative in ophthalmic solutions. • Before applying to skin, remove all traces of soap with water and apply 70% alcohol. • Don't store cotton, wool gauze, or sponges in solution. They absorb benzalkonium chloride and reduce the strength of the solution. • Don't use with occlusive dressings or vaginal packs. • Store in bottles with screw caps. • Incompatible with iodine, silver nitrate, fluorescein, nitrates, peroxide, lanolin, potassium permanganate, aluminum, caramel, kaolin, pine oil, zinc sulfate, zinc oxide, and yellow oxide of mercury. • To prevent rust of metallic instruments stored in benzalkonium chloride, add sodium nitrite to final solution. Change solution weekly. • Available also as 17% concentrate (Zephiran). Even after dilution, this form of Zephiran should be used only on inanimate objects.
None significant.	• Mild antiseptic and astringent. • Not absorbed through intact skin, but in high concentrations, may be absorbed through abraded skin or granulating wounds. • Avoid long-term use. • Ingestion of 5 g (infants) or 20 g (adults) may be fatal.
None significant.	• Bactericidal. Broad spectrum. • Can be used many times a day without causing irritation. • Low potential for producing skin reactions. • Rinse skin thoroughly after use. • Keep out of eyes and ears. • Action is residual. Do not cleanse skin with alcohol after application.
None significant.	• 0.5% solution germicidal against all forms of microorganisms, including spores, in 6 to 12 hours; 10% solution used to disinfect inanimate objects.

(continued on following page)

NAME	INDICATIONS & DOSAGE	SIDE EFFECTS
formaldehyde *(continued)*		
glutaraldehyde Cidex♦	*Cold sterilization of surgical instruments*—cover instruments with 2% solution. *Fumigate hospital and operating rooms*—fog with aerosol.	**Skin:** irritation.
hexachlorophene Germa-Medica "MG," Hexamead-Ph, pHisoHex♦, pHisoScrub, Sept-Soft, Septisol Soy-Dome Cleanser, WescoHEX	*Surgical scrub, bacteriostatic skin cleanser*—use as directed in 0.25% to 3% concentrations.	Note: systemic absorption can cause neurotoxic effects, including irritability, generalized clonic muscular contractions, decerebrate rigidity, convulsions, optic atrophy. (Systemic absorption has occurred only when used on premature infants, mucous membranes, and broken skin and burns.) **Skin:** dermatitis, mild scaling, dryness (especially when combined with excessive scrubbing).
hydrogen peroxide 3% to 6% solution	*Cleansing wound*—use 1.5% to 3% solution. *Mouthwash for necrotizing ulcerative gingivitis*—gargle with 3% solution. *Cleansing douche*—use 2% solution.	**EENT:** excessive use as mouthwash causes "hairy tongue."
iodine solution (2% iodine and 2.4% sodium and iodide in water)♦, tincture (2% iodine and 2.4% sodium iodide in diluted alcohol), Sepp Antiseptic Applicators (2% mild iodine tincture), strong iodine tincture (7% iodine and 5% potassium iodide in diluted alcohol)	*Preoperative disinfection of skin (small wounds and abraded areas)*—apply p.r.n.	**Skin:** irritation, redness, swelling (sign of hypersensitivity).
merbromin Mercurochrome (2% aqueous solution)	*General antiseptic and first-aid prophylactic*— **Adults and children:** apply	**Skin:** sensitization.

♦ Available in U.S. and Canada. ♦♦ Available in Canada only. All other products (no symbol) available in U.S. only. Italicized side effects are common or life-threatening.

INTERACTIONS	NURSING CONSIDERATIONS
	• Not affected by organic matter. • Used with alcohol and sodium nitrite to disinfect instruments and articles that can't tolerate heat (cold sterilization). • Avoid skin or mucous membrane contact with solutions greater than 0.5%. • Always dilute 37% solution.
None significant.	• Excellent disinfectant; broad spectrum of activity against gram-positive and gram-negative bacteria (vegetative and spores), viruses, and fungi. • Use on inanimate objects only. • Comes with activator that must be mixed before use to yield active acidic glutaraldehyde. • Not affected by organic matter. • Whenever possible, use commercially prepared 2% solution rather than diluting the 25% solution.
None significant.	• Use with caution in infants (especially premature infants) and burn patients. These patients tend to absorb hexachlorophene through the skin and may develop neurotoxic effects. • Bacteriostatic agent. Spectrum of activity limited to gram-positive organisms, especially staphylococcus. • Must be used preoperatively for at least 3 days for maximum effectiveness. • After cleaning area, rinse thoroughly (especially the scrotum and perineum). Do not apply alcohol or organic solvents to cleansed area.
None significant.	• Germicidal. • Don't inject into closed body cavities or abscesses; generated gas can't escape. • Dilute concentrate with 1 to 4 parts water. • Useful to remove mucus from inner cannula of tracheostomy tube. • Store tightly capped in cool, dry place. Protect from light and heat. • Do not shake bottle. This causes decomposition.
None significant.	• Microbicidal agent effective against bacteria, fungi, viruses, protozoa, and yeasts. • If skin reaction develops, remove iodine residue from skin and stop use. • To prevent skin irritation, do not cover areas treated with iodine. • Aqueous solution less irritating. • Sodium thiosulfate renders iodine colorless and is used to remove stains. It is also antidote of choice for accidental ingestion.
None significant.	• Bacteriostatic. • Least effective mercurial antiseptic. Its activity is decreased in presence of organic matter.

(continued on following page)

NAME	INDICATIONS & DOSAGE	SIDE EFFECTS
merbromin *(continued)*	p.r.n. as 1% to 2% solution or tincture.	
nitromersol Metaphen	*Disinfection of instruments*— soak in 0.04% solution. *Disinfection of skin*— apply 0.2% to 0.5% solution to area p.r.n. *Irrigation of mucous membranes (eye, urethra)*—instill 0.01% to 0.02% solution as directed. *Skin antiseptic for abrasions*— apply 0.2% solution to area.	**Skin:** erythematous, papular, or vesicular eruptions indicate hypersensitivity; irritation.
oxychlorosene calcium Clorpactin XCB **oxychlorosene sodium** Clorpactin WCS-90	*Topical antiseptic for local infections, preoperative skin cleanser (sodium salt)*—apply as spray, soak, wet dressing, or irrigation as a 4% solution. *Ophthalmic and urologic irrigant (sodium salt)*— 0.1% to 0.2% solution. *Local irrigation during surgery (calcium salt)*—use 0.5% solution.	**Skin:** local irritation.
phenylmercuric nitrate Phe-Mer-Nite	*Preoperative disinfection*—apply p.r.n. as a 0.1% to 0.2% solution.	**Skin:** rash.
poloxamer iodine Prepodyne, SeptoDyne	*Preoperative skin preparation and scrub, wound disinfection*—use as directed.	None reported.
potassium permanganate	*Topical antiseptic*—apply 1:10,000 to 1:500 solution. *Vaginal douche*—instill 1:5,000 to 1:1,000 solution as directed.	**Skin:** solutions greater than 1:5,000 are irritating to skin.
povidone-iodine ACU-dyne, Aerodine, Betadine♦, BPS, Bridine♦♦, Efodine, Final Step, Frepp, Frepp/Sepp, Isodine, Mallisol, Polydine, Proviodine♦♦, Sepp	*Many uses, including preoperative skin preparation and scrub, germicide for surface wounds, postoperative application to incisions, prophylactic application to urinary meatus of catheterized patients, miscellaneous disinfection*— **Adults:** apply p.r.n.	**Skin:** local hypersensitivity reactions.

♦ Available in U.S. and Canada. ♦♦ Available in Canada only. All other products (no symbol) available in U.S. only. Italicized side effects are common or life-threatening.

INTERACTIONS	NURSING CONSIDERATIONS
	• Cleanse injury with soap and water before applying. Let dry. • Stains may be removed with 2% permanganate solution, followed by 5% oxalic acid solution. • Never heat solution. • To prepare 1% solution, dilute with equal parts water.
None significant.	• Contraindicated in hypersensitivity to mercury compounds. • Do not use when aluminum may come in contact with skin. • Incompatible with permanganates, strong acids, and heavy metal salts. • Prepare as needed. Solutions tend to precipitate on standing. • Remove rings when working with solution; the mercury component can damage the precious metals in jewelry.
None significant.	• Effective against bacteria, fungi, viruses, yeast, and spores. • Powder reconstituted in saline solution. • Refrigerate dry crystal until reconstitution. • Oxychlorosene calcium has a special use as a local irrigating agent during surgery for neoplasms, to destroy loose viable neoplastic cells and thereby prevent iatrogenic metastasis. Oxychlorosene sodium is not used for this purpose.
None significant.	• Contraindicated in hypersensitivity to mercurials. • Antiseptic and fungicidal. • Frequent or prolonged use may cause mercury poisoning. • Orange stain removed with soap and water. • Commonly used as a preservative in ophthalmic solutions.
None significant.	• Contraindicated in hypersensitivity to iodines. • Prolonged germicidal action. • Water-soluble solution releases iodine at predetermined rate, causing prolonged action. • Relatively nonirritating to skin.
Iodine: precipitates iodine salt. Do not use together.	• Antiseptic astringent with fungicidal properties. • Germicidal effects reduced by organic matter. • Stains caused by potassium permanganate removed with dilute acids (lemon juice, oxalic acid, or dilute hydrochloric acid). • Never mix with charcoal or give charcoal as antidote. May explode.
None significant.	• Germicidal activity of iodine without irritation to skin and mucous membranes. • Thought to be superior to soap as a disinfectant; less effective than aqueous or alcoholic solutions of iodine. • Treated areas may be bandaged or taped. • Germicidal activity reduced if area cleansed with alcohol or other organic solvents after application of povidone-iodine. • Prolonged, excessive use may lead to systemic absorption and toxicity.

NAME	INDICATIONS & DOSAGE	SIDE EFFECTS
silver protein, mild Argyrol S.S.♦, Silvol, Solargentum	*Topical application for inflammation of eye, nose, throat*— **Adults and children:** apply p.r.n. as a 5% to 25% solution.	**Skin:** argyria in long-term use.
sodium hypochlorite 5% solution (instruments, swimming pools), 0.5% aqueous solution for wounds, Modified Dakin's solution	*Athlete's foot, wound irrigation, disinfection of walls and floors*—apply as directed.	**Skin:** irritation.
thimerosal Aeroaid Thimerosal, Merthiolate	*Preoperative disinfection of skin; antiseptic for open wounds*—apply or instill to affected area daily, b.i.d., or t.i.d. as a 0.1% solution or tincture.	**Skin:** erythematous, vesicular, papular eruptions (indicate hypersensitivity); irritation with tincture.

♦ Available in U.S. and Canada. ♦♦ Available in Canada only. All other products (no symbol) available in U.S. only. Italicized side effects are common or life-threatening.

INTERACTIONS	NURSING CONSIDERATIONS
None significant.	• Store in amber glass bottles; protect from light.
None significant.	• Germicidal and weakly fungicidal. • Interferes locally with thrombin formation, delaying blood clotting. Dissolves necrotic tissue. • Unstable in solution. Make fresh solution and use immediately. • Avoid contact with hair due to its bleaching properties.
None significant.	• Contraindicated in hypersensitivity to mercury-containing compounds. • Do not use when aluminum may come in contact with skin. • Incompatible with permanganate, strong acids, and salts of heavy metals. • Cleanse wound thoroughly before applying tincture. • To prevent skin irritation, allow tincture to dry completely before applying dressing. • Can be instilled into body cavities. • Store in amber glass container.

Emollients, demulcents, and protectants

aluminum paste
calamine
collodion, USP
collodion, flexible
compound benzoin tincture
dexpanthenol
glycerin
hydrophilic lotion
hydrophilic ointment
hydrophilic petrolatum
hydrous wool fat
hydrous wool fat and castor oil
liquid petrolatum
methyl salicylate
oatmeal
para-aminobenzoic acid
petrolatum
silicone
starch
talc (magnesium silicate)
urea or carbamide
vitamins A and D ointment
zinc gelatin

These preparations not only serve as vehicles for other drugs but are also used alone. *Emollients* protect and soften skin and mucous membranes; *demulcents* soothe inflamed or abraded skin and mucous membranes; *protectants* occlude and protect skin, ulcers, and wounds.

Major uses

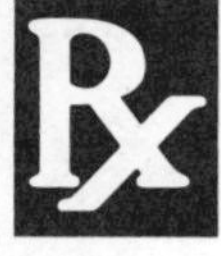

These preparations are used to treat burns, wounds, itching, insect bites, poison ivy, rashes, skin irritation and dryness, mild eczema, sunburn, rheumatic pains, muscle soreness, low back pain, cutaneous ulcers, and varicose veins.

Mechanism of action

• Emollients soften dry skin by preventing evaporation of perspiration.

Methyl salicylate is a counterirritant that increases circulation to the area of application. This causes localized redness and warmth and helps reduce muscle soreness and stiffness.

• Demulcents have analgesic properties to soothe irritation and cool inflammation. Some (such as starch) absorb moisture when secretions are excessive, helping to dry skin.

• Protectants promote healing by reducing irritation and friction.

Talc and other dusting powders are not completely biologically inert and may cause irritation, granulomas, fibrosis, or adhesion.

Flexible collodion is collodion USP, a protectant to which castor oil has been added to improve pliability.

Absorption, distribution, metabolism, and excretion

• Absorption of most of the preparations is confined to the skin: penetration is usually limited to the outer layers. The preparations do not generally reach the systemic circulation.

Methyl salicylate can be absorbed through the skin and, if used in excess, can cause toxicity.

• The preparations are distributed only to the affected areas, and they're usu-

NURSING TIP

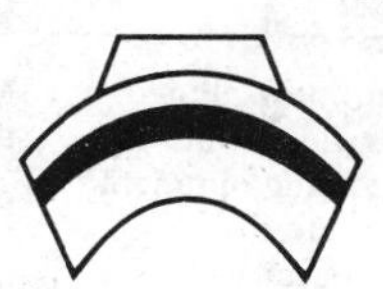

A SOOTHING SKIN CREAM

For an inexpensive cream to heal patients' dry, cracked skin, have your hospital pharmacy make a mixture containing equal parts of Desitin ointment, vitamins A and D ointment, and Nupercainal ointment. Then spoon the mixture into individual containers with lids (denture or stool specimen cups work well).

Before using, ask your patient's doctor if it's all right to apply this mixture to the patient's skin. Also check the patient for hypersensitivity. Then write his name and room number on the lid, seal the container, and place it at the patient's bedside.

Because sterility and bandaging aren't necessary, you can apply the mixture with your ungloved fingers directly on irritated skin. Your patient may want to apply the mixture himself. It's greaseless, so it can be used under clothing. Because the mixture rubs off easily, make a Kardex note to apply it t.i.d. and p.r.n.

Both Desitin and vitamins A and D ointments heal irritated skin, while Nupercainal ointment soothes inflammation and decreases pain. You should see the skin improve within 24 hours, and you may be able to discontinue application within 72 hours.

ally removed topically.

Onset and duration

Onset is generally rapid. Duration depends on the preparation and length of contact with the affected areas.

Combination products

CALADRYL LOTION: diphenhydramine hydrochloride 1%, calamine, camphor, and alcohol 2%.

CALADRYL CREAM: diphenhydramine hydrochloride 1% with calamine.

GER-O-FOAM AEROSOL: methyl salicylate 30%, benzocaine 3%, in oil emulsion.

PANALGESIC: methyl salicylate 50%, aspirin 8%, menthol and camphor 4%, emollient oils 20%, alcohol 18%.

NAME	INDICATIONS & DOSAGE	SIDE EFFECTS
aluminum paste (10% aluminum in zinc oxide ointment with liquid petrolatum)	*Emollient and protectant: colostomy area or other surgical sites*—apply p.r.n.	None.
calamine liniment (15% calamine), lotion (8% calamine), ointment (17% calamine), Rhulihist (3% calamine), Rhulispray (1% calamine)	*Topical astringent and protectant: itching, poison ivy and poison oak, nonpoisonous insect bites, mild sunburn, minor skin irritations*—apply p.r.n.	**Skin:** transient light stinging, irritation, dry skin.
collodion, USP (5% pyroxylin in 1 part alcohol, 3 parts ether) **collodion, flexible** (5% pyroxylin in 1 part alcohol, 3 parts ether plus 20% camphor, 30% castor oil)	*Protectant; vehicle for other medicinal agents; and sealant for small wounds*— apply to dry skin, p.r.n., or use flexible collodion when a flexible noncontracting film is desired.	None.
compound benzoin tincture (10% benzoin in alcohol mixed with glycerin and water) Benzoin Spray	*Demulcent and protectant: cutaneous ulcers, bedsores, cracked nipples, fissures of lips and anus*—apply locally once daily or b.i.d.	None.
dexpanthenol Panthoderm Cream♦ (dexpanthenol 2% in a water-miscible cream base), Panthoderm Lotion	*Epithelial-bed stimulator in emollient base: itching, wounds, insect bites, poison ivy, poison oak, diaper rash, chafing, mild eczema, decubitus ulcers, dry*	None.

♦ Available in U.S. and Canada. ♦♦ Available in Canada only. All other products (no symbol) available in U.S. only. Italicized side effects are common or life-threatening.

INTERACTIONS	NURSING CONSIDERATIONS
Topical enzymes: aluminum may inactivate preparations used to debride wounds. Don't use together.	• Zinc oxide paste can be used as an alternative. • Observe for inflammation or infection since protectants are occlusive layers that retain moisture, exclude air, and trap cutaneous bacteria. • Skin should be cleaned daily or more often as needed. • Emollients and protectants may be used alone, as vehicles for medications, or with other topical medications. Check with doctor.
None significant.	• Contraindicated in hypersensitivity to any of the components. • Watch for sensitivity reactions to calamine. Preparations containing antihistamines can cause sensitivity. • Always shake well before use. • Don't use cotton to apply; it will absorb the solute. Use gauze sponge. • Do not apply to blistered, raw, or oozing areas of the skin. • Toxic if taken internally. • Observe for inflammation or infection since protectants are occlusive layers that retain moisture, exclude air, and trap skin bacteria. • Skin should be cleaned daily or more often as needed. • Emollients, demulcents, protectants may be used alone, as vehicles for medications, or with other topical medications. Check with doctor. • Highly flammable; never use near flame. • May irritate and dry skin. • Keep container tightly closed so solvent won't evaporate.
None significant.	• Observe for inflammation or infection since protectants are occlusive layers that retain moisture, exclude air, and trap cutaneous bacteria. • Skin should be cleaned daily or more often as needed. • Protectants may be used alone, as vehicles for medications, or with other topical medications. Check with doctor. • Camphor in flexible collodion is weakly antiseptic and antipruritic; may irritate and dry skin. • Highly flammable; never use near flame. • Keep container tightly closed so solvent won't evaporate. • Toxic if taken internally. • Avoid excessive inhalation of vapors.
None significant.	• Do not apply to acutely inflamed areas. • Observe for inflammation or infection since protectants are occlusive layers that retain moisture, exclude air, and trap cutaneous bacteria. • Skin should be cleaned daily or more often as needed. • Protectants may be used alone, as vehicles for medications, or with other topical medications. Check with doctor. • For demulcent and expectorant action in laryngitis or croup, use in boiling water and have patient inhale vapors. • Spray is not intended for use as inhalant. • Can be mixed with magnesium-aluminum hydroxide and applied on bedsores.
None significant.	• Contraindicated in wounds of hemophilia patients. • Before each new application *always* thoroughly cleanse affected area, removing all traces of previously applied medication. Observe for inflammation or infection. • Dry lesions respond better than oozing lesions.

(continued on following page)

NAME	INDICATIONS & DOSAGE	SIDE EFFECTS
dexpanthenol *(continued)* (dexpanthenol 2%, menthol 0.1%, and camphor 0.1%)	*lesions*—apply topically, p.r.n.	
glycerin Corn Huskers Lotion (tragacanth 1 g, glycerin 30 ml, propylene glycol 10 ml)	*Emollient and lubricant: rectal tubes and catheters; dry skin, hands*—apply p.r.n.	None.
hydrophilic lotion (white petrolatum 4.2 g, stearyl alcohol 4.2 g, methylparaben 0.004 g, propylparaben 0.002 g, sodium lauryl sulfate 0.167 g, propylene glycol 2 ml, perfume q.s., purified water)	*Protectant and emollient: dry skin, irritation*—apply p.r.n.	None.
hydrophilic ointment Cetaphil, Heb Cream Base, Multibase, Neobase, Unibase, Vanibase (methylparaben 0.025 g, propylparaben 0.015 g, stearyl alcohol 25 g, white petrolatum 25 g, propylene glycol 12 g, sodium lauryl sulfate 1 g, purified water)	*Protectant and emollient: dry skin, oozing lesions*—apply p.r.n.	None.
hydrophilic petrolatum Aquaphor, Hydrosort, Plastibase Hydrophilic, Polysort (cholesterol 3 g, stearyl alcohol 3 g, white wax 8 g, white petrolatum 86 g)	*Protectant and emollient: dry skin, eczema, or psoriasis*—mix with other medicinal ingredients as ordered, and apply p.r.n.	None.
hydrous wool fat Lanolin Lotion (stearic acid 2 g, triethanolamine 0.8 ml, light liquid petrolatum 10 ml, propylparaben 0.2 g, rose water)	*Protectant and emollient*—apply hydrous wool fat p.r.n. *Protection against hydrocarbons, solvents, and cutting oils*—apply hydrous wool fat and castor oil before exposure.	**Skin:** allergic rash.

◆ Available in U.S. and Canada. ◆◆ Available in Canada only. All other products (no symbol) available in U.S. only. Italicized side effects are common or life-threatening.

INTERACTIONS	NURSING CONSIDERATIONS
	• May heal skin lesions in mild eczema and dermatoses.
None significant.	• Applied undiluted to inflamed, dehydrated skin. Paradoxically, excessive use may dry the skin. • Diluted with rose water, glycerin is useful for irritated or dry lips.
None significant.	• Observe for inflammation or infection since protectants are occlusive layers that retain moisture, exclude air, and trap skin bacteria. • Skin should be cleaned daily or more often as needed. • Emollients and protectants may be used alone, as vehicles for medications, or with other topical medications. Check with doctor.
None significant.	• Easily removed with water. • Use when little penetration of medicinal agent is desired. • Observe for inflammation or infection since protectants are occlusive layers that retain moisture, exclude air, and trap skin bacteria. • Skin should be cleaned daily or more often as needed. • Emollients and protectants may be used alone, as vehicles for medications, or with other topical medications. Check with doctor. • This nongreasy ointment is especially suited for application to hairy areas.
None significant.	• Not water soluble; greasy. • Observe for inflammation or infection since protectants are occlusive layers that retain moisture, exclude air, and trap skin bacteria. • Skin should be cleaned daily or more often as needed. • Emollients and protectants may be used alone, as vehicles for medications, or with other topical medications. Check with doctor.
None significant.	• Contraindicated in hypersensitivity to lanolin. • Don't confuse with anhydrous wool fat, which will dry skin if applied alone. • Observe for inflammation or infection since protectants are occlusive layers that retain moisture, exclude air, and trap skin bacteria. • Skin should be cleaned daily or more often as needed.

(continued on following page)

NAME	INDICATIONS & DOSAGE	SIDE EFFECTS
hydrous wool fat *(continued)*		
hydrous wool fat and castor oil (hydrous wool fat 25 g, castor oil 25 g, ceresin wax 5 g, polysorbate 60 5 g, white petrolatum)		
liquid petrolatum Liquid Petrolatum, USP, Light Liquid Petrolatum, NF, Mineral Oil	*Protectant and emollient*—apply locally, full strength, or diluted.	None.
methyl salicylate Banalg, Baumodyne Gel and Ointment, Betula Oil, Gaultheria Oil, Sweet Birch Oil, Wintergreen Oil	*Counterirritant: minor pains of osteoarthritis, rheumatism, sprains, muscle and tendon soreness and tightness, lumbago, sciatica*— **Adults:** apply with gentle massage several times daily. Not recommended for children.	**Skin:** rash, irritation, burning, blistering.
oatmeal Aveeno Colloidal, Aveeno Oilated Bath (with liquid petrolatum and hypoallergenic lanolin)	*Emollient and demulcent: local irritation*—use as a lotion; 1 level tablespoon to a cup of warm water. *Skin irritation, pruritus, common dermatoses, sunburn, dry skin*— **Adults:** 1 packet in tub of warm water. **Children:** 1 to 2 rounded tablespoons in 3 to 4 inches of bath water. **Infants:** 2 or 3 level teaspoons, depending on size of bath.	None.
para-aminobenzoic acid PABA♦, Pabagel♦, Pabanol♦, Pre-Sun♦, PreSun Gel, RV Paba	*Topical protectant: sunburn protection, sun-sensitive skin, slow tanning*— **Adults:** apply evenly to dry skin; follow directions on var-	**Local:** allergic reaction, irritation, sensitization. **Skin:** photocontact dermatitis.

INTERACTIONS	NURSING CONSIDERATIONS
	• Emollients and protectants may be used alone, as vehicles for medications, or with other topical medications. Check with doctor.
None significant.	• Occasionally used with other drugs. • Available in two forms: light mineral oil and heavy mineral oil. • Heavy mineral oil can be used internally as a laxative. Never use light mineral oil as a laxative. Mineral oil used as nose drops can cause lipid pneumonia. • Observe for inflammation or infection since protectants are occlusive layers that retain moisture, exclude air, and trap skin bacteria. • Skin should be cleaned daily or more often as needed. • Emollients and protectants may be used alone, as vehicles for medications, or with other topical medications. Check with doctor.
None significant.	• Never apply directly, undiluted to skin. • Warning: as little as 4 ml ingested by children can cause fatal toxicity; in adults as little as 30 ml. Since GI absorption may be delayed, treat such ingestion with emetic lavage, then a saline cathartic. Continue lavage until no odor of methyl salicylate can be detected in the washings. • Absorbed through skin; prolonged increased application can cause toxicity. Toxic effects include hyperpnea leading to respiratory alkalosis, nausea, vomiting, tinnitus, hyperpyrexia, and convulsions. • Discontinue if rash or redness occurs. Consult doctor if pain or redness persists more than 10 days. • Avoid getting near eyes, open wounds, mucous membranes. • Do not use on sunburned membranes. • Do not apply to broken or irritated skin. • Do not wrap or bandage treated area. • Store in tightly closed container.
None significant.	• Not to be ingested. Don't confuse with oatmeal as food. • Instruct patient to exercise caution to avoid slipping in tub. • Avoid getting in eyes.
None significant.	• Contraindicated in hypersensitivity to any of the components and for persons with damaged or diseased skin. • Discontinue if skin rash occurs. • Encourage slow tanning and short exposure to sun. • Avoid contact with eyes and lids.

(continued on following page)

NAME	INDICATIONS & DOSAGE	SIDE EFFECTS
para-aminobenzoic acid *(continued)* Lipstick, Sunbrella Lotion	ious products for number and time of application, which vary from 2 to 6 hours; reapply after swimming. Not recommended for children.	
petrolatum Vaseline	*Topical protectant and emollient*—use alone or with other drugs, as directed.	None.
silicone Silicone and Zinc Oxide Compound, Silon Spray	*Topical protectant: dermatoses, diaper rash, decubitus ulcers*—apply b.i.d. or t.i.d. in ointment. *Protection against water and corrosive chemicals*—apply before exposure.	None.
starch	*Demulcent: minor skin irritations, pruritus associated with common dermatoses*—mix 2 cups of starch with 4 cups of water, add to tub of water, and soak affected area for 30 minutes.	None.
talc (magnesium silicate)	*Topical lubricant, protectant, drying agent, absorbent dusting powder: irritation such as intertrigo prickly heat*—sprinkle on affected areas p.r.n. for soothing and lubrication.	None.
urea or carbamide Aquacare Dry Skin Cream and Lotion♦, Aquacare/HP Cream and Lotion♦, Aqua Lacten, Artra Ashy Skin Cream, Carmol Ten, Carmol Twenty, Gormel Cream, Nutraplus♦, Rea-Lo, Ultra-Mide, Uremol♦♦, Urtex♦♦	*Emollient: hard, dry skin on hands, elbows, or knees*— **Adults:** apply to affected area b.i.d. or t.i.d., particularly after exposure to sun or wind. Not recommended for children.	**Skin:** transient stinging when applied to irritated or fissured skin.
vitamins A and D ointment A&D, Balmex, Caldesene Medicated, Clocream, Comfortine, Desitin, Primaderm	*Emollient, demulcent, and epithelial-bed stimulant: superficial burns, sunburn, abrasions, slow-healing lesions, chapped skin, diaper rash, skin care of infants or bedridden patients*—apply several times a day.	**Skin:** irritation.

♦ Available in U.S. and Canada. ♦♦ Available in Canada only. All other products (no symbol) available in U.S. only. Italicized side effects are common or life-threatening.

INTERACTIONS	NURSING CONSIDERATIONS
	• Avoid contact with open flame. • May stain clothing. • Observe for inflammation and infection since protectants produce an occlusive layer that retains perspiration, excludes air, and traps cutaneous bacteria, producing sites for anaerobic infections.
None significant.	• Stable, does not become rancid. • Observe for inflammation or infection since protectants are occlusive layers that retain moisture, exclude air, and trap skin bacteria. • Skin should be cleaned daily or more often as needed. • Emollients and protectants may be used alone, as vehicles for medications, or with other topical medications. Check with doctor.
None significant.	• Protect eyes against spray. • Very difficult to remove from skin; resistant to water and soap. • Will not protect against oils or solvents. • Observe for inflammation or infection since protectants are occlusive layers that retain moisture, exclude air, and trap cutaneous bacteria. • Skin should be cleaned daily or more often as needed. • Protectants may be used alone, as vehicles for medications, or with other topical medications. Check with doctor.
None significant.	• Instruct patient to exercise caution to avoid slipping in tub. • Use of cornstarch in intertriginous areas may promote or accelerate a yeast infection since yeast can feed on the sugar.
None significant.	• Don't use on surgical gloves; causes granulation and adhesions in open wounds. • Avoid dust entering eyes or inhalation of talc dust. • Should not be used on open, weeping surfaces; it cakes and crusts.
None significant.	• Contraindicated in viral skin diseases, or in impaired circulation. Use cautiously on face or broken skin. • Wet skin before application. If irritation persists, discontinue. • Avoid contact with eyes. • Emollients produce an occlusive layer that retains perspiration, excludes air, and traps cutaneous bacteria, producing sites for anaerobic infections. Before each new application, *always* thoroughly cleanse affected area, removing all traces of previously applied medication. Observe for inflammation or infection.
None significant.	• Discontinue if skin condition persists or irritation develops. • Observe for inflammation or infection since emollients and demulcents are occlusive layers that retain moisture, exclude air, and trap cutaneous bacteria. • Skin should be cleaned daily or more often as needed. • Emollients and demulcents may be used alone, as vehicles for medications, or with other topical medications. Check with doctor.

NAME	INDICATIONS & DOSAGE	SIDE EFFECTS
zinc gelatin Dome-Paste, Unna's Boot	*Protectant: varicosities, lesions or injuries of lower legs or arms*—heat in hot bath till liquefied, clean skin, dust with talc, and apply gel with paint brush; make three layers, with gauze between each layer; retain 2 weeks. Dome-Paste, in 3″ and 4″ bandages, can be applied directly to arm or leg.	None.

INTERACTIONS	NURSING CONSIDERATIONS
None significant.	• Observe for inflammation and infection since protectants produce an occlusive layer that retains perspiration, excludes air, and traps cutaneous bacteria, producing sites for anaerobic infections. Before each new application *always* thoroughly cleanse affected area, removing all traces of previously applied medication. • Zinc gelatin boot can be removed by unwinding outer bandage and soaking leg or arm in warm water until dressing floats off. Tell patient not to shower or take tub bath with zinc gelatin boot on leg.

PATIENT-TEACHING AID

HOW TO CLEAN AND DRESS YOUR WOUND

Dear Patient:

To ensure the proper healing of your wound or incision, change the dressing as often as your doctor suggested. But if you notice some drainage before the next scheduled change, apply a new dressing immediately. Follow these procedures:

• Before you begin, collect all the materials you'll need and place them within reach: sterile forceps, sterile gloves, sterile dressings, nonperfumed soap, water, and tape.

• If your doctor has asked you to maintain sterile technique, wear sterile gloves, use sterile equipment, and avoid touching the part of the bandage that will cover the wound. In any case, wash your hands carefully before handling the dressings; then handle them carefully and as little as possible.

• Remove soiled dressings and discard carefully in a waterproof bag. Don't contaminate the outside of the bag with soiled dressings.

• If dressings stick to the wound, moisten them with sterile water or hydrogen peroxide before attempting to remove them.

• With a sterile gauze pad, clean the wound with a single circular motion; always wipe from inside to out. Discard the pad after each single circular motion.

• If an ointment was used on the wound, remove it with nonperfumed soap and water; rinse well. Again, always clean and rinse in an in-to-out direction.

• If ordered, apply ointment or other medication to dressing; then apply the dressing to the wound or incision.

• If ordered, apply a protective ointment to the surrounding area.

• If the wound or incision is to be covered, apply a sterile dressing, being careful to handle only the outer top surface of the dressing.

• Secure the dressing with nonallergenic tape, not adhesive tape.

• If you note any changes in the wound, such as redness, swelling, foul odors or pus, notify the doctor immediately.

Keratolytics and caustics

cantharidin
dichloroacetic acid
podophyllum resin
resorcinol
resorcinol monoacetate
salicylic acid
silver nitrate
sulfur
sulfurated lime solution

Keratolytic agents loosen the tightly packed cell products, cell wall, and protein (keratin) that constitute the outer, protective layer (stratum corneum) of the epidermis. They are used in the treatment of benign skin growths and other dermatologic disorders.

By cauterizing tissue at the site of application, caustic agents can destroy moles and warts. Take care when using these agents, however, to protect adjacent skin from their harmful effects.

Major uses

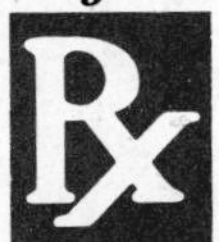

• Keratolytics (cantharidin, resorcinol, salicylic acid, sulfur, and sulfurated lime solution) are used to treat dermatophytosis, warts, corns, and certain acneiform and eczematous dermatoses. In addition, they are used to control fungal infections.

• Caustics (dichloroacetic acid, podophyllum resin, and silver nitrate) destroy warts, condylomata, keratoses, certain types of moles, and hyperplastic tissue.

BEWARE OF TOXICITY FROM PODOPHYLLUM THERAPY

Topical application of podophyllum resin can cause increased side effects and severe systemic toxicity *when an accelerated treatment schedule produces a high cumulative dose.*

Leukopenia and thrombocytopenia developed rapidly in a 15-year-old girl who received three applications of the drug, in combination with benzoin tincture, in 24 hours, to treat condylomata acuminata (genital warts). If your patient is undergoing similarly aggressive treatment, watch for dizziness, nausea, vomiting, abdominal pain, oliguria, anuria, fever, confusion, peripheral neuropathy, lethargy, tachycardia, and tachypnea.

To prevent toxic complications, podophyllum resin should be applied only to small target areas of unbroken skin, and left in contact for no longer than 1 hour. The drug should be withdrawn at the first sign of toxic reaction.

Adapted with permission from Gary P. Stoehr, et al., "Systemic Complications of Local Podophyllin Therapy," *Annals of Internal Medicine,* 89:3:362, September 1978.

Mechanism of action

• Keratolytics soften keratin and loosen cornified epithelium, causing even viable cells to swell, soften, and dissolve.

• Caustics except podophyllum precipitate cell proteins, causing formation of a scab that eventually sloughs off.

Podophyllum inhibits cell division

and other cellular processes, leading to the death of the cell.

Absorption, distribution, metabolism, and excretion

Most of these agents are not appreciably absorbed.

• Cantharidin can be absorbed and may cause severe genitourinary tract irritation.

• Podophyllum can be absorbed through mucous membranes and cause significant toxicity due to cerebral vasoconstriction. For this reason, the use of podophyllum-coated tampons for the treatment of vaginal warts should be discouraged.

Onset and duration

These agents begin to act immediately upon application.

Duration of action and necessity for retreatment depend on the specific agent and the condition.

PATIENT-TEACHING AID

TREATING WARTS OR CORNS

Dear Patient:

The following tips will help you treat your warts or corns.

1. Remember, warts are caused by viruses and can be contagious. Therefore, wash your hands before and after treatment.
2. Gently remove any dead skin with a rough towel, callous file, or pumice stone. Don't use force.
3. Apply petrolatum to the healthy skin surrounding the affected area to protect it from accidental application of the corrosive wart remover.
4. Carefully apply medication only to the wart or corn.
5. Promptly report any change in size or color of a wart to your podiatrist or doctor.
6. To prevent further irritation, make sure shoes fit properly.
7. *Note:* If you are a diabetic or have peripheral vascular disease, don't apply corrosive wart-removing drugs without consulting your podiatrist or doctor.

Combination products

ACNE-AID CREAM: sulfur 2.5%, resorcinol 1.25%, and parachlorometaxylenol 0.375% in a microporous cellulose base.

ACNE-DOME: colloidal sulfur 4% and resorcinol monoacetate 2% in an acid-mantle vehicle.

ACNOMEL CAKE♦: sulfur 4% and resorcinol 1% in a washable base.

ACNOMEL CREAM♦: sulfur 8%, resorcinol 2%, and alcohol 11% in a greaseless base.

BENSULFOID LOTION: fusion of finely divided sulfur (33% by weight) onto colloidal bentonite 6%, resorcinol 2%, zinc oxide 6%, thymol 0.5%, and alcohol 12% in a greaseless base.

CLEARASIL CREAM: benzoyl peroxide 10% and bentonite.

COMPOUND W WART REMOVER: salicylic acid 14%, acetic acid 11%, in castor oil, alcohol, ether, and collodion.

DUOFILM♦: salicylic acid 16.7% and lactic acid 16.7% in flexible collodion.

EXZIT: colloidal sulfur 4% and resorcinol monoacetate 2%.

FOSTEX CAKE♦: sulfur 2% and salicylic acid 2%.

FREEZONE CORN AND CALLUS REMOVER: salicylic acid 13.6%, zinc chloride 2.17%, in castor oil, and collodion, alcohol, and ether.

GETS-IT-LIQUID: salicylic acid, zinc chloride, and collodion in ether and alcohol.

REZAMID LOTION♦: sulfur 5%, resorcinol 2%, parachlorometaxylenol 0.5%, and alcohol 28.5% in a hydroalcoholic lotion base.

SULFORCIN BASE CREAM: sulfur 4% and resorcinol monoacetate 1.5%.

NAME	INDICATIONS & DOSAGE	SIDE EFFECTS
cantharidin Cantharone	**Adults and children:** *Molluscum contagiosum*—coat each lesion. Repeat in a week on new or remaining lesions, this time covering with occlusive tape. Remove tape in 6 to 8 hours. *Palpebral warts*—apply, leave lesion uncovered. *Plantar warts*—pare away keratin, apply generously to affected area, allow to dry, apply protective padding, cover with nonporous tape for a week, then debride. Repeat 3 times, if necessary, on large lesions. *Removal of ordinary and periungual warts and other benign epithelial growths*—apply directly to lesion and cover completely. Allow to dry, then cover with nonporous adhesive tape. Remove tape in 24 hours (or less if extreme pain) and replace with loose bandage. Reapply, if necessary.	**Skin:** annular warts, burning, tingling, extreme tenderness, inflammation.
dichloroacetic acid Bichloracetic Acid	*All types of verrucae; calluses, corns; xanthelasma; ingrown toenails; cysts and benign erosion of the cervix; sebaceous adenoma; infectious granuloma; tattoo marks; epistaxis; spider nevi; tonsil tabs*— **Adults:** applied only by doctor at his discretion.	**Local:** irritation, inflammation of normal skin.
podophyllum resin Podoben	*Venereal warts and granuloma inguinale*— **Adults:** apply podophyllum resin preparation to the lesion, cover with waxed paper, and bandage. Leave covered for 8 to 12 hours, then wash lesion to remove medication. Repeat at weekly intervals.	**Blood:** thrombocytopenia, leukopenia when systemically absorbed. **Local:** irritation of normal skin. **Other:** peripheral neuropathy when systemically absorbed.
resorcinol **resorcinol monoacetate** Euresol, Resorcin	*Acute eczema, urticaria, and other inflammatory skin diseases (1% or 2% concentration in alcohol); acne or seborrhea (5% lotion or 10% soap liniment for scalp); chronic eczema, psoriasis (2% to 10% ointment); acne scarring (45% peeling paste)*— **Adults and children:** apply as directed.	**Skin:** irritation, moderate erythema or scaling. **Other:** darkening of light hair (resorcinol only).

♦ Available in U.S. and Canada. ♦♦ Available in Canada only. All other products (no symbol) available in U.S. only. Italicized side effects are common or life-threatening.

INTERACTIONS	NURSING CONSIDERATIONS
None significant.	• If dropped on normal skin, remove immediately with acetone, alcohol, or tape remover. Scrub with warm, soapy water, and rinse well, as blistering of skin may result. • If dropped on mucous membranes or in eyes, flush well with water to remove precipitated collodion, then continue to flush with water for 15 minutes. • Treat only one or two lesions initially to test patient's sensitivity. • Stop treatment if severe inflammation develops. • If application causes burning, tenderness, or tingling, remove tape and soak area in cool water for 10 to 15 minutes; repeat, if necessary. • If annular warts develop, assure patient that lesions are superficial; re-treat or substitute another procedure. • Does not affect tissue layers below the epidermis and leaves no scar. • Treatment should be supervised by a doctor.
None significant.	• Contraindicated for treatment of malignant or premalignant lesions. • Protect adjacent areas with petrolatum, especially when using 50% solutions. • Sodium bicarbonate is local antidote. • Thoroughly dry area before application. • Warn patient that when solution is applied, treated area will turn from white to red in about 4 hours. • Peeling of skin usually is noticed in 4 days and is completed in a week. • If acid comes in contact with normal skin, wipe off with cotton gauze and flush area with water.
Other keratolytics: may cause extensive damage to the skin. Do not use together.	• Resin is irritating and cytotoxic, and should not be applied to normal skin. Petrolatum can be applied to adjacent areas to protect them during treatment. • Should be applied only by a doctor because of toxicity. • Do not use on extensive areas or for prolonged therapy; may be absorbed systemically. • Warn patient that soreness from local irritation may develop 12 to 48 hours after treatment.
None significant.	• Do not use preparations on or near eyes. • If skin irritation persists, discontinue medication. • Apply lotion with cotton ball to affected area. • When applying the peeling paste, closely observe the patient and site of application until paste is removed. • Use carefully with topical acne preparations because of local irritation.

NAME	INDICATIONS & DOSAGE	SIDE EFFECTS
salicylic acid Calicylic, Keralyt♦, Salactic Liquifilm, Salonil	*Superficial fungal infections, acne, psoriasis, seborrheic dermatitis, other scaling dermatoses, hyperkeratosis, calluses, warts—* **Adults and children:** apply to affected area and place under occlusion at night.	**Skin:** irritation, drying. **Other:** salicylism with percutaneous absorption.
silver nitrate	*Cauterization of mucous membranes, fissures, aphthous lesions (5% to 10% solution); cauterization of granulomatous tissues and warts (solid form)—* **Adults and children:** applied only by doctor at his discretion.	**Local:** *argyria (permanent silver discoloration of skin).*
sulfur Acne-Aid♦, Acnomead, Bensulfoid, EpiClear, Liquimat, Postacne♦, Transact, Xerac	*Acne, ringworm, psoriasis, seborrheic dermatitis, chigger infestation, scabies, favus, staphylococcal folliculitis—* **Adults and children:** apply preparation to affected areas b.i.d., t.i.d., or as directed.	**Local:** excessive drying of skin, blackheads, contact dermatitis.
sulfurated lime solution Vlem-Dome, Vleminckx's solution	*Acne vulgaris, seborrhea—* **Adults and children:** dilute 1 packet in 1 pint hot water and apply as hot dressing for 15 to 20 minutes daily. *Generalized furunculosis—* **Adults and children:** add 30 to 60 ml solution to bath water.	**Local:** may cause excessive drying of skin.

♦ Available in U.S. and Canada. ♦♦ Available in Canada only. All other products (no symbol) available in U.S. only. Italicized side effects are common or life-threatening.

INTERACTIONS	NURSING CONSIDERATIONS
None significant.	• Use with caution in patients with diabetes or peripheral vascular disease. The skin inflammation that may result is difficult to treat. Limit use for children under 12 years. (Do not exceed 1 oz in 24 hours.) • Avoid contact with eyes and mucous membranes. • If excessive skin drying or irritation occurs, apply a bland cream or lotion. • Rinse hands after application (unless they are being treated). • Skin should be hydrated for at least 5 minutes before treatment and washed the morning after treatment. • Most preparations are occlusive, which increases percutaneous absorption. Therefore, do not use on large surface areas for prolonged periods. • Not for use on broken, inflamed, or ulcerated areas.
None significant.	• May cause burns. Avoid accidental contact with skin and eyes. If accidental contact with skin occurs, flush with water for at least 15 minutes; accidental contact with eyes, call doctor at once. • Not to be ingested; may cause altered respiration, coma, convulsions, paralysis, and even death. If ingested, call doctor at once. Give 1 tablespoon salt in warm water; repeat until emesis is clear. Or have patient drink milk or beaten egg whites mixed in warm water. Keep patient warm and lying down. • Warn that silver nitrate stains skin and clothing. • Silver nitrate pencils must be moistened with water before use.
None significant.	• Prolonged use may cause severe contact dermatitis. • When initiating therapy, use sparingly for patients with sensitive skin. • Avoid contact with eyes. If accidental contact occurs, flush with water. • Wash skin thoroughly before application. Tell patient that tingling sensation may be felt upon application. • Skin is more reactive to drug in cold, dry climates, so decrease frequency of application. In hot, humid climates, increase frequency of application. • Do not use on same area with topical acne preparation or preparations containing a peeling agent (for example, benzoyl peroxide); may cause severe irritation. • Do not use on same area with any mercury-containing preparation; may cause a foul odor, irritate the skin, or stain skin black.
None significant.	• Discontinue use if excessive drying or skin irritation develops. • Avoid contact with jewelry, metallic objects, or clothing. • Avoid getting solution in eyes, nose, or mouth. • Fumes are irritating and malodorous (rotten eggs). Ventilate adequately. • Do not use in same area with topical acne preparations; may cause severe irritation. • Do not use in same area with mercury-containing preparations; may cause a foul odor, irritate skin, or turn skin black.

Miscellaneous dermatomucosal agents

ammonium mercury
anthralin
benzoyl peroxide
collagenase
dextranomer
fluorouracil
hydroquinone
methoxsalen
scarlet red
selenium sulfide
streptokinase-streptodornase
sutilains
tretinoin (vitamin A acid, retinoic acid)

Miscellaneous topical drugs include acne and burn products, irritants, rubefacients, antiseptics, enzymes, antimetabolites, and preparations that affect skin pigmentation.

Major uses

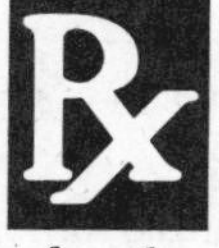

- Ammoniated mercury, anthralin, and selenium sulfide relieve psoriasis, atopic dermatitis, chronic dermatitis and eczema, seborrhea, pruritus, ringworm, and other skin conditions.
- Benzoyl peroxide and tretinoin are used to treat acne vulgaris.
- Collagenase, dextranomer, scarlet red, streptokinase-streptodornase, and sutilains clean, debride, and heal burns, surgical wounds, and ulcerative and pyogenic lesions.
- Fluorouracil is used to treat superficial forms of skin cancer.
- Hydroquinone is used to treat problems of skin hyperpigmentation.
- Methoxsalen accelerates pigmentation.

Mechanism of action

- Ammoniated mercury inhibits sulfhydryl enzymes and combines with amino and other chemical groups.
- Anthralin acts as a local antieczematous irritant.
- Benzoyl peroxide has antimicrobial and keratolytic activity.
- Collagenase is an enzymatic debriding agent that digests undenatured collagen fibers in necrotic tissue and removes substrates for bacterial proliferation. It facilitates access to infected areas by antibiotics, antibodies, and leukocytes.
- Dextranomer is a synthetic polymer that aids in granulation.
- Fluorouracil acts as an antimetabolite. It interferes with DNA synthesis by inhibiting thymidylate synthetase.
- Hydroquinone inhibits tyrosinase, preventing the conversion of tyrosine to melanin.
- Methoxsalen is a potent photosensitizer of the skin that promotes melanin formation by facilitating the action of ultraviolet light. It does not promote pigmentation in the absence of light.
- Scarlet red stimulates proliferation of the basal layer of the skin.
- Selenium sulfide has irritant, antibacterial, and antifungal properties.
- Streptokinase-streptodornase are enzymes produced during growth of certain strains of hemolytic streptococci.

Streptokinase stimulates plasminogen activator; streptodornase hydrolyzes deoxyribonucleoprotein.

• Sutilains is a proteolytic enzyme that selectively digests necrotic tissue.

• Tretinoin (vitamin A acid) is a potent drying and peeling agent.

Absorption, distribution, metabolism, and excretion

These topical drugs may be absorbed systemically if they're used for long periods or applied to large areas of the body.

Onset and duration

These agents begin to act immediately upon application. The duration of action and the necessity for retreatment depend not only on the specific agent but also on the condition being treated.

Combination products

EMERSAL: ammoniated mercury 5% and salicylic acid 2.5%.

LOROXIDE♦: benzoyl peroxide 5.5% and chlorhydroxyquinoline 0.25%.

LOROXIDE HC♦: benzoyl peroxide 5.5%, chlorhydroxyquinoline 0.25%, and hydrocortisone 0.5%.

SULFOXYL REGULAR: benzoyl peroxide 5% and sulfur 2%.

SULFOXYL STRONG: benzoyl peroxide 10% and sulfur 5%.

VANOXIDE♦: benzoyl peroxide 5% and chlorhydroxyquinoline 0.25%.

VANOXIDE-HC♦: benzoyl peroxide 5%, chlorhydroxyquinoline 0.25%, and hydrocortisone 0.5%.

APPLYING TOPICAL DRUGS TO BURNS

Apply topical drugs after hydrotherapy or debridement. Using sterile technique, apply ointment and creams as follows:

• Apply a layer 2 to 4 mm thick directly to the burn eschar and leave it open to air. Reapply as necessary to keep the eschar covered.

• Apply the topical medication to the gauze and then apply the medicated gauze to the burn. Place dry gauze over the dressing, and cover with a stockinette or net dressing, such as Surgifix. Change dressings one to three times a day.

Drug solutions are used in all stages of burn care. Apply in one of the following ways:

• *Wet to dry.* Soak dressings in the solution and apply them to the burn. Apply a dry dressing over them.

• *Wet.* Prepare and apply dressings as described above, but keep them wet by frequent irrigations with the topical solution. Change dressings at least daily. Monitor the patient's temperature for hypothermia due to the cooling effect produced by evaporation from dressings.

For information on applying dextranomer (Debrisan) and silver sulfadiazine (Silvadene) to decubitus ulcers, see next page. For information on psoriasis treatments, see pages 1116-1117.

APPLYING SILVADENE AND DEBRISAN TO DECUBITUS ULCERS

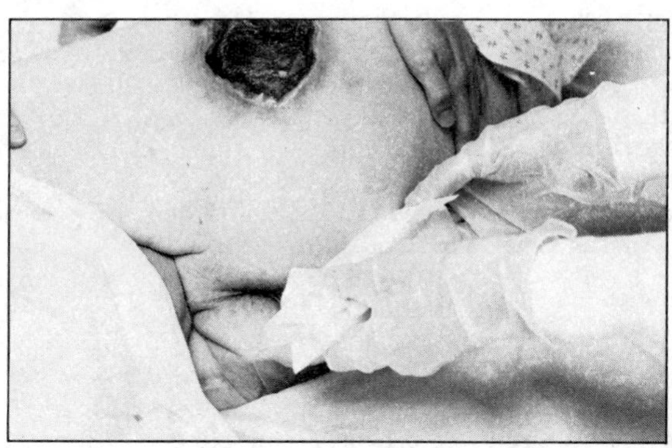

1 First, assemble the equipment. Then, tell your patient what you'll be doing. Place him in a right side-lying position. Protect bed linen with bedsaver pads. Put the plastic bag on the bed, next to your patient.

Open the irrigation set and pour the normal saline solution into the container. Wash your hands and put on the nonsterile gloves. Remove the soiled dressing, as shown, folding soiled sides together.

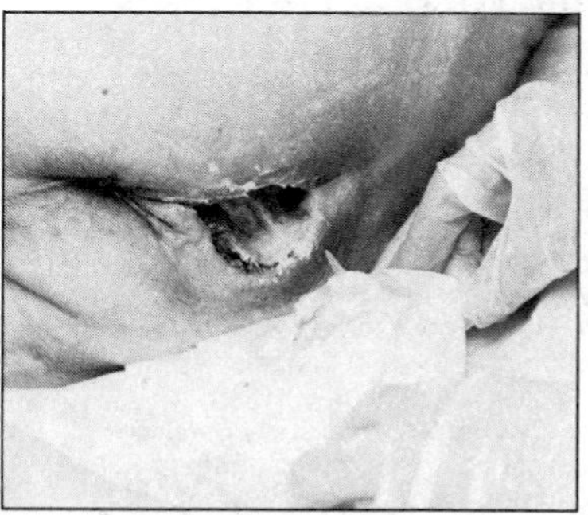

2 Carefully examine the ulcer and the dressing. Check for signs of infection, such as redness, swelling, or excessive drainage. Note the color and amount of drainage (if present). Discard the soiled dressing in the plastic bag.

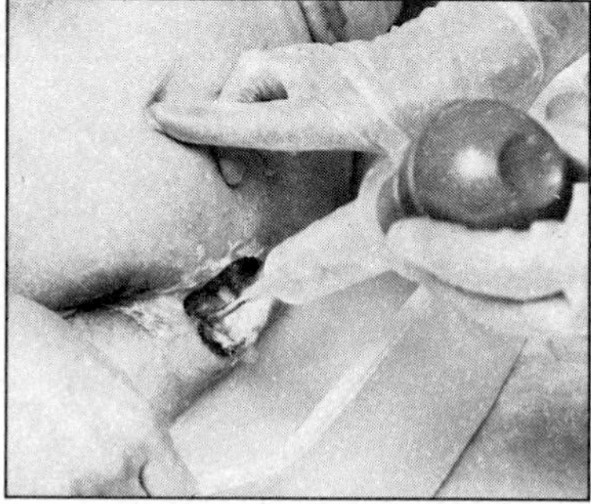

3 Draw up 30 ml of sterile saline solution into the syringe. Place the irrigating container at the ulcer's base. Hold the syringe tip 2″ (5 cm) from the ulcer and flush it with the saline to remove loose debris and old medication. Don't touch syringe tip to ulcer.

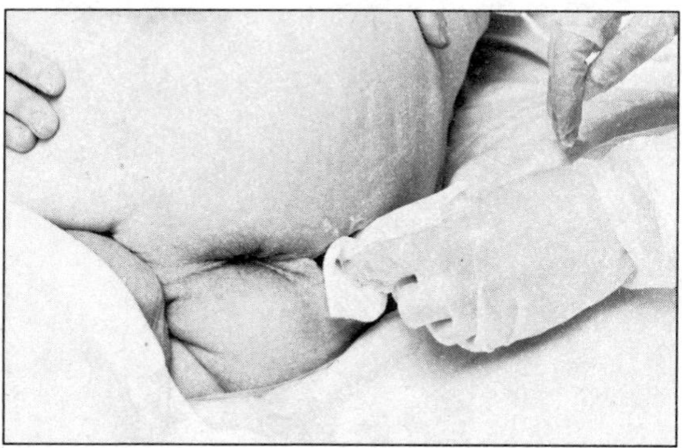

4 Wrap a sterile gauze pad around your finger, using aseptic technique. Then, gently pat the ulcer dry, as the nurse is doing here. Discard the pad in the plastic bag. Remove your gloves and discard them in the plastic bag. Wash your hands thoroughly.

When caring for a patient with a decubitus ulcer, you may initiate wound and skin precautions. If the doctor has ordered silver sulfadiazine (Silvadene) ointment and dextranomer (Debrisan) applied with every dressing change, follow these steps:

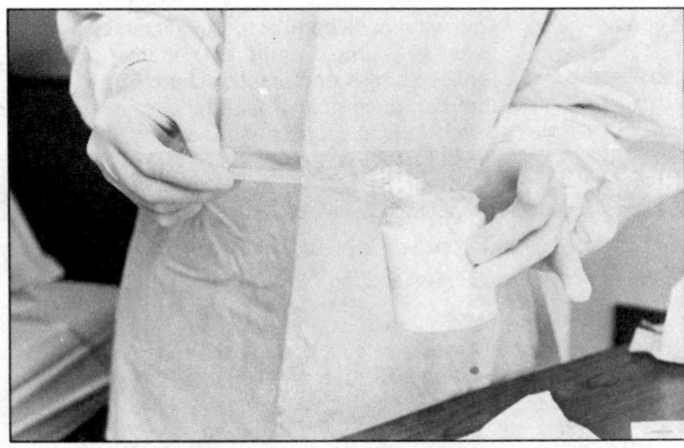

5 Next, open all your sterile supplies, creating a sterile field. Put on your sterile gloves.

Then, holding the Silvadene container in your left hand, use the tongue depressor to scoop the Silvadene out of the container (see photo). Remember, your left hand is now contaminated.

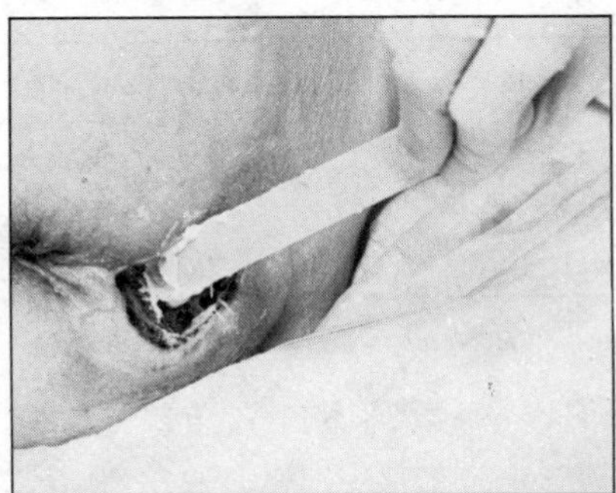

6 Using the tongue depressor, apply the ointment evenly into the ulcer, as shown here.

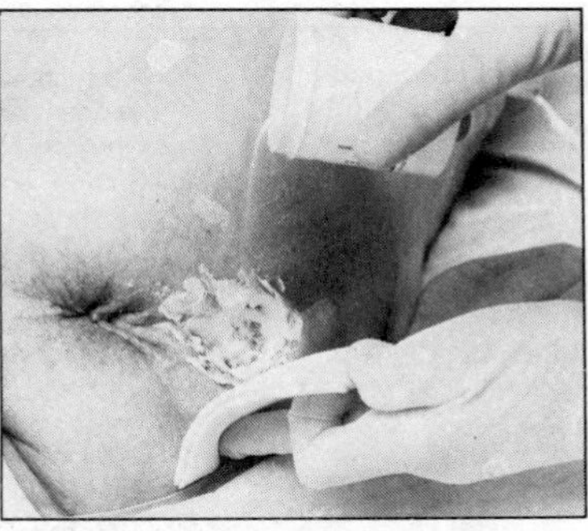

7 As you use your left hand to hold the outer surface of the sterile gauze pad at the base of the decubitus ulcer, pour the Debrisan granules into the ulcer with your right hand. Both of your hands are now contaminated.

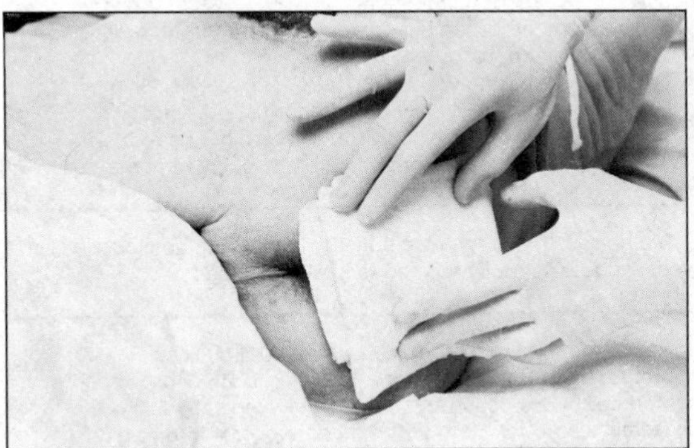

8 Cover the ulcer with sterile gauze pads; touch only the outer surface of the pads. Place the Surgipad over the gauze pads. Tape dressing in place.

Remove gloves. Discard them in the plastic bag. Secure the bag with a fastener, and discard following hospital policy. Wash your hands.

Document the procedure appropriately.

WHAT YOU SHOULD KNOW ABOUT PSORIASIS TREATMENTS

The most common treatments for psoriasis are topical tars, topical corticosteroids, and natural or artificial ultraviolet light. Difficult cases are treated with chemotherapy or photochemotherapy.

The topical drug anthralin is also effective in treating psoriasis; however, it may cause staining, renal toxicity, and erythema of healthy skin adjacent to the psoriatic lesions.

Topical psoralens (such as methoxsalen) are used in combination with ultraviolet light with few side effects. Antihistamines alleviate pruritus, and their sedative effect reduces stress and emotional problems that can accompany psoriasis. Your psychological support and teaching can

TREATMENT	USE/PATIENT GUIDELINES
Topical tars	• Apply to body areas *except* the face and intertriginous areas, such as the groin, axillary spaces, or beneath pendulous breasts. • Apply in downward strokes to prevent folliculitis. • Consult pharmacist when selecting medicated shampoos such as Ionil T or Polytar. Wait at least 10 minutes after scalp application before rinsing. • If scalp medications such as 10% coal tar solution in Nivea Oil are ordered, apply preferably at night. Wearing a disposable shower cap increases penetration.
Topical corticosteroids	• Rub a small amount into lesions two or three times a day. • If a scalp-medicating corticosteroid lotion (such as fluocinolone acetonide [Synalar solution 0.01%]) is ordered, apply preferably at night. Wearing a disposable shower cap increases penetration.
Ultraviolet light (natural)	• Sunbathe daily, using routine precautions, and aim for *slight* skin redness. • Sunbathe 20 to 30 minutes the first day and increase exposure 10 to 20 minutes each day. • Wear a wide-brimmed hat or apply a sunscreen to protect lesion-free face.
Ultraviolet light (artificial)	• Wear goggles. • Limit first treatment to 30 seconds, but increase subsequent daily treatments by 30 seconds, depending on skin tolerance. • Consult doctor for appropriate length of time for maintenance dose (2 to 15 minutes daily). • Stop treatments when skin has been clear 3 to 4 months. • If lesions return, resume treatments. • Protect lesion-free face with towel or sunscreen. Only minimal ultraviolet light is usually needed for face lesions. • If exacerbation occurs, apply topical tar b.i.d. and before treatment. Increase booth time by 30-second increments, as tolerated, if no unusual redness develops.
Chemotherapy	• Methotrexate is administered P.O., I.V., or I.M. as single weekly dose, carefully tailored to individual needs.
Photochemotherapy	• Becoming the chemotherapy treatment of choice. • Methoxsalen (Oxsoralen) is administered P.O., followed 2 hours later by exposure to long-wave ultraviolet light. Should be administered for 10 to 20 treatments over 4 to 8 weeks, then twice monthly for maintenance.

also help the patient cope with his condition.

These treatments don't cure psoriasis, but they reduce its severity by arresting rapid skin-cell reproduction. Psoriatic skin is more permeable than normal skin, allowing topical drugs to enter rapidly. Therefore, local treatments are most effective in early disease stages and less so as the skin barrier returns to normal. Drug penetration is also enhanced by removal of psoriatic plaque before therapy or by the use of occlusive dressings after application.

Health teaching varies, depending on the type of treatment ordered. You can help your patient by giving him the following information:

ADVANTAGES	DISADVANTAGES
• Inexpensive • Gives longest remissions • Alcohol-based tars, such as Estar gel, are nongreasy, so they don't stain clothes or look unsightly. • Tars enhance sun's effects on dark-skinned patients after several days' exposure.	• Water- or oil-miscible bases, such as Aquaphor or Vaseline, are greasy, so patient should wear old clothing after application. • Fair-skinned patients sunburn more easily after application of topical tars.
• Can be applied to ears, face, and intertriginous areas • May be effective on small, new spots and on tough, older plaques	• May cause burning, itching, irritation, hypertrichosis, acneiform eruptions, contact dermatitis. With occlusive dressings, maceration of skin, secondary infection, atrophy, striae, and miliaria are common. • Systemic absorption possible with extensive application and long-term use
• Costs nothing and may be enjoyable • Sun's effects enhanced in dark-skinned patients if used with tars	• Excessive exposure to sun can cause burns that aggravate psoriasis. • Excessive exposure to sun may cause later wrinkling and increases risk of skin cancer. • Inadequate exposure to sun may be subtherapeutic.
• Artificial ultraviolet light is convenient and controlled. (Ultraviolet light booths are found in dermatologists' offices and in clinics and hospitals, and they can be constructed at home. Such booths are also available in some commercial tanning centers, but advise your patients to ask their doctors' permission and guidance before using commercial facilities.) • Quicker, possibly more private than sunbathing, and available year-round. All areas of the body can be exposed if necessary.	• Exposure time requires careful control. • Expensive
• Chemotherapy may be used in serious, widespread psoriasis that doesn't respond well to topical therapy.	• Methotrexate is highly toxic, requiring close monitoring both of blood and of kidney and liver functions during therapy.
• Photochemotherapy may be used in serious, widespread psoriasis that doesn't respond well to topical therapy.	• Expensive • Not available at all hospitals

NAME	INDICATIONS & DOSAGE	SIDE EFFECTS
ammoniated mercury Mercuronate 5% Ointment	*Psoriasis, seborrheic dermatitis, impetigo contagiosa, tinea capitis, and favus*— **Adults and children:** apply to affected area b.i.d. or t.i.d.	None reported.
anthralin Anthra-Derm♦, Lasan	*Psoriasis, chronic dermatitis*— **Adults and children:** apply thinly daily or b.i.d. Concentrations range from 0.1% to 1%; start with lowest and increase, if necessary.	**GU:** possible renal toxicity. **Skin:** erythema on healthy skin.
benzoyl peroxide Benoxyl♦, Benzac, Benzagel♦, Clear by Design, Dermodex, Desquam-X♦♦, Dry and Clear, Epi-Clear Antiseptic, Oxy-5, Oxy-10, Panoxyl♦, Persadox, Persadox HP, Persa-Gel, Xerac BP	*Adjunctive treatment of acne*— **Adults and children:** apply once daily or b.i.d.	**Skin:** transient stinging on application, feeling of warmth, painful irritation.
collagenase Santyl♦	*Debridement of dermal ulcers and severely burned areas*— **Adults and children:** apply ointment (250 units/g) to lesion daily or every other day.	**Skin:** slight erythema of surrounding area, especially if ointment is not confined to lesion. **Other:** hypersensitivity reactions.

♦ Available in U.S. and Canada. ♦♦ Available in Canada only. All other products (no symbol) available in U.S. only. Italicized side effects are common or life-threatening.

INTERACTIONS	NURSING CONSIDERATIONS
None significant.	• Don't apply to large areas of body or use for extended periods of time. Mercury poisoning could result. Signs of mercury poisoning include cloudy urine; headache; dizziness; irritation, soreness, or swelling of gums; nausea; skin rash. • Don't apply to highly inflamed skin, sunburn, or open wounds. • Has no odor. Doesn't stain. • Don't use in same area with topical preparations containing sulfur; may cause foul odor or skin irritation or may stain skin black.
None significant.	• Contraindicated in renal damage. Should not be used on acute or inflammatory eruptions. • Partial excretion in urine may cause renal irritation, casts, and albuminuria. Check urine weekly. • Discontinue if allergic reaction, pustular folliculitis, or renal irritation occurs. • Don't get in eyes. May cause conjunctivitis, keratitis, corneal opacity. • Wear plastic gloves to apply anthralin; wash hands thoroughly after using. • May cause a temporary yellow-brown discoloration to hair, skin, and alkaline urine. May stain clothing. • Avoid applying medication to normal skin by coating the area surrounding the lesion with petrolatum.
Tretinoin: reduced effectiveness of benzoyl peroxide. Do not use together.	• Contraindicated in sensitivity to any of the ingredients. • Don't use on eyelids, mucous membranes, denuded or highly inflamed skin. • Dryness, redness, peeling should occur 3 to 4 days after starting treatment. If these common reactions cause considerable discomfort, discontinue temporarily until they subside. • If painful irritation develops, discontinue use. • Cleanser (4%) may cause bleaching of hair or colored fabric.
Detergents, hexachlorophene, antiseptics (especially those containing heavy metal ions such as mercury or silver), iodine, soaks or acidic solutions containing metal ions such as aluminum acetate (Burow's solution): decreased enzymatic activity. Do not use together.	• Use with caution in debilitated patients, since debriding enzymes may increase risk of bacteremia; watch for signs of systemic infection. • Before application, cleanse lesion with gauze saturated in normal saline, neutral buffer solution, or hydrogen peroxide; use topical antibacterial agent (such as neomycin-bacitracin-polymyxin B) if infection is present. Apply to lesion in powder form before using collagenase. If infection persists, discontinue collagenase until infection is healed. Confine collagenase ointment to area of lesion (Lassar's paste may protect surrounding skin). Apply ointment in thin layers to assure contact with necrotic tissue and complete wound coverage; apply collagenase ointment with tongue depressor on deep wounds; with gauze on shallow wounds. Remove any debris that comes off easily. Remove excess ointment, and cover wound with sterile gauze pad. • Discontinue when sufficient debridement has occurred. • Observe wound to monitor progress of therapy. Appearance of granulation may indicate effectiveness. Notify doctor if inflammation or color of drainage indicates any spread of infection. • Watch for symptoms of protein sensitization (long-term therapy). • If enzymatic action must be stopped for any reason, apply Burow's solution. • Avoid getting ointment in eyes. If this occurs, flush with water at once. • Protect drug from heat.

NAME	INDICATIONS & DOSAGE	SIDE EFFECTS
dextranomer Debrisan	*To clean secreting wounds, such as venous stasis and decubitus ulcers, infected surgical wounds, and burns—* **Adults and children:** apply to affected area daily, b.i.d., or more often, p.r.n. Apply to ⅛- or ¼-inch thickness, and cover with sterile gauze pad.	**Skin:** temporary pain.
fluorouracil Efudex♦, Fluoroplex♦	*Multiple actinic or solar keratoses; superficial basal cell carcinoma—* **Adults and children:** apply cream (5%) or solution (2% or 5%) b.i.d.	**Skin:** erythema, pain, burning, scaling, pruritus, hyperpigmentation, dermatitis, soreness, suppuration, swelling.
hydroquinone Artra Skin Tone Cream, Derma-Blanch, Eldopaque♦, Eldopaque-Forte♦, Eldoquin♦, Eldoquin Forte♦, Esoterica Medicated Cream, Golden Peacock, HQC Kit, Quinnone	*Bleaching of blemished skin, lentigo, chloasma, freckles, old-age spots, and other skin conditions due to increased melanin—* **Adults, and children 12 years and over:** apply 2% to 4% concentration daily or b.i.d.	**Skin:** mild irritation, sensitization, rash.
methoxsalen Oxsoralen♦	*Protect against sunburn, enhance pigmentation, and induce repigmentation in vitiligo—* **Adults, and children over 12 years:** for small, well-defined lesions, apply topically weekly or less often and expose to ultraviolet A light gradually, as directed.	**CNS:** nervousness, insomnia, depression. **GI:** discomfort, nausea, diarrhea. **Hepatic:** hepatic toxicity. **Skin:** edema, erythema, painful blistering, burning, peeling, *photosensitivity.*

♦ Available in U.S. and Canada. ♦♦ Available in Canada only. All other products (no symbol) available in U.S. only. Italicized side effects are common or life-threatening.

INTERACTIONS	NURSING CONSIDERATIONS
None significant.	• Before application, cleanse wound with sterile water, saline solution, or other appropriate solution. Do not dry. • Pack cratered wounds with beads, allowing room for expansion of beads. Cover with dressing to hold beads in place. • When saturated, medication turns gray-yellow and should be removed. • To remove, irrigate with sterile water, saline solution, or other cleansing solution. • Dextranomer beads are not effective in cleaning nonsecreting wounds. When the wound has healed to the point where it is no longer exuding, treatment should be discontinued. • Dextranomer beads are hydrophilic; each gram of beads can absorb 4 ml of exudate. • Keep drug away from moisture; store in well-closed container. • Avoid contact with eyes. • Be careful not to spill beads onto floor, as the resultant slipperiness can be a safety hazard.
None significant.	• Wash hands immediately after handling medication. • Avoid use with occlusive dressings. • Patient should avoid prolonged exposure to sunlight or ultraviolet light. • Apply with caution near eyes, nose, and mouth. • Warn patient that treated area may be unsightly during therapy and for several weeks after therapy is stopped. Complete healing may not occur until 1 or 2 months after treatment is stopped. • Ingestion and systemic absorption may cause leukopenia, thrombocytopenia, stomatitis, diarrhea, or GI ulceration, bleeding, and hemorrhage. • Topical application to large ulcerated areas may cause systemic toxicity. • For basal cell carcinoma, use 5% strength.
None significant.	• Contraindicated in patients with prickly heat, sunburn, irritated skin; or as depilatory. • Don't use near eyes. • If rash or irritation develops, discontinue therapy. • Sensitivity can be tested by applying a small amount of low-concentration medication on skin before treatment is started. Allergic reactions should appear within 24 hours. • Doesn't cause permanent depigmentation. • Advise patient to use opaque sunscreen when outdoors since sun can darken lesions faster than hydroquinone can lighten them.
Photosensitizing agents: do not use together.	• Contraindicated in hepatic insufficiency, porphyria, acute systemic lupus erythematosus, and hydromorphic, polymorphic light eruptions. Use with caution in familial history of sunlight allergy, GI diseases, chronic infection. • Regulate therapy carefully. Overdosage or overexposure to light can cause serious burning or blistering. • Topical treatment should be directly supervised by a doctor. • When applied topically to face or hands, patient should protect area from light (except during treatment exposure) for 24 hours after therapy. • Protect eyes and lips during light exposure treatments. • Monthly liver function tests should be done on patients with vitiligo (especially at beginning of therapy). • Significant changes require 6 to 9 months of therapy.

NAME	INDICATIONS & DOSAGE	SIDE EFFECTS
scarlet red Decubitex Ointment (also contains peruvian balsam, zinc oxide, starch, castor oil, petrolatum, xantham gum, sodium propionate, methylparaben, propylparaben, propylene glycol, and water)	*Aid in management of decubitus ulcers—* **Adults and children:** pour a small amount of 3% hydrogen peroxide or normal saline solution on the affected area. Cleanse thoroughly and apply ointment. Cover with dry sterile gauze.	None reported.
selenium sulfide Exsel♦, Iosel 250, Selsun♦, Selsun Blue, Sul-Blue	*Dandruff, seborrheic scalp dermatitis—* **Adults and children:** massage 1 to 2 teaspoonfuls into clean, wet scalp. Leave on for 2 to 3 minutes. Rinse thoroughly, and repeat application. Apply twice weekly for 2 weeks, then once a week for 2 weeks, or as often as needed to maintain control.	**Skin:** oily or dry scalp and hair, hair discoloration, hair loss, sensitivity reactions.
streptokinase-streptodornase Varidase♦	*Adjunctive treatment of suppurative surface tissues, including ulcers, radiation necrosis, infected wounds, burns, surgical incisions, skin grafts, and whenever clotted blood, or fibrinous or purulent accumulations are undesirable—* **Adults and children:** apply on individual basis, depending on area treated and doctor's instructions.	**Systemic:** fever.
sutilains Travase♦	*Debridement of second- and third-degree burns, adjunctive debridement of decubitus ulcers, pyogenic wounds, or ulcers re-*	**CNS:** local paresthesias. **Skin:** mild pain, bleeding, transient dermatitis.

♦ Available in U.S. and Canada. ♦♦ Available in Canada only. All other products (no symbol) available in U.S. only. Italicized side effects are common or life-threatening.

INTERACTIONS	NURSING CONSIDERATIONS
None significant.	• Change dressing twice daily, especially where seeping and secretions are present. • Ointment should be in contact with newly forming tissue for maximum therapeutic results. Wound should be allowed to "breathe" by being loosely covered. • Using excess ointment or covering the wound completely will retard wound healing. • Use ointment until healing is complete. • In advanced decubitus ulcers, use normal saline solution rather than hydrogen peroxide.
None significant.	• Contraindicated in sulfur hypersensitivity. • Use with caution around areas of acute inflammation or exudation to avoid increased absorption. • If sensitivity reactions occur, discontinue use. • Reduce or prevent hair discoloration by thorough rinsing after treatment. • Avoid contact with eyes. • Highly toxic if ingested. • Wash hands carefully after handling. • Protect from heat.
Detergents, anti-infectives (such as benzalkonium chloride, hexachlorophene, iodine): decreased enzymatic activity. Do not use together.	• Contraindicated in areas of active hemorrhage. • Remove exudates carefully and frequently, especially from closed areas, to avoid pyogenesis. • Not effective on fibrous tissue, mucoproteins, or collagens. • Refrigerated solution stable for 2 weeks. Room temperature solution stable for 24 hours. • Use rubber dams or gauze or nylon dressing to keep medication in constant contact with lesion. • Prolonged use may result in a high antienzyme titer. Dosage may need to be increased. • Product comes as solution or jelly. Mix to dilution ordered. • To make jelly, add 5 ml sterile water for injection or sterile normal saline solution to 125,000-unit vial streptokinase-streptodornase; mix with 15-ml jar of carboxymethyl cellulose (CMC) jelly 4.5%. The resulting mixure contains 5,000 IU SK and 1,250 IU SD/ml or g. • Thoroughly cleanse and irrigate wound area with sterile normal saline solution or water before treatment to remove antiseptics, detergents, and heavy metal antibacterials, which can decrease enzyme activity. • Moisten wound area for optimal enzymatic activity. Dress wound if necessary, but remove waste products frequently. Observe wound to monitor progress of therapy. Appearance of granulation tissue may indicate effectiveness. Notify doctor if inflammation or color of drainage indicates spread of infection. • Avoid getting solution in eyes. If this occurs, flood with water at once. • Protect drugs from heat.
Detergents, anti-infectives (such as benzalkonium chloride, hexachloro-	• Contraindicated in wounds involving major body cavities or containing exposed nerves or nerve tissue, fungating neoplastic ulcers, wounds in women of childbearing age, persons having limited cardiac or pulmonary reserves.

(continued on following page)

NAME	INDICATIONS & DOSAGE	SIDE EFFECTS
sutilains *(continued)*	*sulting from peripheral vascular disease—* **Adults and children:** apply thinly to area extending ¼ to ½ inch beyond area to be debrided. Cover with loose wet dressing t.i.d. or q.i.d.	
tretinoin (vitamin A acid, retinoic acid) Retin-A	*Acne vulgaris (especially grades I, II, and III)—* **Adults and children:** cleanse affected area and lightly apply solution once daily at bedtime.	**Skin:** *feeling of warmth, slight stinging, local erythema, peeling at site,* chapping and swelling, blistering and crusting, temporary hyperpigmentation or hypopigmentation.

♦ Available in U.S. and Canada. ♦♦ Available in Canada only. All other products (no symbol) available in U.S. only. Italicized side effects are common or life-threatening.

INTERACTIONS	NURSING CONSIDERATIONS
phene, iodine, and nitrofurazone), and compounds containing metallic ions (such as silver nitrate and thimerosal): adversely affected enzymatic activity. Do not use together.	• Use cautiously near eyes. If accidental contact occurs, flush eyes repeatedly with large amounts of normal saline solution or sterile water. • Before application, cleanse and irrigate affected area with normal saline solution or sterile water to remove antiseptic or heavy metal antibacterial agents. • May give mild analgesic to reduce painful reactions, but discontinue if pain is severe; also discontinue if bleeding or dermatitis occurs. • For best response, keep affected area moist. • In concomitant use of topical antimicrobial agent, apply sutilains first. • Store at 2° to 10° C. (35.6° to 50° F.).
None significant.	• Contraindicated in hypersensitivity to any tretinoin component. Use with caution in eczema. • If severe local irritation develops, discontinue temporarily and readjust dosage when application is resumed. • Some redness and scaling are normal reactions. • Beneficial effects should be seen within 6 weeks of treatment. • When treatment is stopped, relapses generally occur within 3 to 6 weeks. • Patient should wash face with a mild soap no more than two or three times a day. Warn against using strong or medicated cosmetics, soaps, or other skin cleansers. • Exposure to sunlight or ultraviolet rays should be minimal during treatment. If patient is sunburned, delay therapy until sunburn subsides. • Avoid contact with eyes, mouth, nose, and mucous membranes. • Warn patient not to use topical products containing alcohol, astringents, spices, and lime. These may interfere with action of tretinoin. • Warn patient to wait until skin is completely dry before applying tretinoin.

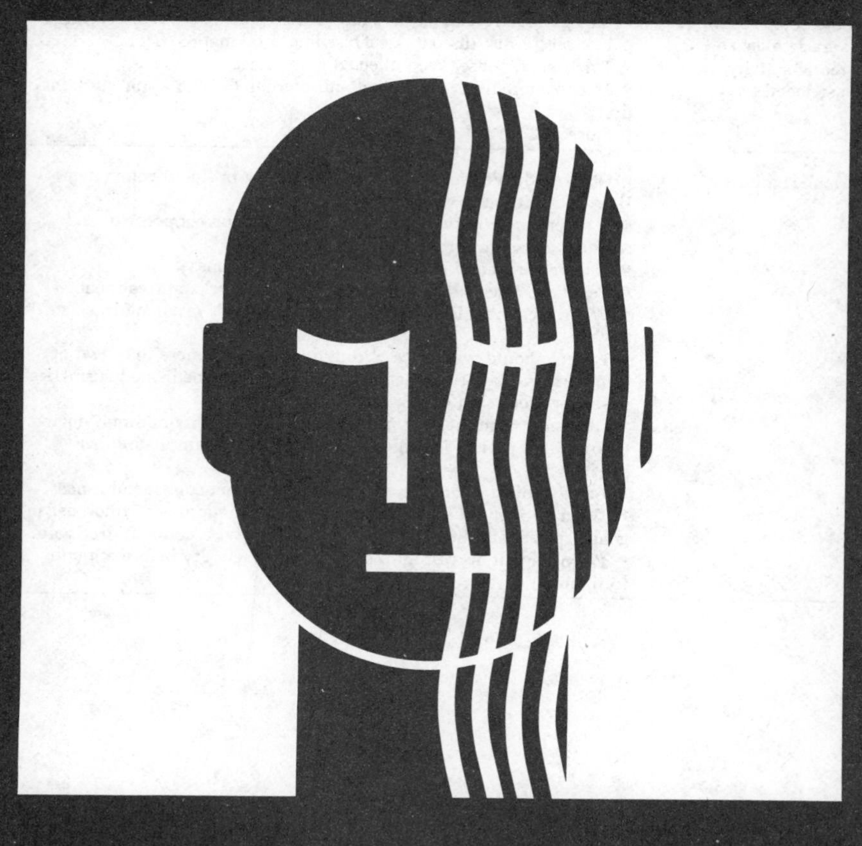

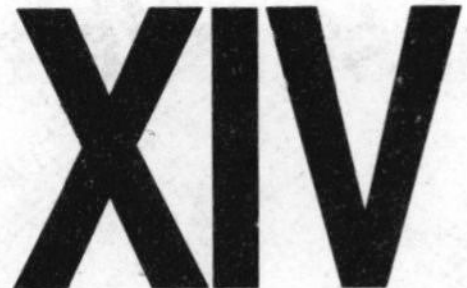

XIV Anesthetic Agents

96 Local anesthetics

bupivacaine hydrochloride
chloroprocaine hydrochloride
dibucaine hydrochloride
etidocaine hydrochloride
lidocaine hydrochloride
mepivacaine hydrochloride
piperocaine hydrochloride
prilocaine hydrochloride
procaine hydrochloride
tetracaine hydrochloride

Local anesthetics block nerve conduction when they're injected locally into nerve tissue in appropriate concentrations. They can act on any part of the central nervous system (CNS) and on any type of nerve cell. First they affect the small, nonmyelinated autonomic fibers; then those mediating cold, warmth, pain, and touch; and finally those mediating motor function. Nerve function is regained in reverse order. (See diagram on p. 1138)

Local anesthetics can be divided into two groups, amides and esters, depending on which type of chemical bond is in the molecule. Amide-derived drugs are bupivacaine, dibucaine, etidocaine, lidocaine, mepivacaine, and prilocaine. Ester derivatives are chloroprocaine, piperocaine, procaine, and tetracaine.

The amide or ester bond affects certain pharmacologic properties such as the duration of action, which, with these agents, can be considered a determinant of toxicity. Dosage varies greatly according to the procedure to be performed, level of anesthesia required, number of neuronal segments to be blocked, tissue vascularity, and patient response. The smallest dose and lowest concentration needed to produce the desired anesthesia should be used.

Major uses

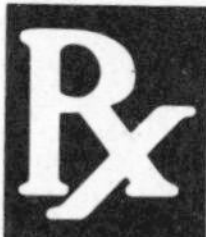

Local anesthetics are used in dental or minor surgical procedures (biopsy, for example). In addition, they furnish regional (nerve

NURSING TIP

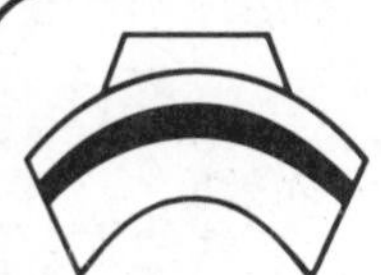

MONITORING THE PATIENT WHO'S RECEIVED A NERVE BLOCK

After receiving a nerve block with a local anesthetic, your patient needs special attention. Be sure to:

- Watch him for anaphylaxis or other reactions to the drug used, such as hives, rash, or seizure activity.
- Protect the extremity in which the drug was given. For example, pad the side rails of the bed, or position and support the arm or leg with pillows.
- Frequently check the patient's circulation and level of sensation (every 15 to 30 minutes, as ordered) until the block is reversed.

block) anesthesia, including spinal, caudal, and epidural anesthesia (in tubal ligation or hernia repair, for example).

Mechanism of action

Local anesthetics block depolarization by interfering with sodium-potassium exchange across the nerve-cell membrane, preventing generation and conduction of the nerve impulse.

When local anesthetics are combined with epinephrine, anesthesia is prolonged because the rate of absorption decreases. The vasoconstriction produced by the epinephrine also helps control local bleeding.

Absorption, distribution, metabolism, and excretion

- Absorption varies according to dose, site of injection, and vasodilation produced by the drug. Epinephrine combined with a local anesthetic decreases absorption.
- The drugs are distributed to all body tissues.
- Esters are hydrolyzed (metabolized) rapidly and almost completely by blood cholinesterases. The remaining drug is metabolized by the liver, and the metabolites are excreted in urine.
- Amides are metabolized primarily in the liver, and the metabolites are excreted in urine.

Onset and duration

The drugs begin to act in less than 15 minutes after application, but duration of action varies.

Epinephrine prolongs duration of effect.

- Bupivacaine, dibucaine, etidocaine, and tetracaine have long durations (3 to 6 hours).
- Chloroprocaine and procaine have short durations (30 to 60 minutes).
- Lidocaine, mepivacaine, piperocaine, and prilocaine provide anesthesia for 1 to 3 hours.

Combination products

None, although epinephrine is added to some solutions to prolong effect.

PREVENTING ROUTE SIDE EFFECTS

Sometimes the route by which a regional anesthetic is administered precipitates complications or side effects. For example, local anesthetics are often injected into the epidural space—commonly in the lumbar area—within the vertebral canal. The epidural route affords easy administration, minimal trauma to the spinal cord, and widespread sympathetic blockade. And because it doesn't puncture the dural space, patients seldom suffer a spinal headache. However, because the epidural space is highly vascular, a high dosage may cause systemic toxic effects. If your patient shows signs of toxicity, such as CNS disturbances, rising blood pressure, and a rapid pulse, call the doctor.

When a local anesthetic is injected directly into the cerebrospinal fluid (CSF), it produces sympathetic blockade. The patient who is anesthetized by the *spinal route* may suffer a spinal headache, caused by CSF leaking around the dural puncture site. He may even experience diplopia and tinnitus. Sitting up may reduce CSF pressure, causing side effects.

You can help. Keep the patient in a horizontal position and, unless contraindicated, be sure he's well hydrated. Give mild analgesics p.r.n. If the patient's headache is severe, consult the doctor. He may inject normal saline solution into the epidural space to prevent further CSF leakage.

NAME	INDICATIONS & DOSAGE	SIDE EFFECTS
bupivacaine hydrochloride Marcaine♦	Available with or without epinephrine. Dosages given are for drug *without* epinephrine. **Epidural:** *Sol.* — *Vol. (ml)* — *Dose (mg)* 0.75% — 10 to 20 — 75 to 150 0.50% — 10 to 20 — 50 to 100 0.25% — 10 to 20 — 25 to 50 **Caudal:** *Sol.* — *Vol. (ml)* — *Dose (mg)* 0.50% — 15 to 30 — 75 to 150 0.25% — 15 to 30 — 37.5 to 75 **Peripheral nerve block:** *Sol.* — *Vol. (ml)* — *Dose (mg)* 0.50% — 5 to 80 — 25 to 400 (max.) May repeat dose q 3 hours. Dose and interval may be increased with epinephrine. Maximum 400 mg daily.	**Skin:** dermatologic reactions. **Other:** edema, status asthmaticus, or *anaphylaxis* and anaphylactoid reactions. Side effects of local anesthetics generally result from high blood levels of the drug. Examples of these are: **CNS:** anxiety, apprehension, nervousness, convulsions followed by drowsiness, unconsciousness, and *respiratory arrest.* **CV:** myocardial depression, *arrhythmias, cardiac arrest.* **EENT:** blurred vision. **GI:** nausea, vomiting.
chloroprocaine hydrochloride Nesacaine (for infiltration and regional anesthesia), Nesacaine-CE (for caudal and epidural anesthesia)	Available only without epinephrine. **Infiltration and nerve block:** *Sol.* — *Vol. (ml)* — *Dose (mg)* 1% — 3 to 20 — 30 to 200 2% — 2 to 40 — 20 to 400 **Caudal and epidural:** *Sol.* — *Vol. (ml)* — *Dose (mg)* 2% to 3% — 15 to 25 — 300 to 750 May repeat with smaller doses q 40 to 50 minutes. Dose and interval may be increased with epinephrine. Maximum adult dose 800 mg, or 1 g when mixed with epinephrine.	**Skin:** dermatologic reactions. **Other:** edema, status asthmaticus, or *anaphylaxis* and anaphylactoid reactions. Side effects of local anesthetics generally result from high blood levels of the drug. Examples of these are: **CNS:** anxiety, apprehension, nervousness, convulsions followed by drowsiness, unconsciousness, and *respiratory arrest.* **CV:** myocardial depression, *arrhythmias, cardiac arrest.* **EENT:** blurred vision. **GI:** nausea, vomiting.
dibucaine hydrochloride Nupercaine	Available only without epinephrine. **Spinal anesthesia:** *Perineum and lower limbs* *Sol.* — *Vol. (ml)* — *Dose (mg)* 0.5% — 0.5 to 1 — 2.5 to 5 *Lower abdomen* *Sol.* — *Vol. (ml)* — *Dose (mg)* 0.5% — 1 to 1.5 — 5 to 7.5 *Upper abdomen* *Sol.* — *Vol. (ml)* — *Dose (mg)* 0.5% — 2 — 10 **Spinal anesthesia:** *Lower extremities as high as pelvis* *Sol.* — *Vol. (ml)* — *Dose (mg)* 1:1,500 — 6 — 4 *(continued)*	**Skin:** dermatologic reactions. **Other:** edema, status asthmaticus, or *anaphylaxis* and anaphylactoid reactions. Side effects of local anesthetics generally result from high blood levels of the drug. Examples of these are: **CNS:** anxiety, apprehension, nervousness, convulsions followed by drowsiness, unconsciousness, and *respiratory arrest.* **CV:** myocardial depression, *arrhythmias, cardiac arrest.* **EENT:** blurred vision. **GI:** nausea, vomiting.

INTERACTIONS	NURSING CONSIDERATIONS
Chloroform, halothane, cyclopropane, trichloroethylene, and related drugs: cardiac arrhythmias may occur when used with bupivacaine *with* epinephrine. Use with extreme caution. *MAO inhibitors, tricyclic antidepressants:* severe, sustained hypertension may occur when used with bupivacaine *with* epinephrine. Use with extreme caution.	• Contraindicated in children under 12 years and for spinal, paracervical block, or topical anesthesia. Use cautiously in debilitated, elderly, or acutely ill patients; and in patients with severe hepatic disease or drug allergies. • Use solutions with epinephrine cautiously in cardiovascular disorders and in body areas with limited blood supply (ears, nose, fingers, toes). • Keep resuscitative equipment and drugs available. • Don't use solution with preservatives for caudal or epidural block. • Onset in 4 to 17 minutes; duration 3 to 6 hours. • Causes less fetal depression than other local anesthetics. • Discard partially used vials without preservatives. • For treatment of anaphylaxis, see inside front cover.
None significant.	• Contraindicated in hypersensitivity to procaine, tetracaine, or other para-aminobenzoic acid derivatives, and for spinal or topical anesthesia. Epidural and caudal contraindicated in CNS disease. Use cautiously in debilitated, elderly, or acutely ill patients; children; and in patients with drug allergies, paracervical block, or cardiovascular disease. • Use solutions with epinephrine cautiously in cardiovascular disorders and in body areas with limited blood supply (ears, nose, fingers, toes). • A 3-ml test dose should be injected at least 10 minutes before giving total dose to check for intravascular or subarachnoid injection. Motor paralysis and extensive sensory anesthesia indicate subarachnoid injection. • Don't use solution with preservatives for caudal or epidural block. • Don't use discolored solution. • Keep resuscitative equipment and drugs available. • Duration 30 to 60 minutes. • Discard partially used vials without preservatives. • For treatment of anaphylaxis, see inside front cover.
None significant.	• Contraindicated in cerebrospinal disease, septicemia, pernicious anemia with spinal cord symptoms, arthritis, pyogenic skin infection in puncture area. Use cautiously in hysteria, chronic backache, headache of long duration, migraine, shock, hypotension, leaking spinal fluid, cardiac decompensation, pleural effusions, increased abdominal pressure, possibility of hemorrhage. • Low spinal solution contraindicated in cesarean section or in presence of blood when doing lumbar puncture. Use low spinal solutions cautiously in patients with cardiac or neurologic disease or back problems and in uncooperative or hysterical patients. • Use solutions with epinephrine cautiously in cardiovascular disorders and in body areas with limited blood supply (ears, nose, fingers, toes). • Keep resuscitative equipment and drugs available. • Don't use for nerve block or infiltration. • Don't use discolored solution. • Used primarily for spinal block and as topical anesthetic. • Onset in 10 to 15 minutes; duration 6 hours.

(continued on following page)

NAME	INDICATIONS & DOSAGE	SIDE EFFECTS
dibucaine hydrochloride *(continued)*	*Lower abdomen* *Sol.* *Vol. (ml)* *Dose (mg)* 1:1,500 10 to 15 6.67 to 10 *Upper abdomen* *Sol.* *Vol. (ml)* *Dose (mg)* 1:1,500 15 to 18 10 to 12	
etidocaine hydrochloride Duranest	Available with or without epinephrine. Doses cited are for drug *with* epinephrine. Dose and interval may be decreased without epinephrine. **Infiltration:** *Sol.* *Vol. (ml)* *Dose (mg)* 0.5% 1 to 80 5 to 400 **Peripheral nerve block:** *Sol.* *Vol. (ml)* *Dose (mg)* 0.5% 5 to 80 25 to 400 1% 5 to 40 50 to 400 **Central neural block:** *Lower limbs, cesarean section, lumbar peridural* *Sol.* *Vol. (ml)* *Dose (mg)* 1% 10 to 30 100 to 300 1.5% 10 to 20 150 to 300 *Vaginal* *Sol.* *Vol. (ml)* *Dose (mg)* 0.5% 10 to 30 50 to 150 1% 5 to 20 50 to 200 **Caudal:** *Sol.* *Vol. (ml)* *Dose (mg)* 0.5% 10 to 30 50 to 150 1% 10 to 30 100 to 300	**Skin:** dermatologic reactions. **Other:** edema, status asthmaticus, or *anaphylaxis* and anaphylactoid reactions. Side effects of local anesthetics generally result from high blood levels of the drug. Examples of these are: **CNS:** anxiety, apprehension, nervousness, convulsions followed by drowsiness, unconsciousness, and *respiratory arrest.* **CV:** myocardial depression, *arrhythmias, cardiac arrest.* **EENT:** blurred vision. **GI:** nausea, vomiting.
lidocaine hydrochloride Ardecaine, Canocaine, Dilocaine, Dolicaine, L-Caine, Nervocaine, Norocaine, Rocaine, Ultracaine, Xylocaine Hydrochloride♦	Available with or without epinephrine. Doses cited are for drug *without* epinephrine except where indicated. **Caudal** *(obstetrics)* **or epidural** *(thoracic):* *Sol.* *Vol. (ml)* *Dose (mg)* 1% 20 to 30 200 to 300 **Caudal** *(surgery):* *Sol.* *Vol. (ml)* *Dose (mg)* 1.5% 15 to 20 225 to 300 **Epidural** *(lumbar anesthesia):* *Sol.* *Vol. (ml)* *Dose (mg)* 1.5% 15 to 20 225 to 300 2% 10 to 15 200 to 300 Maximum dose 200 to 300 mg per hour. *For anesthesia other than spinal*—maximum single adult dose 4.5 mg/kg or 300 mg. *With epinephrine for anesthesia other than spinal*—maximum single adult dose 7 mg/kg or 500 mg. Don't repeat dose more often than q 2 hours.	**Skin:** dermatologic reactions. **Other:** edema, status asthmaticus, or *anaphylaxis* and anaphylactoid reactions. Side effects of local anesthetics generally result from high blood levels of the drug. Examples of these are: **CNS:** anxiety, apprehension, nervousness, convulsions followed by drowsiness, unconsciousness, and *respiratory arrest.* **CV:** myocardial depression, *arrhythmias, cardiac arrest.* **EENT:** blurred vision. **GI:** nausea, vomiting.

♦ Available in U.S. and Canada. ♦♦ Available in Canada only. All other products (no symbol) available in U.S. only. Italicized side effects are common or life-threatening.

INTERACTIONS	NURSING CONSIDERATIONS
	• Discard partially used vials without preservatives. • For toxicity, see APPENDIX, *Drug Toxicities*.
Chloroform, halothane, cyclopropane, trichloroethylene, and related drugs: cardiac arrhythmias may occur when used with etidocaine *with* epinephrine. Use with extreme caution. *MAO inhibitors, tricyclic antidepressants, phenothiazines:* severe, sustained hypertension or hypotension may occur when used with etidocaine solution *with* epinephrine. Use with extreme caution.	• Contraindicated in inflammation or infection in puncture region, children under 14 years, septicemia, severe hypertension, spinal deformities, neurologic disorders, and spinal block. Use cautiously in debilitated, elderly, or acutely ill patients; severe shock; heart block; epidural block in obstetrics; general drug allergies; hepatic and renal disease. • Use solutions with epinephrine cautiously in cardiovascular disease and in body areas with limited blood supply (ears, nose, fingers, toes). • Don't use solution with preservatives for caudal or epidural block. • Keep resuscitative equipment and drugs available. • Onset in 2 to 8 minutes; duration 3 to 6 hours. • For treatment of anaphylaxis, see inside front cover.
Chloroform, halothane, cyclopropane, trichloroethylene, and related drugs: cardiac arrhythmias may occur when used with lidocaine *with* epinephrine. Use with extreme caution. *MAO inhibitors, tricyclic antidepressants:* severe, sustained hypertension may occur when used with lidocaine *with* epinephrine. Use with extreme caution.	• Contraindicated in inflammation or infection in puncture region, septicemia, severe hypertension, spinal deformities, neurologic disorders. Use cautiously in debilitated, elderly, or acutely ill patients; in severe shock; heart block; in obstetrics; general drug allergies; and paracervical block. • Use solutions with epinephrine cautiously in cardiovascular disorders and in body areas with limited blood supply (ears, nose, fingers, toes). • Keep resuscitative equipment and drugs available. • A 2- to 5-ml test dose should be injected at least 5 minutes before giving total dose to check for intravascular or subarachnoid injection. Motor paralysis and extensive sensory anesthesia indicate subarachnoid injection. • Solutions containing preservatives should not be used for spinal, epidural, or caudal block. • Discard partially used vials without preservatives. • For treatment of anaphylaxis, see inside front cover.

(continued on following page)

NAME	INDICATIONS & DOSAGE	SIDE EFFECTS
lidocaine hydrochloride *(continued)*	**Spinal surgical anesthesia:** *Sol.* *Vol. (ml)* *Dose (mg)* 5% with 7.5% dextrose 1.5 to 2 75 to 100 Dose and interval may be increased with epinephrine.	
mepivacaine hydrochloride Carbocaine♦, Cavacaine, Isocaine	Available with or without levonordefrin (vasoconstrictor). Doses cited are for drug *without* levonordefrin. **Nerve block:** *Sol.* *Vol. (ml)* *Dose (mg)* 1% 5 to 20 50 to 200 2% 5 to 20 100 to 400 **Transvaginal block or infiltration** *(maximum dose):* *Sol.* *Vol. (ml)* *Dose (mg)* 1% 40 400 **Paracervical block** *(obstetrics):* *Sol.* *Vol. (ml)* *Dose (mg)* 1% 10 100 Give on each side (200 mg total) per 90-minute period. **Caudal and epidural:** *Sol.* *Vol. (ml)* *Dose (mg)* 1% 15 to 30 150 to 300 1.5% 10 to 25 150 to 375 2% 10 to 20 200 to 400 **Therapeutic block** *(pain management):* *Sol.* *Vol. (ml)* *Dose (mg)* 1% 1 to 5 10 to 50 2% 1 to 5 20 to 100 **Adults:** maximum single dose 7 mg/kg up to 550 mg. Don't repeat more often than q 90 minutes. Maximum total dose 1,000 mg daily. **Children:** maximum dose 5 to 6 mg/kg. In children under 3 years or weighing less than 14 kg, use 0.5% or 1.5% solution only. Dose and interval may be increased with levonordefrin.	**Skin:** dermatologic reactions. **Other:** edema, status asthmaticus, or *anaphylaxis* and anaphylactoid reactions. Side effects of local anesthetics generally result from high blood levels of the drug. Examples of these are: **CNS:** anxiety, apprehension, nervousness, convulsions followed by drowsiness, unconsciousness, and *respiratory arrest.* **CV:** myocardial depression, *arrhythmias, cardiac arrest.* **EENT:** blurred vision. **GI:** nausea, vomiting.
piperocaine hydrochloride Metycaine	**Caudal block** *(obstetrics in women with normal-sized pelvic canals):* *Sol.* *Vol. (ml)* *Dose (mg)* 1.5% 30 450 May give additional 20-ml doses (300 mg) q 30 to 40 minutes, p.r.n. *(continued)*	**Skin:** dermatologic reactions. **Other:** edema, status asthmaticus, *anaphylaxis* and anaphylactoid reactions. Side effects of local anesthetics generally result from high blood levels of the drug. Examples of these are: **CNS:** anxiety, apprehension, nervousness, convulsions followed by

♦ Available in U.S. and Canada. ♦♦ Available in Canada only. All other products (no symbol) available in U.S. only. Italicized side effects are common or life-threatening.

INTERACTIONS	NURSING CONSIDERATIONS
Chloroform, halothane, cyclopropane, trichloroethylene, and related drugs: cardiac arrhythmias may occur when used with mepivacaine *with* levonordefrin. Use with extreme caution. *MAO inhibitors, tricyclic antidepressants:* severe, sustained hypertension may occur when used with mepivacaine *with* levonordefrin. Use with extreme caution.	• Contraindicated in sensitivity to methylparaben, in heart block, or for spinal anesthesia. Use cautiously in debilitated, elderly, or acutely ill patients, or for paracervical block. • Use solutions with levonordefrin cautiously in cardiovascular disease and in body areas with limited blood supply (ears, nose, fingers, toes). • Monitor fetal heart rate when paracervical block used in delivery. • Keep resuscitative equipment and drugs available. • Don't use solutions with preservatives for caudal or epidural block. • Onset in 15 minutes; duration 3 hours. • Discard partially used vials without preservatives. • For treatment of anaphylaxis, see inside front cover.
None significant.	• Contraindicated in hypersensitivity to procaine, tetracaine, or other para-aminobenzoic acid derivatives, CNS diseases, spinal deformities, infection at injection site, extreme obesity, profound anemia, or spinal block, in highly nervous women. • Don't use solutions with preservatives for caudal block. • Keep resuscitative equipment and drugs available. • Effect peaks in 20 to 30 minutes, then decreases over next 10 minutes. • Dilute 2% solutions to 0.5% or 1% with NaCl injection or Ringer's injection. Don't use sterile water for injection. • An 8-ml dose of anesthetic solution should be injected a few min-

(continued on following page)

NAME	INDICATIONS & DOSAGE	SIDE EFFECTS
piperocaine hydrochloride *(continued)*	**Infiltration** *(maximum dose):* *Sol.* *Vol. (ml)* *Dose (mg)* 0.5% 200 1,000 1% 80 800 For dental infiltration, use a 1% to 2% solution. For peripheral or sympathetic nerve block, use 0.5% to 2% solution.	drowsiness, unconsciousness, and *respiratory arrest.* **CV:** myocardial depression, *arrhythmias, cardiac arrest.* **EENT:** blurred vision. **GI:** nausea, vomiting.
prilocaine hydrochloride Citanest♦, Propitocaine	**Infiltration:** *Sol.* *Vol. (ml)* *Dose (mg)* 1% to 2% 20 to 30 200 to 600 **Peripheral nerve block** *(intercostal or paravertebral):* *Sol.* *Vol. (ml)* *Dose (mg)* 1% to 2% 3 to 5 30 to 100 **Peripheral nerve block** *(sciatic [femoral or brachial plexus] or caudal nerve block [surgery]):* *Sol.* *Vol. (ml)* *Dose (mg)* 2% 20 to 30 400 to 600 3% 15 to 20 450 to 600 **Caudal nerve block** *(obstetrics):* *Sol.* *Vol. (ml)* *Dose (mg)* 1% 20 to 30 200 to 300 **Epidural:** *Sol.* *Vol. (ml)* *Dose (mg)* 1% 20 to 30 200 to 300 2% 20 to 30 400 to 600 3% 15 to 20 450 to 600 Maximum single adult dose 8 mg/kg up to 600 mg. In continuous caudal or epidural anesthesia, don't give maximum dose more often than q 2 hours.	**Skin:** dermatologic reactions. **Other:** edema, status asthmaticus, or *anaphylaxis* and anaphylactoid reactions. With 4% solution: swelling and paresthesia of lips and mouth. At maximum dose: methemoglobinemia. Side effects of local anesthetics generally result from high blood levels of the drug. Examples of these are: **CNS:** anxiety, apprehension, nervousness, convulsions followed by drowsiness, unconsciousness, and *respiratory arrest.* **CV:** myocardial depression, *arrhythmias, cardiac arrest.* **EENT:** blurred vision. **GI:** nausea, vomiting.
procaine hydrochloride Novocain♦, Unicaine	**Spinal anesthesia**—before using, dilute 10% solution with 0.9% NaCl injection, sterile distilled water, or cerebrospinal fluid. For hyperbaric technique, use dextrose solution. *Perineum:* use 0.5 ml 10% solution and 0.5 ml diluent injected at fourth lumbar interspace. *Perineum and lower extremities:* use 1 ml 10% solution and 1 ml diluent injected at third or fourth lumbar interspace. *Up to costal margin:* use 2 ml 10% solution and 1 ml diluent injected at second, third, or fourth lumbar interspace. **Epidural block:** *Sol.* *Vol. (ml)* *Dose (mg)* 1.5% 25 375	**Skin:** dermatologic reactions. **Other:** edema, status asthmaticus, or *anaphylaxis* and anaphylactoid reactions. Side effects of local anesthetics generally result from high blood levels of the drug. Examples of these are: **CNS:** anxiety, apprehension, nervousness, convulsions followed by drowsiness, unconsciousness, and *respiratory arrest.* **CV:** myocardial depression, *arrhythmias, cardiac arrest.* **EENT:** blurred vision. **GI:** nausea, vomiting.

♦ Available in U.S. and Canada. ♦♦ Available in Canada only. All other products (no symbol) available in U.S. only. Italicized side effects are common or life-threatening.

INTERACTIONS	NURSING CONSIDERATIONS
	utes before giving total dose to check for subarachnoid injection. Motor paralysis and extensive sensory anesthesia indicate subarachnoid injection. • Discard partially used vials without preservatives. • For treatment of anaphylaxis, see inside front cover.
None significant.	• Contraindicated in methemoglobinemia, severe shock, heart block, infection at injection site, or for spinal block. Use cautiously in debilitated, elderly, or acutely ill patients; children under 10 years; and in general drug sensitivities. • Epidural and caudal contraindicated in CNS disease, spinal deformities, septicemia, severe hypertension, and in children. • Keep resuscitative equipment and drugs available. • Duration 1 to 3 hours. • Don't use solutions with preservatives for caudal or epidural block. • Discard partially used vials without preservatives. • A 5-ml test dose should be injected at least 5 minutes before giving total dose to check for intravascular or subarachnoid injection. Motor paralysis and extensive sensory anesthesia indicate subarachnoid injection. • For treatment of anaphylaxis, see inside front cover.
Echothiophate iodide: reduced hydrolysis of procaine. Use together cautiously.	• Contraindicated in traumatized urethra and in hypersensitivity to chloroprocaine, tetracaine, or other para-aminobenzoic acid derivatives. Use cautiously in hyperexcitable patients, and in patients with CNS diseases, infection at puncture site, shock, profound anemia, cachexia, sepsis, hypertension, hypotension, GI hemorrhage, bowel perforation or strangulation, peritonitis, cardiac decompensation, massive pleural effusions, and increased intra-abdominal pressure. • Contraindications to obstetric use: pelvic disproportion, placenta previa, abruptio placentae, floating fetal head, intrauterine manipulation. • Keep resuscitative equipment and drugs available. • A 1- to 5-ml test dose should be given 5 to 15 minutes before total epidural dose. Motor paralysis and extensive sensory anesthesia indicate subarachnoid injection. • Use solution without preservatives for epidural block. • Onset in 2 to 5 minutes; duration 60 minutes. • Discard partially used vials without preservatives. • For treatment of anaphylaxis, see inside front cover.

(continued on following page)

NAME	INDICATIONS & DOSAGE	SIDE EFFECTS
procaine hydrochloride *(continued)*	**Peripheral nerve block:** *Sol.* *Vol. (ml)* *Dose (mg)* 1% 50 250 2% 25 500 *Infiltration:* use 250 to 600 mg 0.25% to 0.5% solution. Maximum initial dose 1 g. Dose and interval may be increased with epinephrine.	
tetracaine hydrochloride Pontocaine♦	*Low spinal (saddle block) in vaginal delivery:* give 2 to 5 mg as hyperbaric solution (in 10% dextrose). Maximum dose 15 mg. *Perineum and lower extremities:* give 5 to 10 mg. *Prolonged spinal anesthesia (2 to 3 hours):* dilute 1% solution with equal volume of cerebrospinal fluid, or dissolve 5 mg powdered drug in 1 ml cerebrospinal fluid immediately before giving. Give 1 ml/5 seconds. *Up to costal margin:* give 15 to 20 mg.	**Skin:** dermatologic reactions. **Other:** edema, status asthmaticus, or *anaphylaxis* and anaphylactoid reactions. Side effects of local anesthetics generally result from high blood levels of the drug. Examples of these are: **CNS:** anxiety, apprehension, nervousness, convulsions followed by drowsiness, unconsciousness, and *respiratory arrest.* **CV:** myocardial depression, *arrhythmias, cardiac arrest.* **EENT:** blurred vision. **GI:** nausea, vomiting.

♦ Available in U.S. and Canada. ♦♦ Available in Canada only. All other products (no symbol) available in U.S. only. Italicized side effects are common or life-threatening.

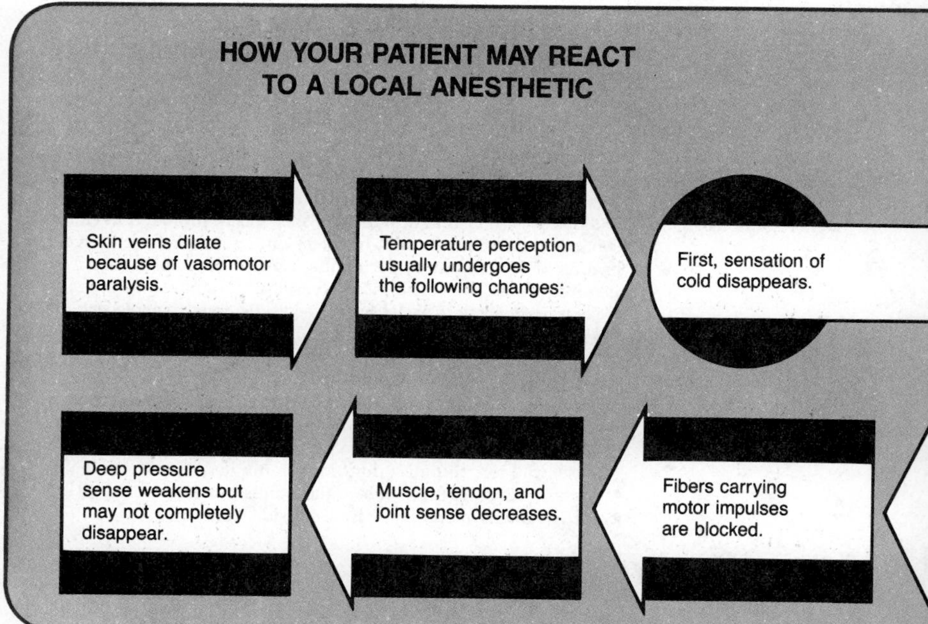

HOW YOUR PATIENT MAY REACT TO A LOCAL ANESTHETIC
Skin veins dilate because of vasomotor paralysis.
Temperature perception usually undergoes the following changes:
First, sensation of cold disappears.
Deep pressure sense weakens but may not completely disappear.
Muscle, tendon, and joint sense decreases.
Fibers carrying motor impulses are blocked.

INTERACTIONS	NURSING CONSIDERATIONS
None significant.	• Contraindicated in infection at injection site, serious CNS diseases, and in hypersensitivity to procaine, chloroprocaine, tetracaine, or other para-aminobenzoic acid derivatives. Use cautiously in shock, profound anemia, cachexia, hypertension, hypotension, peritonitis, cardiac decompensation, massive pleural effusion, increased intracranial pressure, infection, and in highly nervous patients. • Saddle block contraindicated in cephalopelvic disproportion, placenta previa, abruptio placentae, intrauterine manipulation, floating fetal head. • Don't use cloudy, discolored, or crystallized solutions. • Keep resuscitative equipment and drugs available. • 10 times as strong as procaine HCl. • Onset in 15 minutes; duration up to 3 hours. • When cerebrospinal fluid is added to powdered drug or drug solution during spinal anesthesia, solution may be cloudy. • Protect from light; store in refrigerator. • For treatment of anaphylaxis, see inside front cover.

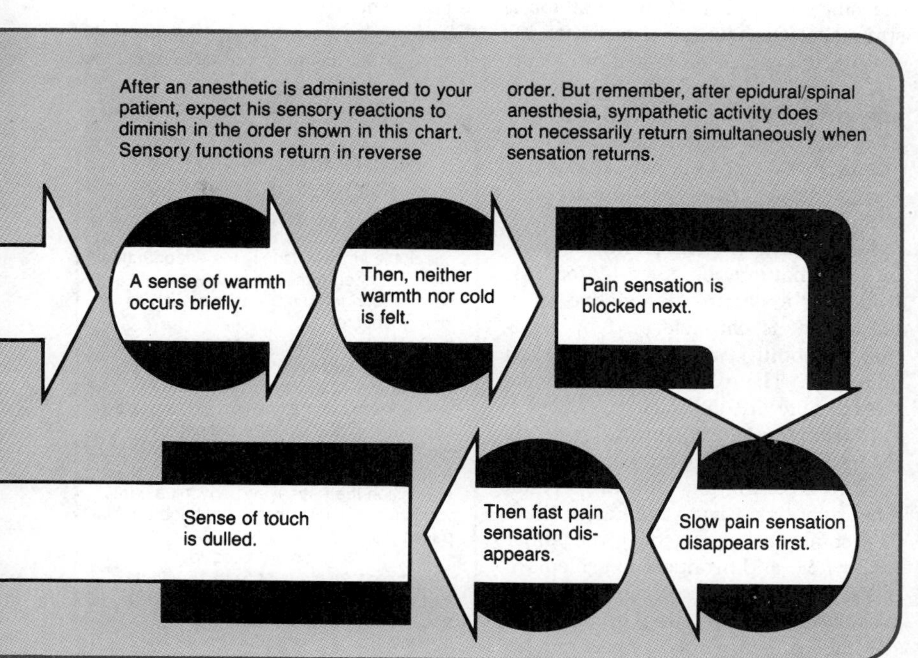

After an anesthetic is administered to your patient, expect his sensory reactions to diminish in the order shown in this chart. Sensory functions return in reverse order. But remember, after epidural/spinal anesthesia, sympathetic activity does not necessarily return simultaneously when sensation returns.
A sense of warmth occurs briefly.
Then, neither warmth nor cold is felt.
Pain sensation is blocked next.
Slow pain sensation disappears first.
Then fast pain sensation disappears.
Sense of touch is dulled.

General anesthetics

fentanyl citrate with droperidol
ketamine hydrochloride
methohexital sodium
thiamylal sodium
thiopental sodium

General anesthetics are central nervous system (CNS) depressants that induce varying degrees of analgesia, depression of consciousness, skeletal muscle relaxation, and reduced reflex activity. There are two types of general anesthetics—inhalation and parenteral. (See the chart on pp. 1142 to 1143 for a summary of inhalation anesthetics.)

With the exception of ketamine and fentanyl with droperidol, these agents are ultra–short-acting barbiturates. They're potent anesthetics, generally administered intravenously, that cause loss of consciousness within seconds and allow pleasant recovery.

Ketamine is a short-acting nonbarbiturate that may be given I.V. or I.M. It induces a state of dissociative anesthesia that is characterized by sedation, immobility, amnesia, and marked analgesia. The patient seems awake but is really unconscious.

Fentanyl, a narcotic analgesic, is chemically related to meperidine. It's used in combination with droperidol, a neuroleptic derivative of haloperidol. The combination can be given either I.V. or I.M. and produces neuroleptanalgesia, a state that resembles the dissociative anesthesia caused by ketamine.

Although general anesthesia can be accomplished with a single drug, a combination of agents is generally used to produce balanced anesthesia. Narcotics, skeletal muscle relaxants, and tranquilizers may be combined with the anesthetic agent.

Major uses

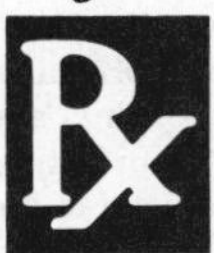

Parenteral general anesthetics induce anesthesia before administration of inhalation anesthetics. They're also used alone for short-term procedures or for basal anesthesia in children.

- Thiopental sodium is also used to control postanesthetic convulsive states.

MANAGING RECOVERY FROM ANESTHESIA

- Immediately on receiving a patient, check his airway. Usually the endotracheal tube has been removed by the anesthesiologist. Watch for complications, such as laryngospasms.
- During the late stages of recovery from anesthesia, you may need to insert an oropharyngeal airway to prevent the tongue from obstructing the air passage. Leave it in place until the patient fully regains consciousness.
- Give oxygen if needed.
- Position the patient so he won't aspirate vomitus or secretions into tracheobronchial passages.
- Suction the patient if needed.
- Monitor vital signs at 5- to 15-minute intervals until the patient is fully reactive.
- Check the position and function of all drains, tubes, and intravenous lines.

STAGES AND SIGNS IN ANESTHESIA

STAGE	PLANES AND CHARACTERISTICS		SITE OF DEPRESSION ON CNS	THIOPENTAL EFFECTS	BARBITURATE EFFECTS
	Analgesia	**Amnesia**			
I Analgesia and amnesia (conscious)	1. None 2. Partial effect 3. Total effect	None Total effect Total effect	Slight-to-moderate depression of cortex	Euphoria, loss of discrimination and inability to interact with the environment	Intercostal and diaphragmatic breathing slows immediately. Patient *may* be quiet or euphoric.
II Dream (unconscious)	Unpredictable reactions; irregular breathing		Predominant control by subcortex	Loss of consciousness	No delirium
III Surgical Light	1. Rhythmical breathing		Moderate depression of subcortex	Hypoactivity to painful stimulus	Vigilance to airway important; assisted respiration indicated
Medium	2. Sensory loss (pauses after expiration grow longer)		Predominant control by midbrain	Loss of somatic response to pain	Same as for light stage
	3. Level of progressive intercostal paralysis				
Deep	4. Level of diaphragmatic breathing (intercostal paralysis complete)		Moderate depression of midbrain	Loss of visceral response to pain	Same as for light stage
IV Medullary paralysis	Respiratory arrest		Moderate depression of pons	Fall in pulse pressure	If continued, cardiac arrest will occur.

Adapted from Etsten and Himwich, *Anesthesiology*, vol. 7 (Philadelphia: J.B. Lippincott Co., 1946) and Possati, et al., *Anesthesia and Analgesia Current Researchers*, vol. 32 (Cleveland: International Anesthesia Research Society, 1953). Used with permission of the publishers.

Mechanism of action

- Barbiturate anesthetics (methohexital, thiamylal, and thiopental) act by depressing the CNS. They inhibit the firing rate of neurons within the ascending reticular activating system.
- Ketamine appears to interrupt association pathways in the brain, causing dissociative anesthesia, a feeling of dissociation from the environment.
- Fentanyl with droperidol acts as a CNS depressant to produce reduced motor activity and analgesia.

Absorption, distribution, metabolism, and excretion

- All barbiturate anesthetics are given by the I.V. route; therefore, absorption is immediate and complete. They are well distributed to body tissues, metabolized in the liver, and excreted in urine.
- Fentanyl with droperidol is well absorbed from I.M. injection sites and distributed widely to body tissues. It is metabolized in the liver and eliminated in urine and in feces.

WHAT YOU SHOULD KNOW ABOUT INHALATION ANESTHETICS

ANESTHETIC	CHARACTERISTICS	SIDE EFFECTS AND INTERACTIONS	NURSING CONSIDERATIONS
cyclopropane	• Potent general inhalation anesthetic; rarely used because it's highly explosive • Rapid induction and recovery • May be given with high levels of oxygen	• Nausea, vomiting, hypotension, delirium, and headaches occur frequently. • Dose of nondepolarizing neuromuscular blockers should be reduced when used with this agent.	• To prevent hypercapnia, control ventilation. • Small doses of narcotics given just before completion of surgery lessen nausea and delirium. • When treating an overdose, maintain an adequate airway and use respiratory assistance.
ether (ethyl ether, diethyl ether)	• Not widely used because it's highly explosive • Produces profound skeletal muscle relaxation • Induction relatively slow; recovery prolonged	• Causes significant nausea and vomiting postoperatively, making recovery unpleasant • Dose of nondepolarizing neuromuscular blockers should be reduced when used with this agent.	• Useful in asthmatic patients because it dilates the bronchioles
halothane (fluothane)	• May be used with N_2O or muscle relaxant • Produces rapid and smooth induction	• Cardiac rate and rhythm changes (bradycardia, nodal rhythm, AV dissociation); decreased cardiac output with resulting hypotension (with high concentrations); ventricular fibrillation (when used with epinephrine and norepi-	• Patient awakens slowly after long procedures on high concentrations. • Check vital signs often. Hyperventilation can rapidly reverse effect. • Keep atropine available to reverse bradycardia. • Record all premedi-

• Ketamine is well absorbed after I.M. injection, widely distributed to body tissues, and metabolized in the liver. The metabolite is excreted primarily in urine, with smaller amounts eliminated in feces.

Onset and duration

• Barbiturate anesthetics have an onset within 30 to 60 seconds after administration. Duration is usually 10 to 30 minutes after the last I.V. dose.

Methohexital furnishes anesthesia for 5 to 15 minutes.

Thiamylal, when administered rectally, produces maximal effects within 30 minutes; its duration of action is about 1 hour.

• Fentanyl begins to work in seconds; its duration of action is 30 to 60 minutes. Onset of droperidol occurs in 3 to 10 minutes; duration is 2 to 4 hours.

• Ketamine has an onset within 30 seconds after I.V. or I.M. administration. Duration, when the drug is given I.V., is 5 to 10 minutes. Duration after I.M. induction is 12 to 25 minutes.

Combination products

None.

ANESTHETIC	CHARACTERISTICS	SIDE EFFECTS AND INTERACTIONS	NURSING CONSIDERATIONS
halothane *(continued)*		nephrine); tachypnea; hepatic dysfunction. • Seldom causes nausea or vomiting; nonirritating to mucous membranes • CNS depressants (including alcohol) potentiate halothane effect.	cations carefully. • Shivering is common in recovery phase.
methoxyflurane (penthrane)	• Often used with N_2O, sodium pentothal, or muscle relaxants • Potent anesthetic; used in short procedures because it's rapidly metabolized	• Nephrotoxic • May enhance adverse renal effects of antibiotics (tetracycline, garamycin, tobramycin, kanamycin) • Seldom causes nausea, vomiting, or arrhythmias • CNS depressants (including alcohol) potentiate effect.	• Prolonged postoperative drowsiness and analgesia are likely. • Check vital signs often. Hyperventilation can rapidly reverse effect. • Record all premedications carefully.
nitrous oxide (N_2O)	• Used for rapid induction • Not a potent anesthetic; must be administered with O_2. • Nonirritating to mucous membranes	• Arterial hypoxemia; poor muscle relaxation • CNS depressants (including alcohol) potentiate N_2O effect.	• To prevent diffusion hypoxia, give O_2 therapy by nasal prongs or mask. • Check vital signs often. Hyperventilation can rapidly reverse effect. • Record all premedications carefully. • Keep ABG kit available.

USE CAUTION WHEN ADMINISTERING NARCOTIC ANALGESICS TO A POSTOPERATIVE PATIENT

If you administer narcotic analgesics to postoperative patients, you should know about the drugs' dangerous additive effects on patients who've had certain anesthetics. These may occur when the patient has been given an anesthetic that contains a narcotic, such as fentanyl citrate with droperidol (Innovar).

If the patient still has some anesthetic in his blood and the narcotic analgesic dose hasn't been reduced, *the combined amount of narcotic could be high enough to cause respiratory depression.*

So always check to see what anesthetics a patient has received, read all warning stickers, and question anything that seems out of order. Your extra caution could save a patient's life.

NAME	INDICATIONS & DOSAGE	SIDE EFFECTS
fentanyl citrate with droperidol Controlled Substance Schedule II Innovar (Each ml contains [in a 1:50 ratio] fentanyl 0.05 mg as a citrate and droperidol 2.5 mg.)	Doses vary depending on application, use of other agents, and patient's age, body weight, and physical status. *Anesthesia*— **Adults:** *Premedication*—0.5 to 2 ml I.M. 45 to 60 minutes before surgery. *Adjunct to general anesthetic*—Induction: 1 ml/20 to 25 lb body weight by slow I.V. to produce neuroleptanalgesia. Maintenance: not indicated as sole agent for maintenance of surgical anesthesia. Used in combination with other measures. To prevent excessive accumulation of the relatively long-acting droperidol component, fentanyl alone should be used in increments of 0.025 to 0.05 mg (0.5 to 1 ml) for maintenance of analgesia. However, during prolonged surgery, additional 0.5- to 1-ml amounts of Innovar may be given with caution. *Diagnostic procedures*—0.5 to 2 ml I.M. 45 to 60 minutes before procedure. In prolonged procedure, give 0.5 to 1 ml I.V. with caution and without a general anesthetic. *Adjunct to regional anesthetic*—1 to 2 ml I.M. or slow I.V. **Children:** Premedication—0.25 ml/20 lb body weight I.M. 45 to 60 minutes before surgery. *Adjunct to general anesthetic*—0.5 ml/20 lb body weight (total combined dose for induction and maintenance). Following induction with Innovar, fentanyl alone in a dose of ¼ to ⅓ of adult dose should be used to avoid accumulation of droperidol. However, during prolonged surgery, additional amounts of Innovar may be administered with caution. Safety of use in children under 2 years has not been established.	**CNS:** emergence delirium and hallucinations, postoperative drowsiness. **CV:** vasodilation, *hypotension*, decreased pulmonary arterial pressure, bradycardia, or tachycardia. **EENT:** blurred vision, *laryngospasms.* **GI:** *nausea, vomiting.* **Respiratory:** *respiratory depression, apnea,* or *arrest.* **Other:** drug dependence, muscle rigidity, chills, *shivering,* twitching, diaphoresis.
ketamine hydrochloride Ketaject, Ketalar♦	*Induce anesthesia for procedures, especially short-term diagnostic or surgical, not requiring skeletal muscle relaxation; before giving other general*	**CNS:** *tonic and clonic movements resembling convulsions, respiratory depression, apnea when administered too rapidly.* **CV:** *increased blood pressure and*

♦ Available in U.S. and Canada. ♦♦ Available in Canada only. All other products (no symbol) available in U.S. only. Italicized side effects are common or life-threatening.

INTERACTIONS	NURSING CONSIDERATIONS
CNS depressants (such as barbiturates, tranquilizers, narcotics, and general anesthetics): additive or potentiating effect. Dosage should be reduced. *MAO inhibitors:* severe and unpredictable potentiation of Innovar. Do not use together or within 2 weeks of MAO inhibitor therapy.	• Contraindicated in intolerance to either component. Use with caution in patients with head injuries and increased intracranial pressure, chronic obstructive pulmonary disease, hepatic and renal dysfunction, bradyarrhythmias, and in elderly or debilitated patients. • Hypotension is a common side effect. However, if blood pressure drops, also consider hypovolemia as a possible cause. Use appropriate parenteral fluids to help restore blood pressure. • Vital signs should be monitored frequently. • Monitor pulmonary artery pressure. • Be aware that respiratory depression, muscular rigidity of respiratory muscles, and respiratory arrest can occur. Have narcotic antagonist and CPR equipment on hand. • Maintain airway. • Postoperative EEG pattern may return to normal slowly. • Postoperatively, if narcotic analgesics are required, use initially in reduced doses, as low as ¼ to ⅓ those usually recommended. • When Innovar is given for anesthesia induction, fentanyl (Sublimaze) should be used for maintenance analgesia during procedure. • Premedication with Innovar has sometimes been associated with patient agitation and refusal of surgery. Administration of diazepam may relieve this. • For toxicity, see APPENDIX, *Drug Toxicities*.

Thyroid hormones: may elevate blood pressure and cause tachycardia. Give cautiously.	• Contraindicated in patients with history of cerebrovascular accident; patients who would be endangered by a significant rise in blood pressure; and those with severe hypertension; severe cardiac decompensation; surgery of the pharynx, larynx, or bronchial tree, unless used with muscle relaxants. Use with caution in chronic alcoholism,

(continued on following page)

NAME	INDICATIONS & DOSAGE	SIDE EFFECTS
ketamine hydrochloride *(continued)*	*anesthetics or to supplement low-potency agents, such as nitrous oxide—* **Adults and children:** 1 to 4.5 mg/kg I.V., administered over 60 seconds; or 6.5 to 13 mg/kg I.M. To maintain anesthesia, repeat in increments of half to full initial dose.	*pulse rate,* hypotension, bradycardia. **EENT:** diplopia, nystagmus, slight increase in intraocular pressure, *laryngospasms, salivation.* **GI:** mild anorexia, nausea, vomiting. **Skin:** transient erythema, measles-like rash. **Other:** *dream-like states, hallucinations, confusion, excitement,* irrational behavior, psychic abnormalities.
methohexital sodium Controlled Substance Schedule IV Brevital Sodium, Brietal Sodium♦♦	*General anesthetic for short-term procedures (oral surgery, gynecologic and genitourinary examinations); reduction of fractures; before electroconvulsive therapy; for prolonged anesthesia when used with gaseous anesthetics—* **Adults and children:** 5 to 12 ml 1% solution (50 to 120 mg) I.V. at 1 ml/5 seconds. Dose required for induction may vary from 50 to 120 mg or more; average about 70 mg. Induction dose provides anesthesia for 5 to 7 minutes. Maintenance—intermittent injection: 2 to 4 ml 1% solution (20 to 40 mg) q 4 to 7 minutes; continuous I.V. drip: administer 0.2% solution (1 drop/second).	**CNS:** *muscular twitching,* headache, emergence delirium. **CV:** *temporary hypotension, tachycardia,* circulatory depression, *peripheral vascular collapse.* **GI:** excessive salivation, *nausea, vomiting.* **Skin:** tissue necrosis with extravasation. **Local:** pain at injection site, injury to nerves adjacent to injection site. **Respiratory:** *laryngospasm, bronchospasm, respiratory depression, apnea.* **Other:** hiccups, coughing, acute allergic reactions, *twitching.* Extended use may cause cumulative effect; may be habit-forming.
thiamylal sodium Controlled Substance Schedule III Surital♦	*General anesthetic for short-term procedures; anesthetic before administering other general anesthetics (dosage individualized to patient's response)—* **Adults:** 3 to 6 ml 2.5% solution I.V. at 1 ml/5 seconds. Additional intermittent injections of 0.5 to 1 ml. Maximum dose 1 g (40 ml 2.5% solution). *Rectal administration before diagnostic procedures—* **Children:** 800 mg to 1 g 5% so-	**CNS:** excitement, headache, emergence delirium. **CV:** hypotension, *circulatory depression,* thrombophlebitis, *hypoxia.* **GI:** nausea, vomiting, excessive salivation. **Skin:** rash, urticaria, tissue necrosis with extravasation. **Respiratory:** *laryngospasm, bronchospasm, respiratory depression, apnea.* **Local:** pain at injection site, in-

♦ Available in U.S. and Canada. ♦♦ Available in Canada only. All other products (no symbol) available in U.S. only. Italicized side effects are common or life-threatening.

INTERACTIONS	NURSING CONSIDERATIONS
	alcohol-intoxicated patients, patients with cerebrospinal fluid pressure elevated before anesthesia. • Discourage giving anything orally at least 6 hours before elective surgery. • Because of rapid induction, patient should be physically supported during administration. • Do not inject barbiturates and ketamine HCl from same syringe, as they are chemically incompatible. • Monitor vital signs before, during, and after anesthesia. • Check cardiac function in patients with hypertension or cardiac depression. • Maintain airway. • Resuscitation equipment should be available and ready for use. • Start supportive respiration if respiratory depression occurs. Use mechanical support if possible rather than administering analeptics. • Keep verbal, tactile, and visual stimulation at a minimum during recovery phase to reduce incidence of emergent reactions. • Hallucinations and excitement can occur on emergence from anesthesia; they can be abated by giving diazepam (if ordered). • A potent hallucinogen that can readily produce dissociative anesthesia (patient feels detached from environment). Dissociative effect and hallucinatory side effects have made this a popular drug of abuse among young people.
None significant.	• Contraindicated in severe hepatic dysfunction, hypersensitivity to barbiturates, or porphyria; in shock or impending shock; and in patients for whom general anesthetics would be hazardous. Use with caution in debilitated patients, in patients with asthma, respiratory obstruction, severe hypertension or hypotension, myocardial disease, congestive heart failure, severe anemia, or extreme obesity. • Maintain pulmonary ventilation. • Avoid extravascular or intra-arterial injections. • Monitor vital signs before, during, and after anesthesia. • Have resuscitative equipment and drugs ready. • Reduce postoperative nausea by having patient fast before administration. • Incompatible with silicone; avoid contact with rubber stoppers or parts of syringes that have been treated with silicone. • Incompatible with lactated Ringer's solution. • Do not mix with acid solutions such as atropine sulfate. • Solvents recommended are 5% glucose solution or isotonic (0.9%) sodium chloride solution instead of distilled water. • Rate of flow must be individualized for each patient. • Solutions may be stored and used as long as they remain clear and colorless. Solutions cannot be heated for sterilization.
None significant.	• Contraindicated in hepatic dysfunction or disease, traumatic or impending shock, porphyria, hypersensitivity to barbiturates, and in those for whom general anesthetics would be hazardous. Use with caution in respiratory disease or obstruction, obesity, marked disturbance of arterial tension, heart failure, anemia, status asthmaticus, endocrine or renal dysfunction, and in debilitated patients. • Maintain airway. • Have resuscitative equipment and drugs ready. • Monitor vital signs before, during, and after anesthesia. • Avoid extravascular or intra-arterial injection. • Incompatible with lactated Ringer's solution or solutions containing bacteriostatic or buffer agents, which tend to cause precipitation. • Don't inject air into solution; may cause cloudiness.

(continued on following page)

NAME	INDICATIONS & DOSAGE	SIDE EFFECTS
thiamylal sodium *(continued)*	lution/22.5 kg body weight. *Supplemental anesthetic—* **Adults:** 0.2% or 0.3% solution continuous I.V. drip. Recovery occurs within 20 to 30 minutes after last injection.	jury to nerves adjacent to injection site. **Other:** hiccups. Extended use can cause cumulative effects; may be habit-forming.
thiopental sodium Controlled Substance Schedule III Pentothal Sodium♦ (injection and rectal suspension)	*Induce anesthesia before administering other anesthetics—* 210 to 280 mg (3 to 4 ml/kg) usually required for average adult (70 kg). *General anesthetic for short-term procedures—* **Adults:** 2 to 3 ml 2.5% solution (50 to 75 mg) administered I.V. only at intervals of 20 to 40 seconds, depending on reaction. Dose may be repeated with caution, if necessary. *Convulsive states following anesthesia*—75 to 125 mg (3 to 5 ml of 2.5% solution) immediately. *Psychiatric disorders (narcoanalysis, narcotherapy)—* 100 mg/minute (4 ml/minute 2.5% solution) until confusion occurs and before sleep. Maximum dose 50 ml/minute. *Basal anesthesia by rectal administration—* **Adults and children:** administer up to 1 g/22.5 kg (50 lb) body weight, or 0.5 ml 10% solution/kg body weight. Maximum 1 to 1.5 g (children weighing 34 kg or more) and 3 to 4 g (adults weighing 91 kg or more). *Note:* Thiopental is rarely administered rectally for basal sedation or anesthesia because of variable absorption from the rectum.	**CNS:** *prolonged somnolence,* retrograde amnesia. **CV:** *myocardial depression, arrhythmias.* **Skin:** tissue necrosis with extravasation. **Respiratory:** *respiratory depression (momentary apnea following each injection is typical), bronchospasm, laryngospasm.* **Local:** pain at injection site. **Other:** sneezing, coughing, *shivering.* May be habit-forming.

INTERACTIONS	NURSING CONSIDERATIONS
	• Sterile water is the preferred solvent for injections. For drip maintenance use 5% glucose or isotonic sodium chloride solution to avoid extreme hypotonicity. • Solutions of atropine sulfate, *d*-tubocurarine, or succinylcholine may be given concurrently but should not be mixed together. • Do not heat solutions for sterilization. Solutions should be stored in refrigerator and used within 6 days. If kept at room temperature, use within 24 hours.
None significant.	• Contraindicated in absence of suitable veins for intravenous administration, hypersensitivity to barbiturates, status asthmaticus, porphyria, respiratory depression or obstruction, decompensated cardiac disease, severe anemia, hepatic cirrhosis, shock, renal dysfunction, increased intracranial pressure, myxedema. • Give test dose (1 to 3 ml 2.5% solution) to assess reaction to drug. • When used as general anesthetic, give atropine sulfate as premedication to diminish laryngeal reflexes and to prevent laryngeal spasm. • Have resuscitative equipment and oxygen ready. • Avoid extravasation and intra-arterial injection. • Maintain airway. • Monitor vital signs before, during, and after anesthesia. • Solutions of atropine sulfate, *d*-tubocurarine, or succinylcholine may be given concurrently but should not be mixed together. • Do not heat solutions for sterilization. Solutions should be stored in refrigerator and used within 6 days. If kept at room temperature, use within 24 hours.

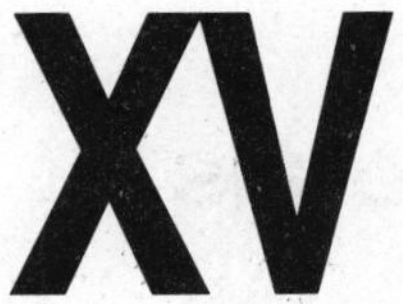

Nutritional Agents

Vitamins and minerals

vitamin A
- oleovitamin A

vitamin B complex
- cyanocobalamin (B_{12})
- cyanocobalamin, hydroxocobalamin (B_{12a})
- folic acid (B_9)
- leucovorin calcium
- niacin (B_3)
- niacinamide
- pyridoxine hydrochloride (B_6)
- riboflavin (B_2)
- thiamine hydrochloride (B_1)

vitamin C
- ascorbic acid

vitamin D
- cholecalciferol (D_3)
- ergocalciferol (D_2)

vitamin E

vitamin K analogs
- menadione/menadiol sodium diphosphate (K_3)
- phytonadione (K_1)

multivitamins

sodium fluoride

trace elements
- chromium
- copper
- iodine
- manganese
- zinc
- zinc sulfate

Vitamins are organic dietary constituents that are necessary for health. Supplied in small amounts, they're important components of enzyme systems that catalyze metabolic reactions. Diseases now known to be caused by vitamin deficiencies include night blindness (vitamin A deficiency), beriberi (thiamine deficiency), pellagra (niacin deficiency), scurvy (ascorbic acid deficiency), and rickets (vitamin D deficiency). Vitamins are categorized as water-soluble (B complex and C) and fat-soluble (A, D, E, and K).

Trace elements are inorganic substances needed in small quantities to maintain homeostasis.

Major uses

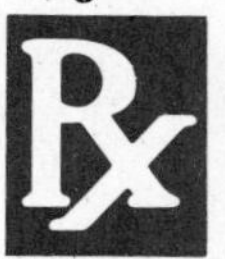

- Vitamins are used to prevent or treat selective or multiple vitamin deficiencies. They're essential to the proper synthesis and metabolism of body protein.
- Trace elements are used to prevent or treat dietary deficiencies and other clinical problems that result from these deficiencies.

Zinc sulfate is also a therapeutic adjunct for various skin disorders, acrodermatitis enteropathica, rheumatoid arthritis, and hypogeusia (reduced sense of taste) when these disorders coexist with low serum zinc levels.

Chromium enhances intracellular transport of insulin and glucose.

Copper is essential for the synthesis of ceruloplasmin, which aids the normal flow of iron from cells to plasma and catalyzes the oxidation of iron from the ferrous to the ferric state.

Iodine aids in the synthesis of the thyroid hormones thyroxine and triiodothyronine.

DIETARY MINERAL REQUIREMENTS AND SOURCES

MINERAL/ NUTRIENT	REQUIRE-MENTS	SOURCES
Calcium	✔	Milk and milk products, green leafy vegetables, citrus fruits, dried peas and beans
Chloride	✔	Table salt
Chromium	✓	Dried brewer's yeast, whole grain cereals, liver
Cobalt	✓	Meats, eggs, dairy products, other sources of vitamin B_{12}
Copper	✓	Unprocessed foods, organ meats, shellfish, nuts, dried legumes
Fluorine	✓	Fluoridated water
Iodine	✓	Iodized salt, seafood
Iron	✓	Liver, meat products, egg yolks, fish, green leafy vegetables, peas, beans, dried fruits, whole grain cereals, iron-enriched foods
Magnesium	✔	Nuts, soybeans, whole grains, molasses, spices, seafood
Manganese	✓	Bran, coffee, tea, nuts, peas, beans
Phosphorus	✔	Cheddar cheese, nuts, meats, poultry, fish, eggs, whole grains
Potassium	✔	Avocados, dried apricots, bananas, meats, fish, chicken, potatoes, molasses, peanut butter, milk
Selenium	✓	Various plant (fruit or vegetable) and animal sources; amount depends on the selenium available in the environment—soil or seawater—before being taken up by the food source
Sodium	✔	Meats, poultry, fish, eggs, milk, processed foods, green olives, salt
Sulfur	✔	Thiamine, pantothenic acid, biotin, lipoic acid
Zinc	✓	Meats, fish, egg yolks, milk

✔ *Macronutrient element:* Required in fairly large amounts in the diet (more than 100 milligrams per day).

✓ *Micronutrient or trace element:* Required in trace amounts in the diet.

Note: Patients should avoid routine intake of recommended upper levels for trace elements. Toxic levels may result from taking only 2 to 3 times the average requirements, which for adults can range from as little as 0.06 mcg for cobalt to 15 mg for zinc.

Sodium fluoride is used to retard tooth decay and may be beneficial in bone disorders.

Manganese is used by enzymes involved in polysaccharide synthesis.

Mechanism of action

- Vitamins act as coenzymes or coen-

RECOMMENDED DAILY DIETARY ALLOWANCES[a]

GROUP	AGE	WEIGHT		HEIGHT		PROTEIN	FAT-SOLUBLE VITAMINS		
	(years)	(kg)	(lb)	(cm)	(in)	(g)	Vitamin A (mcg RE)[b]	Vitamin D (mcg)[c]	Vitamin E (mg α-TE)[d]
Infants	0.0 to 0.5	6	13	60	24	kg × 2.2	420	10	3
	0.5 to 1.0	9	20	71	28	kg × 2.0	400	10	4
Children	1 to 3	13	29	90	35	23	400	10	5
	4 to 6	20	44	112	44	30	500	10	6
	7 to 10	28	62	132	52	34	700	10	7
Males	11 to 14	45	99	157	62	45	1,000	10	8
	15 to 18	66	145	176	69	56	1,000	10	10
	19 to 22	70	154	178	70	56	1,000	7.5	10
	23 to 50	70	154	178	70	56	1,000	5	10
	51 +	70	154	178	70	56	1,000	5	10
Females	11 to 14	46	101	157	62	46	800	10	8
	15 to 18	55	120	163	64	46	800	10	8
	19 to 22	55	120	163	64	44	800	7.5	8
	23 to 50	55	120	163	64	44	800	5	8
	51 +	55	120	163	64	44	800	5	8
Pregnant						+30	+200	+5	+2
Lactating						+20	+400	+5	+3

[a] The allowances are intended to provide for individual variations among most normal persons as they live in the United States under usual environmental stresses. Diets should be based on a variety of common foods in order to provide other nutrients for which human requirements have been less well defined.

[b] Retinol equivalents. 1 retinol equivalent = 1 mcg retinol or 6 mcg/beta-carotene.

[c] As cholecalciferol. 10 mcg cholecalciferol = 400 IU of vitamin D.

[d] alpha-tocopherol equivalents. 1 mg *d*-alpha tocopherol = 1 alpha-TE.

[e] 1 NE (niacin equivalent) is equal to 1 mg of niacin or 60 mg of dietary tryptophan.

[f] The folacin allowances refer to dietary sources as determined by *Lactobacillus casei* assay after treatment with enzymes (conjugases) to make polyglutamyl forms of the vitamin available to the test organism.

[g] The recommended daily allowance for vitamin B_{12} in infants is based on average

zyme precursors to catalyze protein, fat, and carbohydrate metabolism, and to facilitate energy-producing and anabolic reactions.

• Trace elements may act in metalloenzyme units. They participate in synthesis and stabilization of proteins and nucleic acids in subcellular and membrane transport systems.

• Sodium fluoride's mechanism is unknown; however, the fluoride ion in sodium fluoride stabilizes the apatite crystal of bone and teeth. The sodium fluoride compound may also act as a catalyst for bone remineralization.

Absorption, distribution, metabolism, and excretion

• Vitamins are readily absorbed and distributed in the body. Excretion rates of water-soluble vitamins vary with metabolic status, stress, disease, and requirements for tissue repair. Excess water-soluble vitamins are generally metabolized in the liver and rapidly excreted in urine. Fat-soluble vitamins, which require bile and adequate pancreatic secretions for absorption, are

Designed for the maintenance of good nutrition of practically all healthy people in the U.S.A.

WATER-SOLUBLE VITAMINS							MINERALS					
Vitamin C (mg)	Thiamin (mg)	Riboflavin (mg)	Niacin (mg NE)[e]	Vitamin B_6 (mg)	Folacin[f] (mcg)	Vitamin B_{12} (mcg)	Calcium (mg)	Phosphorus (mg)	Magnesium (mg)	Iron (mg)	Zinc (mg)	Iodine (mcg)
35	0.3	0.4	6	0.3	30	0.5[g]	360	240	50	10	3	40
35	0.5	0.6	8	0.6	45	1.5	540	360	70	15	5	50
45	0.7	0.8	9	0.9	100	2.0	800	800	150	15	10	70
45	0.9	1.0	11	1.3	200	2.5	800	800	200	10	10	90
45	1.2	1.4	16	1.6	300	3.0	800	800	250	10	10	120
50	1.4	1.6	18	1.8	400	3.0	1,200	1,200	350	18	15	150
60	1.4	1.7	18	2.0	400	3.0	1,200	1,200	400	18	15	150
60	1.5	1.7	19	2.2	400	3.0	800	800	350	10	15	150
60	1.4	1.6	18	2.2	400	3.0	800	800	350	10	15	150
60	1.2	1.4	16	2.2	400	3.0	800	800	350	10	15	150
50	1.1	1.3	15	1.8	400	3.0	1,200	1,200	300	18	15	150
60	1.1	1.3	14	2.0	400	3.0	1,200	1,200	300	18	15	150
60	1.1	1.3	14	2.0	400	3.0	800	800	300	18	15	150
60	1.0	1.2	13	2.0	400	3.0	800	800	300	18	15	150
60	1.0	1.2	13	2.0	400	3.0	800	800	300	10	15	150
+20	+0.4	+0.3	+2	+0.6	+400	+1.0	+400	+400	+150	[h]	+5	+25
+40	+0.5	+0.5	+5	+0.5	+100	+1.0	+400	+400	+150	[h]	+10	+50

concentration of the vitamin in human milk. The allowances after weaning are based on energy intake (as recommended by the American Academy of Pediatrics) and consideration of other factors, such as intestinal absorption.

[h] The increased requirement during pregnancy cannot be met by the iron content of habitual American diets nor by the existing iron stores of many women; therefore the use of 30 to 60 mg of supplemental iron is recommended. Iron needs during lactation are not substantially different from those of nonpregnant women, but continued supplementation of the mother for 2 to 3 months after parturition is advisable to replenish stores depleted by pregnancy.

Reproduced from *Recommended Dietary Allowances*, 9th ed. (Washington, D.C.: National Academy Press, 1980). Source: Food and Nutrition Board, National Academy of Sciences—National Research Council.

stored for longer periods.

• Vitamins A and E are metabolized largely in the liver and eliminated mainly through the bile in feces.

• Vitamin D has a complex metabolism. Cholecalciferol and ergocalciferol are metabolized in the liver to more active metabolites (25-hydroxy derivatives). In the kidneys, these forms are metabolized to their 1,25-dihydroxy derivatives, which are even more active. Eventually, all vitamin D metabolites are eliminated mainly through the bile in feces.

• Vitamin K's metabolism and excretion are unknown.

• Trace minerals are readily absorbed after oral or parenteral administration and distributed throughout the body. They are excreted largely unchanged in urine.

Onset and duration

Most vitamin and trace element deficiencies respond quickly to therapeutic doses. Duration of action depends on the patient's total metabolic needs.

THE FACTS ABOUT SOME VITAMIN SUPPLEMENTS

Some manufacturers of vitamin pills and mineral pills make certain claims about the wonders of their products. Are their claims justified? Does your patient need to take these pills every morning? And can he take *too much* of a vitamin?

If a person is healthy and eats a balanced diet, including meats, fruits, vegetables, nuts, milk products, cereal grains, and so on, he's probably better off without a vitamin supplement. Taking extra vitamins is an unnecessary expense. And excessive intake of fat-soluble vitamins *can* cause severe toxic effects. (See *Possible Effects of*

VITAMIN	CLAIM
A	• Therapeutic aid for children with schizophrenia or learning disabilities • Effective against warts, acne and other skin diseases, stress ulcers, and respiratory tract infections
B_1 (thiamine)	• Stimulates mental response • Effective against skin diseases, multiple sclerosis, infections, cancer, and impotence
B_6 (pyridoxine)	• Useful in preventing kidney stones • Controls vomiting during pregnancy
B_{12}	• Overcomes the feeling of being run down
C	• Decreases severity of the common cold • Lessens the chance of getting a cold • Effective against atherosclerosis, allergy, mental illness, corneal infection, ulcers, thrombosis, anemia, and pressure sores
D	• Lowers blood cholesterol levels • Prevents and cures osteoporosis in the elderly
E	• Aids in growing hair • Settles skin problems • Reduces arthritis pain • Prevents ulcers • Enhances sexuality
Pantothenic acid	• Retards graying of hair

Combination products

Vitamin A and D combinations
B complex with vitamin C
Multivitamins
Calcium and vitamin products
Fluoride with vitamins

Too Much of a Vitamin, p. 1177.)

Vitamin supplements may be needed by pregnant or lactating women, persons taking antibiotics or oral contraceptives, heavy drinkers, dieters, or smokers. Also, those with intestinal disorders that restrict normal dietary intake or impair absorption may need vitamin supplements. (In any of these cases, the patient should check with his doctor to see what vitamins or minerals he may be lacking.)

The following chart lists some current claims about vitamins and the latest data from the FDA.

FACT	REMARKS
• Needed for new cell growth and healthy tissues • Essential for vision in dim light	• Claims for treatment of schizophrenia are not justified. • Research is proceeding on possible medical uses (for example, treatment of epidermal and bladder cancers, and stress ulcers). • High intake can be toxic; however, the vitamin A in plants is nontoxic.
• Needed for normal digestion, growth, fertility, lactation, nerve tissue growth and function, and carbohydrate metabolism	• Claims are unfounded.
• Utilizes proteins for the body	• Claims are unfounded.
• Helps develop RBCs and in the function of all cells	• Only strict vegetarians need to supplement their diets with this vitamin.
• Produces collagen • Effective against scurvy • Aids tooth and bone formation • Enhances wound healing • Increases resistance to infection	• Studies are inconclusive concerning this vitamin's association with the common cold. Little is known about the effects of massive dosing with this vitamin. • Claims for other medical uses are unfounded. • Evidence suggests that some effects may be detrimental, such as kidney stones and altered laboratory testing for diabetes.
• Aids bone formation	• Claims are unfounded.
• Acts as a supplement in premature infants who've had poor placental transfer of vitamin E • Effective against anemia and skin conditions in infants deficient in this vitamin • Acts as an antioxidant	• Claims are unfounded. • Adequate amounts are supplied by the average American diet. No evidence exists concerning the consequence on humans of low intake of this vitamin. • Some pharmaceutical researchers are investigating other therapeutic uses.
• Supports proper growth and maintenance	• Although persons extremely deficient in this vitamin experience graying of the hair, massive doses will not retard the graying process for most people.

B complex vitamins with iron
Miscellaneous vitamins and minerals
Geriatric supplements with multivitamins and minerals
Multivitamins and minerals with hormones

NAME	INDICATIONS & DOSAGE	SIDE EFFECTS
oleovitamin A Acon, Afaxin♦♦, Alphalin, Aquasol A♦, Dispatabs, Natola	*Severe vitamin A deficiency with xerophthalmia*— **Adults, and children over 8 years:** 500,000 IU P.O. daily for 3 days, then 50,000 IU P.O. daily for 14 days, then maintenance with 10,000 to 20,000 IU P.O. daily for 2 months, followed by adequate dietary nutrition and RDA vitamin A supplements. *Severe vitamin A deficiency*— **Adults, and children over 8 years:** 100,000 IU P.O. or I.M. daily for 3 days, then 50,000 IU P.O. or I.M. daily for 14 days, then maintenance with 10,000 to 20,000 IU P.O. daily for 2 months, followed by adequate dietary nutrition and RDA vitamin A supplements. **Children 1 to 8 years:** 17,500 to 35,000 IU I.M. daily for 10 days. **Infants under 1 year:** 7,500 to 15,000 IU I.M. daily for 10 days. *Maintenance only*— **Children 4 to 8 years:** 15,000 IU I.M. daily for 2 months, then adequate dietary nutrition and RDA vitamin A supplements. **Children under 4 years:** 10,000 IU I.M. daily for 2 months, then adequate dietary nutrition and RDA vitamin A supplements.	Side effects are usually seen only with toxicity (hypervitaminosis A). **Blood:** hypoplastic anemia, leukopenia. **CNS:** irritability, headache, increased intracranial pressure, fatigue, lethargy, malaise. **EENT:** miosis, papilledema, exophthalmos. **GI:** anorexia, epigastric pain, diarrhea. **GU:** hypomenorrhea. **Skin:** alopecia; drying, cracking, scaling of skin; pruritus; lip fissures; massive desquamation; increased pigmentation; night sweating **Hepatic:** jaundice, hepatomegaly. **Other:** skeletal—slow growth, decalcification of bone, fractures, hyperostosis, painful periostitis, premature closure of epiphyses, migratory arthralgia, cortical thickening over the radius and tibia, bulging fontanelles; splenomegaly.
cyanocobalamin (vitamin B_{12}) Anacobin♦♦, Bedoce, Bedoz♦♦, Berubigen, Betalin-12, Bio-12♦♦, Crystimin, Cyanabin♦♦, Cyanocobalamin, Cyano-Gel, DBH-B_{12}, Dodex, Kaybovite, Neo-Vadrin, Pernavite, Poyamin, Redisol♦, Rhodavite, Rubesol, Rubion♦♦, Rubramin♦, Ruvite,	*Vitamin B_{12} deficiency due to inadequate diet, subtotal gastrectomy, or any other condition, disorder, or disease except malabsorption related to pernicious anemia or other gastrointestinal disease*— **Adults:** 25 mcg P.O. daily as dietary supplement, or 30 to 100 mcg S.C. or I.M. daily for 5 to 10 days, depending on severity of deficiency. Maintenance dose: 100 to 200 mcg I.M. once monthly. For subsequent prophylaxis, advise adequate nutrition	**CV:** peripheral vascular thrombosis. **GI:** transient diarrhea. **Skin:** itching, transitory exanthema, urticaria. **Local:** pain, burning at S.C. or I.M. injection sites. **Other:** *anaphylaxis*, anaphylactoid reactions.

INTERACTIONS	NURSING CONSIDERATIONS
Mineral oil, cholestyramine resin: reduced GI absorption of fat-soluble vitamins. If needed, give mineral oil at bedtime.	• Oral administration contraindicated in presence of malabsorption syndrome; if malabsorption is due to inadequate bile secretion, oral route may be used with concurrent administration of bile salts (dehydrocholic acid). Also contraindicated in hypervitaminosis A. Intravenous administration contraindicated except for special water-miscible forms intended for infusion with large parenteral volumes. Intravenous push of vitamin A of any type is also contraindicated (anaphylaxis or anaphylactoid reactions and death have resulted). • Caution: Evaluate intake from fortified foods, dietary supplements, self-administered drugs, and prescription drug sources. • In pregnant women, avoid doses exceeding 6,000 IU daily. • To avoid toxicity, discourage patient self-administration of megavitamin doses without specific indications. Also stress that the patient should not share prescribed vitamins with family or others. If family member feels vitamin therapy may be of value, have him contact his doctor. • Watch for side effects if dosage is high. • Acute toxicity has resulted from single doses of 25,000 IU/kg of body weight; 350,000 IU in infants and over 2,000,000 IU in adults have also proved acutely toxic. • Chronic toxicity in infants (3 to 6 months) has resulted from doses of 18,500 IU daily for 1 to 3 months. In adults, chronic toxicity has resulted from doses of 50,000 IU daily for over 18 months; 500,000 IU daily for 2 months, and 1,000,000 IU daily for 3 days. • Monitor patient closely during vitamin A therapy for skin disorders since high dosages may induce chronic toxicity. • Liquid preparations available if nasogastric administration is necessary. • Record eating and bowel habits. Report abnormalities to doctor. • Adequate vitamin A absorption requires suitable protein intake, bile (give supplemental salts if necessary), concurrent RDA doses of vitamin E, and zinc (multivitamins usually supply zinc, but supplements may be necessary in long-term hyperalimentation). • Absorption is fastest and most complete with water-miscible preparations, intermediate with emulsions, and slowest with oil suspensions. • In severe hepatic dysfunction, diabetes, and hypothyroidism, use vitamin A rather than carotenes for vitamin therapy because the vitamin itself is more easily absorbed and the diseases adversely affect conversion of carotenes into vitamin A. If carotenes are prescribed, dosage should be doubled. • Protect from light.
Neomycin, colchicine, para-aminosalicylic acid and salts, chloramphenicol: malabsorption of vitamin B_{12}. Don't use together.	• Parenteral administration contraindicated in hypersensitivity to vitamin B_{12} or cobalt. Alternate use of large oral doses of vitamin B_{12} is controversial and should not be considered routine; combined with intrinsic factor increases risk of hypersensitive reactions and should be avoided. Therapeutic dose contraindicated before proper diagnosis; vitamin B_{12} therapy may mask folate deficiency. • I.V. administration may cause anaphylactic reactions. Use cautiously and only if other routes are ruled out. • Use cautiously in anemic patients with coexisting cardiac, pulmonary, or hypertensive disease; in patients with early Leber's disease; in patients with severe vitamin B_{12}–dependent deficiencies, especially those receiving cardiotonic glycosides (monitor closely the first 2 to 3 days for hypokalemia, fluid overload, pulmonary edema, congestive heart failure, and hypertension); and in patients with gouty conditions (monitor serum uric acid levels for hyperuricemia).

(continued on following page)

NAME	INDICATIONS & DOSAGE	SIDE EFFECTS
cyanocobalamin (vitamin B_{12}) *(continued)* Sigamine, Sytobex, Vibedoz, Vi-Twel **cyanocobalamin, hydroxocobalamin (vitamin B_{12a})** Alpha Redisol, Alpha-Ruvite, Codroxomin, Droxomin, Neo-Betalin 12, Rubesol-LA, Sytobex-H	and daily RDA vitamin B_{12} supplements. **Children:** 1 mcg P.O. daily as dietary supplement, or 1 to 30 mcg S.C. or I.M. daily for 5 to 10 days, depending on severity of deficiency. Maintenance: at least 60 mcg per month I.M. or S.C. For subsequent prophylaxis, advise adequate nutrition and daily RDA vitamin B_{12} supplements. *Pernicious anemia or vitamin B_{12} malabsorption—* **Adults:** initially, 100 to 1,000 mcg I.M. daily for 2 weeks, then 100 to 1,000 mcg I.M. once monthly for life. If neurologic complications are present, follow initial therapy with 100 to 1,000 mcg I.M. once every 2 weeks before starting monthly regimen. **Children:** 1,000 to 5,000 mcg I.M. or S.C. given over 2 or more weeks in 100-mcg increments; then 60 mcg I.M. or S.C. monthly for life. *Methylmalonic aciduria—* **Neonates:** 1,000 mcg I.M. daily for 11 days with a protein-restricted diet. *Diagnostic test for vitamin B_{12} deficiency without concealing folate deficiency in patients with megaloblastic anemias—* **Adults and children:** 1 mcg I.M. daily for 10 days with diet low in vitamin B_{12} and folate. Reticulocytosis between days 3 and 10 confirms diagnosis of vitamin B_{12} deficiency. *Schilling test flushing dose—* **Adults and children:** 1,000 mcg I.M. in a single dose.	
folic acid (vitamin B_9) Folvite♦, Novofolacid♦♦	*Megaloblastic or macrocytic anemia secondary to folic acid or other nutritional deficiency, hepatic disease, alcoholism, intestinal obstruction, excessive hemolysis—* **Pregnant and lactating women:** 0.8 mg P.O., S.C., or I.M. daily. **Adults, and children over 4 years:** 1 mg P.O., S.C., or I.M. daily for 4 to 5 days. After ane-	**Skin:** allergic reactions (rash, pruritus, erythema). **Other:** *allergic bronchospasms,* general malaise.

♦ Available in U.S. and Canada. ♦♦ Available in Canada only. All other products (no symbol) available in U.S. only. Italicized side effects are common or life-threatening.

INTERACTIONS	NURSING CONSIDERATIONS
	• Don't mix parenteral liquids in same syringe with other medication. Protect from light. • Repository forms add cost without extra effectiveness and may stimulate antibody formation. • Infection, tumors, or renal, hepatic, and other debilitating diseases may reduce therapeutic response. • Deficiencies more common in strict vegetarians and their breast-fed infants. • Stress need for patients with pernicious anemia to return for monthly injections. Although total body stores may last 3 to 6 years, anemia will recur if not treated monthly. • May cause false-positive intrinsic factor antibody test. • Hydroxocobalamin is approved for I.M. use only. Only advantage of hydroxocobalamin over vitamin B_{12} is longer duration. • 50% to 98% of injected dose may appear in urine within 48 hours. Major portion is excreted within first 8 hours. • Closely monitor serum potassium levels for first 48 hours. Give potassium if necessary. • Physically incompatible with dextrose solutions, alkaline or strongly acidic solutions, oxidizing and reducing agents, and many other drugs. • For treatment of anaphylaxis, see inside front cover.
Chloramphenicol: antagonism of folic acid. Monitor for decreased folic acid effect. Use together cautiously.	• Contraindicated in normocytic, refractory, or aplastic anemias; as sole agent in treatment of pernicious anemia (since it may mask neurologic effects); in treatment of methotrexate, pyrimethamine, or trimethoprim overdose; and in undiagnosed anemia (since it may mask pernicious anemia). • Patients with small-bowel resections and intestinal malabsorption may require parenteral administration routes. • Don't mix with other medications in same syringe for I.M. injections. • Protect from light. • May use concurrent folic acid and vitamin B_{12} therapy if supported by diagnosis.

(continued on following page)

NAME	INDICATIONS & DOSAGE	SIDE EFFECTS
folic acid (vitamin B_9) *(continued)*	mia secondary to folic acid deficiency is corrected, proper diet and RDA supplements are necessary to prevent recurrence. **Children under 4 years:** up to 0.3 mg P.O., S.C., or I.M. daily. *Prevention of megaloblastic anemia of pregnancy and fetal damage—* **Women:** 1 mg P.O., S.C., or I.M. daily throughout pregnancy. *Nutritional supplement—* **Adults:** 0.1 mg P.O., S.C., or I.M. daily. **Children:** 0.05 mg P.O. daily. *Treatment of tropical sprue—* **Adults:** 3 to 15 mg P.O. daily. *Test of megaloblastic anemia patients to detect folic acid deficiency without masking pernicious anemia—* **Adults and children:** 0.1 to 0.2 mg P.O. or I.M. for 10 days while maintaining a diet low in folate and vitamin B_{12}. (Reticulosis, reversion to normoblastic hematopoiesis, and return to normal hemoglobin indicate folic acid deficiency.)	
leucovorin calcium (citrovorum factor or folinic acid) Calcium Folinate	*Overdose of folic acid antagonist—* **Adults and children:** P.O., I.M., or I.V. dose equivalent to the weight of the antagonist given. *Leucovorin rescue after high methotrexate dose in treatment of malignancy—* **Adults and children:** dose at doctor's discretion within 6 to 36 hours of last dose of methotrexate. *Toxic effects of methotrexate used to treat severe psoriasis—* **Adults and children:** 4 to 8 mg I.M. 2 hours after methotrexate dose. *Hematologic toxicity due to pyrimethamine therapy—* **Adults and children:** 5 mg P.O. or I.M. daily. *Hematologic toxicity due to trimethoprim therapy—* **Adults and children:** 400 mcg to 5 mg P.O. or I.M. daily. *Megaloblastic anemia due to*	**Skin:** allergic reactions (rash, pruritus, erythema). **Other:** *allergic bronchospasms.*

♦ Available in U.S. and Canada. ♦♦ Available in Canada only. All other products (no symbol) available in U.S. only. Italicized side effects are common or life-threatening.

INTERACTIONS	NURSING CONSIDERATIONS
	• Proper nutrition is necessary to prevent recurrence of anemia. • Peak folate activity occurs in the blood in 30 to 60 minutes. • Hematologic response to folic acid in patients receiving chloramphenicol concurrently with folic acid should be carefully monitored.
None significant.	• Contraindicated in treatment of undiagnosed anemia, since it may mask pernicious anemia. Use cautiously in pernicious anemia; a hemolytic remission may occur while neurologic manifestations remain progressive. • Do not confuse leucovorin (folinic acid) with folic acid. • Follow leucovorin rescue schedule and protocol closely to maximize therapeutic response. Generally, leucovorin should not be administered simultaneously with systemic methotrexate. • Treat overdosage of folic acid antagonists; administer within 1 hour if possible; usually ineffective after 4-hour delay. • Protect from light and heat, especially reconstituted parenteral preparations. • Since allergic reactions have been reported with folic acid, the possibility of allergic reactions to leucovorin should be considered.

(continued on following page)

NAME	INDICATIONS & DOSAGE	SIDE EFFECTS
leucovorin calcium (citrovorum factor or folinic acid) *(continued)*	*congenital enzyme deficiency—* **Adults and children:** 3 to 6 mg I.M. daily, then 1 mg P.O. daily for life. *Folate-deficient megaloblastic anemias—* **Adults and children:** up to 1 mg of leucovorin I.M daily. Duration of treatment depends on hematologic response.	
niacin (vitamin B_3, nicotinic acid) **niacinamide (nicotinamide)** Diacin, Efacin, Lipo-Nicin, Niac, Nico400, Nicobid, Nicocap, Nicolar, Nico-Span, Ni-Span, Vasotherm, Wampocap	*Pellagra—* **Adults:** 10 to 20 mg P.O., S.C., I.M., or I.V. infusion daily, depending on severity of niacin deficiency. Maximum daily dose recommended, 500 mg; should be divided into 10 doses, 50 mg each. **Children:** up to 300 mg P.O. or 100 mg I.V. infusion daily, depending on severity of niacin deficiency. After symptoms subside, advise adequate nutrition and RDA supplements to avoid recurrence. *Hyperlipoproteinemia types III, IV, and V, and as secondary agent in type II—* **Adults:** up to 1 g 3 or 4 times a day. *Peripheral vascular disease and circulatory disorders—* **Adults:** 250 to 800 mg P.O. daily in divided doses.	Most side effects are dose-dependent. **CNS:** dizziness, transient headache. **CV:** *excessive peripheral vasodilation.* **GI:** *nausea, vomiting, diarrhea,* possible activation of peptic ulcer, epigastric or substernal pain. **Hepatic:** hepatic dysfunction. **Metabolic:** hyperglycemia, hyperuricemia. **Skin:** *flushing,* pruritus, dryness.
pyridoxine hydrochloride (vitamin B_6) Bee six, Hexa-Betalin♦, Hexacrest, Hexavibex♦	*Dietary vitamin B_6 deficiency—* **Adults:** 10 to 20 mg P.O., I.M., or I.V. daily for 3 weeks, then 2 to 5 mg daily as a supplement to a proper diet. **Children:** 100 mg P.O., I.M., or I.V. to correct deficiency, then an adequate diet with supplementary RDA doses to prevent recurrence. *Seizures related to vitamin B_6 deficiency or dependency—* **Adults and children:** 100 mg I.M. or I.V. in single dose. *Vitamin B_6-responsive anemias or dependency syndrome (inborn errors of metabolism)—* **Adults:** up to 600 mg P.O., I.M., or I.V. daily until symptoms subside, then 50 mg daily for life. **Children:** 100 mg I.M. or I.V.,	**CNS:** drowsiness, paresthesias.

♦ Available in U.S. and Canada. ♦♦ Available in Canada only. All other products (no symbol) available in U.S. only. Italicized side effects are common or life-threatening.

INTERACTIONS	NURSING CONSIDERATIONS
Antihypertensive drugs of the sympathetic blocking type: may have an additive vasodilating effect and cause postural hypotension. Use together cautiously. Warn patient about postural hypotension.	• Contraindicated in hepatic dysfunction, active peptic ulcer disease, severe hypotension, arterial hemorrhage. Use with caution in patients with gallbladder disease, diabetes mellitus, gout. • Monitor hepatic function and blood glucose early in therapy. • Give with meals to minimize GI side effects. • Timed-release niacin or niacinamide may avoid excessive flushing effects with large doses. Give slow I.V. Explain harmlessness of flushing syndrome to ease patient's mind. • Stress that medication used to treat hyperlipoproteinemia or to dilate peripheral vessels is not "just a vitamin." Explain importance of adhering to therapeutic regimen.
None significant.	• Contraindicated in hypersensitivity to parenteral pyridoxine and in doses larger than 5 mg for patients also receiving levodopa. Caution patient to check dosage, especially in multivitamins. • Protect from light. Do not use injection solution if it contains a precipitate. Slight darkening is acceptable. • Excessive protein intake increases daily pyridoxine requirements. • If sodium bicarbonate is required to control acidosis in isoniazid toxicity, do not mix in same syringe with pyridoxine. • If prescribed for maintenance therapy to prevent deficiency recurrence, stress importance of compliance and of good nutrition. Explain that pyridoxine in combination therapy with isoniazid has a specific therapeutic purpose and is not "just a vitamin." Emphasize need for adhering to therapeutic regimen. • Patients receiving levodopa alone (not with carbidopa) shouldn't take pyridoxine.

(continued on following page)

NAME	INDICATIONS & DOSAGE	SIDE EFFECTS
pyridoxine hydrochloride (vitamin B_6) *(continued)*	then 2 to 10 mg I.M. or 10 to 100 mg P.O. daily. *Prevention of vitamin B_6 deficiency during isoniazid therapy—* **Adults:** 25 to 50 mg P.O. daily. **Children:** at least 0.5 to 1.5 mg daily. **Infants:** at least 0.1 to 0.5 mg daily. If neurologic symptoms develop in pediatric patients, increase dosage as necessary. *Treatment of vitamin B_6 deficiency secondary to isoniazid—* **Adults:** 100 mg P.O. daily for 3 weeks, then 50 mg daily. **Children:** titrate dosages.	
riboflavin (vitamin B_2)	*Riboflavin deficiency or adjunct to thiamine treatment for polyneuritis or cheilosis secondary to pellagra—* **Adults, and children over 12 years:** 5 to 50 mg P.O., S.C., I.M., or I.V. daily, depending on severity. **Children under 12 years:** 2 to 10 mg P.O., S.C., I.M., or I.V. daily, depending on severity. For maintenance, increase nutritional intake and supplement with vitamin B complex.	**GU:** high doses make urine bright yellow.
thiamine hydrochloride (vitamin B_1) Apatate Drops, Betaline S, Betaxin♦♦, Bewon♦, Megamin♦♦, Thia	*Beriberi—* **Adults:** 10 to 500 mg, depending on severity, I.M. t.i.d. for 2 weeks, followed by dietary correction and multivitamin supplement containing 5 to 10 mg daily thiamine for 1 month. **Children:** 10 to 50 mg, depending on severity, I.M. daily for several weeks with adequate dietary intake. *Anemia secondary to thiamine deficiency; polyneuritis secondary to alcoholism, pregnancy, or pellagra—* **Adults:** 100 mg P.O. daily. **Children:** 10 to 50 mg P.O. daily in divided doses. *Wernicke's encephalopathy—* **Adults:** up to 500 mg to 1 g I.V. for crisis therapy, followed by 100 mg b.i.d. for maintenance.	**CNS:** restlessness. **CV:** *hypotension after rapid I.V. injection,* angioneurotic edema, cyanosis. **EENT:** tightness of throat (allergic reaction). **GI:** nausea, hemorrhage, diarrhea. **Skin:** feeling of warmth, pruritus, urticaria, sweating. **Other:** *anaphylactic reactions,* weakness, pulmonary edema.

INTERACTIONS	NURSING CONSIDERATIONS
None significant.	• Protect from light. • Stress proper nutritional habits to prevent recurrence of deficiency. • Riboflavin deficiency usually accompanies other vitamin B complex deficiencies and may require multivitamin therapy.
None significant.	• Contraindicated in hypersensitivity to thiamine products. I.V. push contraindicated, except when treating life-threatening myocardial failure in "wet beriberi." Use with caution in I.V. administration of large doses (to prevent anaphylactic reactions); skin-test patients with history of hypersensitivity before therapy. Have epinephrine on hand to treat anaphylaxis should it occur after a large parenteral dose. • Use parenteral administration only when P.O. route is not feasible. • Clinically significant deficiency can occur in approximately 3 weeks of totally thiamine-free diet. Thiamine deficiency usually requires concurrent treatment for multiple deficiencies. • Doses larger than 30 mg t.i.d. may not be fully utilized by body. When body tissues are saturated with thiamine, it is excreted in urine as pyrimidine. • If beriberi occurs in a breast-fed infant, both mother and child should be treated with thiamine. • Unstable in alkaline solutions; should not be used with materials that yield alkaline solutions. • For treatment of anaphylaxis, see inside front cover.

(continued on following page)

NAME	INDICATIONS & DOSAGE	SIDE EFFECTS
thiamine hydrochloride (vitamin B_1) *(continued)*	*"Wet beriberi," with myocardial failure—* **Adults and children:** 100 to 500 mg I.V. for emergency treatment.	
ascorbic acid (vitamin C) Adenex♦♦, Ascorbajen, Ascorbicap, Ascorbineed, Ascoril♦♦, Best-C, Cecon, Cemill, Cenolate, Cetane, Cevalin, Cevi-Bid, Ce-Vi-Sol♦, Cevita, Chew-Cee, C-Ject, C-Long, C-Syrup-500, Liqui-Cee, Megascorb♦♦, Redoxon♦♦, Saro-C, Solucap C, Tega-C, Vitacee, Viterra C	*Frank and subclinical manifestations of scurvy—* **Adults:** 100 mg to 2 g, depending on severity, P.O., S.C., I.M., or I.V. daily, then at least 50 mg daily for maintenance. **Children:** 100 to 200 mg, depending on severity, P.O., S.C., I.M., or I.V. daily, then at least 35 mg daily for maintenance. **Infants:** 50 to 100 mg P.O., I.M., I.V., or S.C. daily. *Extensive burns, delayed fracture or wound healing, postoperative wound healing, severe febrile or chronic disease states—* **Adults:** 200 to 500 mg S.C., I.M., or I.V. daily. **Children:** 100 to 200 mg P.O., S.C., I.M., or I.V. daily. *Prevention of vitamin C deficiency in those with poor nutritional habits or increased requirements—* **Adults:** at least 45 to 50 mg P.O., S.C., I.M., or I.V. daily. **Pregnant or lactating women:** at least 60 mg P.O., S.C., I.M., or I.V. daily. **Children:** at least 40 mg P.O., S.C., I.M., or I.V. daily. **Infants:** at least 35 mg P.O., S.C., I.M., or I.V. daily. *Potentiation of methenamine in urine acidification—* **Adults:** 4 to 12 g daily in divided doses. *Preoperatively in patients undergoing gastrectomy—* **Adults:** 1 g daily for 4 to 7 days.	**CNS:** faintness or dizziness with fast I.V. administration. **GI:** diarrhea, epigastric burning. **GU:** acid urine, oxaluria, renal calculi. **Skin:** discomfort at injection site.
vitamin D (cholecalciferol: vitamin D_3; ergocalciferol: vitamin D_2) Calciferol, Deltalin, Drisdol♦, Radiostol♦♦, Radiostol Forte♦♦	*Rickets and other vitamin D deficiency diseases—* **Adults:** 12,000 IU P.O. or I.M. daily initially, increased as indicated by response up to 500,000 IU daily in most cases and up to 800,000 IU daily for vitamin D–resistant rickets. **Children:** 1,500 to 5,000 IU P.O. or I.M. daily for 2 to	Side effects listed are usually seen in vitamin D toxicity only. **CNS:** headache, dizziness, ataxia, weakness, somnolence, decreased libido, overt psychosis, convulsions. **CV:** calcifications of soft tissues, including the heart. **EENT:** dry mouth, metallic taste, rhinorrhea, conjunctivitis (cal-

♦ Available in U.S. and Canada. ♦♦ Available in Canada only. All other products (no symbol) available in U.S. only. Italicized side effects are common or life-threatening.

INTERACTIONS	NURSING CONSIDERATIONS
None significant.	• Use cautiously in G-6-PD deficiency to avoid possibility of hemolytic anemia. • Avoid rapid I.V. administration. • Protect solution from light. • Discourage self-administration for colds; harmful side effects are possible. • I.V. form used investigationally in some cancer centers as adjunct to treat some forms of cancer.
Mineral oil, cholestyramine resin: inhibited GI absorption of oral vitamin D. Space doses. Use together cautiously.	• Contraindicated in hypercalcemia, hypervitaminosis A, renal osteodystrophy with hyperphosphatemia. • If I.V. route is necessary, use only water-miscible solutions intended for dilution in large-volume parenterals. Use cautiously in cardiac patients, especially if they are receiving cardiotonic glycosides. • Monitor eating and bowel habits; dry mouth, nausea, vomiting, metallic taste, and constipation can be early signs of toxicity. • Patients with hyperphosphatemia require dietary phosphate restrictions and binding agents to avoid metastatic calcifications and renal calculi.

(continued on following page)

NAME	INDICATIONS & DOSAGE	SIDE EFFECTS
vitamin D (cholecalciferol: vitamin D_3; ergocalciferol: vitamin D_2) *(continued)*	4 weeks, repeated after 2 weeks, if necessary. Alternatively, a single dose of 600,000 IU. Monitor serum calcium daily to guide dosage. After correction of deficiency, maintenance includes adequate dietary nutrition and RDA supplements. *Hypoparathyroidism*— **Adults and children:** 50,000 to 200,000 IU P.O. or I.M. daily, with 4 g calcium supplement.	cific), photophobia, tinnitus. **GI:** anorexia, nausea, constipation, diarrhea. **GU:** polyuria, albuminuria, hypercalciuria, nocturia, impaired renal function, renal calculi. **Metabolic:** hypercalcemia, hyperphosphatemia. **Skin:** hyperthermia, pruritus, widespread soft-tissue calcification. **Other:** bone and muscle pain, bone demineralization, weight loss.
vitamin E Aquasol E♦, D-Alpha-E, Daltose♦♦, E-Ferol, Eprolin, Epsilan-M, Hy-E-Plex, Kell-E, Lethopherol, Maxi-E, Pertropin, Solucap E, Tocopher-Caps, Tokols, Viterra E	*Vitamin E deficiency in premature infants and in patients with impaired fat absorption*— **Adults:** 60 to 75 IU, depending on severity, P.O. or I.M. daily. Maximum 300 IU daily. **Children:** 1 mg equivalent per 0.6 g of dietary unsaturated fat P.O. or I.M. daily.	None reported.
menadione/ menadiol sodium diphosphate (vitamin K_3) Kappadione, Synkavite♦♦, Synkayvite	*Hypoprothrombinemia secondary to vitamin K malabsorption or drug therapy, or when oral administration is desired and bile secretion is inadequate*— **Adults:** 2 to 10 mg menadione P.O. or 5 to 15 mg menadiol sodium diphosphate P.O. or parenterally, titrated to patient's requirements.	**CNS:** headache, kernicterus. **GI:** nausea, vomiting. **Skin:** allergic rash, pruritus, urticaria. **Local:** pain, hematoma at injection site.
phytonadione (vitamin K_1) AquaMephyton♦, Konakion♦, Mephyton♦	*Hypoprothrombinemia secondary to vitamin K malabsorption, drug therapy, or excess vitamin A*— **Adults:** 2 to 25 mg, depending on severity, P.O. or parenterally,	**CNS:** dizziness, convulsive movement. **CV:** transient hypotension after I.V. administration, rapid and weak pulse, cardiac irregularities. **GI:** nausea, vomiting.

♦ Available in U.S. and Canada. ♦♦ Available in Canada only. All other products (no symbol) available in U.S. only. Italicized side effects are common or life-threatening.

INTERACTIONS	NURSING CONSIDERATIONS
	• Dosage range between therapeutic and toxic effects is narrow. When high therapeutic doses are used, frequent serum and urine calcium, potassium, and urea determinations should be made. • Malabsorption due to inadequate bile or hepatic dysfunction may require addition of exogenous bile salts to oral vitamin D. • Protect solution from light. • This vitamin is fat soluble. Warn patient of the dangers of increasing dosage without consulting the doctor. Also, discourage sharing of this drug: it is not "just a vitamin" and can have serious toxic effects. • Patients taking vitamin D should restrict their intake of magnesium-containing antacids.
Mineral oil, cholestyramine resin: inhibited GI absorption of oral vitamin E. Space doses. Use together cautiously.	• Water-miscible forms more completely absorbed in GI tract than other forms. • Adequate bile is essential for absorption. • Requirements increase with rise in dietary polyunsaturated acids. • May protect other vitamins against oxidation. • Used for a variety of disorders with mixed successes and failures. Dosages not established. • Megadoses can cause thrombophlebitis. • This vitamin is fat soluble. Discourage patient from self-medication with megadoses, as they can cause undesirable side effects.
Mineral oil, cholestyramine resin: inhibited GI absorption of oral vitamin K. Space doses. Use together cautiously.	• Contraindicated in treatment of oral anticoagulant overdose; in treatment of hereditary hypoprothrombinemia (because vitamin K_3 can paradoxically worsen it); in patients with hepatocellular disease, unless it is caused by biliary obstruction; or in treatment of heparin-induced bleeding. Use cautiously during last weeks of pregnancy to avoid toxic reactions in newborns and in G-6-PD deficiency to avoid hemolysis. In severe bleeding, do not delay other measures such as giving fresh frozen plasma or whole blood. Use large doses cautiously in severe hepatic disease. • Failure to respond to vitamin K_3 may indicate coagulation defects. • Excessive use of vitamin K_3 may temporarily defeat oral anticoagulant therapy. Higher doses of oral anticoagulant or interim use of heparin may be required. • Protect parenteral products from light. • When I.V. route must be used, rate shouldn't exceed 1 mg/minute. • Effects of I.V. injections more rapid but shorter lived than S.C. or I.M. injections. • Monitor prothrombin time to determine dosage effectiveness. • Observe for signs of side effects and report them to doctor. • Use caution in handling bulk menadione powder. It is irritating to the skin and the respiratory tract. • Leafy vegetables are high in vitamin K content and may alter warfarin needs. • This vitamin is fat soluble.
Mineral oil, cholestyramine resin: inhibited GI absorption of oral vitamin K. Use together cautiously.	• Contraindicated in hereditary hypoprothrombinemia; bleeding secondary to heparin therapy or overdose; hepatocellular disease, unless it is caused by biliary obstruction (vitamin K can paradoxically worsen the hypoprothrombinemia). Oral administration contraindicated if bile secretion is inadequate, unless supplemented with bile salts. Use cautiously, if at all, during last weeks of pregnancy to avoid

(continued on following page)

NAME	INDICATIONS & DOSAGE	SIDE EFFECTS
phytonadione (vitamin K_1) *(continued)*	repeated and increased up to 50 mg, if necessary. **Children:** 5 to 10 mg P.O. or parenterally. **Infants:** 2 mg P.O. or parenterally. I.V. injection rate for children and infants should not exceed 3 mg/m²/minute or a total of 5 mg. *Hypoprothrombinemia secondary to effect of oral anticoagulants—* **Adults:** 2.5 to 10 mg P.O., S.C., or I.M., based on prothrombin time, repeated, if necessary, 12 to 48 hours after oral dose or 6 to 8 hours after parenteral dose. In emergency, give 10 to 50 mg slow I.V., rate not to exceed 1 mg/minute, repeated q 4 hours, as needed. *Prevention of hemorrhagic disease in neonates—* **Neonates:** 0.5 to 1 mg S.C. or I.M. immediately after birth, repeated in 6 to 8 hours, if needed, especially if mother received oral anticoagulants or long-term anticonvulsant therapy during pregnancy. *Differentiation between hepatocellular disease or biliary obstruction as source of hypoprothrombinemia—* **Adults and children:** 10 mg I.M. or S.C. *Prevention of hypoprothrombinemia related to vitamin K deficiency in long-term parenteral nutrition—* **Adults:** 5 to 10 mg S.C. or I.M. weekly. **Children:** 2 to 5 mg S.C. or I.M. weekly. *Prevention of hypoprothrombinemia in infants receiving less than 0.1 mg/liter vitamin K in breast milk or milk substitutes—* **Infants:** 1 mg S.C. or I.M. monthly.	**Skin:** sweating, flushing, erythema. **Local:** pain, swelling, and hematoma at injection site. **Other:** bronchospasms, dyspnea, cramp-like pain, *anaphylaxis and anaphylactoid reactions, usually after rapid I.V. administration.*
multivitamins Available by many brand names. Contain vitamins A, B complex, C, D, and	*Prevention of vitamin deficiencies in patients with inadequate diets or increased daily requirements; treatment of multiple vitamin deficiencies and*	• Multivitamin preparations with ordinary doses of each component are usually nontoxic. • Megavitamin combinations may promote significant accumulation

INTERACTIONS	NURSING CONSIDERATIONS
	toxic reactions in newborns; in G-6-PD deficiency to avoid hemolysis. Use large doses cautiously in severe hepatic disease. • Failure to respond to vitamin K may indicate coagulation defects. • In severe bleeding, don't delay other measures such as fresh frozen plasma or whole blood. • Protect parenteral products from light. Wrap infusion container with aluminum foil. • Effects of I.V. injections more rapid but shorter lived than S.C. or I.M. injections. • Monitor prothrombin time to determine dosage effectiveness. • Observe for signs of side effects and report them to the doctor. • Phytonadione therapy for hemorrhagic disease in infants causes fewer adverse reactions than do other vitamin K analogs. • Check brand name labels for administration route restrictions. • Administer I.V. by slow infusion (over 2 to 3 hours). Mix in normal saline solution, dextrose 5% in water, or dextrose 5% in normal saline solution. Observe patient closely for signs of flushing, weakness, tachycardia, and hypotension; may progress to shock. • Leafy vegetables are high in vitamin K content and may alter warfarin needs. • This vitamin is fat soluble. • For treatment of anaphylaxis, see inside front cover.
Refer to each component of the multivitamin combination.	• A single discovered vitamin deficiency usually coexists with others. After initial deficiencies are corrected, stress need for adequate nutrition and multivitamin supplements, if appropriate. • Tell patient about possible interactions of vitamins in combinations and what precautions to take to avoid problems.

(continued on following page)

NAME	INDICATIONS & DOSAGE	SIDE EFFECTS
multivitamins *(continued)* E in varying amounts.	*prevention of recurrence; additions to parenteral nutrition solutions to meet patient's normal or increased requirements to reduce cost and facilitate patient compliance with therapy for multiple vitamin deficiencies*— **Adults and children:** dosage depends on nature and severity of deficiencies and composition of multivitamin preparation.	of fat-soluble vitamins, with resultant toxicity. • Multivitamins containing therapeutic doses of folic acid may mask pernicious anemia. Unless prescribed otherwise by doctor, patient should avoid folic acid in undiagnosed but suspected pernicious anemia. • Other side effects depend on specific components and concentrations in each multivitamin preparation.
sodium fluoride Flo-Tabs, Fluor-A-Day ♦♦, Fluoritabs, Flura-Drops, Karidium♦, Luride Lozi-Tabs, Pediaflor, Pedi-Dent♦, Studafluor	*Aid in the prevention of dental caries*— Oral— **Children 3 years and under:** 0.5 mg daily. **Children over 3 years:** 1 mg daily. Topical— **Children 6 to 12 years:** 5 ml. **Adults, and children over 12 years:** 10 ml. Use once daily after thoroughly brushing teeth and rinsing mouth. Rinse around and between teeth for 1 minute, then spit out.	**CNS:** headaches, weakness. **GI:** gastric distress. **Skin:** hypersensitivity reactions such as atopic dermatitis, eczema, and urticaria.
trace elements chromium, copper, iodine (as iodide), manganese, zinc	*Prevention of individual trace element deficiencies in patients receiving long-term hyperalimentation*— *Chromium*— **Adults:** 10 to 15 mcg I.V. daily. **Children:** 0.14 to 0.20 mcg/kg I.V. daily. *Copper*— **Adults:** 0.5 to 1.5 mg I.V. daily. **Children:** 0.05 to 0.2 mg/kg I.V. daily. *Iodine*— **Adults:** 1 mcg/kg I.V. daily. *Manganese*— **Adults:** 1 to 3 mg I.V. daily. *Zinc*— **Adults:** 2 to 4 mg I.V. daily. **Children:** 0.05 mg/kg I.V. daily.	None reported.
zinc sulfate Orazinc	*Treatment of zinc deficiency or adjunct to treatment of disorders related to low serum zinc levels, including oral and decubitus leg ulcers, acne, granu-*	**GI:** distress and irritation, nausea, vomiting with high doses.

INTERACTIONS	NURSING CONSIDERATIONS
	• Stress need to follow doctor's orders regarding daily dosages and follow-up therapy. • Avoid excessive use of large-volume parenteral solutions of multivitamin supplements containing fat-soluble vitamins to prevent hypervitaminosis. I.V. solutions of water-soluble multivitamins may be used more freely. • Chewable flavored multivitamins available for children. Prevent use of these drugs as candy. • Liquid preparations may contain varying percentages of alcohol. Check label; alert patient to content. • Warn against overdosing. Encourage patient to eat a well-balanced diet. Stress hazards of self-administered megadoses of vitamins. These medications are drugs, not just harmless vitamins. Explain possible side effects. • Store vitamins in a cool place in light-resistant containers to limit loss of potency.
None significant.	• Contraindicated when fluoride intake from drinking water exceeds 0.7 ppm; sodium-free diets. • Chronic toxicity (fluorosis) may result from prolonged use of higher than recommended doses. • Intended for use only where community water supplies are not fluoridated. • Advise patient to notify dentist if tooth mottling occurs. • Tablets may be dissolved in mouth, chewed, or swallowed whole. • Drops may be administered orally undiluted or mixed with fluids or food. • Topical forms (rinses and gels) should not be swallowed. Most effective when used immediately after brushing teeth. • Tell patient to dilute drops or rinses in plastic containers rather than glass. • Used investigationally in the treatment of osteoporosis.
None significant at recommended dosages.	• Check trace element serum levels of patients who have received total parenteral nutrition for 2 months or longer. Give supplement if ordered. Call doctor's attention to low serum levels of these elements. • Normal serum levels are 0.07 to 0.15 mg/ml copper; 0.05 to 0.15 mg/100 ml zinc; 4 to 20 mcg/100 ml manganese. • Solutions of trace elements are compounded by pharmacy for addition to total parenteral nutrition solutions according to various formulas. One common trace element solution is Shil's solution, which contains copper 1 mg/ml, iodide 0.06 mg/ml, manganese 0.4 mg/ml, and zinc 2 mg/ml.
None significant.	• Therapeutic benefits result only if patient is zinc-deficient. • Normal serum levels may not reliably show absence of zinc deficiency. • Results may not appear for 6 to 8 weeks in zinc-depleted patients. • If nausea or other GI side effects occur, decreasing dosage to

(continued on following page)

NAME	INDICATIONS & DOSAGE	SIDE EFFECTS
zinc sulfate *(continued)*	*lomata of the ear, rheumatoid arthritis, idiopathic hypogeusia, anosmia; also, as adjunct to vitamin A therapy when patient fails to respond to vitamin A alone and in acrodermatitis enteropathica*— **Adults:** 200 to 220 mg P.O. t.i.d. (equivalent to 135 to 150 mg elemental zinc daily, 9 times the adult RDA of 15 mg daily). **Children:** dosages not established. RDA is 0.3 mg/kg daily.	

INTERACTIONS	NURSING CONSIDERATIONS
	100 mg b.i.d. may help, since zinc is thought to irritate gastric mucosa. • Brown bread and dairy products may hinder zinc absorption.

POSSIBLE EFFECTS OF TOO MUCH OF A VITAMIN

Many people believe that taking megadoses of vitamins—doses much higher than recommended—promotes good health, vitality, youthfulness, and well-being. But taking such megadoses, especially of the fat-soluble vitamins A, D, and E, can be harmful unless supervised by a doctor. In some cases, less severe effects of vitamin overdose, such as diarrhea and headaches, may appear first. But more severe effects may result if vitamin overdosage isn't remedied.

Here are some possible effects of excessive vitamin intake:

Vitamin A *(continued daily intake of more than 50,000 IU)*
- Dry, coarse, scaly skin
- Fissures in the lips
- Pruritus
- Sore mouth and tongue
- Clubbed fingers
- Rash or pigmentation
- Insomnia
- Low-grade fever
- Headaches
- Bone pain and stunted bone growth
- Painful swelling under the skin
- Urinary frequency
- Hypoplastic anemia
- Leukopenia
- Liver and spleen enlargement (with possibly permanent liver damage)
- Increased intracranial pressure

Vitamin D *(continued daily intake of more than 50,000 IU)*
- Weakness
- Fatigue
- Headache
- Nausea and vomiting
- Hypercalcemia
- Calcified soft tissues
- Osteoporosis
- Kidney stones
- Rapid deterioration in kidney function
- Retarded mental and physical growth in children

Vitamin C *(continued daily intake of more than 2,000 mg)*
- Diarrhea
- Kidney stones
- Scurvy in infants soon after birth (when megadoses were taken by mother during pregnancy)
- Interference with vitamin B_{12} absorption

Niacin *(nicotinic acid)*
- Flushing
- Pruritus
- Rash
- Heartburn
- Nausea and vomiting
- Ulcer activation
- Hypotension
- Tachycardia
- Syncope
- Hyperglycemia
- Abnormal liver function and possibly jaundice

Note: The FDA has proposed that some minerals not be made available over the counter because deficiency is rare. Other minerals—copper, iodine, iron, potassium, and manganese—can be dangerous at two to ten times their recommended dose.

99 Calorics

amino acid solution
corn oil
dextrose (D-glucose)
essential crystalline amino acid solution
fat emulsions
fructose (levulose)
invert sugar
medium-chain triglycerides

Calorics are nutrients that furnish calories for metabolic energy, promote protein synthesis, and prevent essential fatty acid deficiency.

Major uses

Rx Calorics supply calories to establish a positive nitrogen balance. Each caloric component provides energy for the patient's basal metabolic expenditure.

• Amino acids are used to supply protein for the protein-depleted patient.
• Carbohydrates (dextrose, fructose, and invert sugar) are a source of energy for central nervous system functions, hematopoiesis, and renal metabolism.

Fructose and invert sugar also furnish partial fluid replacement.

• Fat emulsions contain the essential fatty acids linoleic and linolenic acids. These are useful both as calorie sources and as treatment of essential fatty acid deficiency. Linoleic acid also prevents dermatologic scaling.

Medium-chain triglycerides are used as an oral calorie source in patients who suffer from fat malabsorption.

Mechanism of action

• Amino acids are used for protein synthesis of the viscera and skeletal muscle in the protein-depleted patient.
• I.V. carbohydrates minimize glyconeogenesis and promote anabolism in patients who can't receive sufficient oral caloric intake. I.V. solutions of dextrose, fructose, and invert sugar supply the energy equivalent of 3.4 kcal/g.
• Fat emulsions, administered I.V., contribute essential fatty acids and a denser calorie source (1.1 kcal/ml) than proteins or carbohydrates.

Medium-chain triglycerides provide a denser oral calorie source than proteins or carbohydrates in the patient who absorbs fat poorly.

Absorption, distribution, metabolism, and excretion

Calorics are rapidly absorbed and utilized by the body.

• Carbohydrates are, as the renal threshold is exceeded, excreted in the urine.
• The essential fatty acids are metabolized to water and carbon dioxide and are excreted through the urine and perspiration.
• Amino acids are not excreted as such. The nitrogen portion of the amino acid molecule, however, is excreted in urine as urea nitrogen.

Onset and duration

• Anabolism may develop 1 to 5 days after initiation of total parenteral nutrition, which is meant to exceed the patient's basal energy expenditure. Daily replenishment will ensure continued anabolism.

Combination products

DEXTROSE 2½%, 5%, 10% and sodium chloride 0.45%.

DEXTROSE 2½%, 5%, 10% and sodium chloride 0.9%.

DEXTROSE 3⅓% and sodium chloride 0.3%.

DEXTROSE 5% and sodium chloride 0.11%, 0.2%, 0.33%.

POTASSIUM CHLORIDE 10 mEq, 20 mEq, 27 mEq, 30 mEq, 40 mEq, in 5% dextrose in water.

POTASSIUM CHLORIDE 10 mEq, 20 mEq, 30 mEq, 40 mEq in 5% dextrose, and 0.2% sodium chloride.

POTASSIUM CHLORIDE 10 mEq, 20 mEq, 30 mEq, 40 mEq in 5% dextrose, and 0.45% sodium chloride.

DEXTROSE 5% WITH ELECTROLYTE #75: 50 g/L dextrose, 40 mEq/L Na^+, 35 mEq/L K^+, 40 mEq/L Cl^-, 15 mEq/L phosphate, and 20 mEq/L lactate.

ISOLYTE M WITH 5% DEXTROSE: 50 g/L dextrose, 40 mEq/L Na^+, 35 mEq/L K^+, 40 mEq/L Cl^-, 15 mEq/L phosphate, and 20 mEq/L acetate.

ISOLYTE G WITH 5% DEXTROSE: 50 g/L dextrose, 63 mEq/L Na^+, 17 mEq/L K^+, and 150 mEq/L Cl^-.

IONOSOL G IN 10% DEXTROSE: 100 g/L dextrose, 63 mEq/L Na^+, 17 mEq/L K^+, and 151 mEq/L Cl^-.

ISOLYTE G WITH 10% DEXTROSE: 100 g/L dextrose, 63 mEq/L Na^+, 17 mEq/L K^+, and 150 mEq/L Cl^-.

DEXTROSE 2.5% IN HALF-STRENGTH RINGER'S: 25 g/L dextrose, 74 mEq/L Na^+, 2 mEq/L K^+, 2 mEq/L Ca^{++}, and 78 mEq/L Cl^-.

DEXTROSE 5% IN RINGER'S: 50g/L dextrose, 147 mEq/L Na^+, 4 mEq/L K^+, 4 mEq/L Ca^{++}, and mEq/L 155 Cl^-.

DEXTROSE 2½% IN HALF-STRENGTH LACTATED RINGER'S: 25 g/L dextrose, 65 mEq/L Na^+, 2 mEq/L K^+, 1 mEq/L Ca^{++}, 54 mEq/L Cl^-, and 14 mEq/L lactate.

DEXTROSE 2½% IN LACTATED RINGER'S: 25 g/L dextrose, 130 mEq/L Na^+, 4 mEq/L K^+, 3 mEq/L Ca^{++}, 109 mEq/L Cl^-, and 28 mEq/L lactate.

DEXTROSE 5% IN LACTATED RINGER'S: 50 g/L dextrose, 130 mEq/L Na^+, 4 mEq/L K^+, 3 mEq/L Ca^{++}, 109 mEq/L Cl^-, and 28 mEq/L lactate.

DEXTROSE 10% IN LACTATED RINGER'S: 100 g/L dextrose, 130 mEq/L Na^+, 4 mEq/L K^+, 3 mEq/L Ca^{++}, 109 mEq/L Cl^-, and 28 mEq/L lactate.

DEXTROSE 5% IN ACETATED RINGER'S: 50 g/L dextrose, 130 mEq/L Na^+, 4 mEq/L K^+, 3 mEq/L Ca^{++}, 109 mEq/L Cl^-, and 28 mEq/L acetate.

DEXTROSE 5% WITH ELECTROLYTE #48: 50 g/L dextrose, 25 mEq/L Na^+, 20 mEq/L K^+, 3 mEq/L Mg^{++}, 22 mEq/L Cl^-, 3 mEq/L phosphate, and 23 mEq/L lactate.

IONOSOL MB IN 5% DEXTROSE: 50 g/L dextrose, 25 mEq/L Na^+, 20 mEq/L K^+, 3 mEq/L Mg^{++}, 22 mEq/L Cl^-, 3 mEq/L phosphate, and 23 mEq/L lactate.

IONOSOL B IN 5% DEXTROSE: 50 g/L dextrose, 57 mEq/L Na^+, 25 mEq/L K^+, 5 mEq/L Mg^{++}, 49 mEq/L Cl^-, 13 mEq/L phosphate, and 25 mEq/L lactate.

POLYONIC M-56 IN 5% DEXTROSE: 50 g/L dextrose, 40 mEq/L dextrose, 40 mEq/L Na^+, 13 mEq/L K^+, 3 mEq/L Mg^{++}, 40 mEq/L Cl^-, and 16 mEq/L acetate.

PLASMA-LYTE 56 IN 5% DEXTROSE: 50 g/L dextrose, 40 mEq/L Na^+, 13 mEq/L K^+, 3 mEq/L Mg^{++}, 40 mEq/L Cl^-, and 16 mEq/L acetate.

ISOLYTE P WITH 5% DEXTROSE: 50 g/L dextrose, 25 mEq/L Na^+, 20 mEq/L K^+, 3 mEq/L Mg^{++}, 22 mEq/L Cl^-, 3 mEq/L phosphate, and 23 mEq/L acetate.

ISOLYTE S WITH 5% DEXTROSE: 50 g/L dextrose, 140 mEq/L Na^+, 5 mEq/L K^+, 3 mEq/L Mg^{++}, 98 mEq/L Cl^-, and 27 mEq/L acetate.

PLASMA-LYTE 148 IN DEXTROSE: 50 g/L dextrose, 140 mEq/L Na^+, 5 mEq/L K^+, 3 mEq/L Mg^{++}, 98 mEq/L Cl^-, and 27 mEq/L acetate.

POLYONIC R-148 IN 5% DEXTROSE: 50 g/L dextrose, 140 mEq/L Na^+, 5 mEq/L K^+, 3 mEq/L mg^{++}, 98 mEq/L Cl^-, and 27 mEq/L acetate.

NAME	INDICATIONS & DOSAGE	SIDE EFFECTS
amino acid solution (crystalline amino acid solution) Aminosyn, Travasol♦, Veinamine	*Total, supportive, or supplemental and protein-sparing parenteral nutrition when gastrointestinal system must rest during healing, or when patient can't, shouldn't, or won't eat at all or eat enough to maintain normal nutrition and metabolism—* **Adults:** 1 to 1.5 g/kg I.V. daily. **Children:** 2 to 3 g/kg I.V. daily. Individualize dosage to metabolic and clinical response as determined by nitrogen balance and body weight corrected for fluid balance. Add electrolytes, vitamins, and nonprotein caloric solutions as needed.	**CNS:** mental confusion, unconsciousness, headache, dizziness. **CV:** hypervolemia related to congestive heart failure (in susceptible patients), *pulmonary edema,* exacerbation of hypertension (in predisposed patients). **GI:** nausea, vomiting. **GU:** glycosuria, osmotic diuresis. **Hepatic:** fatty liver. **Metabolic:** *rebound hypoglycemia* (when long-term infusions are abruptly stopped), *hyperglycemia,* metabolic acidosis, alkalosis, hypophosphatemia, *hyperosmolar syndrome, hyperosmolar-hyperglycemic-nonketotic syndrome,* hyperammonemia, *electrolyte imbalances,* and dehydration (if hyperosmolar solutions used). **Skin:** chills, flushing, feeling of warmth. **Local:** tissue sloughing at infusion site due to extravasation, *catheter sepsis, thrombophlebitis, thrombosis.* **Other:** allergic reactions.
corn oil Lipomul♦	*As energy source—* **Adults:** 45 ml P.O. b.i.d. to q.i.d. after or between meals, alone or with proteins, milk, or other energy sources. **Children:** 30 ml P.O. daily to q.i.d. after or between meals, alone or with proteins, milk, or other energy sources.	**GI:** nausea, vomiting, diarrhea.
dextrose (D-glucose)	*Fluid replacement and caloric supplementation in patient who can't maintain adequate oral intake or who is restricted from doing so—* **Adults and children:** dosage depends on fluid and caloric requirements. Use peripheral I.V. infusion of 2.5%, 5%, or 10% solution, central I.V. infusion of 20% solution for minimal fluid	**CNS:** mental confusion, unconsciousness in hyperosmolar syndrome. **CV:** (with fluid overload) pulmonary edema, exacerbated hypertension, and congestive heart failure in susceptible patients. *Prolonged or concentrated infusions may cause phlebitis, sclerosis of vein, especially with peripheral route of administration.*

♦ Available in U.S. and Canada. ♦♦ Available in Canada only. All other products (no symbol) available in U.S. only. Italicized side effects are common or life-threatening.

INTERACTIONS	NURSING CONSIDERATIONS
None significant.	• Contraindicated in patients with severe uncorrected electrolyte or acid-base imbalances, in hyperammonemia, and in decreased circulating blood volume. Use cautiously in renal insufficiency or failure, cardiac disease, and hepatic impairment. Long-term use for infants and children must be closely monitored. • Monitor serum electrolytes, magnesium, glucose, BUN, renal and hepatic function. Check serum calcium levels frequently to avoid bone demineralization in children. • If long-term therapy is needed, doctor may order trace element and vitamin supplements. Avoid overuse of fat-soluble vitamins A and D—can cause toxic hypervitaminosis. • Refrigerate solution until ½ hour before it will be infused. • Don't mix medications, except electrolytes, vitamins, and trace elements with hyperalimentation solution without first consulting pharmacist. • Control infusion rate carefully with infusion pump. • If infusion rate falls behind, do not attempt to "catch up." Notify doctor. • Check infusion site frequently for erythema, inflammation, irritation, tissue sloughing, necrosis, and phlebitis. Change I.V. sites routinely to prevent irritation and infection. I.V. catheter is usually introduced into subclavian vein. • Watch closely for signs of fluid overload. Notify doctor promptly. • Some crystalline amino acid solutions contain large amounts of acetates and lactates; use cautiously in patients with alkalosis or hepatic insufficiency. • Most side effects are due to mixing amino acids with hypertonic dextrose solutions. • Check fractional urines every 6 hours for glycosuria (if present, the doctor may order insulin coverage). • Assess body temperature every 4 hours; elevation may indicate sepsis, infection. • If patient has chills, fever, or other signs of sepsis, replace I.V. tubing and bottle and send them to the laboratory to be cultured. • For additional information on hyperalimentation, see Chapter 7, PARENTERAL AND ENTERAL NUTRITION.
Griseofulvin: increased GI absorption of griseofulvin. Space doses.	• Contraindicated in gallbladder calculi or complete GI obstructions. Use cautiously in steatorrhea, partial GI obstruction, enterostomies, hepatic cirrhosis, portacaval shunts. • To minimize nausea, diarrhea, and vomiting, give more frequent, smaller doses with meals or mixed with milk.
None significant.	• Contraindicated in hyperglycemia, diabetic coma, intracranial or intraspinal hemorrhage, delirium tremens. Use cautiously in cardiac or pulmonary disease, hypertension, renal insufficiency, urinary obstruction, or hypovolemia. • Control infusion rate carefully. Maximal rate for dextrose infusion is 0.5 g/kg/hour. Use infusion pump when infusing dextrose with amino acids for total parenteral nutrition. • Never infuse concentrated solutions rapidly; can cause hyperglycemia, fluid shift. • Never stop abruptly. If necessary, have 10% dextrose solution available to treat hypoglycemia if rebound hyperinsulinemia occurs.

(continued on following page)

NAME	INDICATIONS & DOSAGE	SIDE EFFECTS
dextrose *(continued)*	needs. Use 50% solution to treat insulin-induced hypoglycemia. Solutions from 40% to 70% are used diluted in admixtures, normally with amino acid solutions, for total parenteral nutrition given through a central vein.	**GU:** glycosuria, osmotic diuresis. **Metabolic:** (with rapid infusion of concentrated solution or prolonged infusion) hyperglycemia, hypervolemia, hyperosmolarity. Rapid termination of long-term infusions may cause hypoglycemia from rebound hyperinsulinemia. **Skin:** sloughing and tissue necrosis, if extravasation occurs with concentrated solutions.
essential crystalline amino acid solution Nephramine	*Management of potentially reversible renal decompensation*— **Adults:** 0.3 to 0.5 g/kg I.V., up to 26 g total daily (250 ml with 500 ml 70% dextrose injection), and infuse through central I.V. line at initial rate of 20 to 30 ml/hour, increased in steps of 10 ml/hour every 24 hours, to a maximum of 60 to 100 ml/hour. Individualize dose and infusion rate to tolerance for glucose, fluid, and nitrogen. Add electrolytes and vitamins as needed. **Children:** up to 1 g/kg daily, individualized to patient's tolerance for glucose, fluid, and nitrogen. Add electrolytes, trace elements, and vitamins as needed.	**CNS:** mental confusion, dizziness, unconsciousness, headache. **CV:** hypervolemia related to congestive heart failure (in susceptible patients), *pulmonary edema,* exacerbation of hypertension (in predisposed patients). **GI:** nausea, vomiting. **GU:** glycosuria, osmotic diuresis. **Metabolic:** *rebound hypoglycemia* (when long-term infusions are abruptly stopped), *hyperglycemia,* metabolic acidosis, alkalosis, hypophosphatemia, hyperosmolar syndrome, *hyperosmolar-hyperglycemic-nonketotic syndrome,* hyperammonemia, *electrolyte imbalances,* and dehydration (if hyperosmolar solutions used). **Skin:** chills, flushing, feeling of warmth. **Local:** tissue sloughing at infusion site due to extravasation, *catheter sepsis, thrombophlebitis.* **Other:** allergic reactions.
fat emulsions Intralipid♦, Liposyn	**Intralipid:** *Source of calories adjunctive to total parenteral nutrition*— **Adults:** 1 ml/minute I.V. for 15 to 30 minutes. If no adverse reactions, increase rate to deliver 500 ml over 4 hours. Infuse	**Early reactions of fat overload:** **Blood:** hyperlipemia, hypercoagulability, rarely thrombocytopenia in neonates. **CNS:** headache, sleepiness, dizziness. **EENT:** pressure over eyes.

INTERACTIONS	NURSING CONSIDERATIONS
	• Monitor serum glucose carefully. Prolonged therapy with 5% dextrose solution can cause depletion of pancreatic insulin production and secretion. • Take care to prevent extravasation. Check injection site frequently to prevent irritation, tissue sloughing, necrosis, and phlebitis. • Watch closely for signs of fluid overload, especially if fluid intake is restricted. • Monitor intake/output and weight carefully, especially when renal function is impaired. • Check vital signs frequently. Report side effects promptly. • Don't give dextrose solutions without saline with blood transfusions; may cause clumping of red blood cells.
None significant.	• Contraindicated in severe uncorrected electrolyte or acid-base imbalances, hyperammonemia, and decreased circulating blood volume. • Monitor serum electrolytes, magnesium, glucose, BUN, renal and hepatic function. Check serum calcium levels frequently to avoid bone demineralization in children. • In long-term therapy, doctor may order trace element and vitamin supplements. Avoid overuse of fat-soluble vitamins. • Refrigerate solution until ½ hour before it will be infused. • Don't mix medications, except electrolytes, vitamins, and trace elements with hyperalimentation solution without first consulting pharmacist. • Control infusion rate carefully with infusion pump. • If infusion rate falls behind, do not attempt to "catch up." Notify doctor. • Check infusion site frequently for erythema, inflammation, irritation, tissue sloughing, necrosis, and phlebitis. Change I.V. sites routinely to prevent irritation. I.V. catheter is usually placed in subclavian vein. • Watch closely for signs of fluid overload. Notify doctor promptly. • Essential amino acid solution is used identically to other crystalline amino acid solutions, except that it contains only the essential amino acids. By controlling amino acid content, patients with impaired renal function have decreases in blood urea nitrogen level, minimized deterioration of serum potassium, magnesium, and phosphorus balances. May lead to earlier return of renal function in patients with potentially reversible acute renal failure and may decrease morbidity associated with acute renal failure. • Most side effects due to mixing essential crystalline amino acid solution with hypertonic dextrose solutions. • Check fractional urines every 6 hours for glycosuria (if present, the doctor may order insulin coverage). • Assess body temperature every 4 hours; elevation may indicate sepsis, infection. • If patient has chills, fever, or other signs of sepsis, replace I.V. tubing and bottle and send them to the laboratory to be cultured. • For additional information on hyperalimentation, see Chapter 7, PARENTERAL AND ENTERAL NUTRITION.
None significant.	• Contraindicated in hyperlipemia, lipid nephrosis, and acute pancreatitis accompanied by hyperlipemia. Use cautiously in severe hepatic disease, pulmonary disease, anemia, blood coagulation disorders, or patients with possible danger of fat embolism. • Never mix with electrolytes or other nutrient products or dilute manufactured fat emulsions. Infusion may be piggybacked into another I.V. line, but do not place additives in the fat emulsion bottle.

(continued on following page)

NAME	INDICATIONS & DOSAGE	SIDE EFFECTS
fat emulsions *(continued)*	only 1,500-ml unit the first day. Total daily dose should not exceed 2.5 g/kg (25 ml/kg 10% emulsion). **Children:** 0.1 ml/minute for 10 to 15 minutes. If no adverse reactions, increase rate to deliver 10 ml/kg over 4 hours. Daily dose should not exceed 4 g/kg (40 ml/kg 10% emulsion). Equals 60% of daily caloric intake. Protein-carbohydrate hyperalimentation should supply remaining 40%. *Fatty acid deficiency—* **Adults and children:** 8% to 10% of total caloric intake I.V. **Liposyn:** *Prevention of fatty acid deficiency—* **Adults:** 500 ml I.V. twice weekly. Infuse initially at a rate of 1 ml/minute for 30 minutes. Rate may be increased but should not exceed 500 ml over 4 to 6 hours. **Children:** 5 to 10 ml/kg I.V. daily. Infuse initially at a rate of 0.1 ml/minute for 30 minutes. Rate may be increased but should not exceed 100 ml/hour.	**GI:** nausea, vomiting. **Skin:** flushing, diaphoresis. **Local:** irritation at infusion site. **Other:** fever, dyspnea, chest and back pains, cyanosis, allergic reactions, deposition of I.V. fat. **Delayed reactions:** **Blood:** thrombocytopenia, leukopenia, leukocytosis. **CNS:** focal seizures. **CV:** shock. **Hepatic:** transient increased liver function test, hepatomegaly. **Other:** fever, splenomegaly.
fructose (levulose)	*Source of carbohydrate calories primarily when fluid replacement is also indicated and as a dextrose substitute for patients with diabetes—* **Adults and children:** dosage depends on caloric needs. I.V. infusion rate should not exceed 1 g/kg/hour. Single liter 10% solution yields 375 calories.	**CV:** increased pulse rate, precipitation or exacerbation of congestive heart failure in susceptible patients, *pulmonary edema.* **Hepatic:** hepatomegaly. **Metabolic:** metabolic acidosis, hypervolemia. **Local:** extravasation at infusion site may cause sloughing of skin, thrombophlebitis. **Other:** increased respiratory rate.
invert sugar Travert	*Nonelectrolyte fluid replacement and caloric supplementation solution—* **Adults and children:** dosage depends on patient's age, weight, clinical need. I.V. infusion rate should not exceed 1 g/kg/hour. Single liter 5% invert sugar yields 375 calories.	**CNS:** mental confusion. **CV:** increased pulse rate, precipitation or exacerbation of congestive heart failure in susceptible patients, *pulmonary edema,* hypertension. **GU:** glycosuria, osmotic diuresis. **Metabolic:** metabolic acidosis, hypervolemia, hyperglycemia, hypoglycemia. **Local:** extravasation at infusion site may cause sloughing of skin, thrombophlebitis. **Other:** increased respiratory rate.

INTERACTIONS	NURSING CONSIDERATIONS
	• Do not use an in-line filter when administering this drug because the fat particles are larger than the 0.22-micron cellulose filter. • Discard fat emulsion if it separates or becomes oily. Intralipid may be refrigerated, although refrigeration is not essential. Liposyn needs no refrigeration. • Avoid rapid infusion. Use an infusion pump to regulate rate. • Check injection site daily. Report signs of inflammation or infection promptly. • Watch closely for side effects, especially during first half hour of infusion. • Monitor serum lipids closely when patient is receiving fat emulsion therapy. Lipemia must clear between dosing. • Check platelet count frequently in neonates receiving fat emulsions I.V. • Monitor hepatic function carefully in long-term use. • Intralipid and Liposyn differ mainly by their fatty acid components.
None significant.	• Contraindicated in hereditary fructose intolerance or in patients receiving therapy for hypoglycemia. Use cautiously in cardiac disease, hypertension, pulmonary disease, hypervolemia, renal insufficiency, or urinary tract obstructions. • Control infusion rate carefully. Make sure rate does not exceed 1 g/kg/hour in infants. • Change infusion sites regularly to avoid irritation with prolonged therapy. Take care to avoid extravasation. • Watch closely for signs of fluid overload, pulmonary edema, or congestive heart failure. • May be safely used in patients with diabetes.
None significant.	• Contraindicated in hereditary fructose intolerance, hyperglycemia, diabetic coma, intracranial or intraspinal hemorrhage, or delirium tremens. Use cautiously in cardiac disease, hypertension, pulmonary disease, hypervolemia, renal insufficiency, or urinary tract obstructions. • Control infusion rate carefully. Make sure rate does not exceed 1 g/kg/hour in infants. • Change infusion sites regularly to avoid irritation with prolonged therapy. Take care to avoid extravasation. • Watch closely for signs of fluid overload, pulmonary edema, or congestive heart failure. Monitor blood pressure frequently. • May be safely used in patients with diabetes. • Monitor serum glucose closely. Prolonged therapy can cause depletion of pancreatic insulin production and secretion.

(continued on following page)

NAME	INDICATIONS & DOSAGE	SIDE EFFECTS
invert sugar *(continued)*		
medium-chain triglycerides M.C.T. Oil♦	*Inadequate digestion or absorption of food fats*— **Adults:** 15 ml P.O. t.i.d. to q.i.d.	**CNS:** reversible coma and precoma in susceptible patients. **GI:** *nausea, vomiting, diarrhea.*

INTERACTIONS	NURSING CONSIDERATIONS
	• Don't stop abruptly. If necessary, have 10% dextrose available to prevent rebound hyperinsulinemia and subsequent hypoglycemia. • Monitor intake/output and weight closely, especially if renal function is impaired. • Check vital signs frequently. Tell doctor promptly if side effects develop.
None significant.	• Contraindicated in advanced hepatic disease. • To minimize GI side effects, give smaller doses more frequently with meals or mixed with fruit juice or salad dressing. • More easily absorbed than long-chain fats; not dependent on bile salts for emulsification. • Rapid metabolism provides quick energy. • May be useful in obesity control and in lowering cholesterol levels. Also used in patients with short-bowel syndrome.

DRUG ALERT

I.V. LIPIDS CAN THREATEN PREMATURE INFANTS

The risks of I.V. lipids can equal and even outweigh potential benefits for premature infants. Because a number of infants have died following this treatment, each patient must be carefully evaluated before receiving these emulsions.

Evidence indicates that I.V. lipids sharply increase susceptibility to infection, a particular hazard for the unstable premature infant. I.V. lipids also appear to cause life-threatening fat buildup in the pulmonary capillaries, even when infusion rates are well under the recommended maximum and when serum tests show no lipemia.

Infants who are preterm and small for gestational age have diminished ability to metabolize lipids and shouldn't receive more than the recommended dosage of 4 g/kg/day. To decrease the chance of I.V. fat overload, the doctor may decide to order less than this maximum recommended dose. Infusion should be as slow as possible, not exceeding the recommended rate of 1 g/kg/4 hours (0.25 g/kg/hour).

When initiating the infusion, watch the infant closely for signs of acute hypersensitivity: dyspnea, tachypnea, wheezing, palpitations, cyanosis, fever, shivering, and vomiting. If any occur, stop the infusion and notify the doctor immediately.

Carefully monitor the infant's serum triglycerides and plasma free fatty acid levels to determine whether infused fat is being eliminated from the infant's circulation. If lipemia doesn't clear before the next infusion is to be administered, notify the doctor immediately.

Premature infants with a bilirubin level greater than 5 mg/100 ml shouldn't receive I.V. fat emulsions.

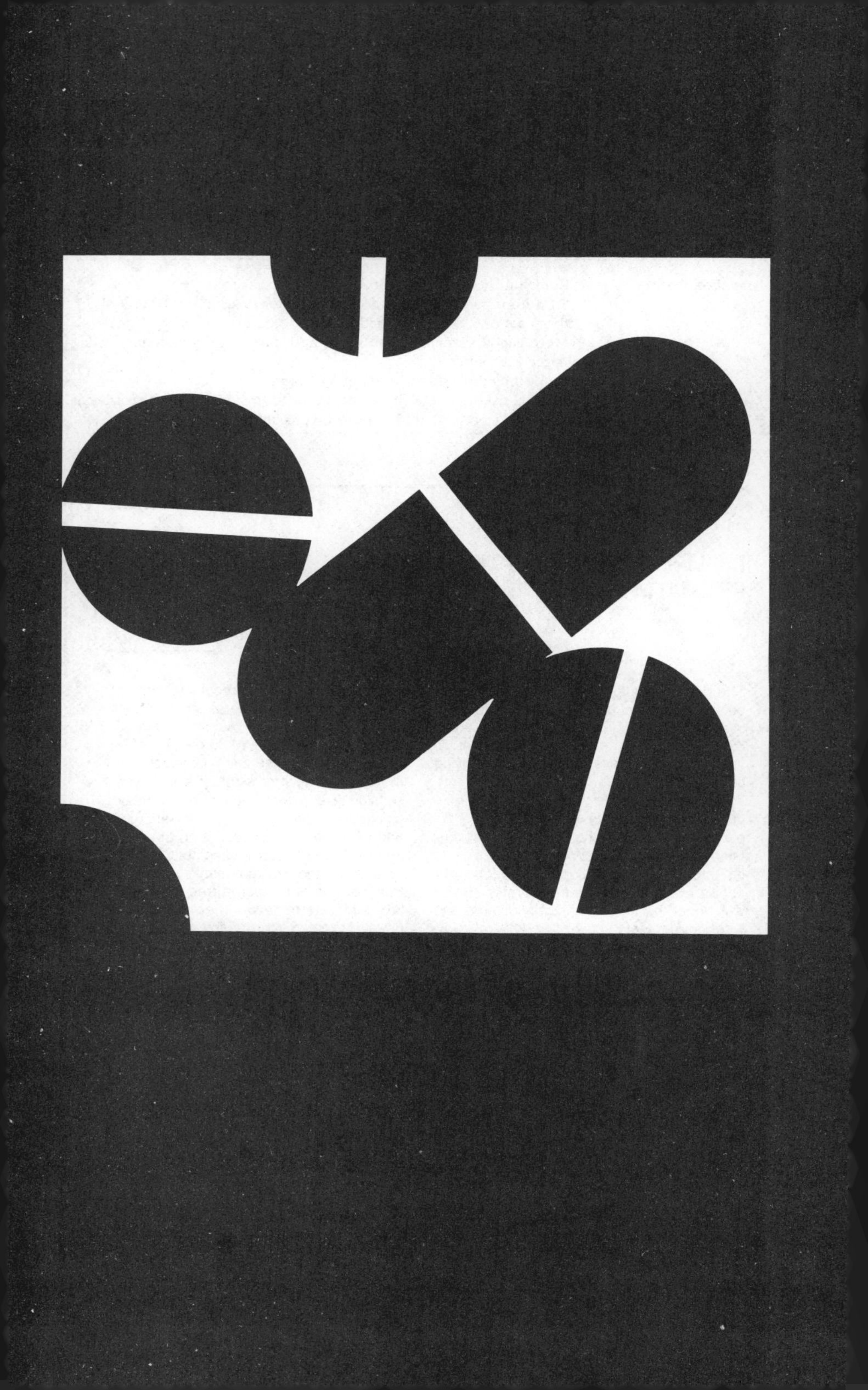

XVI Miscellaneous Drug Categories

100 Immune serums

antirabies serum, equine
hepatitis B immune globulin, human
immune serum globulin
rabies immune globulin, human
Rh_O (D) immune globulin, human
tetanus immune globulin, human

Immune serums provide passive immunity against various infectious diseases or suppress antibody formation, as in Rh incompatibility. Immune serum globulins are obtained from hyperimmunized human or animal donors, or pooled plasma. These products are then purified and standardized. Immune serums are effective only for prophylaxis.

Major uses

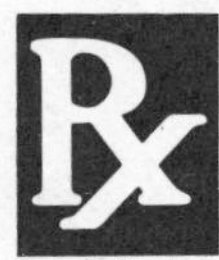

Immune serums prevent various infectious diseases; they may relieve symptoms after suspected exposure (postexposure prophylaxis). They also prevent formation of active antibodies, as in Rh_o-negative, D^u-negative mothers who deliver Rh_o-positive or D^u-positive infants, or in transfusion accidents.

Mechanism of action

Immune serums contain preformed protective substances (antibodies) from the serum of human beings or animals, especially horses, that have been immunized by injection with the organisms or toxins of diseases. These antibodies, therefore, combat specific diseases.

Absorption, distribution, metabolism, and excretion

Not applicable.

Onset and duration

Onset of passive immunity is immediate but duration is temporary, generally lasting about 3 to 4 weeks after immunization.

Combination products

None.

COMPARING ACTIVE AND PASSIVE IMMUNITY

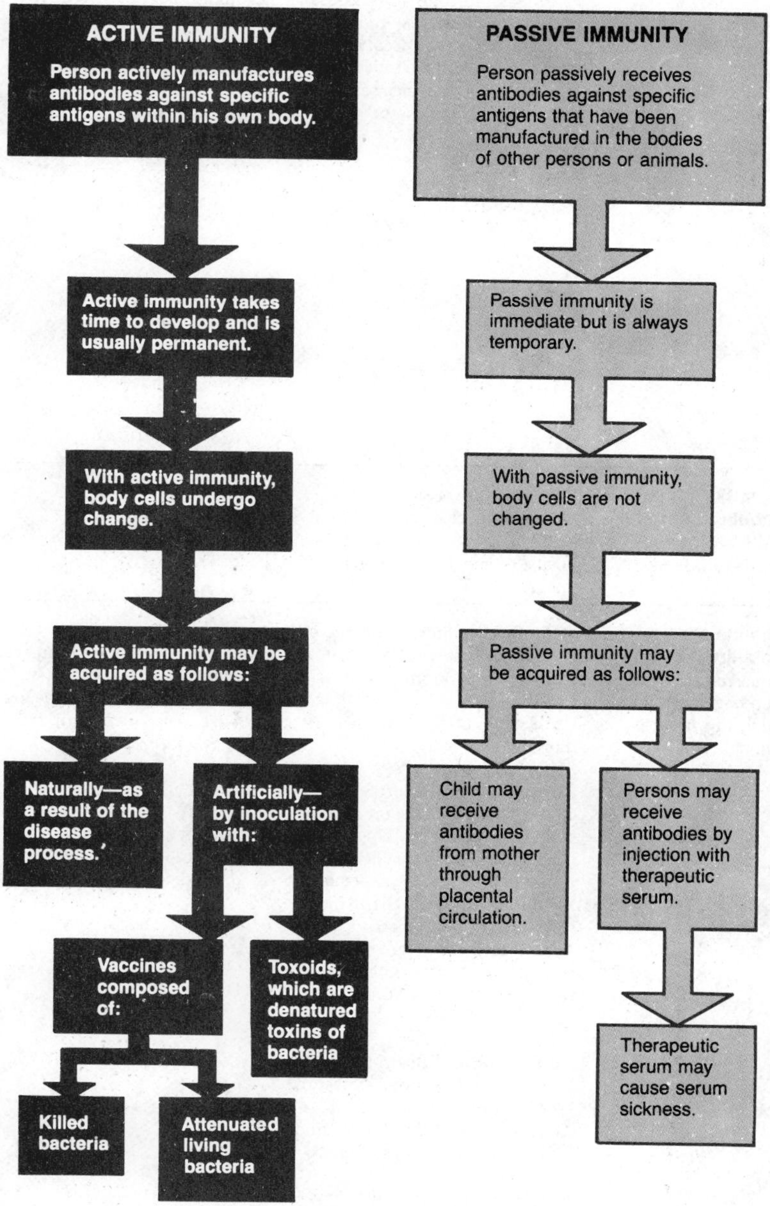

ACTIVE IMMUNITY

Person actively manufactures antibodies against specific antigens within his own body.

Active immunity takes time to develop and is usually permanent.

With active immunity, body cells undergo change.

Active immunity may be acquired as follows:

- Naturally—as a result of the disease process.
- Artificially—by inoculation with:
  - Vaccines composed of:
    - Killed bacteria
    - Attenuated living bacteria
  - Toxoids, which are denatured toxins of bacteria

PASSIVE IMMUNITY

Person passively receives antibodies against specific antigens that have been manufactured in the bodies of other persons or animals.

Passive immunity is immediate but is always temporary.

With passive immunity, body cells are not changed.

Passive immunity may be acquired as follows:

- Child may receive antibodies from mother through placental circulation.
- Persons may receive antibodies by injection with therapeutic serum.
  - Therapeutic serum may cause serum sickness.

Used with permission from Joan Luckmann and Karen C. Sorensen, *Medical-Surgical Nursing* (Philadelphia: W.B. Saunders Co., 1980).

NAME	INDICATIONS & DOSAGE	SIDE EFFECTS
antirabies serum, equine	*Rabies exposure*— **Adults and children:** 40 to 55 units/kg at time of first dose of rabies vaccine. Use half dose to infiltrate wound area. Give remainder I.M. Don't give rabies vaccine and antirabies serum in same syringe or at same site.	**Local:** pain at injection site. **Systemic:** within 6 to 12 days serum sickness occurs in 15% to 25% of patients. Symptoms are skin eruptions, arthralgia, pruritus, lymphadenopathy, fever, headache, malaise, abdominal pain, *anaphylaxis.*
hepatitis B immune globulin, human H-BIG, HyperHep, Hep-B-Gammagee	*Hepatitis B exposure*— **Adults and children:** 0.06 ml/kg I.M. within 7 days after exposure. Repeat 28 days after exposure.	**Systemic:** *anaphylaxis.*
immune serum globulin Gamastan, Gammagee, Gammar, Gamulin, Immu-G, Immuglobin	*Agammaglobulinemia or hypogammaglobulinemia*— **Adults:** 30 to 50 ml I.M. monthly. **Children:** 20 to 40 ml I.M. monthly. *Hepatitis A exposure*— **Adults and children:** 0.02 to 0.04 ml/kg I.M. as soon as possible after exposure. Up to 0.1 ml/kg may be given after prolonged or intense exposure. *Serum hepatitis post-transfusion*— **Adults and children:** 10 ml I.M. within 1 week after transfusion and 10 ml I.M. 1 month later. *Measles exposure*— **Adults and children:** 0.02 ml/kg within 6 days after exposure. *Modification of measles*— **Adults and children:** 0.04 ml/kg I.M. within 6 days after exposure. *Measles vaccine complications*— **Adults and children:** 0.02 to 0.04 ml/kg I.M.	**Skin:** urticaria. **Local:** pain, erythema, muscle stiffness. **Systemic:** angioedema, headache, malaise, fever, nephrotic syndrome, *anaphylaxis.*

♦ Available in U.S. and Canada. ♦♦ Available in Canada only. All other products (no symbol) available in U.S. only. Italicized side effects are common or life-threatening.

INTERACTIONS	NURSING CONSIDERATIONS
None significant.	• In hypersensitivity to equine serum, use rabies immune globulin, human, instead. If unavailable, desensitize before giving. Consult doctor or pharmacist. • Do sensitivity test on all patients before giving. Dilute serum 1:100 or 1:1,000 with 0.9% sodium chloride for injection. Inject intradermally on inner forearm. Inject other arm with 0.1 ml of 0.9% sodium chloride for injection intradermally as control. Read within 20 minutes. Positive reaction: wheal 10 mm or more and erythematous flare 20 × 20 mm. • Use only when rabies immune globulin, human, not available. • Obtain history of animal bite, allergies (especially to equine serum and to eggs), and reaction to immunization. • Epinephrine solution 1:1,000 should always be available when administering this drug. • This immune serum provides immediate passive immunity (short-term). • Do not confuse this drug with rabies vaccine, which is a suspension of attenuated or killed microorganisms used to confer long-term active immunity. These two drugs are often administered together prophylactically after exposure to known or suspected rabid animals. • Ask patient when he received last tetanus immunization, since many doctors order a booster at this time. • For treatment of anaphylaxis, see inside front cover.
None significant.	• Buttocks or deltoid areas preferred injection sites. • Nurse should receive immunization if exposed to hepatitis B (for example, needle-stick, direct contact). • Obtain history of allergies and reaction to immunization. • For treatment of anaphylaxis, see inside front cover.
None significant.	• Obtain history of allergies and reaction to immunization. • Have drugs available for anaphylactic reaction. • Divide dose of more than 10 ml, and inject into different sites, preferably buttocks. Do not inject more than 3 ml per injection site. • Do not give for hepatitis A exposure if 6 weeks or more have elapsed since exposure or after onset of clinical illness. • For treatment of anaphylaxis, see inside front cover.

(continued on following page)

NAME	INDICATIONS & DOSAGE	SIDE EFFECTS
immune serum globulin *(continued)*	*Poliomyelitis exposure—* **Adults and children:** 0.3 to 0.4 ml/kg I.M. within 7 days after exposure. *Chickenpox exposure—* **Adults and children:** 0.2 to 1.3 ml/kg I.M. as soon as exposed. *Rubella exposure in first trimester of pregnancy—* **Women:** 0.2 to 0.4 ml/kg I.M. as soon as exposed.	
rabies immune globulin, human Hyperab	*Rabies exposure—* **Adults and children:** 20 IU/kg at time of first dose of rabies vaccine. Use half dose to infiltrate wound area. Give remainder I.M. Don't give rabies vaccine and rabies immune globulin in same syringe or at same site.	**Local:** pain, redness, induration at injection site. **Other:** slight fever, *anaphylaxis.*
Rh_O (D) immune globulin, human Gamulin R, HypRho-D, MICRhoGAM, RhoGam	*Rh exposure—* **After abortion, miscarriage, ectopic pregnancy, or delivery:** transfusion unit or blood bank determines fetal packed red blood cell volume entering woman's blood, then gives one vial I.M. if fetal packed RBC volume is less than 15 ml. More than one vial I.M. may be required if there is large fetomaternal hemorrhage. Must be given within 72 hours after delivery or miscarriage. *Transfusion accidents—* **Adults and children:** consult blood bank or transfusion unit at once. Must be given within 72 hours. *Postabortion or postmiscarriage to prevent Rh antibody formation—* **Women:** consult transfusion unit or blood bank. Ideally should be given within 3 hours, but may be given up to 72 hours after abortion or miscarriage.	**Local:** discomfort at injection site. **Other:** slight fever.

INTERACTIONS	NURSING CONSIDERATIONS
None significant.	• Repeated doses contraindicated after rabies vaccine is started. • Use only with rabies vaccine and immediate local treatment of wound. Give regardless of interval between exposure and initiation of therapy. • Obtain history of animal bite, allergies, reaction to immunization. • Corticosteroids decrease resistance to infection and decrease antibody response to vaccine. Stop corticosteroids after possible rabies exposure. • This immune serum provides passive immunity. • Do not confuse this drug with rabies vaccine, which is a suspension of attenuated or killed microorganisms used to confer active immunity. These two drugs are often given together prophylactically after exposure to known or suspected rabid animals. • Ask the patient when he received his last tetanus immunization, since many doctors order a booster at this time. • For treatment of anaphylaxis, see inside front cover.
None significant.	• Contraindicated in Rh_o (D)-positive or D^u-positive patients and those previously immunized to Rh_o (D) blood factor. • Immediately after delivery, send a sample of infant's cord blood to laboratory for type and crossmatch. Confirm mother is Rh_o (D)-negative and D^u-negative. Infant must be Rh_o (D)-positive or D^u-positive. • Give only to postpartum mother, not infant. • Obtain history of allergies and reaction to immunization. • MICRhoGAM recommended for every woman undergoing abortion or miscarriage up to 12 weeks' gestation unless she is Rh_o (D)-positive or D^u-positive, has Rh antibodies, or the father and/or fetus is Rh-negative. • For I.M. use only. • Store at 2° to 8° C. (36° to 46° F.). Do not freeze. • This immune serum provides passive immunity to the woman exposed to Rh_o-positive fetal blood during pregnancy. Prevents formation of maternal antibodies (active immunity), which would endanger future Rh_o-positive pregnancies. • Explain to the patient how drug protects future Rh_o-positive infants (see Rh isoimmunization diagram).

NAME	INDICATIONS & DOSAGE	SIDE EFFECTS
tetanus immune globulin, human Homo-Tet, Hu-Tet, Hyper-Tet, Immu-Tetanus, T-I-Gammagee	*Tetanus exposure*— **Adults and children:** 250 units I.M. *Tetanus treatment*— **Adults and children:** single doses of 3,000 to 6,000 units have been used, but optimal dosage schedules not established. Do not give at same site as toxoid.	**Local:** pain, stiffness, erythema. **Other:** slight fever, allergy, *anaphylaxis.*

INTERACTIONS	NURSING CONSIDERATIONS
None significant.	• Use tetanus immune globulin only if wound is over 24 hours old or patient has had less than two previous tetanus toxoid injections. • Obtain history of injury, tetanus immunizations, last tetanus toxoid injection, allergies, and reaction to immunization. • Thoroughly cleanse and remove all foreign matter from wound. • This immune serum provides passive immunity. Antibodies remain at effective levels for 3 weeks or longer, which is several times the duration of antitoxin-induced antibodies. Protects the patient for the incubation period of most tetanus cases. • Human globulin is not a substitute for tetanus toxoid, which should be given at the same time to produce active immunization. • Do not confuse this drug with tetanus toxoid. • For treatment of anaphylaxis, see inside front cover.

THE FACTS ABOUT RH ISOIMMUNIZATION

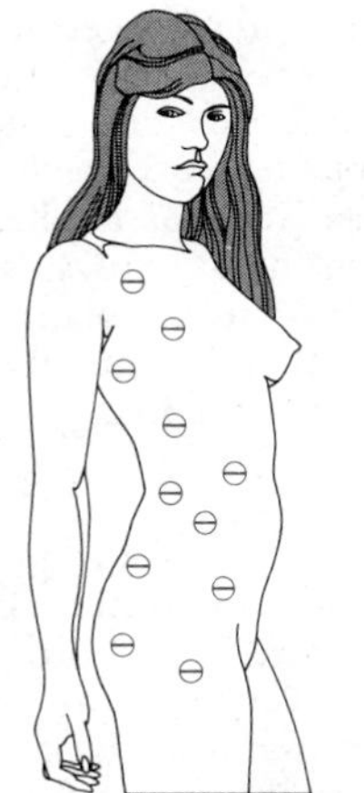

1. Rh-negative woman prepregnancy.

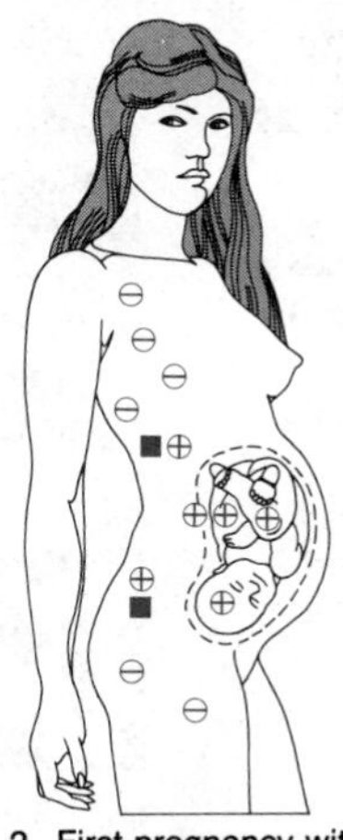

2. First pregnancy with Rh-positive fetus.

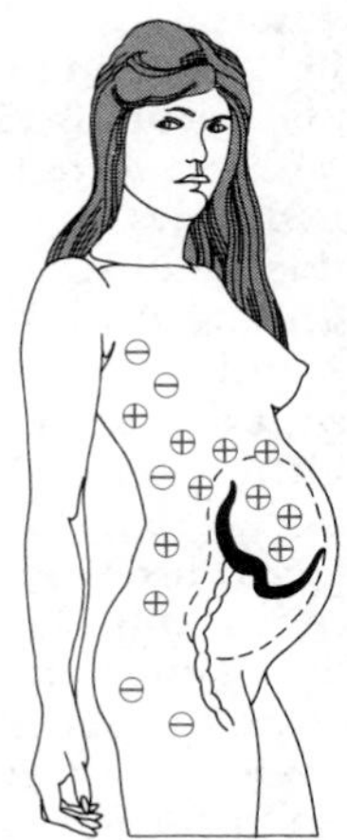

3. Placental separation.

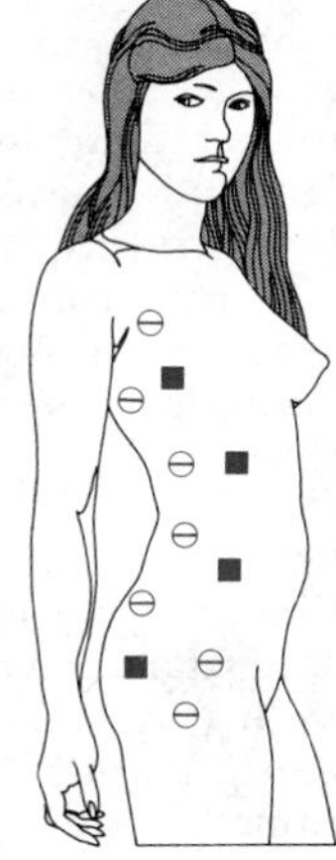

4. Postdelivery, mother becomes sensitized to Rh-positive blood and develops anti-Rh-positive antibodies (darkened squares).

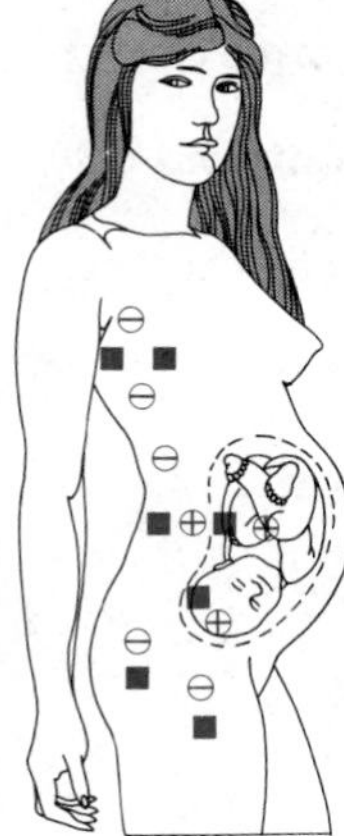

5. During next pregnancy with Rh-positive fetus, maternal anti-Rh-positive antibodies enter fetal circulation, attach to Rh-positive RBCs, and subject them to hemolysis.

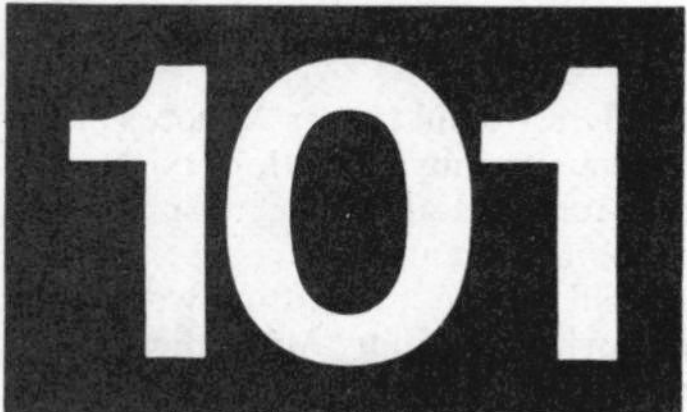

Vaccines and toxoids

BCG vaccine
cholera vaccine
diphtheria and tetanus toxoids, adsorbed
diphtheria and tetanus toxoids and pertussis vaccine (DPT)
diphtheria toxoid, adsorbed, pediatric
influenza virus vaccine, trivalent
influenza virus, trivalent types A and B
measles, mumps, and rubella virus vaccine, live
measles (rubeola) and rubella virus vaccine, live attenuated
measles (rubeola) virus vaccine, live attenuated
meningitis vaccines
mumps virus vaccine, live
plague vaccine
pneumococcal vaccine, polyvalent
poliovirus vaccine, live, oral, trivalent
rabies vaccine (duck embryo), dried, killed virus
rabies vaccine, human diploid cell (HDCV)
rubella and mumps virus vaccine, live
rubella virus vaccine, live attenuated (RA 27/3)
smallpox vaccine
staphylococcus toxoid
tetanus toxoid, adsorbed
tetanus toxoid fluid
typhoid vaccine
typhus vaccine
yellow fever vaccine

Vaccines and toxoids provide active immunity against certain bacterial and viral diseases. Vaccines contain killed or attenuated living microorganisms that stimulate the formation of antibodies. Toxoids contain exotoxins (heat-labile, proteinaceous toxins formed by bacteria and secreted outside the bacterial cell). These substances are chemically changed to make them nontoxic, but they retain the ability to stimulate antitoxin (antibody) formation.

Major uses

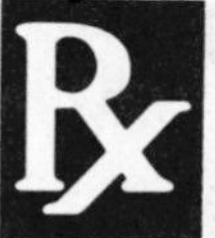

Vaccines and toxoids prevent certain infectious diseases and childhood diseases. They also prevent diseases that are transmitted through injury or animal bite, such as tetanus and rabies.

Mechanism of action

Vaccines and toxoids initiate formation of specific antibodies by stimulating the host's antigen-antibody mechanism, providing active, acquired immunity. (Active immunity can be induced by exposure to an infectious disease or to one of its antigens, or by vaccination.)

Onset and duration

Onset of active immunity is not immediate. Antibody production doesn't reach immunity-providing levels for a few days to a few weeks. Duration of immunity is long, lasting for years.

IMMUNIZATIONS FOR TRAVELERS

Dear Patient:

When planning a trip abroad, you need to know which immunizations are required by the countries you'll visit. Legal requirements for entry and epidemiologic conditions in different countries may vary. Here are some general guidelines:

VACCINE	WHO SHOULD RECEIVE
Tetanus and diphtheria	Everyone, whether traveling or not, should have a booster injection every 10 years.
Polio	Travelers not previously immunized should receive primary immunization series; previously immunized travelers to rural/remote areas of tropical or developing countries should receive one additional dose of vaccine.
Measles	Persons born after 1957 who haven't received vaccine and don't have a history of infection
Hepatitis A	Travelers to developing countries who are going beyond normal tourist routes or staying 3 months or longer
Yellow fever	Travelers to infected areas (check with local health department); some countries require vaccination for travelers from infected areas.
Typhoid	Travelers to rural areas of tropical countries and any area of outbreak
Plague	Travelers to interior regions of Vietnam, Democratic Kampuchea, and the Lao People's Democratic Republic
Typhus	Travelers to remote highland areas of Bolivia, Ecuador, Guatemala, Mexico, Peru, Burundi, Ethiopia, and Rwanda, or mountainous areas of Asia
Rabies	Travelers anticipating contact with possibly infected animals
Cholera	Not generally recommended for tourists, but some countries require it for travelers from infected areas
Smallpox	Many countries require evidence of vaccination for entry.
Malaria chemoprophylaxis	Travelers to malarious areas should make sure adequate chemoprophylaxis is available.

For more information write for Health Information for International Travel, *by the Center for Disease Control (U.S. Government Printing Office, Washington, D.C. 20402).*

NAME	INDICATIONS & DOSAGE	SIDE EFFECTS
BCG vaccine	*Tuberculosis exposure, cancer immunotherapy—* **Adults and children:** 0.1 ml intradermally. **Newborns:** 0.05 ml intradermally.	**Local:** lymphangitis, lymph node and skin abscess, ulceration at site of injection (2 to 3 weeks after injection), lupus reaction. **Other:** urticaria of trunk and limbs, *anaphylaxis.*
cholera vaccine	*Primary immunization—* **Adults, and children over 10 years:** 2 doses of 0.5 ml I.M. or 1 ml S.C., 1 week to 1 month before traveling in cholera area. Booster: 0.5 ml q 6 months as long as protection is needed. **Children 5 to 10 years:** 0.3 ml I.M. or S.C. **Children 6 months to 4 years:** 0.2 ml I.M. or S.C. Boosters of same dose should be given q 6 months as long as protection needed.	**Systemic:** malaise, fever, flushing, urticaria, tachycardia, hypotension, headache, *anaphylaxis.* **Local:** erythema, swelling, pain, induration.
diphtheria and tetanus toxoids, adsorbed	*Primary immunization—* **Adults, and children 7 years and over:** use adult strength; 0.5 ml I.M. 4 to 6 weeks apart for 2 doses and a third dose 1 year later. Booster: 0.5 ml I.M. q 10 years. **Children under 7 years:** use pediatric strength; 0.5 ml I.M. 4 to 8 weeks apart for 2 doses and a third dose 6 to 12 months later. Booster: 0.5 ml when starting school.	**Systemic:** chills, fever, malaise, *anaphylaxis.* **Local:** stinging, edema, erythema, pain, induration.
diphtheria and tetanus toxoids and pertussis vaccine (DPT) Tri-Immunol,	*Primary immunization—* **Children 6 weeks to 6 years:** 0.5 ml I.M. 2 months apart for 3 doses and a fourth dose 1 year later. Booster: 0.5 ml I.M. when	**Systemic:** slight fever, chills, malaise, *convulsions, encephalopathy, anaphylaxis.* **Local:** soreness, redness, expected nodule remaining several weeks.

♦ Available in U.S. and Canada. ♦♦ Available in Canada only. All other products (no symbol) available in U.S. only. Italicized side effects are common or life-threatening.

INTERACTIONS	NURSING CONSIDERATIONS
Isoniazid (INH): inhibited multiplication of BCG. Avoid using together.	• Contraindicated in patients with hypogammaglobulinemia, positive tuberculin reaction (when meant for use as immunoprophylactic after exposure to tuberculosis), immunosuppression, fresh smallpox vaccination, and burns, and in those receiving corticosteroid therapy. Use cautiously in chronic skin disease. Inject in area of healthy skin only. • Obtain history of allergies and reaction to immunization. • Vaccine is of no value as immunoprophylactic in patients with positive tuberculin test. • Keep epinephrine 1:1,000 available to treat anaphylaxis. • Recommended injection site is over insertion of deltoid muscle. • Do not shake vial following reconstitution. • Expected lesion forms in 7 to 10 days. • Live vaccine; destroy by autoclaving or formaldehyde solution before disposal. • Patient should have tuberculin skin test 2 to 3 months after BCG vaccination to determine success of vaccine. • Use of BCG has shown some value in treatment of various cancers such as leukemia, some lung cancers, malignant melanoma, multiple myeloma, and some breast tumors. Currently, researchers are trying to find ways of augmenting the immune system's response to cancer. They hope to stimulate the body to destroy tumor cells. • For treatment of anaphylaxis, see inside front cover.
None significant.	• Contraindicated in corticosteroid therapy or in immunosuppression. Defer in acute illness. • Obtain history of allergies and reaction to immunization. • Keep epinephrine 1:1,000 available. • May be given intradermally, but I.M. and subcutaneous routes give higher levels of protection. • For treatment of anaphylaxis, see inside front cover.
None significant.	• Contraindicated in immunosuppression, radiation, or corticosteroid therapy. Defer in respiratory illness or polio outbreaks, or acute illness except in emergency. Use single antigen during polio risks. In children under 6 years, use only when diphtheria, tetanus, and pertussis toxoid combination is contraindicated because of pertussis component. • Verify strength (pediatric or adult) of toxoid used. • Don't use hot or cold compresses; may increase severity of local reaction. • Obtain history of allergies and reaction to immunization. • Keep epinephrine 1:1,000 available. • Give in site not previously used for vaccines or toxoids. • For treatment of anaphylaxis, see inside front cover.
None significant.	• Contraindicated in corticosteroid therapy or immunosuppression. Defer in acute illness. • Stop immunization if CNS disorder occurs. Immunization may be continued with diphtheria and tetanus toxoids without pertussis component at doses of 0.05 to 0.1 ml.

(continued on following page)

NAME	INDICATIONS & DOSAGE	SIDE EFFECTS
diphtheria and tetanus toxoids and pertussis vaccine (DPT) *(continued)* Triogen, Triple Antigen	starting school. Not advised for adults, or children over 6 years.	
diphtheria toxoid, adsorbed, pediatric	*Diphtheria immunization—* **Children under 6 years:** 0.5 ml I.M. 6 to 8 weeks apart for 2 doses and a third dose 1 year later. Booster: 0.5 ml I.M. at 5- to 10-year intervals. Not advised for adults or for children over 6 years; instead, use adult strength of diphtheria toxoid (usually combined with tetanus toxoid).	**Systemic:** fever, malaise, urticaria, tachycardia, flushing, pruritus, hypotension, aches and pains, *anaphylaxis.* **Local:** erythema, pain, induration, expected nodule persistent for several weeks.
influenza virus vaccine, trivalent Fluax♦♦, Fluogen♦, Fluzone-Connaught **influenza virus, trivalent types A & B**	*Brazil, Bangkok, and Singapore influenza prophylaxis—* **Adults 28 years and over:** 0.5 ml whole or split virus I.M. Use adult formula. **Youths 13 to 27 years:** 0.5 ml whole or split virus I.M. Repeat dose in 4 weeks. Those who received the 1979 or 1980 vaccine require only 1 dose. **Children 3 to 12 years:** give 0.5 ml split virus I.M. Repeat dose in 4 weeks unless child received 1979 or 1980 vaccine. **Children 6 to 35 months:** 0.25 ml split virus I.M. Repeat dose in 4 weeks unless child received 1979 or 1980 vaccine. Recommendations are for 1981 only. Must check yearly for new recommendations.	**Systemic:** *fever, malaise, myalgia, Guillain-Barré syndrome, anaphylaxis.* **Local:** erythema, induration. Side effects occur most often in children and in others not exposed to influenza viruses.
measles, mumps, and rubella virus vaccine, live M-M-R-II♦	*Immunization—* **Children 12 months to puberty:** 1 vial (1,000 units) S.C.	**Systemic:** fever, rash, regional lymphadenopathy, urticaria, *anaphylaxis.* **Local:** erythema.

♦ Available in U.S. and Canada. ♦♦ Available in Canada only. All other products (no symbol) available in U.S. only. Italicized side effects are common or life-threatening.

INTERACTIONS	NURSING CONSIDERATIONS
	• DPT injection may be given at same time as trivalent oral polio vaccine (TOPV). • Obtain history of allergies and reaction to immunization. • Keep epinephrine 1:1,000 available. • Not to be used for active infection. • Don't give subcutaneously. • Shake before using. Refrigerate. • For treatment of anaphylaxis, see inside front cover.
None significant.	• Contraindicated in immunosuppression, radiation or corticosteroid therapy, children under 12 months with cerebral damage. Defer in acute illness or polio outbreak, except in emergency. • Don't use hot or cold compresses; may intensify local reaction. • Obtain history of allergies and reaction to immunization. • Keep epinephrine 1:1,000 available to treat anaphylaxis. • Shake vial well before using. Store in refrigerator. • For treatment of anaphylaxis, see inside front cover.
None significant.	• Contraindicated in egg allergy. Defer in acute respiratory or other active infection, or when there is risk of poliomyelitis infection. • Obtain history of allergies, especially to eggs, and reaction to immunization. • Give injections in deltoid or midlateral thigh. • Keep epinephrine 1:1,000 available. • Recommended for patients with chronic disease, metabolic disorders, and those over 65 years of age. • Fever, malaise, and myalgia begin 6 to 12 hours after vaccination and persist 1 to 2 days. • Allergic reactions, which occur immediately, are extremely rare. • Paralysis associated with Guillain-Barré syndrome is uncommon, but patient should be made aware of risk as compared to risk of influenza and its complications. • For treatment of anaphylaxis, see inside front cover.
Immune serum globulin, whole blood, plasma: antibodies in serum may interfere with immune response. Don't use vaccine within 3 months of transfusion.	• Contraindicated in immunosuppression; cancer; blood dyscrasias; corticosteroid or radiation therapy; gamma globulin disorders; fever; active, untreated tuberculosis. Use cautiously in hypersensitivity to neomycin, chickens, ducks, eggs, or feathers. Defer immunization in acute illness. • Presence of maternal antibodies may prevent response in children under 12 months. • Treat fever with antipyretics. • Store in refrigerator; protect from light. Solution may be used if red, pink, or yellow, but must be clear. • Use only diluent supplied. Discard 8 hours after reconstituting. • Obtain history of allergies, especially to ducks, rabbits, antibiotics, and reaction to immunization. • Inject in outer aspect of upper arm. Don't give I.V. • Keep epinephrine 1:1,000 available.

NAME	INDICATIONS & DOSAGE	SIDE EFFECTS
measles (rubeola) and rubella virus vaccine, live attenuated M-R-Vax-II	*Immunization—* **Children 15 months to puberty:** 1 vial (1,000 units) S.C.	**Systemic:** fever, rash, lymphadenopathy, *anaphylaxis.*
measles (rubeola) virus vaccine, live attenuated Attenuvax♦, M-Vac	*Immunization—* **Adults, and children 15 months or over:** 0.5 ml (1,000 units) S.C.	**Systemic:** fever, rash, lymphadenopathy, *anaphylaxis,* febrile convulsions in susceptible children, anorexia, leukopenia. **Local:** erythema, swelling, tenderness.
meningitis vaccines Meningovax-C, Meningovax-A/C, Menomune-A, Menomune-C, Menomune-A/C	*Meningococcal meningitis prophylaxis—* **Adults, and children over 2 years:** 0.5 ml S.C. Use vaccine group C or A, except in highly endemic areas; in these areas use A/C combination. **Children 3 months to 2 years:** 0.5 ml S.C. Use vaccine group A.	**Systemic:** headache, malaise, chills, fever, cramps, *anaphylaxis.* **Local:** pain, erythema, induration.
mumps virus vaccine, live Mumpsvax♦	*Immunization—* **Adults, and children over 12 months:** 1 vial (5,000 units) S.C.	**Systemic:** *slight fever,* rash, malaise, mild allergic reactions.

♦ Available in U.S. and Canada. ♦♦ Available in Canada only. All other products (no symbol) available in U.S. only. Italicized side effects are common or life-threatening.

INTERACTIONS	NURSING CONSIDERATIONS
Immune serum globulin, whole blood, plasma: antibodies in serum may interfere with immune response. Don't use vaccine within 3 months of transfusion. *Tuberculin skin test:* may temporarily decrease response to test. Defer skin testing.	• Contraindicated in immunosuppression; cancer; blood dyscrasias; corticosteroid or radiation therapy; gamma globulin disorders; fever; active, untreated tuberculosis. Use cautiously in hypersensitivity to neomycin, chickens, ducks, eggs, or feathers, and when there is a history of febrile seizures or in cerebral injury. Defer immunization in acute illness. • Do not give within 1 month of other live virus vaccines, except oral poliovirus vaccine. • Store in refrigerator and protect from light. Solution may be used if red, pink, or yellow, but must be clear (with no precipitation). • Use only diluent supplied. Discard 8 hours after reconstituting. • Inject in outer aspect of upper arm. Don't inject I.V. • For treatment of anaphylaxis, see inside front cover.
Immune serum globulin, whole blood, plasma: antibodies in serum may interfere with immune response. Don't use vaccine within 3 months of transfusion. *Tuberculin skin test:* may temporarily decrease response to test. Defer skin testing.	• Contraindicated in immunosuppression; cancer; blood dyscrasias; corticosteroid or radiation therapy; gamma globulin disorders; active, untreated tuberculosis; fever. Use with caution in hypersensitivity to neomycin, chickens, eggs, or feathers. Defer in acute illness or after administration of blood or plasma. • Warn patient to avoid pregnancy for 3 months after vaccination. • Do not give I.V. • Obtain history of allergies, especially to eggs, and reaction to immunization. • Keep epinephrine 1:1,000 available. • Store in refrigerator and protect from light. Solution may be used if red, pink, or yellow, but must be clear (with no precipitation). • Use only diluent supplied. Discard 8 hours after reconstituting. • May be given with oral poliovirus vaccine. • For treatment of anaphylaxis, see inside front cover.
None significant.	• Contraindicated in immunosuppression. Defer in acute illness. • Tell patient to avoid pregnancy for 3 months after vaccination. • Obtain history of allergies and reaction to immunization. • Do not give I.V. • Keep epinephrine 1:1,000 available. • For treatment of anaphylaxis, see inside front cover.
Immune serum globulin, whole blood, plasma: antibodies in serum may interfere with immune response. Don't use vaccine within 3 months of transfusion. *Tuberculin skin test:* may temporarily decrease response to test. Defer skin testing.	• Contraindicated in immunosuppression; cancer; blood dyscrasias; corticosteroid or radiation therapy; gamma globulin disorders; active, untreated tuberculosis; pregnancy. Use cautiously in hypersensitivity to neomycin, chickens, ducks, eggs, or feathers. Defer in acute illness and for 3 months following transfusions or immune serum globulin. • Keep epinephrine 1:1,000 available. • Mumpsvax should not be given less than 1 month before or after immunization with other live virus vaccines, with the exception of Attenuvax, Meruvax, and/or monovalent or trivalent live, oral poliovirus vaccine, which may be administered simultaneously. • The vaccine will not offer protection when given after exposure to natural mumps. • Not recommended for infants younger than 12 months because retained maternal mumps antibodies may interfere with the immune response. • Stress importance of avoiding pregnancy for 3 months after immunization. If necessary, provide contraceptive information. • Treat fever with antipyretics.

(continued on following page)

NAME	INDICATIONS & DOSAGE	SIDE EFFECTS
mumps virus vaccine, live *(continued)*		
plague vaccine	*Primary immunization and booster—* **Adults, and children over 11 years:** 1 ml I.M. followed by 0.2 ml in 1 to 3 months, then 0.2 ml 3 to 6 months after second injection. Booster: 0.1 to 0.2 ml q 6 months while in plague area. **Children under 1 year:** 1/5 adult primary or booster dose. **Children 1 to 4 years:** 2/5 adult primary or booster dose. **Children 5 to 10 years:** 3/5 adult primary or booster dose.	**Systemic:** malaise, headache, slight fever, lymphadenopathy, *anaphylaxis.* **Local:** swelling, induration, erythema.
pneumococcal vaccine, polyvalent Pneumovax♦, Pnu-Imune	*Pneumococcal immunization—* **Adults, and children 2 years or over:** 0.5 ml I.M. or S.C. Not recommended for children under 2 years.	**Systemic:** *slight fever, anaphylaxis.* **Local:** severe local reaction can occur when revaccination takes place within 3 years.
poliovirus vaccine, live, oral, trivalent Orimune	*Poliovirus immunization—* **Adults, and children over 6 weeks:** two drops or 0.5 ml P.O. in 5 ml of water or simple syrup, or on sugar cube. Repeat dose in 8 weeks. Give third dose at 18 months. Booster: two drops or 0.5 ml P.O.	None reported.
rabies vaccine (duck embryo), dried, killed virus	*Postexposure immunization for domestic animal bite—* **Adults and children:** 1 ml S.C.	**Systemic:** peripheral neuritis, dorsolumbar myelitis, acute idiopathic polyneuritis, acute enceph-

♦ Available in U.S. and Canada. ♦♦ Available in Canada only. All other products (no symbol) available in U.S. only. Italicized side effects are common or life-threatening.

INTERACTIONS	NURSING CONSIDERATIONS
	• Don't give I.V. • Store in refrigerator and protect from light. Solution may be used if red, pink, or yellow, but must be clear. • Use only diluent supplied. Discard 8 hours after reconstituting. • Obtain history of allergies, especially to antibiotics, and reaction to immunization. • For treatment of anaphylaxis, see inside front cover.
None significant.	• Contraindicated in immunosuppression. Defer in respiratory infection. • Deltoid area preferred injection site. • Obtain history of allergies and reaction to immunization. • Keep epinephrine 1:1,000 available. • For treatment of anaphylaxis, see inside front cover.
None significant.	• Check immunization history carefully to avoid revaccination within 3 years. • Inject in deltoid or midlateral thigh. Don't inject I.V. • Keep refrigerated. Reconstitution or dilution not necessary. • Treat fever with mild antipyretics. • Protects against 14 pneumococcal types, which account for 80% of pneumococcal disease. • Obtain history of allergies and reaction to immunization. • Keep epinephrine 1:1,000 available. • For treatment of anaphylaxis, see inside front cover.
Immune serum globulin, whole blood, plasma: antibodies in serum may interfere with immune response. Don't use vaccine within 3 months of transfusion.	• Contraindicated in immunosuppression, cancer, immunoglobulin abnormalities, and in radiation, antimetabolite, alkylating agent, or corticosteroid therapy. Defer in acute illness, vomiting, or diarrhea. • Use with caution in siblings of child with known immunodeficiency syndrome. • This vaccine not effective in modifying or preventing existing or incubating poliomyelitis. • Check the parents' immunization history when they bring in child for vaccine; this is a good time for parents to receive boosters. • Keep frozen until used. Once thawed, if unopened, may store refrigerated up to 30 days. Opened vials may be refrigerated up to 7 days. Thaw before administration. • Color change from pink to yellow has no effect on the efficiency of the vaccine. Yellow color results from vaccine being stored at low temperatures. • Obtain history of allergies and reaction to immunization. • Not for parenteral use.
None significant.	• Stop corticosteroids during immunization period. • When postexposure immunization is indicated, pregnancy is not a contraindication.

(continued on following page)

NAME	INDICATIONS & DOSAGE	SIDE EFFECTS
rabies vaccine (duck embryo) dried, killed virus *(continued)*	daily for 14 days in the abdomen on alternate sides. *Postexposure immunization for wild animal bite—* **Adults and children:** 2 ml S.C. daily for 7 days, then 1 ml daily for 7 more days. Supplemental doses may be needed after initial therapy. *Preexposure immunization (for patients constantly exposed to rabies)—* **Adults and children:** 1 ml S.C. weekly for 3 weeks, then fourth dose 6 months later; or 1 ml S.C. 1 month apart for 2 doses, then third dose 7 months after second. Booster (for patients constantly exposed to rabies): 1 ml q 1 to 2 years.	alomyelitis, fever, weakness, stiff neck, respiratory distress, *anaphylaxis.* **GI:** *nausea, vomiting, diarrhea, abdominal cramps.* **Skin:** urticaria. **Local:** *stinging, pain, erythema, induration,* lymphadenopathy.
rabies vaccine, human diploid cell (HDCV)	*Postexposure antirabies immunization—* **Adults and children:** 5 1-ml doses of HDCV I.M. (for example, in the deltoid region). Give first dose as soon as possible after exposure; give an additional dose on each of days 3, 7, 14, and 28 after first dose.	**Systemic:** headache, nausea, abdominal pain, muscle aches, dizziness. **Local:** *pain, erythema, swelling or itching at injection site.*
rubella and mumps virus vaccine, live Biavax-II	*Measles and mumps immunization—* **Adults, and children over 12 months:** 1 vial (1,000 units) S.C.	**Systemic:** fever, rash, thrombocytopenic purpura, urticaria, arthritis, arthralgia, polyneuritis, *anaphylaxis.* **Local:** pain, erythema, induration, lymphadenopathy.
rubella virus vaccine, live attenuated (RA 27/3) Meruvax-II♦	*Measles immunization—* **Adults, and children over 12 months:** 1 vial (1,000 units) S.C. or I.M.	**Systemic:** fever, rash, thrombocytopenic purpura, urticaria, arthritis, arthralgia, polyneuritis, *anaphylaxis.* **Local:** pain, erythema, induration, lymphadenopathy.

♦ Available in U.S. and Canada. ♦♦ Available in Canada only. All other products (no symbol) available in U.S. only. Italicized side effects are common or life-threatening.

INTERACTIONS	NURSING CONSIDERATIONS
	• Immediate, thorough cleaning of wound is the best way to prevent rabies. • Rabies immune globulin may be given at time of first vaccine dose to provide immediate protection. • Use of this drug confers active immunity. • Use 23G or 24G, ½″ to ¾″ needle. • Obtain history of allergies, especially to eggs, ducks, or proteins, and reaction to immunization. • Keep epinephrine 1:1,000 available. • For treatment of anaphylaxis, see inside front cover.
None significant.	• Stop corticosteroids during immunization period. • When postexposure immunization is indicated, pregnancy is not a contraindication. • Persons with a history of hypersensitivity should be given rabies vaccine with caution. Persons allergic to duck embryo vaccine are less likely to be allergic to HDCV. • Keep epinephrine 1:1,000 available. • HDCV is the preferred rabies vaccine because of its presumed greater efficacy and because fewer adverse reactions are known to be associated with it. • Contact state health department or Merieux Institute (1-800-327-2842) on vaccine availability. • For treatment of anaphylaxis, see inside front cover.
Immune serum globulin, whole blood, plasma: antibodies in serum may interfere with immune response. Don't give vaccine within 3 months of transfusion. *Tuberculin skin test:* may temporarily decrease response to test. Defer skin testing.	• Contraindicated in immunosuppression; cancer; blood dyscrasias; corticosteroid or radiation therapy; gamma globulin disorders; active, untreated tuberculosis; fever; pregnancy. Use with caution in hypersensitivity to neomycin, chickens, ducks, eggs, or feathers. Defer in acute illness and after administration of immune serum globulin, blood, or plasma. • Stress importance of avoiding pregnancy for 3 months after immunization. If necessary, provide contraceptive information. • Store in refrigerator and protect from light. Solution may be used if red, pink, or yellow, but must be clear. • Use only diluent supplied. Discard 8 hours after reconstituting. • Obtain history of allergies, especially to ducks, rabbits, and antibiotics, and reaction to immunization. • Inject into outer aspect of upper arm. Don't inject I.V. • Keep epinephrine 1:1,000 available. • For treatment of anaphylaxis, see inside front cover.
Immune serum globulin, whole blood, plasma: antibodies in serum may interfere with immune response. Don't use	• Contraindicated in immunosuppression; cancer; blood dyscrasias; corticosteroid or radiation therapy; gamma globulin disorders; active, untreated tuberculosis; fever. Use cautiously in hypersensitivity to neomycin, chickens, ducks, eggs, or feathers. Defer in acute illness and after administration of human immune serum globulin, blood, or plasma.

(continued on following page)

NAME	INDICATIONS & DOSAGE	SIDE EFFECTS
rubella virus vaccine, live attenuated (RA 27/3) *(continued)*		
smallpox vaccine Dryvax	*Immunization—* **Adults:** deposit drop of vaccine on cleansed site and make series of multiple pressures with sharp needle through drop. Use only for laboratory personnel working with virus.	**Systemic:** encephalopathy, transverse myelitis, acute infection, polyneuritis, eczema vaccinatum, eye infection, rash, *anaphylaxis,* fever. **Local:** necrosis, pustule (expected), infection.
staphylococcus toxoid	*Prophylaxis and treatment of recurrent boils, carbuncles, pustular acne (when combined with antibiotics)—* **Adults and children:** administer a graded series of I.M. or S.C. injections based on results of sensitivity testing. Give injections q 2 to 7 days, utilizing two dilutions supplied.	**Systemic:** hypersensitivity, *anaphylaxis.*
tetanus toxoid, adsorbed Tet Tox Adsorbed	*Primary immunization—* **Adults and children:** 0.5 ml (adsorbed) I.M. 4 to 6 weeks apart for 2 doses, then third	**Systemic:** slight fever, chills, malaise, aches and pains, flushing, urticaria, pruritus, tachycardia, hypotension, *anaphylaxis.*

♦ Available in U.S. and Canada. ♦♦ Available in Canada only. All other products (no symbol) available in U.S. only. Italicized side effects are common or life-threatening.

INTERACTIONS	NURSING CONSIDERATIONS
vaccine within 3 months of transfusion. *Tuberculin skin test:* may temporarily decrease response to test. Defer skin testing.	• Stress importance of avoiding pregnancy for 3 months after immunization. If necessary, provide contraceptive information. • Store in refrigerator and protect from light. Solution may be used if red, pink, or yellow, but must be clear. • Use only diluent supplied. Discard 8 hours after reconstituting. • Obtain history of allergies, especially to ducks and rabbits, and reaction to immunization. • Inject into outer aspect of upper arm. Don't inject I.V. • Keep epinephrine 1:1,000 available. • For treatment of anaphylaxis, see inside front cover.
Immune serum globulin, whole blood, plasma: antibodies in serum may interfere with immune response. Don't use vaccine within 3 months of transfusion. *Methotrexate:* may interfere with immune response. Don't use together.	• Contraindicated in wounds or burns, skin disorders (for example, eczema), immunosuppression, antimetabolite and radiation therapy, and pregnancy. Also contraindicated in patients with active infections and in those with leukemia, lymphomas, or other malignant neoplasms affecting the bone marrow or lymphatic system. Weigh risks against benefits. Use cautiously in hypersensitivity to chickens, eggs, or feathers, or to neomycin or other antibiotic preservatives in this vaccine (polymyxin B, streptomycin, chlortetracycline). • Don't expose site to direct sunlight for several days or to water for 2 hours. Don't cover site initially. In pustular stage, loose dressing may be applied. Warn patient against touching site: may spread lesion and cause secondary infection. • Obtain history of allergies—especially to chickens or beef, and antibiotics—and reaction to immunization. • Do not inject. • Reconstituted solution may be stored for 3 months under refrigeration. • A successful primary vaccination shows a typical jennerian vesicle. If none is observed, vaccination procedures should be checked and vaccination repeated with a different lot of vaccine until a successful result is obtained. • After revaccination, two responses are possible. A "major reaction" is the formation of a vesicular or pustular lesion of an area of definite palpable induration, which indicates virus multiplication has most likely taken place and revaccination is successful. Any other reaction is regarded as "equivocal." When an equivocal reaction is observed, revaccination procedures should be checked and revaccination repeated with another lot of vaccine. • Keep epinephrine 1:1,000 available. • For treatment of anaphylaxis, see inside front cover.
None significant.	• Use with antibiotics. • Give test dose first. • Obtain history of allergies and reaction to immunization. • Keep epinephrine 1:1,000 available. • For treatment of anaphylaxis, see inside front cover.
None significant.	• Contraindicated in immunosuppression and immunoglobulin abnormalities. Defer in acute illness and polio outbreaks, except in emergencies. • For prevention, not treatment, of tetanus infections.

(continued on following page)

NAME	INDICATIONS & DOSAGE	SIDE EFFECTS
tetanus toxoid *(continued)* **tetanus toxoid fluid** Tet Tox Fluid	dose 1 year after the second. *Primary immunization—* **Adults and children:** 0.5 ml (fluid) I.M. or S.C. 4 to 8 weeks apart, for 3 doses, then fourth dose of 0.5 ml 6 to 12 months after third dose. Booster: 0.5 ml I.M. at 10-year intervals.	**Local:** erythema, induration, nodule.
typhoid vaccine	*Primary immunization—* **Adults, and children over 10 years:** 0.5 ml S.C.; repeat in 4 weeks. Booster: same dose as primary immunization q 3 years. **Children 6 months to 10 years:** 0.25 ml S.C.; repeat in 4 weeks. Booster: same dose as primary immunization q 3 years.	**Systemic:** *fever,* malaise, headache, nausea, *anaphylaxis.* **Local:** swelling, pain, inflammation.
typhus vaccine	*Immunization against louse-borne epidemic typhus—* **Adults:** 0.5 ml Lederle vaccine or 1 ml Lilly vaccine S.C.; repeat in 4 weeks. **Children under 10 years:** 0.25 ml Lederle vaccine or 0.5 ml Lilly vaccine S.C.; repeat in 4 weeks.	**Systemic:** fever, malaise, *anaphylaxis.* **Local:** pain, induration, erythema.
yellow fever vaccine	*Primary vaccination—* **Adults, and children over 6 months:** 0.5 ml S.C. Booster: repeat 0.5 ml S.C. q 10 years.	**Systemic:** fever, malaise, *anaphylaxis.*

INTERACTIONS	NURSING CONSIDERATIONS
	• Determine date of last tetanus immunization. • Don't use hot or cold compresses; may increase severity of local reaction. • Obtain history of allergies and reaction to immunization. • Keep epinephrine 1:1,000 available. • Adsorbed form produces longer duration of immunity. Fluid form provides quicker booster effect in patients actively immunized previously. • Do not confuse this drug with tetanus immune globulin, human. • For treatment of anaphylaxis, see inside front cover.
None significant.	• Contraindicated in corticosteroid therapy. Defer in acute illness. • Treat fever with antipyretics. • Do not give intradermally. • Obtain history of allergies and reaction to immunization. • Keep epinephrine 1:1,000 available. • Store at 2° to 10° C. (35.6° to 50° F.). • Shake thoroughly before withdrawal from vial. • For treatment of anaphylaxis, see inside front cover.
None significant.	• Contraindicated in corticosteroid therapy and in egg hypersensitivity. Defer in acute illness. • Use for classic epidemic typhus, not endemic forms. • Obtain history of allergies, especially to eggs, and past reaction to immunization. • Keep epinephrine 1:1,000 available. • For treatment of anaphylaxis, see inside front cover.
None significant.	• Contraindicated in gamma globulin deficiency, immunosuppression, cancer, corticosteroid or radiation therapy, allergies to chickens or eggs, and in pregnancy. Also contraindicated in infants under 6 months except in high-risk areas. • Reconstitute with sodium chloride injection that contains no preservatives (preservatives decrease potency of vaccine). • Must be kept frozen. Shake well before using. Use within 1 hour after reconstitution. Discard remainder. • Obtain history of allergies, especially to eggs, and reaction to immunization. • Don't give within 1 month of other live virus vaccines. • Keep epinephrine 1:1,000 available. • For treatment of anaphylaxis, see inside front cover.

Antitoxins and antivenins

black widow spider antivenin
botulism antitoxin, bivalent equine
crotaline antivenin, polyvalent
diphtheria antitoxin, equine
***Micrurus fulvius* antivenin**
tetanus antitoxin (TAT), equine

Antitoxins and antivenins bind to and neutralize toxins and venoms. The preparations are made from blood of horses inoculated with specific toxins.

Major uses

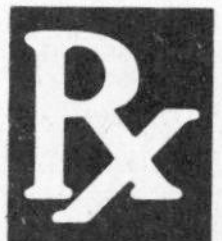

- Antitoxins are used to prevent and treat bacterial toxin infections.
- Antivenins are used to treat symptoms of insect and spider bites, and snakebites.

Mechanism of action

- Antitoxins provide passive immunity. This type of immunity is acquired by inoculation with purified, concentrated antibodies formed in the blood of horses immunized by specific toxins.
- Toxins and venoms are bound to and neutralized by the specific antitoxin or antivenin.

Absorption, distribution, metabolism, and excretion

Not applicable.

Onset and duration

Onset is immediate, but duration of immunity hasn't been determined.

Combination products

None.

HOW TO USE AN EMERGENCY ANAPHYLAXIS KIT

Dear Patient:

This emergency anaphylaxis kit contains all you need to combat an allergic reaction from an insect bite or sting: prefilled syringe with two doses of epinephrine, alcohol swabs, tourniquet, and antihistamine tablets. If you've been stung:

1. Notify the doctor immediately.

2. Remove the insect's stinger. Don't push, pinch, squeeze, or drive the stinger farther into the skin. If you can't remove the stinger quickly, go immediately to step 3.

A

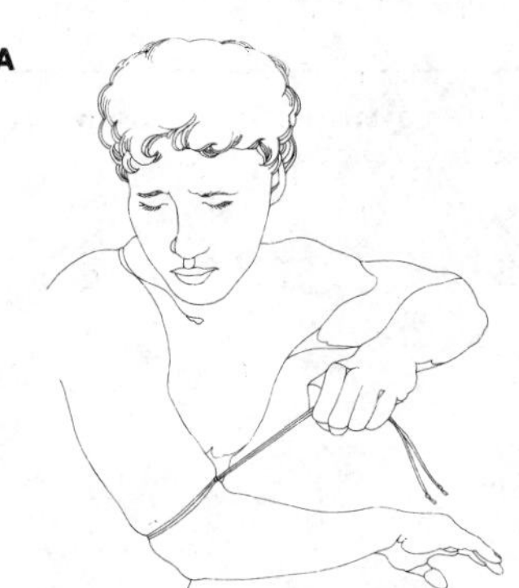

3. If you were stung on the arm or leg, apply the tourniquet between the sting and your torso, and tighten it (A). *(Note:* Loosen the tourniquet slightly every 10 minutes to maintain circulation.) If you were stung on the face, neck, or a place where you can't apply a tourniquet, apply ice to the affected area.

4. Use an alcohol swab to clean a 4″ area of skin above the tourniquet.

5. Remove the needle cover from the prefilled syringe. Expel air from the syringe by pointing the needle upward and carefully pushing the plunger until a bead of liquid forms on the needle tip.

6. Insert the whole needle straight down

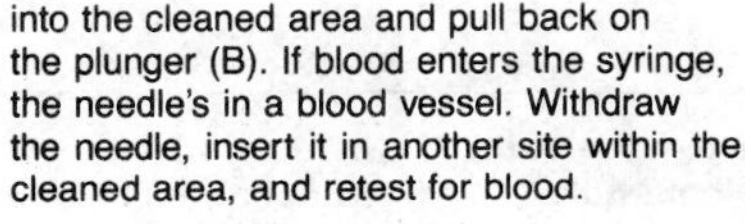

into the cleaned area and pull back on the plunger (B). If blood enters the syringe, the needle's in a blood vessel. Withdraw the needle, insert it in another site within the cleaned area, and retest for blood.

B

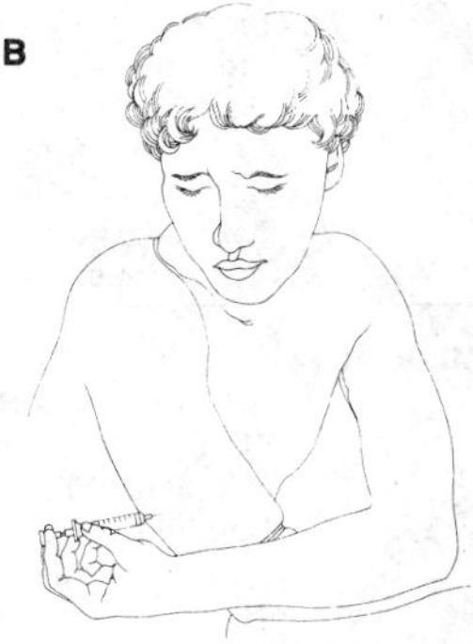

7. When you're sure the needle's not in a blood vessel, depress the plunger and inject the prescribed dose of epinephrine. Guidelines: Adults, and children over age 12—up to 0.5 ml; children ages 7 to 12—0.2 ml; children ages 2 to 6—0.15 ml; infants to age 2—0.05 to 0.1 ml.

8. Chew and swallow antihistamine tablets. Guidelines: Adults, and children over age 12—4 tablets; children under age 12—2 tablets.

9. Apply ice or meat tenderizer to the affected area, if available. Keep warm. Avoid exertion.

10. If you see no improvement in 10 minutes, prepare the syringe for a second injection. Rotate the plunger one quarter turn to the right, to align with the rectangular slot in the syringe. Repeat steps 4 through 7.

11. See the doctor or go to your hospital emergency department as soon as you finish this procedure.

NAME	INDICATIONS & DOSAGE	SIDE EFFECTS
black widow spider antivenin Antivenin *(Latrodectus mactans)*♦	*Black widow spider bite—* **Adults and children:** 2.5 ml I.M. in deltoid. Second dose may be needed.	**Systemic:** hypersensitivity, *anaphylaxis, neurotoxicity.*
botulism antitoxin, bivalent equine	*Botulism—* **Adults and children:** 1 vial I.V. stat and q 4 hours, p.r.n., until patient's condition improves. Dilute antitoxin 1:10 in 5% or 10% dextrose in water or normal saline solution before giving. Give first 10 ml of dilution over 5 minutes; after 15 minutes, rate may be increased.	**Systemic:** hypersensitivity, *anaphylaxis,* serum sickness (urticaria, pruritus, fever, malaise, arthralgia) may occur in 5 to 13 days.
crotaline antivenin, polyvalent	*Crotalid (rattlesnake) bites—* **Adults and children:** initially, 10 to 50 ml or more I.M. or S.C., depending on severity of bite and patient's response. If large amount of venom, 70 to 100 ml I.V. directly into superficial vein. Subsequent doses based on patient's response; may give 10 ml q ½ to 2 hours, p.r.n. If bite is in extremity, inject part of initial dose at various sites around limb above swelling; don't inject in finger or toe. The smaller the patient, the larger the initial dose.	**Systemic:** hypersensitivity, *anaphylaxis.*
diphtheria antitoxin, equine	*Diphtheria prevention—* **Adults and children:** 1,000 to 5,000 units I.M. *Diphtheria treatment—* **Adults and children:** 20,000 to 80,000 units or more slow I.V. Additional doses may be given in 24 hours. I.M. route may be used in mild cases.	**Systemic:** hypersensitivity, *anaphylaxis,* serum sickness (urticaria, pruritus, fever, malaise, arthralgia) may occur in 7 to 12 days.
***Micrurus fulvius* antivenin**	*Eastern and Texas coral snake bite—* **Adults and children:** 3 to 5 vials slow I.V. through running I.V. of 0.9% normal saline	**Systemic:** hypersensitivity, *anaphylaxis.*

♦ Available in U.S. and Canada. ♦♦ Available in Canada only. All other products (no symbol) available in U.S. only. Italicized side effects are common or life-threatening.

INTERACTIONS	NURSING CONSIDERATIONS
None significant.	• If possible, hospitalize patient. • Immobilize patient; splint bitten limb to prevent spread of venom. • Test for sensitivity before giving. • Epinephrine 1:1,000 should be available in case of adverse reaction. • Venom is neurotoxic and may cause respiratory paralysis and convulsions. Watch patient carefully for 2 to 3 days. • Obtain accurate patient history of allergies, especially to horses, and reaction to immunization. • Earliest possible use of the antivenin is recommended for best results. • Antivenin may also be given I.V. in severe cases (as when the patient is in shock). Drug is given in 10 to 50 ml of saline solution over a 15-minute period. • For treatment of anaphylaxis, see inside front cover.
None significant.	• Test for sensitivity before giving. • Epinephrine 1:1,000 should be available in case of adverse reaction. Bivalent antitoxin contains antibodies against types A and B *Clostridium botulinum.* Antitoxins against all other types available only from Center for Disease Control in Atlanta, Georgia. • Obtain accurate patient history of allergies, especially to horses, and reaction to immunization. • Earliest possible use of antitoxin is recommended for best results. • For treatment of anaphylaxis, see inside front cover.
Antihistamines: enhanced toxicity of crotaline venoms. Don't use together.	• Test for sensitivity before giving. • Immobilize patient immediately. Splint bitten extremity. • Epinephrine 1:1,000 should be available in case of adverse reaction. • Type and crossmatch as soon as possible since hemolysis from venom prevents accurate crossmatching. • Early use of antivenin recommended for best results. • Watch patient carefully for delayed allergic reaction or relapse. • Because children have less resistance and less body fluid to dilute venom, they may need twice the adult dose. • Obtain accurate patient history of allergies, especially to horses, and reaction to immunization. • Discard unused reconstituted drug. • For treatment of anaphylaxis, see inside front cover.
None significant.	• Test for sensitivity before giving. • Epinephrine 1:1,000 should be available in case of adverse reaction. • Obtain accurate patient history of allergies, especially to horses, and reaction to immunization. • Therapy should be started immediately, without waiting for culture and sensitivity reports, if patient has clinical symptoms of diphtheria (sore throat, fever, tonsillar membrane). • Refrigerate antitoxin at 2° to 10°C. (35.6° to 50° F.). May be warmed to 32.2° to 35° C. (90° to 95° F.), never higher. • For treatment of anaphylaxis, see inside front cover.
None significant.	• Test for sensitivity before giving. • Immobilize patient or splint bitten limb to prevent spread of venom. • If possible, hospitalize patient. • Early use of antivenin recommended for best results.

(continued on following page)

NAME	INDICATIONS & DOSAGE	SIDE EFFECTS
***Micrurus fulvius* antivenin** *(continued)*	solution. Give first 1 to 2 ml over 3 to 5 minutes, and watch for signs of allergic reaction. If no signs develop, continue injection. Up to 10 vials may be needed. Not effective for Sonoran or Arizona coral snake bites.	
tetanus antitoxin (TAT), equine	*Tetanus prophylaxis—* **Patients over 29.5 kg:** 3,000 to 5,000 units I.M. or S.C. **Patients under 29.5 kg:** 1,500 to 3,000 units I.M. or S.C. *Tetanus treatment—* **All patients:** 10,000 to 20,000 units injected into wound. Give additional 40,000 to 200,000 units I.V. Start tetanus toxoid at same time but at different site and with a different syringe.	**Local:** pain, numbness, skin eruptions. **Systemic:** joint pain, hypersensitivity, *anaphylaxis.*

♦ Available in U.S. and Canada. ♦♦ Available in Canada only. All other products (no symbol) available in U.S. only. Italicized side effects are common or life-threatening.

INTERACTIONS	NURSING CONSIDERATIONS
	• Venom is neurotoxic and may cause respiratory paralysis. Watch patient carefully for 24 hours. Be ready to take supportive measures. Epinephrine 1:1,000 should be available in case of adverse reaction. • Obtain accurate patient history of allergies, especially to horses, and reaction to immunization. • For treatment of anaphylaxis, see inside front cover.
None significant.	• Test for sensitivity before giving. • Use only when tetanus immune globulin (human) not available. • Obtain accurate patient history of allergies, especially to horses, and reaction to immunization. If respiratory difficulty develops, give 0.4 ml of 1:1,000 solution epinephrine HCl. • Preventive dose should be given to those who have had two or fewer injections of tetanus toxoid and who have tetanus-prone injuries more than 24 hours old. • For treatment of anaphylaxis, see inside front cover.

PATIENT PREPARATION

TEST FOR HYPERSENSITIVITY

Antitoxin and antivenin preparations frequently cause hypersensitivity. All patients, therefore, should receive a test dose of the drug either intradermally or ophthalmically, regardless of past history of negative sensitivity.

Intradermal test

• Dilute serum 1:10 with 0.9% sodium chloride for injection. Inject 0.02 ml of diluted serum intradermally on inner aspect of forearm. As a control, inject the other arm with 0.02 ml of 0.9% sodium chloride for injection.

• Observe for 20 minutes. If a wheal 10 mm or larger develops at the test site, surrounded by an erythematous flare 20 mm × 20 mm, the test is positive for hypersensitivity.

• If the skin test is positive, give an ophthalmic test.

Ophthalmic test

• Dilute serum 1:10 with 0.9% sodium chloride for injection. Instill one drop of dilution into conjunctival sac.

• Observe for 20 minutes. Hyperemia and congestion of the mucous membranes are a positive test for hypersensitivity.

• If the skin test is positive and the eye test is negative, the patient may be desensitized before antitoxin or antivenin is administered.

Note: Always have epinephrine 1:1,000 on hand when administering antitoxins or antivenins, even though test dose results are negative. The patient can develop hypersensitivity at any time during therapy.

103 Acidifiers and alkalinizers

Acidifiers
ammonium chloride
dilute hydrochloric acid

Alkalinizers
sodium bicarbonate
sodium lactate
tromethamine

Acidifiers and alkalinizers may correct acid-base imbalances in metabolic disorders. In severe metabolic alkalosis, acidifiers may be given to lower blood pH. In metabolic acidosis, alkalinizers raise blood pH.

Major uses

Rx

- Acidifiers are used to treat metabolic alkalosis. Ammonium chloride also acidifies the urine.
- Alkalinizers are used to treat metabolic acidosis. Sodium bicarbonate and sodium acetate may also alkalinize the urine. This blocks tubular reabsorption of acidic drugs and increases their excretion. Alkalinizing the urine can be part of the treatment of aspirin or phenobarbital overdose.

Mechanism of action

- Acidifiers increase free hydrogen ion (H^+) concentration.
- Alkalinizers decrease free hydrogen ion concentration. Sodium bicarbonate restores the buffering capacity of the body. Sodium lactate is metabolized to sodium bicarbonate before it can produce a buffering effect. Tromethamine combines with hydrogen ions and associated acid anions; the resulting salts are excreted by the kidneys.

Absorption, distribution, metabolism, and excretion

- Ammonium chloride and sodium bicarbonate are rapidly and well absorbed orally. Sodium lactate, dilute hydrochloric acid, and tromethamine are administered I.V. Ammonium chloride and sodium bicarbonate can be administered either orally or I.V.
- Ammonium chloride and sodium lactate are metabolized in the liver.
- Ammonium chloride is excreted in urine.
- Tromethamine is not metabolized and is excreted in urine.

Onset and duration

Onset is rapid after oral administration and immediate after I.V. administration. Duration of action varies, depending on use and underlying disease.

Combination products

None.

THE REGULATORS OF BLOOD pH

The body regulates its pH through three mechanisms, as shown here:

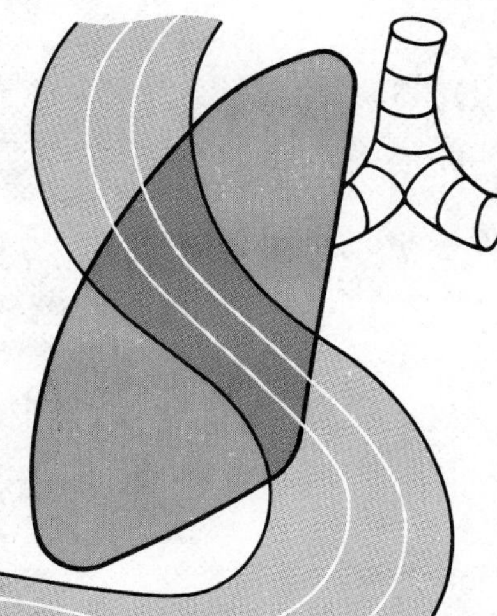

• *The lungs* act within minutes to regulate the volatile carbonic acid in the blood through exhalation or retention of carbon dioxide. If there is an excess of H^+ and the blood is too acidic, the patient may *hyper*ventilate to get rid of excess acid. If there is an inadequate amount of H^+ and blood is too alkaline, the patient may *hypo*ventilate to store CO_2 (which forms carbonic acid) and restore the pH to normal.

• *Blood buffers* neutralize excess acids or alkalies that form as a result of metabolic processes. In plasma, pH is determined by the ratio of bicarbonate to carbonic acid—the principal buffer pair. The ratio of carbonic acid to base bicarbonate is usually 1:20, but this ratio changes as one shifts into the other to help offset changes in hydrogen ion concentration.

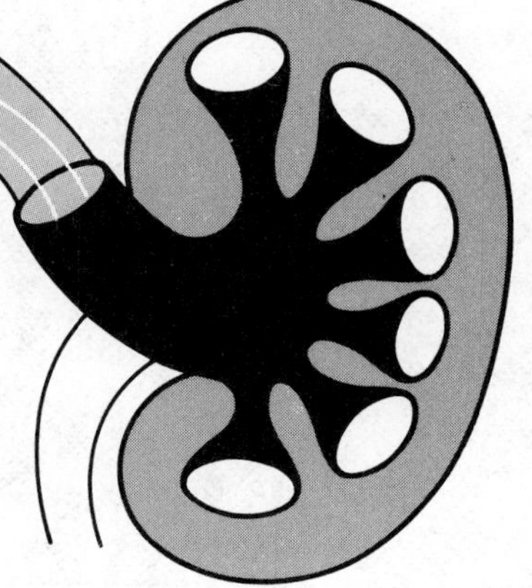

• *The kidneys* take hours or days to play their part in acid-base regulation, but they secrete or retain hydrogen or bicarbonate ions until the pH balance is exactly normal.

Remember that you cannot effectively evaluate serum electrolytes without knowing the blood pH. This is because small changes in pH greatly affect the movement of electrolytes across the cell membrane and cause dramatic changes in the serum levels. Normal blood pH is 7.35 to 7.45.

For information on how to recognize acidosis and alkalosis, see chart on next page.

HOW TO RECOGNIZE ACIDOSIS AND ALKALOSIS

CONDITION	POSSIBLE CAUSES	SYMPTOMS
Respiratory acidosis (primary carbon dioxide excess)	Diseases that impair carbon dioxide elimination by the lungs (emphysema); respiratory depressant drugs (narcotics, barbiturates, sedatives); breathing excessive carbon dioxide; breath-holding	Lethargy, weakness, shallow and irregular respirations, disorientation, headache, cyanosis
Respiratory alkalosis (primary carbon dioxide deficit)	Excessive mechanical ventilation, hyperventilation, CNS disease, hysteria, anxiety, persistent fever, congestive heart failure, pulmonary embolism, early salicylate intoxication	Hyperreflexia, blurred vision, tetany, vertigo, muscle cramps, sighing, diaphoresis
Metabolic acidosis (primary bicarbonate deficit)	Renal disease, starvation, diabetic ketosis, lactic acidosis, severe diarrhea, biliary fistulas, ingestion of substances such as methyl alcohol, salicylates, paraldehyde, or ethylene glycol	Kussmaul's respiration, restlessness, disorientation, stupor
Metabolic alkalosis (primary bicarbonate excess)	Vomiting, diuretics, hyperadrenocorticism, hyperaldosteronism, nasogastric suction, ingestion of sodium bicarbonate or other alkali	Weakness, apathy, leg cramps, paresthesias

SIGNS	BLOOD GAS LEVELS			NURSING CONSIDERATIONS
	pH	HCO_3	pCO_2	
Hypoventilation, asterixis, tachycardia	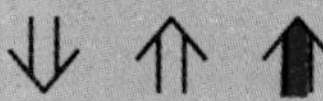 ↓	↑	↑ (shaded)	• The most common treatment is directed at improving ventilation. • Expect to see an elevated plasma bicarbonate level as a compensatory mechanism in patients with chronic obstructive lung disease. • Observe patients with emphysema for signs of CO_2 narcosis and remember not to precipitate this severe complication by giving excessive oxygen therapy to such patients.
Hyperventilation, latent tetany, positive Chvostek's sign, convulsions	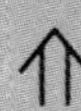 ↑	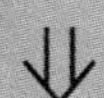 ↓	 ↓ (shaded)	• Treatment is directed at underlying disorder. • Try to reassure and calm a patient who is hyperventilating. Rebreathing exhaled air from a paper bag can increase carbon dioxide levels in these patients. • Respirator should be checked hourly and adjusted to deliver optimal ventilation without overventilating the patient.
Shock, coma, tachypnea, almond odor from mouth	 ↓	 ↓ (shaded)	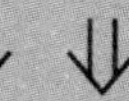 ↓	• Treatment is directed at underlying disorder. • In patients with diabetes, expect a drop in blood pressure, stupor, and possible coma. Monitor vital signs carefully. Draw stat blood glucose. • Secondary or compensatory metabolic alkalosis can result from the body's compensatory mechanisms to increase bicarbonate levels.
Signs of potassium depletion, tetany, respiratory depression, arrhythmia	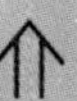 ↑	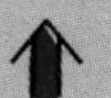 ↑ (shaded)	↑	• Treatment is directed at underlying condition. • Volume and potassium depletion should be corrected. • This condition, most commonly seen after acute vomiting or nasogastric suctioning, is the result of hydrogen ion loss from the hydrochloric acid of digestive juices. • Can also occur in patients who ingest sodium bicarbonate regularly (for example, to relieve acid stomach). • Monitor heart for arrhythmias due to potassium loss through body compensatory mechanisms.

KEY: ↓ = decreased ↑ = increased. Shaded arrows indicate the primary abnormality.

NAME	INDICATIONS & DOSAGE	SIDE EFFECTS
ammonium chloride	*Metabolic alkalosis*— **Adults and children:** 4 mEq/kg slow I.V. or calculated by amount of chloride deficit. Infusion rate: 0.9 to 1.3 ml/minute 2.14% solution. Do not exceed 2 ml/minute. Hypodermoclysis has been used in infants and young children. One half calculated volume should be given, then patient should be reassessed. *As an acidifying agent*—4 to 12 g P.O. daily in divided doses.	Side effects usually result from ammonia toxicity or too rapid I.V. administration. **CNS:** headache, confusion, progressive drowsiness, excitement alternating with coma, hyperventilation, *calcium-deficient tetany, twitching, hyperreflexia, EEG abnormalities.* **CV:** bradycardia. **GI:** (with oral dose) *gastric irritation, nausea, vomiting,* thirst, anorexia, retching. **GU:** glycosuria. **Metabolic:** *acidosis, hyperchloremia, hypokalemia,* hyperglycemia. **Skin:** rash, pallor. **Local:** pain at injection site. **Other:** irregular respirations with periods of apnea.
dilute hydrochloric acid	*Metabolic alkalosis*— pharmacy prepares (0.1 normal HCl solution in sterile water) 100 mEq hydrogen and 100 mEq chloride/liter.	None confirmed.
sodium bicarbonate	*Cardiac arrest*— **Adults and children:** as a 7.5% or 8.4% solution, 1 to 3 mEq/kg I.V. initially; may repeat in 10 minutes. Further doses based on blood gases. If blood gases unavailable, use 0.5 mEq/kg q 10 minutes until spontaneous circulation returns. **Infants up to 2 years:** 4.2% solution, I.V. infusion. Rate not to exceed 8 mEq/kg/day. *Metabolic acidosis*— **Adults and children:** dose depends on blood CO_2 content, pH, and patient's clinical condition. Generally, 2 to 5 mEq/kg I.V. infused over 4- to 8-hour period. *Systemic or urinary alkalinization*— **Adults:** 325 mg to 2 g P.O. q.i.d.	**GI:** gastric distention, belching, flatulence. **GU:** renal calculi or crystals. **Metabolic:** (with overdose) alkalosis, hypernatremia, hyperkalemia, hyperosmolarity.
sodium lactate	*Alkalinize urine*— **Adults:** 30 ml of a $\frac{1}{6}$ molar solution/kg of body weight given in divided doses over 24 hours. *Metabolic acidosis*— **Adults:** usually given as $\frac{1}{6}$ mo-	**Metabolic:** (with overdose) alkalosis, hypernatremia, hyperkalemia, hyperosmolarity.

INTERACTIONS	NURSING CONSIDERATIONS
Spironolactone: systemic acidosis. Use together cautiously.	• Contraindicated in severe hepatic or renal dysfunction. Use cautiously in pulmonary insufficiency or cardiac edema and in infants. • Give after meals to decrease GI side effects. Enteric-coated tablets may also minimize GI symptoms but are absorbed erratically. • Pain of I.V. injection may be lessened by decreasing infusion rate. • Determine CO_2 combining power and serum electrolytes before and during therapy to prevent acidosis. • Monitor urine pH and output. Diuresis is normal for first 2 days. • Dilute concentrated solutions (21.4%, 26.75%) to 2.14% before giving. • Monitor rate and depth of respirations frequently. • Hypodermoclysis should be into lateral aspect of thigh. Stop infusion immediately if pain occurs.
None significant.	• Not available commercially; prepared in pharmacy. • Administer I.V. solution slowly through a central venous line. • Monitor pH, blood gases, and electrolytes at 4- to 6-hour intervals.
None significant.	• No contraindications for use in life-threatening emergencies. Contraindicated in hypertension, in patients with tendency toward edema, in patients who are losing chlorides by vomiting or from continuous GI suction, in patients receiving diuretics known to produce hypochloremic alkalosis, and in patients on salt restriction or with renal disease. • May be added to other I.V. fluids. • Parenteral bicarbonate solutions will precipitate calcium salts. Do not mix in same infusion fluid. I.V. bolus injections should be given only through running I.V. lines free of calcium salts. See Chapter 6, UNDERSTANDING INTRAVENOUS SOLUTION COMPATIBILITY. • Because sodium bicarbonate inactivates catecholamines such as epinephrine and norepinephrine, do not mix with I.V. solutions of these agents. • To avoid risk of alkalosis, determine blood pH, Pa_{O_2}, Pa_{CO_2}, and electrolytes. Keep doctor informed of laboratory results. • Tell patient not to take with milk. May cause hypercalcemia, alkalosis, and possibly renal calculi.
None significant.	• Contraindicated in severe hepatic disease, respiratory alkalosis, and acidosis associated with congenital heart disease with persistent cyanosis. • Monitor serum electrolytes to avoid alkalosis and hyperkalemia.

(continued on following page)

NAME	INDICATIONS & DOSAGE	SIDE EFFECTS
sodium lactate *(continued)*	lar injection (167 mEq lactate/ liter). Dosage depends on degree of bicarbonate deficit.	
tromethamine Tham♦	*Metabolic acidosis (associated with cardiac bypass surgery or with cardiac arrest)*— **Adults:** dose depends on bicarbonate deficit. Calculate as follows: ml of 0.3 M tromethamine solution required = wt in kg × bicarbonate deficit (mEq/liter). Additional therapy based on serial determinations of existing bicarbonate deficit. **Children:** calculate dose as above. Give slowly over 3 to 6 hours. Additional therapy based on degree of acidosis. Total 24-hour dose should not exceed 33 to 40 ml/kg.	**CNS:** respiratory depression. **Metabolic:** hypoglycemia, hyperkalemia (with decreased urinary output). **Local:** venospasm; intravenous thrombosis; inflammation, necrosis, and sloughing if extravasation occurs.

INTERACTIONS	NURSING CONSIDERATIONS
None significant.	• Contraindicated in anuria, uremia, chronic respiratory acidosis, pregnancy (except acute, life-threatening situations). Use cautiously in renal disease or poor urinary output. Monitor EKG and serum K^+ in these patients. • To prevent blood pH from rising above normal, adjust dose carefully. • Give slowly through large needle (18G to 20G) into largest antecubital vein or by indwelling catheter. • Before, during, and after therapy, make the following determinations: blood pH; carbon dioxide tension; bicarbonate, glucose, and electrolyte levels. • Mechanical ventilation should be readily available. Use when giving drug to patient with associated respiratory acidosis. • Except in life-threatening situations, do not use longer than 1 day. • If extravasation occurs, infiltrate area with 1% procaine and hyaluronidase 150 units; may reduce vasospasm and dilute remaining drug in local area. • Concentration of tromethamine should not exceed 0.3 M.

104 Uricosurics

probenecid
sulfinpyrazone

Uricosurics are renal tubular blocking agents. By inhibiting active reabsorption of uric acid at the proximal convoluted tubule, they promote excretion of uric acid. This action then lowers uric acid levels in the blood. (For information on allopurinol and colchi-

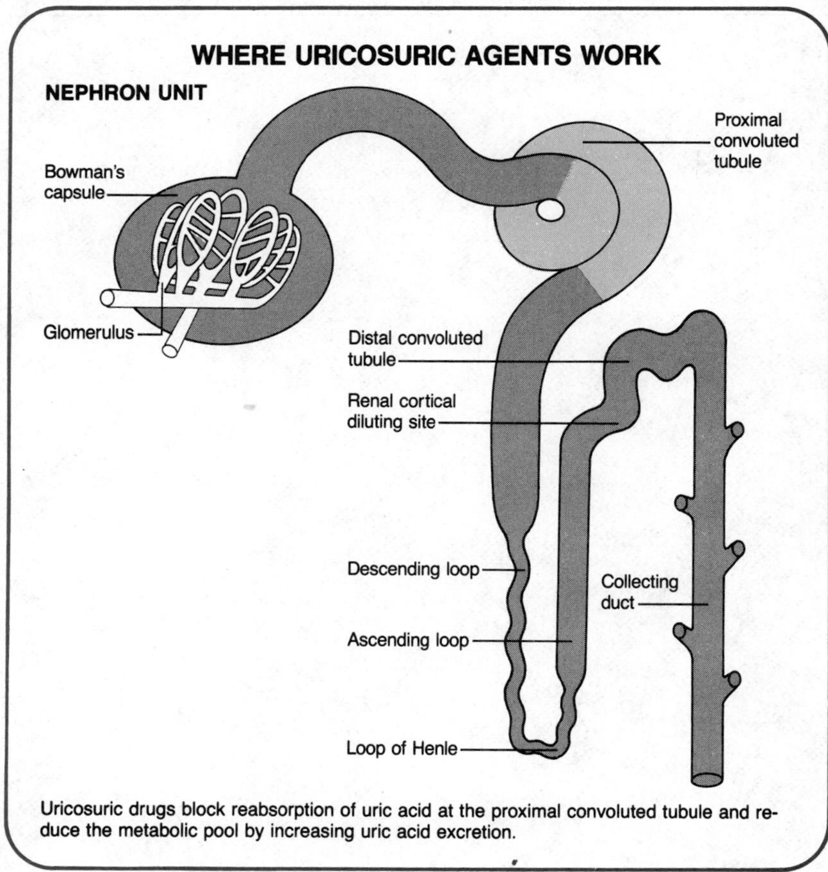

Uricosuric drugs block reabsorption of uric acid at the proximal convoluted tubule and reduce the metabolic pool by increasing uric acid excretion.

cine, which are not uricosuric agents but are used in gout, see Chapter 111, UNCATEGORIZED DRUGS.)

Major uses

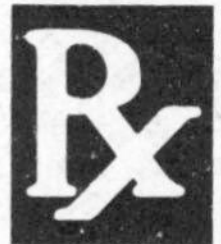

Both uricosurics are used for maintenance therapy in chronic gouty arthritis and tophaceous gout.

- Probenecid is used as an adjunct in penicillin antibiotic therapy by increasing antibiotic blood concentrations.
- Sulfinpyrazone also inhibits platelet aggregation. Some studies have found it useful for patients with myocardial infarction.

Mechanism of action

Uricosurics block renal tubular reabsorption of uric acid, increasing excretion. (See illustration on the opposite page.) They also inhibit active renal tubular secretion of many weak organic acids (for example, penicillins and cephalosporins).

Absorption, distribution, metabolism, and excretion

- The drugs are rapidly and completely absorbed from the gastrointestinal tract after oral administration.
- Probenecid is 95% bound to plasma proteins; sulfinpyrazone is 98% bound to plasma proteins.
- Probenecid and sulfinpyrazone are metabolized in the liver and excreted in urine. A small amount of sulfinpyrazone is also eliminated in feces.

Onset and duration

- Onset (appearance in blood and uric-acid clearance) occurs 30 minutes after oral administration.
- Probenecid's effect on penicillin begins after 2 hours. Blood levels peak 2 to 4 hours after administration.

The drug's duration of action is 4 to 10 hours.

- Sulfinpyrazone blood levels peak 1 to 2 hours after ingestion. Duration of action is also 4 to 10 hours.

UNDERSTANDING THE ANTURANE CONTROVERSY

Every year about 8% of American heart attack victims discharged from the hospital to recuperate die within 12 months. Three fourths of these deaths occur during the first 6 months—most of them caused by arrhythmias that produce sudden death.

Several research studies have attempted to discover which drugs, if any, could prevent these lethal arrhythmias during the high-risk period of 6 months after a heart attack.

One group of researchers thought sulfinpyrazone (Anturane) might decrease the number of sudden deaths since it's been effective in preventing platelets from sticking together and clogging blood vessels. Consequently, a study was conducted involving more than 1,600 patients in 26 medical centers in the United States and in Canada. This was known as the Anturane Reinfarction Trial.

Patients entered the double-blind study 25 to 35 days after they had had their heart attacks. The Anturane reinfarction researchers concluded, after 2 years of study, that Anturane reduced the overall number of sudden deaths by 43%.

After reviewing the study's conclusions, the FDA turned down the manufacturer's request for permission to label and advertise Anturane for the prevention of sudden death after heart attack because it felt the study's claimed reduction in sudden deaths had been exaggerated.

Evaluation of research methodology showed several factors that may have biased the study in favor of Anturane. Experts who reviewed the data found some deaths misclassified, and most of the misclassified deaths favored the study hypothesis.

What all this means for your patient is that *Anturane is no miracle cure for post–heart-attack deaths.* Although Anturane may be helpful, there's some doubt about its real effectiveness. Its use for prevention of sudden death after heart attack remains unapproved.

Combination products

COLBENEMID: probenecid 500 mg and colchicine 0.5 mg.

PROBEN-C: probenecid 500 mg and colchicine 0.5 mg.

NAME	INDICATIONS & DOSAGE	SIDE EFFECTS
probenecid Benemid♦, Benn, Benuryl♦♦, Probalan, Probenimead, Robenecid	*Adjunct to penicillin or cephalosporin therapy—* **Adults, and children over 50 kg:** 500 mg P.O. q.i.d. **Children 2 to 14 years (under 50 kg):** initially, 25 mg/kg P.O., then 40 mg/kg divided q.i.d. *Single-dose treatment of gonorrhea—* **Adults:** 3.5 g ampicillin P.O. with 1 g probenecid P.O. given together; or 1 g probenecid P.O. 30 minutes before dose of 4.8 million units of aqueous penicillin G procaine I.M., injected at 2 different sites. *Treatment of hyperuricemia of gout, gouty arthritis—* **Adults:** 250 mg P.O. b.i.d. for first week, then 500 mg b.i.d., to maximum of 2 g daily. Maintenance: 500 mg daily for 6 months.	**Blood:** *hemolytic anemia.* **CNS:** headache, dizziness. **CV:** hypotension. **GI:** anorexia, nausea, vomiting, *gastric distress.* **GU:** urinary frequency. **Skin:** dermatitis, pruritus. **Other:** flushing, sore gums, fever.
sulfinpyrazone Anturan♦♦, Anturane	*Inhibition of platelet aggregation, increase of platelet survival time in treatment of thromboembolic disorders, angina, myocardial infarction, transient cerebral ischemic attacks, peripheral arterial atherosclerosis—* **Adults:** 200 mg P.O. q.i.d. *Maintenance therapy for common gout: reduction, prevention of joint changes and tophi formation—* **Adults:** 100 to 200 mg P.O. b.i.d. first week, then 200 to 400 mg P.O. b.i.d. Maximum 800 mg daily.	**GI:** *nausea, dyspepsia,* epigastric pain, blood loss, reactivation of peptic ulcers. **Skin:** rash.

♦ Available in U.S. and Canada. ♦♦ Available in Canada only. All other products (no symbol) available in U.S. only. Italicized side effects are common or life-threatening.

INTERACTIONS	NURSING CONSIDERATIONS
Salicylates: inhibited uricosuric effect of probenecid, causing urate retention. Do not use together.	• Contraindicated in blood dyscrasias; acute gout attack; penicillin therapy in presence of known renal impairment; gouty nephropathy; urinary tract stones or obstruction; azotemia, hyperuricemia secondary to cancer chemotherapy, radiation, or myeloproliferative neoplastic diseases. Use cautiously with peptic ulcer or renal impairment. • Usually preferred over sulfinpyrazone because probenecid produces fewer, less severe GI and hematologic side effects. • Contains no analgesic or anti-inflammatory agent, and is of no value during acute gout attacks. • Suitable for long-term use; no cumulative effects or tolerance. • Not effective with chronic renal insufficiency (glomerular filtration rate less than 30 ml/minute). • Periodic BUN and renal function studies recommended in long-term therapy. • May increase frequency, severity, and length of acute gout attacks during first 6 to 12 months of therapy. Prophylactic colchicine is given during first 3 to 6 months. • Tell patient to avoid alcohol; it increases urate level. • Force fluids to maintain minimum daily output of 2 to 3 liters. Alkalinize urine with sodium bicarbonate or potassium citrate ordered by doctor. These measures will prevent hematuria, renal colic, urate stone development, and costovertebral pain. • Give with milk, food, or antacids to minimize GI distress. Continued disturbances might indicate need to lower dose. • Restrict foods high in purine: anchovies, liver, sardines, kidneys, sweetbreads, peas, lentils. • Instruct patient and family that drug must be taken regularly as ordered or gout attacks may result. Tell him to visit doctor regularly so blood levels can be monitored and dosage can be adjusted if necessary. Lifelong therapy may be required in patients with hyperuricemia. • May produce false-positive glucose tests with Benedict's solution or Clinitest, but not with glucose oxidase method (Clinistix, Diastix, Tes-Tape). • Decreases urinary excretion of 17-ketosteroids, phenolsulfonphthalein (PSP), Bromsulphalein (BSP), aminohippuric acid, and iodine-related organic acids, interfering with laboratory procedures. • For treatment of anaphylaxis, see inside front cover.
Probenecid: inhibited renal excretion of sulfinpyrazone. Use together with caution. *Salicylates:* inhibited uricosuric effect of sulfinpyrazone. Do not use together.	• Contraindicated in hypersensitivity to pyrazole derivatives (including oxyphenbutazone, phenylbutazone); active peptic ulcer; gouty nephropathy; urolithiasis or urinary obstruction; bone marrow depression; azotemia, hyperuricemia secondary to cancer chemotherapy, radiation, or myeloproliferative neoplastic diseases; and during or within 2 weeks after gout attack. Use cautiously in diminished hepatic or renal function. • Use in treating thromboembolic conditions is investigational and is most often directed at prevention of recurrent myocardial infarction. • Recommended for patients unresponsive to probenecid. Suitable for long-term use; no cumulative effects or tolerance. • Contains no analgesic or anti-inflammatory agent, and is of no value during acute gout attacks. • Periodic BUN, CBC, and renal function studies advised during long-term use. • May increase frequency, severity, and length of acute gout attacks during first 6 to 12 months of therapy; prophylactic colchicine is given during first 3 to 6 months. • Therapy, especially at start, may lead to renal colic and formation of uric acid stones. Until acid levels are normal (about 6 mg/100 ml), monitor intake and output closely.

(continued on following page)

NAME	INDICATIONS & DOSAGE	SIDE EFFECTS
sulfinpyrazone *(continued)*		

♦ Available in U.S. and Canada. ♦♦ Available in Canada only. All other products (no symbol) available in U.S. only. Italicized side effects are common or life-threatening.

INTERACTIONS	NURSING CONSIDERATIONS
	• Force fluids to maintain minimum daily output of 2 to 3 liters. Alkalinize urine with sodium bicarbonate or other agent ordered by doctor. • Give with milk, food, or antacids to minimize GI disturbances. • Restrict foods high in purine: anchovies, liver, sardines, kidneys, sweetbreads, peas, lentils. • Instruct patient and family that drug must be taken regularly as ordered or gout attacks may result. Tell him to visit doctor regularly so blood levels can be monitored and dosage adjusted if necessary. • Lifelong therapy may be required in patients with hyperuricemia. • Decreases urinary excretion of aminohippuric acid and phenolsulfonphthalein (PSP), interfering with laboratory procedures. • Alkalinizing agents are used therapeutically to increase sulfinpyrazone activity, preventing urolithiasis. • Warn patient not to take any aspirin-containing medications. • Monitor patients taking oral hypoglycemic agents; these drugs' effects may be potentiated by sulfinpyrazone, causing hypoglycemia.

105 Enzymes

bromelains
chymotrypsin
fibrinolysin and desoxyribonuclease
hyaluronidase
papain
streptokinase-streptodornase
trypsin

Enzymes are complex proteins that induce chemical changes without being changed themselves. Although several enzyme groups are used therapeutically, only those that reduce inflammation or debride necrotic tissue are described in this chapter.

Enzymes can be given orally, topically, locally, subcutaneously, or intramuscularly. They work best in a moist environment but are destroyed by heat or cold. They are also inactivated by detergents, antiseptics, and heavy-metal compounds. Enzymes furnish adjunctive therapy only, so other medical or surgical management is necessary to cure or alleviate underlying causes of tissue necrosis and inflammation.

Major uses

Rx

- Bromelains, chymotrypsin, papain, and trypsin (proteolytic enzymes) are used as adjunctive therapy for inflammation and edema from accidental or surgical trauma.
- Fibrinolysin and desoxyribonuclease—in topical applications only—remove necrotic debris and exudate from wounds.
- Hyaluronidase increases absorption and dispersion of infusions and locally injected drugs such as anesthetics.
- Streptokinase-streptodornase (a mixture of bacterial enzymes) dissolves blood clots and the fibrinous portion of exudate.

Mechanism of action

Enzymes reverse the decreased tissue permeability that develops with inflammation and edema. In this way, they restore flow of blood and other body fluids, and facilitate drainage and tissue repair.

They degrade protein of blood clots, necrotic tissue, and purulent exudate, which may block free flow of body fluids and impede resolution of inflammation and edema.

They digest protein matter, cleaning wounds by liquefaction and dissolution.

Absorption, distribution, metabolism, and excretion

The extent of absorption of these enzymes cannot be measured. Their distribution, metabolism, and excretion are unknown.

Onset and duration

Unknown.

Combination products

CHYMORAL ENTERIC-COATED TABLETS: 50,000 units enzymatic activity; trypsin and chymotrypsin in ratio of 6:1.

CHYMORAL-100: 100,000 units enzymatic activity; trypsin and chymotrypsin in ratio of 6:1.
GRANULEX AEROSOL: trypsin 0.1 mg, balsam Peru 72.5 mg, and castor oil 650 mg per 0.82 ml.
ORENZYME BITABS ENTERIC-COATED TABLETS: 100,000 units trypsin and 8,000 units chymotrypsin.
ORENZYME ENTERIC-COATED TABLETS♦: 50,000 units trypsin and 4,000 units chymotrypsin.

NURSING TIP

PROMOTING EFFECTIVE ENZYME THERAPY FOR DECUBITUS ULCERS

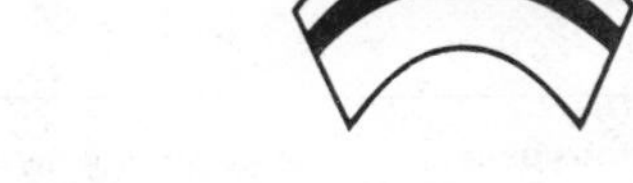

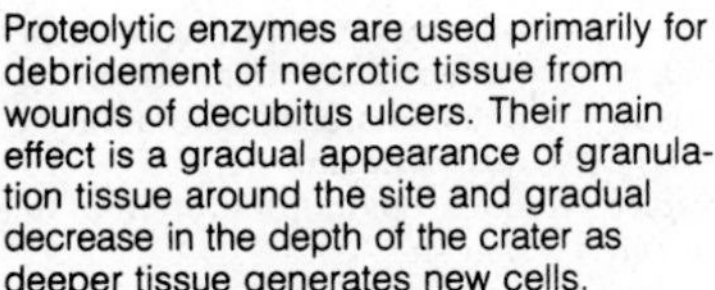

Proteolytic enzymes are used primarily for debridement of necrotic tissue from wounds of decubitus ulcers. Their main effect is a gradual appearance of granulation tissue around the site and gradual decrease in the depth of the crater as deeper tissue generates new cells.

Enzyme therapy has many limitations. Because enzymes are proteins, they need a high degree of purification before administration. Even then, they may be antigenic and cause toxic reactions. Another drawback is that protein-digesting enzymes of the gastrointestinal tract tend to inhibit proteolytic enzyme activity. Despite these limitations, enzymes have been proven useful.

However, effective treatment with enzymes requires certain supportive measures, depending on the underlying cause—stasis, trauma, or infection.

- Use sterile technique in caring for the patient with decubitus ulcers.
- Use a heat lamp and air exposure between dressings to promote drying and increase the blood supply to the ulcerated area.
- Provide oxygen saturation by inserting an oxygen catheter through a paper-cup tent over decubitus ulcers. This promotes healing by producing a drying effect.
- Use enzymes carefully according to the progress of the wound or decubitus area. Remember that denuding necrotic areas may expose capillaries and cause bleeding at the site.
- Place the patient on a flotation pad to protect pressure points on the body.
- Turn the patient frequently.
- Give regular back rubs and gently massage all pressure areas of the body.
- Monitor adequate food and fluid intake to speed recovery.

NAME	INDICATIONS & DOSAGE	SIDE EFFECTS
bromelains Ananase	*Adjunct to reduce inflammation and edema, ease pain, and speed tissue repair of traumatic injuries (contusions, sprains, strains, dislocations), cellulitis, furunculosis, ulcerations*— **Adults:** initially, 100,000 units P.O. q.i.d., then 50,000 units t.i.d. or q.i.d. for maintenance.	**Blood:** bleeding tendencies. **GI:** mild diarrhea, nausea, vomiting. **GU:** menorrhagia, metrorrhagia. **Other:** fever, hypersensitivity reactions (rash, urticaria).
chymotrypsin Avazyme	*Adjunct in general, rectal, oral, and dental surgery*— **Adults:** preoperatively, 2,500 units I.M.; then 2,500 units once or twice daily, as indicated. *Adjunct in treatment of respiratory conditions (asthma, bronchitis, rhinitis, sinusitis)*— **Adults:** 2,500 to 5,000 units I.M. once or twice weekly; more often if needed. **Children:** ½ adult dose. *Chronic or recurrent inflammation (peptic ulcer, ulcerative colitis, phlebitis, thrombophlebitis, dermatologic conditions)*— **Adults:** 2,500 to 5,000 units I.M. once or twice weekly. Tablet containing 10,000 units may be given buccally q.i.d. alone or in conjunction with I.M. therapy. *Relief of episiotomy symptoms*— **Adults:** 5,000 units I.M. repeated twice at 12-hour intervals. Tablet containing 20 mg (20,000 units) may be given P.O. q.i.d. *Pelvic inflammatory diseases*— **Adults:** 2,500 units daily for 7 days; repeat course if needed.	**Blood:** increased bleeding tendencies. **GI:** nausea, vomiting, diarrhea with oral administration. **GU:** hematuria, albuminuria, menorrhagia. **Local:** pain, induration at injection site. **Other:** chills, dizziness, fever, rapid dissolution of animal-origin sutures, *hypersensitivity reactions (rash, urticaria, itching, anaphylaxis).*
fibrinolysin and desoxyribonuclease Elase♦	*Debridement of inflammatory and infected lesions (surgical wounds, ulcerative lesions, second- and third-degree burns, circumcision, episiotomy, cervicitis, vaginitis, abscesses, fistulas, and sinus tracts)*— **Intravaginally:** 5 ml ointment may be inserted using applicator supplied, once daily for vaginitis or cervicitis. **Topical use:** apply ointment 30 units fibrinolysin, 20,000 units desoxyribonuclease/30 g at	**Local:** hyperemia with high doses.

♦ Available in U.S. and Canada. ♦♦ Available in Canada only. All other products (no symbol) available in U.S. only. Italicized side effects are common or life-threatening.

INTERACTIONS	NURSING CONSIDERATIONS
Alkaline solutions, antacids: dissolve enteric coating of tablet. Do not use within 1 hour of bromelains.	• Contraindicated in hypersensitivity to pineapple or pineapple products. Use cautiously with anticoagulant therapy and in patients with blood-clotting abnormalities, including hemophilia; hepatic or renal disease; and systemic infection. • Obtain history of allergies. Watch for hypersensitivity reactions and discontinue drug immediately if any occur. • Destruction of enteric coating may decrease effectiveness. Tablets must be swallowed whole; do not crush or break. • Observe wound to monitor progress of therapy. Appearance of granulation tissue may indicate effectiveness. Notify doctor if inflammation or color of drainage indicates spread of infection. • Protect from heat.
Alkaline solutions, antacids: dissolve enteric coating of tablet. Do not use within 1 hour of oral administration of chymotrypsin.	• Contraindicated in hypersensitivity to trypsin or to sesame oil (injectable form), septicemia, severe generalized or localized infection, and blood coagulation disorders such as hemophilia. Use with caution in severe hepatic or renal disease. • Parenteral administration: Do not give I.V. Test for sensitivity before giving. Inject deep into gluteal muscle; rotate sites. Watch for hypersensitivity reactions, including changes in blood pressure and pulse rate. Watch for pain, induration at injection site. Stop if reaction occurs. • Avoid getting in eyes. If drug does get into eyes, flood with water at once. • Protect from heat. • For treatment of anaphylaxis, see inside front cover.
None significant.	• Contraindicated for parenteral use. • Dense, dry eschar must be removed surgically before enzymatic debridement. Enzyme must be in constant contact with substrate. Accumulated necrotic debris must be removed periodically. • Clean wound with water or peroxide and dry gently; cover with thin layer of Elase. Cover with nonadhering dressing. • Change dressing at least once a day. Flush away necrotic debris and reapply ointment. • Solution as wet dressing: Mix 1 vial of Elase powder with 10 to 50 ml saline solution; saturate strips of fine gauze with solution. Pack ulcerated area with Elase gauze. Allow gauze to dry in contact with ulcerated lesion for about 6 to 8 hours. Remove dried gauze and repeat 3 to 4 times daily. • Solution as irrigating agent: Drain cavity and replace Elase every

(continued on following page)

NAME	INDICATIONS & DOSAGE	SIDE EFFECTS
fibrinolysin and desoxyribonuclease *(continued)*	intervals as long as enzyme action is desired. *Irrigating agent for infected wounds, empyema cavities, abscesses, otorhinolaryngologic wounds, subcutaneous hematomas*—dilution for irrigation depends on extent and severity of wound: 25 units fibrinolysin powder, 15,000 units desoxyribonuclease per 30-ml vial.	
hyaluronidase Wydase♦	*Adjunct to increase absorption and dispersion of other injected drugs*— **Adults and children:** 150 units to injection medium containing other medication. *Hypodermoclysis*— **Adults, and children over 3 years:** 150 units injected S.C. before clysis or injected into clysis tubing near needle for each 1,000 ml clysis solution. *Subcutaneous urography*— **Adults and children:** with patient prone, give 75 units S.C. over each scapula, followed by injection of contrast medium at same sites.	**Skin:** rash, urticaria. **Local:** irritation.
papain Panafil, Papase♦	*Prevention of inflammation and edema in surgical procedures*— **Adults and children:** 10,000 to 20,000 units P.O. or buccally 1 to 2 hours before surgery, then 20,000 units q.i.d. for up to 5 days. *Treatment of inflammation and burns, enzymatic debridement, promotion of normal healing and deodorization of surface lesions, particularly in local infection, necrosis, fibrinous or purulent debris, sloughing*— **Adults and children:** apply ointment 10% directly to lesion 1 to 2 times daily. Cover with gauze.	**Blood:** increased bleeding tendencies. **GI:** nausea, vomiting, diarrhea with oral administration. **Local:** tingling at site of buccal absorption, occasional itching or stinging with first application of ointment. **Other:** fever, hypersensitivity reactions (rash, urticaria, pruritus).
streptokinase-streptodornase Varidase♦	*Anti-inflammatory agent to relieve pain, swelling, tenderness, erythema; management of edema and localized extravasation of blood from infection, trauma, certain dental condi-*	**GI:** nausea, vomiting, diarrhea with oral administration. **Skin:** rash, urticaria.

♦ Available in U.S. and Canada. ♦♦ Available in Canada only. All other products (no symbol) available in U.S. only. Italicized side effects are common or life-threatening.

INTERACTIONS	**NURSING CONSIDERATIONS**
	6 to 10 hours to reduce amount of by-product accumulation and to minimize loss of enzyme activity. Although parenteral use is contraindicated, Elase is used as an irrigating agent in certain specific conditions. • Prepare solution just before use. Discard after 24 hours.
Local anesthetics: increased potential for toxic local reaction. Use together cautiously.	• Use with caution in patients with blood-clotting abnormalities, severe hepatic or renal disease. • Do not inject into acutely inflamed or cancerous areas. • In hypodermoclysis, adjust dose, rate of injection, and type of solution to patient response. • Administration precautions: Skin-test for sensitivity. Avoid injecting into diseased areas (may spread infection). Observe injection site for local reactions. • Avoid getting solution in eyes. If solution does get into eyes, flood with water at once. • Protect from heat. Do not use cloudy or discolored solution.
With topical use, detergents and antiseptics (benzalkonium chloride, hexachlorophene, iodine, hydrogen peroxide): decreased enzymatic activity. Do not use together.	• Contraindicated in hypersensitivity to papaya fruit. Oral administration contraindicated in anticoagulant therapy; blood-clotting abnormalities, including hemophilia; and systemic infections. Use cautiously in severe hepatic or renal disease. • Instruct patient on proper route to be used. Oral tablets may be swallowed with water or chewed. • Before treatment, thoroughly cleanse and irrigate wound area with sterile normal saline solution or water to remove antiseptics, detergents, and heavy-metal antibacterials, which can decrease enzyme activity. Don't use hydrogen peroxide, as it inactivates topical papain. Moisten area for optimal enzymatic activity. Apply ointment in thin layers to assure contact with necrotic tissue. Cover with gauze. • Irrigate lesion with mild cleansing solution (not hydrogen peroxide) at each redressing. • Observe wound to monitor progress of therapy. Appearance of granulation tissue may indicate effectiveness. Notify doctor if inflammation or color of drainage indicates spread of infection. • Avoid getting ointment in eyes. If it does get into eyes, flood with water at once. • Protect drug from heat.
None significant.	• Contraindicated in active hemorrhage; decreased level of fibrinogen; acute cellulitis without suppuration; or risk of reopening preexisting bronchopleural fistulas, especially in active tuberculosis. Use P.O. and I.M. forms with caution in severe renal disease, depressed hepatic function or hepatic disease, or abnormalities of blood-clotting mechanism.

(continued on following page)

NAME	INDICATIONS & DOSAGE	SIDE EFFECTS
streptokinase-streptodornase *(continued)*	*tions*—dose and route of administration are determined by patient's response, location of lesion, ease of drainage or aspiration, size of cavity, and ability of cavity to expand. Higher doses than those stated may be advisable in severe cases. **Adults and children:** 1 tablet containing 10,000 IU streptokinase (SK) and 2,500 IU streptodornase (SD) q.i.d. for 4 to 6 days; 0.5 ml P.O. of injectable solution (5,000 IU SK) I.M. b.i.d.	
trypsin	*In general and oral surgical procedures to reduce inflammation, accelerate reabsorption of edema, facilitate restoration of local tissue circulation; to reduce inflammation and edema of bronchial mucosa; as adjunct in treatment of phlebothrombosis, thrombophlebitis, iritis, iridocyclitis, chorioretinitis, cutaneous ulcerative conditions*— **Adults:** 50,000 to 100,000 units P.O. q.i.d.; or 12,500 units I.M. daily or for severe conditions b.i.d. for 1 to 2 days, then 12,500 units daily. Solution for wet dressings: 10,000 units in each ml normal saline solution or water for injection. Apply new dressings when dry. Ointment: 5,000 units/g once daily or b.i.d. Inhalation: 125,000 units dissolved in 3 ml saline solution or water inhaled at least once daily.	**Blood:** increased bleeding tendencies. **CNS:** dizziness, fainting. **EENT:** rhinorrhea, sneezing, with aerosol inhalation. **GI:** nausea, vomiting, diarrhea, abdominal pain. **GU:** albuminuria, hematuria. **Skin:** rash, pruritus, urticaria. **Local:** pain and induration, local irritation. **Other:** febrile reactions, angioneurotic edema, rapid dissolution of sutures of animal origins, *anaphylaxis*.

INTERACTIONS	NURSING CONSIDERATIONS
	• Do not give I.V. • If infection is present, consider concomitant antimicrobial therapy with compatible agent, such as tetracycline, penicillin, streptomycin. • I.M. use: Add 2 ml sterile water for injection or sterile normal saline solution to 25,000-unit vial streptokinase-streptodornase (result is solution of 5,000 IU SK per 0.5 ml). Inject deep I.M., preferably into gluteal muscle. Store remaining solution for up to 2 weeks in refrigerator or 24 hours at room temperature. • Avoid getting solution in eyes. If solution does get into eyes, flood with water at once. • Protect from heat. • Streptokinase and streptodornase are antigenic; antienzymes may develop following prolonged therapy or acute hemolytic streptococcal infections. High antienzyme titer apparently not harmful, but dosage may have to be increased to overcome its effect.
With topical use, detergents and antiseptics (benzalkonium chloride, hexachlorophene, iodine, hydrogen peroxide): decreased enzymatic activity. Do not use together.	• Contraindicated in patients with history of allergic reactions to parenteral enzyme therapy. Use with extreme caution in severe hepatic or renal disease, abnormalities of blood-clotting mechanism. • Test for possible hypersensitivity reactions before I.M. administration. Observe for 30 minutes after I.M. administration. Have epinephrine 1:1,000 available. • Do not apply to actively bleeding areas, ocular lesions, or to ulcerated carcinomas. • Do not give I.V. • Enteric-coated tablets must be swallowed whole; do not crush or break. • Give deep I.M. in gluteal muscle, alternating sites. • Follow nasal inhalation with water or saline spray. Have patient take several swallows of water to remove large droplets from oropharynx. • Store in tightly closed container. Protect from heat. • For treatment of anaphylaxis, see inside front cover.

106 Oxytocics

carboprost tromethamine
dinoprost tromethamine
dinoprostone
ergonovine maleate
methylergonovine maleate
oxytocin citrate, buccal
oxytocin, synthetic injection
oxytocin, synthetic nasal
sodium chloride 20% solution

Oxytocics stimulate the smooth muscle of the uterus during childbirth. They are especially useful in the last stage of labor (Stage III), in which the placenta is sloughed and expelled. Generally, oxytocics should be avoided in stages I and II since they increase the risk of uterine rupture.

Major uses

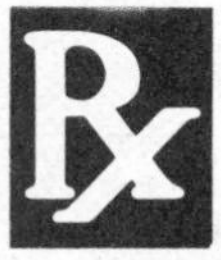

- Carboprost, dinoprost, dinoprostone, and sodium chloride induce therapeutic abortion in the second trimester.
- Ergonovine and methylergonovine correct postpartum uterine atony.
- Ergonovine, methylergonovine, and oxytocins control postpartum bleeding.
- Oxytocins induce labor or intensify uterine contractions at term.
- Oxytocin, synthetic nasal preparation, stimulates contraction of the myoepithelium in the mammary glands, facilitating milk ejection in lactating females.

Mechanism of action

- Carboprost, dinoprost, and dinoprostone (prostaglandins) produce strong, prompt contractions of uterine smooth muscle, possibly mediated by calcium and cyclic 3',5'-adenosine monophosphate. Endocrine levels also influence contractions. These drugs promote cervical dilation and softening, and exert uterine effects by direct stimulation of the myometrium.
- Ergonovine and methylergonovine (ergot alkaloids) increase motor activity of the uterus by direct stimulation. A gravid uterus responds markedly even to small doses.
- Oxytocin may act as a hormone in potent and selective stimulation of uterine and mammary gland smooth muscle. It produces uterine contractions of the same intensity, duration, and frequency as those in spontaneous labor. Oxytocin may stimulate contractions of uterine smooth muscle by increasing the sodium permeability of uterine myofibrils.
- Sodium chloride 20% solution may damage decidual cells, causing release of prostaglandins and leading to fetal death and abortion.

Absorption, distribution, metabolism, and excretion

- Carboprost, dinoprost, and dinoprostone diffuse slowly into maternal blood after administration and are widely distributed in maternal and fetal tissues. They concentrate in fetal liver and are rapidly metabolized in maternal lungs and liver. They're excreted within 24 hours, mainly in urine.

• Ergonovine and methylergonovine are rapidly absorbed after oral or I.M. administration and are slowly metabolized in the liver. Metabolism in neonates may be prolonged.
• Oxytocin is inactivated by trypsin in the gastrointestinal tract; tissue peptidases inactivate most of the drug when it is administered buccally. Oxytocin is distributed to extracellular fluid, and small amounts may reach the fetal circulation. The drug has a short half-life (3 to 5 minutes), which is reduced late in pregnancy and in lactation. The liver and kidneys destroy most of the drug. Only small amounts are excreted unchanged in urine.
• Sodium chloride undergoes little or no systemic absorption. It appears to concentrate in the decidual and fetal parts of the placenta. Some of the drug diffuses into the maternal blood and is excreted in urine.

Onset and duration

• Carboprost, dinoprost, and dinoprostone begin to act promptly. Their action is dose-dependent, with sensitivity increasing at term. Contractions usually begin within 10 to 15 minutes after administration and may continue 10 to 30 minutes after the drug is stopped. In most patients, abortion occurs within 30 hours.
• Ergonovine and methylergonovine produce uterine contractions immediately after I.V. administration and within 5 to 15 minutes after oral or I.M. administration. Contractions may continue 3 or more hours after oral or I.M. administration, and 45 minutes after I.V. administration. Small doses produce increased contractions followed by a normal degree of relaxation; larger doses produce more forceful contractions but increase resting tonus.
• Oxytocin produces uterine contractions within several minutes; they continue 2 to 3 hours.
• A sodium chloride 20% solution that produces a sodium concentration in amniotic fluid of at least 2.2 mEq/ml usually induces abortion within 50 hours. Instillation may be repeated in 48 hours. If the patient fails to respond to the second dose, other abortifacient methods should be tried.

Combination products

None.

WHEN OXYTOCIN IS USED TO INDUCE LABOR

The hormone oxytocin stimulates uterine contractions and initiates labor naturally. But when *synthetic* oxytocin is used to induce labor, the contractions are, in many cases, stronger and longer, with shorter relaxation periods between. Thus, synthetic oxytocin should only be used when medically indicated and *not* for the convenience of the doctor or the mother. Unfortunately, oxytocin is used to induce labor in 40% to 50% of deliveries, yet it may be needed in less than 2%.

These problems may occur when using synthetic oxytocin to induce labor:
• The baby may be stressed before its first breath. Frequent strong contractions diminish the baby's ability to restore its supply of oxygen between contractions because uterine blood flow is shut off during each strong contraction. Be especially alert for signs of fetal distress.
• Studies show that when oxytocin is given to women in labor, 25% show some asphyxiation patterns. When oxytocin and epidural anesthetic are used together, 50% of the women show asphyxiation patterns.
• The need for pain-killing drugs or anesthetic is probably higher with oxytocin, because the contractions are stronger.
• Oxytocin's rate of success is only 85%. Thus, labor sometimes stops abruptly, leaving the mother with a partially dilated cervix. This is a disappointing and potentially frightening experience for the woman who is sent home in this condition and told to return when labor begins normally. Such patients require extra health teaching and emotional support.

Adapted from Dr. Silvia Feldman, *Choices in Childbirth* (New York: Grosset & Dunlap, 1978), with permission from the publisher.

NAME	INDICATIONS & DOSAGE	SIDE EFFECTS
carboprost tromethamine Prostin/M15	*Abort pregnancy between 13th and 20th weeks of gestation*—initially, 250 mcg is administered deep I.M. Subsequent doses of 250 mcg should be administered at intervals of 1½ to 3½ hours, depending on uterine response. Increments in dosage may be increased to 500 mcg if contractility is inadequate after several 250 mcg doses. Total dose should not exceed 12 mg.	**GI:** *vomiting, diarrhea.* **Other:** *fever.*
dinoprost tromethamine Prostin F_2 Alpha	*Abort second trimester pregnancy*—1 ml of amniotic fluid is withdrawn by transabdominal intra-amniotic catheter. If no blood is present in tap, 40 mg of dinoprost is injected directly into amniotic sac. Initially, 5 mg is given very slowly (1 mg/minute), and patient is watched for adverse reactions. Then, remainder is injected. If abortion not completed in 24 hours, another 10 to 40 mg may be given. Uterine activity may continue 10 to 30 minutes after drug is stopped.	**CNS:** dizziness, fainting. **GI:** *nausea, vomiting, diarrhea,* abdominal cramps, epigastric pain. **Other:** bronchospasm, wheezing.
dinoprostone Prostin E_2♦	*Abort second trimester pregnancy, evacuate uterus in cases of missed abortion, intrauterine fetal deaths up to 28 weeks of gestation, or benign hydatidiform mole*—insert 20 mg suppository high into posterior vaginal fornix. Repeat q 3 to 5 hours until abortion is complete.	**CNS:** *headache.* **CV:** hypotension (in large doses). **GI:** *nausea, vomiting, diarrhea.* **GU:** vaginal pain, vaginitis. **Other:** fever, shivering, chills.
ergonovine maleate Ergotrate Maleate♦	*Prevent or treat postpartum and postabortion hemorrhage due to uterine atony or subinvolution*—0.2 mg I.M. q 2 to 4 hours, maximum 5 doses; or 0.2 mg I.V. (only for severe uterine bleeding or other life-threatening emergency) over 1 minute while blood pressure and uterine contractions are	**CNS:** dizziness, headache. **CV:** hypertension, chest pain. **EENT:** tinnitus. **GI:** *nausea, vomiting.* **GU:** uterine cramping. **Other:** sweating, dyspnea, hypersensitivity.

♦ Available in U.S. and Canada. ♦♦ Available in Canada only. All other products (no symbol) available in U.S. only. Italicized side effects are common or life-threatening.

INTERACTIONS	NURSING CONSIDERATIONS
None significant.	• Contraindicated in patients with pelvic inflammatory disease or active cardiac, pulmonary, renal, or hepatic disease. Use cautiously in patients with a history of asthma; hypertension; cardiovascular, renal, or hepatic disease; anemia; jaundice; diabetes; epilepsy. • I.M. injection of this drug is technically less difficult and poses fewer potential risks than other prostaglandin abortifacients. • Carboprost can be used without concern that expulsion of vaginal suppositories may occur in the presence of profuse vaginal bleeding. • Live birth may result. • Should be used only in a hospital setting by trained personnel.
Alcohol (I.V. infusions of 500 ml of 10% over 1 hour): inhibited uterine activity. *I.V. oxytocin:* cervical perforation, especially in primigravida patients or in those with inadequately dilated cervices. Use with caution.	• Contraindicated in patients with pelvic inflammatory disease. Use with caution in cardiovascular, renal, or hypertensive disease; asthma; glaucoma; or epilepsy. • Observe and record character and amount of vaginal bleeding. • Live birth may result. • Other measures may be required if dinoprost fails to terminate pregnancy completely. Utilization of hypertonic saline solution should be delayed until uterine contractions stop. • Monitor vital signs. Report rapid fall in blood pressure or hypertonic uterine contractions. • Instruct patient to remain in prone position. • After abortion, observe patient frequently for cervical injuries. • Store at 2° to 8° C. (35.6° to 46.4° F.). Discard 24 months after manufacture date. • Should be used only in hospital setting by trained personnel.
None significant.	• Contraindicated in patients with pelvic inflammatory disease or history of pelvic surgery, incisions, uterine fibroids, or cervical stenosis. Use with caution in asthma, epilepsy, anemia, diabetes, hyper- or hypotension, jaundice, or cardiovascular, renal, or hepatic disease. • Live birth may result. • Warm dinoprostone suppositories in their wrapping to room temperature. • After insertion of suppository, patient should remain supine for 10 minutes. • Store suppositories in freezer at temperature no higher than −20° C. (−4° F.). • Should be administered only when critical-care facilities are readily available. • Dinoprostone-induced fever is self-limiting and transient. Treat with water or alcohol sponging and increased fluid intake rather than with aspirin, which has not proved effective. • Abortion should be complete within 30 hours.
Regional anesthetics, dopamine, I.V. oxytocin: excessive vasoconstriction. Use together cautiously.	• Contraindicated for induction or augmentation of labor, before delivery of placenta, in threatened spontaneous abortion, and in patients with allergy or sensitivity to ergot preparations. Use cautiously in hypertension, cardiac disease, venoatrial shunts, mitral valve stenosis, obliterative vascular disease, sepsis, and hepatic or renal impairment. • Monitor blood pressure, pulse rate, and uterine response. Report sudden changes in vital signs, frequent periods of uterine relaxation, and/or character and amount of vaginal bleeding. • Hypocalcemia may decrease patient response. If patient is not also taking digitalis, cautious administration of calcium gluconate I.V.

(continued on following page)

NAME	INDICATIONS & DOSAGE	SIDE EFFECTS
ergonovine maleate *(continued)*	monitored. I.V. dose may be diluted to 5 ml with 0.9% sodium chloride injection. After initial I.M. or I.V. dose, may give 0.2 to 0.4 mg P.O. q 6 to 12 hours for 2 to 7 days. Decrease dose if severe uterine cramping occurs.	
methylergonovine maleate Methergine	*Prevent and treat postpartum hemorrhage due to uterine atony or subinvolution*—0.2 mg I.M. q 2 to 5 hours for maximum of 5 doses; or I.V. (excessive uterine bleeding or other emergencies) over 1 minute while blood pressure and uterine contractions are monitored. I.V. dose may be diluted to 5 ml with 0.9% sodium chloride injection. Following initial I.M. or I.V. dose, may give 0.2 to 0.4 mg P.O. q 6 to 12 hours for 2 to 7 days. Dose may be decreased if severe cramping occurs.	**CNS:** dizziness, headache. **CV:** hypertension, transient chest pain, dyspnea, palpitation. **EENT:** tinnitus. **GI:** *nausea, vomiting.* **Other:** sweating, hypersensitivity.
oxytocin citrate, buccal Pitocin Citrate♦	*Induction of labor*—1 tablet (200 USP units) in alternate cheeks until firm, regular uterine contractions, 40 to 60 seconds long, q 3 minutes, are achieved. Repeat q 30 minutes until 15 tablets (3,000 units) have been given over 24 hours, or until delivery is imminent or anesthetic is administered. Average dose to complete labor, 1,700 units; same number of tablets are used to maintain labor once induced.	***Maternal*** **CV:** hypertension; premature ventricular contractions; hypotension; increase in heart rate, venous return, cardiac output; *arrhythmias in large doses.* **GI:** nausea, vomiting. **GU:** uterine hypertonicity, spasm, tetanic contraction or rupture, postpartum hemorrhage. **Local:** parabuccal irritation. ***Fetal*** **CV:** bradycardia, cardiac arrhythmias. **Hepatic:** jaundice. **Other:** hypoxia, intracranial hemorrhage due to overstimulation of uterus during labor, birth canal trauma.

♦ Available in U.S. and Canada. ♦♦ Available in Canada only. All other products (no symbol) available in U.S. only. Italicized side effects are common or life-threatening.

INTERACTIONS	NURSING CONSIDERATIONS
	may produce desired oxytocic action. • Contractions begin 5 to 15 minutes after P.O. administration; immediately after I.V. injection. May continue 3 hours or more after P.O. or I.M. administration; 45 minutes after I.V. injection. • Store in tightly closed, light-resistant container. Discard if discolored. • Store I.V. solutions below 8° C. (46.4° F.). Daily stock may be kept at cool room temperature for 60 days. • Keep patient warm. • Have drug ready for immediate use if it is to be given postpartum.
Regional anesthetics, dopamine, I.V. oxytocin: excessive vasoconstriction. Use together cautiously.	• Contraindicated for induction of labor; before delivery of placenta; in patients with hypertension, toxemia, or sensitivity to ergot preparations; in threatened spontaneous abortion. Use with caution in sepsis, obliterative vascular disease, hepatic or renal disease, hypertension, cardiac disease, venoatrial shunts, mitral valve stenosis. • Monitor and record blood pressure, pulse rate, uterine response; and report any sudden change in vital signs or frequent periods of uterine relaxation, and character and amount of vaginal bleeding. • Contractions begin 5 to 15 minutes after P.O. administration; 2 to 5 minutes after I.M. injection; immediately following I.V. injection. May continue 3 hours or more after P.O. or I.M. administration; 45 minutes after I.V. injection. • Store in tightly closed, light-resistant containers. Discard if discolored. • Store I.V. solutions below 8° C. (46.4° F.). Daily stock may be kept at room temperature for 60 to 90 days.
Cyclopropane anesthetics: increased risk of hypotension or bradycardia. Use together cautiously. *Thiopental anesthetics:* delayed induction time. Adjust dose. *Vasoconstrictors (vasopressors):* severe hypertension if oxytocin is used within 3 to 4 hours of vasoconstrictor. Monitor patient closely.	• Contraindicated in control and management of third stage of labor; to expel placenta; to control postpartum bleeding; in unconscious or postpartum patients; in management of inevitable, incomplete, or missed abortion, abruptio placentae, placenta previa, fetal distress, or other obstetric emergencies. Use cautiously in prematurity, previous major cervical or uterine surgery (including cesarean section), grand multiparity, invasive cervical carcinoma, overdistention of uterus, history of uterine sepsis. • In eclampsia, if delivery isn't imminent within 12 hours after oxytocin is started, cesarean section is recommended. • Used to induce or reinforce labor only when pelvis is known to be adequate, when fetal maturity is assured, when fetal position is favorable and vaginal delivery is indicated. • May be hazardous in patients with cardiac disease or in those receiving spinal or epidural anesthetic. • Should be given only in hospital setting and under qualified supervision. • Buccal administration is more difficult to control than I.M. or I.V. route; can be given by different routes sequentially but never at the same time. • Monitor uterine contractions, heart rate, blood pressure, intrauterine pressure, and character and volume of blood loss. • Monitor and record fetal heart beat. • Patient may rinse mouth with cold water before tablet is placed in parabuccal space. For maximum buccal absorption, patient should avoid disturbing tablet. A tablet swallowed accidentally is not harmful, but the digestive process destroys its oxytocic action. • Report contractions above 50 mm Hg measured by electronic monitor. • Store at temperature lower than 25° C. (77° F.).

NAME	INDICATIONS & DOSAGE	SIDE EFFECTS
oxytocin, synthetic injection Oxytocin♦, Pitocin♦, Syntocinon♦, Uteracon	*Induction or stimulation of labor*—initially, 1 ml (10 units) ampul in 1,000 ml of 5% dextrose injection or 0.9% sodium chloride solution I.V. infused at 1 to 2 milliunits/minute. Increase rate at 15- to 30-minute intervals until normal contraction pattern is established. Maximum 1 to 2 ml (20 milliunits)/minute. Decrease rate when labor is firmly established. *Reduction of postpartum bleeding after expulsion of placenta*—10 to 40 units added to 1,000 ml of 5% dextrose in water or 0.9% sodium chloride solution infused at rate necessary to control bleeding. *Facilitate threatened abortion*—10 to 40 units (1 to 4 ml) oxytocin added to 1,000 ml of 5% dextrose in water, normal saline solution, or other nonhydrating solution; infused at rate necessary to control uterine atony.	***Maternal*** **Blood:** afibrinogenemia; may be related to increase in postpartum bleeding. **CNS:** subarachnoid hemorrhage resulting from hypertension; *convulsions or coma resulting from water intoxication.* **CV:** hypotension; increased heart rate, systemic venous return, and cardiac output; arrhythmia. **GI:** nausea, vomiting. **Other:** hypersensitivity, tetanic contractions, abruptio placentae, impaired uterine blood flow, and increased uterine motility. ***Fetal*** **Blood:** increased risk of hyperbilirubinemia. **CV:** bradycardia, tachycardia, premature ventricular contractions. **Other:** *anoxia, asphyxia.*
oxytocin, synthetic nasal	*To promote initial milk ejection; may be useful in relieving postpartum breast engorgement*—one spray or three drops into one or both nostrils 2 or 3 minutes before breast-feeding or pumping breasts.	None reported.
sodium chloride 20% solution	*To induce fetal death and abortion in second trimester of pregnancy (beyond 16th week of gestation)*—after transabdominal tap of amniotic sac, at least 1 ml of fluid is withdrawn and examined. If no blood is found, 250 ml of amniotic fluid may be aspirated and 250 ml (maximum dose) of sodium chloride solution instilled over 20 to 30 minutes, while patient is observed for adverse reactions. Sodium chloride instillation may be repeated in 48 hours if membranes are still intact. I.V. infusion of oxytocin or intra-amniotic dinoprost tromethamine may be given to patients who fail to respond to second dose after oxytocic action of saline solution has ceased.	**Blood:** mild, self-limiting disseminated intravascular coagulation; coagulation changes, including decreased platelet count, hematocrit, fibrinogen, and factors V and VIII; increased plasma volume, fibrin levels, and thrombin, PT, and PTT times. Occur within first 12 to 24 hours. **CV:** *pulmonary embolism,* pneumonia. **GU:** *cortical necrosis of kidneys,* cervical laceration and perforation, cervicovaginal fistula, and uterine rupture reported in primigravida patients receiving concomitant I.V. oxytocin before cervix is adequately dilated. **Local:** infection at injection site. **Other:** fever, flushing.

INTERACTIONS	NURSING CONSIDERATIONS
Cyclopropane anesthetics: less pronounced bradycardia; more severe hypotension than occurs with oxytocin alone. Use together cautiously. *Thiopental anesthetics:* delayed induction reported. May require dosage adjustment. *Vasoconstrictors:* severe hypertension if oxytocin is given within 3 to 4 hours of vasoconstrictor in patient receiving caudal block anesthetic. Monitor patient closely.	• Contraindicated in cases of cephalopelvic disproportion or where delivery requires conversion, as in transverse lie; fetal distress, when delivery isn't imminent; severe toxemia; and other obstetric emergencies. Use cautiously in history of cervical or uterine surgery, grand multiparity, uterine sepsis, traumatic delivery, or overdistended uterus, and in primipara over 35 years. Use with extreme caution during first and second stages of labor, since cervical laceration, uterine rupture, and maternal and fetal death are reported. • Used to induce or reinforce labor only when pelvis is known to be adequate, when vaginal delivery is indicated, when fetal maturity is assured, and when fetal position is favorable. Should be used only in hospital where critical-care facilities and doctor are immediately available. • Don't give simultaneously by more than one route. • Incompatible with fibrinolysis, norepinephrine, prochlorperazine edisylate, protein hydrolysate, and warfarin sodium. • Rotate bottle gently to distribute drug in diluted solution. • Monitor and record uterine contractions, heart rate, blood pressure, intrauterine pressure, fetal heart rate, and character and volume of blood loss. • Store at temperature below 25° C. (77° F.), but do not freeze. • Oxytocin produces antidiuretic effect; monitor intake/output. • If contractions occur less than 2 minutes apart and if contractions above 50 mm Hg are recorded, or if contractions last 90 seconds or longer, stop infusion, turn patient on her side, and notify doctor. • Oxygen administration may be necessary. • Not recommended for I.M. use.
None significant.	• Instruct patient to clear nasal passages first. With patient's head in vertical position, hold squeeze bottle upright and eject solution into patient's nostril. • Support patient's wish to breast-feed with quiet, nonstressful environment, and encouragement.
Indomethacin: may prolong abortion if used within 4 to 6 hours after intra-amniotic instillation of sodium chloride solution. Defer indomethacin dose. *Oxytocin:* intense uterine contractions and increased risk of uterine rupture or cervical laceration. Don't use together.	• Contraindicated in blood disorders or in actively contracting or hypertonic uterus. Use with extreme caution in cardiac disease, hypertension, epilepsy, renal impairment, uterine incision, or pelvic adhesions, or in history of pelvic surgery. • Should be done only by doctors trained in amniocentesis when critical-care facilities are immediately available. • Monitor constantly for signs of accidental intravascular, endometrial, or intraperitoneal injection. Procedure usually painless. If patient complains of pain, burning, feeling of heat, thirst, severe headache, mental confusion, distress, tinnitus, numbness of fingertips, or anxiety, stop instillation at once. Inadvertent I.V. injection can cause hypernatremia, myometrial necrosis, with secondary vomiting, cerebral blood clots, cardiovascular collapse, and death. • Patient should drink at least 2 liters of water on day of procedure to improve salt excretion. • General anesthetics or sedatives should not be used during administration of hypertonic saline solution.

107 Spasmolytics

aminophylline
or theophylline ethylenediamine
dyphylline
flavoxate hydrochloride
oxtriphylline
oxybutynin chloride
theophylline
theophylline sodium glycinate

Spasmolytics check or relieve smooth-muscle spasms. The xanthine derivatives (theophylline and its salts, and dyphylline) are direct-acting bronchodilators; that is, they act directly on the smooth muscle of the respiratory tract. The theophylline salts include oxtriphylline, theophylline, theophylline ethylenediamine (aminophylline), and theophylline sodium glycinate.

These drugs are mainstays of therapy for chronic obstructive pulmonary disease (COPD) and especially acute bronchial asthma. They are usually combined with various sympathomimetics in a total treatment program. In addition to exerting bronchodilating actions, they also act as mild diuretics.

Flavoxate and oxybutynin, unlike the xanthine derivatives, act on the genitourinary system rather than the respiratory system.

Major uses

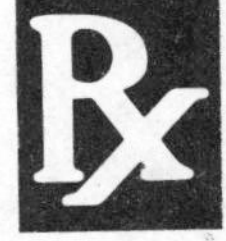

• Flavoxate and oxybutynin relieve symptoms of certain bladder disorders, including uninhibited neurogenic bladder.
• Xanthine derivatives relieve acute bronchial asthma and reverse bronchospasm associated with asthma, bronchitis, and emphysema.

Mechanism of action

• Flavoxate has a direct spasmolytic effect on smooth muscles of the urinary tract. It also provides some local anesthesia and analgesia.
• Oxybutynin has both a direct spasmolytic effect and an atropine-like effect on urinary tract smooth muscles; it has little or no effect on smooth muscles of blood vessels. It increases urinary bladder capacity and provides local anesthesia and analgesia.
• Of the xanthine derivatives, theophylline and its salts competitively inhibit phosphodiesterase, the enzyme that degrades cyclic adenosine monophosphate (AMP). This increases intracellular cyclic AMP, which in turn causes relaxation of the smooth muscle of the bronchial airways and pulmonary blood vessels. This action relieves bronchospasm and increases vital capacity.

Dyphylline presumably has the same mechanism of action as theophylline, but this has not been proven.

Absorption, distribution, metabolism, and excretion

• Flavoxate's metabolism has not been determined, but the drug is excreted by the kidneys.
• Oxybutynin is metabolized probably by the liver. Its metabolites are excreted by the kidneys.
• Xanthine derivatives have delayed

WHAT YOU SHOULD KNOW ABOUT AMINOPHYLLINE

The usual loading dose for aminophylline is 5 to 6 mg/kg, followed by an infusion of 0.4 to 0.6 mg/kg/hour. Keep the patient's history in mind as you check his prescribed dose to be sure it's within the proper range.

Since the patient may suffer convulsions if the drug infuses too fast, use an I.V. infusion pump to administer it. If a pump isn't available, use a minidripper.

Never place a total daily aminophylline dose in one 24-hour I.V. container. Instead, divide the dose into separate containers, for example, four infusions of 6 hours each. This way, the patient won't be in as much danger if the contents accidentally infuse too fast.

The patient will respond to the drug almost immediately. Since you can monitor both the drip rate and the patient's reaction to the drug, you can easily watch for side effects.

Be sure to:

- Check pulse rate and blood pressure.
- Monitor heart rate to detect cardiac arrhythmias. If you do detect arrhythmias, stop the infusion and call the doctor.
- Record the patient's fluid intake and output. Since aminophylline has a diuretic effect, your patient could become dehydrated.
- Make sure a bedpan is nearby.

The usual therapeutic blood levels of aminophylline are between 10 and 20 mcg/ml. If the patient's blood levels rise above 20 mcg/ml, he may exhibit symptoms of drug toxicity—anorexia, nausea, vomiting, abdominal pain, and nervousness. If you detect these effects, notify the doctor. You should monitor the patient's blood levels after the first hour of administration, then after 12 hours and 24 hours, and finally, once every 3 days. If your patient demonstrates a toxic symptom, check his blood levels immediately.

Another caution: Since the patient's breathing difficulty will make him restless, check the I.V. site frequently; his restlessness may dislodge the I.V.

After 3 days of I.V. aminophylline, most patients improve enough to proceed to oral drug therapy.

FLOW RATES FOR AMINOPHYLLINE INFUSIONS

DOSE (every 6 hr)	FLOW RATE*
100 mg	9 ml/hr
150 mg	14 ml/hr
200 mg	19 ml/hr
250 mg	23 ml/hr
300 mg	28 ml/hr
350 mg	33 ml/hr
400 mg	37 ml/hr

*1 g/500 ml *or* 2 g/1,000 ml

Courtesy of Temple University Hospital, Philadelphia, Pa.

absorption after oral administration if there is food in the stomach. Absorption is delayed and incomplete when the drugs are given by rectal suppository. They are distributed to body fluids and tissues, metabolized in the liver, then excreted in urine.

The drugs may accumulate in elderly patients and in those with hepatic dysfunction, cor pulmonale, and CHF.

Onset and duration

- Onset of flavoxate and oxybutynin takes place 30 to 60 minutes after administration. Blood levels peak in 3 to 6 hours, and duration of action is 6 to 10 hours.
- Because xanthine derivatives vary widely in onset and duration, individual responses must be carefully observed. Blood levels of 10 to 20 mcg/ml are usually needed to produce optimal bronchodilation. I.V. administration supplies the highest and most rapid concentration. Blood levels usually peak about 1 to 2 hours after administration of capsules or uncoated tablets; extended-release forms, about 4 hours; retention enemas, 1 to 2 hours; and rectal suppositories, 3 to 5 hours.

NAME	INDICATIONS & DOSAGE	SIDE EFFECTS
aminophylline or theophylline ethylenediamine Aminodur Dura-Tab, Aminophyl♦♦, Aminophyllin, Corophyllin♦♦, Lixaminol, Mini-Lix, Phyllocontin, Somophyllin	*For treatment of acute and chronic bronchial asthma, bronchospasm; also used for Cheyne-Stokes respiration, pulmonary vasodilator—* Oral: **Adults:** 500 mg stat; then 250 to 500 mg q 6 to 8 hours. **Children:** 7.5 mg/kg stat; then 3 to 6 mg/kg q 6 to 8 hours. I.V.: inject very slowly, minimum time of 4 to 5 minutes; do not exceed 25 mg/minute infusion rate. Loading dose: 5.6 mg/kg over 30 minutes. Maintenance dose: **Adults:** 0.3 to 0.9 mg/kg/hour I.V. by continuous infusion. **Children less than 9 years:** 1 mg/kg/hour. I.M.: **Adults:** 500 mg. Painful. Not recommended. Rectal: **Adults:** 500 mg suppository or by retention enema q 6 to 8 hours.	**CNS:** *restlessness, dizziness,* headache, *insomnia,* lightheadedness, *convulsions.* **CV:** *palpitations, sinus tachycardia,* extrasystoles, flushing, marked hypotension, increase in respiratory rate. **GI:** *nausea, vomiting, anorexia,* bitter aftertaste, dyspepsia, heavy feeling in stomach. **Skin:** urticaria. **Local:** *rectal suppositories may cause irritation.*
dyphylline Airet, Air-Tabs, Brophylline, Coeurophylline♦♦, Dilin♦, Dilor, Dyflex, Dylline, Emfabid, Lufyllin, Neothylline, Protophylline♦♦	*For relief of acute and chronic bronchial asthma and reversible bronchospasm associated with chronic bronchitis and emphysema—* **Adults:** 200 to 800 mg P.O. q 6 hours; or 250 to 500 mg I.M. injected slowly at 6-hour intervals. **Children over 6 years:** 4 to 7 mg/kg P.O. daily, in divided doses.	**CNS:** *restlessness, dizziness,* headache, *insomnia,* lightheadedness, *convulsions.* **CV:** *palpitations, sinus tachycardia,* extrasystoles, flushing, marked hypotension, increase in respiratory rate. **GI:** *nausea, vomiting, anorexia,* bitter aftertaste, dyspepsia, heavy feeling in stomach. **Skin:** urticaria.

♦ Available in U.S. and Canada. ♦♦ Available in Canada only. All other products (no symbol) available in U.S. only. Italicized side effects are common or life-threatening.

INTERACTIONS	NURSING CONSIDERATIONS
Alkali-sensitive drugs: reduced activity. Do not add to I.V. fluids containing aminophylline. *Propranolol and nadolol:* antagonism. Propranolol and nadolol may cause bronchospasm in sensitive patients. Use together cautiously. *Troleandomycin, erythromycin:* decreased hepatic clearance of theophylline; elevated theophylline levels. Monitor for signs of toxicity. *Barbiturates:* enhanced metabolism and decreased theophylline blood levels. Monitor for decreased aminophylline effect.	• Contraindicated in hypersensitivity to xanthine compounds (caffeine, theobromine); preexisting cardiac arrhythmias, especially tachyarrhythmias. Use cautiously in young children; in elderly patients with congestive heart failure or other cardiac or circulatory impairment, cor pulmonale, hepatic disease; in patients with active peptic ulcer, since it may increase volume and acidity of gastric secretions; and in hyperthyroidism or diabetes mellitus. • Individuals metabolize xanthines at different rates. Adjust dose by monitoring response, tolerance, pulmonary function, and theophylline blood levels: therapeutic level = 10 to 20 mcg/ml; toxicity seen over 20 mcg/ml. • Plasma clearance may be decreased in patients with congestive heart failure, hepatic dysfunction, or pulmonary edema. Smokers show accelerated clearance. Dose adjustments necessary. • I.V. drug administration can cause burning; dilute with dextrose in water solution. • Monitor vital signs; measure and record intake/output. Expected clinical effects include improvement in quality of pulse and respiration. • Warn elderly patient of dizziness, common side effect at start of therapy. • GI symptoms may be relieved by taking oral drug with full glass of water at meals, although food in stomach delays absorption. Enteric-coated tablets may also delay and impair absorption. No evidence that antacids reduce GI side effects. • Suppositories slowly and erratically absorbed; retention enemas may be absorbed more rapidly. Rectally administered preparations can be given when patient cannot take drug orally. Schedule after evacuation, if possible; may be retained better if given before meal. Advise patient to remain recumbent 15 to 20 minutes after insertion. • Question patient closely about other drugs used. Warn that over-the-counter remedies may contain ephedrine in combination with theophylline salts; excessive CNS stimulation may result. Tell him to check with doctor before taking *any* other medications. • Before giving loading dose, check that patient has not had recent theophylline therapy. • Supply instructions for home care and dosage schedule. Some patients may require round-the-clock dosage schedule. • Warn patients with allergies that exposure to allergens may exacerbate bronchospasm. • For symptoms and treatment of toxicity, see APPENDIX, *Drug Toxicities.*
None significant.	• Contraindicated in hypersensitivity to xanthine compounds (caffeine, theobromine); preexisting cardiac arrhythmias, especially tachycardias. Use cautiously in young children; in elderly patients with congestive heart failure, any impaired cardiac or circulatory function, cor pulmonale, renal or hepatic disease; in patients with peptic ulcer, hyperthyroidism, or diabetes mellitus. • I.V. use not recommended. • Dyphylline is metabolized faster than theophylline; dosage intervals may have to be decreased to ensure continual therapeutic effect. Higher daily doses may be needed. • Dose should be decreased in renal insufficiency. • Monitor vital signs; measure and record intake/output. Expected clinical effects include improvement in quality of pulse and respiration. • Warn elderly patient of dizziness, a common side effect. • Gastric irritation may be relieved by taking oral drug after meals; no evidence that antacids reduce this side effect. May produce less

(continued on following page)

NAME	INDICATIONS & DOSAGE	SIDE EFFECTS
dyphylline *(continued)*		
flavoxate hydrochloride Urispas	*Symptomatic relief of dysuria, frequency, urgency, nocturia, incontinence, and suprapubic pain associated with urologic disorders—* **Adults, and children over 12 years:** 100 to 200 mg P.O. q.i.d.	**CNS:** *mental confusion* (especially in elderly), nervousness, dizziness, headache, drowsiness, difficulty with concentration. **CV:** tachycardia, palpitations. **EENT:** *dry mouth and throat, blurred vision,* disturbed eye accommodation. **GI:** abdominal pain, constipation (with high doses), nausea, vomiting. **Skin:** urticaria, dermatoses. **Other:** fever.
oxtriphylline Choledyl♦, Theophylline Choline♦♦	*To relieve acute bronchial asthma and reversible bronchospasm associated with chronic bronchitis and emphysema—* **Adults, and children over 12 years:** 200 mg P.O. q 6 hours. **Children 2 to 12 years:** 4 mg/kg P.O. q 6 hours. Increase as needed to maintain therapeutic levels of theophylline (10 to 20 mcg/ml).	**CNS:** *restlessness, dizziness,* headache, *insomnia,* lightheadedness, *convulsions.* **CV:** *palpitations, sinus tachycardia,* extrasystoles, flushing, marked hypotension, increase in respiratory rate. **GI:** *nausea, vomiting, anorexia,* bitter aftertaste, dyspepsia, heavy feeling in stomach. **Skin:** urticaria.
oxybutynin chloride Ditropan	*Antispasmodic for neurogenic bladder—* **Adults:** 5 mg P.O. b.i.d. to t.i.d. to maximum of 5 mg q.i.d. **Children over 5 years:** 5 mg P.O. b.i.d. to maximum of 5 mg t.i.d.	**CNS:** *drowsiness,* dizziness, insomnia, *dry mouth,* flushing. **CV:** *palpitations, tachycardia.* **EENT:** *transient blurred vision,* mydriasis, cycloplegia. **GI:** nausea, vomiting, *constipation,* bloated feeling. **GU:** impotence, suppression of lactation, *urinary hesitance or retention.* **Skin:** urticaria, severe allergic reactions in patients sensitive to anticholinergics. **Other:** decreased sweating, fever.

♦ Available in U.S. and Canada. ♦♦ Available in Canada only. All other products (no symbol) available in U.S. only. Italicized side effects are common or life-threatening.

INTERACTIONS	**NURSING CONSIDERATIONS**
	gastric discomfort than theophylline. • Discard dyphylline ampul if precipitate is present. Protect from light. • Question patient closely about other drugs used. Warn that over-the-counter remedies may contain ephedrine in combination with theophylline salts; excessive CNS stimulation may result. Tell him to check with doctor before taking *any* other medications. • Supply instructions for home care and dosage schedule. • For symptoms and treatment of toxicity, see APPENDIX, *Drug Toxicities.*
None significant.	• Contraindicated in pyloric or duodenal obstruction, obstructive intestinal lesions or ileus, achalasia, GI hemorrhage, obstructive uropathies of lower urinary tract. Use cautiously in patients suspected of having glaucoma. • Check history for other drug use before giving drugs with anticholinergic side effects. • Warn about possible drowsiness, mental confusion, and blurred vision. • Tell the patient to report adverse effects or lack of response to drug. • For symptoms and treatment of toxicity, see APPENDIX, *Drug Toxicities.*
Erythromycin, troleandomycin: decreased hepatic clearance of theophylline; increased plasma level. Monitor for signs of toxicity. *Barbiturates:* enhanced metabolism and decreased theophylline blood levels. Monitor for decreased effect. *Propranolol and nadolol:* antagonism. May cause bronchospasms in sensitive patients. Use together cautiously.	• Contraindicated in hypersensitivity to xanthines (caffeine, theobromine); preexisting cardiac arrhythmias, especially tachyarrhythmias. • Tell patient to report GI distress, palpitations, irritability, restlessness, nervousness, or insomnia; may indicate excessive CNS stimulation. • Administer drug after meals and at bedtime. • Store at 15° to 30° C. (59° to 86° F.). Protect elixir from light, tablets from moisture. • Equivalent to 64% anhydrous theophylline. • Monitor therapy carefully. • Combination products that contain ephedrine not recommended; excessive CNS stimulation may result (nervousness, tremors, akathisia). • For symptoms and treatment of toxicity, see APPENDIX, *Drug Toxicities.*
None significant.	• Contraindicated in myasthenia gravis, GI obstruction, adynamic ileus, megacolon, severe or ulcerative colitis; in elderly or debilitated patients with intestinal atony; and in patients with obstructive uropathy. Use cautiously in elderly patients; in patients with autonomic neuropathy, reflux esophagitis, or hepatic or renal disease. • May aggravate symptoms of hyperthyroidism, coronary artery disease, congestive heart failure, cardiac arrhythmias, tachycardia, hypertension, or prostatic hypertrophy. • Therapy should be stopped periodically to determine whether patient can get along without it. Minimizes tendency toward tolerance. • Rapid onset of action, peaks at 3 to 4 hours, lasts 6 to 10 hours. • Neurogenic bladder should be confirmed by cystometry before oxybutynin is given. Evaluate patient response to therapy periodically by cystometry.

(continued on following page)

NAME	INDICATIONS & DOSAGE	SIDE EFFECTS
oxybutynin chloride *(continued)*		
theophylline Accurbron, Adophyllin, Aerolate, Aqualin, Asthmophylline♦♦, Bronkodyl, Elixicon, Elixophyllin♦, Labid, Lanophyllin, Liquophylline, Norophylline, Optiphyllin, Oralphyllin, Physpan, Quibron BID, Slo-Phyllin, Somophyllin♦, Theo-dur, Theo-Lix, Theo II, Theobid, Theocap, Theoclear, Theolair♦, Theolixir♦, Theolline, Theon, Theophyl♦, Theo-Span, Theostat, Theotal, Theovent **theophylline sodium glycinate** Acet-Am♦♦, Panophylline Forte, Synophylate, Theocyne♦♦, Theo-tort	*Prophylaxis and symptomatic relief of bronchial asthma, bronchospasm of chronic bronchitis and emphysema—* **Adults:** 100 to 200 mg P.O. q 6 hours; or 250 to 500 mg rectally q 8 to 12 hours. **Children:** 50 to 100 mg P.O. q 6 hours, not to exceed 10 to 12 mg/kg/24 hours, in divided doses q 8 to 12 hours. Oral timed-release form given q 8 to 12 hours. *Symptomatic relief of bronchial asthma, pulmonary emphysema, and chronic bronchitis—* **Adults:** 330 to 660 mg (sodium glycinate) P.O. q 6 to 8 hours, after meals. **Children over 12 years:** 220 to 330 mg (sodium glycinate) P.O. q 6 to 8 hours. **Children 6 to 12 years:** 330 mg (sodium glycinate) P.O. q 6 to 8 hours. **Children 3 to 6 years:** 110 to 165 mg (sodium glycinate) P.O. q 6 to 8 hours. **Children 1 to 3 years:** 55 to 110 mg (sodium glycinate) P.O. q 6 to 8 hours.	**CNS:** *restlessness, dizziness,* headache, *insomnia,* lightheadedness, *convulsions.* **CV:** *palpitations, sinus tachycardia,* extrasystoles, flushing, marked hypotension, increase in respiratory rate. **GI:** *nausea, vomiting, anorexia,* bitter aftertaste, dyspepsia, heavy feeling in stomach. **Skin:** urticaria.

♦ Available in U.S. and Canada. ♦♦ Available in Canada only. All other products (no symbol) available in U.S. only. Italicized side effects are common or life-threatening.

INTERACTIONS	NURSING CONSIDERATIONS
	• Rule out partial intestinal obstruction in patients with diarrhea, especially those with colostomy or ileostomy, before giving oxybutynin. • If urinary tract infection is present, patient should receive antibiotics concomitantly. • Warn patient that drug may impair alertness or vision. • Since oxybutynin suppresses sweating, its use during very hot weather may precipitate fever or heatstroke. • Store in tightly closed containers at 15° to 30° C. (59° to 86° F.). • For symptoms and treatment of toxicity, see APPENDIX, *Drug Toxicities*.
Erythromycin, troleandomycin: decreased hepatic clearance of theophylline; increased plasma levels. Monitor for signs of toxicity. *Barbiturates:* enhanced metabolism and decreased theophylline blood levels. Monitor for decreased effect. *Propranolol and nadolol:* antagonism. May cause bronchospasms in sensitive patients. Use together cautiously.	• Contraindicated in hypersensitivity to xanthine compounds (caffeine, theobromine); preexisting cardiac arrhythmias, especially tachyarrhythmias. Use cautiously in young children; in elderly patients with congestive heart failure or other circulatory impairment, cor pulmonale, renal or hepatic disease; and in patients with peptic ulcer, hyperthyroidism, or diabetes mellitus. • Individuals metabolize xanthines at different rates; determine dose by monitoring response, tolerance, pulmonary function, and theophylline plasma levels: therapeutic level = 10 to 20 mcg/ml. • Monitor vital signs; measure and record intake/output. Expected clinical effects include improvement in quality of pulse and respiration. • Warn elderly patients of dizziness, a common side effect at start of therapy. • GI symptoms may be relieved by taking oral drug with full glass of water after meals, although food in stomach delays absorption. • Question patient closely about other drugs used. Warn that over-the-counter remedies may contain ephedrine in combination with theophylline salts; excessive CNS stimulation may result. Tell him to check with doctor before taking *any* other medications. • Supply instructions for home care and dosage schedule. • Daily dosage may need to be decreased in patients with congestive heart failure or hepatic disease, or in elderly patients, since metabolism and excretion may be decreased. Monitor carefully, using blood levels, observation, examination, and interview. Give drug around the clock, using sustained-release product at bedtime. • Be careful not to confuse sustained-release dosage forms with standard-release dosage forms.

NURSING TIP

A WARNING ABOUT AMINOPHYLLINE SUPPOSITORIES

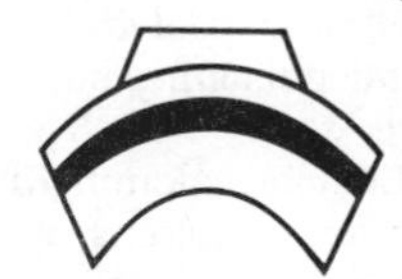

Recent studies indicate that absorption of aminophylline in suppository form is slow and unreliable. Your patient would have to retain the suppository at least 6 hours to achieve maximum absorption!

Blood concentrations of the drug fall below the therapeutic level desired. And rectal suppositories take longer than oral forms to attain maximum blood concentrations.

So only use suppositories in special, short-term situations and when the oral form of the drug is poorly tolerated or impossible to administer.

Administer aminophylline I.V. in all acute or emergency situations.

Heavy metal antagonists

deferoxamine mesylate
dimercaprol
edetate calcium disodium
edetate disodium
D-penicillamine

Heavy metal antagonists prevent or reverse formation of complexes that heavy metals make with organic compounds in the body. Heavy metals such as antimony, arsenic, cadmium, copper, iron, lead, mercury, and thallium can form insoluble metal complexes that interfere with normal functions, poisoning the central nervous system, gastrointestinal tract, and various organs, especially the kidneys. By combining with the heavy metals, the antagonists neutralize their toxic effects.

Major uses

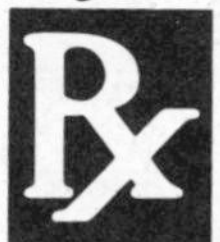

• Deferoxamine is used in treatment of acute iron intoxication, chronic iron poisoning, and iron storage diseases.
• Dimercaprol is used to treat heavy metal poisoning such as Wilson's disease.
• Edetate calcium disodium is effective for symptoms of heavy metal poisoning.
• Edetate disodium is used to treat heavy metal poisoning and hypercalcemia.
• D-penicillamine relieves Wilson's disease and rheumatoid arthritis. It also prevents formation of kidney stones in cystinuria.

Mechanism of action

Heavy metal antagonists act as chelating agents to react with and neutralize calcium, cysteine, and heavy metals such as iron and copper. These substances bind more easily to heavy metal antagonists than to body tissues. The resulting complex (chelate) is stable, soluble, and easily excreted in urine.
• D-penicillamine's action on rheumatoid arthritis is unknown but is

CARING FOR PATIENTS WITH CYSTINURIA: SOME GUIDELINES

To prevent the formation of calculi:
Make sure your patient drinks large amounts of fluid during the day. Suggest that he drink 16 oz (approximately 500 ml) of fluid before he goes to bed and another 16 oz if he awakes during the night, since urine tends to be most concentrated and acidic at this time.

To determine whether your patient has calculi:
Your patient should have X-rays taken regularly. His doctor will decide how often these X-rays are necessary.

To lessen the likelihood of calculi formation:
Advise your patient to avoid foods containing methionine, such as rich meat soups and broths, milk, eggs, cheese, and peas. Methionine is a major forerunner of cystine.
Note: Children and pregnant women should not adhere to this diet because of its low protein content.

PATIENT-TEACHING AID

WHAT YOU SHOULD KNOW ABOUT WILSON'S DISEASE

Dear Patient:

In addition to the medication your doctor has prescribed, here are some ways you can help control your condition:

- Avoid foods that contain copper, such as chocolate, nuts, shellfish, mushrooms, liver, molasses, broccoli, and cereals enriched with copper. Read product labels for contents, especially if these foods have minerals added or are fortified.
- Use distilled or demineralized water if your drinking water contains more than 0.1 mg of copper/liter. (You can get this information from the local water authority or public health agency.)
- Except when you're taking supplemental iron, take sulfurated potash or Carbo-Resin with your meals to minimize your absorption of copper.
- Make sure any vitamin preparations you take are copper-free.
- Continue your medication therapy as ordered. It may take 1 to 3 months before your neurologic symptoms begin to subside. This is normal, so don't be discouraged or stop therapy before the benefits have a chance to occur.

probably due to inhibited collagen formation.

Absorption, distribution, metabolism, and excretion

- D-penicillamine is the only drug that's well absorbed when given orally. The others must be given parenterally.
- All the drugs are distributed to all body tissues, except edetate calcium disodium, which doesn't penetrate cerebrospinal fluid or red cells.
- All the drugs are excreted primarily unchanged in urine, except dimercaprol and D-penicillamine. These two drugs are metabolized in the liver and then eliminated in urine and feces.

Onset and duration

- Onset of action for deferoxamine and for edetate disodium hasn't been determined.
- Dimercaprol begins to act 30 to 60 minutes after I.M. administration.
- Edetate calcium disodium takes effect approximately 1 hour after I.V. administration.
- D-penicillamine, when given orally, begins to work after about 1 hour.
- Duration of action varies with the ratio of heavy metal antagonist to metal present and also with renal function.

Combination products

None.

NAME	INDICATIONS & DOSAGE	SIDE EFFECTS
deferoxamine mesylate Desferal♦	*Acute iron intoxication—* **Adults and children:** 1 g I.M. or I.V. followed by 500 mg I.M. or I.V. for two doses, q 4 hours; then 500 mg I.M. or I.V. q 4 to 12 hours. Infusion rate shouldn't exceed 15 mg/kg/hour. *Chronic iron overload and in patients requiring multiple transfusions—* **Adults and children:** 500 mg to 1 g I.M. daily and 2 g slow I.V. infusion in separate solution along with each unit of blood transfused. Maximum dose 6 g daily. I.V. infusion rate shouldn't exceed 15 mg/kg/hour. S.C.: 1 to 2 g administered q 8 to 24 hours.	**Local:** pain and induration at injection site. *After rapid I.V. administration: erythema, urticaria, hypotension.* **With long-term use:** sensitivity reaction (cutaneous wheal formation, pruritus, rash, *anaphylaxis), diarrhea, leg cramps, fever, tachycardia, blurred vision, dysuria, abdominal discomfort.*
dimercaprol BAL in Oil♦	**Adults and children:** *Severe arsenic or gold poisoning*—3 mg/kg deep I.M. q 4 hours for 2 days, then q.i.d. on 3rd day, then b.i.d. for 10 days. *Mild arsenic or gold poisoning*—2.5 mg/kg deep I.M. q.i.d. for 2 days, then b.i.d. on 3rd day, then once daily for 10 days. *Mercury poisoning*—5 mg/kg deep I.M. initially, then 2.5 mg/kg daily or b.i.d. for 10 days. *Acute lead encephalopathy or lead level more than 100 mcg/ml*— 4 mg/kg deep I.M. injection, then q 4 hours with edetate calcium disodium (12.5 mg/kg I.M.). Use separate sites. Maximum dose 5 mg/kg per dose.	**CNS:** pain or tightness in throat, chest, or hands; headache; paresthesias; muscle pain or weakness. **CV:** *transient increase in blood pressure, returns to normal in 2 hours; tachycardia.* **EENT:** blepharospasm, conjunctivitis, lacrimation, rhinorrhea, excessive salivation. **GI:** halitosis; nausea; vomiting; burning sensation in lips, mouth, and throat. **GU:** renal damage if alkaline urine not maintained. **Metabolic:** decreased iodine uptake. **Local:** sterile abscess, pain at injection site. **Other:** fever (especially in children), sweating, pain in teeth.
edetate calcium disodium Calcium Disodium Versenate♦, Calcium EDTA	*Lead poisoning—* **Adults:** 1 g/250 to 500 ml of 5% dextrose in water or 0.9% normal saline solution I.V. over 1 to 2 hours daily or q 12 hours for 3 to 5 days; repeat after 2 days if indicated. Maximum dose 50 mg/kg daily. **Children:** 35 mg/kg I.M. daily divided q 8 to 12 hours. Maximum dose 50 mg/kg daily. *Acute lead encephalopathy or lead levels above 100 mcg/ml—* **Adults and children:** 12.5 mg/kg with dimercaprol 4 mg/kg	**CNS:** headache, paresthesias, numbness. **CV:** cardiac arrhythmias, hypotension. **GI:** anorexia, nausea, vomiting. **GU:** *proteinuria, hematuria; nephrotoxicity with renal tubular necrosis leading to fatal nephrosis in excessive dose.* **Other:** arthralgia, myalgia, hypercalcemia. **4 to 8 hours after infusion:** sudden fever and chills, fatigue, excessive thirst, sneezing, nasal congestion.

INTERACTIONS	NURSING CONSIDERATIONS
None significant.	• Contraindicated in severe renal disease or anuria. Use cautiously in impaired renal function. • Monitor intake/output carefully. • I.M. route preferred. • Use I.V. only when patient has cardiovascular collapse or shock. For I.V. use, dissolve as for I.M. use; dilute in normal saline solution, 5% dextrose in water, or lactated Ringer's solution. • If giving I.V., change to I.M. as soon as possible. • For reconstitution, add 2 ml of sterile water for injection to each ampul. Make sure drug is completely dissolved. Reconstituted solution good for 1 week at room temperature. Protect from light. • Warn patient urine may be red. • Have epinephrine 1:1,000 readily available in case of allergic reaction. • For treatment of anaphylaxis, see inside front cover.
^{131}I uptake thyroid tests: decreased; don't schedule patient for this test during course of dimercaprol therapy. *Iron:* formed toxic metal complex; concurrent therapy contraindicated.	• Contraindicated in hepatic dysfunction (except postarsenical jaundice), acute renal insufficiency. • Don't use for iron, cadmium, or selenium toxicity. Complex formed is highly toxic, even fatal. • Ephedrine or antihistamine may prevent or relieve mild side effects. • Ineffective in arsine gas poisoning. • Solution with slight sediment usable. • Keep urine alkaline to prevent renal damage. Oral $NaHCO_3$ may be ordered. • Don't give I.V.; give by deep I.M. route only. The injection site can be massaged after drug is given. • Drug has an unpleasant, garlic-like odor. • Be careful when preparing and administering drug not to let drug come in contact with skin, as it may cause a skin reaction.
None significant.	• Contraindicated in severe renal disease or anuria. • I.V. use contraindicated in lead encephalopathy; may increase intracranial pressure. Use I.M. route instead. • Force fluids to facilitate lead excretion in all patients except those with lead encephalopathy. • Monitor intake/output, urinalysis, BUN, and EKGs. • To avoid toxicity, use with dimercaprol. • Oral form available but use discouraged because of poor GI absorption; often used ineffectively as prophylaxis against lead exposure; can even increase lead absorption from GI tract. • Procaine HCl may be added to I.M. solutions to minimize pain. Watch for local reactions. • Avoid rapid I.V. infusions. I.M. route preferred. • Do not confuse this drug with edetate disodium, which is used for the emergency treatment of hypercalcemia.

(continued on following page)

NAME	INDICATIONS & DOSAGE	SIDE EFFECTS
edetate calcium disodium *(continued)*	deep I.M. after initial dose of dimercaprol 4 mg deep I.M. Use separate sites. After first dose, reduce to 3 mg/kg for 2 to 7 days.	
edetate disodium Disodium EDTA, Disotate, Endrate, Sodium Versenate	*Hypercalcemic crisis—* **Adults and children:** 15 to 50 mg/kg slow I.V. infusion. Dilute in 500 ml of 5% dextrose in water or 0.9% normal saline solution. Give over 3 to 4 hours. Maximum adult dose 3 g/day; maximum children's dose 70 mg/kg/day.	**CNS:** circumoral paresthesias, numbness, headache, malaise, fatigue, muscle pain or weakness. **CV:** hypertension, thrombophlebitis. **GI:** nausea, vomiting, diarrhea, anorexia, abdominal cramps. **GU:** in excessive doses—nephrotoxicity with urgency, nocturia, dysuria, polyuria, proteinuria, renal insufficiency and failure, tubular necrosis. **Metabolic:** *severe hypocalcemia,* decreased magnesium. **Local:** pain at site of infusion, erythema, dermatitis.
D-penicillamine Cuprimine♦, Depen	*Wilson's disease—* **Adults:** 250 mg P.O. q.i.d. before meals. Adjust dose to achieve urinary copper excretion of 0.5 to 1 mg daily. **Children:** 20 mg/kg daily P.O. divided q.i.d. before meals. Adjust dose to achieve urinary copper excretion of 0.5 to 1 mg daily. *Cystinuria—* **Adults:** 250 mg P.O. q.i.d. before meals. Adjust dose to achieve urinary cystine excretion of less than 100 mg daily when renal calculi present, or 100 to 200 mg daily when no calculi present. Maximum adult dose is 5 g daily. **Children:** 30 mg/kg daily P.O. divided q.i.d. before meals. Adjust dose to achieve urinary cystine excretion of less than 100 mg daily when renal calculi present, or 100 to 200 mg daily when no calculi present. *Rheumatoid arthritis—*	**Blood:** *leukopenia, eosinophilia, thrombocytopenia, monocytosis, granulocytopenia,* elevated sedimentation rate, lupus erythematosus-like syndrome. **EENT:** tinnitus. **GI:** *nausea, vomiting, anorexia.* **GU:** *nephrotic syndrome, glomerulonephritis.* **Hepatic:** hepatotoxicity. **Metabolic:** *decreased pyridoxine (may cause optic neuritis),* decreased zinc and mercury. **Skin:** friability, especially at pressure spots; wrinkling; erythema; urticaria; ecchymoses. **Other:** *reversible taste impairment, especially of salts and sweets;* hair loss. *About ⅓ of patients develop allergic reactions (rash, pruritus, fever), arthralgia, lymphadenopathy.* With long-term use, myasthenia gravis syndrome.

♦ Available in U.S. and Canada. ♦♦ Available in Canada only. All other products (no symbol) available in U.S. only. Italicized side effects are common or life-threatening.

INTERACTIONS	NURSING CONSIDERATIONS
None significant.	• Contraindicated in anuria, known or suspected hypocalcemia, or significant renal disease; active or healed tubercular lesions; history of seizures or intracranial lesions; generalized arteriosclerosis associated with aging. Use cautiously in limited cardiac reserve, incipient congestive heart failure, hypokalemia, diabetes. • Avoid rapid I.V. infusion; profound hypocalcemia may occur. • Monitor EKG and test renal function frequently. • Obtain serum calcium levels after each dose. • Keep I.V. calcium available. • Keep patient in bed for 15 minutes after infusion to avoid postural hypotension. • Don't use to treat lead toxicity; use edetate calcium disodium instead. • Record I.V. site used, and try to avoid repeated use of the same site, as this increases likelihood of thrombophlebitis. • Generalized systemic reactions may occur 4 to 8 hours after drug administration; these include fever, chills, back pain, emesis, muscle cramps, and urinary urgency. Report such reactions to doctor. Treatment is usually supportive. Symptoms generally subside within 12 hours. • Do not confuse this drug with edetate calcium disodium, which is used to treat lead poisoning. • Edetate disodium not currently drug of choice for treatment of hypercalcemia; other treatments are safer and more effective.
Oral iron: decreased effectiveness of D-penicillamine. If used together, give at least 2 hours apart.	• Contraindicated in pregnant women with cystinuria. Use cautiously in penicillin allergy; cross sensitivity may occur. • Report to doctor if fever or other allergic reactions occur. • Patient should receive pyridoxine daily. • Handle patients carefully to avoid skin damage. • Dose should be given on empty stomach to facilitate absorption of drug. • Patient should drink large amounts of fluid, especially at night. • Tell patient that therapeutic effect may be delayed up to 3 months. • Monitor CBC, and renal and hepatic function regularly throughout therapy (every 2 weeks for the first 6 months, then monthly). • Hold drug and notify doctor if WBC falls below 3,500/mm^3 and/or platelet count falls below 100,000/mm^3 (these are indications to stop drug). A progressive decline in platelet or WBC in three successive blood tests may necessitate temporary cessation of therapy, even if these counts are within normal limits. • Advise patient to report fever, sore throat, chills, bruising, increased bleeding time; may be early signs of granulocytopenia. • Provide appropriate health teaching for patients with Wilson's disease and cystinuria. See patient-teaching aid, p. 1259.

(continued on following page)

NAME	INDICATIONS & DOSAGE	SIDE EFFECTS
D-penicillamine *(continued)*	**Adults:** 250 mg P.O. daily initially, with increases of 250 mg q 2 to 3 months if necessary. Maximum dose 1 g daily.	

♦ Available in U.S. and Canada. ♦♦ Available in Canada only. All other products (no symbol) available in U.S. only. Italicized side effects are common or life-threatening.

DRUG ADVANCES

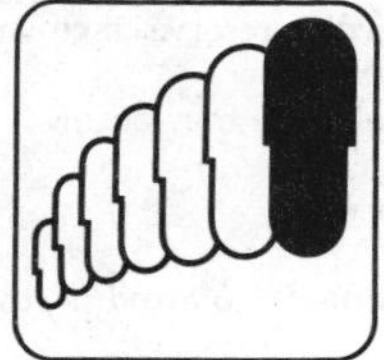

PENICILLAMINE: ANOTHER WEAPON AGAINST RHEUMATOID ARTHRITIS

Besides the traditional salicylates and other anti-inflammatory agents, rheumatoid arthritis sufferers now have an alternative drug treatment—penicillamine, or D-penicillamine. Formerly, this drug's primary use was to treat two rather uncommon diseases: cystinuria and Wilson's disease. First tried in 1963 on patients with rheumatoid arthritis, penicillamine proved through 15 years of clinical trials to be a potentially useful drug for treating this disease.

Although penicillamine is in the same chemical family as the antibiotic penicillin, penicillamine has no antibiotic activity. But because the two drugs are chemically similar, patients allergic to penicillin may also be allergic to penicillamine.

Penicillamine has many side effects, and if used inappropriately, it can cause serious toxicity. Some patients develop

INTERACTIONS	NURSING CONSIDERATIONS

maculopapular and pruritic rashes, usually during the first month of therapy. If a rash occurs, the doctor may discontinue this treatment—at least temporarily—until the rash subsides. Then he may resume penicillamine therapy at a lower dose. Watch for a rash while the patient's taking penicillamine. Nephritis, neutropenia, thrombocytopenia, systemic lupus erythematosus, and myasthenia gravis are other uncommon but severe side effects of penicillamine.

Hypogeusia (altered taste) is a common side effect; patients report that salt and sweet tastes are muted. Usually this effect diminishes as therapy progresses. Nausea, vomiting, and anorexia are also usual complaints.

Oral iron therapy can interfere with penicillamine absorption in the gastrointestinal tract. So, if your patient's taking iron, space the doses at least 2 hours apart to minimize this effect. Remember, penicillamine increases the body's need for pyridoxine (vitamin B_6), so make sure the patient takes any prescribed multivitamins.

The patient should receive the lowest possible effective dose of penicillamine. Advise the patient to tell the doctor if he feels the current dose isn't effective. Gradually increasing the dose helps lessen the frequency and severity of side effects.

A patient should respond to penicillamine therapy in 6 to 12 weeks. If the patient's condition doesn't improve after 6 months, the doctor will probably stop this treatment and try another approach. Fortunately, penicillamine usually provides some relief, even for patients with the most resistant cases of rheumatoid arthritis.

109 Gold salts

aurothioglucose
gold sodium thiomalate

Gold, the precious metal, has been used in the treatment of arthritis since 1929. Since the early 1960s, numerous studies have confirmed the effectiveness of gold therapy (also known as chrysotherapy), so its use has been increasing.

The drugs are actually gold *salts* that contain about 50% gold; the gold is attached to sulphur molecules.

Although the drugs can retard juvenile and adult rheumatoid arthritis in the early stages, they have little value in advanced stages of the disease. Unfortunately, gold therapy often produces serious side effects and must be discontinued.

Although gold salts do not possess analgesic properties, they can produce remissions. Many rheumatologists believe that gold salts constitute the drugs of choice after aspirin. These drugs may also retard the advance of new erosive lesions.

In patients who can tolerate gold injections without developing severe toxic reactions, about 75% show symptomatic improvement; 20% to 25% of these show disease remission.

Major uses

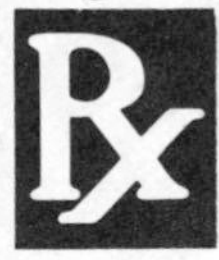

Gold salts are used to treat active rheumatoid arthritis that has not responded adequately to salicylates, penicillamine, rest, and physical therapy.

Mechanism of action

The exact mechanism of action is unknown. Anti-inflammatory effects in the active stage of rheumatoid arthritis are probably due to inhibition of sulfhydryl systems, which alters cellular metabolism. Gold salts may also alter enzyme function and immune response, and suppress phagocytic activity.

Absorption, distribution, metabolism, and excretion

- Aurothioglucose, in oil suspension, is absorbed slowly and irregularly after I.M. injection.
- Gold sodium thiomalate is well absorbed after I.M. injection.
- Gold salts are widely distributed to body tissues. Arthritic joints contain two to two and a half times as much gold as uninvolved joints.
- The metabolism of gold salts is unclear. In all likelihood, however, the compounds are *not* reduced to the element gold.
- The drugs are excreted slowly, mostly in urine. A small amount, however, is eliminated in feces. After a cumulative dose of 1 g, urinary excretion of gold can be detected for as long as 1 year.

Onset and duration

Although action may not begin for 8 to 12 weeks after administration, it may last long after therapy is stopped, depending on the patient's response.

Combination products

None.

ABOUT RHEUMATOID ARTHRITIS

Rheumatoid arthritis (RA), which is often treated with gold compounds, is a chronic systemic disease characterized by a fluctuating, progressive inflammation and destruction of the joints.

CLINICAL FEATURES

- History of persistent painful morning stiffness that may last for hours (in other forms of arthritis, stiffness may last only a short while)
- Spindle-shaped joint swelling
- Subcutaneous nodules (small non-tender masses over pressure points)
- Swelling of ulnar side of the wrist
- Signs of muscle wasting, weight loss, erythema of palms, malaise
- Fatigue occurring at same time each day regardless of previous activity level
- Elevated erythrocyte sedimentation rate
- Presence of rheumatoid factor in the serum (in about 30% of patients with RA)

TREATMENT

Long-term management aims to relieve pain, arrest the inflammatory process, and prevent further joint damage by means of:

- *Team evaluation* (nurse, doctor, physical therapist, social worker, dietitian)
- *Drug therapy:* Teach patient to watch for and report side effects of salicylates, anti-inflammatory agents, corticosteroids, antimalarial agents, cytotoxic and immunosuppressive agents, chelating agents, and gold compounds.
- *Specialized physical and occupational therapy:* Teach the importance of continuing prescribed ranges-of-motion and specialized exercises. Assess tolerance for physical activities, including activities of daily living.
- *Prescribed rest:* 8 to 12 hours of sleep a night and a rest period during the day (total body rest or rest of the involved joints). To achieve correct resting and sleeping positions, patient should use a firm mattress; a small pillow, to avoid flexion contractures of the neck; and a footboard, to avoid footdrop. He should avoid using pillows under the knees.
- *Diets:* For weight reduction or increased protein intake.
- *Orthopedic appliances:* Special shoes, splints, and soft collars can ease pain, prevent fatigue, and provide proper alignment.

PATIENT TEACHING

Some specific advice for patients with RA:

- Avoid fatigue: Try to rest 5 to 10 minutes out of each hour. Plan your work. Work slowly but at an even pace. Sit whenever possible. Alternate sitting and standing tasks. Use good posture.
- Avoid undue stress on the joints: Use the largest joint available for a given task. Support weak or painful joints. Avoid holding objects for long periods; hold objects parallel to knuckles. Use hands toward the center of the body. Slide—don't lift—objects. Avoid bending and climbing.
- Use aids for dressing—long-handled shoehorn, reacher, elastic shoelaces. Whenever possible, sit to dress. Use a zipper-pull for long or difficult zippers; avoid back zippers. Use a button hook for manipulating buttons. Arrange closets efficiently. Keep like items and items usually worn together, hanging together.
- Be skeptical of anyone offering cures. Arthritis quacks defraud patients of millions of dollars annually in the United States.

Compare the hands illustrated here. Note that the cartilage spaces in the arthritic hand have narrowed. The gold compounds given to treat the arthritis have concentrated in the joints.

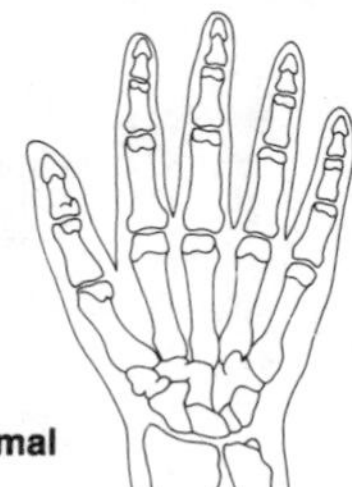

Normal

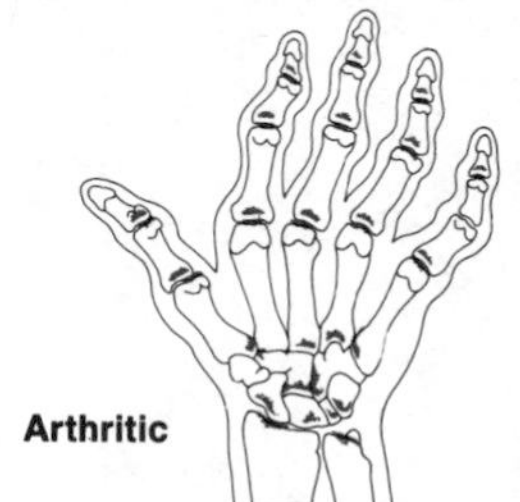

Arthritic

NAME	INDICATIONS & DOSAGE	SIDE EFFECTS
aurothioglucose Solganal	*Rheumatoid arthritis*— **Adults:** initially, 10 mg (aurothioglucose) I.M., followed by 25 mg for second and third doses at weekly intervals. Then, 50 mg weekly until 1 g has been given. If improvement occurs without toxicity, continue 25 to 50 mg at 3- to 4-week intervals indefinitely as maintenance therapy. **Children 6 to 12 years:** ¼ usual adult dose. Alternatively, 1 mg/kg I.M. once weekly for 20 weeks.	Adverse reactions to gold are considered severe and potentially life-threatening. Report any side effect to the doctor at once. **Blood:** *thrombocytopenia* (with or without purpura), *aplastic anemia, agranulocytosis,* leukopenia, eosinophilia. **CNS:** *dizziness,* syncope, sweating. **CV:** bradycardia. **EENT:** corneal gold deposition, corneal ulcers. **GI:** *metallic taste, stomatitis,* difficulty swallowing, nausea, vomiting. **GU:** *albuminuria, proteinuria, nephrotic syndrome,* nephritis, acute tubular necrosis. **Hepatic:** hepatitis, jaundice. **Skin:** *rash and dermatitis in 20% of patients. (If drug is not stopped, may lead to fatal exfoliative dermatitis.)* **Other:** *anaphylaxis,* angioneurotic edema.
gold sodium thiomalate Myochrysine♦	*Rheumatoid arthritis*— **Adults:** initially, 10 mg (gold sodium thiomalate) I.M., followed by 25 mg in 1 week. Then, 50 mg weekly until 14 to 20 doses have been given. If improvement occurs without toxicity, continue 50 mg q 2 weeks for 4 doses; then, 50 mg q 3 weeks for 4 doses; then, 50 mg q month indefinitely as maintenance therapy. If relapse occurs during maintenance therapy, resume injections at weekly intervals. **Children:** 1 mg/kg/week I.M. for 20 weeks. If response is good, may be given q 3 to 4 weeks indefinitely.	

♦ Available in U.S. and Canada. ♦♦ Available in Canada only. All other products (no symbol) available in U.S. only. Italicized side effects are common or life-threatening.

INTERACTIONS	NURSING CONSIDERATIONS
None significant.	• Contraindicated in patients with severe uncontrollable diabetes, renal disease, hepatic dysfunction, marked hypertension, heart failure, systemic lupus erythematosus, Sjögren's syndrome, skin rash, and drug allergies or hypersensitivities. Use cautiously with other drugs that cause blood dyscrasias. • Indicated only in active rheumatoid arthritis that has not responded adequately to salicylates, D-penicillamine, rest, and physical therapy. • Most side effects are readily reversible if drug is stopped immediately. • Administer all gold salts I.M., preferably intragluteally. Color of drug is pale yellow; don't use if it darkens. • Observe patient for 30 minutes after administration because of possible anaphylactic reaction. • Inform patient that benefits of therapy may not appear for 6 to 8 weeks or longer. • Gold therapy may alter liver function studies. • Aurothioglucose is a suspension. Immerse vial in warm water and shake vigorously before injecting. • When giving gold sodium thiomalate, advise patient to lie down and to remain recumbent for 10 to 20 minutes after injection. • Complete blood counts including platelet estimation should be performed before every second injection for the duration of therapy. • Dermatitis is the most common side effect of these drugs. Advise patient to report any skin rashes or problems immediately. Pruritus often precedes dermatitis and should be considered a warning of impending skin reactions. Any pruritic skin eruption while a patient is receiving gold therapy should be considered a reaction until proven otherwise. Therapy is stopped until reaction subsides. • Stomatitis is the second most common side effect of gold therapy. Advise patient that stomatitis is often preceded by a metallic taste. This warning should be reported to the doctor immediately. • Advise patient of the importance of close medical follow-up and the need for frequent blood and urine tests during therapy. • Urine should be analyzed for protein and sediment changes before each injection. • Platelet counts should be performed if patient develops purpura or ecchymoses. • If side effects are mild, some rheumatologists may order resumption of gold therapy after 2 to 3 weeks' rest. • Dimercaprol should be kept on hand to treat acute toxicity. • For treatment of anaphylaxis, see inside front cover.

THE LATEST BREAKTHROUGH: ORAL GOLD

Auranofin, a new gold drug, may increase compliance in patients with rheumatoid arthritis on gold therapy. Why? Because it can be administered orally.

Until now, all gold compounds have been parenteral preparations that are administered I.M. Gold therapy patients received a weekly injection of 50 mg. This injection was painful and the large dose often damaged the kidneys. But since auranofin is administered orally, it's painless and able to be taken daily in a smaller single dose. So far, only minor side effects, such as diarrhea and skin irritations, have been observed. Investigations are now underway to determine what, if any, long-term toxicities of oral gold there may be.

Patients who don't respond to I.M. gold therapy may respond to oral gold therapy. These results suggest auranofin may work by a different mechanism than parenteral drugs.

10 Diagnostic skin tests

histoplasmin
Old tuberculin
tuberculin purified protein derivative

Diagnostic skin tests are used to assess immunocompetence. They contain bacterial, fungal, or viral antigens not previously encountered by a patient (new antigens) that evaluate primary immune response. The tests also use common antigens previously encountered by a patient (recall antigens) to evaluate his secondary immune response.

When antigens combine with previously formed antibodies to cause an antigen-antibody response, they produce an immediate hypersensitivity (anaphylactic) reaction. Diagnostic skin tests indicate delayed hypersensitivity reactions. Delayed hypersensitivity reactions are mediated by T-cells reacting to the antigen.

Reactions are read as significant positive or negative according to size of induration (varies with specific test). Positive reactions (erythema and induration in 24 to 48 hours, followed by resolution of the reactions) may indicate an intact cellular immune response due to past or possibly active infection, or a nonspecific inflammatory response.

Negative reactions mean active infection is highly unlikely. False-positive and false-negative reactions may occur, so skin tests alone are not diagnostic.

A patient's inability to react to a battery of common antigens (anergy) suggests that he is immunodeficient.

Major uses

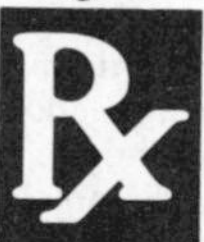

Skin tests are used to:
- diagnose and differentiate infectious diseases
- determine immunity to infectious diseases
- help evaluate a patient's response to immunotherapy
- identify diminished or delayed hypersensitivity or anergy in a patient.

Purified protein derivative is one of the substances used to assess immunocompetence in patients with cancer.

Mechanism of action

Skin tests cause antigen-antibody reactions and nonspecific inflammatory reactions.

Absorption, distribution, metabolism, and excretion

Not applicable.

Onset and duration

Not applicable.

Combination products

None.

HOW TO PERFORM AND INTERPRET THE MANTOUX (PPD) TEST FOR TUBERCULOSIS

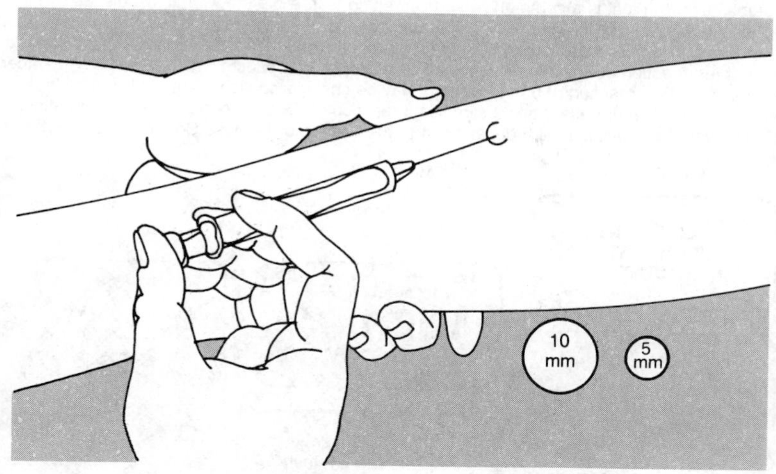

1. Check the label of the PPD vial for drug strength and expiration date. (PPD is available in three strengths, containing 1, 5, or 250 tuberculin units. The intermediate strength, containing 5 tuberculin units, is the one most often used for diagnostic testing.)

2. Use an easy-to-read tuberculin syringe with a 25G needle.

3. After you draw the PPD into the syringe, administer it within 5 minutes (it can be absorbed by glass and plastic).

4. After cleansing the site with alcohol, allow the skin to dry and then inject the PPD in the upper third of the patient's ventral forearm, just beneath the skin's surface (intradermal injection). Be sure the needle bevel is facing up.

5. A wheal—a pale elevation of skin—6 to 10 mm in diameter should appear immediately.

6. If no wheal forms, the injection may have been too deep. Reinject the PPD at a site at least 2″ (5 cm) from the first site, or on the other arm.

7. To interpret the skin test, measure the area of induration (hardening or thickening of tissues) at 48 and 72 hours. *(Note:* Erythema isn't generally considered evidence of an active or dormant infection.)

An induration of 10 mm or greater indicates a significant reaction. (This was formerly called a positive reaction.) Significance of a reaction is determined not only by the size of the reaction but by circumstances. For example, a reaction of 5 mm or more may be considered significant in a person who has an immediate family member with tuberculosis.

8. Record the results for the attending doctor.

Note: A significant PPD reaction usually results in patients previously vaccinated with bacille Calmette-Guérin (BCG) vaccine. If you know a patient has received BCG vaccine, don't administer the PPD test. Also, a false-negative reaction can occur in an anergic patient (who can't react to any skin tests) or in an immunosuppressed patient.

Tuberculosis diagnosis must be confirmed by chest X-ray and/or positive sputum smear. (See next page.)

Source: Center for Disease Control criteria, and American Thoracic Surgeons Society statement on tuberculosis skin test reactions, August 1981

WHAT TO DO WHEN YOUR PATIENT HAS A SIGNIFICANT REACTION TO TB SKIN TESTING

A tuberculin skin test is a commonly used screening test. A patient with active disease shows a significant reaction; however, a significant reaction is *not* diagnostic of TB. A significant reaction is 10 mm or more induration. Significance of a reaction is determined not only by the size of the reaction but by circumstances. For example, in a patient who has a family member with active TB, a reaction of 5 mm or more may be considered significant. Follow the steps in this flow chart if your patient has a significant reaction to TB testing. For further information, contact your local public health department or the Center for Disease Control, Atlanta, Ga.

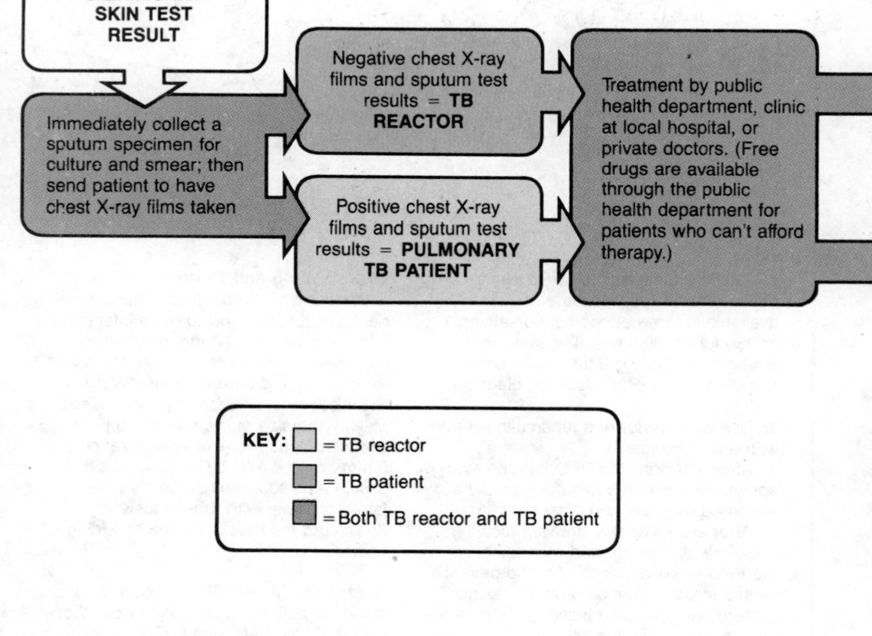
SIGNIFICANT SKIN TEST RESULT
Immediately collect a sputum specimen for culture and smear; then send patient to have chest X-ray films taken
Negative chest X-ray films and sputum test results = TB REACTOR
Positive chest X-ray films and sputum test results = PULMONARY TB PATIENT
Treatment by public health department, clinic at local hospital, or private doctors. (Free drugs are available through the public health department for patients who can't afford therapy.)
KEY:
= TB reactor
= TB patient
= Both TB reactor and TB patient

Source: Center for Disease Control Criteria and American Thoracic Surgeons Society Standards, August, 1981.

If reactor is over age 35, no drug treatment is given unless patient has close contact with pulmonary TB patient; has diabetes, Hodgkin's disease, leukemia, silicosis; is receiving immunosuppressive or steroid therapy; or has had a gastrectomy.

If reactor is under age 35, has negative sputum tests, and abnormal chest X-ray films without presence of active disease, chemoprophylaxis with isoniazid is strongly recommended, especially if the patient is receiving steroids; has close contact with pulmonary TB patient; has diabetes, Hodgkin's disease, leukemia, silicosis; is receiving immunosuppressive therapy; or has had a gastrectomy.

If reactor is under age 6, chemoprophylaxis with isoniazid is mandatory.

For TB patient, drug treatment with isoniazid and rifampin must continue for a minimum of 9 months, even when patient's sputum culture is negative after 3 months. Reinforce patient compliance.

Family members should receive skin tests.

Provide drug treatment. Explain to the patient that he will be in isolation for the first 3 days of therapy. Teach him how to use the drug and maintain a proper diet. Make sure he understands that his skin test will always show a significant reaction even though he may no longer have TB. This is because the skin test detects not only the presence of active disease, but also the presence of sensitized lymphocytes that the individual may have developed as a result of exposure to or immunization against the disease. Sputum cultures and chest X-ray films are definitive for active disease.

Perform routine sputum cultures and chest X-rays.
(Hospitalized patient: every day)
(Outpatient: if sputum is positive, every month; if negative, every few months depending on the clinical situation)

TB patient should have a periodic follow-up for 1 year after therapy is discontinued and regular checkups thereafter, as determined by his doctor.

If symptoms return, seek help from doctor or public health department.

NAME	INDICATIONS & DOSAGE	SIDE EFFECTS
histoplasmin♦	*Suspected histoplasmosis*— **Adults and children:** 0.1 ml of 1:100 dilution intradermally on inner forearm. Use tuberculin syringe with 26G or 27G, ⅜" needle.	**Local:** urticaria, ulceration or necrosis in highly sensitive patients. **Other:** shortness of breath, sweating, *anaphylaxis.*
Old tuberculin Old Tuberculin Test♦; Tuberculin, Mono-Vacc Test; Old Tuberculin Tine Test	*Diagnosis of tuberculosis*— **Adults and children:** 10 tuberculin units (0.1 ml of 1:1,000) Old tuberculin intradermally on inner forearm. In suspected tuberculosis, use 1 tuberculin unit first. Use tuberculin syringe with 26G or 27G, ⅜" needle. Multiple-puncture test: cleanse skin thoroughly with alcohol; make skin taut on inner forearm; press points firmly into selected site.	**Local:** hypersensitivity (vesiculation, ulceration, necrosis). **Other:** *anaphylaxis.*
tuberculin purified protein derivative Aplisol, Aplitest, Sclavo test-PPD, Sterneedle, Tuberculin PPD-Heaf, Tuberculin PPD-Stabilized, Tubersol	*Diagnosis of tuberculosis, evaluation of immunocompetence in patients with cancer*— **Adults and children:** 5 tuberculin units (0.1 ml) intradermally on inner forearm. Suspected sensitivity dose is 1 tuberculin unit. Patients failing to react to 5 tuberculin units should be tested with 250 tuberculin units. First strength equals 1 tuberculin unit/0.1 ml; intermediate strength, 5 tuberculin units/0.1 ml. Second strength equals 250 tuberculin units/ 0.1 ml. Use tuberculin syringe with 26G or 27G, ⅜" needle. Multiple-puncture test: cleanse	**Local:** pain, pruritus, vesiculation, ulceration, necrosis. **Other:** *anaphylaxis.*

INTERACTIONS	NURSING CONSIDERATIONS
None significant.	• Read test at 24 to 48 hours. Induration of 5 mm or more is positive response. • Reaction may be depressed in patients with malnutrition or immunosuppression. • Cross-reaction may occur with other fungi (for example, *Candida albicans, Blastomyces dermatitides).* • Obtain accurate history of allergies and reactions to skin tests. • Keep epinephrine 1:1,000 available. • Cold packs or topical corticosteroids may relieve pain and itching if severe local reaction occurs. • For treatment of anaphylaxis, see inside front cover.
None significant.	• Contraindicated in known tuberculin-positive reactors. • False-positive reaction can occur in sensitive patients. • Reaction may be depressed in patients with malnutrition or immunosuppression. • Read test in 48 to 72 hours. An induration of 10 mm or greater indicates a significant reaction (formerly called positive reaction). Significance of a reaction is determined not only by the size of the reaction but by circumstances. For example, a reaction of 5 mm or more may be considered significant in a person who has a TB patient in his immediate family. Likewise, a reaction of 2 mm or more may be considered significant in pediatric patients. The amount of induration at the site determines the significance of the reaction, and not the amount of redness at the site. • Multiple-puncture test: 1- to 2-mm induration is significant. • Old Tuberculin Tine Test equals 5 tuberculin units purified protein derivative. • Obtain accurate history of allergies, especially to acacia (contained in tine test as stabilizer), and reactions to skin tests. • Keep epinephrine 1:1,000 available. • Subcutaneous injection invalidates test results. Bleb must form on skin upon intradermal injection. • Corticosteroids and other immunosuppressives may suppress skin test reaction. • Cold packs or topical corticosteroids may relieve pain and itching if severe local reaction occurs after test. • For treatment of anaphylaxis, see inside front cover.
None significant.	• Contraindicated in known tuberculin-positive reactors; severe reactions may occur. Use cautiously with active tuberculosis. • Read test in 48 to 72 hours. An induration of 10 mm or greater indicates a significant reaction (formerly called positive reaction). Significance of a reaction is determined not only by the size of the reaction but by circumstances. For example, a reaction of 5 mm or more may be considered significant in a person who has a TB patient in his immediate family. Likewise, a reaction of 2 mm or more may be considered significant in pediatric patients. The amount of induration at the site determines the significance of the reaction, and not the amount of redness at the site. • Multiple-puncture test: vesiculation is significant reaction; induration of less than 2 mm without vesiculation is not significant. • One tuberculin unit may give false-negative test result; 250 tuberculin units may give false-positive test result. • Obtain accurate history of allergies and reactions to skin tests. • Reaction may be depressed in malnutrition, immunosuppression, or viral infections (up to 4 weeks postinfection).

(continued on following page)

NAME	INDICATIONS & DOSAGE	SIDE EFFECTS
tuberculin purified protein derivative *(continued)*	skin thoroughly with alcohol; make skin taut on inner forearm; press points firmly into selected site.	

◆ Available in U.S. and Canada. ◆◆ Available in Canada only. All other products (no symbol) available in U.S. only. Italicized side effects are common or life-threatening.

INTERACTIONS	NURSING CONSIDERATIONS
	• Antigen adsorbed by plastic. Use at once after drawing into plastic syringe. • Keep epinephrine 1:1,000 available. • Subcutaneous injection invalidates test results. Bleb must form on skin upon intradermal injection. • Cold packs or topical corticosteroids may relieve pain and itching if severe local reaction occurs. • Never give initial test with second test strength (250 tuberculin units). • A tine test (multiple-puncture test) is available for rapid screening. • Corticosteroids and other immunosuppressives may suppress skin test reaction. • Significant response at the injection site in patients with cancer indicates immunocompetence (the patient can respond to a challenge of his immune system). These patients have a better chance of responding to immunotherapy. • For treatment of anaphylaxis, see inside front cover.

DIAGNOSTIC SKIN TESTS: GLOSSARY OF TERMS

Anergy: diminished or absent sensitivity reaction to a specific antigen

Antigen: any substance capable of stimulating the production of antibodies and/or sensitized lymphocytes, under appropriate conditions

Cellular immune response: production of lymphocytes by the T cells of the thymus in response to an antigen

Delayed hypersensitivity: a slowly developed increase in cellular immune response to a specific antigen

Humoral immune response: production of antibodies by the thymus-independent B cells in response to an antigen

Immunity: state of resistance to antigens or foreign microorganisms due to the development of antibodies and/or sensitized lymphocytes

Immunocompetence: ability to develop an immune response to an antigen

Immunodeficiency: an inadequate humoral and/or cellular immune response that is mediated by the response of humoral antibodies or immune lymphoid cells

Immunotherapy: administration of preformed antibodies (serum or gamma globulin) to a patient for the production or enhancement of immunity

Nonspecific inflammatory response: a localized, protective reaction to foreign substances in the body tissues. This reaction destroys, dilutes, or sequesters both the affected tissue and the affecting agent

Primary immune response: the immune response to initial antigen stimulation, characterized by a latent period (ranging from several days to two weeks) before a specific antibody is developed

Secondary immune response (also called anamnestic response, booster response, memory response, recall response, and second-set response): the rapid reappearance of an antibody in the blood after administration of an antigen to which patient had previously developed a primary immune response

111 Uncategorized drugs

adenosine phosphate
allopurinol
amantadine hydrochloride
bromocriptine mesylate
clomiphene citrate
colchicine
cromolyn sodium
diazoxide, oral
dimethyl sulfoxide 50% (DMSO)
disulfiram
levodopa
levodopa-carbidopa
methoxsalen
pralidoxime chloride
ritodrine hydrochloride

For information on alprostadil, see APPENDIX, *New Drugs*.

These drugs, with diverse uses, don't fall into the preceding classes of drugs.

Major uses

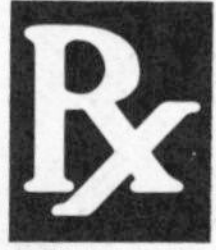

• Adenosine phosphate is a therapeutic adjunct for varicose veins and thrombophlebitis; it is also used to treat symptoms of bursitis, tendinitis, tenosynovitis, intractable pruritus, and multiple sclerosis.

• Allopurinol lowers blood and urine uric acid levels in primary gout.

• Amantadine alleviates idiopathic parkinsonism, parkinsonian syndrome, and drug-induced extrapyramidal reactions.

• Bromocriptine is used in short-term treatment of amenorrhea or galactorrhea associated with hyperprolactinemia. It also prevents postpartum galactorrhea.

• Clomiphene induces ovulation in anovulatory women who want to become pregnant.

• Colchicine relieves attacks of gouty arthritis.

• Cromolyn is a therapeutic adjunct for severe, chronic bronchial asthma.

• Oral diazoxide is used to treat hypoglycemia, particularly in infants and children.

• Dimethyl sulfoxide is instilled into the urinary bladder for symptomatic relief of interstitial cystitis.

• Disulfiram is an adjunct in the treatment of chronic alcoholism.

• Levodopa and levodopa-carbidopa are therapeutic for symptoms of idiopathic parkinsonism and parkinsonian syndrome resulting from encephalitis lethargica, carbon monoxide poisoning, chronic manganese poisoning, and cerebral arteriosclerosis.

• Methoxsalen is effective in the repigmentation of idiopathic vitiligo.

• Pralidoxime is an antidote for poisoning by pesticides and organophosphorus chemicals. It is also used to treat overdose of anticholinesterase drugs given in myasthenia gravis.

• Ritodrine is used in the management of preterm labor.

Mechanism of action

• Adenosine phosphate may correct biochemical imbalance or deficiency at the cellular level. Therapeutic effects may also result from the drug's vasodilation and ability to reduce tissue edema and inflammation.

PATIENT-TEACHING AID

HOW TO TAKE YOUR BASAL BODY TEMPERATURE

Dear Patient:

You are currently taking clomiphene to induce ovulation. Knowing when ovulation has occurred is helpful in both planning and avoiding pregnancy. You can determine when your ovulatory (fertile) period is by taking your basal body temperature every morning. To do so:

- Use a basal body temperature thermometer. This measures temperature between 96° F. and 100° F. and is calibrated by tenths of a degree, enabling easier identification of slight temperature changes that occur during your cycle.
- Take your temperature each morning before getting out of bed, since physical activity changes basal temperature. You may take your temperature by the oral, rectal, vaginal, or axillary route. But you should use the same route each day.
- After taking your temperature, shake down the thermometer for the next day. Even shaking the thermometer when you awake can change your basal body temperature.
- Plot your daily temperatures on a monthly graph, like the one shown here. Note any conditions that might affect your basal temperature, such as colds or other infections, sleeplessness, or emotional upset.

The basal body temperature graph shows the time of ovulation and indicates your fertile period. Basal temperature dips slightly at the time of ovulation, then rises approximately 1°. The temperature stays at this level until 3 or 4 days before the next cycle begins. The probable time of ovulation in this basal temperature graph is day 13; note the drop in temperature followed by elevation. An elevated temperature sustained past the time of the next normal menstrual flow suggests pregnancy has occurred.

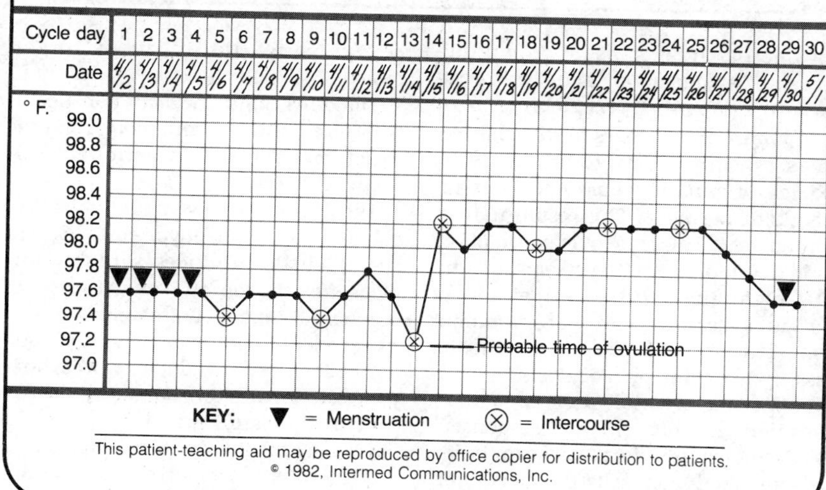

- Allopurinol reduces uric-acid production by inhibiting the biochemical reactions preceding its formation.
- Amantadine increases dopamine release in animal brain, but its exact mechanism of action in humans is unknown.
- Bromocriptine inhibits secretion of

DRUG ERROR

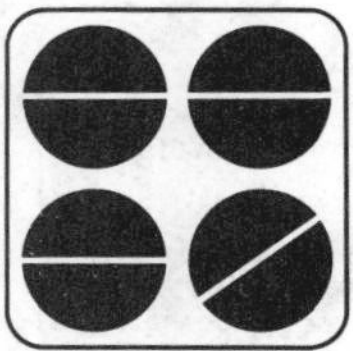

BE CAREFUL WHEN GIVING DISULFIRAM TO PATIENTS ON OTHER MEDICATIONS

A nurse made this potentially dangerous mistake during her first experience with a patient receiving disulfiram: The patient was also taking an antipsychotic medication—mesoridazine besylate (Serentil). The nurse, following hospital policy to give elixirs instead of tablets whenever possible, gave him Serentil elixir.

When she checked on the patient a half hour after administering the antipsychotic, his face was flushed, his blood pressure was elevated, and he was complaining of palpitations, light-headedness, and nausea.

At first, the nurse thought the patient had been drinking, but he adamantly denied this. Then she thought he might have inadvertently taken some medication containing alcohol. So she asked, "How about cough medicine?"

As soon as she said these words, the nurse realized what had happened. She had given the patient an elixir—which contains 12% alcohol.

Luckily, the patient's alcohol reaction was mild, but if the alcohol content in the elixir had been higher, he might have had a more serious reaction, such as disorientation or unconsciousness. Even fatal reactions have occurred in patients who drank alcoholic beverages while taking disulfiram.

After this experience, the hospital issued a written policy stating that patients on disulfiram should receive *only tablet forms* of all medications.

Note: When you recognize a disulfiram-alcohol reaction, take the usual measures to restore blood pressure and to treat shock; administer oxygen, I.V. antihistamine or I.V. ephedrine sulfate. (Advise your patient to carry medication identification noting these emergency measures.)

prolactin. It acts as a dopamine-receptor antagonist by activating postsynaptic dopamine receptors.

• Clomiphene appears to stimulate release of pituitary gonadotropins, follicle-stimulating hormone, and luteinizing hormone. This results in maturation of the ovarian follicle, ovulation, and development of the corpus luteum.

• Colchicine inhibits migration of granulocytes to an area of inflammation. It decreases lactic acid production associated with phagocytosis and interrupts the cycle of urate crystal deposition and inflammatory response.

• Cromolyn inhibits the degranulation of sensitized mast cells that occurs after a patient's exposure to specific antigens. It also inhibits release of histamine and slow-reacting substance of anaphylaxis (SRS-A).

• Oral diazoxide inhibits release of insulin from the pancreas and decreases peripheral utilization of glucose.

• Dimethyl sulfoxide acts nonspecifically as an anti-inflammatory agent. Its exact mechanism of action is unknown.

• Disulfiram blocks oxidation of alcohol at the acetaldehyde stage. Excess acetaldehyde produces a highly unpleasant reaction in the presence of even small amounts of alcohol.

• Levodopa and levodopa-carbidopa act as follows: Levodopa is decarboxylated to dopamine, countering the depletion of striatal dopamine in extrapyramidal centers, which is thought to produce parkinsonism. Carbidopa inhibits the peripheral decarboxylation of levodopa without affecting levodopa's metabolism within the central nervous system (CNS). Therefore, more levodopa is available to be decarboxylated to dopamine in the brain.

- Methoxsalen may enhance melanogenesis, either directly or secondarily, to an inflammatory process.
- Pralidoxime reactivates cholinesterase that has been inactivated by organophosphorus pesticides and related compounds. It permits degradation of accumulated acetylcholine and facilitates normal functioning of neuromuscular junctions.
- Ritodrine is a beta-receptor agonist that stimulates the $beta_2$-adrenergic receptors in uterine smooth muscle, inhibiting contractility.

Absorption, distribution, metabolism, and excretion

- Allopurinol is well absorbed orally from the gastrointestinal (GI) tract. Most of it is metabolized in the liver to the active metabolite oxypurinol. This metabolite, as well as some unchanged drug, is excreted in urine.
- Amantadine is well absorbed from the GI tract. It is largely excreted unchanged in urine.
- Bromocriptine is poorly absorbed from the GI tract. Metabolized by the liver, it is eliminated in urine and—through the bile—in feces.
- Clomiphene is well absorbed from the GI tract and metabolized largely in the liver. About 50% of the drug is eliminated in feces within 5 days; the remaining unchanged drug and metabolites are either recirculated in the enterohepatic vascular network or stored in body fat.
- Colchicine is well absorbed from the GI tract when given orally. It is metabolized in the liver and eliminated in both urine and feces.
- Cromolyn is absorbed into the systemic circulation after its inhalation into the lungs. The drug is excreted unchanged in urine and bile. Small amounts are swallowed and eliminated in feces.
- Oral diazoxide is well absorbed from the GI tract. Most of it is excreted unchanged in urine.
- Dimethyl sulfoxide's absorption is unknown. It is metabolized in the liver

PATIENT-TEACHING AID

PREVENTING ANTABUSE-ALCOHOL REACTIONS

Dear Patient:

The doctor has prescribed Antabuse (disulfiram) to help you stop drinking alcoholic beverages. Most patients tolerate the drug well, but you may suffer such side effects as drowsiness, fatigue, impotence, headache, skin eruptions, and metallic aftertaste. These effects will disappear after about 2 weeks of therapy, as your body adjusts to the drug.

Antabuse interferes with the breakdown of alcohol in your body. Should you take a drink, toxic levels of acetaldehyde will accumulate and produce a rapid, intense, and unpleasant reaction. *Caution: A severe reaction could be fatal.* Be aware of the hidden alcohol content of common substances. Don't use alcohol in food, sauces, or vinegar; apply alcohol-containing shampoos, liniments, or lotions (such as after-shave); or take alcohol-containing medications, such as Paregoric, Comtrex, Nyquil, Nervine, or liquid vitamins. Metronidazole and paraldehyde may also cause a reaction. If you have a reaction, you may experience severe nausea and vomiting, hypotension, rapid pulse rate and respirations, flushed face, bloodshot eyes, throbbing in head and neck, sweating, thirst, weakness, confusion, blurred vision.

An Antabuse reaction may last as long as there's alcohol in the blood. You may have an Antabuse-alcohol reaction up to 2 weeks after you've stopped taking the drug.

If you're undergoing Antabuse therapy, always carry an identification card in case of an emergency. It should state that you're receiving Antabuse; the symptoms and treatment of an Antabuse-alcohol reaction; and your doctor's name, address, and phone number.

THERAPEUTIC ACTIVITY

THERAPEUTIC ACTIVITY OF UNCATEGORIZED DRUGS

DRUG	ONSET	DURATION
adenosine phosphate	5 to 30 minutes	1 to 2 hours
allopurinol	30 to 60 minutes	Blood and urine uric acid levels fall within 2 to 3 days, but full effect may not be seen for 1 week. Uric acid returns to pretreatment levels slowly.
amantadine	10 to 15 minutes	Up to 24 hours; acidification of urine increases excretion rate.
bromocriptine	2 hours	4 to 5 hours
clomiphene	Unknown	Unknown
colchicine	Pain alleviated within 12 hours after P.O. administration and completely gone usually within 24 to 48 hours after P.O. and 4 to 12 hours after I.V. administration.	Blood levels fall 1 to 2 hours after oral dose, then rise due to recycling; drug found in leukocytes 9 days after single I.V. dose.
cromolyn	Immediately on inhalation	3 to 4 hours
diazoxide	Within 1 hour	8 hours
dimethyl sulfoxide	Unknown	Unknown
disulfiram	Rapidly absorbed from gastrointestinal tract, but full effect may not be seen for 12 hours.	Slowly eliminated; about 20% remains in body after 1 week; sensitization to alcohol may last 6 to 12 days after last dose.
levodopa and levodopa-carbidopa	Rapidly absorbed (10 to 15 minutes), especially when stomach is empty.	5 to 24 hours
methoxsalen	1 hour; peaks in 2 hours	8 hours
pralidoxine	2 to 5 minutes	Short-acting; repeated doses every 3 to 4 hours may be needed.
ritodrine	I.V.: immediate P.O.: 30 minutes	Depends on amount of uterine activity (generally 2 to 6 hours)

to dimethyl sulfone and dimethyl sulfide. Dimethyl sulfone is excreted in urine and feces; dimethyl sulfide is excreted in the breath and through the skin.

- Disulfiram is well absorbed from the GI tract. It is metabolized in the liver and excreted slowly in urine. About 20% of the drug remains in the body for 1 week or longer.
- Levodopa and levodopa-carbidopa are well absorbed from the GI tract. Levodopa's penetration into the CNS is enhanced when carbidopa is administered concurrently. Levodopa is metabolized (decarboxylated) to dopamine in the peripheral tissues and the GI tract. Eventually dopamine itself is metabolized in the liver and excreted in urine. Carbidopa is not extensively metabolized; most of it is excreted unchanged in urine.
- Methoxsalen is well absorbed from the GI tract, metabolized in the liver, and excreted in urine.
- Pralidoxime is variably and incompletely absorbed from the GI tract and after I.M injection. It is largely metabolized in the liver and excreted in urine both as a metabolite and as the unchanged compound.
- Ritodrine is poorly absorbed orally but is completely bioavailable after I.V. infusion. The drug is excreted in urine within 24 hours.

Onset and duration

The chart on the opposite page summarizes the therapeutic activity of the drugs described in this chapter.

Combination products

COLBENEMID: probenecid 500 mg and colchicine 0.5 mg.

PROBENECID WITH COLCHICINE: probenecid 500 mg and colchicine 0.5 mg.

NAME	INDICATIONS & DOSAGE	SIDE EFFECTS
adenosine phosphate Adenocrest, Adenyl, Cobalasine, My-B-Den	*To relieve edema, pruritus, dermatitis, and erythema of varicose veins; symptomatic treatment of bursitis, tendinitis, intractable pruritus—* **Adults:** 20 to 100 mg I.M. (extended-release) daily for 3 or 4 days, reduced to same dosage every other day. Depending on patient response, reduce dose to 20 mg once or twice weekly; or 20 mg I.M. daily to t.i.d. (simple aqueous solution); or every hour for 5 doses for first 3 days, followed by 20 mg daily as needed; or 100 mg in aqueous solution injected as single dose daily for 3 days, followed by 100 mg on alternate days thereafter as needed. *Sublingual dose to supplement I.M. injection—* **Adults:** 20 mg sublingually q hour, 5 to 7 doses per day for 4 to 7 days. Maintenance dose: 40 to 100 mg daily sublingually, adjusted to patient response.	**CNS:** dizziness, headache. **CV:** *palpitations, hypotension, dyspnea.* **GI:** epigastric discomfort, nausea, diarrhea. **Skin:** erythema, flushing. **Other:** *anaphylaxis; local reaction at injection site; may increase symptoms of bursitis or tendinitis.*
allopurinol Lopurin, Zyloprim♦	*Gout, primary or secondary to hyperuricemia; secondary to diseases such as acute or chronic leukemia, polycythemia vera, multiple myeloma, and psoriasis—* Dosage varies with severity of disease; can be given as single dose or divided, but doses larger than 300 mg should be divided. **Adults:** mild gout, 200 to 300 mg P.O. daily; severe gout with large tophi, 400 to 600 mg P.O. daily. Same dose for maintenance in secondary hyperuricemia. *Hyperuricemia secondary to malignancies—* **Children 6 to 10 years:** 300 mg P.O. daily. **Children under 6 years:** 150 mg P.O. daily. *Impaired renal function—* **Adults:** 200 mg daily if creatinine clearance is 10 to 20 ml/minute; 100 mg daily if creatinine is less than 10 ml/minute; 100 mg more than 24 hours apart if clearance is less than	**Blood:** *agranulocytosis,* anemia, *aplastic anemia.* **CNS:** drowsiness. **EENT:** cataracts, retinopathy. **GI:** nausea, vomiting, diarrhea, abdominal pain. **Hepatic:** altered liver function tests. **Skin:** *rash, usually maculopapular; exfoliative,* urticarial, and purpuric lesions; erythema multiforme; severe furunculosis of nose; ichthyosis, *toxic epidermal necrolysis.*

♦ Available in U.S. and Canada. ♦♦ Available in Canada only. All other products (no symbol) available in U.S. only. Italicized side effects are common or life-threatening.

INTERACTIONS	NURSING CONSIDERATIONS
None significant.	• Contraindicated in myocardial infarction and cerebral hemorrhage. Use cautiously in patients with history of allergy or asthma. Obtain accurate history of allergies before giving first dose. • Anaphylactic reactions have occurred following use of gelatin I.M. solution. Discontinue if patient complains of dyspnea or tightness in chest. • Don't give I.V. • Place sublingual tablets under tongue. Warn patient not to mix with food or water, or to swallow excessively until dissolved. • I.M. extended-release in gelatin vehicle: warm solution before using. Inject into gluteal muscle, using 22G to 20G 1″ to 1½″ needle. • Assess patient for reduction of edema, inflammation. • For treatment of anaphylaxis, see inside front cover.
Uricosuric agents: additive effect; may be used to therapeutic advantage.	• Contraindicated in hypersensitivity and in patients with idiopathic hemochromatosis; and in patients who have developed reactions to it. Use cautiously in hepatic or renal disease. • Obtain accurate patient history; note possible allergies with other drug use before first dose. • Discontinue at first sign of skin rash, which may precede severe hypersensitivity reaction, or any other adverse reaction. Warn patient to report all side effects immediately. • Monitor intake/output; daily urinary output of at least 2 liters and maintenance of neutral or slightly alkaline urine are desirable. Patient should be encouraged to drink plenty of fluids while taking this drug unless otherwise contraindicated. • Periodically check CBC, hepatic and renal function, especially at start of therapy. • Acute gouty attacks may occur in first 6 weeks of therapy; concurrent use of colchicine may be prescribed prophylactically. • Minimize GI side effects by administering with meals or immediately after. • Evaluate effectiveness, using serum uric acid levels. Goal is to lower serum level to 6 mg/100 ml, usually within 7 to 10 days; to gradually reduce size of tophi, with no new deposits within 6 months; and to relieve joint pain and increase mobility. • Allopurinol may predispose patient to ampicillin-induced skin rash. • Allopurinol may cause rash even weeks after discontinuation of drug. • Since drug may cause drowsiness, advise patient to refrain from driving car or performing tasks requiring mental alertness until CNS response to drug is known.

(continued on following page)

NAME	INDICATIONS & DOSAGE	SIDE EFFECTS
allopurinol *(continued)*	3 ml/minute. *To prevent acute gouty attacks—* **Adults:** 100 mg daily; increase at weekly intervals by 100 mg without exceeding maximum (800 mg), until serum uric acid level falls to 6 mg/100 ml or less. *To prevent uric acid nephropathy during cancer chemotherapy—* **Adults:** 600 to 800 mg P.O. daily for 2 to 3 days, with high fluid intake.	
amantadine hydrochloride Symmetrel♦	*To treat drug-induced extrapyramidal reactions—* **Adults:** 100 mg P.O. b.i.d., up to 300 mg daily in divided doses. Patients may benefit from as much as 400 mg daily, but doses over 200 mg must be closely supervised. *To treat idiopathic parkinsonism, parkinsonian syndrome—* **Adults:** 100 mg P.O. b.i.d.; in patients who are seriously ill or receiving other antiparkinsonism drugs, 100 mg daily for at least 1 week, then 100 mg b.i.d., p.r.n.	**CNS:** depression, fatigue, confusion, *dizziness,* psychosis, hallucinations, anxiety, irritability, *ataxia, insomnia,* weakness, headache. **CV:** peripheral edema, *orthostatic hypotension,* congestive heart failure. **GI:** anorexia, nausea, constipation, vomiting, dry mouth. **GU:** urinary retention. **Skin:** *livedo,* dermatitis.
bromocriptine mesylate Parlodel♦	*To treat amenorrhea and galactorrhea associated with hyperprolactinemia—* 2.5 mg P.O. b.i.d. or t.i.d. with meals for 14 days; and for no more than 6 months. *Prevention of postpartum lactation—* 2.5 mg b.i.d. with meals for 14 days. Treatment may be extended for up to 21 days, if necessary.	**CNS:** *dizziness,* headache, fatigue, nervousness. **EENT:** nasal congestion, tinnitus, blurred vision. **GI:** *nausea,* vomiting, abdominal cramps, constipation, diarrhea.

♦ Available in U.S. and Canada. ♦♦ Available in Canada only. All other products (no symbol) available in U.S. only. Italicized side effects are common or life-threatening.

INTERACTIONS	NURSING CONSIDERATIONS
None significant.	• Use cautiously in epilepsy or seizures, with congestive heart failure, renal impairment, peripheral edema, hepatic disease, eczematoid dermatitis, uncontrolled psychosis, or severe psychoneurosis. • Don't stop abruptly, since this might precipitate a parkinsonian crisis; taper off gradually. • Warn elderly patients about orthostatic hypotension. Suggest they change position slowly, dangle legs before getting up, and lie down if they feel faint or dizzy. Advise elderly males to sit down to urinate, especially at night. • Last daily dose should be given as early as possible to avoid insomnia. • Warn patient that drug may produce dizziness, blurred vision, impaired coordination; activities requiring mental alertness should be resumed gradually. • Advise patient to report decrease in drug's effectiveness to doctor.
None significant.	• Contraindicated in hypersensitivity to ergot derivatives. • Patient should be examined carefully for pituitary tumor (Forbes-Albright syndrome). Use of bromocriptine will not affect tumor size (cause tumor to regress) although it may alleviate amenorrhea or galactorrhea. • May lead to early postpartum conception. Test for pregnancy every 4 weeks or whenever period is missed after menses are reinitiated. • Advise patient to use contraceptive methods other than oral contraception during treatment. • Safe use of bromocriptine during pregnancy has not been established; therefore this drug is not indicated in treatment of infertility. • "First-dose phenomenon" occurs in 1% of patients. Sensitive patients may collapse for 15 to 60 minutes but can usually tolerate subsequent treatment without ill effects. • Incidence of adverse effects is high (68%); however, most are mild to moderate, and only 6% of patients discontinue drug for this reason. Nausea is the most common side effect. • Recurrence rates when used to treat amenorrhea or galactorrhea associated with hyperprolactinemia are high (70% to 80%). • Advise the patient that it may take 6 to 8 weeks or longer for menses to be reinstated and galactorrhea to be suppressed. • Should be given with meals. • Giving last daily dose at bedtime with a snack may help decrease nausea and dizziness. • Has been used investigationally in management of parkinsonism.

NAME	INDICATIONS & DOSAGE	SIDE EFFECTS
clomiphene citrate Clomid♦	*To induce ovulation*—50 to 100 mg P.O. daily for 5 days, starting any time; or 50 to 100 mg P.O. daily starting on day 5 of menstrual cycle (first day of menstrual flow is day 1). Repeat until conception occurs or until 3 courses of therapy are completed.	**CNS:** headache, restlessness, insomnia, dizziness, lightheadedness, depression, fatigue, tension. **CV:** hypertension. **EENT:** blurred vision, diplopia, scotomata, photophobia (signs of impending visual toxicity). **GI:** nausea, vomiting, bloating, distention, increased appetite, weight gain. **GU:** urinary frequency and polyuria; ovarian enlargement and cyst formation, which regress spontaneously when drug is stopped. **Metabolic:** hyperglycemia. **Skin:** urticaria, rash, dermatitis. **Other:** *hot flashes,* reversible alopecia, *breast discomfort.*
colchicine Colchicine, Novocolchine♦♦	*To prevent acute attacks of gout as prophylactic or maintenance therapy*— **Adults:** 0.5 or 0.6 mg P.O. daily; or 1 to 1.8 mg P.O. daily for more severe cases. *To prevent attacks of gout in patients undergoing surgery*— **Adults:** 0.5 to 0.6 mg P.O. t.i.d. 3 days before and 3 days after surgery. *To treat acute gout, acute gouty arthritis*— **Adults:** initially, 1 to 1.2 mg P.O., then 0.5 or 0.6 mg q hour, or 1 to 1.2 mg q 2 hours until pain is relieved or until nausea, vomiting, or diarrhea ensues. Or 2 mg I.V. followed by 2 mg I.V. in 12 hours if necessary. Total I.V. dose over 24 hours not to exceed 4 mg. *Note:* Give I.V. by slow I.V. push over 2 to 5 minutes. Avoid extravasation. Don't dilute colchicine injection with 0.9% sodium chloride or 5% dextrose injection, or any other fluid that might change pH of colchicine solution. If lower concentration of colchicine injection needed, dilute with sterile water for injection. However, if diluted solution becomes turbid, don't inject.	**Blood:** *aplastic anemia and agranulocytosis with prolonged use;* nonthrombocytopenic purpura. **CNS:** peripheral neuritis. **GI:** *nausea, vomiting, abdominal pain, diarrhea.* **Skin:** urticaria, dermatitis. **Local:** severe local irritation if extravasation occurs. **Other:** alopecia.

♦ Available in U.S. and Canada. ♦♦ Available in Canada only. All other products (no symbol) available in U.S. only. Italicized side effects are common or life-threatening.

INTERACTIONS	NURSING CONSIDERATIONS
None significant.	• Contraindicated in thrombophlebitis, thromboembolic disorders, or history of these conditions; cancer of breast or reproductive organs; undiagnosed abnormal genital bleeding; ovarian cyst; hepatic disease or dysfunction. Use cautiously in hypertension, mental depression, migraines, seizures, diabetes mellitus, or gonadotropin sensitivity. Report development or worsening of these conditions to doctor. May require stopping drug. • Patient with visual disturbances should report symptoms to doctor at once. • Tell patient possibility of multiple births exists with this drug. Risk increases with higher doses. • Teach patient to take basal body temperature and chart on graph to ascertain whether ovulation has occurred. • Advise patient to stop drug and contact doctor immediately if abdominal symptoms or pain occurs because these indicate ovarian enlargement or ovarian cyst. • Reassure patient that response (ovulation) generally occurs after the first course of therapy. If pregnancy does not occur, course of therapy may be repeated twice. • Since drug may cause dizziness or visual disturbances, caution patient not to perform hazardous tasks until response to drug is known. • Advise patient to stop drug and contact doctor immediately if she suspects she is pregnant (drug may have teratogenic effect).
None significant.	• Use cautiously in hepatic dysfunction, cardiac disease, renal disease, GI disorders, and in aged or debilitated patients. • Reduce dosage if weakness, anorexia, nausea, vomiting, or diarrhea appears. First sign of acute overdosage may be GI symptoms, followed by vascular damage, muscle weakness, ascending paralysis. Delirium and convulsions may occur without patient losing consciousness. • Do not administer I.M. or subcutaneously; severe local irritation occurs. • As maintenance therapy, give with meals to reduce GI effects. May be used with uricosuric agents. • Baseline lab studies, including CBC, should precede therapy and be repeated periodically. • Monitor fluid intake/output. Keep output at 2,000 ml daily. • Store in tightly closed, light-resistant container. • Change needle before making direct I.V. injection.

NAME	INDICATIONS & DOSAGE	SIDE EFFECTS
cromolyn sodium Intal♦, Rynacrom♦♦	*Adjunct in treatment of severe perennial bronchial asthma—* **Adults, and children over 5 years:** contents of 20 mg capsule to be inhaled q.i.d. at regular intervals.	**CNS:** dizziness, headache. **EENT:** *irritation of the throat and trachea, cough, bronchospasm following inhalation of dry powder; esophagitis;* nasal congestion; pharyngeal irritation; wheezing. **GI:** nausea. **GU:** dysuria, urinary frequency. **Skin:** rash, urticaria. **Other:** joint swelling and pain, lacrimation, swollen parotid gland, angioedema.
diazoxide, oral Proglycem	*Management of hypoglycemia due to a variety of conditions resulting in hyperinsulinism—* **Adults and children:** 3 to 8 mg/kg/day P.O., divided into 3 equal doses q 8 hours. **Infants and newborns:** 8 to 15 mg/kg/day P.O., divided into 2 or 3 equal doses q 8 to 12 hours.	**Blood:** *leukopenia, thrombocytopenia.* **CV:** *cardiac arrhythmias.* **EENT:** diplopia. **GI:** nausea, vomiting. **Metabolic:** sodium and fluid retention, ketoacidosis and hyperosmolar nonketotic coma, hyperuricemia. **Other:** *severe hypertrichosis (hair growth) in 25% of adults and higher percentage of children.*
dimethyl sulfoxide 50% (DMSO) Rimso-50	*Symptomatic relief of interstitial cystitis—* **Adults:** instill 50 ml directly into bladder with catheter or syringe; allow to remain for 15 minutes. Repeat every 2 weeks until maximum symptomatic relief is obtained. Thereafter, the time intervals between therapy may be increased.	**Other:** *garlic-like taste in mouth,* hypersensitivity.

♦ Available in U.S. and Canada. ♦♦ Available in Canada only. All other products (no symbol) available in U.S. only. Italicized side effects are common or life-threatening.

INTERACTIONS	NURSING CONSIDERATIONS
None significant.	• Contraindicated in acute asthma attacks and status asthmaticus. • Not to be taken orally; insert capsule into inhaler provided; follow manufacturer's directions. • Watch for recurrence of asthmatic symptoms when dosage is decreased, especially when corticosteroids are also used. • Use only when acute episode has been controlled, airway is cleared, and patient is able to inhale. • Patient considered for cromolyn therapy should have pulmonary function tests to show significant bronchodilator-reversible component to his airway obstruction. • Teach correct use of inhaler: insert capsule in device properly, exhale completely before placing mouthpiece between lips, then inhale deeply and rapidly with steady, even breath; remove inhaler from mouth, hold breath a few seconds, and exhale. Repeat until all powder has been inhaled. For an example of inhalational technique, see the patient-teaching aid, *How to Use an Inhaler,* in Chapter 39, ADRENERGICS. • Store capsules at room temperature in a tightly closed container; protect from moisture and temperatures higher than 40° C. (104° F.). • Instruct patient to avoid excessive handling of capsule. • Esophagitis may be relieved by antacids or a glass of milk.
Thiazide diuretics: may potentiate hyperglycemic, hyperuricemic, and hypotensive effects. Monitor appropriate lab values.	• Contraindicated in thiazide hypersensitivity and functional hypoglycemia. • Oral diazoxide does not significantly lower blood pressure. • A nondiuretic congener of thiazide diuretics. • Most important use is in management of hypoglycemia due to hyperinsulinism in infants and children. • Monitor urine regularly for glucose and ketones; report any abnormalities to doctor. • If not effective after 2 or 3 weeks, drug should be stopped. • Hair growth on arms and forehead is a common side effect that will subside when drug treatment is completed. Reassure patient. • Available in capsules and oral suspension.
None significant.	• Chronic use of DMSO has been associated with ophthalmic changes. Eyes should be examined periodically. • After retention of Rimso-50 for 15 minutes, it's expelled by spontaneous voiding. • Administration of oral analgesics of opium and belladonna suppositories before instillation can reduce bladder spasm in sensitive patients. • Lidocaine jelly or similar local anesthetic should be applied to urethra before insertion of catheter to avoid spasm. • Warn patient before administration that he may experience some discomfort as the drug is introduced into the bladder. Reassure patient that this generally subsides with repeated administration. • Warn patient that he may experience a garlic-like taste several minutes after administration which may persist for several hours. • Not for I.M. or I.V. injection. • Patients on DMSO therapy should have liver and renal function tests and complete blood counts every 6 months while receiving drug. • Safety of DMSO in pregnancy has not been established. Use only if potential maternal benefits outweigh potential risks to fetus. • Safety and effectiveness of DMSO in children not yet established. • Used investigationally as a topical treatment for arthritis-inflamed joints.

NAME	INDICATIONS & DOSAGE	SIDE EFFECTS
disulfiram Antabuse♦, Cronetal, Ro-Sulfiram	*Adjunct in management of chronic alcoholism—* **Adults:** maximum of 500 mg q morning for 1 to 2 weeks. Can be taken in evening if drowsiness occurs. Maintenance: 125 to 500 mg daily (average dose 250 mg) until permanent self-control is established. Treatment may continue for months or years.	**CNS:** drowsiness, headache, fatigue, neuritis. **EENT:** optic neuritis. **GI:** metallic or garlic-like aftertaste. **GU:** impotence. **Skin:** acneiform or allergic dermatitis. **Other:** *"disulfiram reaction," which may include flushing, throbbing headache, dyspnea, nausea, copious vomiting, sweating, thirst, chest pain, palpitations, hyperventilation, hypotension, syncope, anxiety, weakness, blurred vision, confusion. In severe reactions, respiratory depression, cardiovascular collapse, arrhythmias, myocardial infarction, acute congestive heart failure, convulsions, unconsciousness, and even death can occur.*
levodopa Bendopa, Bio Dopa, Dopar, Larodopa♦, Levopa♦, Parda, Rio-Dopa	*Treatment of idiopathic parkinsonism and parkinsonian syndrome resulting from encephalitis lethargica; carbon monoxide and chronic manganese intoxication; and cerebral arteriosclerosis—* administered orally with food in dosages carefully adjusted to individual requirements, tolerance, response. **Adults:** initially, 0.5 to 1 g P.O. daily, given b.i.d., t.i.d., or q.i.d. with food; increase by no more than 0.75 g daily q 3 to 7 days, until usual maximum of 8 g is reached. Larger dose requires close supervision.	**Blood:** hemolytic anemia, leukopenia. **CNS:** *choreiform, dystonic, dyskinetic movements; involuntary grimacing, head movements, myoclonic body jerks, ataxia, tremors, muscle twitching; bradykinetic episodes; psychiatric disturbances, memory loss, nervousness, anxiety, disturbing dreams, euphoria, malaise, fatigue; severe depression, suicidal tendencies, dementia, delirium, hallucinations (may necessitate reduction or withdrawal of drug).* **CV:** *orthostatic hypotension,* cardiac irregularities, flushing, hypertension, phlebitis. **EENT:** blepharospasm, blurred

INTERACTIONS	**NURSING CONSIDERATIONS**
Isoniazid (INH): ataxia or marked change in behavior. Avoid use. *Metronidazole:* psychotic reaction. Do not use together. *Paraldehyde:* toxic levels of the acetaldehyde. Do not use together. *Alcohol:* disulfiram reaction.	• Contraindicated in alcohol intoxication, psychoses, myocardial disease, coronary occlusion, or those receiving metronidazole, paraldehyde, alcohol, or alcohol-containing preparations. Use cautiously in diabetes mellitus, hypothyroidism, epilepsy, cerebral damage, nephritis, hepatic cirrhosis or insufficiency, abnormal EEG, multiple drug dependence. • Used only under close medical and nursing supervision. Patient should clearly understand consequences of disulfiram therapy and give permission. Drug should be used only in patients who are cooperative and well motivated, and who are receiving supportive psychiatric therapy. • Complete physical exam and lab studies, including CBC, SMA-12, and transaminase, should precede therapy and be repeated regularly. • If compliance is questionable, crush tablets and mix with juice or other liquid; observe patient. • Warn patient to avoid all sources of alcohol: sauces, cough syrups. Even external application of liniments, shaving lotion, back-rub preparations may precipitate disulfiram reaction. Tell him that alcohol reaction may occur as long as 2 weeks after single dose of disulfiram; the longer patient remains on drug, the more sensitive he will become to alcohol. • Patient should wear a bracelet or carry a card supplied by drug manufacturer identifying him as disulfiram user. Cards may be obtained from Ayerst Laboratories, 685 Third Ave., New York, N.Y. 10017. *Note:* Mild reactions may occur in sensitive patients with blood alcohol level of 5 to 10 mg/100 ml; symptoms are fully developed at 50 mg/100 ml; unconsciousness usually occurs at 125 to 150 mg/100 ml level. Reaction may last ½ hour to several hours, or as long as alcohol remains in blood. • Caution patient's family that disulfiram should never be given to the patient without his knowledge; severe reaction or death could result if such a patient then ingested alcohol. • Reassure patient that disulfiram-induced side effects, such as drowsiness, fatigue, impotence, headache, peripheral neuritis, and metallic- or garlic-like taste, subside after about 2 weeks of therapy. *Caution:* Warn patient to ingest no alcohol or alcohol-containing products for at least 12 hours before administering.
Anticholinergic drugs, tricyclic antidepressants, benzodiazepines, clonidine, papaverine, phenothiazines and other antipsychotics, and phenytoin: watch for decreased levodopa effect. *Pyridoxine:* reduced efficacy of levodopa. Examine vitamin preparations for content of vitamin B_6 (pyridoxine). *Antacids, propranolol:* may increase levodopa effect. Use	• Contraindicated in narrow-angle glaucoma, melanoma, or undiagnosed skin lesions. Use cautiously in cardiovascular, renal, hepatic, pulmonary disorders; in those with peptic ulcer, psychiatric illness, myocardial infarction with residual arrhythmias; and in patients with bronchial asthma, emphysema, and endocrine disease. • Carefully monitor patients also receiving antihypertensive medication, hypoglycemic agents. Stop MAO inhibitors at least 2 weeks before therapy is begun. • Adjust dosage according to patient's response and tolerance. Observe and monitor vital signs, especially while adjusting dose. Report significant changes. • Instruct patient to report adverse reactions and therapeutic effects. • Warn of possible dizziness and orthostatic hypotension, especially at start of therapy. Patient should change position slowly and dangle legs before getting out of bed. Elastic stockings may control this side effect in some patients. • Muscle twitching and blepharospasm (twitching of eyelids) may be an early sign of drug overdosage; report immediately. • Patients on long-term use should be tested regularly for diabetes

(continued on following page)

NAME	INDICATIONS & DOSAGE	SIDE EFFECTS
levodopa *(continued)*		vision, diplopia, mydriasis or miosis, widening of palpebral fissures, activation of latent Horner's syndrome, oculogyric crises, nasal discharge. **GI:** *nausea, vomiting, anorexia;* weight loss may occur at start of therapy; constipation; flatulence; diarrhea; epigastric pain; hiccups; sialorrhea; dry mouth; bitter taste. **GU:** urinary frequency, retention, incontinence; darkened urine; excessive and inappropriate sexual behavior; priapism. **Hepatic:** hepatotoxicity. **Other:** dark perspiration, hyperventilation.
levodopa-carbidopa (combination) Sinemet♦	*Treatment of idiopathic Parkinson's disease, postencephalitic parkinsonism, and symptomatic parkinsonism; carbon monoxide and manganese intoxication—* **Adults:** 3 to 6 tablets of 25 mg carbidopa/250 mg levodopa daily given in divided doses. Do not exceed 8 tablets of 25 mg carbidopa/250 mg levodopa a day. Optimum daily dosage must be determined by careful titration for each patient.	**Blood:** hemolytic anemia. **CNS:** *choreiform, dystonic, dyskinetic movements; involuntary grimacing, head movements, myoclonic body jerks, ataxia,* tremors, muscle twitching; bradykinetic episodes; psychiatric disturbances, memory loss, nervousness, anxiety, disturbing dreams, euphoria, malaise, fatigue; severe depression, suicidal tendencies, dementia, delirium, hallucinations (may necessitate reduction or withdrawal of drug). **CV:** *orthostatic hypotension,* cardiac irregularities, flushing, hypertension, phlebitis. **EENT:** blepharospasm, blurred vision, diplopia, mydriasis or miosis, widening of palpebral fissures, activation of latent Horner's syndrome, oculogyric crises, nasal discharge. **GI:** nausea, vomiting, anorexia, weight loss may occur at start of therapy; constipation; flatulence; diarrhea; epigastric pain; hiccups; sialorrhea; dry mouth; bitter taste.

INTERACTIONS	NURSING CONSIDERATIONS
together cautiously.	and acromegaly; repeat blood tests, liver and kidney function studies periodically. • Advise patient and family that multivitamin preparations, fortified cereals, and certain over-the-counter medications may contain pyridoxine (vitamin B_6), which can reverse the effects of levodopa. • If therapy is interrupted for long period, drug should be adjusted gradually to previous level. • Therapeutic response usually occurs following each dose and disappears within 5 hours but varies considerably. • Patient who must undergo surgery should continue levodopa as long as oral intake is permitted, generally 6 to 24 hours before surgery. Drug should be resumed as soon as patient is able to take oral medication. • Protect from heat, light, moisture. If preparation darkens, it has lost potency and should be discarded. • Coombs' test occasionally becomes positive during extended use. Expect uric acid elevations with colorimetric method, but not with uricase method. • Alkaline phosphatase, SGOT, SGPT, LDH, bilirubin, BUN, and PBI show transient elevations in patients receiving levodopa; WBC, hemoglobin, and hematocrit show occasional reduction. • Combination of levodopa-carbidopa usually reduces amount of levodopa needed by 75%, thereby reducing incidence of side effects. • Pills may be crushed and mixed with applesauce or baby food fruits for patients who have difficulty swallowing pills. • Warn patient and family not to increase drug dose without the doctor's orders (they may be tempted to do this as disease symptoms of parkinsonism progress). Daily dose should not exceed 8 g.
Papaverine, diazepam, clonidine, phenothiazines: may antagonize antiparkinson actions. Use together cautiously.	• Contraindicated in narrow-angle glaucoma, melanoma, or undiagnosed skin lesions. Use cautiously in cardiovascular, renal, hepatic, pulmonary disorders; in history of peptic ulcer, psychiatric illness, myocardial infarction with residual arrhythmias; and in bronchial asthma, emphysema, and endocrine disease. • Carefully monitor patients also receiving antihypertensive medication, hypoglycemic agents. Discontinue MAO inhibitors at least 2 weeks before therapy is begun. • Dosage is adjusted according to patient's response and tolerance to drug. Therapeutic and adverse reactions occur more rapidly with levodopa-carbidopa than with levodopa alone. Observe and monitor vital signs, especially while dosage is being adjusted; report significant changes. • Instruct patient to report adverse reactions and therapeutic effects. • Warn patient of possible dizziness and orthostatic hypotension, especially at start of therapy. Patient should change position slowly and dangle legs before getting out of bed. Elastic stockings may control this side effect in some patients. • Muscle twitching and blepharospasm (twitching of eyelids) may be an early sign of drug overdosage; report immediately. • Patients on long-term therapy should be tested regularly for diabetes and acromegaly; blood tests, liver and kidney function studies should be repeated periodically. • If patient is being treated with levodopa, discontinue at least 8 hours before starting levodopa-carbidopa. • This combination drug usually reduces the amount of levodopa needed by 75%, thereby reducing the incidence of side effects. • Pyridoxine (vitamin B_6) does not reverse the beneficial effects of Sinemet. Multivitamins can be taken without fear of losing control of

(continued on following page)

NAME	INDICATIONS & DOSAGE	SIDE EFFECTS
levodopa-carbidopa *(continued)*		**GU:** urinary frequency, retention, incontinence; darkened urine; excessive and inappropriate sexual behavior; priapism. **Hepatic:** hepatotoxicity. **Other:** dark perspiration, hyperventilation.
methoxsalen Oxsoralen♦	*To induce repigmentation in vitiligo—* **Adults, and children over 12 years:** 20 mg P.O. daily, 2 to 4 hours before carefully timed exposure to ultraviolet light.	**CNS:** nervousness, insomnia, depression. **GI:** *discomfort, nausea, diarrhea.* **Skin:** edema, erythema, painful blistering, burning, peeling.
pralidoxime chloride Protopam♦	*Antidote for organophosphate poisoning—* **Adults:** I.V. infusion of 1 to 2 g in 100 ml of saline solution over 15 to 30 minutes. If pulmonary edema is present, give drug by slow I.V. push over 5 minutes. Repeat in 1 hour if muscle weakness persists. Additional doses may be given cautiously. I.M. or S.C. injection can be used if I.V. is not feasible; or 1 to 3 g P.O. q 5 hours. **Children:** 20 to 40 mg/kg I.V. *To treat cholinergic crisis in myasthenia gravis—* **Adults:** 1 to 2 g I.V., followed by increments of 250 mg I.V. q 5 minutes.	**CNS:** dizziness, headache, drowsiness, excitement, and manic behavior following recovery of consciousness. **CV:** tachycardia. **EENT:** blurred vision, diplopia, impaired accommodation, laryngospasm. **GI:** nausea. **Other:** muscular weakness, muscle rigidity, hyperventilation.

INTERACTIONS	NURSING CONSIDERATIONS
	disease symptoms associated with parkinsonism. • If therapy is interrupted temporarily, the usual daily dosage may be given as soon as patient resumes oral medication. • Available as tablets with carbidopa-levodopa in a 1 to 10 ratio (Sinemet 10/100 and Sinemet 25/250); also in a 1 to 4 ratio (Sinemet 25/100). • Sinemet 25/100 may reduce many side effects seen with 1 to 10 ratio strengths. • Carbidopa (Lodosyn) as a single agent is available from Merck Sharp & Dohme upon doctor's request. • Warn patient and family not to increase dose without doctor's order.
Photosensitizing agents: do not use together. May increase toxicity.	• Contraindicated in hepatic insufficiency, porphyria, acute lupus erythematosus, hydromorphic and polymorphic light eruptions. Use with caution in familial history of sunlight allergy, GI diseases, or chronic infection. • Regulate therapy carefully. Overdosage or overexposure to light can cause serious burning or blistering. • Drug should be taken orally with meals or milk. • During light exposure treatments, protect eyes and lips. • Monthly liver function tests should be done on patients with vitiligo (especially at beginning of therapy).
None significant.	• Contraindicated in poisoning with Sevin, a carbamate insecticide, since it increases drug's toxicity. Use with extreme caution in renal insufficiency or myasthenia gravis (overdosage may precipitate myasthenic crisis); also in patients with history of asthma or peptic ulcer. • Use in hospitalized patients only; have respiratory and other supportive measures available. Obtain accurate medical history and chronology of poisoning if possible. Give drug as soon as possible after poisoning. • I.V. preparation should be given slowly, as dilute solution. • Initial measures should include removal of secretions, maintenance of patent airway, and artificial ventilation if needed. • Drug relieves paralysis of respiratory muscles but is less effective in relieving depression of respiratory center. • Atropine along with pralidoxime should be given I.V., 2 to 4 mg, if cyanosis is not present. If cyanosis is present, atropine should be given I.M. Give atropine every 5 to 10 minutes until signs of atropine toxicity appear (flushing, tachycardia, dry mouth, blurred vision, excitement, delirium, hallucinations); maintain atropinization for at least 48 hours. • Dilute with sterile water without preservatives. • Not effective against poisoning due to phosphorus, inorganic phosphates, or organophosphates with no anticholinesterase activity. • Difficult to distinguish toxic effects produced by atropine, or organophosphate compounds, from pralidoxime. Observe patient for 48 to 72 hours if poison ingested. Delayed absorption may occur from lower bowel. • Caution patients who are being treated for organophosphate poisoning to avoid contact with insecticides for several weeks after treatment with this drug. • Patients with myasthenia gravis treated for overdose of cholinergic drugs should be observed closely for signs of rapid weakening. These patients can pass quickly from a cholinergic crisis to a myasthenic crisis and require more cholinergic drugs to treat the myasthenia. Keep edrophonium (Tensilon) available in such situations for establishing differential diagnosis.

NAME	INDICATIONS & DOSAGE	SIDE EFFECTS
ritodrine hydrochloride Yutopar	*Management of preterm labor—* **Intravenous therapy:** dilute 150 mg (3 ampuls) in 500 ml fluid yielding a final concentration of 0.3 mg/ml. Usual initial dose is 0.1 mg/minute, to be gradually increased according to the results by 0.05 mg/minute q 10 minutes until desired result obtained. Effective dosage range usually lies between 0.15 and 0.35 mg/minute. **Oral maintenance:** 1 tablet (10 mg) may be given approximately 30 minutes before termination of intravenous therapy. Usual dosage for first 24 hours of oral maintenance is 10 mg q 2 hours. Thereafter, usual dose is 10 to 20 mg q 4 to 6 hours. Total daily dose should not exceed 120 mg.	Intravenous— **CNS:** nervousness, anxiety, headache. **CV:** *dose-related alterations in blood pressure, palpitations,* EKG changes. **GI:** nausea, vomiting. **Other:** erythema. Oral— **CNS:** tremor. **CV:** palpitations. **GI:** nausea, vomiting. **Skin:** rash.

♦ Available in U.S. and Canada. ♦♦ Available in Canada only. All other products (no symbol) available in U.S. only. Italicized side effects are common or life-threatening.

INTERACTIONS	NURSING CONSIDERATIONS
Corticosteroids: may produce pulmonary edema in mother. When these drugs are used concomitantly, monitor closely.	• Contraindicated before 20th week of pregnancy. • Contraindicated in the following conditions: antepartum hemorrhage, eclampsia, intrauterine fetal death, chorioamnionitis, maternal cardiac disease, pulmonary hypertension, maternal hyperthyroidism, uncontrolled maternal diabetes mellitus. • Because cardiovascular responses are common and more pronounced during intravenous administration, cardiovascular effects, including maternal pulse rate and blood pressure and fetal heart rate, should be closely monitored. • Monitor amount of fluids administered intravenously, to avoid circulatory overload. • Ritodrine decreases intensity and frequency of uterine contractions. • Don't use intravenous ritodrine if solution is discolored or contains a precipitate.

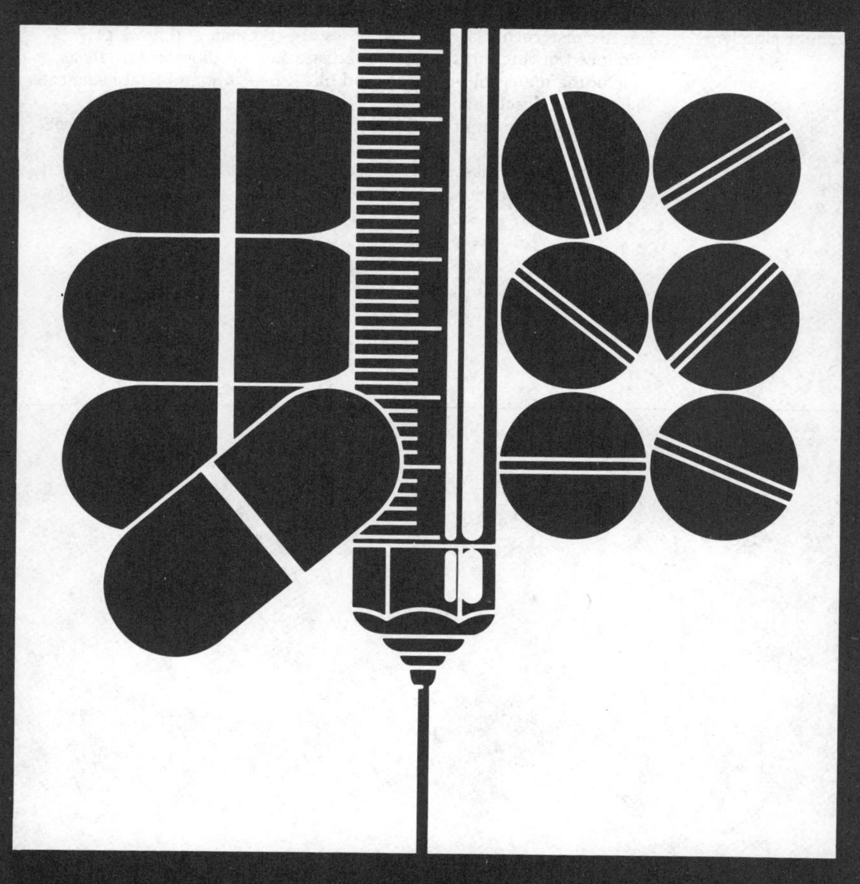

XVII Appendices and Index

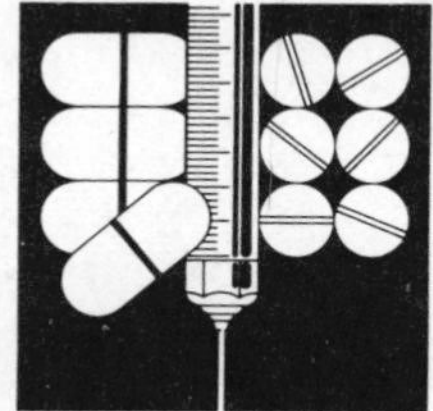

New drugs

NAME	INDICATIONS & DOSAGE	SIDE EFFECTS
albuterol Proventil, Ventolin (See chapter 39 for information about other adrenergics.)	*Relief of bronchospasm in patients with reversible obstructive airway disease—* **Adults, and children 12 years or older:** 1 to 2 inhalations q 4 to 6 hours. More frequent administration or a greater number of inhalations is not recommended. Not recommended for children under age 12.	**CNS:** *tremor, nervousness,* dizziness, insomnia. **CV:** tachycardia, palpitations, hypertension. **EENT:** drying and irritation of nose and throat. **GI:** heartburn, nausea, vomiting.
alprazolam Xanax Controlled Substance Schedule IV (See chapter 32 for information about other tranquilizers.)	*Anxiety and tension—* **Adults:** Usual starting dose is 0.25 to 0.5 mg t.i.d. Maximum total daily dosage is 4 mg in divided doses. In elderly or debilitated patients, usual starting dose is 0.25 mg b.i.d. or t.i.d.	**CNS:** *drowsiness, lightheadedness,* headache, confusion. **CV:** transient hypotension. **EENT:** dry mouth. **GI:** nausea, vomiting, discomfort.
alprostadil Prostin VR Pediatric	*Palliative therapy for temporary maintenance of patency of ductus arteriosus until surgery can be performed—* **Infants:** 0.1 mcg/kg/minute by I.V. infusion. When therapeutic response is achieved, reduce infusion rate to give lowest dosage that will maintain response. Maximum dosage is 0.4 mcg/kg/minute. Alternatively, administer through umbilical artery catheter placed at ductal opening.	**Blood:** disseminated intravascular coagulation. **CNS:** seizures. **CV:** *flushing,* bradycardia, hypotension, tachycardia. **GI:** diarrhea. **Other:** *apnea, fever, sepsis.*

♦ Available in U.S. and Canada. ♦♦ Available in Canada only. All other products (no symbol) available in U.S. only. Italicized side effects are common or life-threatening.

INTERACTIONS	NURSING CONSIDERATIONS
Propranolol and other beta blockers: blocked effect of albuterol and vice versa. Monitor patient carefully if used together.	• Use cautiously in patients with cardiovascular disorders, including coronary insufficiency and hypertension; in patients with hyperthyroidism or diabetes mellitus; and in patients who are unusually responsive to adrenergics. • Warn patient about the possibility of paradoxical bronchospasm. If this occurs, the drug should be discontinued immediately. • Albuterol reportedly produces less cardiac stimulation than other sympathomimetics, especially isoproterenol. • Albuterol is also known by the generic name of salbutamol. • Teach patient how to administer metered dose correctly. Have him shake container; exhale through nose; administer aerosol while inhaling deeply on mouthpiece of inhaler; hold breath for a few seconds, then exhale slowly. Tell him to allow 2 minutes between inhalations. • Store drug in light-resistant container.
Cimetidine: possible increased sedation. Monitor patient carefully if used together.	• Contraindicated in acute narrow-angle glaucoma, psychosis, and anxiety-free psychiatric disorders. • Reduce dosage in elderly or debilitated patients. • Do not withdraw drug abruptly. Abuse or addiction is possible. Withdrawal symptoms may occur. • Warn patient not to combine drug with alcohol or other depressants, and also to avoid activities that require alertness and psychomotor coordination until response to drug is determined. • Caution patient against giving medication to others. • Drug should not be prescribed for everyday stress. • Drug is not for long-term use (more than 4 months). • Warn patient not to continue drug without doctor's approval. • Alprazolam is the first of a new type of benzodiazepine, known as a triazolo-benzodiazepine. It's more rapidly metabolized and excreted than most of the other drugs in the benzodiazepine class and has a lower incidence of lethargy than other drugs of this class.
None reported.	• Contraindicated in neonatal respiratory distress syndrome. • Because drug inhibits platelet aggregation, use cautiously in neonates with bleeding tendencies. • Monitor arterial pressure by umbilical artery catheter, auscultation, or Doppler transducer. Slow rate of infusion if arterial pressure falls significantly. • In infants with restricted pulmonary bloodflow, measure drug's effectiveness by monitoring blood oxygenation. In infants with restricted systemic bloodflow, measure drug's effectiveness by monitoring systemic blood pressure and blood pH. • Drug must be diluted before being administered. Fresh solution must be prepared daily. Discard any solution more than 24 hours old. • Apnea and bradycardia may reflect drug overdose. If the signs occur, stop infusion immediately.

NAME	INDICATIONS & DOSAGE	SIDE EFFECTS
amiloride hydrochloride Midamor (See chapter 63 for information about other diuretics.)	*Hypertension; or edema associated with congestive heart failure, usually in patients who are also taking thiazide or other potassium-wasting diuretics*— **Adults:** Usual dosage is 5 mg P.O. daily. Dosage may be increased to 10 mg daily, if necessary. As much as 20 mg daily can be given.	**CNS:** *headache,* weakness, dizziness. **CV:** orthostatic hypotension. **GI:** *nausea, anorexia, diarrhea, vomiting,* abdominal pain, constipation. **GU:** *impotence.* **Metabolic:** *hyperkalemia.*
aminoglutethimide Cytadren (See chapter 75 for information about other antineoplastics that alter hormonal balance.)	*Suppression of adrenal function in Cushing's syndrome and adrenal cancer*— **Adults:** 250 mg P.O. q.i.d. at 6-hour intervals. Dosage may be increased in increments of 250 mg daily every 1 to 2 weeks to a maximum total daily dose of 2 g.	**Blood:** transient leukopenia, *severe pancytopenia.* **CNS:** *drowsiness,* headache, dizziness. **CV:** hypotension, tachycardia. **Endocrine:** adrenal insufficiency, masculinization, hirsutism. **GI:** *nausea, anorexia.* **Skin:** *morbilliform skin rash,* pruritus, urticaria. **Other:** fever, myalgia.
atenolol Tenormin (See chapter 22 for information about other antihypertensives.)	*Treatment of hypertension*— **Adults:** initially, 50 mg P.O. daily single dose. Dosage may be increased to 100 mg once daily after 7 to 14 days. Dosages greater than 100 mg are unlikely to produce further benefit.	**CNS:** *fatigue, lethargy,* vivid dreams, hallucinations. **CV:** *bradycardia, hypotension, congestive heart failure,* peripheral vascular disease. **GI:** nausea, vomiting, diarrhea. **Metabolic:** hypoglycemia without tachycardia. **Skin:** rash. **Other:** fever.

♦ Available in U.S. and Canada. ♦♦ Available in Canada only. All other products (no symbol) available in U.S. only. Italicized side effects are common or life-threatening.

INTERACTIONS	NURSING CONSIDERATIONS
None significant.	• Contraindicated with elevated serum potassium levels (greater than 5.5 mEq/liter). Don't administer to patients receiving other potassium-sparing diuretics, such as spironolactone and triamterene. Also contraindicated in anuria. • Use cautiously in patients with renal impairment, because potassium retention is increased. • Risk of hyperkalemia is greater when a potassium-wasting drug is not taken concurrently. When amiloride is taken this way, be sure to monitor daily potassium levels. • Discontinue immediately if potassium level exceeds 6.5 mEq/liter. • Warn patient to avoid excessive ingestion of potassium-rich foods. • Administer amiloride with or after meals to prevent nausea.
None significant.	• May cause adrenal hypofunction, especially under stressful conditions such as surgery, trauma, or acute illness. Patients may need hydrocortisone and mineralocorticoid supplements in these situations. Monitor patients carefully. • Monitor blood pressure frequently. Advise patient to stand up slowly in order to minimize orthostatic hypotension. • May decrease thyroid hormone production. Monitor thyroid function studies. • Perform baseline hematologic studies and monitor CBC periodically. • Warn patient that drug can cause drowsiness and dizziness. Advise him to avoid activities that require alertness and good psychomotor coordination until response to drug has been determined. • Tell patient to report if skin rash persists for more than 5 to 8 days. Reassure patient that drowsiness, nausea, and loss of appetite will diminish within 2 weeks after start of aminoglutethimide therapy. Tell patient to notify doctor if these symptoms persist. • Also used to produce medical adrenalectomy in patients with metastatic breast cancer.
Insulin, hypoglycemic drugs (oral): can alter dosage requirements in previously stabilized diabetics. Observe patient carefully. *Cardiac glycosides:* excessive bradycardia and increased depressant effect on myocardium. Use together cautiously.	• Contraindicated in sinus bradycardia and greater than first degree conduction block, and cardiogenic shock. • Use cautiously in patients with cardiac failure. • Similar to metoprolol, atenolol is a cardioselective beta blocker. Atenolol can be used in patients with bronchospastic diseases such as asthma and emphysema, but should be used cautiously–especially with 100-mg dose. • Dosage should be reduced if patient has renal insufficiency. • Once-a-day dosage encourages patient compliance. Advise patient to take the drug at a regular time every day. Drug can be dispensed in a 28-day calendar pack. • Always check patient's apical pulse before giving this drug; if slower than 60 beats/minute, hold drug and call doctor. • Monitor blood pressure frequently. If patient develops severe hypotension, administer a vasopressor. • Don't discontinue abruptly; can exacerbate angina and myocardial infarction. • Teach patient about his disease and therapy. Explain the importance of taking this drug, even when he's feeling well. Warn patient not to discontinue drug suddenly, but to call doctor if unpleasant side effects develop. • This drug masks common signs of shock and hypoglycemia.

NAME	INDICATIONS & DOSAGE	SIDE EFFECTS
bacampicillin Spectrobid (See chapter 14 for information about other penicillins.)	*Upper and lower respiratory tract infections due to streptococci, pneumococci, staphylococci, and* Hemophilus influenzae; *urinary tract infections due to* Escherichia coli, Proteus mirabilis, *and* Streptococcus faecalis; *skin infections due to streptococci and susceptible staphylococci—* **Adults, and children weighing more than 25 kg:** 400 to 800 mg P.O. q 12 hours. *Gonorrhea—* Usual dosage is 1.6 g plus 1 g probenecid given as a single dose. Not recommended for children under 25 kg.	**Blood:** anemia, thrombocytopenia, thrombocytopenic purpura, eosinophilia, leukopenia. **GI:** *nausea,* vomiting, *diarrhea,* glossitis, stomatitis. **Other:** *hypersensitivity (erythematous maculopapular rash, urticaria, anaphylaxis),* overgrowth of nonsusceptible organisms.
beclomethasone dipropionate Beconase Nasal Inhaler Vancenase Nasal Inhaler (See chapter 86 for information about other oral and nasal agents.)	*Relief of symptoms of seasonal or perennial rhinitis—* **Adults, and children 12 years or older:** Usual dosage is one spray (42 mcg) in each nostril 2 to 4 times daily (total dosage 168 to 336 mcg daily). Most patients require one spray in each nostril t.i.d. (252 mcg daily). Not recommended for children under age 12.	**CNS:** headache. **EENT:** *mild transient nasal burning and stinging,* nasal congestion, sneezing, epistaxis, watery eyes. **GI:** nausea and vomiting. **Other:** development of local fungal infections.
calcifediol Calderol (See chapter 62 for information about other parathyroid and parathyroid-like agents.)	*Treatment and management of metabolic bone disease associated with chronic renal failure—* **Adults:** initially, 300 to 350 mcg P.O. weekly, given on a daily or alternate-day schedule. Dosage may be increased at 4-week intervals. Optimal dose must be carefully determined for each patient.	Vitamin D intoxication associated with hypercalcemia: **CNS:** headache, somnolence. **EENT:** conjunctivitis, photophobia, rhinorrhea. **GI:** nausea, vomiting, constipation, metallic taste, dry mouth. **GU:** polyuria. **Other:** weakness, bone and muscle pain.

♦ Available in U.S. and Canada. ♦♦ Available in Canada only. All other products (no symbol) available in U.S. only. Italicized side effects are common or life-threatening.

INTERACTIONS	NURSING CONSIDERATIONS
Probenecid: increased blood levels of bacampicillin or other penicillins. Probenecid is often used for this purpose. *Chloramphenicol, erythromycin, tetracyclines:* antibiotic antagonism. Administer penicillins at least 1 hour before bacteriostatic antibiotics.	• Use cautiously in patients with other drug allergies, especially to cephalosporins (possible cross-allergenicity). • Obtain cultures for sensitivity tests before first dose. Unnecessary to wait for results before beginning therapy. • Before giving bacampicillin or any other penicillin, ask patient if he's had any previous allergic reactions to the drug. However, a negative history of penicillin allergy is no guarantee against a future allergic reaction. • Bacampicillin is especially formulated to produce high blood levels of antibiotic when administered twice daily. • Diarrhea may occur less frequently with bacampicillin than with ampicillin. • Tell patient to take medication even after he feels better until the entire quantity prescribed is taken. • Tell patient to call the doctor if rash, fever, or chills develop. A rash is the most common allergic reaction. • With prolonged therapy, bacterial or fungal superinfection may occur, especially in the elderly or the debilitated, and in those with low resistance to infection due to immunosuppressors or irradiation. Close observation is essential. • Check expiration date. Warn patient against using leftover penicillin products for a new illness or sharing penicillin with family and friends. • Unlike ampicillin, bacampicillin may be taken with meals without fear of diminished drug absorption. Give with food to prevent GI distress.
None reported.	• Use cautiously, if at all, in patients with active or quiescent respiratory tract tubercular infections, or in untreated fungal, bacterial, or systemic viral or ocular herpes simplex infections. • Use cautiously in patients who have recently had nasal septal ulcers or nasal surgery or trauma. • Recommended dosages will not suppress hypothalamic-pituitary-adrenal (HPA) function. Warn patient not to exceed this dosage. • Indicated when conventional treatment (antihistamines, decongestants) fails. • Beclomethasone is not effective for active exacerbations. Nasal decongestants or oral antihistamines may be needed instead. • Advise patient to use drug regularly, as prescribed; its effectiveness depends on regular use. • Explain that the therapeutic effects of this corticosteroid, unlike those of decongestants, are not immediate. Most patients achieve benefit within a few days, but some may need 2 to 3 weeks for maximum benefit. • If symptoms don't improve within 3 weeks or if nasal irritation persists, patient should stop drug and notify doctor.
Cholestyramine: may impair absorption of calcifediol. Monitor calcium levels.	• Contraindicated in hypercalcemia or vitamin D toxicity. Withhold all preparations containing vitamin D in patients taking calcifediol. Use cautiously in patients on digitalis because hypercalcemia may precipitate cardiac arrhythmias. • Monitor serum calcium; serum calcium times serum phosphate should not exceed 70. During titration, serum calcium levels should be determined at least weekly. If hypercalcemia occurs, calcifediol should be discontinued but resumed after serum calcium returns to normal. • Advise patient to adhere to diet and calcium supplementation, and

(continued on following page)

NAME	INDICATIONS & DOSAGE	SIDE EFFECTS
calcifediol *(continued)*		
calcium polycarbophil Mitrolan (See chapter 47 for information about other antidiarrheals.)	*Diarrhea associated with irritable bowel syndrome, as well as acute nonspecific diarrhea (tablets must be chewed before swallowing)—* **Adults:** 1 g P.O. q.i.d. as required. Maximum 6 g in 24-hour period. **Children 6 to 12 years:** 500 mg P.O. t.i.d. as required. Maximum 3 g in 24-hour period. **Children 3 to 6 years:** 500 mg P.O. b.i.d. as required. Maximum 1.5 g in 24-hour period. *Constipation (tablets must be chewed before swallowing)— (See chapter 48 for information about other laxatives.)* **Adults:** 1 g P.O. q.i.d. as required. Maximum 6 g in 24-hour period. **Children 6 to 12 years:** 500 mg P.O. t.i.d. as required. Maximum 3 g in 24-hour period. **Children 3 to 6 years:** 500 mg P.O. b.i.d. as required. Maximum 1.5 g in 24-hour period.	**GI:** abdominal fullness and increased flatus, intestinal obstruction. **Other:** laxative dependence in long-term or excessive use.
cefotaxime Claforan (See chapter 15 for information about other cephalosporins.)	*Treatment of serious infections of the lower respiratory and urinary tracts, gynecological infections, bacteremia, septicemia, and skin infections. Among susceptible microorganisms are streptococci, including* Streptococcus pneumoniae *and* Staphylococcus pyogenes; Staphylococcus aureus *(penicillinase- and nonpenicillinase-producing);* Staphylococcus epidermidis; Escherichia coli; Klebsiella *species;* Hemophilus influenzae; Enterobacter *species;* Proteus *species; and* Peptostreptococcus *species—* **Adults:** usual dose is 1 g I.V. or I.M. q 6 to 8 hours. Up to 12 g daily can be administered in life-threatening infections.	**Blood:** transient neutropenia, eosinophilia, hemolytic anemia. **CNS:** headache, malaise, paresthesias, dizziness. **GI:** nausea, anorexia, vomiting, diarrhea, glossitis, dyspepsia, abdominal cramps, tenesmus, anal pruritus, oral candidiasis (thrush). **GU:** nephrotoxicity, genital pruritus and moniliasis. **Skin:** *maculopapular and erythematous rashes, urticaria.* **Local:** *at injection site–pain, induration, sterile abscesses, temperature elevation, tissue slough; phlebitis and thrombophlebitis with I.V. injection.* **Other:** hypersensitivity, dyspnea.

♦ Available in U.S. and Canada. ♦♦ Available in Canada only. All other products (no symbol) available in U.S. only. Italicized side effects are common or life-threatening.

INTERACTIONS	NURSING CONSIDERATIONS
	avoid nonprescription drugs. • Patient should receive adequate daily intake of calcium—1,000 mg RDA. • Most patients respond to doses between 50 and 100 mcg daily or between 100 and 200 mcg on alternate days.
None significant.	• Contraindicated in patients with signs of GI obstruction. • Don't use for more than 2 days in a row. • Don't use in place of specific therapy for underlying cause of the diarrhea. • Advise patient to chew tablets thoroughly before swallowing. When used as an antidiarrheal, tell patient *not* to drink a glass of water afterward. When used for constipation, tell patient to drink a full glass of water with each dose. • For episodes of severe diarrhea, the dose may be repeated every half hour, but maximum daily dosage should not be exceeded. • Rectal bleeding or failure to respond to therapy may indicate need for surgery. • Use for short-term treatment. • Before giving for constipation, determine if patient has adequate fluid intake, sufficient exercise, and proper diet. Tell him that dietary sources of bulk include bran and other cereals, fresh fruit, and vegetables. • Not absorbed systemically; nontoxic. • Bulk laxative; increases bulk and water content of stool.
Probenecid: may inhibit excretion and increase blood levels of cefotaxime. Use together cautiously.	• Contraindicated in hypersensitivity to other cephalosporins. Use cautiously in patients with impaired renal function and in those with history of sensitivity to penicillin. Ask patient if he's had any reaction to previous cephalosporin or penicillin therapy before administering first dose. • Prolonged use may result in overgrowth of nonsusceptible organisms. Careful observation of patient for superinfection is essential. • Obtain cultures for sensitivity tests before therapy, but therapy may begin pending results of cultures and sensitivity tests. • Cefotaxime is the first of the so-called third-generation cephalosporins. It's said to have increased antibacterial activity against gram-negative microorganisms. • Some doctors may prescribe cefotaxime in clinical situations in which they formerly prescribed aminoglycosides. However, this drug is not effective against infections caused by *Pseudomonas* organisms. • For I.V. use, reconstitute with at least 10 ml sterile water for injection. Reconstituted solutions may be further diluted with sterile water for injection; 0.9% sodium chloride; 5% or 10% dextrose; 5% dextrose and 0.9% sodium chloride; 5% dextrose and 0.45% sodium chloride injection; 5% dextrose and 0.2% sodium chloride injection and lactated Ringer's solution.

(continued on following page)

NAME	INDICATIONS & DOSAGE	SIDE EFFECTS
cefotaxime *(continued)*	Total daily dosage is same for I.M. or I.V. administration and depends on susceptibility of organism and severity of infection. In patients with impaired renal function, doses or frequency of administration must be modified according to degree of renal impairment, severity of infection, susceptibility of organism, and blood levels of drug. Should be injected deep I.M. into a large muscle mass, such as gluteus or lateral aspect of thigh.	
cinoxacin Cinobac (See chapter 18 for information about other urinary tract antiseptics.)	*Treatment of initial and recurrent urinary tract infections caused by susceptible strains of* Escherichia coli, Klebsiella, Enterobacter, Proteus mirabilis, Proteus vulgaris, *and* Proteus morgani, Serratia, *and* Citrobacter— **Adults, and children 12 years or older:** 1 g daily, in two to four divided doses for 7 to 14 days. Not recommended for children under age 12.	**CNS:** *dizziness, headache,* drowsiness, insomnia, convulsions. **EENT:** sensitivity to light. **GI:** *nausea, vomiting, abdominal pain,* diarrhea. **Skin:** rash, urticaria, pruritus.
clocortolone pivalate Cloderm (See chapter 89 for information about other topical corticosteroids.)	*Inflammation of corticosteroid-responsive dermatoses, such as atopic dermatitis, contact dermatitis, seborrheic dermatitis*— **Adults and children:** apply cream sparingly to affected areas t.i.d. and rub in gently.	**Skin:** burning, itching, irritation, dryness, folliculitis, hypopigmentation, striae, acneiform eruptions, perioral dermatitis, hypertrichosis, allergic contact dermatitis. *With occlusive dressings: secondary infection, maceration, atrophy, striae, miliaria.*

INTERACTIONS	NURSING CONSIDERATIONS
Probenecid: may decrease urinary levels of cinoxacin by inhibiting renal tubular secretion. Monitor for increased toxicity and reduced antibacterial effectiveness.	• Contraindicated in patients who are hypersensitive to nalidixic acid. Use cautiously in patients with impaired renal and hepatic function. • Not effective against *Pseudomonas,* enterococci, or staphylococci. • Obtain clean-catch urine specimen for culture and sensitivity before starting therapy and repeat p.r.n. • High urine levels permit twice-daily dosing. • Report CNS side effects to doctor immediately. They indicate serious toxicity and usually mean that administration of drug should be stopped. • Cinoxacin should be taken with meals to help decrease GI side effects. • Resistant bacteria may emerge with this drug. • Warn patient about photophobic effects of drug, and advise him to avoid very bright sunlight.
None significant.	• Use cautiously in viral skin diseases, such as varicella, vaccinia, herpes simplex; fungal infections; skin tuberculosis; impaired circulation. • Avoid application in or near eyes. • Systemic absorption especially likely with occlusive dressings, prolonged treatment, or extensive body surface treatment. • Stop drug and notify doctor if patient develops signs of systemic absorption or hypersensitivity, skin irritation or ulceration, or infection. (If antifungals or antibiotics are being used with corticosteroids and infection does not respond immediately, corticosteroids should be stopped until infection is controlled.) • Before applying, gently wash skin. To prevent damage to skin, rub in medication gently, leaving a thin coat. When treating hairy sites, part hair and apply direct to lesion. • Occlusive dressing: apply cream heavily, then cover with a thin, pliable, nonflammable plastic film; seal to adjacent normal skin with hypoallergenic tape. Minimize adverse reactions by using occlusive dressing intermittently. • For patient with eczematous dermatitis who may develop irritation with adhesive material, hold dressing in place with gauze, elastic bandages, or stockings. • Notify doctor and remove occlusive dressing if body temperature rises. • Occlusive dressings are generally not used in presence of infections or with weeping or exudative lesions.

(continued on following page)

NAME	INDICATIONS & DOSAGE	SIDE EFFECTS
clocortolone pivalate *(continued)*		
flunisolide Nasalide Nasal Solution (See chapter 86 for information about other oral and nasal agents.)	*Relief of symptoms of seasonal or perennial rhinitis—* **Adults:** Starting dose is 2 sprays (50 mcg) in each nostril b.i.d. Total daily dose is 200 mcg. If necessary, dose may be increased to 2 sprays in each nostril t.i.d. Maximum total daily dosage is 8 sprays in each nostril (400 mcg daily). **Children 6 to 14 years:** Starting dose is 1 spray (25 mcg) in each nostril t.i.d. or 2 sprays (50 mcg) in each nostril b.i.d. Total daily dose is 150 to 200 mcg. Maximum total daily dose is 4 sprays in each nostril (200 mcg daily). Not recommended for children under age 6.	**CNS:** headache. **EENT:** *mild, transient nasal burning and stinging,* nasal congestion, sneezing, epistaxis, watery eyes. **GI:** nausea, vomiting. **Other:** development of local fungal infections.
halazepam Paxipam Controlled Substance Schedule IV (See chapter 32 for information about other tranquilizers.)	*Relief of anxiety and tension—* **Adults:** Usual dose is 20 to 40 mg P.O. t.i.d. or q.i.d. Optimal daily dosage is generally 80 to 160 mg. Daily doses up to 600 mg have been given. In elderly or debilitated patients, initial dosage is 20 mg once or twice daily.	**CNS:** *drowsiness, lethargy, hangover,* fainting. **CV:** transient hypotension. **EENT:** dry mouth. **GI:** nausea and vomiting, discomfort.
isosorbide Ismotic (See chapter 84 for information about other miscellaneous ophthalmics.)	*Short-term reduction of intraocular pressure due to glaucoma—* **Adults:** initially, 1.5 g/kg P.O. Usual dosage range is 1 to 3 g/kg P.O.	**CNS:** vertigo, light-headedness, lethargy. **GI:** gastric discomfort, diarrhea, anorexia. **Metabolic:** hypernatremia, hyperosmolality.
ketoconazole Nizoral (See chapter 10 for	*Treatment of systemic candidiasis, chronic mucocandidiasis, oral thrush, candiduria, coccidi-*	**CNS:** headache, nervousness, dizziness. **GI:** *nausea, vomiting,* abdominal

◆ Available in U.S. and Canada. ◆◆ Available in Canada only. All other products (no symbol) available in U.S. only. Italicized side effects are common or life-threatening.

INTERACTIONS	NURSING CONSIDERATIONS
	• Change dressings as ordered by doctor. Inspect skin for infection, striae, and atrophy. Discontinue drug and notify doctor if these occur. • Treatment should be continued for a few days after clearing of lesions to prevent recurrence. • Instruct patient to report signs of drug sensitivity.
None reported.	• Use cautiously, if at all, in patients with active or quiescent respiratory tract tubercular infections or in untreated fungal, bacterial, or systemic viral, or ocular herpes simplex infections. • Use cautiously in patients who have recently had nasal septal ulcers or nasal surgery or trauma. • Recommended dosages will not suppress hypothalamic-pituitary-adrenal (HPA) function. Warn patient not to exceed this dosage. • Indicated when conventional treatment (antihistamines, decongestants) fails. • Flunisolide is not effective for acute exacerbations. Nasal decongestants or oral antihistamines may be needed instead. • Advise patient to use drug regularly, as prescribed; its effectiveness depends on regular use. • Explain that the therapeutic effects of this corticosteroid, unlike those of decongestants, are not immediate. Most patients achieve benefit within a few days, but some may need 2 to 3 weeks for maximum benefit. • If symptoms don't improve within 3 weeks or if nasal irritation persists, patient should stop drug and notify doctor.
Cimetidine: possible increased sedation. Monitor carefully.	• Contraindicated in acute narrow-angle glaucoma, psychosis, and anxiety-free psychiatric disorders. Use with caution in hepatorenal impairment. • Reduce dosage in elderly or debilitated patients. • Do not withdraw drug abruptly. • Abuse and addiction are possible. Withdrawal symptoms may occur. • Warn patient not to combine drug with alcohol or other depressants, and also to avoid activities that require alertness and psychomotor coordination until response to drug is determined. • Caution patient against giving medication to others. • Drug should not be prescribed for everyday stress. • Halazepam is not for long-term use (more than 4 months). • Warn patient not to continue the drug without the doctor's approval.
None significant.	• Contraindicated in anuria due to severe renal disease, severe dehydration, frank or impending acute pulmonary edema, and hemorrhagic glaucoma. • Repetitive doses should be used cautiously in patients with diseases associated with salt retention, such as congestive heart failure. • Pour over cracked ice, and tell patient to sip the medication. This procedure improves palatability. • Especially useful for rapid reduction in intraocular pressure.
Antacids, anticholinergics, cimetidine: decreased absorption of	• Contraindicated in patients with fungal meningitis since ketoconazole penetrates poorly into the cerebrospinal fluid. • Ketoconazole is not effective in patients with achlorhydria. The

(continued on following page)

NAME	INDICATIONS & DOSAGE	SIDE EFFECTS
ketoconazole *(continued)* information about other antifungals.)	*oidomycosis, histoplasmosis, chromomycosis, and paracoccidioidomycosis—* **Adults, and children over 40 kg:** initially, 200 mg P.O. daily single dose. Dosage may be increased to 400 mg once daily in patients who don't respond to lower dosage. **Children (20 to 40 kg):** 100 mg (½ tablet) daily single dose. **Children (less than 20 kg):** 50 mg (¼ tablet) daily single dose.	pain, diarrhea, constipation. **Hepatic:** mild, reversible hepatitis. **Skin:** itching.
meclocycline sulfosalicylate Meclan (See chapter 87 for information about other local anti-infectives.)	*Treatment of acne vulgaris—* **Adults and adolescents:** apply to affected area b.i.d. morning and evening. Less frequent application may be used depending on patient's response.	**Skin:** *stinging and burning on application,* skin irritation, slight yellowing of treated skin (especially in patients with light complexions). Treated skin areas fluoresce under ultraviolet light.
mezlocillin sodium Mezlin (See chapter 14 for information about other penicillins.)	*Systemic infections caused by susceptible strains of gram-positive and especially gram-negative organisms* (Proteus, Pseudomonas aeruginosa)— **Adults:** 200 to 300 mg/kg daily I.V. or I.M. given in 4 to 6 divided doses. Usual dose is 3 g q 4 h or 4 g q 6 h. For very serious infections, up to 24 g daily may be administered. **Children to age 12:** 50 mg/kg q 4 h by I.V. infusion or direct I.V. injection.	**Blood:** *bleeding with high doses,* neutropenia, eosinophilia, leukopenia, *thrombocytopenia.* **CNS:** *convulsions,* neuromuscular irritability. **GI:** nausea, diarrhea. **Local:** pain at injection site, vein irritation, phlebitis. **Metabolic:** *hypokalemia.* **Other:** *hypersensitivity (edema, fever, chills, rash, pruritus, urticaria, anaphylaxis),* overgrowth of nonsusceptible organisms.

INTERACTIONS	NURSING CONSIDERATIONS
ketoconazole. Wait at least 2 hours after ketoconazole dose before administering these drugs.	drug requires acidity for dissolution and absorption. • Instruct patient to dissolve each tablet in 4 ml aqueous solution of 0.2 N hydrochloric acid; and, to avoid contact with teeth, to sip the mixture through a straw (glass or plastic). Tell patient to follow with a glass of water. • Make sure patient understands that treatment should be continued until all clinical and laboratory tests indicate that active fungal infection has subsided. If drug is discontinued too soon, infection will reoccur. Minimum treatment for candidiasis is 7 to 14 days. Minimum treatment for other systemic fungal infections is 6 months. • Ketoconazole represents a major advance since it is the most effective oral antifungal drug available and it produces the least side effects.
None significant.	• Contraindicated in hypersensitivity to any of the components. • Onset of beneficial response usually within 2 weeks of start of treatment. • If condition doesn't improve or worsens, medication should be discontinued and therapy reevaluated. • Prolonged use may result in overgrowth of nonsusceptible organisms. • Patient may continue use of cosmetics. • Yellow-skin staining is generally worse when excessive amounts are applied. • Drug fluoresces under black light.
Gentamicin, tobramycin: chemically incompatible. Don't mix together in I.V. solution. Give 1 hour apart. *Chloramphenicol erythromycin, tetracyclines:* antibiotic antagonism. Give penicillins at least 1 hour before bacteriostatic antibiotics.	• Use cautiously in patients hypersensitive to drugs, especially to cephalosporins (possible cross-hypersensitivity), and those with bleeding tendencies, uremia, hypokalemia. • Obtain cultures for sensitivity tests before starting therapy. Unnecessary to wait for culture and sensitivity results before starting therapy. • Before giving penicillin, ask patient if he's had allergic reactions to this drug. A negative history of penicillin allergy, however, is no guarantee against future allergic reaction. • Dosage should be altered in patients with impaired hepatorenal functions. • Check CBC frequently. Drug may cause thrombocytopenia. • Monitor serum potassium level. • Patient with high serum level of this drug may have convulsions. Take seizure precautions. • When giving I.V., mix with 5% dextrose in water or other suitable I.V. fluids. • Give I.V. intermittently to prevent vein irritation. Change site every 48 hours. • Large doses may cause increased yeast growths. Report symptoms to doctor. • Almost always used with another antibiotic, such as gentamicin. • With prolonged therapy, superinfections may occur, especially in the elderly or debilitated, or those with low resistance to infection due to immunosuppressors or irradiation. Monitor patient closely. • Check drug expiration date. • Compared with similar antibiotics such as carbenicillin and ticarcillin, mezlocillin is less likely to cause hypokalemia. • Drug may be better suited to patients on salt-free diets than car-

(continued on following page)

NAME	INDICATIONS & DOSAGE	SIDE EFFECTS
mezlocillin sodium *(continued)*		
moxalactam disodium Moxam (See chapter 15 for information about other cephalosporins.)	*Treatment of serious infections of lower respiratory and urinary gynecologic infections, bacteremia, septicemia, and skin infections.* *Susceptible microorganisms include* Streptococcus pneumoniae *and* Staphylococcus pyogenes; Staphylococcus aureus *(penicillinase- and nonpenicillinase-producing);* Staphylococcus epidermidis; Escherichia coli; Klebsiella; Hemophilus influenzae; Enterobacter; Proteus; *some* Pseudomonas *species; and* Peptostreptococcus. **Adults:** Usual daily dose is 2 to 6 g I.M. or I.V. administered in divided doses q 8 h for 5 to 10 days, or up to 14 days. Up to 12 g/day may be needed in life-threatening infections or in infections due to less susceptible organisms. **Children:** 50 mg/kg I.M. or I.V. q 6 to 8 hours. **Neonates:** 50 mg/kg I.M. or I.V. q 8 to 12 hours. Total daily dosage is same for I.M. or I.V. administration and depends on susceptibility of organism and severity of infection. In patients with impaired renal function, doses or frequency of administration must be modified according to degree of impairment, severity of infection, susceptibility of organism, and blood levels of drug. Should be injected deep I.M. into a large muscle mass, such as gluteus or lateral aspect of thigh.	**Blood:** transient neutropenia, eosinophilia, hemolytic anemia. **CNS:** headache, malaise, paresthesias, dizziness. **GI:** nausea, anorexia, vomiting, diarrhea, glossitis, dyspepsia, abdominal cramps, tenesmus, pruritus ani, oral candidiasis (thrush). **GU:** nephrotoxicity, genital pruritus, moniliasis. **Skin:** *maculopapular and erythematous rashes, urticaria.* **Local:** *pain at injection site, induration, sterile abscesses, tissue sloughing; phlebitis and thrombophlebitis with I.V. injection.* **Other:** *hypersensitivity,* dyspnea, elevated temperature.
nifedipine Procardia (See chapter 21 for information about other antiarrhythmics.)	*Management of vasospastic (also called Prinzmetals or variant angina) and classic chronic stable angina pectoris—* **Adults:** Starting dose is 10 mg P.O. t.i.d. Usual effective dose range is 10 to 20 mg t.i.d. Some patients may require up to 30 mg q.i.d. Maximum daily dose is 180 mg.	**CNS:** *dizziness, light-headedness, flushing, headache,* weakness, syncope. **CV:** peripheral edema, hypotension, palpitations. **EENT:** nasal congestion. **GI:** *nausea, heartburn,* diarrhea. **Other:** muscle cramps, dyspnea.

INTERACTIONS	NURSING CONSIDERATIONS
	benicillin and ticarcillin (contains 1.85 mEq Na^+/g of mezlocillin). • For treatment of anaphylaxis, see inside front cover.
Ethyl alcohol: may cause a disulfiram-like reaction. Warn patients not to drink alcohol for several days after discontinuing moxalactam. *Probenecid:* may inhibit excretion and increase blood levels of moxalactam. Use together cautiously.	• Contraindicated in hypersensitivity to other cephalosporins. Use cautiously in patients with impaired renal function and in those with history of sensitivity to penicillin. Before administering first dose, ask patient if he's had any reaction to cephalosporin or penicillin therapy. • Prolonged use may result in overgrowth of nonsusceptible organisms. Monitor patient closely for superinfection. • Obtain cultures for sensitivity tests before therapy. Unnecessary to wait for culture and sensitivity results before starting therapy. • Moxalactam is one of the third generation cephalosporins. It's said to have increased antibacterial activity against gram-negative organisms. • Some doctors may prescribe moxalactam in clinical situations in which they formerly prescribed aminoglycosides. However, the drug is not as potent against *Pseudomonas* infections. • For direct intermittent I.V. administration, add 10 ml of sterile water for injection, 5% dextrose injection, or 0.9% NaCl injection/g of moxalactam.
Propranolol (and other beta blockers): may cause heart failure. Use together cautiously.	• Use cautiously in patient with congestive heart failure or hypotension. • Monitor blood pressure regularly, especially of patient who is also taking beta blockers or antihypertensives. • Patient may briefly develop anginal exacerbation when beginning drug therapy or at times of dosage increase. Reassure him that this symptom is temporary. • Although rebound effect hasn't been observed when drug is stopped, dosage should still be reduced slowly under doctor's supervision. • If patient is kept on nitrate therapy while drug dosage is being ti-

(continued on following page)

NAME	INDICATIONS & DOSAGE	SIDE EFFECTS
nifedipine *(continued)*		
pyrethrins Rid, A-200 Pyrinate, Pyrin-Aid, Pyrinyl, Barc, TISIT, Triple X (See chapter 88 for information about other pediculicides.)	*Treatment of infestations of head, body, and pubic (crab) lice and their eggs*— **Adults and children:** apply to hair, scalp, or other infested area until entirely wet. Allow to remain for 10 minutes, but no longer. Wash thoroughly with warm water and soap, or shampoo. Remove dead lice and eggs with fine-toothed comb. Treatment may be repeated, if necessary, but don't exceed 2 applications within 24 hours.	**Skin:** *irritation with repeated use.*
scopolamine Transderm-V (See chapter 49 for information about other antiemetics.)	*Prevention of nausea and vomiting associated with motion sickness*— **Adults:** One Transderm-V system (a circular flat unit) programmed to deliver 0.5 mg of scopolamine over 3 days (72 hours), applied to the skin behind the ear several hours before the antiemetic is required. Not recommended for children.	**CNS:** *drowsiness,* restlessness, disorientation, confusion. **EENT:** *dry mouth,* transient impairment of eye accommodation.
temazepam Controlled Substance Schedule IV Restoril (See chapter 29 for information about other sedatives.)	*Insomnia*— **Adults:** 15 to 30 mg P.O. at bedtime.	**CNS:** *drowsiness, dizziness, lethargy,* disturbed coordination, daytime sedation, confusion. **GI:** anorexia, diarrhea.

◆ Available in U.S. and Canada. ◆◆ Available in Canada only. All other products (no symbol) available in U.S. only. Italicized side effects are common or life-threatening.

INTERACTIONS	NURSING CONSIDERATIONS
	trated, urge him to continue his compliance. Sublingual nitroglycerin, especially, may be taken as needed when anginal symptoms are acute. • Nifedipine is the first oral calcium blocker commercially available.
None significant.	• Contraindicated when skin is raw or inflamed. Notify doctor immediately if skin irritation develops; tell patient to discontinue drug and to wash it off skin. Use cautiously in infants and small children. • Do not apply to open areas or acutely inflamed skin, or to face, eyes, mucous membranes, or urethral meatus. After accidental contact with eyes, flush with water and notify doctor. • Warn parents not to let infants or children suck their fingers after drug application. • Discourage repeated use, which can lead to skin irritation and possible systemic toxicity. • Topical corticosteroids may be needed if dermatitis develops from scratching. • Instruct patient to change and sterilize (boil, launder, dry clean, or apply very hot iron) all clothing and bed linen after drug is washed off. • Products containing pyrethrins are available without prescription. Some authorities consider pyrethrins and gamma benzene hexachloride (Kwell) equally effective for lice infestation.
None significant.	• Use cautiously in patients with glaucoma, pyloric obstruction, or urinary bladder neck obstruction. • Wash and dry hands thoroughly before applying the system on dry skin behind the ear. After removing the system, discard it, then wash both the hands and application site thoroughly. • If the system becomes displaced, remove and replace it with another system on a fresh skin site in the postauricular area. • A patient brochure is available with this product; tell patient to request it from the pharmacist. • Warn patient against driving and other activities that require alertness until response to drug is determined. • Sugarless hard candy may help minimize dry mouth. • Transderm-V is effective if applied 2 to 3 hours before experiencing motion, but more effective if used 12 hours before. Therefore, advise patient to apply system the night before a planned trip. • Transdermal method of administration releases a controlled therapeutic amount of scopolamine.
None significant.	• Use cautiously in patients with impaired hepatic or renal function; in patients with mental depression or suicidal tendencies; and in patients with history of drug abuse. Use caution and low end of dosage range for elderly or debilitated patients. • Prevent hoarding or self-overdosing by patients who are depressed, suicidal, or drug-dependent, or who have a history of drug abuse. Warn against combining with alcohol and against hazardous activity requiring alertness or skill. • Remove cigarettes of bedridden patient receiving drug. • Supervise walking; raise bed rails, especially for elderly patients. • One of the newer benzodiazepine derivatives. • May produce less residual sedative effects (hangover) the next day than flurazepam and diazepam. Relatively short-acting.

NAME	INDICATIONS & DOSAGE	SIDE EFFECTS
timolol maleate Blocadren (See chapter 22 for information about other antihypertensives.)	*Hypertension—* **Adults:** Initial dosage is 10 mg P.O. b.i.d. Usual daily maintenance dosage is 20 to 40 mg. Maximum daily dosage is 60 mg. Drug is used either alone or in combination with diuretics. *Myocardial infarction—* **Adults:** Recommended dosage for long-term prophylaxis in survivors of acute myocardial infarction (MI) is 10 mg P.O. b.i.d.	**CNS:** *fatigue, lethargy,* vivid dreams, hallucinations, dizziness. **CV:** *bradycardia, hypotension, congestive heart failure (CHF),* peripheral vascular disease. **GI:** nausea, vomiting, diarrhea. **Metabolic:** hypoglycemia without tachycardia. **Skin:** rash. **Other:** *increased airway resistance,* fever.
tobramycin Tobrex (See chapter 77 for information about other ophthalmic anti-infectives.)	*Treatment of external ocular infections caused by susceptible bacteria—* **Adults and children:** in mild to moderate infections, instill 1 or 2 drops into the affected eye q 4 hours. In severe infections, instill 2 drops into the infected eye hourly.	**Eye:** burning or stinging upon instillation. **Other:** hypersensitivity.

♦ Available in U.S. and Canada. ♦♦ Available in Canada only. All other products (no symbol) available in U.S. only. Italicized side effects are common or life-threatening.

INTERACTIONS	NURSING CONSIDERATIONS
Insulin, hypoglycemic drugs (oral): can alter requirements for these drugs in previously stabilized diabetics. Monitor for hypoglycemia. *Cardiac glycosides:* excessive bradycardia and increased depressant effect on myocardium. Use together cautiously.	• Contraindicated in diabetes mellitus, asthma, allergic rhinitis; during ethyl ether anesthesia; in sinus bradycardia and heart block greater than first degree; in cardiogenic shock; in right ventricular failure secondary to pulmonary hypertension. Use with caution in CHF and respiratory disease, and in patients taking other antihypertensives. • Always check patient's apical pulse rate before giving this drug. If you detect extremes in pulse rates, withhold medication and call the doctor immediately. • Monitor blood pressure frequently. If patient develops severe hypotension, notify doctor. He may prescribe a vasopressor. • Instruct patient about the disease and therapy. Explain the importance of taking drug exactly as prescribed, even when he's feeling well. Tell patient not to discontinue drug suddenly: abrupt discontinuation can exacerbate angina and MI. Tell patient to call doctor if unpleasant side effects develop. • This drug masks common signs of shock and hypoglycemia. • If patient is taking the drug for hypertension, warn him not to increase the dosage without first consulting his doctor. At least 7 days should intervene between increases in dosage. • Timolol is the first beta blocker approved for use in post-MI patients. Like other beta blockers, it prolongs survival of MI patients.
Tetracycline-containing eye preparations: incompatible with tyloxapol, an ingredient in Tobrex. Don't use together.	• Prolonged use may result in overgrowth of nonsusceptible organisms, including fungi. • Always wash hands before and after instilling solution. • Warn patient to avoid sharing washcloths and towels with family members. • Tell patient to watch for signs of sensitivity, such as itching lids or constant burning. Patient who develops such signs should discontinue drug and notify doctor immediately. • Warn patient not to touch tip of dropper to eye or surrounding tissue. • Show patient how to instill.

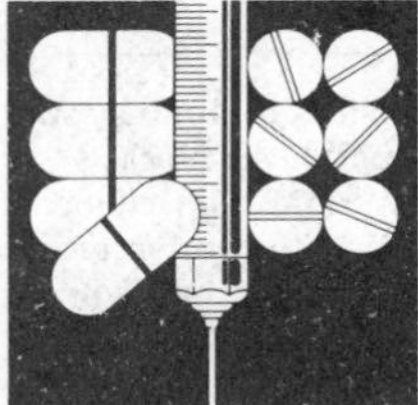

Drug toxicities

Drug toxicity—unlike anaphylaxis, which results from hypersensitivity—follows overdosage, or ingestion of a drug meant for external use. Cumulative toxicity may result from long-term use of a drug that is slowly excreted. The information that follows tells you how to identify, treat, and reverse toxic reactions with specific antidotes; and how to relieve their symptoms with other drugs or with supportive measures. Generally, the doses cited are recommended for adults. With some exceptions, children's doses should be calculated individually. (Supportive treatment of toxicity is covered in the tabular information for each drug.)

ACETAMINOPHEN

Symptoms to watch for:

• In the first 3 to 4 hours after ingestion: nausea, vomiting, anorexia, and sweating are likely, but some patients have no symptoms.

• 24 to 36 hours after ingestion, the patient may still be asymptomatic; liver enzyme levels may begin to rise.

• Hepatic toxicity may develop 2 to 5 days after ingestion. Watch for vomiting, right upper quadrant tenderness, elevated SGOT, SGPT, and serum bilirubin levels, and increased prothrombin time (PT). Hypoglycemia is possible.

How to confirm toxicity:

• Monitor SGOT, SGPT, and serum bilirubin levels, and PT.

• Monitor serum acetaminophen levels. Levels over 300 mcg/ml 4 hours after ingestion are associated with severe hepatic damage; levels under 120 mcg/ml 4 hours after ingestion usually mean hepatic damage is unlikely.

What to do:

• Stop drug.

• Induce emesis with 15 to 30 ml of ipecac syrup or do gastric lavage.

Important: Do not give ipecac syrup if the patient is unconscious.

• Supportive measures include parenteral fluids, fresh frozen plasma, or clotting factors.

• Immediately begin therapy with acetylcysteine (Mucomyst), the direct antidote to acetaminophen overdose: Give 140 mg/kg P.O. of the 20% acetylcysteine (Mucomyst) solution; then give 70 mg/kg P.O. q 4 hours for a total of 17 doses (total dosage, 1330 mg/kg). Acetylcysteine solution may be diluted to a 5% concentration with a soft drink (cola, ginger ale, and so forth) to make it more palatable.

ANTICHOLINERGICS (INCLUDING TRICYCLIC ANTIDEPRESSANTS)

Anisotropine methylbromide, atropine sulfate, belladonna leaf, benztropine mesylate, biperiden hydrochloride, biperiden lactate, chlorphenoxamine hydrochloride, clidinium bromide, cycrimine hydrochloride, dicyclomine hydrochloride, diphemanil methylsulfate, ethopropazine hydrochloride, flavoxate hydrochloride, glycopyrrolate, hexocyclium methylsulfate, homatropine methylbromide, hyoscyamine sulfate, isopropamide iodide, mepenzolate bromide, methantheline bromide, methixene hydrochloride, methscopolamine bromide, orphenadrine hydrochloride, oxybutynin chloride, oxyphencyclimine hydrochloride, oxyphenonium bromide, procylidine hydrochloride, propantheline bromide, scopolamine hydrobromide, thiphenamil hydrochloride, tridihexethyl chloride, trihexyphenidyl hydrochloride. Diphenoxylate hydrochloride with atropine sulfate may cause anticholinergic as well as narcotic-like toxicity. Remember: Other drugs, such as antihistamines and phenothiazines, also have secondary anticholinergic actions.

Symptoms to watch for:

CNS: confusion, excitement, convulsions, coma.

CV: increased heart rate (may occur with therapeutic doses).

EENT: dilated pupils, blurred vision,

increased intraocular tension, and dry mouth (all may occur with therapeutic doses).
GI: dysphagia.
GU: urinary retention.
Skin: hot, dry, and red.
Other: rapid respirations, muscle stiffness, and fever.
What to do:
• Stop drug.
• Maintain airway and respirations.
• Induce emesis with 15 to 30 ml of ipecac syrup or do gastric lavage.
Important: Don't give ipecac syrup if patient is unconscious. Give activated charcoal 5 to 50 g, or 5 to 10 times estimated weight of ingested drug.
• Give saline laxative (e.g., 200 ml magnesium citrate).
• Give antidote: physostigmine salicylate can reverse life-threatening central and peripheral effects of anticholinergics. Dilute each mg in 5 ml normal saline. Give 0.5 to 4 mg I.M. or I.V. slowly every 2 hours. Keep atropine sulfate available for treating possible physostigmine salicylate toxicity (symptoms are bradycardia, convulsions, and severe bronchoconstriction). Remember that physostigmine is contraindicated in hypotension.
• Monitor EKG.
• If the patient has fever, sponge with wet towels.
• If the patient shows excitement, delirium, or convulsions, give small doses of short-acting barbiturate (sodium pentobarbital).
• Catheterize patient unable to void.
• Darken patient's room, or use pilocarpine eye drops for dilated pupils.

BARBITURATES AND PRIMIDONE

Amobarbital, amobarbital sodium, aprobarbital, barbital, butabarbital sodium, hexobarbital, mephobarbital, metharbital, pentobarbital, pentobarbital sodium, phenobarbital, phenobarbital sodium, secobarbital, secobarbital sodium, talbutal. Primidone is not a barbiturate, but symptoms and treatment of primidone toxicity are similar to those of barbiturate toxicity.
Symptoms to watch for: (All indicate acute toxicity):
CNS: headache, confusion, ataxia, CNS depression ranging from sleepiness to coma (may be preceded by excitement and hallucinations).
CV: hypotension.
GU: crystalluria (in primidone toxicity), low urinary output.
EENT: ptosis, miosis, mydriasis in severe poisoning.
Skin: cyanosis, especially in ear lobes, nose, or fingers; occasional blisters or bullous lesions.
Other: slow, shallow breathing; flaccid muscles; hypothermia, hyperthermia; shock.
How to confirm toxicity:
• Positively identify ingested drug.
• Measure and identify barbiturates in blood, urine, or gastric contents.
• Monitor for potentially lethal blood levels:
—phenobarbital, 80 mcg/ml or higher
—amobarbital and butabarbital, 50 mcg/ml or higher
—secobarbital and pentobarbital, 30 mcg/ml or higher
What to do:
• Stop drug.
• Maintain adequate airway. Perform endotracheal suction every hour unless pulmonary edema develops (in which case endotracheal suction is contraindicated).
• Maintain adequate oxygen intake and carbon dioxide removal.
• Begin gastric lavage (most effective when started within 2 hours of ingestion). Use cuffed endotracheal tube.
• Delay absorption with activated charcoal. Dose: 5 to 10 times estimated weight of ingested drug.
• Barbiturate toxicity has no specific antidote. Don't give analeptic drugs such as caffeine.
• Maintain blood pressure by infusing 5% plasma or low molecular weight dextran I.V. Monitor central venous pressure. If fluid infusion doesn't maintain blood pressure, give metaraminol or levarterenol.
• Elevate patient's head 15 degrees to help prevent cerebral edema.
• Turn patient at least every 2 hours.
• Give up to 40 ml/kg fluids daily if renal function is adequate. Maintain daily urine output at 15 to 30 ml/kg.
• Monitor sodium, potassium, and chloride levels daily.
• In phenobarbital toxicity, forced alkaline diuresis with sodium bicarbonate and osmotic diuretic may be useful.
• Treat hypothermia by applying blankets. Avoid too-rapid warming.
• Dialysis is indicated in severe barbiturate poisoning or inadequate renal function.
• Frequently monitor patient's pulse rate, temperature, color of skin, reflexes, and response to painful stimuli.

CARDIOTONIC GLYCOSIDES

Deslanoside, digitalis leaf, digitoxin, digoxin, gitalin, lanatoside, ouabain.

Symptoms to watch for:

CNS: headache, weakness, lassitude, fatigue, somnolence, memory loss, dizziness, ataxia, confusion, aphasia, neuralgias, paresthesias, muscle pain and weakness, fainting, seizures, stupor, coma, apathy, depression, personality changes, irritability, restlessness, insomnia, nightmares, euphoria, mania, giddiness, excitement, agitation, belligerence, violent behavior, delusions, hallucinations, psychosis, delirium.
CV: premature ventricular beats (most common in adults), paroxysmal and nonparoxysmal nodal rhythms, atrioventricular dissociation; paroxysmal atrial tachycardia with AV block (most common in children).

How to confirm toxicity:

- Monitor EKG. Watch for premature ventricular contractions, paroxysmal atrial tachycardia with AV block, nonparoxysmal AV nodal tachycardia, sinus bradycardia, atrial fibrillation, ventricular tachycardia or fibrillation, sinus arrest, SA block, premature atrial contraction, premature AV nodal contraction, and junctional tachycardia with escape rhythms.
- Monitor blood levels: 2 ng/ml of digoxin and 35 ng/ml of digitoxin may indicate toxicity.

What to do:

- Stop drug.
- Treat arrhythmias. If patient has marked hypokalemia and atrial, junctional, or ventricular tachycardia, give potassium chloride: adults, 40 mEq/liter of 5% dextrose in water, maximum 20 mEq/hour; children, potassium chloride 0.5 mEq/kg in 5% dextrose in water. Don't use potassium in patients with hyperkalemia, impaired kidney function, second and third degree AV block, or SA block. Throughout, monitor EKG to end the potassium infusion promptly when hypokalemia is corrected and to avoid overcorrection to hyperkalemia by watching for signs of potassium toxicity (peaking T waves).

  If patient is not hypokalemic, use *phenytoin.* The loading dose is up to 15 mg/kg I.V. at 50 mg/minute; maintenance, 5 to 7 mg/kg I.V. q 12 hours at a rate not to exceed 50 mg/minute. Don't use phenytoin in patients with second and third degree AV block, SA block, or marked sinus bradycardia. If phenytoin is contraindicated, infuse 1 mg/kg lidocaine hydrochloride as an I.V. bolus, at 25 to 50 mg/minute followed by constant infusion of 1 to 4 mg/minute. Use lidocaine hydrochloride with caution in patients with congestive heart failure. Lidocaine is contraindicated in patients with second and third degree AV block, SA block, and marked sinus bradycardia.

  In patients with atrial tachycardia with AV block and premature ventricular contractions, give 1 to 3 mg propranolol by slow I.V. infusion (1 mg/minute). Repeat after 2 minutes, if needed. Wait 4 hours before giving subsequent doses. Propranolol is contraindicated in patients with asthma, marked sinus bradycardia, SA block, second and third degree AV block, cardiogenic shock, heart failure, or pulmonary hypertension. Occasionally, quinidine and procainamide are also useful. The patient with second or third degree AV block, SA block, and marked sinus bradycardia may need an artificial pacemaker.
- Remember, all patients with cardiotonic glycoside toxicity need constant EKG monitoring.
- Keep in mind that many of the arrhythmias that cardiotonic glycosides effectively treat closely resemble the arrhythmias that result from cardiotonic glycoside toxicity, and that patients with congestive heart failure often complain of nausea and vomiting. So whenever you see these symptoms in a patient receiving cardiotonic glycosides, and you can't positively rule out toxicity, withhold the drug temporarily if the patient's clinical condition permits.

CHOLINERGIC (PARASYMPATHETIC) DRUGS

Ambenonium chloride, edrophonium chloride, neostigmine bromide, neostigmine methylsulfate, physostigmine salicylate, and pyridostigmine bromide.

Symptoms to watch for: (All indicate cholinergic crisis)

CNS: incoordination, blurred vision, weakness, fasciculation, paralysis; agitation and restlessness with extreme overdosage of neostigmine bromide, neostigmine methylsulfate, and pyridostigmine bromide; agitation, restlessness, dizziness, and mental confusion with extreme overdosage of ambenonium chloride.
CV: hypotension, cardiospasm, bradycardia, and tachycardia.
EENT: miosis, and lacrimation.
GI: nausea, vomiting, and diarrhea.
Other: salivation, sweating, muscle

cramps, bronchospasm, and dyspnea.

What to do:

- Stop drug.
- Maintain adequate respirations; if necessary, use mechanical ventilation with repeated bronchial aspiration.
- Give atropine sulfate I.V. Atropine should be used in adequate doses to reverse the cholinergic effects of these drugs. Adequate atropinization is indicated by complete clearing of bronchial and pulmonary rales. Dosage: adults, 2-5 mg I.V.; children, 0.05 mg/kg.
- To reduce ganglionic and skeletal side effects of physostigmine salicylate, may give slow infusion of pralidoxime chloride I.V. Dosage: adults, 1 to 2 g in 100 ml normal saline over 15 to 30 minutes; children, 20 to 40 mg/kg.

BETHANECHOL CHLORIDE

Symptoms to watch for:

CNS: headache.

CV: circulatory collapse, hypotension, and cardiac arrest after I.M. or I.V. administration; substernal pressure or pain, transient complete heart block, and orthostatic hypotension.

GI: bloody diarrhea after I.M. or I.V. administration; abdominal cramps, nausea, and vomiting.

Skin: flushing.

Other: shock after I.M. or I.V. administration; salivation, sweating, fainting, bronchoconstriction.

What to do:

- Stop drug immediately.
- Give 0.4 to 0.6 mg atropine sulfate subcutaneously or I.V. every 4 to 6 hours.
- For severe cardiovascular reactions or bronchoconstriction, give 0.2 to 1 ml epinephrine 1:1000.

HEPARIN SODIUM

Symptoms to watch for:

- Bleeding, especially in elderly women, postoperative patients, or after recent trauma.

How to recognize it:

- Watch for partial thromboplastin time or activated clotting time greater than 2 1/2 times control value accompanied by signs of bleeding.
- Monitor for decreased red blood cell count, hematocrit, or hemoglobin.

What to do:

- Stop heparin immediately.
- If necessary, give heparin antagonist protamine sulfate by slow I.V. injection over 1 to 3 minutes. Usually, 1 mg protamine sulfate will neutralize 90 units of heparin.
- Protamine sulfate doses may have to be repeated, based on clotting tests. However, repeat protamine doses cautiously, because large doses may act as an anticoagulant. Don't exceed 50 mg protamine sulfate in a 10-minute period.

INSULIN AND ORAL HYPOGLYCEMIC AGENTS (ANTIDIABETIC DRUGS)

Acetohexamide, chlorpropamide, insulin (all forms), tolazamide, and tolbutamide.

Symptoms to watch for: (All indicate hypoglycemia)

- Parasympathetic phase—hunger, nausea, belching, bradycardia, and mild hypotension.
- Decreased cerebral function phase—lethargy, frequent yawning, decreased spontaneity of conversation, and inability to do simple calculations.
- Sympathetic phase—increased systolic and mean blood pressure, sweating, and tachycardia.
- Coma with or without convulsions.

Confirming diagnostic measures:

- Monitor blood for hypoglycemia: (serum glucose level less than 50 mg/100 ml).

What to do:

- For mild hypoglycemia, if patient is alert, give 120 ml (4 oz.) of an oral carbohydrate, such as orange juice or other sweetened juices, cola, or ginger ale q 5 to 10 minutes until symptoms of hypoglycemia disappear. Alternately may give 0.5 to 2 mg glucagon I.M.
- For comatose patients or those not responding to or refusing oral carbohydrates, give 50 ml of 50% dextrose I.V., or 0.5 to 2 mg glucagon I.M. if not used previously. Keep airway open. Prevent tongue-biting.
- If patient doesn't respond to above treatment, repeat 50% dextrose dose twice; then start 10% dextrose by continuous I.V. infusion (at rate of 20 drops/minute). Monitor blood glucose level.

LITHIUM CARBONATE, LITHIUM CITRATE

Symptoms to watch for:

CNS: seizures, impaired consciousness, transitory neurologic asymmetries similar to those produced by cerebral hemorrhage; tremors, fasciculations, stiff

neck, ataxia, seizures, restlessness, confusion, stupor, and coma.
CV: arrhythmias, pulse deficit, and hypotension.
EENT: widely opened eyes, transient vertical nystagmus, and tinnitus.
GI: dry mouth.
GU: urinary incontinence.
Other: irregular or deep respirations; gasping and grunting with hyperextension of arms and legs, allergic vasculitis, and fecal incontinence.

What to do:

- Stop drug.
- Use gastric suction.
- Monitor lithium serum levels (should not exceed 2 mEq/liter in acute treatment phase; or 1.5 mEq/liter in maintenance phase).
- Replace fluids and electrolytes as necessary.
- Increase lithium excretion by:
  —forced osmotic diuresis, using up to 200 g mannitol I.V. (5% to 10% solution). Maintain urinary output of 100 to 500 ml/hour and a positive fluid balance.
  —alkalization of urine with 325 mg to 2 g sodium bicarbonate P.O. q.i.d., or 30 ml/kg sodium lactate by slow I.V. infusion daily.
  —administration of caffeine, aminophylline, and sometimes acetozolamide.

METHAQUALONE

Symptoms to watch for:

Blood: nasal or GI bleeding.
CNS: hypertonia, hyperreflexia, muscle twitching, convulsions, coma, and delirium.
CV: tachycardia.
EENT: dilated pupils.
GI: vomiting.
GU: renal insufficiency.
Other: pulmonary and cutaneous edema, shock, and hepatic damage.

What to do:

- Stop drug.
- If patient is not convulsing, induce emesis with 15 to 30 ipecac syrup or do gastric lavage. **Important:** Do not give ipecac syrup if the patient is unconscious.
- Delay absorption with activated charcoal. Dose: 5 to 10 times estimated weight of ingested drug or 1 g/kg of patient's body weight.
- Adults: For prolonged convulsions, give a neuromuscular blocker such as tubocurarine, 1 unit/kg of body weight I.V. slowly over 60 to 90 seconds. Initial dose should be 20 units (3 mg) less than dose calculated by body weight. Assist respirations.
- Hemodialysis may be useful.

METHYPRYLON

Symptoms to watch for:

CNS: coma, excitation, convulsions, delirium, hallucinations, somnolence, and confusion.
CV: hypotension.
EENT: constricted pupils.
Other: fever, hypothermia, and respiratory depression.

What to do:

- Stop drug.
- Induce emesis with 15 to 30 ml ipecac syrup or do gastric lavage. **Important:** Do not give ipecac syrup if patient is unconscious.
- Delay absorption with activated charcoal. Dose: 5 to 10 times estimated weight of ingested drug or 1 g/kg of patient's body weight.
- Supportive measures.
- Give norepinephrine 8 to 12 mcg/minute by I.V. infusion adjusted to maintain normal blood pressure. To dilute, add 4 mg levarterenol to 1 liter 5% dextrose in water.
- To treat convulsions and excitation, give short-acting barbiturate, such as thiopental sodium, 75 to 124 mg I.V.
- Severe overdosage may require hemodialysis.

NARCOTICS

Phenanthrene derivatives: codeine, codeine phosphate, codeine sulfate, hydrocodone bitartrate, hydromorphone hydrochloride, hydromorphone sulfate, levorphanol tartrate, morphine sulfate, opium alkaloids (concentrated), oxycodone, oxymorphone hydrochloride. Morphine sulfate is the prototype of this class.

Phenylpiperidine derivatives: anileridine hydrochloride, fentanyl citrate, and meperidine hydrochloride. Meperidine hydrochloride is the prototype of this class.

Diphenoxylate hydrochloride with atropine sulfate may cause meperidine-like toxicity as well as anticholinergic toxicity.

Symptoms to watch for:

CNS: respiratory depression, which may progress to Cheyne-Stokes respiration; apnea; CNS depression, ranging from stupor to profound coma; muscle tremors and twitches; delirium; disorientation; hallucinations; and (with meperidine derivatives) occasional grand mal

epileptic seizures.
CV: bradycardia, hypotension, cyanosis, circulatory collapse, cardiac arrest, and (with meperidine derivatives) possible tachycardia.
EENT: miosis (with morphine derivatives and methadone), mydriasis (with meperidine derivatives).
GI: dry mouth (with meperidine derivatives).
Other: cold, clammy skin; hypothermia; and flaccid skeletal muscles.

Confirming diagnostic measures:

- Make a positive identification of ingested drug, if possible.
- Note symptoms:
  —coma, pinpoint pupils, and depressed respirations indicative of morphine derivative and methadone toxicity. Keep in mind that in terminal narcosis or severe hypoxia, morphine and methadone toxicity may cause mydriasis.
  —coma, dilated pupils, depressed respirations indicative of meperidine derivative toxicity.
- Analyze urine, blood, gastric contents, or all three body fluids for narcotics.

What to do:

- Stop drug.
- Establish airway; ventilate as needed.
- Induce emesis with 15 to 30 ml ipecac syrup or do gastric lavage, especially within first 2 hours of ingestion.

Important: Do not give ipecac syrup if the patient is unconscious or shows signs of CNS depression.

- Give naloxone (Narcan). Dosage: in adults, 0.4 mg I.V., I.M., or subcutaneously repeated after 2 to 3 minutes up to 3 times, as needed; in children, 0.01 mg/kg I.V., I.M., or subcutaneously repeated after 2 to 3 minutes up to 3 times, as needed.
- Keep in mind that a narcotic antagonist (naloxone, for example) may precipitate acute withdrawal syndrome in patients who are physically addicted to narcotics.
- Maintain body warmth.
- Maintain adequate fluid intake.
- Treat shock with oxygen, I.V. fluids, and vasopressors as needed.
- Monitor vital signs and level of consciousness frequently.

ORAL ANTICOAGULANTS

Anisindione, dicumarol, phenindione, phenprocoumon, warfarin potassium, and warfarin sodium.

Symptoms to watch for:

- Minor bleeding, such as purpura, hematoma, epistaxis, or hematuria. Red-orange discoloration of urine with anisindione and phenindione may be mistaken for hematuria.
- Major bleeding, such as GI or intracranial bleeding, intrapulmonary, adrenal, or retroperitoneal bleeding, hemarthroses, and bleeding into pericardial space are also possible but less common.
- Skin necrosis and the sudden onset of painful ecchymoses, usually on the lower half of the body or on the breast, with coumarin derivatives.

How to confirm toxicity:

- Watch for PT greater than twice control value.
- Monitor for decreased red blood cell count, hematocrit, or hemoglobin.
- Test for blood in stools (Hematest, Hemoccult).

What to do:

- Stop anticoagulant and control bleeding immediately.
- Give antidote, vitamin K_1 (phytonadione) 2.5 to 10 mg I.M., subcutaneously, or by slow I.V. injection. Repeat in 6 to 8 hours if necessary. If patient is not bleeding but has elevated PT, you may give 2.5 to 10 mg phytonadione P.O. May repeat in 12 to 48 hours. In emergency, you may give 10 to 50 mg by slow I.V.; maximum rate 1 mg/minute. Repeat q 4 hours as needed.
- You may give fresh frozen plasma or fresh whole blood to replace clotting factors. In major bleeding, fresh frozen plasma is necessary since onset of phytonadione begins after 6 to 8 hours.

PHENOTHIAZINES

Acetophenazine maleate, butaperazine maleate, carphenazine maleate, chlorpromazine hydrochloride, dimethothiazine mesylate, fluphenazine decanoate, fluphenazine enanthate, fluphenazine hydrochloride, mesoridazine besylate, methdilazine hydrochloride, perphenazine, piperacetazine, prochlorperazine, prochlorperazine edisylate, prochlorperazine maleate, promazine hydrochloride, promethazine hydrochloride, thiethylperazine maleate, thioridazine, trifluoperazine, triflupromazine, trimeprazine tartrate.

Symptoms to watch for:

CNS: restlessness, confusion, excitement in early or mild intoxication; convulsions; depression ranging from drowsiness to coma; areflexia; parkinsonian-like extrapyramidal symptoms (tremors, rigidity, akinesia, shuffling gait, postural abnormalities, pill-rolling movements, masklike facies,

and excessive salivation); dystonic and dyskinesic extrapyramidal symptoms; dystonia most common in children; dyskinesia most common in adults (disordered tonicity of muscles and torsion spasms, opisthotonos, drooping of the head, protrusion of tongue, mandibular tics, and stiff neck); difficult swallowing and breathing (accompanied by profuse sweating, pallor, and fever); akathisia (extreme motor restlessness; and continual moving of hands, mouth, and body).
CV: hypotension, tachycardia, EKG changes, cardiac arrhythmias, cyanosis, and vasomotor collapse.
EENT: miosis.
GI: dry mouth.
Other: hypothermia, and sudden apnea.

What to do:

- Stop drug.
- Maintain airway; promote adequate ventilation.
- Gastric lavage is effective up to several hours after drug is ingested.
- Delay absorption with activated charcoal. Dose: 5 to 10 times estimated weight of ingested drug or 1 g/kg of patient's body weight.
- Don't induce emesis; dystonic reactions may cause aspiration of vomitus.
- Treat severe dystonia and dyskinesia with 2 mg benztropine mesylate I.V. followed by 1 to 2 mg P.O. b.i.d. to prevent recurrence; or diphenhydramine hydrochloride 25 to 50 mg deep I.M. or I.V.
- Treat parkinsonian reactions with benztropine mesylate 0.5 to 6 mg P.O. daily; with trihexyphenidyl hydrochloride 2.5 mg P.O. daily to t.i.d.; with biperiden hydrochloride or lactate 2 mg t.i.d. to q.i.d.; or with 2 to 2.5 mg procyclidine hydrochloride P.O. t.i.d., increased to 60 mg daily, if necessary. Don't use levodopa.
- Attempt to treat akathisia with antiparkinson drugs as above; treatment is often ineffective.
- If stimulants are needed, use amphetamines, ephedrine, or caffeine and sodium benzoate. Don't use pentylenetetrazol or other stimulants, which may cause convulsions.
- Observe patient for orthostatic hypotension; monitor blood pressure in supine and standing positions. Instruct ambulatory patient to rise from bed slowly and dangle feet for a few minutes before standing.
- Treat severe hypotension with slow I.V. infusion of norepinephrine 8 to 12 mcg/minute. Adjust to maintain normal blood pressure. To dilute, add 4 mg norepinephrine to 1 liter of 5% dextrose in water. Or use phenylephrine hydrochloride 0.1 to 0.5 mg added to 500 ml of 5% dextrose in water, at a rapid rate initially, then slowed to maintain blood pressure at desired level. Do not use epinephrine; it may paradoxically lower blood pressure.
- Stay with patient and give reassurance that symptoms will subside.

PROPOXYPHENE SALTS

Symptoms to watch for:

CNS: stupor, coma, and convulsions.
CV: EKG abnormalities, and circulatory collapse.
EENT: miosis.
Metabolic: nephrogenic diabetes insipidus.
Other: respiratory depression, pulmonary edema, and cyanosis.

Confirming diagnostic measures:

- Watch for EKG abnormalities.

What to do:

- Stop drug.
- Maintain airway.
- Give antidote, naloxone hydrochloride (Narcan). Dosage: in adults, 0.4 mg I.V., I.M., or subcutaneously, repeated after 2 to 3 minutes up to 3 times, as needed; in children, 0.01 mg/kg I.V. or I.M. Doses may be repeated in 2 to 3 minutes.
- Induce emesis with 15 to 30 ml ipecac syrup or do gastric lavage. **Important:** Do not give ipecac syrup if the patient is unconscious.
- Delay absorption with activated charcoal. Dose: 5 to 10 times estimated weight of ingested drug or 1 g/kg of patient's body weight.
- Use supportive measures as needed (oxygen, I.V. fluids, and vasopressors).

SALICYLATES

Symptoms to watch for:

- Mild toxicity—burning pain in mouth, throat, or abdomen; slight to moderate hyperpnea; lethargy; vomiting; tinnitus; hearing loss; and dizziness.
- Moderate toxicity—ecchymoses, restlessness, incoordination, dehydration, fever, sweating, delirium, excitability, marked lethargy, and severe hyperpnea.
- Severe toxicity—sodium, potassium, and bicarbonate loss and metabolic acidosis in young children; coma; convulsion; cyanosis; oliguria; uremia; pulmonary edema; respiratory failure;

and severe hyperpnea.

• Small doses of methyl salicylate are potentially fatal in children.

Confirming diagnostic measures:

• Monitor blood salicylate levels for 6 hours after ingestion. (**Note:** Salicylamide is not determined by serum salicylate analysis.) Look for the following salicylate levels in adults:

—no intoxication: less than 45 mg/dl
—mild intoxication: 45 to 65 mg/dl
—moderate intoxication: 65 to 90 mg/dl
—severe intoxication: 90 to 120 mg/dl

Blood levels of 120 mg/dl or more are usually fatal.

• Blood levels may continue to rise for 6 to 10 hours after overdose.

What to do:

• Stop drug.
• Induce emesis with 15 to 30 ml ipecac syrup. **Important:** Do not give ipecac syrup if the patient is unconscious.
• If patient shows CNS depression, do gastric lavage and protect airway.
• Delay absorption with activated charcoal. Dose: 5 to 10 times estimated weight of ingested drug or 1 g/kg of patient's body weight.
• Give a saline cathartic (e.g., magnesium citrate 200 ml).
• For hypotension, give I.V. fluids according to the patient's acid/base and electrolyte status.
• For respiratory depression, give artificial respiration with oxygen.
• For hypoglycemia, give dextrose I.V.
• Maintain fluid balance with 5% dextrose in water with sodium chloride. Begin management with the following dosages, adjusting according to results of physical and lab exams.

—in mild salicylate intoxication, give 100 ml/kg fluids P.O.
—in severe intoxication, give 400 ml 5% dextrose in water/m^2 body surface area, with 5 mEq sodium chloride/dl and 2.5 mEq sodium bicarbonate/dl.
—when adequate urine flow is established, decrease sodium dose by 50% and add potassium chloride.

• For acidosis, initially give 2 to 5 mEq sodium bicarbonate/kg by slow I.V. infusion over 24 to 48 hours.
• For bleeding due to hypoprothrombinemia give phytonadione (vitamin K_1), 25 mg/day I.M. or I.V.
• For impaired renal function, use dialysis to remove salicylates.
• For hyperpyrexia, sponge patient with tepid water. Don't use alcohol.
• Continue monitoring serum sodium, potassium, glucose, blood gases, and salicylate levels.

SPASMOLYTICS

Aminophylline, dyphilline, oxtriphylline, papaverine, theophylline, theophylline sodium glycinate.

Symptoms to watch for:

CNS: headache, insomnia, irritability, restlessness, convulsions (especially in infants and small children), hyperreflexia, fasciculations, coma, and fainting.
CV: tachycardia, marked hypotension, and circulatory failure.
EENT: tinnitus and flashing lights.
GI: nausea, vomiting, epigastric pain, hematemesis, and diarrhea.
GU: albuminuria and microhematuria.
Skin: cyanosis.
Other: dehydration, extreme thirst, tachypnea, respiratory arrest, and fever.

What to do:

• Stop drug.
• Induce emesis with 15 to 30 ml ipecac syrup or do gastric lavage. **Important:** Do not give ipecac syrup if the patient is unconscious.
• Delay absorption with activated charcoal. Dose: 5 to 10 times estimated weight of ingested drug or 1 g/kg of patient's body weight.
• Give I.V. fluids and oxygen and use additional supportive measures to prevent hypotension and maintain fluid and electrolyte balance.
• Monitor serum levels until drug concentration is below 20 mcg/ml.

BENZODIAZEPINE TRANQUILIZERS

Symptoms to watch for:

CNS: confusion, coma, somnolence, and diminished reflexes.
CV: possible hypotension.
Other: possible depression.

What to do:

• Stop drug.
• Maintain airway; promote oxygen intake and carbon dioxide removal.
• Monitor respirations, pulse, and blood pressure.
• Induce emesis with 15 to 30 ml ipecac syrup or do gastric lavage. **Important:** Do not give ipecac syrup if the patient is unconscious.
• Delay absorption with activated charcoal. Dose: 5 to 10 times estimated weight of ingested drug or 1 g/kg of patient's body weight.

U.S. AND CANADIAN SUBSTANCE ABUSE AND POISON INFORMATION SERVICES

STATE (U.S.)	SUBSTANCE ABUSE AGENCY	POISON INFORMATION CENTER
Alabama	Division of Mental Illness and Substance Abuse, Department of Mental Health, 135 S. Union St., Montgomery 36130 (205) 834-4350	Southeast Alabama Medical Center, Ashford Hwy., Dothan 36302 (205) 793-8800 West Alabama Poison Control Center, Druid City Hospital, 809 University Blvd., Tuscaloosa 35404 (205) 345-0600
Alaska	Office of Alcoholism and Drug Abuse, Pouch H-05-F, 231 Franklin, Juneau 99811 (907) 586-6201	Fairbanks Memorial Hospital, 1605 Cowles, Fairbanks 99701 (907) 456-7182 Providence Hospital, 3200 Providence Dr., Anchorage 99504 (907) 274-6535/6536
Arizona	Division of Behavioral Health Services, Alcohol Section, 2500 E. Van Buren St., Phoenix 85008 (602) 244-1331 Division of Behavioral Health Services, Drug Abuse Section, 2500 E. Van Buren St., Phoenix 85008 (602) 244-1331	St Luke's Hospital, 525 N. 18th St., Phoenix 85006 (602) 253-3334 College of Pharmacy, University of Arizona, Arizona Health Science Center, Tucson 85724 (602) 626-6016 / (800) 362-0101 (within state only)
Arkansas	Office of Alcohol and Drug Abuse Prevention, 1515 W. 7th Ave., Suite 310, Little Rock 72202 (501) 371-2603	University of Arkansas, Medical Center, 4301 W. Markham St., Little Rock 72201 (501) 661-6161
California	Department of Alcohol and Drug Program, 111 Capital Mall, Sacramento 95814 (916) 445-1940	Los Angeles Co. Medical Association, Regional Poison Information Center, 1925 Wilshire Blvd., Los Angeles 90057 (213) 484-5151 San Francisco Bay Area Poison Control Center, San Francisco General Hospital, Room 1E86, 1001 Potrero Ave., San Francisco 94110 (415) 666-2845
Colorado	Colorado Department of Health, Alcohol and Drug Abuse Division, 4210 E. 11th Ave., Denver 80220 (303) 320-6137	Rocky Mountain Poison Center, W. 8th Ave. and Cherokee St., Denver 80204 (303) 629-1123
Connecticut	Alcohol and Drug Abuse Commission, 999 Asylum Ave., Hartford 06105 (203) 566-4145	Connecticut Poison Center, University of Connecticut Health Center, Farmington 06032 (203) 674-3456
Delaware	Bureau of Alcoholism and Drug Abuse, 1901 N. DuPont Hwy., Newcastle 19720 (302) 421-6101	Delaware Poison Information Service, Inc., 501 W. 14th St., Wilmington 19899 (302) 655-3389

The agencies and centers listed in this appendix are valuable community resources. They can furnish you and your patient with educational information on substance abuse rehabilitation and poison prevention programs.

STATE (U.S.)	SUBSTANCE ABUSE AGENCY	POISON INFORMATION CENTER
District of Columbia	Alcohol and Drug Abuse Planning Division, 601 Indiana Ave., Washington 20004 (202) 724-5641	National Capital Poison Center, Georgetown Hospital, 3800 Reservoir Rd., N.W. Washington 20007 (202) 625-3333
Florida	Alcoholic Rehabilitation Program, 1309 Winewood Blvd., Tallahassee 32301 (904) 488-0900 Drug Abuse Program, 1309 Winewood Blvd., Tallahassee 32301 (904) 488-0900	Jackson Memorial Hospital, 1611 N.W. 12th Ave., Miami 33136 (305) 325-7429 Poison Control Center, Shands Hospital, Box J316—JHMHC, Gainesville 32610 (904) 392-3389
Georgia	Division of Mental Health and Mental Retardation, Alcohol and Drug Section, 618 Ponce de Leon Ave., Atlanta 30365 (404) 894-4785	Athens General Hospital, 1199 Prince Ave., Athens 30613 (404) 543-5215 Georgia Poison Control Center, Box 26066, 80 Butler St., S.E., Atlanta 30335 (404) 588-4400 / (404) 525-3323 (teletype for deaf)
Hawaii	Alcohol and Drug Abuse Branch, 1270 Queen Emma St., Honolulu 96813 (808) 548-7655	Hawaii Poison Center, 1319 Punahou St., Honolulu 96826 (808) 941-4411
Idaho	Bureau of Substance Abuse, 450 W. State St., Boise 83720 (208) 334-4368	St. Anthony Hospital, 650 N. 7th St., Pocatello 83201 (206) 232-2733
Illinois	Department of Mental Health and Developmental Disabilities, Alcohol Division, 160 N. LaSalle St., Chicago 60601 (312) 793-2907 Illinois Dangerous Drugs Commission, 300 N. State St., 15th Floor, Chicago 60610 (312) 822-9860	Cook County Children's Hospital, 700 S. Wood St., Chicago 60612 (312) 633-7777
Indiana	Department of Mental Health, Division of Addiction Services, 429 Pennsylvania Ave., Indianapolis 46204 (317) 232-7816	Indiana Poison Control Center, 1001 W. 10th St., Indianapolis 46202 (317) 630-7351 Methodist Hospital of Indiana, Inc., 1604 N. Capitol Ave., Indianapolis 46202 (317) 927-3033
Iowa	Department of Substance Abuse, Suite 202, Insurance Exchange Building, 505 5th Ave., Des Moines 50319 (515) 281-3641	University of Iowa Hospital's Poison Control Center, Iowa City 52242 (319) 356-2922

U.S. AND CANADIAN SUBSTANCE ABUSE AND POISON INFORMATION SERVICES *(continued)*

STATE (U.S.)	SUBSTANCE ABUSE AGENCY	POISON INFORMATION CENTER
Kansas	Alcohol and Drug Abuse Section, Biddle Building, 2700 W. 6th St., Topeka 66606 (913) 296-3925	University of Kansas Medical Center, 39th and Rainbow Blvd., Kansas City 66103 (913) 588-6633
Kentucky	Bureau for Health Services, Substance Abuse Branch, 275 E. Main St., Frankfort 40601 (502) 564-2880	Central Baptist Hospital, 1740 S. Limestone, Lexington 40503 (606) 278-3411 (8 a.m. to 9 p.m.) Kentucky Poison Control Center, Norton-Kosair Children's Hospital, 200 E. Chestnut St., Louisville 40202 (502) 589-8222
Louisiana	Office of Mental Health and Substance Abuse, 655 N. 5th St., P.O. Box 4049, Baton Rouge 70821 (504) 342-2545	Charity Hospital, P.O. Box 35070, 1532 Tulane Ave., New Orleans 70140 (504) 568-5222
Maine	Bureau of Rehabilitation, Office of Alcoholism and Drug Abuse Prevention, 32 Winthrop St., Augusta 04330 (207) 289-2781	Maine Medical Center, Emergency Division, 22 Bramhall St., Portland 04102 (207) 871-0111 (switchboard) (800) 442-6305 (within state only)
Maryland	Alcoholism Control Administration, 201 W. Preston St., Baltimore 21201 (301) 383-2781 Drug Abuse Administration, 201 W. Preston St., Baltimore 21201 (301) 383-7404	University of Maryland, School of Pharmacy, 636 W. Lombard St., Baltimore 21201 (301) 528-7701/ (800) 492-2414 (within state only)
Massachusetts	Division of Alcoholism, 755 Boylston St., Boston 02116 (617) 727-1960 Division of Drug Rehabilitation, 160 N. Washington St., Boston 02114 (617) 727-8614	Massachusetts Poison Control Systems, 300 Longwood Ave., Boston 02115 (617) 232-2120 / (800) 682-9211 (within state only)
Michigan	Office of Substance Abuse Services, 3500 N. Logan St., P.O. Box 30035, Lansing 48909 (517) 373-8600	University Hospital, 1405 E. Ann St., Ann Arbor 48104 (313) 764-5102 (poison center) (313) 763-0243 (drug information) Western Michigan Poison Center, 1840 Wealthy, S.E. Grand Rapids 49506 (616) 774-7854 / (800) 632-2727 (within state only)
Minnesota	Department of Public Welfare, Chemical Dependency Program Division, 658 Cedar St., St. Paul 55155 (612) 296-3991	Hennepin Co. Medical Center, 701 Park Ave., Minneapolis 55415 (612) 347-3141

STATE (U.S.)	SUBSTANCE ABUSE AGENCY	POISON INFORMATION CENTER
Mississippi	Department of Mental Health, Division of Alcohol and Drug Abuse, Robert E. Lee Building, Jackson 39201 (601) 354-7031	University Medical Center, 2500 N. State St., Jackson 39216 (601) 354-7660
Missouri	Department of Mental Health, Division of Alcohol and Drug Abuse, 2002 Missouri Blvd., Jefferson City 65102 (314) 751-4942	Cardinal Glennon Memorial Hospital for Children, 1465 S. Grand Blvd., St. Louis 63104 (314) 772-5200 Children's Mercy Hospital, 24th and Gillham Rd., Kansas City 64108 (816) 234-3434
Montana	Department of Institutions, Alcohol and Drug Abuse Division, 1539 11th Ave., Helena 59620 (406) 449-2827	Department of Health/Environmental Sciences, Helena 59601 (800) 525-5042 (within state only)
Nebraska	Division of Alcoholism and Drug Abuse, P.O. Box 94728, Lincoln 68509 (402) 471-2851	Children's Memorial Hospital, Poison Control Center, 8301 Dodge St., Omaha 68114 (402) 553-5400 / (800) 642-9999 (within state only)
Nevada	Bureau of Alcohol and Drug Abuse, King St., Carson City 89710 (702) 885-4790	Washoe Medical Center, 77 Pringle Way, Reno 89520 (702) 785-4129/4140 (night line)
New Hampshire	Office of Alcohol and Drug Abuse Prevention, Health and Welfare Building, Hazen Dr., Concord 03301 (603) 271-4627/4630	New Hampshire Poison Center, Mary Hitchcock Hospital, 2 Maynard St., Hanover 03755 (603) 643-4000 / (800) 562-8236 (within state only)
New Jersey	Division of Alcoholism, CN 362, Trenton 08625 (609) 292-8947 Division of Narcotic and Drug Abuse Control, 129 E. Hanover St., Trenton 08608 (609) 292-5760	Medical Center at Princeton, 253 Witherspoon St., Princeton 08540 (609) 734-4554 Newark Beth Israel Medical Center, 201 Lyons Ave., Newark 07112 (201) 926-7240/41/42/43
New Mexico	Behavioral Services Division, Substance Abuse Bureau, P.O. Box 968, Santa Fe 87504 (505) 827-5271	New Mexico Poison/Drug Information Center, University of New Mexico, Albuquerque 87131 (505) 843-2551
New York	Division of Alcoholism and Alcohol Abuse, 194 Washington Ave., Albany 12210 (518) 474-5417 Division of Drug Abuse Services, Executive Park, S., Albany 12203 (518) 457-7629	Buffalo Children's Hospital, 219 Bryant Street, Buffalo, 14222 (716) 878-7654 Nassau County Medical Center, 2201 Hempstead Tpke., East Meadow 11554 (516) 542-2323

U.S. AND CANADIAN SUBSTANCE ABUSE AND POISON INFORMATION SERVICES *(continued)*

STATE (U.S.)	SUBSTANCE ABUSE AGENCY	POISON INFORMATION CENTER
North Carolina	Division of Mental Health and Mental Retardation Services, Alcohol and Drug Abuse Section, 325 N. Salisbury St., Raleigh 27611 (919) 733-4670	Mercy Hospital, 2001 Vail Ave., Charlotte, 28207 (704) 379-5827 New Hanover Memorial Hospital, 2431 S. 17th Street, Wilmington 28401 (919) 343-7046
North Dakota	Mental Health/Mental Retardation Services, Division of Alcoholism and Drug Abuse, State Capitol Building, Bismarck 58505 (701) 224-2767	Bismarck Hospital, 300 N. 7th St., Bismarck 58501 (701) 223-4357
Ohio	Division of Alcoholism, 246 N. High St., Columbus 43215 (614) 466-3425 Bureau of Drug Abuse, 65 S. Front St., Columbus 43215 (614) 466-9015	Drug/Poison Information Center, University of Cincinnati Medical Center, 7701 Medical Science Bldg., 231 Bethesda Ave., Cincinnati 45267 (513) 872-5111
Oklahoma	Division of Alcoholism, P.O. Box 53277, Capitol Station, Oklahoma City 73152 (405) 521-0044 Drug Abuse Division, P.O. Box 53277, Capitol Station, Oklahoma City 73152 (405) 521-0044	Oklahoma Children's Memorial Hospital, P.O. Box 26307, 940 N.E. 13th St., Oklahoma City 73126 (405) 271-5454
Oregon	State Alcohol and Drug Program Office, Mental Health Division, 2575 Bittern St., N.E., Salem 97310 (503) 378-2163	University Hospital North, Room 2519, University of Oregon, Health Sciences Center, Portland 97201 (503) 225-8968
Pennsylvania	Governor's Council on Drug and Alcohol Abuse, 2101 N. Front St., Harrisburg 17120 (717) 787-9857	Philadelphia Poison Information, 321 University Ave., Philadelphia 19104 (215) 823-7460 (toxicology) (215) 922-5523 (emergency) Pittsburgh Poison Center, 125 DeSoto St., Pittsburgh 15213 (412) 682-6669
Rhode Island	Division of Substance Abuse, Administration Building, General Hospital, Rhode Island Medical Center, Cranston 02920 (401) 464-2091	Rhode Island Poison Center, Rhode Island Hospital, 593 Eddy St., Providence 02902 (401) 277-4000
South Carolina	Commission on Alcohol and Drug Abuse, 3700 Forest Dr., Columbia 29204 (803) 758-2521	Medical University of South Carolina, 171 Ashley Ave., Charleston 29401 (803) 792-4201

STATE (U.S.)	SUBSTANCE ABUSE AGENCY	POISON INFORMATION CENTER
South Dakota	Division of Alcoholism, Joe Foss Building, Pierre 57501 (605) 773-4806 Division of Drugs and Substances Control, Joe Foss Building, Pierre 57501 (605) 773-3123	McKennan Hospital, 800 E. 21st St., Sioux Falls 57101 (605) 336-3894 / (800) 952-0123 (within state only)
Tennessee	Department of Mental Health and Mental Retardation, Alcohol and Drug Abuse Services, James K. Polk Building, 505 Deaderick St., Nashville 37219 (615) 741-1921	Vanderbilt University Hospital, 21st Ave., S., Nashville 37232 (615) 322-6435
Texas	Texas Commission on Alcoholism, Sam Houston State Office Building, 8th Floor 201 E. 14th St., Austin 78701 (512) 475-2725 Department of Community Affairs, Drug Abuse Prevention Division, P.O. Box 13166, Austin 78711 (512) 475-6351	W.I. Cook Children's Hospital, 1212 W. Lancaster Ave., Fort Worth 76102 (817) 336-6611
Utah	Division of Alcoholism and Drugs, 150 W. North Temple, Room 350, P.O. Box 2500, Salt Lake City 84110 (801) 533-6532	Intermountain Regional Poison Control Center, 50 N. Medical Dr., Salt Lake City, 84132 (801) 581-2151
Vermont	Department of Social and Rehabilitative Services, Alcohol and Drug Abuse Division, 103 S. Main St., Waterbury 05676 (802) 241-2170	Vermont Poison Center, Medical Center Hospital of Vermont, Colchester Ave., Burlington 05401 (802) 658-3456
Virginia	Department of Mental Health and Mental Retardation, Division of Substance Abuse, 109 Governor St., Richmond 23219 (804) 786-5313	Medical College of Virginia Hospital Pediatric OPD, Box 522 MCV Station, Richmond 23298 (804) 786-9123
Washington	Bureau of Alcoholism and Substance Abuse, Mail Stop OB-44W, Olympia 98504 (206) 753-3073	Children's Orthopedic Hospital and Medical Center, P.O. Box 5371, 4800 Sandpoint Way, N.E., Seattle 98105 (206) 634-5252
West Virginia	Department of Health, Alcoholism and Drug Abuse Program, State Capitol, 1800 Washington St., East Charleston 25305 (304) 348-2276	Charleston Area Medical Center (CAMS), Charleston 25325 (800) 642-3625 (within state only)

U.S. AND CANADIAN SUBSTANCE ABUSE AND POISON INFORMATION SERVICES *(continued)*

STATE (U.S.)	SUBSTANCE ABUSE AGENCY	POISON INFORMATION CENTER
Wisconsin	Bureau of Alcohol and Other Drug Abuse, P.O. Box 7851, Madison 53707 (608) 266-2717	University Hospital, 600 Highland Ave., Madison 53792 (608) 262-3702
Wyoming	Alcohol and Drug Abuse Programs, Hathaway Building, Cheyenne 82002 (307) 777-7115	Wyoming Poison Center, DePaul Hospital, 2600 E. 18th St., Cheyenne 82001 (307) 635-9256 / (800) 442-2704 (within state only)
Puerto Rico	Department of Addiction Control Services, State Alcohol Program, Box B-Y, Rio Piedras Station, Rio Piedras 00928 (809) 763-5014 State Drug Abuse Program, Box B-Y, Rio Piedras Station, Rio Piedras 00928 (809) 763-8957/7575	
PROVINCE (CANADA)	**SUBSTANCE ABUSE AGENCY**	**POISON INFORMATION CENTER**
Alberta	(Head office) Alberta Alcoholism and Drug Abuse Commission, 6th Floor, Pacific Plaza, 10909 Jasper Ave., Edmonton T5J 3M9 (403) 427-4263 (Edmonton office) Alcoholism and Drug Abuse Commission, 108th St., Edmonton T5K 2J5 (403) 430-9942	Poison Treatment Center, University Hospital, Edmonton T6G 2B7 (403) 432-8822
British Columbia	Drug and Alcohol Programs Commission, P.O. Box 50, 805 W. Broadway, Vancouver V5Z 1K1 (604) 873-0263 Greater Victoria Drug and Alcohol Rehabilitation Society, Suite 202 Maynard Ct., 733 Johnson St., Victoria V8W 1M8 (604) 388-4312	Royal Jubilee Hospital, 1900 Fort St., Victoria V8R 1J8 (604) 595-9211
Manitoba	Alcoholism Foundation of Manitoba, West Bow Mall, 1580 Dublin Ave., Winnipeg R3E 0L4 (204) 453-1044 (Manitoba office) Manitoba Treatment Center, 100 Nassau St., Winnipeg R3E 0L4	St. Boniface General Hospital, 409 Tache Ave., Winnipeg R2H 2A6 (204) 233-8563 (switchboard) (204) 237-2264 (emergency)

PROVINCE (CANADA)	SUBSTANCE ABUSE AGENCY	POISON INFORMATION CENTER
New Brunswick	The Alcoholism and Drug Dependency Commission of New Brunswick, P.O. Box 6000, 103 Church St., Fredricton E3B 5H1 (506) 453-2136	Dr. Evere Chelmers Hospital, Tiestman St., Fredricton E3B 5H1 (506) 452-5400
Newfoundland and Labrador	Alcohol and Drug Addiction Foundation of Newfoundland, P.O. Box 4554, St. John's, Newfoundland A1C 6C8 (709) 579-4041	The Dr. Chas. A. Janeway Child Health Center, Newfoundland Dr., St. John's, Newfoundland A1A 1R8 (709) 778-4222 Capt. William Jackman Memorial Hospital, Booth Ave., Labrador City, Labrador (709) 944-2632
Northwest Territories	Alcohol and Drug Program, Department of Social Services, Government of the Northwest Territories, 5th Floor, Precambrian Building, Yellowknife X1A 2L9 (403) 873-7155	Stanton Yellowknife Hospital, Box 10, Franklin Ave., Yellowknife X0E 1H0 (403) 873-3444
Nova Scotia	Nova Scotia Commission on Drug Dependency, 5668 South St., Halifax B3J 1A6 (902) 424-4270	The Izaak Walton Killam Hospital for Children, University Ave., Halifax B3H 1V7 (902) 424-6111
Ontario	Addiction Research Foundation, 39 Russell St., Toronto M5S 2S1 (416) 595-6000	East General and Orthopaedic Hospital, 825 Coxwell Ave., Toronto M4C 3E7 (416) 461-8272 Hospital for Sick Children, 555 University Ave., Toronto M5G 1X8 (416) 979-1900
Prince Edward Island	Addiction Foundation of Prince Edward Island, P.O. Box 37, Charlottetown C1A 7K2 (902) 892-4265	Charlottetown Hospital, Haviland St., Charlottetown C1A 3S8 (902) 894-5561
Quebec		Hôpital Sainte Justine, 3175 Ct., Ste.-Catherine Rd., W., Montreal H3T 1C5 (514) 731-4931 X291
Saskatchewan	The Alcoholism Commission of Saskatchewan, 3475 Albert St., Regina S4S 6X6 (306) 565-2345	Regina General Hospital, 1440 14th Ave., Regina S4P 0W5 (306) 359-4444
Yukon Territory	Alcohol and Drug Services, Government of the Yukon Territory, P.O. Box 2703, Whitehorse Y1A 2C6	

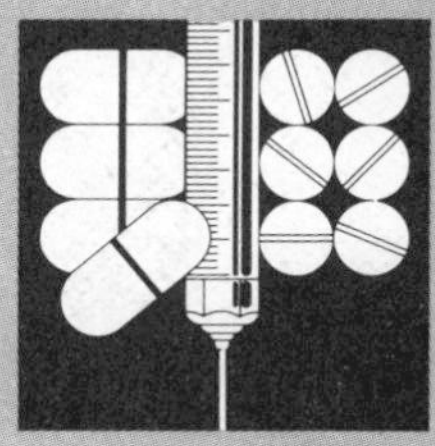

A guide to drugs for cardiovascular emergencies

NAME	INDICATIONS AND DOSAGE
atropine sulfate	*Atrioventricular block, junctional or escape rhythms, and severe nodal or sinus bradycardia—* *Bolus:* 0.5 to 1.0 mg I.V. Dose may be repeated every 5 minutes up to 2 mg.
bretylium tosylate Bretylol	*Ventricular fibrillation—* *Bolus:* 5 to 10 mg/kg of body weight I.V. Repeat every 15 to 30 minutes up to 30 mg/kg of body weight. *Maintenance dose I.V.:* 500 mg in 500 ml dextrose in water (5%) or normal saline solution at 1 to 2 mg/minute. *Maintenance dose I.M.:* 5 to 10 mg/kg of body weight undiluted. Repeat in 1 to 2 hours, if necessary.
calcium chloride	*Asystole—* *Bolus:* 0.5 to 1 g I.V. Available as 1 g = 10 ml. Don't exceed rate of 1 ml/minute.
dopamine hydrochloride Intropin ♦	*Cardiogenic shock, hypotension, and hypovolemic shock—* 5 to 20 mcg/kg of body weight/minute by I.V. infusion, up to 50 mcg/kg of body weight/minute
epinephrine hydrochloride Adrenalin Chloride	*Cardiac and circulatory failure and hypotensive states—* 0.5 to 1 mg I.V. bolus or 4 mg/500 cc of I.V. solution at 1 to 8 mcg/minute; 0.1 to 0.2 mg intracardiac *Severe allergic reactions—* 0.1 to 0.5 ml of 1:1,000 subcutaneously or I.M. Repeat every 10 to 15 minutes as needed, or 0.1 to 0.25 ml of 1:1,000 I.V. *Note:* 1 mg = 1 ml of 1:1,000 or 10 ml of 1:10,000

♦ Available in U.S. and Canada. ♦♦ Available in Canada only. All other products (no symbol) available in U.S. only. Italicized side effects are common or life-threatening.

NURSING CONSIDERATIONS

- Undesirable effects: *Dry mouth, mental confusion, palpitations, tachycardia, and urinary retention*
- Contraindicated in tachycardia.
- Monitor heart rate and rhythm to determine the drug's effects.
- Store in amber or light-resistant container.
- Antidote for atropine overdose is physostigmine salicylate.
- Doses lower than 0.5 mg can cause paradoxical bradycardia.

- Undesirable effects: *Bradycardia; severe hypotension accompanied by symptoms such as dizziness, syncope, and vertigo;* severe nausea and vomiting (with too-rapid infusion); and ventricular irritability
- Contraindicated in digitalis-induced arrhythmia.
- Monitor vital signs (especially blood pressure) every 15 minutes until stable.
- If blood pressure drops precipitously, keep patient on complete bed rest and administer vasopressors.
- Keep patient supine until tolerance to hypotension develops.

- Undesirable effects: *Bradycardia,* hypercalcemia, syncope, and tingling sensations
- Use cautiously in patient with cor pulmonale, respiratory acidosis, respiratory failure, or in patients receiving digitalis.
- Monitor EKG when administering drug I.V.
- Don't confuse calcium chloride with calcium gluconate.

- Undesirable effects: Anginal-type pain, ectopic beats, *hypotension,* pallor, palpitations, respiratory distress, diaphoresis, tremors, vasoconstriction, vomiting, and widening of QRS intervals.
- Contraindicated in uncorrected tachyarrhythmia, ventricular fibrillation, or arterial embolism.
- Drug deteriorates. Discard after 24 hours or sooner if it becomes discolored or contains a precipitate.
- Administer by infusion pump.
- Monitor vital signs, checking for cardiac conduction abnormalities every 15 minutes. Report changes to the doctor.
- Measure hourly urinary output.
- Mix with I.V. solution just before administering.
- Don't mix with other drugs in alkaline solution (sodium bicarbonate, for example).

- Undesirable effects: Cerebral hemorrhage, diaphoresis, *hyperglycemia,* hypertension, precordial pain, pulmonary edema, *tachycardia,* tremors, *ventricular fibrillation,* and widened pulse pressure
- Use with extreme caution in patients in shock (other than anaphylactic) or with ventricular fibrillation or degenerative heart disease.
- Watch for changes in heart rate if drug is given with propranolol hydrochloride.
- Don't expose to light, heat, or air.
- If the drug is given I.V., take and record baseline blood pressure and pulse before beginning therapy. Monitor patient closely until desired effect is obtained, then every 5 minutes until stable. After the patient's condition is stable, monitor blood pressure every 15 minutes.
- If the patient's blood pressure rises sharply, reduce I.V. flow rate and alert the doctor. (He may order rapid-acting vasodilators to counteract pressor effects of large doses of the drug.)
- Massage site after I.M or subcutaneous administration to prevent vasoconstriction and necrosis. Phentolamine hydrochloride may be injected locally to neutralize effects.

(continued on following page)

DRUGS FOR CARDIOVASCULAR EMERGENCIES *(continued)*

NAME	INDICATIONS AND DOSAGE
epinephrine hydrochloride *(continued)*	
isoproterenol hydrochloride Isuprel ♦	*Asystole and bradyarrhythmia—* 0.02 to 0.06 mg I.V., then 0.01 to 0.2 mg I.V. or 5 mcg/minute I.V. *Shock—* 0.5 to 5 mcg/minute by continuous infusion
lidocaine hydrochloride Xylocaine ♦	*Acute ventricular arrhythmia secondary to myocardial infarction or cardiotonic glycosides, life-threatening premature ventricular contractions, and ventricular tachycardia—* *Bolus:* 50 to 100 mg (1 to 1.5 mg/kg of body weight) I.V. at 25 to 50 mg/minute. Maximum dose is 200 mg; Maximum dose is 100 mg in elderly or lightweight patients and those with congestive heart failure or hepatic disease. Repeat bolus every 3 to 5 minutes (two to four times) until arrhythmia subsides or side effects develop. *Infusion:* 2 to 4 g/500 ml dextrose in water (5%) at 1 to 4 mg/minute.
norepinephrine injection (formerly levarterenol bitartrate) Levophed ♦	*Hypotension—* 8 to 12 mcg/minute I.V. infusion; then adjust to maintain normal blood pressure
procainamide hydrochloride Pronestyl ♦	*Supraventricular and ventricular arrhythmias—* 100 mg every 5 minutes until arrhythmia subsides, then 2 to 6 mg/minute in continuous I.V. infusion
sodium bicarbonate	*Cardiac arrest—* *Bolus:* 1 to 3 mEq/kg of body weight I.V. Dose may be repeated in 10 minutes. Further dose is based on arterial blood gas values. *Metabolic disorders—* 2 to 5 mEq I.V. over 4 to 8 hours

♦ Available in U.S. and Canada. ♦♦ Available in Canada only. All other products (no symbol) available in U.S. only. Italicized side effects are common or life-threatening.

NURSING CONSIDERATIONS

- Drug deteriorates. Discard after 24 hours or sooner if it becomes discolored or contains a precipitate.
- Don't mix with other drugs in alkaline solution (sodium bicarbonate, for example). Use dextrose in water solution (5%) or normal saline, or combination of the two. Mix with solution just before administering.

- Undesirable effects: Bronchial edema; chest pain; hypertension, which may be followed by hypotension; *palpitations;* tachycardia; tremors; and vomiting
- Contraindicated in patients with preexisting arrhythmia induced by digitalis toxicity.
- Use cautiously in patients with cardiac failure or limited cardiac reserve.
- Closely monitor vital signs and urinary output. If heart rate exceeds 110 beats/minute (BPM), slow or discontinue the infusion. *Note:* A heart rate over 60 BPM can trigger ventricular arrhythmia in a patient with complete heart block.
- Draw blood to obtain arterial blood gas values. When drug is given for shock, monitor blood pressure, central venous pressure, and EKG. Measure hourly urinary output. Adjust infusion rate accordingly.
- If precordial distress or anginal pain occurs, stop the infusion immediately.
- Propranolol inhibits beta-adrenergic effects of isoproterenol. Give together cautiously.
- Administer by microdrip I.V. tubing or infusion pump.
- Drug deteriorates. Discard after 24 hours or sooner if it becomes discolored or contains a precipitate.

- Undesirable effects: Accelerated ventricular rate, *anaphylaxis,* bradycardia, *cardiac or respiratory depression or arrest, cardiovascular collapse,* convulsions, dysphagia, *hypotension, tremors,* twitching, and vomiting
- Contraindicated in complete or second-degree heart block.
- Use cautiously in the elderly and in patients with congestive heart failure or renal or hepatic disease.
- Draw blood to monitor cardiac enzymes, blood urea nitrogen, and creatinine.
- Monitor heart rate and blood pressure.
- Administer by infusion pump. *Note:* Patients must be monitored at all times.
- Expect additive cardiac depressant effects when the drug is administered with phenytoin.

- Undesirable effects: *Decreased urinary output, headache, metabolic acidosis,* severe hypertension, and *ventricular tachycardia and fibrillation*
- Use cautiously in patients with hypertension, hyperthyroidism, or severe heart disease.
- Report decreased urinary output to the doctor immediately.
- If prolonged I.V. therapy is necessary, change injection site frequently.
- When stopping the drug, slow the infusion rate gradually. Continue to monitor vital signs, even after stopping. Watch for possible precipitous drop in blood pressure.
- Keep emergency drugs on hand to reverse effects of norepinephrine: atropine for reflex bradycardia; propranolol for arrhythmias; and phentolamine for increased vasopressor effects.

- Undesirable effects: *Bradycardia, nausea and vomiting, and severe hypotension*
- Use cautiously in patients with congestive heart failure or conduction disturbances.
- Use an infusion pump or a microdropper and timer to monitor the infusion precisely. *Note:* Patients receiving such infusion must be monitored at all times.
- Monitor blood pressure and EKG continuously during I.V. administration. Watch for prolonged Q-T and Q-R intervals, heart block, or increased arrhythmias. If they occur, withhold drug, obtain rhythm strip, and notify the doctor immediately.
- Keep patient supine for I.V. administration.

- Undesirable effects: Alkalosis and hypernatremia
- Drug may be added to I.V. solution unless solution contains dopamine hydrochloride, epinephrine hydrochloride, or norepinephrine injection.
- Don't infuse through I.V. line containing calcium; drug will precipitate.
- During administration, draw blood for arterial blood gas values and electrolyte measurements.

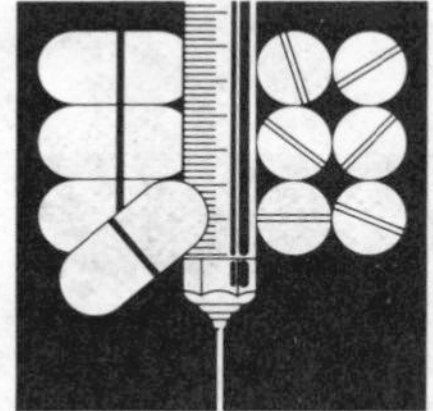

Diagnostic imaging agents

The two types of diagnostic imaging agents are contrast imaging agents and radioactive imaging agents. This introduction describes their characteristic properties, potential adverse reactions, and precautions associated with their use. The table that follows summarizes the more common imaging agents and specifies their diagnostic uses, special preparation required, and relevant nursing considerations.

Contrast imaging agents

Contrast imaging agents—also known as radiopaque dyes or drugs—are impenetrable by X-rays. Thus, they allow radiologic visualization of internal structures, such as the gallbladder, the kidneys, and the gastrointestinal (GI) tract. Depending on the structure to be studied, contrast imaging agents may be instilled directly into a site such as the spinal tract or the uterus; or they may be given orally. Some agents have an affinity for a certain organ or tissue and, when given orally, can localize radiopacity to a definite segment of the GI tract; or they can be absorbed and excreted as, for example, by the gallbladder.

Except for barium sulfate, all contrast imaging agents are iodinated organic compounds and are either fat or water soluble. Because iodinated contrast agents can interfere with thyroid function tests (for example, thyroid uptake studies), such tests should always *precede* radiologic examination.

Varied adverse effects

Most contrast imaging agents exert adverse effects, ranging from minor discomfort to anaphylactic reaction. Such common effects include abdominal cramps, diarrhea, flushing, iodine hypersensitivity, nausea, vomiting, and pruritus. The most common effect of barium sulfate, for example, is constipation.

Although the incidence of iodine hypersensitivity related to contrast agents is low, be sure to ask the patient about previous X-ray procedures and if he had any reactions to them. If the patient has a history of iodine hypersensitivity, alternative tests should be performed, if possible. However, when iodinated contrast agents are required, despite known iodine hypersensitivity, administration of antihistamines and low doses of corticosteroids for several days before the test can minimize adverse reactions.

Hypersensitivity and other severe reactions to contrast imaging agents are most likely to develop after parenteral administration. For example, such administration can induce the sickling phenomenon in a patient with sickle cell disease. In all patients, such administration may induce anaphylactic reaction, with bronchospasm and shock. So, observe carefully for any adverse reactions. Keep in mind that sneezing, wheezing, and tissue swelling are often the first signs of a severe anaphylactic reaction. To treat such reactions promptly, be sure that an antihistamine (preferably diphenhydramine), epinephrine, steroids, and resuscitative equipment for treating shock or other cardiovascular emergency are readily available. In some patients, administration of iodinated contrast agents induces serum sickness (characterized by fever, rash, and pruritus) that develops after 3 to 8 days.

Iodinated contrast agents should be used cautiously in patients with acute hepatorenal disease because of their diminished capacity to excrete these drugs. Similarly, they should be used cautiously in patients with suspected or known pheochromocytoma, because they may trigger hypertensive crisis.

Radioactive imaging agents

Radioactive imaging agents—also called radiopharmaceuticals—are used primarily for diagnosis but may also be used for treatment. These agents contain radionuclides, or radioisotopes—radioactive counterparts of naturally occurring elements. Radionuclides occur naturally or can be prepared in nuclear reactors called atomic piles or in cyclotrons. These atomic reactors rearrange the nuclear configurations, making the nuclei unstable and causing them to emit rays or particles. This discharge of radiant energy is called radioactivity.

Radionuclides have the same chemical properties as the more stable elements. They are taken up and metabolized by organs and tissues exactly as their nonradioactive forms.

Most radionuclides emit gamma rays, which are like X-rays except that they are produced in the nucleus rather than by collision with orbital electrons. Since gamma rays are highly penetrating, they can—after ingestion—be detected externally with special instruments. Their high penetration and ease of measurement make radionuclides effective as diagnostic tracers. Measuring the emitted radiation can help evaluate a metabolic pathway, indicate the size of an organ, or pinpoint the site of disease.

Three diagnostic methods typically use radioactive imaging agents: biochemical concentration, dilution techniques, and flow or diffusion measurements. In *biochemical concentration,* the concentration of a radionuclide in a body structure reflects the structure's function or metabolic condition. *Dilution techniques* measure blood volume and total body water. *Flow or diffusion measurements* evaluate cardiac output, pulmonary ventilation, and peripheral vascular disorders.

Margin of safety

The doses of radiation emitted by radioactive imaging agents are well within tolerable limits of exposure to radiation. The small quantities used produce no pharmacologic effects or hypersensitivity. Actually, the radiation exposure during radioactive imaging is often lower than that during a routine X-ray. Nevertheless, unnecessary exposure to even these low levels of radiation must be avoided. Children, and persons of reproductive age should receive the *minimum* effective dose; patients who are pregnant should receive radioactive imaging agents only when their use is unavoidable.

Radiation precautions

Federal guidelines mandate the maximum permissible doses for occupational exposure to radiation. These guidelines require that all persons exposed to radiation must wear film badges that measure and record the level of exposure. Such precautions are most critical during exposure to gamma rays, because gamma rays penetrate so deeply into body tissues. Potential exposure to gamma radiation necessitates a shield of high-density material, such as lead, and strict observance of safety rules. Such rules restrict work to the greatest possible distance from the source of radiation and limit exposure to the shortest possible time.

To prevent contamination from radioactive spillage, all work with unsealed radioactive materials should be done on disposable and absorbent materials. Radioactive substances should always be mixed under a hood by workers who wear masks to prevent inhalation of radioactive particles. Such workers should also wear disposable rubber or plastic gloves and wash their hands frequently. They must also carefully segregate radioactive wastes from uncontaminated wastes and dispose of them safely. They should never eat or smoke in potentially contaminated areas.

DIAGNOSTIC IMAGING AGENTS

AGENT AND DIAGNOSTIC USE	PATIENT PREPARATION	NURSING CONSIDERATIONS
Contrast Imaging Agents		
acetrizoate sodium Cystokon, Pyelokon-R, Salpix		
Excretory urography, nephrography, nephrotomography, retrograde pyelography, hysterosalpingography	Nothing by mouth after midnight before examination	Administered by slow I.V. infusion. Drug has been used for a variety of diagnostic procedures but has been largely replaced by better-tolerated compounds.
barium sulfate *Oral:* Baridol, Barosperse, Barotrast, and Oratrast among others		
Esophagography, upper gastroenterography	No solid foods after dinner the evening before examination; nothing by mouth after midnight, after initial film, and before 3-hour delayed film	Constipation is common if barium is not completely evacuated; laxatives may be necessary.
Rectal: Baridol, Barosperse, and Barotrast among others		
Lower gastroenterography, or barium enema	Liquid dinner before examination, no solids thereafter; laxative late afternoon of day before examination or Dulcolax after meals; soapsuds enema morning of examination; enema or suppository immediately before examination	Barium in the peritoneal cavity can cause peritonitis and dense intestinal adhesions that may require surgery. *Note:* Do not confuse barium *sulfate* with barium *sulfide* or barium *sulfite;* the latter two are poisons.
diatrizoate meglumine or **diatrizoate sodium** *Oral or rectal:* Hypaque Sodium		
Esophagography, upper and lower gastroenterography	No solid foods after dinner evening before examination; nothing by mouth after midnight, after initial film, and before 3-hour delayed film.	Agent is acceptable substitute if patient is allergic to barium sulfate. If used for examination of lower bowel (enema), preparation same as for barium enema.
Transurethral: Cystografin		
Retrograde cystourethrography	A laxative the night before test, and a low-residue diet the day before test are recommended.	After sterile catheterization, bladder should be filled to capacity with Cystografin. Reflux of solution or bladder discomfort indicates full bladder.
Rectal: Gastrografin		
Lower gastroenterography	Liquid dinner before examination, no solids thereafter; laxative (citrate of magnesia or X-Prep) late afternoon of day before examination, or Dulcolax after meals; soapsuds enema morning of examination; enema or suppository immediately before examination	May give orally for upper gastrointestinal (GI) tract examinations. Follow standard upper GI examination preparation. Drug is a good substitute for barium. Suggested enema dilution for adults is 240 ml of drug in 1,000 ml tap water; for children over age 5, 90 ml of drug in 500 ml of water.

AGENT AND DIAGNOSTIC USE	PATIENT PREPARATION	NURSING CONSIDERATIONS
diatrizoate meglumine or **diatrizoate sodium** *(continued)*		
I.V. push: Cardiografin, Renografin, Reno-M-60, Renovist*		
Angiocardiography, angiography, translumbar aortography, venography	Nothing by mouth after midnight; light sedative and local anesthetic required; light anesthetic may be required.	Examination may be performed in OR, especially if left-sided cardiac catheterization is to be performed. Special consent form may be required; check institution protocol.
Arthrography, diskography	Local anesthetic or sedative required.	Inadvertent injection into subarachnoid space can cause fatal convulsions.
Cerebral angiography	Light sedative required; nothing by mouth from midnight before examination.	Check institution protocol for special consent form requirements.
Computerized tomography (CT scan)	Depends on area to be scanned	Patient must lie completely still for test. Special consent form may be required.
Direct cholangiography	None	Examination carried out during surgery under general anesthetic.
Hysterosalpingography	Preexamination douche, emptying of bladder, and sedative required.	Patient may be nervous and require reassurance.
Splenoportography	Prior GI series and hematologic survey required; nothing by mouth for several hours before test; mild sedation given; local anesthetic usually necessary.	Special consent may be required.
Localization of placenta	Variable	1 ml of drug is injected by doctor or radiologist into amnionic sac. Not a routine test but may be used to diagnose placenta previa in patient with painless bleeding during third trimester.
Neoplastic effusions	Depends on location and type of effusion	Drug is instilled by doctor or radiologist into the pleural (25 to 30 ml), peritoneal (25 to 60 ml), or tumor cavity after aspiration of most of the fluid. Test permits delineation of tumor mass and assessment of cavity size and distribution of fluids within. Not a routine test. *Note:* Do not mix diphenhydramine or promethazine hydrochloride with either form of diatrizoate; precipitate will form. Protect drug from light.
Continuous I.V. infusion: Reno-M-30		
Excretory urography	Laxative the night before test, and low-residue diet the day before test are recommended.	Urography contraindicated in patients with anuria.

* Several forms of Renografin and Renovist available. Drug selected depends on test. Not all forms of drug appropriate for all tests.

DIAGNOSTIC IMAGING AGENTS *(continued)*

AGENT AND DIAGNOSTIC USE	PATIENT PREPARATION	NURSING CONSIDERATIONS
diatrizoate meglumine or **diatrizoate sodium** *(continued)*		
Urethral instillation: Reno-M-60		
Retrograde pyelography	Low-residue diet the day before test, and laxative the night before test are recommended. Nothing by mouth after midnight.	Post-test oliguria or anuria may develop.
ethiodized oil Ethiodol		
Lymphangiography	Local anesthetic and subcutaneous injection of 1 to 2 ml of 1% Patent Blue dye into first and second interdigital spaces of foot is done by radiologist.	Agent is injected slowly through lymphatic vessels. Penetration of venous system and pulmonary capillaries by agent can cause cerebral, hepatic, and pulmonary emboli as well as foreign-body granulomas.
iocetamic acid Cholebrine		
Oral cholecystography	Normal diet permitted 1 to 2 days before examination and fat-free meal immediately before administration of drug the evening before test. Nothing by mouth except water 10 to 15 hours before examination.	Encourage patient with mild-to-moderate renal impairment to take fluids. Agent is contraindicated in severe hepatorenal disease. Laxatives may prevent proper absorption.
iodipamide meglumine Cholografin		
Cholangiography, cholecystography	Low-residue diet for day before examination. Nothing by mouth except water after midnight. Either castor oil 4 to 6 hours before, or neostigmine at time of examination is given to dispel gas from bowel.	Infuse agent slowly (about 10 minutes). Agent appears in bile within 10 to 15 minutes. *Note:* Don't mix diphenhydramine or promethazine hydrochloride with this drug; precipitate will form. For I.V. use only. Protect from light and heat.
iopanoic acid Telepaque		
Oral cholecystography	Normal diet (i.e., with some fats) permitted 1 to 2 days before examination; fat-free meal immediately before administration of drug evening before examination. Nothing by mouth except water after midnight. An enema may be given before the test to remove gas from bowel.	Administer agent 12 to 14 hours before examination. Urge patient with mild-to-moderate renal impairment to take fluids. Contraindicated in patient with uricosuria or severe hepatorenal disease. Concomitant administration of drugs that cause stomach emptying can impair absorption.
iophendylate Pantopaque		
Myelography	Premedication with sedative or tranquilizer, and local anesthetic is necessary.	Special consent form required. Agent is given intrathecally by radiologist or doctor; after instilla-

AGENT AND DIAGNOSTIC USE	PATIENT PREPARATION	NURSING CONSIDERATIONS
iophendylate *(continued)*		tion, needle is left in place to remove agent at end of test. Test may be done in OR. Patient may have to lie flat for several hours after test to prevent postexamination headache. Contraindicated when lumbar puncture (LP) contraindicated and within 14 days of previous LP.
iothalamate meglumine or **iothalamate sodium** Angio-Conray, Conray-280*, Conray-325, Conray-420, Conray-480, Retro-Conray		
Peripheral angiography, venography	Premedication with sedative or tranquilizer, and local anesthetic needed; general anesthetic may be needed. Nothing by mouth from midnight before test.	Check institution protocol for special consent form requirements. Examination may be performed in OR or special procedures room.
Cerebral angiography	Premedication with sedative or tranquilizer, and local anesthetic needed; light general anesthetic may be required; nothing by mouth after midnight before test.	Check institution protocol for special consent form requirements. Examination may be performed in OR.
Excretory urography	Low-residue diet and laxative the day before examination; fluids must be restricted.	Monitor intake and output following test. *Note:* Drug incompatible with promethazine hydrochloride (Sparine); precipitate will form.
ipodate calcium or **ipodate sodium** Oragrafin Calcium, Oragrafin Sodium		
Oral cholecystography, oral cholangiography	Normal diet (i.e., with some fats) permitted 1 to 2 days before examination; fat-free meal immediately before administration of drug evening before examination. Mild laxative may be given but is usually not necessary. Nothing by mouth except water after ingestion of agent and until examination is completed.	Neither form is agent of choice for cholangiography; rapid cholangiography is possible 1 hour after ingestion. If necessary, a repeat dose is given the evening of the first test; give no more than 12 capsules in 24 hours. Ipodate calcium is more rapidly absorbed that ipodate sodium. Carefully monitor blood pressure of patient with heart disease. Keep patient with hyperuricemia well hydrated to prevent urate crystalluria, uric acid nephropathy, and renal failure. Use with caution in patient with known sensitivity to iodine and iodinated compounds.
methiodal sodium Skiodan		
Retrograde pyelography, I.V. pyelography	Nothing by mouth, including fluids, after midnight before ex-	Heat redissolves precipitated crystals. Retrograde pyelography

* Numbers indicate solution strength. Not all solutions are suitable for all examinations.

DIAGNOSTIC IMAGING AGENTS *(continued)*

AGENT AND DIAGNOSTIC USE	PATIENT PREPARATION	NURSING CONSIDERATIONS
methiodal sodium *(continued)*	amination; local anesthetic may be required.	can cause oliguria, anuria, and renal shutdown. I.V. injection of drug produces diuretic effect.
metrizoate sodium Isopaque 440, Triosil		
Peripheral arteriography, cerebral angiography	Premedication with sedative or tranquilizer is necessary. Nothing by mouth after midnight before tests.	*For cerebral angiography only:* Inadvertent injection into subarachnoid space can cause fatal convulsions.
Excretory urography	Fluid restriction 12 to 15 hours before examination; laxative can dispel gas from bowel; sedative may be needed.	Assess urinary function by monitoring postexamination output.
tyropanoate sodium Bilopaque		
Oral cholecystography	Normal diet (i.e., with some fats) permitted 1 to 2 days before examination; fat-free meal immediately before administration of drug evening before examination. Nothing by mouth except water. Withhold tobacco and chewing gum. Laxative or enema can be given to dispel gas from bowel. Sedative may be required.	Agent is contraindicated in patients with severe gastrointestinal or hepatorenal disease; these conditions reduce drug's absorption. Concomitant administration of drugs that produce stomach-emptying may impair tyropanoate absorption.
Radioactive imaging agents		
chromated Cr 51 erythrocytes Chromalbin		
Determinations of red cell mass and survival, and blood volume	None	Blood transfusions just before test or significant blood loss during test can cause inaccurate results.
cyanocobalamin Co 57 Racobalamin-57, Cyanocobalamin Co 57, Rubratope-57		
Determination of vitamin B_{12} absorption	Nothing by mouth	Immediately after administration of agent, 24-hour urine collection started; 48-hour collection is required for patients with renal failure. Two hours after administration of agent, patient should receive 1 mg of vitamin B_{12} I.M. X-ray studies using barium interfere with test results; do not give laxatives on day of test.
ferrous citrate Fe 59 Ferrous Citrate Fe 59		
Determination of iron turnover capability	None	Blood transfusions just before test or significant blood loss during test can cause inaccurate results.

AGENT AND DIAGNOSTIC USE	PATIENT PREPARATION	NURSING CONSIDERATIONS
gallium citrate Ga 67 Imaging of abscesses and tumors	Laxative on evening before test and enema on day of test are required.	Test should be performed 24 to 48 hours after administration of agent; barium in bowel can interfere with test.
indium chloride In 111 Imaging of abscesses, bone marrow, and tumors	None	Test should be performed 24 to 48 hours after administration of agent; barium in bowel can interfere with test.
indium DTPA In 111 Imaging of cerebrospinal fluid pathway	Sedative may be required; local anesthetic is applied at injection site.	Check institution protocol for special consent form requirements. Agent administered intrathecally. Patient may have to lie flat for several hours after test to prevent spinal headache. Barium in bowel can interfere with test. Test may be performed in OR or special procedures room.
iodinated I 125 serum albumin Albumotope I-125 Determination of plasma and blood volumes, detection of thrombi	Premedication and local anesthetic required if drug is administered intrathecally for study of hydrocephalus.	Useful for ventricular scanning in hydrocephalus; consent form may be required.
iodinated I 131 serum albumin Albumotope I-131 Determination of plasma and blood volumes, detection of thrombi	Premedication and local anesthetic required if drug is administered intrathecally for study of hydrocephalus.	Useful for ventricular scanning in hydrocephalus; consent form may be required.
iodohippurate sodium I 131 Hippuran-131, Hippuran I 131, Hipputope Determination of kidney function	Patient should be well hydrated on day of test.	Patient should receive 8 to 10 drops saturated solution of potassium iodide (SSKI) bid for 2 days after administration of agent. Renal X-ray studies on day of test can interfere with results.
rose bengal sodium I 131 Robengatope, Sodium Rose Bengal I 131 Determination of gallbladder patency and liver function	Depends on type of testing to be done	Test can be performed on patient with history of iodine hypersensitivity. Patient should receive 8 to 10 drops of SSKI bid for 2 days

DIAGNOSTIC IMAGING AGENTS *(continued)*

AGENT AND DIAGNOSTIC USE	PATIENT PREPARATION	NURSING CONSIDERATIONS
rose bengal sodium I 131 *(continued)*		after administration of agent. Tell patient stool will be red until drug is completely eliminated.
selenium Se 75 Selenomethionine Se 75, Sethotope		
Determination of pancreatic function; organ scanning	Nothing by mouth 8 hours before test, then high-protein, low-carbohydrate breakfast immediately before administration of agent (pancreatic function).	Barium in bowel can interfere with test.
sodium iodide I 131 Iodotope, Iodotope Therapeutic, Oriodide-131, Oriodide-131-H, Radiocaps-131, Theriodide-131		
Determination of thyroid uptake measurement and imaging	For detection of recurrent thyroid carcinoma, thyroid hormone should be discontinued or thyroid-stimulating hormone administered I.M. (10 units daily) for 3 days before test.	High doses destroy thyroid cells and are used to treat thyroid cancer; iodinated I 131 has an affinity for thyroid tissue anywhere in the body, as in metastasis; radioactivity of I 131 then destroys thyroid cells. Diagnostic test performed 2 hours after administration of agent. Ingestion of iodinated contrast agents and iodine-containing drugs before test can interfere with results. Urine contains radioactive material for several days after test; dispose of properly.
sodium pertechnetate Tc 99m		
Imaging of brain, Meckel's diverticulum, and thyroid function	Sodium or potassium perchlorate given immediately before administration of agent in test for brain function to prevent agent's uptake by choroid plexus and salivary and thyroid glands; perchlorate not given for thyroid or Meckel's diverticulum tests.	Patient's urine contains low levels of radioactive material; wear disposable gloves when disposing of urine.
technetium Tc 99m Imidoacetic acid		
Imaging of gallbladder patency and liver function	Variable	Patient must lie very still during test.
technetium Tc 99m albumin aggregated		
Imaging of CSF leakage and blood pooling, especially during cardiac cycle	Sedative may be needed before lumbar puncture for instillation of agent; local anesthetic necessary.	Patient may have to lie flat for several hours after lumbar puncture, to prevent spinal headache.

AGENT AND DIAGNOSTIC USE	PATIENT PREPARATION	NURSING CONSIDERATIONS
technetium Tc 99m albumin macroaggregated		
Imaging of lung perfusion, detection of thrombi	Variable	Following I.V. injection of tracer, particles become trapped in lung and define ischemic areas. Check institution protocol for special consent form requirements.
technetium Tc 99m erythrocytes		
Determination of red cell mass and survival, and blood volume; blood pool imaging, especially during cardiac cycle	Variable	Blood transfusions just before test or significant blood loss during test can cause inaccurate results.
technetium Tc 99m glucoheptonate		
Imaging of brain and of kidney function	Variable	Patient must lie still during test; sedative may be necessary for uncooperative patient.
technetium Tc 99m phosphate complexes		
Imaging of acute myocardial infarction (MI) and bone marrow integrity	Sedative may be required if patient can't remain supine during test (about 45 minutes).	Detection of acute MI is accurate only 2 to 10 days after symptoms develop. Patient's urine contains radioactive material; wear disposable gloves when disposing of urine.
technetium Tc 99m sulfur colloid		
Imaging of bone marrow integrity, and liver and spleen function	Variable	Barium in bowel can interfere with liver and spleen tests.
thallium Tl 201 chloride		
Imaging of myocardial infarction (MI)	Variable	Agent can detect MI in patient at any age. Can differentiate between old and new infarcts.
xenon Xe 133		
Imaging of lung ventilation	Explain to patient that drug will be injected I.V.	Xenon Xe 133 is given I.V.; xenon gas is rapidly excreted by the lungs; radioactivity is measured by external detectors over chest.
ytterbium TB 169 DTPA		
Imaging of cerebrospinal fluid pathway	Sedative may be required; local anesthetic applied at injection site.	Agent administered intrathecally. Patient may have to lie flat several hours after test to prevent spinal headache.

DRUGS THAT INFLUENCE LABORATORY TEST VALUES

The following list of selected drugs summarizes their effects on results of clinical laboratory tests. These effects can result not only from direct interference with the laboratory procedure employed, but from the drugs' pharmacologic properties as well.

An example of procedural interference is seen in ascorbic acid's effect on SMA 12/60 measurement of the serum bilirubin level. The presence of ascorbic acid falsely elevates the serum bilirubin level in blood samples analyzed by the SMA 12/60, but

TEST / DRUG	TEST RESULT BLOOD	TEST RESULT URINE
Aldolase, serum		
aminocaproic acid	▲	
clofibrate	▲	
corticotropin (I.M.)	▲	
ethyl alcohol	▲	
narcotic analgesics (overdose)	▲	
probucol	▼	
Alkaline phosphatase, serum		
albumin infusions	▲	
anticonvulsants	▲	
clofibrate	▼	
Ammonia, blood		
acetazolamide	▲	
ammonium chloride	▲	
asparaginase	▲	
barbiturates	▲	
chlorthalidone	▲	
diphenhydramine	▼	
ethyl alcohol	▲	
furosemide	▲	
kanamycin	▼	
Lactobacillus acidophilus	▼	
lactulose	▼	
levodopa	▼	
mercurial diuretics	▲	
narcotic analgesics	▲	
neomycin	▼	
thiazide diuretics	▲	
Amylase, serum		
asparaginase	▲	
azathioprine	▲	
calcium infusion	▲	
chlorthalidone	▲	
contraceptives, oral	▲	
contrast media, iodinated	▲	
corticosteriods	▲	
cyproheptadine	▲	
ethacrynic acid	▲	
ethyl alcohol	▲	
furosemide	▲	
histamine	▲	
indomethacin	▲	
isoniazid	▲	
methyldopa	▲	
oxyphenbutazone	▲	
pancreatic extracts	▲	
para-aminosalicylic acid	▲	
pentazocine	▲	
procainamide	▲	
rifampin	▲	
salicylates	▲	
sulfasalazine	▲	
sulfamethizole	▲	
tetracyclines	▲	
thiazide diuretics	▲	
Antiglobulin (Coombs') test, direct		
amphotericin B	+	
ampicillin	+	

KEY: ▲ = increased by drug; ▼ = decreased by drug; + = positive effect; ☒ = variable effect; □ = no effect

not in samples analyzed by other methods. An example of pharmacologic interference is the effect of thiazide diuretics on the serum potassium level. Thiazides promote exaggerated excretion of potassium, which, in turn, may lead to hypokalemia.

Obviously, many other factors can also influence the results of laboratory tests. Nevertheless, the following information should help you evaluate how drugs may affect your patient's laboratory tests and therapy.

TEST / DRUG	TEST RESULT BLOOD	TEST RESULT URINE
Antiglobulin (Coombs') test, direct *(continued)*		
cephalosporins	+	
chlorpropamide	+	
cyclophosphamide	+	
ethosuximide	+	
hydralazine	+	
indomethacin	+	
isoniazid	+	
levodopa	+	
mefenamic acid	+	
mephenytoin	+	
methadone	+	
methyldopa	+	
methysergide	+	
penicillins	+	
phenacetin	+	
phenothiazines	+	
phenylbutazone	+	
phenytoin	+	
quinidine	+	
quinine	+	
rifampin	+	
tolbutamide	+	
Bilirubin, serum		
ascorbic acid	▲ or ▼	
barbiturates	▼	
contrast media, iodinated	▲	
epinephrine	▲	
ethyl alcohol	▼	
fat emulsion	▲	
iron dextran	▲	
isoproterenol	▲	
Bilirubin, serum *(continued)*		
levodopa	▲	
methyldopa	▲	
monoamine oxidase inhibitors	▲	
novobiocin	▲	
oxytocic agents	▲	
rifampin	▲	
Bilirubin, urine		
ethoxazene		+
mefenamic acid		+
phenazopyridine		+
phenothiazines		+
Catecholamines, urine		
aminophylline		▲
antidepressants, tricyclic		▲
caffeine		▲
clonidine		▼
contrast media, iodinated		▼
epinephrine inhalation		▲
ethyl alcohol		▲
glucagon		▲
guanethidine		▼
insulin		▲
isoproterenol		▲
levodopa		▲
methenamine compounds		▲
methyldopa		▲
nitroglycerin		▲
quinidine		▲
quinine		▲

DRUGS THAT INFLUENCE LABORATORY TEST VALUES *(continued)*

TEST / DRUG	TEST RESULT BLOOD	TEST RESULT URINE
Catecholamines, urine *(continued)*		
reserpine		▼
sympathomimetics		▲
tetracyclines		▲
vitamin B complex		▲
Ceruloplasmin, serum		
estrogens	▲	
methadone	▲	
phenytoin	▲	
Cholinesterase, serum		
contraceptives, oral	▼	
cyclophosphamide	▼	
echothiophate iodide	▼	
monoamine oxidase inhibitors	▼	
pancuronium bromide	▼	
phenothiazines	▼	
Corticosteroids, plasma		
calcium gluconate	▲	
dextroamphetamine	▲	
estrogens	▲	
ethyl alcohol	▲	
heparin	▲	
lithium carbonate	▼	
methamphetamine	▲	
methoxamine	▲	
nicotine	▲	
spironolactone	▲	
vasopressin	▲	
Creatine phosphokinase (CPK), serum		
aminocaproic acid	▲	
amphetamines (I.V.)	▲	
amphotericin B	▲	
ampicillin (I.M.)	▲	
barbiturates (I.M.)	▲	
carbenicillin (I.M.)	▲	
chlorpromazine (I.M.)	▲	
chlorthalidone	▲	
clindamycin (I.M.)	▲	
clofibrate	▲	
digitalis glycosides (I.M.)	▲	
ethyl alcohol	▲	
insulin	▲	
lidocaine (I.M.)	▲	
methyldopa	▲	
morphine	▲	
penicillamine	▲	
phenmetrazine (I.V.)	▲	
tubocurarine	▲	
Gamma glutamyl transferase (transpeptidase), serum		
aminoglycosides	▲	
barbiturates	▲	
benzodiazepines	▲	
clofibrate	▼	
contraceptives, oral	▼	
ethyl alcohol	▲	
phenytoin	▲	
streptokinase	▲	

KEY: ▲ = increased by drug; ▼ = decreased by drug; + = positive effect; ☒ = variable effect; ☐ = no effect

TEST / DRUG	TEST RESULT BLOOD	TEST RESULT URINE
Glucose, blood		
acetaminophen	▼	
acetazolamide	▲	
amphetamines	▼	
anabolic steroids	▼	
antidepressants, tricyclic	▲	
arginine (L-arginine)	▲	
benzodiazepines	▲	
caffeine	▲	
chlorthalidone	▲	
clofibrate	▼	
clonidine	▲	
corticosteroids	▲	
cyproheptadine	▼	
dextrans	▲	
dextrothyroxine	▲	
diazoxide	▲	
epinephrine	▲	
ethacrynic acid	▲	
fenfluramine	▼	
furosemide	▲	
guanethidine	▼	
haloperidol	▼	
heparin	▲	
indomethacin	▲	
levodopa	▲	
lithium carbonate	▲	
marijuana	▼	
monoamine oxidase inhibitors	▼	
morphine	▲	
nalidixic acid	▲	
nicotinic acid	▲	
nitrofurantoin	▲	
oxytetracycline	▼	
pentamidine	▼	
phenolphthalein	▲	

TEST / DRUG	TEST RESULT BLOOD	TEST RESULT URINE
Glucose, blood *(continued)*		
phenothiazines	▲	
phenytoin	▲	
propranolol	▼	
propoxyphene	▼	
reserpine	▲	
salicylates	▲ or ▼	
thiabendazole	▲	
thiazide diuretics	▲	
triamterene	▲	
tromethamine	▼	
Glucose, urine		
ascorbic acid		▲
carbamazepine		▲
cephalosporins		▲
chloral hydrate		▲
chloramphenicol		▲
corticosteroids		▲
dextrothyroxine		▲
EDTA		▲
furazolidone		▲
isoniazid		▲
levodopa		▲ or ▼
lithium carbonate		▲
metaxalone		▲
methyldopa		▲
morphine		▲
nalidixic acid		▲
nicotinic acid		▲
nitrofurantoin		▲
para-aminosalicylic acid		▲
penicillin G		▲
phenacetin		▲
phenazopyridine		▼
phenothiazines		▲
probenecid		▲
sulfonamides		▲

DRUGS THAT INFLUENCE LABORATORY TEST VALUES *(continued)*

TEST / DRUG	TEST RESULT BLOOD	TEST RESULT URINE
Glucose, urine *(continued)*		
tetracyclines		▲
thiazide diuretics		▲
Growth hormone, serum		
amphetamines	▲	
bromocriptine	▲	
levodopa	▲	
methysergide	▼	
metyrapone	▲	
nicotine	▲	
nicotinic acid	▲	
5-Hydroxyindoleacetic acid (5-HIAA), urine		
antidepressants, tricyclic		▼
caffeine		▲
corticotropin		▼
ethyl alcohol		▼
fluorouracil		▲
guaifenesin		▲
heparin		▼
isoniazid		▼
levodopa		▼
melphalan		▲
methamphetamine		▲
methocarbamol		▲
methyldopa		▼
monoamine oxidase inhibitors		▼
phenmetrazine		▲
phenothiazines		▼
reserpine		▲
Ketones, urine		
insulin		▲
isoniazid		▲
Ketones, urine *(continued)*		
isopropyl alcohol		▲
paraldehyde		▲
Lactate (lactic acid), blood		
epinephrine	▲	
ethyl alcohol	▲	
fructose	▲	
glucose infusions	▲	
isoniazid	▲	
lactate infusions	▲	
methylene blue	▼	
morphine	▼	
nitrofurantoin	▲	
phenformin*	▲	
sodium bicarbonate	▲	
sodium nitroprusside	▲	
streptozocin	▲	
Lipids, serum		
allopurinol	▲	
anabolic steroids	▲	
antidiabetic drugs	▼	
bromide	▲	
chlortetracycline	▼	
cholestyramine	▼	
clofibrate	▼	
colchicine	▼	
contraceptives, oral	▲	
dextrothyroxine	▼	
disulfiram	▲	
epinephrine	▲	
estrogens	▲	
ethyl alcohol	▲	

KEY: ▲ = increased by drug; ▼ = decreased by drug; + = positive effect; ☒ = variable effect; ☐ = no effect

TEST / DRUG	TEST RESULT BLOOD	TEST RESULT URINE
Lipids, serum *(continued)*		
furosemide	▲	
glucagon	▼	
heparin	▼	
kanamycin	▼	
levodopa	▲	
lincomycin	▲	
metyrapone	▼	
miconazole	▲	
neomycin	▼	
nicotinic acid	▼	
norepinephrine	▲	
para-aminosalicylic acid	▼	
paromomycin	▼	
penicillamine	▲	
pentylenetetrazol	▼	
phenothiazines	▲	
phenytoin	▲	
salicylates	▼	
sitosterols	▼	
Magnesium, serum		
aminoglycosides	▼	
ammonium chloride	▲	
calcium salts	▼	
contraceptives, oral	▼	
ethacrynic acid	▲	
ethyl alcohol	▼	
insulin	▲	
lithium carbonate	▲	
magnesium products	▲	
mercurial diuretics	▲	
triamterene	▲	
vitamin D	▲	
Phenolsulfonphthalein (PSP), urine		
danthron		▲
ethoxazene		▲
penicillins		▼
phenolphthalein		▲
salicylates		▼
sulfonamides		▼
thiazide diuretics		▼
Potassium, serum		
aminocaproic acid	▲	
aminosalicylic acid	▼	
amphotericin B	▼	
ampicillin	▼	
antineoplastic agents	▲	
carbenicillin	▼	
chlorthalidone	▼	
corticosteroids	▼	
ethacrynic acid	▼	
furosemide	▼	
glucagon	▲	
glucose	▼	
indomethacin	▲	
insulin	▼	
isoniazid	▲	
laxatives	▼	
levodopa	▼	
lithium carbonate	▼	
mannitol infusions	▲	
penicillin G potassium	▲	
penicillin G sodium	▼	
polymixin B	▼	
salicylates	▼	

* Formerly a major cause of lactic acidosis; no longer approved for use in diabetes.

DRUGS THAT INFLUENCE LABORATORY TEST VALUES *(continued)*

TEST / DRUG	TEST RESULT BLOOD	TEST RESULT URINE
Potassium, serum *(continued)*		
salt substitutes	▲	
spironolactone	▲	
succinylcholine	▲	
thiazide diuretics	▼	
triamterene	▲	
Prolactin, serum		
apomorphine	▼	
carbidopa	▲	
cimetidine	▲	
contraceptives, oral	▲	
ergot alkaloids	▼	
estrogens	▲	
ethyl alcohol	▲	
haloperidol	▲	
levodopa	▼	
methyldopa	▲	
metoclopramide	▲	
monoamine oxidase inhibitors	▲	
phenothiazines	▲	
reserpine	▲	
thiothixene	▲	
Protein, urine		
acetazolamide		▲
amphotericin B		▲
bacitracin		▲
cephalosporins		▲
colistin		▲
corticosteroids		▲
dextrans		▲
gold salts		▲
griseofulvin		▲
isoniazid		▲
kanamycin		▲
levodopa		▲
Protein, urine *(continued)*		
lithium carbonate		▲
mefenamic acid		▲
metaxalone		▲
methicillin		▲
nafcillin		▲
neomycin		▲
para-aminosalicylic acid		▲
paramethadione		▲
penicillamine		▲
penicillins		▲
phenindione		▲
phenylbutazone		▲
polymixin B		▲
probenicid		▲
salicylates		▲
sodium bicarbonate		▲
streptomycin		▲
sulfonamides		▲
sulfones		▲
thiabendazole		▲
tolbutamide		▲
tolmetin		▲
trimethadione		▲
Steroids, urine		
aminoglutethimide		▼
calcium gluconate		▼
carbamazepine		▼
cephalosporins		▲
chlordiazepoxide		▲
chlorthalidone		▲
contraceptives, oral		▼
corticosteroids		▼

KEY: ▲ = increased by drug; ▼ = decreased by drug; + = positive effect; ⊠ = variable effect; □ = no effect

TEST / DRUG	TEST RESULT BLOOD	/ URINE
Steroids, urine *(continued)*		
corticotropin		▲
ethacrynic acid		▼
gonadotropins		▲
hydrochloro-thiazide		▼
meprobamate		▲
methenamine compounds		▲
nalidixic acid		▲
penicillin G		▲
pentazocine		▼
phenytoin		▼
probenecid		▼
propoxyphene		▼
pyrazinamide		▼
reserpine		▼
salicylates (large doses)		☒ or ☐
sodium chloride		▲
troleandomycin		▲
Sulfobromo-phthalein (BSP) excretion		
anabolic ste-roids	▲	
barbiturates	▲	
contraceptives, oral	▲	
ethoxazene	▲	
heparin	▲	
meperidine	▲	
methadone	▲	
phenazopyridine	▲	
phenolphthalein	▲	
probenecid	▲	
sulfonamides	▲	
Thyroid function, serum PBI		
anabolic steroids	▼	
Thyroid function, serum PBI *(continued)*		
androgens	▼	
bromides	▲	
corticosteroids	▲ or ▼	
dextrothyroxine	▲	
diiodohydroxy-quin	▲	
estrogens	▲	
ethionamide	▼	
gold salts	▼	
inorganic io-dides	▲	
iodochlorhy-droxyquin	▲	
levodopa	▲	
mercurial diuret-ics	▼	
methadone	▲	
methimazole	▼	
para-aminosali-cylic acid	▼	
phenothiazines	▼	
phenylbutazone	▼	
phenytoin	▼	
propranolol	▼	
propylthiouracil	▼	
pyrazinamide	▲	
resorcinol	▼	
salicylates	▼	
sodium nitro-prusside	▼	
sulfonamides	▼	
thiazide diuret-ics	▼	
thyroid, desic-cated	▲	
thyroxine	▲	
triiodothyronine	▼	
Uric acid, serum		
acetazolamide	▲	

DRUGS THAT INFLUENCE LABORATORY TEST VALUES *(continued)*

TEST / DRUG	TEST RESULT BLOOD	TEST RESULT URINE
Uric acid, serum *(continued)*		
acetohexamide	▼	
aminophylline	▲	
anticholinergics	▼	
ascorbic acid	▲	
azathioprine	▼	
chlorprothixene	▼	
chlorthalidone	▲	
clofibrate	▼ or ☐	
corticosteroids	▼	
coumarin	▼	
diazoxide	▲	
epinephrine	▲	
ethacrynic acid	▲	
ethambutol	▲	
ethyl alcohol	▲	
fenoprofen	▼	
furosemide	▲	
gentamicin	▲	
glucose	▼	
griseofulvin	▼	
guaifenesin	▼	
levodopa	▲	
lithium carbonate	▼	
mannitol	▼	
mecamylamine	▲	
mercurial diuretics	▲	
methotrexate	▲	
nicotinic acid	▲	
norepinephrine	▲	
phenothiazines	▲	
phenylbutazone	▼	
pyrazinamide	▲	
quinethazone	▲	
salicylates	☒	
saline infusions	▼	
spironolactone	☐	
thiazide diuretics	▲	
triamterene	▲	
Urobilinogen, urine		
acetazolamide		▲
ammonium chloride		▼
ascorbic acid		▼
Vanillylmandelic acid (VMA), urine		
anileridine		▲
chlorpromazine		▼
clonidine		▼
disulfiram		▼
epinephrine		▲
guanethidine		▼
imipramine		▼
insulin (large doses)		▲
isoproterenol		▲
levodopa		▲
lithium carbonate		▲
methocarbamol		▲
monoamine oxidase inhibitors		▼
morphine		▼
nitroglycerin		▲
norepinephrine		▲
para-aminosalicylic acid		▲
pentobarbital		▼
reserpine		▲
salicylates		▲

KEY: ▲ = increased by drug
▼ = decreased by drug
+ = positive effect
☒ = variable effect
☐ = no effect

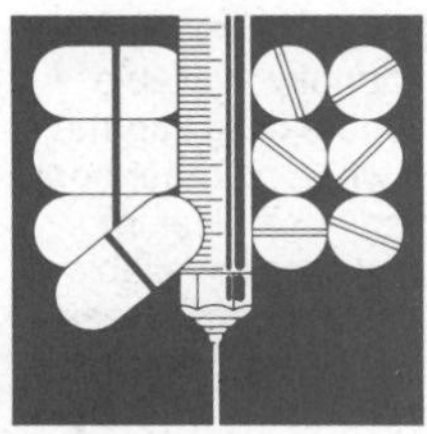

Selected references and further reading

An annotated guide

I General Drug Information and Pharmacology

Bergersen, Betty: *Pharmacology in Nursing,* 14th ed. St. Louis: C.V. Mosby Co., 1979.

Outlines current concepts of pharmacology and their relationship to clinical patient care. A discussion of individual drugs follows the pharmacologic principles in each chapter. A widely used, comprehensive nursing pharmacology text.

Gilman, Alfred G., et al.: *The Pharmacological Basis of Therapeutics,* 6th ed. New York: Macmillan Pub. Co., 1980.

Generally recognized as the standard pharmacology reference. Emphasizes biochemical and physiologic reasons for drug action and effect, rather than on-the-floor drug use. A required text for medical and pharmacy students.

Melmon, K.L., and Morrelli, H.F.: *Clinical Pharmacology: Basic Principles in Therapeutics,* 2nd ed. New York: Macmillan Pub. Co., 1978.

Primarily for clinical pharmacologists and progressive doctors, this rather advanced book concentrates on clinical application of therapeutic principles, integrating pharmacology, physiology, and pathophysiology. Arranged according to diseases and disorders, the text discusses different therapeutic treatment options.

Rodman, Morton J., and Smith, Dorothy W.: *Pharmacology and Drug Therapy in Nursing,* 2nd ed. Philadelphia: J.B. Lippincott Co., 1979.

In this text, drugs are classified according to system, site, or mode of action. Each chapter contains pharmacology principles, drug subclasses and individual drugs, and drug digests on the most frequently used and/or prototype drugs of the class. Includes pathophysiology and nursing implications. One of the most widely used nursing pharmacology texts.

Wiener, Matthew B., et al.: *Clinical Pharmacology and Therapeutics in Nursing.* New York: McGraw-Hill Book Co., 1979.

A basic pharmacology textbook in which drug therapy is integrally related to the nursing process of holistic care. Includes pharmacologic principles and individual drugs classified by their system or effect. Each chapter concludes with a nursing process approach to patient care for the class of drugs, and case studies.

II Clinical Drug References

Books

Albanese, Joseph A.: *Nurse's Drug Reference.* New York: McGraw-Hill Book Co., 1979.

Drug monographs listed alphabetically by generic name. Each monograph contains basic drug information, including classification; trade names; legal status; pharmacologic mechanism, use and dosage ranges; dispensing and patient instructions; contraindications and warnings; nursing implications; and drug and laboratory test interactions.

AMA Drug Evaluations, 4th ed. Chicago: American Medical Association, 1980.

A joint effort of the AMA Department of Drugs and the American Society for Clinical Pharmacology and Therapeutics. Includes individual drug monographs and general subject introductions. Unbiased opinions of pharmacology experts rather than manufacturers.

American Hospital Formulary Service, 2 vols. Bethesda, Md.: American Society of Hospital Pharmacists, 1982.

Known as the "formulary" to many health-care professionals, this two-volume loose-leaf set is a fixture in many hospital nursing stations and pharmacies. It was originally designed to assist pharmacy and therapeutics committees in preparing their own formularies. Although some basic pharmacology is discussed, this book is primarily a clinical reference for dosages, indications, interactions, adverse reactions, and so on. Updated five or six times a year; supplements sent to subscribers.

Facts and Comparisons. St. Louis: Facts and Comparisons, Inc., 1982.

An independent publication containing unbiased drug information available in a loose-leaf binder or as an annual hardbound book. Although it's similar to the *Physicians' Desk Reference* in that its drug monographs are based on approved package inserts, it has some important advantages. First, the drug manufacturer's information is rewritten so that it's more understandable. Second, investigational (unapproved) uses are included, when appropriate. Third, many more drugs are covered. Updated monthly; supplements mailed to subscribers.

Handbook of Nonprescription Drugs, 6th ed. Washington, D.C.: American Pharmaceutical Association, 1979.

This book is the best reference for over-the-counter drugs. Includes hard-to-find, practical information on such topics as hemorrhoid, dermatologic, dental, and other external-use products; discussions of gastrointestinal drugs—such as laxatives, antidiarrheals, and emetics/antiemetics—are particularly worthwhile and well explained. Comprehensive product listings describe the amounts of active ingredients and inert substances in the product.

Loebl, Suzanne, and Spratto, George: *The Nurse's Drug Handbook.* New York: John Wiley & Sons, Inc., 1980.

Essentially a drug reference book that also covers basic pharmacologic principles, administering drugs, promoting patient compliance, and calculating dosages. Drugs classified according to system. Drug monographs include drug use, action and interaction, dosage and administration, contraindications and laboratory interference data, and nursing implications.

Martindale: The Extra Pharmacopeia, 27th ed. London: The Pharmaceutical Press, 1977.

Worldwide in scope, this large volume is probably the most comprehensive book for drug information available. Describing an abundance of internationally available drugs, *Martindale* is where drug information pharmacists look when no other book is helpful. It's particularly useful for information about drugs that aren't available in the United States. Contains uses, precautions, and toxic effects of drugs; also has technical chemical and stability information. International trade names and generic synonyms are listed for every drug.

Nursing82 Drug Handbook. Springhouse, Pa.: Intermed Communications, Inc., 1982.

A portable drug reference book, with drugs classified according to pharmacologic action or site of action. Information includes mechanisms of drug action, generic and trade names, indications and dosages, side effects, interactions, and nursing considerations. Commonly occurring and life-threatening side effects italicized.

Physicians' Desk Reference, 36th ed. Oradell, N.J.: Medical Economics Co., 1982.

Contains selected package inserts of drug products, with complete prescribing information and information about FDA-approved uses for drugs. Full-color drug identification section, organized by manufacturer, and several indexes.

Schmidt, R. Marilyn, and Margolin, Solomon: *Harpers Handbook of Therapeutic Pharmacology.* New York: Harper & Row Publishers, 1981.

Essentially a drug reference book with limited pharmacology. Drug information arranged primarily by organ system. Monographs include clinical uses, pharmacology, special precautions, adverse effects, and clinical guidelines.

United States Pharmacopeia Dispensing Information (USP-DI). Rockville, Md.: United States Pharmacopeial Convention, Inc., 1981.

The agency that has published the standard for drug quality and purity (United States Pharmacopeia) started publishing this practical book in 1980. This yearly publication contains monographs of the most commonly used drugs. *USP-DI* concentrates on information necessary to monitor safe and effective use of a drug *after* it's prescribed—pharmacologic action, precautions, side effects, and so on. Second half of the book contains advice for the patient, written in lay language, that can be reproduced and given to patients.

Newsletters

Inpharma. New York: ADIS Press.

Weekly abstracts from current international drug literature. *Inpharma* focuses on drug uses (approved and investigational), interactions, adverse reactions, and clinical pharmacology. Also lists new drug products and extensive references to various drug-related subjects.

The Medical Letter on Drugs and Therapeutics. New Rochelle, N.Y.: Medical Letter, Inc.

This nonprofit newsletter evaluates new drugs, new uses for established drugs, and other topical clinical drug therapy issues. Its distinguished editorial board and its no-advertisement policy assure nonbiased editorial content. Because it's issued biweekly, information is up to date. Used by many informed practitioners when making drug therapy decisions and by many hospital formulary committees when choosing drugs for their hospital formularies.

Nurse's Drug Alert. New York: M.J. Powers & Co.

This monthly newsletter for nurses summarizes selected drug articles from major journals. Each summary is followed by a paragraph describing relevant nursing implications.

III Special Topics

Drug Interaction and Incompatibility

Hansten, Philip D.: *Drug Interactions,* 4th ed. Philadelphia: Lea & Febiger, 1979.

Considered by many to be *the* most reliable and practical guide to the evaluation of drug interactions. Hansten specifies in bold type which interactions are of major clinical significance and have definitive documentation. These interactions, if unmonitored, are potentially harmful to the patient. Hansten also identifies those interactions that are less well documented or are less potentially harmful to the patient, and those with the least documentation and/or clinical significance. Another attractive feature of the book is a section covering drug effects on clinical laboratory test results.

Trissel, L.A.: *Handbook on Injectable Drugs,* 2nd ed. Washington, D.C.: American Society of Hospital Pharmacists, 1980.

The most complete reference available on the compatibility or incompatibility of injectables (includes 188 commercially available drugs and 47 investigational drugs). Each monograph not only lists drugs that are compatible with one another, but explains why or why not, plus the reasons for conditional compatibility whenever possible. Each conclusion regarding compatibility or incompatibility is referenced to the original source. This book is indispensable in nursing units where I.V. solutions are mixed.

Patient-Teaching References

Canadian Self-Medication: A Reference for the Health Professions. Ottawa: Canadian Pharmaceutical Association, 1980.

This reference book, originally designed for community pharmacists, is also useful for nurses who work in ambulatory-care settings. Discusses nonprescription drugs that can be used in the treatment of various common (and relatively minor) disorders. Contains typical questions the practitioner should ask a patient seeking drug recommendations, with various options for nonprescription treatment. The book also lists many over-the-counter products available in Canada and gives complete directions for their use.

Medication Teaching Manual: A Guide for Patient Counseling, 2nd ed. Washington, D.C.: Society of Hospital Pharmacists, 1980.

Easy-to-understand monographs about commonly prescribed drugs in question-and-answer format. In language the patient can understand, answers are given on why, when, and how the drug is used, and what the patient should do if he forgets to take a dose.

Smith, D.L.: *Medication Guide for Patient Counseling.* Philadelphia: Lea & Febiger, 1980.

Similar to but more comprehensive in scope than the *Medication Teaching Man-*

ual, this book describes useful drug information in lay terms. Most drugs commonly used in the United States and Canada are included as well as some trade names in each country. Early chapters point out the best ways to communicate with patients about their medications. Helpful tips on how to give both verbal and written drug counseling.

Drug Therapy in Children

The Harriet Lane Handbook: A Manual for House Officers, 8th ed. Chicago: Yearbook Medical Publishers, 1978.

Originally intended for pediatric medical residents practicing at Johns Hopkins Hospital, this pocket-sized manual has rapidly become an indispensable guide for all clinicians involved with pediatrics. Drug monographs contain dosages and concise, authoritive remarks about drugs commonly used in children. Diagnostic test information and other useful data, such as growth tables, are included.

Pagliaro, L.A., and Levin, R.H.: *Problems in Pediatric Drug Therapy.* Hamilton, Ill.: Drug Intelligence Publications, 1979.

This pocket-sized reference contains concise, referenced, and accessible pharmacologic and clinical information concerning the use and effects of drugs on a fetus, an infant, and a child. Includes teratogenesis, drugs excreted in breast milk, adverse drug reactions in children, pediatric poisoning, and drug dosing in neonates and children. Wealth of clinical data makes this a useful book for pediatric nurse practitioners.

Yaffe, Sumner J., ed.: *Pediatric Pharmacology.* New York: Grune & Stratton, Inc., 1980.

This multiauthored book covers a wide range. After a discussion of basic principles of drug action in children, specialists cover subjects such as antimicrobials, anticonvulsants, and drugs used in asthma. Such topics as "Drugs and Pregnancy" and "Drugs in the Newborn" are particularly worthwhile. Emphasis in this book is on clinical application of the drugs—not diseases.

Drug Therapy in the Elderly

Ebersole, P., and Hess, P.: "Drug Use and Abuse," *Toward Healthy Aging.* St. Louis: C.V. Mosby Co., 1981.

This chapter in a book designed especially for nurses deals with general aspects of drug use and abuse in the elderly. Heavy emphasis on drug interactions, including a helpful chart listing reasons for every interaction. Another chart suggests ways a nurse can prevent or minimize these drug interactions through proper drug administration. Also includes recommendations for fostering better drug use and compliance, tips for patient education, and a discussion of psychoactive drugs and drugs of abuse (including alcohol).

Green, B.: "The Politics of Psychoactive Drug Use in Old Age," *The Gerontologist,* 18:525, Nov. 6, 1978.

Explores some of the reasons for overuse of many drugs in the geriatric population. Discusses the tendency for doctors to overprescribe medication, especially drugs such as tranquilizers, cerebral vasodilators, and so on. Suggests that such conditions as senility, depression, agitation, and confusion should in many cases not even be treated with drugs. Also examines the subtle influence of drug advertisements in medical journals.

Vestal, R.E.: "Drug Use in the Elderly: A Review of Problems and Special Considerations," *Drugs* 16:358, 1978.

Focuses on the physiologic changes in bodily functions of the elderly patient and how these affect the pharmacologic action of various drug classes. Some of the drug classes discussed are cardiac glycosides, diuretics, antiarrhythmics, antihypertensives, anticoagulants, and many others. Offers several basic principles for monitoring the action of drugs in the elderly and techniques to enhance compliance. An excellent review.

Other Selected References

Eliopoulos, C.: "Geriatric Pharmacology," *Gerontological Nursing.* New York: Harper & Row Publishers, 1979.

Gotz, B.E., and Gotz, V.P.: "Drugs and the Elderly," *American Journal of Nursing,* 78:1347, 1978.

Nandy, K., ed.: *Geriatric Psychopharmacology.* New York: Elsevier/North Holland, 1979.

Drug Calculations for Nurses

Dison, Norma: *Simplified Drugs and Solutions for Nurses.* St. Louis: C.V. Mosby Co., 1980.

A programmed learning text for nurses. Emphasizes basic arithmetic and how to set up problems for solution; weights and measures and conversion of temperature from centigrade to Fahrenheit and vice versa; computations, conversions from one system of measure to another, calculation of pediatric dosages and I.V. flow rates. Includes exercise problems for the student, with answers at the end of the text.

Keane, Claire B., and Fletcher, Sybil M.: *Drugs and Solutions: A Programmed Introduction.* Philadelphia: W.B. Saunders Co., 1980.

A programmed learning text prepared for those who need to calculate drug doses and prepare solutions for administration to patients. Content is organized into short units (frames), with questions and answers; each chapter concludes with a posttest. Content includes basic systems of measure, basic arithmetic, computation of doses by various methods, I.V. flow rate computation, pediatric dosages, preparing solutions, and temperature conversions from centigrade to Fahrenheit and vice versa. The text ends with a final examination.

Other Selected References

McHenry, Ruth W.: *Self-teaching Tests in Arithmetic for Nurses.* St. Louis: C.V. Mosby Co., 1980.

Richardson, Lloyd I., Jr.: *The Mathematics of Drugs and Solutions with Clinical Applications.* New York: McGraw-Hill Book Co., 1980.

Nutritional Support

Elwyn, D.H.: "Nutritional Requirements of Adult Surgical Patients," *Critical Care Medicine,* 8:9, 1980.

An in-depth review of guidelines for substrate administration, along with descriptions of their deficiency states and the adverse effects of overfeeding.

Fischer, J.E., ed.: *Total Parenteral Nutrition.* Boston: Little, Brown & Co.,1976.

The best single source book for information on nutritional support; covers setting up a team, the functions of each team member, and nutritional support in patients with major concurrent medical problems.

Grant, J.P.: *Handbook of Total Parenteral Nutrition.* Philadelphia: W.B. Saunders Co., 1980.

Good summary of total parenteral nutrition based on literature and personal experience. Includes principles of patient selection; catheter insertion and maintenance; preparation and administration of solutions; and recognition, prevention, and management of potential complications.

Heymsfield, S.B., et al.: "Enteral Hyperalimentation: An Alternative to Central Venous Hyperalimentation," *Annals of Internal Medicine,* 90, 1979.

Reviews the indications, selection of feeding mixtures, and mechanical and chemical aspects and monitoring of enteral alimentation.

Managing I.V. Therapy. Nursing Photobook. Springhouse, Pa.: Intermed Communications, Inc., 1980.

A basic summary of all types of I.V. therapy, including hyperalimentation. Therapy indications, methods of administration, types of solutions administered, and the planning and administration of nursing care for patients receiving hyperalimentation are included. Photostory approach to care activities, such as tubing and dressing changes, allows the nurse to see how these procedures are done. Simple, step-by-step approach; good reference for students and those who wish to review procedures.

Michel, L., Serrano, A., and Malt, R.A.: "Current Concepts: Nutritional Support of Hospitalized Patients," *New England Journal of Medicine,* 304:1147, 1981.

A brief review of current assessment, substrate requirements, and complications of nutritional support. Covers parenteral and enteral therapy.

Mullen, J.L., Crosby, L.O., and Rombeau, J.L., eds.: "Symposium on Surgical Nutrition," *Surgical Clinics of North America,* 61:427, June 1981.

Summary of state of the art of clinical nutritional care by leaders in the field. Covers history, assessment, requirements, metabolism, techniques, and nutritional support in various medical/surgical conditions.

Ota, D.M., Imbembo, A.L., and Zuidema, G.D.: "Total Parenteral Nutrition," ***Surgery,*** 83:503, 1978.

A review of the caloric and nutritional requirements of patients, methodology of parenteral nutrition, metabolic and septic complications of total parenteral nutrition.

Chemotherapy and Oncology

Dorr, Robert T., and Fritz, William L.: ***Cancer Chemotherapy Handbook.*** New York: Elsevier, 1980.

A comprehensive compilation of all relevant information on approved and investigational chemotherapeutic drugs. Introductory chapters present basic cell kinetics and principles of chemotherapy. Following chapters include information on drug classes; individual drug monographs, with research, pharmacologic, and clinical information; side effects; and legal aspects of chemotherapy. This book can be highly technical, but it's an excellent reference and possibly the most definitive chemotherapy text currently available.

Herrmann, C.: "Immunology: The Method to Our Madness," ***Cancer Nursing,*** 2:359, Oct. 1979.

An excellent article on the basic principles of immunology and the nurse's role in this type of therapy. A bit technical, but explanations are understandable.

Horton, John, and Hill, George J., II: ***Clinical Oncology.*** Philadelphia: W.B. Saunders Co., 1977.

A comprehensive clinical oncology text encompassing all aspects of neoplasia from tumor growth to staging and treatment. Chemotherapy is just one of the treatment modalities discussed, and the most common types of neoplastic diseases are covered. Intended primarily for doctors but also useful for nurses.

Johnston, Susan, and Patt, Yehuda A.: "Caring for the Patient on Intraarterial Chemotherapy... Are You Ready?" ***Nursing81,*** 11:108, Nov. 1981.

Covers the definition, administration techniques, indications for therapy, complications, and nursing care of patients receiving intraarterial chemotherapy. Comprehensive, up-to-date, and clear explanation.

Koren, Mary Elaine, and Herrmann, Christy Simo: "Cancer Immunotherapy: What, Why, When, How," ***Nursing81,*** 11:34, Jan. 1981.

An easy-to-understand article on the basic principles of immunotherapy. Explains assessment of immune status; results are depicted in full-color photos. Discusses the nurse's role and gives clinical nursing examples.

Marino, Lisa Begg: ***Cancer Nursing.*** St. Louis: C.V. Mosby Co., 1981.

A comprehensive framework for cancer nursing is presented in this text, which deals with all aspects of neoplastic disease and treatment. Discusses the biologic, emotional, social, ethical, and economic issues inherent in cancer diagnosis and treatment. Also highlights the nurse's role in caring for the cancer patient and the unique contributions to cancer care made by nurses. Gives excellent, practical clinical advice as well as nursing strategies for dealing with the problems associated with such intensive and emotionally draining clinical situations.

Rubin, Philip, ed.: ***Clinical Oncology,*** 5th ed. An American Cancer Society Publication. Rochester, N.Y.: University of Rochester School of Medicine and Dentistry, 1980.

This paperbound text is a concise summary of neoplastic diseases and their treatment. Generally intended for doctors, it's an excellent quick reference for nurses as well. Some chapters of the book are specifically written for nurses. Includes the basics of neoplastic disease and the principles of all treatment modalities, including chemotherapy, as well as most neoplastic diseases.

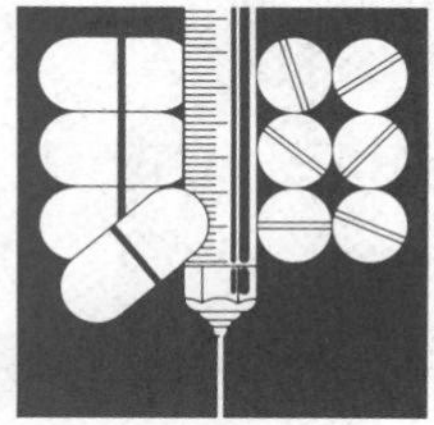

Acknowledgments

CHAPTER 6 ***Understanding intravenous solution incompatibility***
p. 74—Photographs by Paul A. Cohen

CHAPTER 7 ***Parenteral and enteral nutrition therapy***
p. 99—Illustration adapted from photograph courtesy of C.V. Mosby Co., St. Louis, Mo.

CHAPTER 71 ***Nursing implications of chemotherapy***
p. 908—Photographs 1, 3, and 4 courtesy of Joseph L. Konzelman, DDS, Emory University School of Dentistry, Atlanta, Ga.; photograph 2 courtesy of Samuel Dreizen, DDS, MD, University of Texas, Houston, Tex.

CHAPTER 82 ***Topical ophthalmic anesthetics***
p. 997—Photographs by Paul A. Cohen

CHAPTER 88 ***Scabicides and pediculicides***
p. 1039—Patient-teaching aid adapted from Lawrence Charles Parish and Joseph A. Witkowski, "Head Lice: Epidemic in the Schoolroom," *Drug Therapy,* October 1980, with permission from the publisher.

CHAPTER 95 ***Miscellaneous dermatomucosal agents***
pp. 1114-1115—Photographs by Paul A. Cohen

CHAPTER 101 ***Vaccines and toxoids***
p. 1199—Patient-teaching aid adapted from "Immunization for Travelers," *The Medical Letter,* July 13, 1979, with permission from the publisher.

We'd like to thank these community pharmacists who helped us obtain the tablets and capsules photographed in the full-color DRUGS OF ABUSE section: William Balas, RPh; Mark Cohen, RPh; John McVan, RPh; Seymour Margolis, RPh.

Index

A

Boldface page numbers = major entries   c = chart   i = illustration   p = photograph

B

B

C

C

Boldface page numbers = major entries c = chart i = illustration p = photograph

D

Boldface page numbers = major entries c = chart i = illustration p = photograph

E

E

F

G

H

I

J

Boldface page numbers = major entries c = chart i = illustration p = photograph

M

M

Boldface page numbers = major entries c = chart i = illustration p = photograph

M

N

O

O

P

Boldface page numbers = major entries   c = chart   i = illustration   p = photograph

P

Boldface page numbers = major entries c = chart i = illustration p = photograph

Q

S

S

Boldface page numbers = major entries c = chart i = illustration p = photograph

S

T

Boldface page numbers = major entries c = chart i = illustration p = photograph

T

U

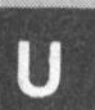

V

W

X

Y

Z

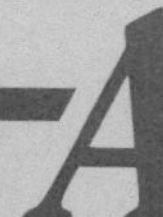

LCOHOL AND FOOD INTERACTIONS WITH SELECTED DRUGS

Drugs listed are those whose interactions are major and well documented, or moderate, that is, potentially harmful.

DRUG	INTERACTION	POSSIBLE EFFECT
Anticoagulants, oral (Chap. 67) anisindione, dicumarol, phenindione, phenprocoumon, warfarin		▲ or ▼ Prothrombin time
Antidepressants, tricyclic (Chap. 31) amitriptyline, desipramine, doxepin, imipramine, nortriptyline, protriptyline, trimipramine		▼ Psychomotor skills
Antidiabetic agents (Chap. 58) acetohexamide, chlorpropamide, tolazamide, tolbutamide		▲ Hypoglycemia in fasting patients ▼ Hypoglycemia in chronic alcoholism. Disulfiram-type reaction*
Antihistamines (Chap. 43) azatadine, brompheniramine, carbinoxamine, chlorpheniramine, clemastine, cyproheptadine, dexchlorpheniramine, dimethindene, dimethothiazine, diphenhydramine, diphenpyraline, doxylamine, methdilazine, promethazine, trimeprazine, tripelennamine, triprolidine		▲ CNS depression
Barbiturates (Chap. 29) amobarbital, aprobarbital, barbital, butabarbital, hexobarbital, mephobarbital, pentobarbital		▲ CNS depression (acute alcoholics) ▼ Sedative effect (chronic alcoholics)
Benzodiazepines (Chap. 32) chlordiazepoxide, clorazepate, diazepam, hydroxyzine, lorazepam, oxazepam, prazepam		▲ CNS depression ▼ Psychomotor skills
MAO inhibitors (Chaps. 22, 31) pargyline, phenelzine, tranylcypromine	*Tell patient to avoid* avocados, Chianti wine, chicken livers, chocolate, meats prepared with tenderizers, pickled herring, processed cheese, yeast extract	▲ Hypertensive crisis ▲ Intracranial bleeding
Narcotic analgesics (Chap. 27) alphaprodine, anileridine, Brompton's cocktail, codeine, fentanyl, hydromorphone, levorphanol, meperidine, methadone, morphine, oxycodone, oxymorphone, pentazocine, propoxyphene		▲ CNS depression (acute alcoholics)
Salicylates (Chap. 25) aspirin, choline magnesium trisalicylate, choline salicylate, magnesium salicylate, salicylamide, salsalate, sodium salicylate, sodium thiosalicylate		▲ GI bleeding
Tetracyclines (Chap. 16) demeclocycline, doxycycline, methacycline, minocycline, oxytetracycline, tetracycline	*Tell patient to avoid* milk and other dairy products	▼ Blood absorption of drug